IMPORTANT

HERE IS YOUR REGISTRATION CODE TO ACCESS MCGRAW-HILL PREMIUM CONTENT AND MCGRAW-HILL ONLINE RESOURCES

For key premium online resources you need THIS CODE to gain access. Once the code is entered, you will be able to use the web resources for the length of your course.

Access is provided only if you have purchased a new book.

If the registration code is missing from this book, the registration screen on our website, and within your WebCT or Blackboard course will tell you how to obtain your new code. Your registration code can be used only once to establish access. It is not transferable.

To gain access to these online resources

1. **USE** your web browser to go to: **http://www.mhhe.com/payne9e**
2. **CLICK** on "First Time User"
3. **ENTER** the Registration Code printed on the tear-off bookmark on the right
4. After you have entered your registration code, click on "Register"
5. **FOLLOW** the instructions to setup your personal UserID and Password
6. **WRITE** your UserID and Password down for future reference. Keep it in a safe place.

If your course is using WebCT or Blackboard, you'll be able to use this code to access the McGraw-Hill content within your instructor's online course.

To gain access to the McGraw-Hill content in your instructor's WebCT or Blackboard course simply log into the course with the user ID and Password provided by your instructor. Enter the registration code exactly as it appears to the right when prompted by the system. You will only need to use this code the first time you click on McGraw-Hill content.

These instructions are specifically for student access. Instructors are not required to register via the above instructions.

The McGraw-Hill Companies

McGraw Hill **Higher Education**

Thank you, and welcome to your McGraw-Hill Online Resources.

13 Digit: 978-0-07-302815-6
10 Digit: 0-07-302815-0
t/a **Understanding Your Health**

REGISTRATION CODE

V39U-BG7P-7BPK-7Y7R-78RY

Understanding Your Health

Understanding Your Health

Ninth Edition

Wayne A. Payne, Ed.D.

Dale B. Hahn, Ph.D.

Ellen B. Lucas, Ph.D.

All of Ball State University,
Muncie, Indiana

Boston   Burr Ridge, IL   Dubuque, IA   Madison, WI   New York   San Francisco   St. Louis
Bangkok   Bogotá   Caracas   Kuala Lumpur   Lisbon   London   Madrid   Mexico City
Milan   Montreal   New Delhi   Santiago   Seoul   Singapore   Sydney   Taipei   Toronto

The McGraw·Hill Companies

 Higher Education

A Division of the McGraw-Hill Companies

UNDERSTANDING YOUR HEALTH
Published by McGraw-Hill, a business unit of The McGraw-Hill Companies, Inc., 1221
Avenue of the Americas, New York, NY, 10020. Copyright © 2007 by The McGraw-Hill
Companies, Inc. All rights reserved. No part of this publication may be reproduced or
distributed in any form or by any means, or stored in a database or retrieval system,
without the prior written consent of The McGraw-Hill Companies, Inc., including, but not
limited to, in any network or other electronic storage or transmission, or broadcast for
distance learning.
Some ancillaries, including electronic and print components, may not be available to
customers outside the United States.

This book is printed on acid-free paper.

1 2 3 4 5 6 7 8 9 0 VNH/VNH 0 9 8 7 6

ISBN-13: 978-0-07-302807-1
ISBN-10: 0-07-302807-X

Vice president and editor-in-chief: *Emily Barrosse*
Publisher: *William R. Glass*
Sponsoring editor: *Christopher Johnson*
Director of development: *Kate Engelberg*
Developmental editor: *Nadia Bidwell for Van Brien & Associates*
Executive marketing manager: *Pamela S. Cooper*
Media producer: *Ron Nelms*
Production editor: *Mel Valentín*
Senior production supervisor: *Carol A. Bielski*
Senior designer: *Kim Menning*
Cover design: *Yuo Riezebas*
Interior design: *Jeanne Calabrese/Glenda King*
Art editor: *Ayelet Arbel*
Photo researcher: *Alexandra Ambrose*
Art director: *Jeanne Schreiber*
Typeface: *10.5/12 Minion*
Compositor: *GTS-LA Campus*
Printer: *Von Hoffman*
Cover image: © *The McGraw-Hill Companies/Christopher Kerrigan, photographer*

The credits section for this book begins on page C-1 and is considered an extension of the
copyright page.

Library of Congress Cataloging-in-Publication Data
Payne, Wayne A.
    Understanding your health/Wayne A. Payne, Dale B. Hahn, Ellen B. Mauer.—9th ed
        p. cm.
    ISBN 0-07-302807-X (alk. paper)
    1. Health. 2. College students—Health and hygiene. I. Hahn, Dale B. II. Mauer, Ellen.
III. Title.
RA777.3.P39 2006
613′.0434—dc22

                                                                2005058375

www.mhhe.com

*To all our students, with the hope that the
decisions they make will be healthy ones.*

contents in brief

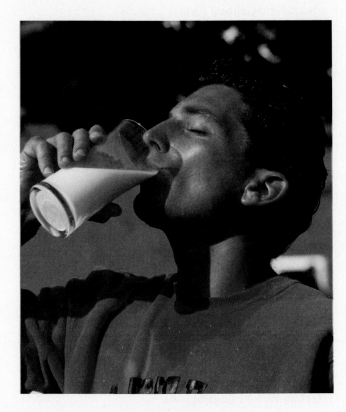

Part Two: The Body 99

Part Five: Sexuality and Reproduction   439

Part Six: Consumer and Safety Issues 533

Part Seven: Completing Life's Journey 623

Preface

As a health educator, you already know that personal health is one of the most exciting courses a college student will take. Today's media-oriented college students are aware of the critical health issues of the new millennium. They hear about environmental issues, substance abuse, sexually transmitted diseases, fitness, and nutrition virtually every day. The value of the personal health course is its potential to expand students' knowledge of these and other health topics. Students will then be able to examine their attitudes toward health issues and modify their behavior to improve their health and perhaps even prevent or delay the onset of certain health conditions.

Understanding Your Health accomplishes this task with a carefully composed, well-documented text that addresses the health issues most important to both instructors and students. As health educators, we understand the teaching issues you face daily in the classroom and have written this text with your concerns in mind.

Hallmarks of the Text

Several unique themes and features set *Understanding Your Health* apart from other personal health texts. These successful features continue to define *Understanding Your Health* in its ninth edition.

A Text for All Students

This book is written for college students in a wide variety of settings, from community colleges to large four-year universities. The content is carefully constructed to be meaningful to students of all ages. We have paid special attention to the increasing numbers of nontraditional-age students (those over age 25) who have decided to pursue a college education. *Understanding Your Health* continues to encourage students of all ages and backgrounds to achieve their goals.

Two Central Themes

Throughout the text, two central themes—the multiple dimensions of health and the developmental tasks— offer students a foundation for understanding their own health and achieving positive behavior change. The multiple dimensions of health are introduced in Chapter 1 and revisited in each part opener, where they are discussed in the context of the chapters that follow. The developmental tasks are also introduced in Chapter 1, where they are applied to young, middle, and older adulthood.

Flexible Organization

The ninth edition of *Understanding Your Health* has 21 chapters. The first stands alone as an introductory chapter that explains the focus of the book. The arrangement of the remaining chapters follows the recommendations of both the users of previous editions of the book and reviewers for this edition. Of course, professors can choose to cover the chapters in any sequence that suits the needs of their courses.

Wellness and Disease Prevention

Throughout this new edition, students are continually urged to be proactive in shaping their future health. Even the chapter titles invite students to take control of their health behavior.

Integrated Presentation of Aging

Topics of interest to midlife and older adults are integrated into appropriate chapters according to subject. This organization allows both traditional-age and nontraditional-age students to learn about the physical and emotional changes that take place as we age.

Separate Coverage of Cancer and Chronic Conditions

Rapid developments in cancer prevention, diagnosis, and treatment warrant a single comprehensive chapter on cancer, in which we present the latest research and information.

In addition, *Understanding Your Health* features a separate chapter in which more than 20 of the most common chronic conditions are discussed.

Technology: The Key to Teaching and Learning

Just a quick glance through the pages of *Understanding Your Health* shows that technology is woven throughout every chapter, both in the content and in the chapter pedagogy. Similarly, the package of supplements that accompanies the text emphasizes technology while acknowledging that printed materials also have merit. Together, the text and its supplements offer the ideal approach to teaching and learning—one that integrates the best tools that technology has to offer, challenging both instructors and students to reach higher.

Updated Coverage: New and Expanded Topics

As experienced health educators and authors, we know how important it is to provide students with the most current information available. The ninth edition of *Understanding Your Health* has been thoroughly updated with the latest information, statistics, and findings. Throughout each chapter, we have incorporated new examples and discussions, from information on newly available prescription drugs and medications (Chapters 2, 3, 11, and 12), to the latest information on dieting and supplements (Chapters 5, 6, and 16).

Another exciting change to this edition of *Understanding Your Health* is the addition of a new chapter, Chapter 21, Accepting Dying and Death. Written by coauthor Ellen B. Lucas, Ph.D., this chapter presents information about the psychological stages of death; coping with grief and the loss of friends, parents, and children; hospice care; euthanasia; and physician-assisted suicide. The chapter also offers important practical advice for preparing advance health care directives.

In addition to these topics, we have once again included chapter-ending "As We Go To Press" boxes in relevant chapters. These unique boxes allow us to comment on breaking news right up to press time, ensuring that the most current issues in health are addressed. For example, in Chapter 2 we discuss the concern and controversy over prescription antidepressants for children, and in Chapter 21 we touch on the growing trend of cryogenic freezing.

Following is a sampling of topics that are either completely new to this edition or are covered in greater depth than in the previous edition:

Chapter 1: Shaping Your Health

- Traditional definitions of health
- Composition and role of health
- Leading causes of death for Americans under 80 years of age

Chapter 2: Achieving Psychological Health

- Advertising psychological medications
- How to say "sorry" and mean it
- Personality types
- Attention Deficit Disorder

Chapter 3: Managing Stress

- New technological stressors
- Stress is different for different populations
- Yoga
- Antidotes to anger

Chapter 4: Becoming Physically Fit

- Anterior and posterior musculature charts

Chapter 5: Understanding Nutrition and Your Diet

- Low-carb diets
- New USDA food guidelines
- Food and spirituality
- Phytochemicals
- Sample 2,000-calorie menu
- Updated fast-food choices
- Food pyramids of other cultures

Chapter 6: Maintaining a Healthy Weight

- Reality television and body image
- Religion and dieting
- Dieting myths
- Childhood obesity
- Clothing sizes around the world
- Surgical intervention

Chapter 7: Making Decisions about Drug Use

- Effects of Methamphetamine abuse
- Warning signs of a meth lab
- Ritalin and Adderall abuse on campus

Chapter 8: Taking Control of Alcohol Use

- Dangers of drinking games
- Alcohol absorption and race

Chapter 9: Rejecting Tobacco Use

- Smoking statistics by state
- Carcinogenic agents
- Sexual dysfunction and infertility
- Employment-related consequences of smoking
- International smoking bans

Chapter 10: Enhancing Your Cardiovascular Health

- Hypertension
- Cholesterol levels
- Updated statistics on cardiovascular disease

Chapter 11: Living with Cancer

- Updated statistics on cancer
- Cancer screening guidelines
- Genetic markers
- Role of self-examination in the detection of breast cancer
- Solar UV index

Chapter 12: Managing Chronic Conditions

- Categorization of chronic conditions
- Expanded discussion of diabetes
- Changing pharmaceutical choices in treating IBDs
- Expanded discussion of multiple sclerosis
- Revised classification for Alzheimer's

Chapter 13: Preventing Infectious Diseases

- Immunization schedule
- 2004–2005 influenza vaccine shortage
- Lyme disease
- Bird influenza
- Updated HIV/AIDS statistics

Chapter 14: Exploring the Origins of Sexuality

- Irregular menstrual cycles
- Changing diet to improve fibrocystic breast condition
- Gender preference

Chapter 15: Understanding Sexual Behavior and Relationships

- Same-sex marriage
- Comparison of drug treatments for erectile dysfunction
- Expanded coverage of transgendered people

Chapter 16: Managing Your Fertility

- Contraceptive effectiveness table
- Standard Days method of periodic abstinence
- Abstinence as birth control
- New methods of contraception
- Side effects of emergency hormonal contraception
- New method of female sterilization (the Essure coil)
- Partial birth abortion

Chapter 17: Becoming a Parent

- Gay and lesbian adoption
- Therapeutic cloning
- Infertility and adoption

Chapter 18: Becoming an Informed Health Care Consumer

- The Internet
- Alternative forms of health care
- Self-diagnosis
- Lack of health insurance
- Medicare prescription drug coverage
- The FDA's drug approval process

Chapter 19: Protecting Your Safety

- Identity theft
- Driving distractions

Chapter 20: The Environment and Your Health

- Media hype
- Religious perspectives on the Human-Environment relationship
- Non-ionizing radiation
- Polycyclic aromatic hydrocarbons
- Ionizing radiation
- Species extinction and the loss of natural habitats

Chapter 21: Accepting Dying and Death

- Definitions of death
- Psychological stages of death
- Advance health care directives
- Coping with specific causes of death
- Euthanasia
- Physician-assisted suicide
- Near-death experiences
- Interacting with dying people
- Discussing death with children
- Hospice care
- Death rituals

Student-Friendly Chapter Pedagogy

Each chapter of *Understanding Your Health* is rich with pedagogical features that offer a variety of ways to address new and emerging health issues and to pique student interest in particular topics.

Chapter Objectives

Each chapter begins with a set of clear objectives that help students distill the most important concepts in the pages that follow.

Taking Charge of Your Health

Located at the end of each chapter, these bulleted lists invite students to put the knowledge and information they've gleaned from the chapter to work in their everyday lives. Cross-referencing the text with Internet links and real-world situations allows students to see how what they've learned can be applied in their own lives.

Eye on the Media

Face it—a student's world revolves around media of all types, especially the Web. Students get most of their health information not from instructors and textbooks but from television, self-help books, popular news magazines, the Web, and the radio. To meet students on this familiar ground, we've included Eye on the Media boxes, which take a critical look at these media sources of health information.

Discovering Your Spirituality

Spirituality has become an important focus in health courses. Discovering Your Spirituality boxes highlight the spiritual dimension of health and its effect on overall wellness. The boxes cover topics such as body image,

living well with cancer or a chronic infectious disease, making decisions about sex, and having an enjoyable social life without abusing alcohol or other drugs.

Considering Complementary Care

This feature highlights nontraditional approaches to health care. Topics include the use of herbal supplements, biofeedback, meditation, and dietary aids. Students are encouraged to critique these approaches, weighing their possible advantages and disadvantages. Although methods that are known to be dangerous are clearly identified as such, students are invited to consider new approaches that are becoming more accepted because they show promising results. An underlying theme is patient responsibility coupled with a physician's advice.

Talking Points

Interspersed throughout each chapter, Talking Points offers students opportunities to explore how they might start a dialogue about specific health-related issues and situations.

Changing for the Better

These unique question-and-answer boxes show students how to put health concepts into practice. Each box begins with a real-life question, followed by helpful tips and practical advice for initiating behavior change and staying motivated to follow a healthy lifestyle.

Learning from Our Diversity

These boxes expose students to alternative viewpoints and highlight what we can learn from the differences that make us unique. Topics include the Mediterranean Food Pyramid, the male contraceptive pill, and special issues related to infectious disease among older adults.

Star Boxes

In each chapter, special material in Star boxes encourages students to delve into a particular topic or closely examine an important health issue.

Personal Assessments

Each chapter contains at least one Personal Assessment inventory. These self-assessment exercises serve three important functions: to capture students' attention, to serve as a basis for introspection and behavior change, and to provide suggestions for carrying the applications further.

Definition Boxes

Key terms are set in boldface type and defined in corresponding boxes. Pronunciation guides are provided where appropriate. Other important terms in the text are set in italics for emphasis. Both approaches facilitate student vocabulary comprehension.

Chapter Summaries

Each chapter concludes with a bulleted summary of key concepts and their significance or application. The student can then return to any topic in the chapter for clarification or study.

Review Questions

A set of questions appears at the end of each chapter to aid the student in review and analysis of chapter content.

Comprehensive Health Assessment

The Comprehensive Health Assessment at the end of Chapter 1 allows students to take a close look at their current state of health, typical health behavior, and risk factors. Using this assessment, students can pinpoint trouble spots in their own health behavior and find out what they can do to reduce their risk of disease or other health conditions. At the end of the semester, they can take a look at their previous answers to see how their behavior changed as they learned more about health and wellness issues.

Health Reference Guide

The updated Health Reference Guide at the back of the book lists many commonly used health resources. Internet addresses, phone numbers, and mailing addresses of various organizations and government agencies are provided as available. The guide is perforated and laminated, making it durable enough for students to keep for later use.

Vegetarian Food Pyramid

Many students now follow or are considering a vegetarian diet. To help them understand how such a diet meets nutrient needs, we have printed a vegetarian food pyramid along with the USDA Food Guide Pyramid in Chapter 5.

Comprehensive Glossary

At the end of the text, all terms defined in boxes, as well as pertinent italicized terms, are merged into a comprehensive glossary.

Appendixes

Understanding Your Health includes four appendixes that are valuable resources for the student:

- **First Aid.** This updated appendix outlines important general first-aid measures, such as what to do when someone is choking, bleeding, or in shock. It includes a special section on recognition and first-aid treatment of epileptic seizures.
- **Body Systems.** The systems of the human body have been clearly and accurately rendered in this appendix to make difficult anatomical concepts easier for students to understand.
- **Canadian Health.** Written by Canadian health educator Don Morrow, this section provides a comprehensive overview of the health promotion movement in Canada. It presents the historical background of the movement, including an explanation of important documents such as *A New Perspective on the Health of Canadians,* the *Ottawa Charter for Health Promotion,* and the theoretical model of *A Framework for Health Promotion.* It also discusses the *Action Statement for Health Promotion in Canada,* current provincial perspectives, recent initiatives, and future directions.
- **Canada's Food Guide to Healthy Eating.** This well-known and respected guide offers an interesting comparison with the USDA Food Guide Pyramid.

Supplements

An extensive supplements package is available to qualified adopters to enhance the teaching-learning process. We have made a concerted effort to produce supplements of extraordinary utility and quality. This package has been carefully planned and developed to help instructors derive the greatest benefit from the text. We encourage instructors to examine them carefully. Many of the products can be packaged with the text at a discounted price. Beyond the following brief descriptions, additional information about these supplements is available from your McGraw-Hill sales representative.

Integrated Instructor's Resource CD

Organized by chapter, the Instructor's Resource CD includes resources to help you teach your course. The CD will work in both Windows and Macintosh environments and includes the following elements:

- **Course Integrator Guide.** This guide includes all the useful features of an instructor's manual, such as learning objectives, suggested lecture outlines, suggested activities, media resources, and Web links. It also integrates the text with all the related resources McGraw-Hill offers, such as the Online Learning Center, the HealthQuest CD-ROM, and the Health and Human Performance Discipline Page. The guide also includes references to relevant print and broadcast media.

- **Test Bank.** This file includes more than 1,000 questions, including multiple-choice, true/false, and short essay. It has been rewritten to enhance clarity, and it now includes critical thinking questions and more applications questions.
- **Computerized Test Bank.** McGraw-Hill's Computerized Testing is the most flexible and easy-to-use electronic testing program available in higher education. The program allows instructors to create tests from book-specific test banks and to add their own questions. It accommodates a wide range of question types, and multiple versions of the test can be created. The program is available for Windows, Macintosh, and Linux environments.
- **PowerPoint.** A complete set of PowerPoint lecture slides for the course is included on the Instructor's Resource CD, as well as on the instructor's portion of the Online Learning Center. This presentation, ready to use in class, was prepared by a professional in the field of health and fitness. It corresponds to the content in each chapter of *Understanding Your Health*, making it easier for you to teach and ensuring that your students can follow your lectures point by point. You can modify the presentation as much as you like to meet the needs of your course.

Online Learning Center

The Online Learning Center to accompany this text offers a number of additional resources for both students and instructors. Many study tools are open to all students. Premium content such as assessments and PowerWeb require student registration using the pass code that comes free with new books. Visit this Web site to find useful materials such as the following:

For the instructor

- Downloadable PowerPoint presentations
- Course Integrator Guide

For the student

- Self-scoring chapter quizzes and online study guides
- Flash cards and crossword puzzles for learning key terms and their definitions
- Learning objectives
- Interactive activities

- Web links for study and exploration of topics in the text
- Online labs
- Wellness worksheets
- PowerWeb
- Newsfeeds
- Student success strategies

HealthQuest CD-ROM, by Bob Gold and Nancy Atkinson

The HealthQuest CD-ROM helps students explore their wellness behavior using state-of-the-art interactive technology. Students can assess their current health status, determine their risks, and explore options for positive lifestyle change. Tailored feedback gives students a meaningful and individualized learning experience without using valuable classroom time. Modules include the Wellboard (a health self-assessment); Stress Management and Mental Health; Fitness; Nutrition and Weight Control; Communicable Diseases; Cardiovascular Health; Cancer; Tobacco, Alcohol, and Other Drugs. An online Instructor's Manual presents ideas for incorporating HealthQuest into your course.

Fitness and Nutrition Log

This logbook helps students track their diet and exercise programs. It serves as a diary to help students monitor their behaviors. It can be packaged with any McGraw-Hill textbook for a small additional fee.

PowerWeb

www.dushkin.com/online

The PowerWeb Web site is a reservoir of course-specific articles and current events. Students can visit PowerWeb to take a self-scoring quiz, complete an interactive exercise, click through an interactive glossary, or check the daily news. An expert in each discipline analyzes the day's news to show students how it relates to their field of study.

PowerWeb is part of the Online Learning Center. Students are also granted full access to Dushkin/McGraw-Hill's Student Site, where they can read study tips, conduct Web research, learn about different career paths, and follow links on the Web.

Wellness Worksheets

This collection of activities and assessments helps students become more involved in their own wellness and better prepared to implement behavior change programs.

It includes over 120 assessments under the topics of General Wellness and Behavior Change; Stress Management; Psychological and Spiritual Wellness; Intimate Relationships and Communication; Sexuality; Addictive Behaviors and Drug Dependence; Nutrition; Physical Activity and Exercise; Weight Management; Chronic Diseases: Cardiovascular Disease and Cancer; Infectious Diseases: Aging, Dying and Death; Consumer Health; Personal Safety; and Environmental Health. They are available online in the premium content or may be packaged with the text at minimal cost.

NutritionCalc Plus

http://nutritioncalc.mhhe.com

NutritionCalc Plus (ISBN 0-07-292084-X) is a dietary analysis program with an easy-to-use interface that allows users to track their nutrient and food group intakes, energy expenditures, and weight control goals. It generates a variety of reports and graphs for analysis, including comparisons with the Food Guide Pyramid and the latest Dietary Reference Intakes (DRIs). The database includes thousands of ethnic foods, supplements, fast foods, and convenience foods, and users can add their own foods to the food list. NutritionCalc Plus is available on CD-ROM or in an online version.

Video Library

The McGraw-Hill Video Library contains many quality videotapes, including selected videos from the *Films for Humanities* series and all the videos from the award-winning *Healthy Living: Road to Wellness* series. Digitized video clips are also available (see Healthy Living Video Clips CD-ROM). The library also features *Students on Health,* a unique video filmed on college campuses across the country that includes eight brief segments, 8 to 10 minutes long, featuring students involved in discussion and role play on health issues. Finally, an additional video—*McGraw-Hill Health Video*—is available. This video features brief clips on a wide range of topics of interest in personal health courses. Contact your McGraw-Hill sales representative to discuss eligibility to receive videos.

PageOut: The Course Web Site Development Center

www.pageout.net

PageOut, free to instructors who use a McGraw-Hill textbook, is an online program you can use to create your own course Web site. PageOut offers the following features:

- A course home page
- An instructor home page
- A syllabus (interactive and customizable, including quizzing, instructor notes, and links to the text's Online Learning Center)
- Web links
- Discussions (multiple discussion areas per class)
- An online gradebook
- Links to student Web pages

Contact your McGraw-Hill sales representative to obtain a password.

Course Management Systems

www.mhhe.com/solutions

Now instructors can combine their McGraw-Hill Online Learning Center with today's most popular course management systems. Our Instructor Advantage program offers customers access to a complete online teaching website called the Knowledge Gateway, prepaid, toll-free phone support, and unlimited e-mail support directly from WebCT and Blackboard. Instructors who use 500 or more copies of a McGraw-Hill textbook can enroll in our Instructor Advantage Plus program, which provides on-campus, hands-on training from a certified platform specialist. Consult your McGraw-Hill sales representative to learn what other course management systems are easily used with McGraw-Hill online materials.

Classroom Performance System

Classroom Performance System (CPS) brings interactivity into the classroom/ lecture hall. It is a wireless response system that gives instructors and students immediate feedback from the entire class. The wireless response pads are essentially remotes that are easy to use and that engage students. CPS is available for both IBM and Mac computers.

Primis Online

www.mhhe.com/primis/online

Primis Online is a database-driven publishing system that allows instructors to create content-rich textbooks, lab manuals, or readers for their courses directly from the Primis Web site. The customized text can be delivered in print or electronic (eBook) form. A Primis eBook is a digital version of the customized text (sold directly to students as a file downloadable to their computer or accessed online by a password). *Understanding Your Health,* ninth edition, is included in the database.

EZ Test

McGraw-Hill's EZ Test is a flexible and easy-to-use electronic testing program. The program allows instructors to create tests from book-specific items. It accommodates a wide range of question types, and instructors may add their own questions. Multiple versions of the test can be created, and any test can be exported for use with course management systems such as WebCT, BlackBoard, and PageOut. EZ Test Online is a new service that gives you a place to easily administer your EZ Test-created exams and quizzes online. The program is available for Windows and Macintosh environments.

You Can Make a Difference: Be Environmentally Responsible, Second Edition, by Judith Getis

This handy text is organized around the three parts of the biosphere: land, water, and air. Each section contains descriptions of the environmental problems associated with that part of the biosphere. Immediately following the problems, or challenges, are suggested ways in which individuals and communities can help solve or alleviate them.

Annual Editions

Annual Editions is an ever-enlarging series of more than 70 volumes, each designed to provide convenient, low-cost access to a wide range of current, carefully selected articles from some of the most important magazines, newspapers, and journals published today. The articles, drawn from more than 400 periodical sources, are written by prominent scholars, researchers, and commentators. All *Annual Editions* have common organizational features, such as annotated tables of contents, topic guides, unit overviews, and indexes. In addition, a list of annotated Web sites is included. An Instructor's Resource Guide with testing suggestions for each volume is available to qualified instructors.

Taking Sides

www.dushkin.com/takingsides

McGraw-Hill/Dushkin's *Taking Sides* series currently consists of 22 volumes, with an instructor's guide with testing material available for each volume. The *Taking Sides* approach brings together the arguments of leading social and behavioral scientists, educators, and contemporary commentators, forming 18–20 debates, or issues, that present the pros and cons of current controversies in an area of study. An Issue Introduction that precedes the two opposing viewpoints gives students the proper context and historical background for each debate. After reading the debate, students are given other viewpoints to consider in the Issue Postscript, which also offers recommendations for further reading. *Taking Sides* fosters critical thinking in students and encourages them to develop a concern for serious social dialogue.

Acknowledgments

The publisher's reviewers made excellent comments and suggestions that were very useful to us in writing and revising this book. Their contributions are present in every chapter. We would like to express our sincere appreciation for both their critical and comparative readings.

For the Ninth Edition:
Denise Colaianni
Western Connecticut State University

William Ebomoyi
University of Northern Colorado

Heidi Fuller
Salem State College

Kim Hyatt
Weber State University

John Kowalczyk
University of Minnesota

Janis McWayne
Francis Marion University

Dave Oster
Jefferson College

Lana Zinger
Queensborough Community College

For the Eighth Edition:
Srijana Bajracharya
Ithaca College

Steve G. Gabany
Indiana State University

Rosann L. Poole
Tallahassee Community College

Kerry J. Redican
Virginia Polytechnic Institute and State University

Andrew L. Shim
Southwestern College

Lucille Talbot
William Paterson University

For the Seventh Edition:
Charles R. Baffi
Virginia Tech

M. Basti
Cuesta College

Susan T. Burge
Cuyahoga Community College

Karen Camarata
Eastern Kentucky University

Kim Clark
California State University, San Bernardino

David P. Diaz
Cuesta College

Mark Doherty
University of Louisiana-Monroe

Bridget Driscoll
California State University, Fullerton

Boyd Foster
Eastern Washington University

Sara Geist
Ohio University

Stephen Green
Mississippi State University

Kathryn Hilgenkamp
Coastal Carolina University

Kimberley Hyatt
Weber State University

Laurie Merges
Kent State University

Ron Murray
University of Virginia

Bill E. Pride
Arizona State University

DawnElla Rust
Stephen F. Austin State University

M. Ann Smith
Chadron State College

Charles Tucker
Valdosta State University

Karen Vail-Smith
East Carolina University

Kathy Webster
California State University, Fullerton

Holly Willey
Mississippi State University

For the Sixth Edition:
Srijana Bajracharya
University of Maine-Presque Isle

Gary Chandler
Gardner-Webb University

Patricia Cost
Weber State University

John Downey
Long Beach City College

Emogene Fox
University of Central Arkansas

Jolynn Gardner
Anoka Ramsey Community College

Ann Wertz Garvin
University of Wisconsin-Whitewater

Patricia Gordon
Arkansas Tech University

Rene Gratz
University of Wisconsin-Milwaukee

Loretta Herrin
Benedict College

Norm Hoffman
Bakersfield College

Carol Johnson
University of Richmond

Susan MacLaury
Kean University

Lori Marti
Mankato State University

Randy McGuire
Eastern Kentucky University

Phyllis Murray
Eastern Kentucky University

Carol Parker
University of Central Oklahoma

Alan Peterson
Gordon College

Kerry Redican
Gordon College

McKay Rollins
Brigham Young University

For the Fifth Edition:
Lori Dewald
Shippensburg University

Chester A. Halterman
Northern Virginia Community College

Richard Hurley
Brigham Young University

John Janowiak
Appalachian State University

Jacquelynn K. Lott
Antelope Valley College

Rosalie D. Marinelli
University of Nevada

For the Fourth Edition:
Rosemary C. Clark
City College of San Francisco

Marianne Frauenknecht
Western Michigan University

Nancy Geha
Eastern Kentucky University

Jeffrey Hallam
Ohio State University

Dawn Larsen
Mankato State University

Loretta M. Liptak
Youngstown State University

Bruce M. Ragon
Indiana University

For the Third Edition:
Charles A. Bish
Slippery Rock University

G. Robert Bowers
Tallahassee Community College

Donald L. Calitri
Eastern Kentucky University

Shae L. Donham
Northeastern Oklahoma State University

P. Tish K. Doyle
University of Calgary

Judy C. Drolet
Southern Illinois University-Carbondale

Dalen Duitsman
Iowa State University

Mary A. Glascoff
East Carolina University

Sonja S. Glassmeyer
California Polytechnic State University-San Luis Obispo

Health Education Faculty
Cerritos College

Norm Hoffman
Bakersfield College

C. Jessie Jones
University of New Orleans

Jean M. Kirsch
Mankato State University

Duane Knudson
Baylor University

Doris McLittle-Marino
University of Akron

Juli Lawrence Miller
Ohio University

Victor Schramske
Normandale Community College

Janet M. Sermon
Florida A&M University

Myra Sternlieb
DeAnza College

Mark G. Wilson
University of Georgia

Focus Group Participants:
Danny Ballard
Texas A&M University

Robert C. Barnes
East Carolina University

Jacki Benedik
University of Southwestern Louisiana

Kathie C. Garbe
Youngstown State University

Virginia Peters
University of Central Oklahoma

Les Ramsdel
Eastern Kentucky University

James Robinson III
University of Northern Colorado

Linda Schiller-Moening
North Hennepin Community College

For the Second Edition:
Dan Adame
Emory University

Judith Boone Alexander
Evergreen Valley College

Judy B. Baker
East Carolina University

Robert C. Barnes
East Carolina University

Loren Bensley
Central Michigan University

Ernst Bleichart
Vanier College

Shirley F. B. Carter
Springfield College

Vivien C. Carver
Youngstown State University

Cynthia Chubb
University of Oregon

Janine Cox
University of Kansas

Dick Dalton
Lincoln University

Sharron K. Deny
East Los Angeles College

Emogene Fox
University of Central Arkansas

George Gerrodette
San Diego Mesa College

Ray Johnson
Central Michigan University

James W. Lochner
Weber State College

Linda S. Myers
Slippery Rock University

Virginia Peters
University of Central Oklahoma

James Robinson III
University of Northern Colorado

Merwin S. Roeder
Kearney State College

James H. Rothenberger
University of Minnesota

Ronald E. Sevier
El Camino Community College

Reza Shahrokh
Montclair State College

Albert Simon
University of Southwestern Louisiana

Dennis W. Smith
University of North Carolina-Greensboro

Loretta R. Taylor
Southwestern College

For the First Edition:
Stephen E. Bohnenblust
Mankato State University

Neil Richard Boyd, Jr.
University of Southern Mississippi

William B. Cissell
East Tennessee State University

Victor A. Corroll
University of Manitoba

Donna Kasari Ellison
University of Oregon Umpqua Community College

Neil E. Gallagher
Towson State University

Susan C. Girratano
California State University-Northridge

Raymond Goldberg
State University of New York College at Cortland

Marsha Hoagland
Modesto Junior College

Carol Ann Holcomb
Kansas State University

Sharon S. Jones
Orange Coast College

Daniel Klein
Northern Illinois University

Susan Cross Lipnickey
Miami University of Ohio

Gerald W. Matheson
University of Wisconsin-La Crosse

Hollis N. Matson
San Francisco State University

David E. Mills
University of Waterloo

Peggy Pederson
Montana State University

Valerie Pinhas
Nassau Community College

Jacy Showers
Formerly of Ohio State University

Parris Watts
University of Missouri-Columbia

Wayne E. Wylie
Texas A&M University

Special Acknowledgments

Authors do not exist in isolation. To publish successful textbooks, an entire team of professionals must work together for a significant amount of time. During the past three decades, we have worked with many talented people to publish 17 successful textbooks.

For this edition of *Understanding Your Health*, we used the professional expertise and writing talents of a team of four contributing authors. Leonard Kaminsky, Ph.D., Professor and Coordinator of Ball State University's Adult Fitness and Cardiac Rehabilitation Programs, took on the task of revising and updating Chapter 4 (Becoming Physically Fit) and Chapter 10 (Enhancing Your Cardiovascular Health). Chapter 7 (Making Decisions About Drug Use) and Chapter 8 (Taking Control of Alcohol Use) were revised by Alison Cockerill, M.S., Health Educator in the Ball State Student Health Center. Robert Pinger, Ph.D., Professor and Chairperson of the Department of Physiology and Health Science at Ball State, revised Chapter 19 (Protecting Your Safety). And Chapter 20, The Environment and Your Health, was written by David LeBlanc, Ph.D., Professor of Biology at Ball State University. We thank these contributors for their professional dedication to this book and their personal commitment to the health of college students with whom they work on a daily basis.

We remain grateful to Vicki Malinee, who saw us through nine book projects. This latest edition of *Understanding Your Health* also bears the imprint of Nick Barrett, Executive Editor, Health and Human Performance.

His infectious enthusiasm for *Understanding Your Health* and his positive vision for the future of our personal health texts make us especially proud to be McGraw-Hill authors.

Special recognition goes to Pam Cooper, Executive Marketing Manager, who is as energetic a person as we have seen in college publishing. We are confident that her experience, expertise, and talent will allow this book to reach many of our teaching colleagues.

We are also grateful to those who worked behind the scenes at McGraw-Hill on the production of this book. Lynda Huenefeld made a major contribution to the development of both the book and its supplements package. Project Manager Mel Valentín juggled this book and its brief version simultaneously with remarkable grace and good humor, all the while keeping watch over every detail and deadline. Senior Designer Kim Menning created an exciting, dynamic new look for the ninth edition. And Photo Research Coordinator Alexandra Ambrose culled a fine selection of colorful, thought-provoking images.

Finally, we would like to thank our families for their continued support and love. More than anyone else, they know the energy and dedication it takes to write and revise textbooks. To them we continue to offer our sincere admiration and loving appreciation.

Wayne A. Payne
Dale B. Hahn
Ellen B. Lucas

A Visual Guide to Understanding Your Health

Whether you're trying to get in shape, looking for sound health advice, trying to interpret the health information you see in the media, or just working toward a good grade, *Understanding Your Health* is designed to help you succeed. Here's a brief guide to some of the useful and eye-opening features you'll find inside.

Chapter Objectives

Each chapter opens with a set of clear learning goals; check them out before you begin reading the chapter, and use them for review once you've completed it.

Eye on the Media

Curious about all those ads you see for various drugs? Wondering about the reliability of the health information you find on the Internet? This feature investigates the way that written, broadcast, and electronic media shape our perceptions about health, health care, and wellness.

---

chapter thirteen

Preventing Infectious Diseases

Chapter Objectives

On completing this chapter, you will be able to:

■ describe the movement of a cold virus through each link in the chain of infectious disease.

■ explain why persons with HIV/AIDS do not generally progress beyond the clinical stage of their disease.

■ develop and then implement a plan to protect (or enhance) your immune system.

■ assess your own immunizations status, and make arrangements for any additional immunizations such as flu shots.

■ understand and describe the importance of frequent hand washing, particularly during the cold and flu season.

■ recognize the importance of testing dead birds found on campus or in your neighborhood for the presence of the West Nile virus.

■ identify those forms of hepatitis that are potentially sexually transmitted, in comparison to those that are not.

■ take proper precautions to protect yourself from HIV/AIDS and other sexually transmitted diseases.

Eye on the Media

From Fear to Hope—AIDS in the News

In the early days of news coverage about AIDS, magazines like *Time* and *Newsweek* ran articles called: "The AIDS Epidemic," "Epidemic of Fear," "Plague Mentality," "Fear of Sex," "The Growing Threat," "A Spreading Scourge," "The New Untouchables," "AIDS Spreading Panic Worldwide," "A Grim Race Against the Clock," and "The Lost Generation." The titles reflected fear of the unknown, a new killer disease.

When the case of Kimberley Bergalis broke into the news in 1991, a routine visit to the dentist was suddenly fraught with risk. Bergalis was the first American to die of AIDS after being infected by her dentist, Dr. David Acer. Four of Acer's other patients became infected with AIDS—all traced back to Acer. The public's reaction was near-hysteria. *Time* ran an article called "Should You Worry About Getting AIDS from Your Dentist?" People started asking their dentists (and other doctors) about their use of sterile precautions and even whether they had been tested for HIV.

By 1996, when the "cocktail" approach to AIDS treatment started showing remarkably good results, Magic Johnson was on the cover of both *Time* and *Newsweek* the same week. After more than 4 years of retirem─── ─ pro ───tball—and the ann── ───

Some People Immune?" and "What—I'm Gonna Live?" Doctors, too, are feeling more positive about the disease. As one AIDS specialist said: "I go to work feeling like there's something I can do for my patients."

For people with HIV/AIDS in the most highly developed countries, the future holds different things. For some, who can't afford to tolerate the new drugs, it's still a matter of waiting to die. Others feel that they've been given a second chance. They can think about having relationships again—something many put on hold when they learned they were HIV positive.

Most people with HIV/AIDS are buying time—hoping for the big breakthrough, the cure for AIDS. They're trying new drug treatments, hoping that one treatment won't disqualify them from the next one. They're watching TV news, reading the newspapers, and using the Internet with greater attention. Will protease-inhibiting drugs be the answer? Are the even newer antiviral medications the breakthrough hoped fo─ ──ccine on ─he horizon?

Changing for the Better

Healthy Restaurant Eating

How do you control portion sizes, make healthy choices, and know how food is prepared when eating out?

More than 35 percent of all food that Americans eat is eaten away from home, at restaurants, school, and other public places. Eating out creates unique challenges in keeping to your commitment to healthy eating. For example, waiting for your table to be ready while you're already feeling hungry and then having a basket of chips put in front of you while you wait for your order can derail the best of intentions. Also all-you-can-eat buffets practically beg you to overeat to "get your money's worth." What are some ways to make healthy choices when eating out?

Eat as you would ~ ~ at home. We tend to ~

- Don't starve yourself before going out to eat in preparation to overeat. Allow yourself plenty of time, taking into consideration how long you will need to wait for your table, wait to order, and be served so that you don't go when you are too hungry and then are starving by the time the food arrives.
- Ask how the food is prepared and the kinds of sauces accompanying the food, including vegetables. Choose lower-fat items that are described as: poached, roasted, stir-fried, broiled, or steamed. Avoid foods that are: breaded, fried, marinated, pan-fried, sautéed, au gratin, or scalloped. Consider terms like alfredo, basted, batter-dipped, buttery, creamy, and crispy to be red flags indicating high-fat ~

Changing for the Better
Learn to put health concepts into practice by following these useful tips. This feature provides practical advice for making positive changes and staying motivated to follow a healthy lifestyle.

TALKING POINTS What fast-food restaurants are your favorites? Are you surprised at any of the information in this chapter regarding your favorite meals? Will you change your order next time you visit a fast-food restaurant?

Talking Points
Throughout each chapter, you'll find these tips for starting a dialogue about sensitive health topics.

Discovering Your Spirituality

Harnessing the Spirit: The Saga of Lance Armstrong

In the summer of 1999, American cyclist Lance Armstrong made one of the most amazing sports comebacks in history. Armstrong won the Tour de France, the most grueling cycling event in the world. In October 1996, Armstrong had been diagnosed with advanced testicular cancer and was given less than a 50% chance of survival. At the time of the diagnosis, the cancer had already spread to Armstrong's abdomen, lungs, and brain.

After being diagnosed with cancer, but before starting aggressive therapy, Armstrong declared himself "a cancer survivor, not a cancer victim." He convinced himself, his family, and his medical support team that he could beat the long odds facing him. He even established the Lance Armstrong Foundation (www.laf.org) before he had surgery and chemotherapy. He battled through his therapy without giving up the hope that the cancer would be defeated.

Miraculously, Armstrong's cancer disappeared. He then stunned the cycling world by returning to active training and planning a comeback that included competing for the 1999 Tour de France title. As Armstrong's physical condition improved and his training regimen became more demanding, cycling enthusiasts believed that Armstrong m~ be able to ~ete in—~ ~rtainly not ~ —the ~

Discovering Your Spirituality
A healthy body and a healthy mind go hand in hand. This feature will help you tap into your spiritual side to improve your self-esteem, foster good relationships with others, and jump-start your physical health.

Considering Complementary Care

Hypnotism: A Solution for Smokers?

On at least one occasion each year a "professional" hypnotist visits the community in which we (the authors) live. A large advertisement appears in the local paper a day or two before his visit to identify his location (usually a motel conference room) and the problems (obesity and smoking) that his brand of hypnosis proves effective against. The cost of a one-time session generally ranges between $30 (for one condition) and $50 (for both conditions), with a discount for groups of two or more preregistered persons. Effective rates are generally stated to be 97.5% for weight reduction and 98% for smoking abatement. The term "effective" is, of course, never defined.

In terms of smoking abatement, what about the services of a clinically trained and hospital-based psychologist who specializes in the use of hypnosis? Does hypnosis of this type have efficacy in smoking abatement—either as a sole treatment modality or in combination with other therapies?

In an attempt to answer this question, a Med-Line search using the key word "hypnosis" was conducted with the following results. In the time period between January and August 2000, 68 studies addressing the clinical application of hypnosis were published in the medical literature. Of these, three studies were related to the use of hypnosis in smoking abatement ~ ~he three studies ~ ~lved the ~a-anal~ ~rlier st~ ~he basis ~

for smoking cessation." They did acknowledge that hypnosis is "possibly efficacious," but only when cognitive/behavioral and educational intervention that often accompanies hypnosis is included in the study.[1] The authors of the second and smallest (9 earlier studies) of the current studies concluded that they were unable to show "that hypnotherapy has a greater effect on 6-month quit rates than did other interventions or no treatment."[2] A recent Med-line review of hypnosis-based smoking-cessation studies shows that very few were undertaken since 2000. Again, results that were reported were, at best, cautiously optimistic, but in most studies the number of persons treated was small, sessions were few in number, and self-reporting was the principal means of assessing results.

Authors of the various, Med-line studies all concluded that more and better designed studies on hypnosis-based smoking cessation were needed.

Searches involving the Web sites of The National Center for Complementary and Alternative Medicine and American Psychological Association failed to identify studies related to hypnosis and smoking cessation.

~ IP, Lynn SJ. Hypnosis and ~ ~ed approaches to smokin~ ~examination of ~ ~on 48(2): 19~

Considering Complementary Care
Interested in nontraditional approaches to health care? What really works? What's really safe? This feature invites you to take a critical look at alternative approaches to health care and make up your own mind.

Learning from Our Diversity

These unique boxes invite you to explore the rich diversity of your own campus, and to gain perspective on the way such characteristics as age, racial/ethnic background, physical abilities, and sexual orientation can shape individuals' lives and well-being.

Learning from our Diversity
Breast Cancer: A Rare Diagnosis in Men

With all the attention given to breast cancer in women—in the news, by physicians, and by research foundations—you may be surprised to learn that men are also diagnosed with this condition. For every 100 women who develop breast cancer, however, only one case is reported among men. Estimates for the year 2005 suggest that no more than 1,690 American men will develop breast cancer. When compared to the 211,240 cases anticipated in women during the same year, the rarity of breast cancer in men becomes apparent.

The typical male breast cancer victim is usually older than 60 and often has a family history of the disease. The BRCA2 tumor suppressor mutation within the   In some

conditions, such as various forms of liver disease, also result in higher levels of estrogen and, eventually, a greater risk of male breast cancer.

In most ways male breast cancer is very similar in type to that seen in women. Infiltrating ductal cancer, ductal carcinoma in situ, and a form of cancer arising from the ducts immediately beneath the nipple (Paget's disease) have been reported. Because of this close similarity to female breast cancer, medical management of male breast cancer closely parallels that seen in women. Surgery (a modified radical mastectomy), chemotherapy, external radiation, and hormonal therapy are used alone or in combination. The latter therapy may include not only   the influence   on-sensitive

---

Personal Assessment

Do you eat too much fat? What's the best method of birth control for you if you are sexually active? Are you a perfectionist? Each chapter in *Understanding Your Health* includes an assessment to help you learn the answers to these and many other questions.

personal assessment

how stressed are you?

A widely used life-stress scale called the Social Readjustment Rating Scale by Holmes and Rahe has been used to determine the degree of stress that you are experiencing because of life events over the past year. It also projects your chances of developing an illness- or stress-related health condition. Stress can lead to some serious health problems, and the more stress you have in your life, the more vulnerable you are to being susceptible to illness. Let's see how you score.

Life-Stress Scale

Check off the events that have happened to you **within the last year.** Then add up your total number of stress units for each life-stress event. The number on the right-hand side represents the amount, duration, and severity of change required to cope with each item. See the point scale at the end of the inventory to determine the health risk associated with your stress level.

Life Event	Value	Score
Death of a partner	100	___
Divorce	73	___
Relationship separation	65	___
Jail term	63	___
Death of a family member	63	___
Personal injury/illness	53	___
Marriage	50	___
Fired from job	47	___
Reconciliation with partner	45	___
Retirement	45	___
Illness—family member	44	___
Pregnancy	40	___
Sexual difficulties	39	___
Addition of a family m	39	___
Change in finan	38	

Begin or end school	26	___
Partner begins/stops working	26	___
Change in living conditions	25	___
Change in personal habits	24	___
Trouble with supervisor	23	___
Change in work hours	20	___
Change in residence	20	___
Change in schools	20	___
Change in recreation	19	___
Change in church activities	19	___
Change in social activities	18	___
Mortgage/loan less than $10,000	17	___
Change in sleeping habits	16	___
Change in family visits	15	___
Change in eating habits	15	___
Vacation	13	___
Christmas	12	___
Minor violations of the law	11	___

TOTAL SCORE ___

What Is Your Health Risk?

Note that positive events such as outstanding personal achievements, vacations, and Christmas can be as stressful as negative ones. Think of events in your life that are not listed on this inventory. For example, where would you put running in a marathon or going on a diet?

⇒ If your score was 150 points or less . . .
You are on reasonably safe and healthy ground. You have about a one-in-three chance of a health change in the next 2 years.

⇒ If your score was between 150–300 points . . .
You have about a 50/50 chance of developing an illness due to stress in the ne

Understanding Your Health

chapter one

Shaping Your Health

Chapter Objectives

On completing this chapter, you will be able to:

▌understand how your health affects your lifestyle.

▌recognize how the delivery of health care influences definitions of health.

▌detail some of the health concerns outlined by the Institute of Medicine and Healthy People 2010.

▌suggest additional reasons why health behavior change is difficult, beyond those outlined in your textbook.

▌speculate on strategies for encouraging health behavior change.

▌list Prochaska's six stages of change.

▌describe and compare the range of traditional and nontraditional students on your campus.

▌describe the developmental tasks of adulthood, and assess your current or past level of progress in mastering them.

▌monitor your own activities, and list the dimensions of health from which resources are drawn.

▌compare wellness and health promotion, noting both the differences and the similarities between the two concepts.

▌describe your textbook's new definition of health, and compare it with definitions from episodic health care and health promotion.

Eye on the Media

Where Does Our Health Information Come From?

Today our health information comes from a variety of media—some more reliable than others. Eye on the Media will appear in each chapter of this text, highlighting the important issue of which ones are good (in other words, valid and reliable) sources for learning about health.

Radio and Television

When you think of radio, the first thing that may come to mind is your favorite music. But two areas of radio are especially important for news and information: talk radio and public radio networks, such as National Public Radio (NPR) and Public Radio International (PRI). Talk radio raises the question of validity of information. For example, if you're listening to a talk show about HIV exposure, the perceptions and opinions of the host (which may be strong or even extreme) are an important part of the show. When this point of view is combined with the opinions of callers, whose "facts" may come from unauthoritative sources, what you're hearing is probably not solid information. It's certainly not a good basis for making your health decisions.

NPR and PRI, however, take a scholarly approach to news, featuring experts who do not always agree on an issue. In general, the news reports on NPR and PRI are long enough to present an in-depth, balanced treatment of health-related topics.

Television too, is often an important source of health information. Coverage ranges from brief health-related segments on national or local news programs to entire cable programs devoted to health topics, such as those seen on the Learning and Discovery channels. While these programs can be timely and accurate, television also provides an array of "Infomericals" promoting health products that should be evaluated more critically.

Newspapers and Magazines

Let's assume that most people read only one or two newspapers a day—their local paper and perhaps a national newspaper such as the *New York Times* or *USA Today.* If so, the health information they are receiving is typically from wire services like the Associated Press; it is condensed and simplified but accurate within these limitations. When health-related information in newspapers is accompanied by illustrations and identification of the original source (such as a professional journal), it is more helpful to the reader.

Unlike newspapers, magazines are so diverse in terms of ownership, intended audience, and standards of validity that it is difficult to determine the reliability of their health-related content. In general, the national news magazines, such as *Time* and *Newsweek,* are very careful about the accuracy of their reporting, often including primary (original) sources. Their content is considered "state of the art." In contrast, the checkout-lane tabloids, such as the *Globe* and the *National Enquirer,* are known for printing stories with "health" content that few readers take seriously. Between these two extremes is a wide array of general content magazines, such as the *Saturday Evening Post,* and health-oriented

Eye on the Media *continued*
magazines, such as *Prevention,* that vary greatly in validity and reliability.

Professional Journals

Your college library probably offers a broad selection of professional journals. Through these publications, the members of an academic discipline share the latest developments and issues in their field with their colleagues and other readers. Because the study of health is so multifaceted, drawing on different disciplines for information, health-related journals are plentiful. The vast majority of articles that appear in publications such as the *New England Journal of Medicine* and the *Journal of the American Dietetic Association* are peer-reviewed. This means that professionals in the particular field review and judge the content of a submitted article to determine whether or not it should be published. Then, if a study being reported was not carefully controlled, or if its underlying theory seems to be flawed, the article is returned to the author(s) for refinement. This process greatly reduces the risk of publishing invalid information. Currently, journals are beginning to appear in fields such as complementary (alternative) health care. When reading such publications, you need to consider whether they are backed by a peer-review process.

Government Documents

Each year various departments of the federal government, particularly the Department of Health and Human Services (DHHS), release the results of research being done under the oversight of its many divisions and agencies.

These documents, such as the annual *Surgeon General's Report on Smoking and Health,* become the source of much of the health-related news reported by other media sources, including textbooks and professional journals. These publications generally can be purchased through the U.S. Government Printing Office. They are also available through urban public libraries and large university libraries. With few exceptions, the information in these publications is reviewed by the most respected authorities in each field.

Books

Books continue to be a vast source of information on health-related topics. Today's health books, in addition to academic health textbooks such as *Understanding Your Health,* fall into three categories: reference books, medical encyclopedias, and single-topic trade (retail) books.

Included in the category of reference books are important professional publications such as *The Merck Manual* and the *Physicians' Desk Reference.* These books, intended for professionals in various health fields, contain the most current information on specific aspects of health. Although these books can be purchased by the general public, their content is technical and complex, and their language is often difficult for nonprofessional readers to follow.

More valuable to the typical American household are the various medical (health) encyclopedias, such as *The Johns Hopkins Home Medical Handbook* and *The Mayo Clinic Family Health Book.* Such books usually include a wide array of medical conditions

and offer valuable information about health promotion and disease prevention. Their clear writing styles and highly valid information make these books excellent home references.

Single-topic health-related trade books, such as those about diets and health problems, are readily available from retail outlets such as bookstores and Internet stores. Like magazines, these books are difficult to assess because of their quantity and the varying backgrounds of the authors. Some are very sound in terms of content and philosophy. Others may be misleading and may contain advice that could be dangerous to your health. Included in this group are self-help books, the best-selling health books of all.

The Internet

By the year 2007, according to Forrester Research, it is projected that nearly 85 percent of American households will have direct access to the Internet. Internet access is also available through libraries, educational institutions, and the workplace. With just a few clicks, you can reach many health-related Web sites that offer a wide range of health information. Chat rooms provide a forum for individuals to share their personal health experiences. Because the Internet is such an important source of health information for both professionals and the general public, this textbook highlights helpful Web sites in all chapters. To learn about criteria for assessing the validity and reliability of Internet information, see Chapter 18.

Source: Forrester Research. *83.4% U.S. households connected by 2007.* April 23, 2004, www.itfacts.biz/index.php?id=105ml-3A.

"Take care of your health, because you'll miss it when it's gone," younger people hear often from their elders. This simple and heartfelt advice is given in the belief that young people take their health for granted and assume that they will always maintain the state of health and wellness they now enjoy. Observation and experience should, however, remind all of us that youth is relatively brief, and health is always changing—often in a downward direction. In fact, as health deteriorates, our ability to participate in meaningful life activities can be compromised or even lost. Consider, for example, how failing health might affect the following activities:

- Your ability to pursue an education or a career
- Your opportunity to socialize with friends and family
- The chance to travel—for business, relaxation, or adventure
- The opportunity to meet and connect with new people
- The ability to conceive or the opportunity to parent children

- Participation in hobbies or recreational activities
- Your enjoyment of a wide range of foods
- The opportunity to live independently

Quality-of-life issues such as these are your parents' and grandparents' focus when they advise you to take care of your health. As you will learn in this chapter, health is intertwined with activities such as these—indeed, your authors will present a new definition of health specifically related to accomplishing these important life tasks. But first, we review a few familiar perceptions of health, each of which is concerned primarily with illness and death, and we discuss strategies for changing health behaviors.

Definitions of Health

By the time they reach college age, most Americans are familiar with the many ways in which health care is provided. Following are some easily recognizable examples, all of which serve to reinforce our traditional definitions of health. Note that these examples involve the cure or management of illness and the extension of life, indicated by concerns about **morbidity** and **mortality.**

We present a new definition of health near the end of the chapter. This new definition should be viewed as a partner to the following traditional examples of health care. The principal difference relates to the new definition's developmental focus rather than a focus on traditional concerns about morbidity and mortality.

Episodic Health Care

The vast majority of Americans use the services of professional health care providers during periods (*episodes*) of illness and injury, that is, when we are "unhealthy." We consult providers, seeking a diagnosis that will explain why we are not feeling well. Once a problem is identified, we expect to receive effective treatment from the practitioners that will lead to our recovery (the absence of illness) and a return to health. If we are willing to comply with the care strategies prescribed by our practitioners, we should soon be able to define ourselves as "healthy" once again.

The familiarity of episodic health care is evident in the 890 million times that Americans visited physicians during 2002. Although some of these visits were for preventive health care (see discussion in the following section), the vast majority were in conjunction with illness. When viewed according to racial group, Whites averaged 3.4 visits, Blacks 2.5, and Asians 2.3 visits during that year.[1] A similar reporting in 2000 indicated that Native Americans made only 0.8 visits that year.[2]

 TALKING POINTS Would you be hesitant to talk to your doctor about health advice you found on the Internet? How would you approach the subject?

Factors That Affect Well-Being

Which factors do today's adults associate with the ability to feel good about their lives? Check the list below for the answers given to this question. Note that virtually no respondent makes direct reference to being free of illness and disease or to living long into the future. Rather, respondents are more aligned with a personally defined sense of being adequately independent, self-sufficient, responsible, respected by others, and nurturing.

- A sense of *personal satisfaction* (82%) was identified as the most important feeling that should be experienced during adulthood.

- A sense of *being in control* of one's life (80%) was the second most identified index of adult well-being.

- A sense that one was a partner in a *good marriage* (78%) appeared as the third most important component of living well as an adult.

- A sense that one was *competent at one's job* (69%) placed employment in fourth position—important but clearly below the factors listed above. Also, note that *making a lot of money* was selected by only 25% as being of primary importance in defining adult life satisfaction.

- A sense that one's *children were (or would be) successful* was cited by 63% of the adults sampled as an important factor in feeling a sense of well-being.

Having studied these responses, you also may appreciate more fully the meaning we assign to having a sense of well-being and the role health plays in making it possible.

Preventive or Prospective Medicine

Simple logic suggests that it makes more sense to prevent illness than to deal with it through episodic health (medical) care. This philosophy characterizes **preventive or prospective medicine.** Unfortunately, however, many physicians say they have little time to practice preventive medicine because of the large number of episodically sick people who fill their offices every day.

Key Terms

morbidity pertaining to illness and disease

mortality pertaining to death

preventive or prospective medicine physician-centered medical care in which areas of risk for chronic illnesses are identified so that they might be lowered

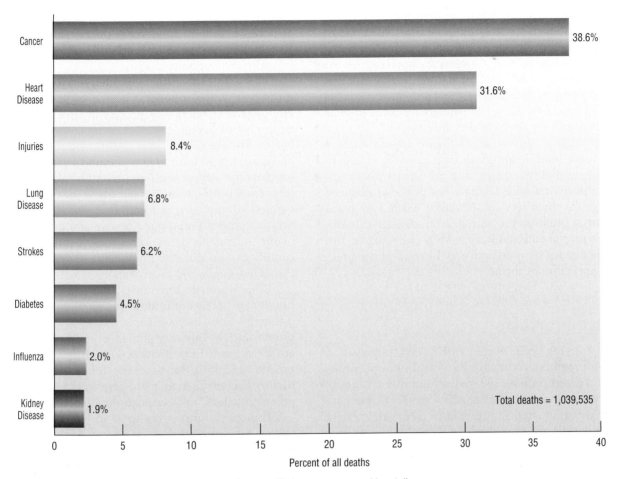

Figure 1-1 Top eight causes of death. 2004 marked the first year that cancer surpassed heart disease as the leading cause of death for Americans under the age of 80.

Sources: *Estimated Cancer Cases and Deaths by Sex, for All Sites,* U.S., 2005. American Cancer Society, 2005; Deaths: Final data for 2002, *National Vital Statistics Report,* National Center for Health Statistics, October 12, 2004.

When physicians do practice preventive or prospective medicine, they first attempt to determine their patient's level of risk for developing particular conditions. They make this assessment by identifying **risk factors** (and **high-risk health behaviors**) with a variety of observational techniques and screening tests, some of which may be invasive (taking tissues from the body such as a biopsy or blood draw). Additionally, an important tool in assessing risk is an accurate family health history, something that over one-third of all adults cannot adequately provide to their health care providers.[3] So important is a health history that the federal government has established a Web site to assist us in becoming familiar with our family's health history (www.hhs.gov/familyhistory). Certainly, if you identify any of the conditions shown in Figure 1-1, share them with your primary care physician.[4]

It is disconcerting to report that important medical information, including laboratory reports, comprehensive drug inventories, and family health histories, are often missing from medical files. A 2003 study involving primary care physician medical records suggests that perhaps one out of every seven patient files is missing information important to providing comprehensive health care.[5]

Key Terms

risk factor a biomedical index such as serum cholesterol level or a behavioral pattern such as smoking, associated with a chronic illness

high-risk health behavior a behavioral pattern, such as smoking, associated with a high risk of developing a chronic illness

Once they have identified levels of risk in patients, health practitioners try to lower those risk levels through patient education, lifestyle modification, and, when necessary, medical intervention. Continued compliance on the part of the patients will result in a lower level of risk that will continue over the years. Note that preventive medicine is guided by practitioners, and patients are expected to be compliant with the direction they are given.

Although preventive medical care appears to be a much more sensible approach than episodic care is in reducing morbidity and mortality, third-party payers (insurance plans) traditionally have not provided adequate coverage for these services. Managed health care plans that earn a profit by preventing sickness, such as health maintenance organizations, or HMOs (see Chapter 18), should be much more receptive to the concept and practice of preventive medicine.

Health Promotion

Throughout the United States, YMCA/YWCA-sponsored wellness programs, commercial fitness clubs, and corporate fitness centers offer risk-reduction programs under the direction of qualified instructors, many of whom are university graduates in disciplines such as exercise science, wellness management, and **health promotion.** Using approaches similar to those employed in preventive medicine, these nonphysician health professionals attempt to guide their clients toward activities and behaviors that will lower their risk of chronic illness. Unlike preventive medicine, with its sometimes invasive assessment procedures and medication-based therapies, health promotion programs are not legally defined as medical practices and thus do not require the involvement of physicians. In addition, the fitness focus, social interaction, and healthy lifestyle orientation these programs provide tend to mask the emphasis on preventing chronic illness that would be the selling point of such efforts if they were undertaken as preventive medicine. In fact, it is likely that people receiving health promotion in these settings do not recognize it as such. Rather, they are submitting to assessments and listening to health-related information only as incidental parts of personal goals, such as losing weight, preparing for their first marathon, or simply meeting friends for lunch-hour basketball.

Community Health Promotion

In addition to the practices just described, a group-oriented form of health promotion is offered in many communities. This approach to improving health through risk reduction is directed at empowering community groups, such as church congregations or a neighborhood association, so they can develop, operate, and financially sustain their own programs with little direct involvement of health promotion specialists.[6,7]

The key to successful community-based health promotion is **empowerment.**[8] In the context of health, empowerment refers to a process in which individuals or groups of people gain increasing control over their health. To take control over health matters, individuals and groups must learn to move beyond a variety of barriers that once were restrictions on health enhancement. In this sense, people learn to take charge of their lives, regardless of any current forces that discourage positive health changes. Empowered people and groups do not blame individuals or environmental realities for health conditions but focus on producing constructive change through dialogue and collaboration.

Empowerment programs have produced positive health consequences for individuals and groups that traditionally have been underserved by the health care system, such as minority populations. Once such people are given needed information, inroads into the political process, and skills for accessing funding sources, they become better able to plan, implement, and operate programs tailored to their unique health needs.

Perhaps no greater challenge in establishing health-related empowerment is that related to the devastating tsunami that occurred on December 26, 2004, in the Indian Ocean basin. In addition to coping with a death toll approaching 200,000 and the displacement of entire communities, much of the effort and resources needed to rebuild viable communities will eventually need to be transitioned from professionally staffed international relief organizations into the hands of the local people. When successful, these empowerment programs stand as excellent examples of the fact that people can make a difference when they become empowered.

Having learned about the sources of our familiar and traditional definitions of health, recall that a new and unique definition of health is presented later in the chapter.

Key Terms

health promotion movement in which knowledge, practices, and values are transmitted to people for use in lengthening their lives, reducing the incidence of illness, and feeling better

empowerment the nurturing of an individual's or group's ability to be responsible for their own health and well-being

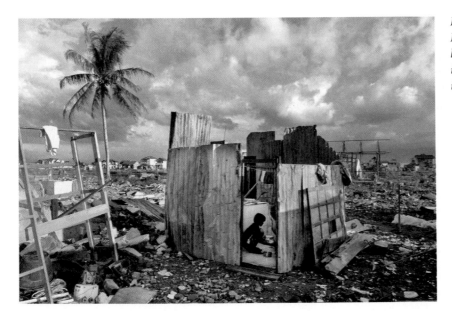

Recovery from the disastrous tsunami of December 26, 2004, will not be complete until local residents are adequately empowered by internationally-based assistance and expertise in the rebuilding of their homes and lives.

Federal Programs to Improve the Health of People in the United States

To identify all the health-related concerns identified by members of the health community would be a monumental undertaking far beyond the scope of this book. However, in 2003, the Institute of Medicine released a list of priority health concerns that they believe need particular attention.[9] Among these priority concerns are these:

- treatment of asthma
- coordination of care for the 60 million or more persons with chronic health conditions
- reduction in the development of diabetes
- development of evidence-based cancer screening
- enhanced rates of immunization, particularly for flu and pneumonia
- improved detection of depression, which is now inadequately diagnosed and treated
- aggressively promoted prevention of cardiovascular disease, presently the second leading killer of American adults under the age of 80
- reduction of tobacco dependence through cessation and prevention of smoking
- widened availability of prenatal care

While improvements in these areas are greatly needed, the Institute of Medicine has no specific programs in place at this time to address them. In comparison, well-established

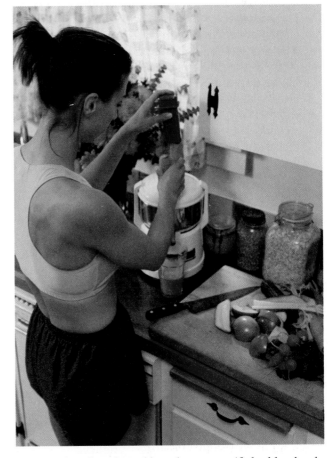

Many students have been able to change a specific health-related behavior, such as replacing poor eating habits with nutritious food choices.

As if being a student is not enough, I'm experiencing a growing sense of concern about health problems that are occurring in my family. I don't want to have some of the problems that family members are now experiencing, so what should I be doing to sustain my current level of good health?

Prescriptions for good health usually place considerable importance on *risk reduction*. Health care professionals stress the importance of identifying behavioral patterns and biomedical indexes that suggest the potential for illness or death. Each of us has the opportunity to receive information, counseling, behavior change strategies, and medical therapies designed to lower our risk. The extent to which we act on this opportunity is our degree of *compliance*.

Some risk factors cannot be reduced. For example, gender, race, age, and genetic predisposition make developing certain conditions more likely. Being aware of these risk factors is important.

To refocus on good health, concentrate on these actions, which can reduce risk factors:

- *Refrain from using tobacco in any form.* This rule is so critically important that the surgeon general of the United States has identified smoking as the single most important reversible factor contributing to illness and early death.
- *If you drink alcohol, do so in moderation.* This is particularly important for people who must drive or operate machinery, women who are pregnant or planning to become pregnant, and people taking certain medications.
- *Engage in regular exercise designed to train the cardiorespiratory system as well as maintain muscle strength.* You can use a wide array of exercises as the basis of a fitness program, and you can develop specific programs around recommendations about frequency, duration, and intensity of activity.
- *Familiarize yourself with the newly adopted Dietary Guidelines for Americans* (Chapter 5). Strong emphasis is now being placed on controlling portion size, increasing the amount of fruits and vegetables in our diets, and exercising daily.
- *Develop effective coping techniques for use in moderating the effects of stress.* Effective coping can reduce the duration of physiological challenge the body faces during periods of unexpected change. Remember, however, that some forms of coping can themselves be sources of additional stress.
- *Maintain normal body weight.* Persons who are excessively overweight or underweight may experience abnormal structural or functional changes, predispose themselves to chronic illnesses, and unnecessarily shorten their lives. Lifelong weight management is preferable to intermittent periods of weight gain and loss.
- *Receive regular preventive health care from competent professionals.* This care should include routine screening and risk-reducing lifestyle management, early diagnosis, and effective treatment if needed.
- *Maintain an optimistic outlook.* Anger, cynicism, and a pessimistic outlook on life can erode the holistic basis on which high-level health is built. Several chronic conditions, including cardiovascular diseases and cancers, occur more frequently in persons who lack a positive outlook on their own lives and life in general.
- *Establish a personally meaningful belief system.* Over the course of long life the presence of such a system and the supportive spiritual community usually associated with it may prove to be the most beneficial health resource we can possess.

InfoLinks

www.cdc.gov/nccdphp/index.htm

and ongoing programs, Healthy People 2000 and Healthy People 2010, have established specific goals and objectives to improve the health of Americans in many of these areas. A brief descripton of these ongoing programs follows.

In 1991 the U.S. Department of Health and Human Services document titled *Healthy People 2000: National Health Promotion and Disease Prevention Objectives*[10] outlined a strategic plan for promoting the health of the American public. The plan included 300 health objectives in 22 priority areas. Forty-seven of the 300 objectives were defined as "sentinel" ones, that is, particularly significant goals that could be used to measure the progress of the 1990s health promotion objectives.

Progress toward achieving the objectives was assessed near the middle of the decade and reported in a document titled *Healthy People 2000: Midcourse Review and 1995 Revisions.*[11] Although progress was reported in some areas, little or no progress was reported in many. Subsequently, a new plan, called *Healthy People 2010: Understanding and Improving Health,*[12] was formulated, refined, and is now being implemented.[13]

Healthy People 2010: Understanding and Improving Health is a health promotion program intended to be implemented at all levels, ranging from individual involvement through multinational cooperative efforts, including *Health for All in the 21st Century,*[14] a World Health Organization health promotion initiative. Although the goals of *Healthy People 2000: National Health Promotion and Disease Prevention Objectives* and *Healthy People 2010: Understanding and Improving Health* are similar, the latter focuses on the projected needs of the United States during the first decade of the new century.

Central to the design of *Healthy People 2010: Understanding and Improving Health* are two paramount goals: (1) increasing quality and years of life and (2) eliminating health disparities in areas such as gender, race, and ethnicity, as well as income and education level. These goals in turn provide 28 more focused objectives. Progress in accomplishing these objectives is anticipated through the manipulation of the behavioral, biological, and environmental determinants of health as they relate to 10 of the leading health indicators: (1) physical activity, (2) weight management, (3) tobacco use, (4) substance abuse, (5) responsible sexual behavior, (6) mental health, (7) injury and violence, (8) environmental quality, (9) immunization, and (10) access to health care.

The success of *Healthy People 2010: Understanding and Improving Health* will not be known until nearer the end of the decade. However, if its goals are ultimately reached, Americans can anticipate improved quantity and quality of life.

Changing Health-Related Behavior

Although some health concerns can be successfully addressed through local, state, national, or international efforts, such as those just outlined, most are ultimately based on the willingness and ability of persons to change aspects of their own behavior.

Why Behavior Change Is Often Difficult

Several factors can strongly influence a person's desire to change high health-risk behaviors, including these:

1. A person must know that a particular behavioral pattern is clearly associated with (or even causes) a particular health problem. For example: cigarette smoking is the primary cause of lung cancer.
2. A person must believe (accept) that a behavioral pattern will make (or has made) him susceptible to this particular health problem. For example: my cigarette smoking will significantly increase my risk of developing lung cancer.
3. A person must recognize that risk-reduction intervention strategies exist and that should she adopt these in a compliant manner she too will reduce her risk for a particular health condition. For example: smoking-cessation programs exist, and following such a program could help me quit smoking.
4. A person must believe that benefits of newly adopted health-enhancing behaviors will be more reinforcing than the behaviors being given up. For example: the improved health, lowered risk, and freedom from dependence resulting from no longer smoking are better than the temporary pleasures provided by smoking.
5. A person must feel that significant others in his life truly want him to alter his high-risk health behaviors and will support his efforts. For example: my friends who are cigarette smokers will make a concerted effort to not smoke in my presence and will help me avoid being around people who smoke.

When one or more of the conditions listed above is not in place, the likelihood that persons will be successful in reducing health-risk behaviors is greatly diminished.

Stages of Change

The process of behavioral change unfolds over time and progresses through defined stages.[15,16] James Prochaska, John Norcross, and Carol DiClemente outlined six predictable stages of change. They studied thousands of individuals who were changing long-standing problems such as alcohol abuse, smoking, and gambling. While these people used different strategies to change their behavior, they all proceeded through six consistent stages of change in the process referred to as **Prochaska's Stages of Change.**[17]

Precontemplation Stage

The first stage of change is called *precontemplation,* during which persons might think about making a change but ultimately find it too difficult and avoid making it. For example, during this phase a smoker might tell friends, "Eventually I will quit" but have no real intention of stopping within the next six months.

Contemplation Stage

For many, however, progress toward change begins as they move into a *contemplation* stage, during which they might develop the desire to change but have little understanding of how to go about it. Typically, they see themselves taking action within the next six months.

Preparation Stage

Following the contemplation stage, a *preparation* stage begins, during which change begins to appear to be not only desirable but possible as well. A smoker might begin making plans to quit during this stage, setting a quit date for the very near future (a few days to a month) and perhaps enrolling in a smoking-cessation program.

> **Key Terms**
>
> **Prochaska's Stages of Change** the six predictable stages— precontemplation, contemplation, preparation, action, maintenance, and termination—people go through in establishing new habits and patterns of behavior

Keys to Longer Living

Experts generally agree on basic lifestyle characteristics that support greater longevity and, we hope, a higher quality of life. Small adjustments that promote this improvement include:

- Testing your cholesterol level regularly and taking a 30-minute brisk walk every day.

- Wearing a seat belt in the car and a helmet while riding a bicycle, motorcycle, or while skating.

- Substituting olive oil for butter.

- Quitting smoking, or at least reducing the amount of tobacco used daily. Lung cancer is the most frequent cause of cancer-related death in the United States.

- Avoiding sun exposure from 11 A.M. until 2 P.M., when UV radiation is most dangerous. Stay inside during those peak hours, and always wear sunscreen outdoors.

- Asking questions of your doctor or pharmacist about concerns, test results, diagnosis, and treatments. It is often helpful to take someone with you to important appointments.

- Don't worry! Even if everyone were overly cautious, we would still not live in a risk-free world—unnecessary worry can stress the mind and body.

Action Stage

Plans for change are implemented during the *action* stage, during which changes are made and sustained for a period of about six months.

Maintenance Stage

The fifth stage is the *maintenance* stage, during which new habits are consolidated and practiced for an additional six months.

Termination Stage

The sixth and final stage is called *termination,* which refers to the point at which new habits are well established, and so efforts to change are complete.

Today's Health Concerns

To this point in the chapter we have identified some health concerns and addressed the desirability of health-related behavior change. Earlier in the chapter we looked at those illnesses that are the major causes of death that afflict people in the United States. However, in spite of astonishing progress on many fronts, we continue to face a number of serious health challenges from those and other illnesses. Heart disease, cancer, accidents, drug use, and mental illness all are important concerns for each of us, even if we are not

directly affected by them. Also becoming increasingly troublesome are the complex problems of environmental pollution, violence, health care costs, and the international scope of the HIV/AIDS epidemic, as well as other sexually transmitted diseases. Figure 1-1 on page 5 lists the eight leading causes of death in the United States expressed as a percentage of all deaths. Table 1.1 depicts the leading causes of death at various age levels. World hunger, overpopulation, and the

Table 1.1 Leading Causes of Death in the United States by Age Group, 2002

In data collected by the American Cancer Society comparing 2003–2004 deaths from cancer and heart disease, cancer was found to have surpassed heart disease for the first time as the leading cause of death for Americans under 80 years of age (see Figure 1-1). However, note the preponderance of heart disease deaths over cancer deaths in persons 85 and over.

1–4 Years	Number of Deaths
Unintentional injuries	1,641
Birth defects	530
Cancer	402
5–14 Years	
Unintentional injuries	2,718
Cancer	1,017
Homicide	356
15–24 Years	
Unintentional injuries	15,912
Homicide	5,214
Suicide	4,010
25–44 Years	
Unintentional injuries	29,279
Heart disease	20,948
Cancer	19,957
45–64 Years	
Cancer	143,018
Heart disease	124,230
Unintentional injuries	23,020
65–84 Years	
Heart disease	431,486
Cancer	311,819
Stroke	76,811
85 and over	
Heart disease	339,409
Cancer	29,182
Stroke	66,412

Source: "Deaths: Final Data for 2002," *National Vital Statistics Report,* National Center For Health Statistics, October 12, 2004.

threat of domestic and international terrorism are other health-related issues that will affect us, as well as the generations that follow.

The health concerns just mentioned are by no means unmanageable. Fortunately, we as individuals can reduce the likelihood of encountering many of these conditions by making choices in the way we live our lives. On a personal level, we can decide to pursue a plan of healthful living to minimize the incidence of illness and disease and to extend life.

Health: More Than the Absence of Illness?

What exactly is health? Is it simply the absence of disease and illness, as Western medicine has held for centuries—or does health embrace other elements we ought to consider now that the 21st century has begun?

Rather routinely national news magazines (and other media) feature articles describing advances in modern medicine.[18,19] These articles describe vividly in words and images the impressive progress being made in fields such as drug research, gene manipulation, computer-aided surgery, and the role of diet in health. Because of articles like this that relate health to medical care, most of us continue to hold to our traditional perception of health as (1) the virtual absence of disease and illness (low levels of morbidity) and (2) the ability to live a long life (reduced risk of mortality). However, in striving to be fully "health educated" in the new century, perhaps we need to consider a broader definition that more accurately reflects the demands associated with becoming functional and satisfied persons as we transition through each adult stage of life—*young adulthood, middle adulthood,* and, finally, *older adulthood.* With this in mind, look forward to another definition of health—one that recognizes the importance of the more familiar definitions of health but is focused on the demands of our own growth and development. However, before looking at this new perception of health and its relationship to life stages (as labeled above), let's meet the readers of this book, today's college students, each of whom falls into one of the adult life stages.

Today's College Students

Readers of this textbook are college students, but they are also young adults, middle-age adults, or even older adults. In some cases their decision to be a student has placed them in settings far different from those being experienced by other people their age. For many students, college classes are sandwiched in between other obligations—for example, full-time job, parenting, community involvement, even the care of older parents. Some might be the first members of their families to pursue higher education. Many students come from economic, racial, or ethnic backgrounds quite different from those of the majority of their classmates. Thus, today there is no one type of college student, but all students are progressing through life in predictable yet unique ways.

Traditional-Age Undergraduate College Students

Statistics indicate that more than 15.8 million students were enrolled in degree-granting U.S. colleges and universities in 2001.[20] Nearly 57 percent of these students were women. In 2001, minority students made up approximately 25 percent of U.S. college students, and foreign students totaled 4 percent. Approximately 60 percent of students attended college on a full-time basis.

Because nearly 62 percent of all undergraduates are traditional-age students, this book is directed first at these students. However, because of significant growth in the proportion of older students, we also address a variety of life experiences and developmental tasks that are appropriate to these students. Unquestionably, the nontraditional-age students in our classes help our traditional-age students understand the wide and varied role that health plays throughout the life cycle.

 TALKING POINTS You are in charge of a campus event for students of various ages from several culture groups. How would you go about finding out what would make the event attractive to students with backgrounds different from your own?

Nontraditional-Age Undergraduate College Students

In 2001, nearly 38.5 percent of U.S. undergraduate college students were classified as **nontraditional-age students.**[20] Included in this vast overlapping group are part-time students, military veterans, students returning to college,

Learning from Our Diversity

Back to the Future: Nontraditional-Age Students Enrich the College Experience

To anyone who's visited a U.S. college campus in the last 15 years, it's abundantly clear that the once typical college student—White, middle class, between the ages of 18 and 24—is no longer in a majority on campus. In most institutions of higher learning, today's student body is a rich tapestry of color, culture, language, ability, and age. Wheelchair-accessible campuses roll out the welcome mat for students with disabilities; the air is filled with the sound of a dozen or more languages spoken by students from virtually every part of the world; students in their 60s chat animatedly with classmates young enough to be their grandchildren.

Of all the trends that are changing the face of college enrollment in the United States, perhaps the most significant is the increasing diversity in the age of students now on campus. Older students today are both a common and welcome sight in colleges and universities across the country. Many women cut short their undergraduate education—or defer graduate school—to marry and raise children. Divorcees, widows, and women whose children are grown often return to college, or enroll for the first time, to prepare for professional careers. And increasingly, both men and women are finding it desirable, if not essential, to further

their education as a means of either keeping their current job or qualifying for a higher position.

Just as children are enriched by the knowledge and experience of their grandparents and other older relatives, so too is today's college classroom a richer place when many of the seats are filled by students of nontraditional age. Without being didactic or preachy, older students can provide valuable guidance and direction to younger classmates who may be uncertain of their career path, or who may be wrestling with decisions about marriage and parenthood. In doing so, nontraditional-age students can gain helpful insights about young people's feelings, attitudes, challenges, and aspirations.

Among the many important benefits of today's increasingly diverse college campus, surely one of the most significant is the enhanced opportunity for intergenerational communication and understanding made possible by the growing numbers of students of nontraditional age.

In your classes, how would you characterize the interactions between traditional-age students and those of nontraditional age? In what ways are they enriching each other's college experience?

---

single parents, older adults, and evening students. These students enter the classroom with a wide assortment of life experiences and observations. Most of these students are 25 to 40 years old. (Read the Learning from Our Diversity box for a closer look at nontraditional-age students.)

Many nontraditional-age students are trying to juggle an extremely demanding schedule. The responsibilities of managing a job, a schedule of classes, and perhaps a family present formidable challenges. Performing these tasks on a limited budget compounds the difficulty. For many of these students, concerns over paying next month's rent, caring for aging parents, and finding affordable child care are among the challenges that confront them.

We want to make this textbook meaningful for both traditional-age and nontraditional-age students. Much of the information we present applies to both categories of students. We ask nontraditional-age students to do two things as you read this book: (1) reflect on your own young adult years and (2) examine your current lifestyle to see how the decisions you made as a younger adult are affecting the quality of your life now. Also, as a nontraditional-age student, you may have young adult children whose lives you can observe in light of the information you will find in this book.

Minority Students

Although enrollment patterns at colleges and universities vary, the overall number of minority students is increasing. In 2001, approximately 25 percent of all college students were minority students, with African Americans, Hispanic Americans, and Asian Americans representing the largest groups of minority students.[21] These students bring a rich variety of cultural influences and traditions to today's college environment.

Students with Disabilities

People with reported disabilities are another rapidly growing student population, currently constituting 9.3 percent of all undergraduates.[22] Improved diagnostic, medical, and rehabilitation procedures coupled with improved educational accommodations have opened up opportunities for these students at an increasing rate. In addition to students who have evident disabilities, such as blindness, deafness, or a physical disability requiring use of a wheelchair, an increasing number of students with "hidden" disabilities are on campus—students with learning disabilities (including attention deficit disorders), those with managed psychiatric and emotional problems, and those recovering from alcohol and substance abuse. Interestingly, many students with

What Is Complementary Medicine?

In addition to the episodic and preventive forms of medical care described earlier, a variety of other forms of health care, both curative and preventive, are moving more progressively into the medical care mainstream. Among these are chiropractic, reflexology, homeopathy, naturopathy, and herbalism (see Chapter 18), to mention but a few. Although the established medical community has long scoffed at these practices as being unscientific and ineffective, they are increasingly attractive to a growing segment of the population. Initially referred to collectively as *alternative* forms of health care, and more recently as *complementary* forms of care, today they are increasingly referred to as *integrative* forms of health care. This last term suggests a fusion (or integration) of various forms of care into traditional treatment/prevention approaches.

The increasing acceptance of integrative forms of health care is also seen in two relatively recent developments. The first is the formation in the mid-1990s of an Office of Complementary and Alternative Medicine within the National Institutes of Health. This office has been charged with the objective and systematic study of selected forms of nontraditional care. Clinical trials of various types are ongoing; they include *treatment trials, supportive care trials, prevention trials, screening trials* (early-detection trials), and *diagnostic trials*, all employing forms of alternative or complementary treatments. Subsequent assessments will be released as they are completed.

A second expression of the growing popularity of integrative forms of health care is the increasing tendency of health insurance companies and HMOs (Health Maintenance Organizations; see Chapter 18) to provide reimbursement of services from providers of nontraditional care. Today approximately 65 percent of all HMOs and several major insurance companies provide coverage for selective forms of integrative care.

As impressive as the "rush to coverage" described above might appear, consumers of medical care services should remember that at this time relatively little carefully controlled research is available on the *efficacy* (effectiveness) of most forms of integrative care.

In spite of cautionary notes such as this, the *popularity* of alternative medical services for improving, maintaining, or restoring health is beyond dispute. A study conducted in 2002 by the Institute of Medicine found that prayer (for self and others), supplement use, relaxation breathing techniques, group prayer, meditation, chiropractic, yoga, and massage were all employed. Prayer, in various settings, was by the far the most widely employed.

---

reported "hidden disabilities" often do not consider themselves to be disabled.[23]

TALKING POINTS When controversial subjects are discussed in class, do you think that your opinions (or how you present them) are affected by the fact that students of different cultural backgrounds are involved in the discussion?

Developmental Tasks of Young Adulthood

Because most of today's undergraduate college students range between the ages of 18 and perhaps 40, we address several areas of growth and development (defined as *developmental tasks*) that characterize the lives of people in this age group. When people sense that they are making progress in some or all of these areas, they are likely to report a sense of life satisfaction or, as we describe it, a sense of well-being.

Forming an Initial Adult Identity

For most of childhood and adolescence, most young people are seen by adults in their neighborhood or community as someone's son or daughter. With the onset of young adulthood, that stage has almost passed; both young people and society are beginning to look at each other in new ways.

As emerging adults, most young people want to present a unique identity to society. Internally they are constructing perceptions of themselves as the adults they wish to be; externally they are formulating the behavioral patterns that will project this identity to others.

Completion of this first developmental task is necessary for young adults to establish a foundation on which to mature identity during later stages of adulthood. As a result of their experiences in achieving an initial adult identity, they become capable of answering the central question of young adulthood: "Who am I?" Most likely, many nontraditional-age students also ask themselves this question as they progress through college and anticipate the changes that will result from completing a high level of formal education.

Establishing Independence

In contemporary society the primary responsibility for socialization during childhood and adolescence is assigned to the family and school, and less formally to the peer group. For nearly two decades these groups function as the primary contributors to a young person's knowledge, values, and behaviors. By young adulthood, however, students of traditional college age should be demonstrating the desire to move away from the dependent relationships that have existed between themselves and these socializing agents.

 TALKING POINTS What does being an adult mean to you at this point? How would you explain this to your best friend?

Travel, new relationships, marriage, military service, and, of course, college have been traditional avenues for disengagement from the family. Generally, the ability and the willingness to follow one or more of these paths helps a young adult establish independence. Success in these endeavors depends on the willingness to use a variety of resources that we will explore later.

Assuming Responsibility

The third developmental task in which traditional-age college students are expected to progress is the assumption of increasing levels of responsibility. Young adults have a variety of opportunities to assume responsibility. College-age young adults may accept responsibility voluntarily, such as when they join a campus organization or establish a new friendship. Other responsibilities are placed on them when professors assign term papers, when dating partners exert pressure on them to conform to their expectations, or when employers require consistently productive work. In other situations they may accept responsibility for doing a particular task not for themselves but for the benefit of others. As important and demanding as these areas of responsibility are, a more fundamental responsibility awaits young adults: the responsibility of maintaining and improving their health and the health of others.

Broadening Social Skills

The fourth developmental task of the young adult years is broadening the range of appropriate and dependable social skills. Adulthood ordinarily involves "membership" in a variety of groups that range in size from a marital pair to a community organization or a multinational corporation. These memberships require the ability to function in many different social settings and with a wide variety of people.

The college experience traditionally has prepared students very effectively in this regard, but interactions in friendships, work relationships, or parenting may require that they make an effort to grow and develop beyond levels they achieved by belonging to a group made up largely of agemates. Young adults need to refine a variety of social skills, including communication, listening, and conflict management.

Nurturing Intimacy

The task of nurturing intimacy usually begins in young adulthood and continues through midlife. During this time it is developmentally important to establish one or more intimate relationships. Most people in this age group are viewing intimacy in its broadest sense as a deeply close, sharing relationship. Intimacy may unfold in the context of dating relationships, close friendships, and certainly mentoring relationships.

Involvement in intimate relationships varies, with some people having many relationships and others having only one or two. The number does not matter. From a developmental standpoint, what matters is that we have others with whom to share our most deeply held thoughts and feelings as we attempt to validate our own unique approach to living. In the absence of a willingness or an ability to pursue intimacy, a sense of emotional isolation can develop.

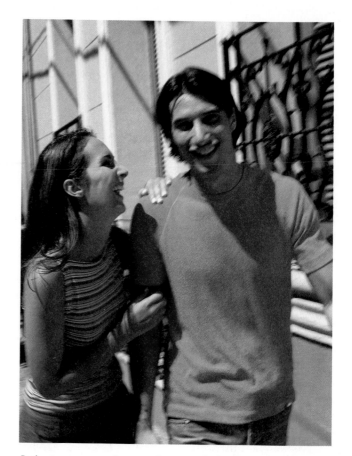

Intimacy can occur in many forms, including traditional dating relationships.

Related Developmental Tasks of Young Adulthood

In addition to the five developmental tasks of young adulthood just described, two additional areas of growth and development seem applicable to 18- to 24-year-olds. These include *obtaining entry-level employment* and *developing parenting skills.*

For at least the last 65 years, students in increasing numbers have pursued a college education in large part to gain entry into many occupations and professions. Students of today certainly anticipate that a college degree will open doors for their first substantial employment or entry-level employment.

In many respects employment needs go beyond those associated purely with money. Employment provides the opportunity to assume new responsibilities in which the skills learned in college can be applied and expanded. Employment also involves taking on new roles (such as colleague, mentor, mentee, or partner) that may play an important part in the way we define ourselves for the remainder of our lives. In addition, employment provides a new, more independent arena in which friendships (intimacy) can be pursued. By no means least important, entry-level employment provides the financial foundation on which we can establish independence.

For many people, young adulthood also marks the entry to parenthood, one of the most important responsibilities anyone can choose to assume. The multitude of decisions associated with this lifetime commitment will, naturally, shape the remainder of one's life. Examples of these decisions are whether to parent or not and, if so, when to begin, how many children to have, how long to wait between children, and what role parenting will play in the context of overall adulthood. The ability to make sound decisions and to develop the skills and insights necessary to parent effectively may be the most challenging aspect of growth and development that confronts young adults.

Developmental Tasks of Middle Adulthood

If you are a traditional-age student, have you wondered what it would be like to be 20 or 30 years older than you are now? What would you be doing, feeling, and thinking if you were the age of your parents? What are your parents thinking about and trying to accomplish as they move through their midlife years?

One thought that probably recurs all too often is the reality of their eventual death. Their awareness that they will not live forever is a subtle but profoundly influential force that can cause them to be restless, to renew attention to their spirituality, and to be more highly motivated to master the developmental tasks of middle adulthood. This motivation and the awareness of the reality of death combine to produce the dynamic concept of being at "the prime of life"—a time when there seems to be a great deal to accomplish and a diminishing amount of time in which to accomplish it.

Achieving Generativity

In a very real sense, people in middle adulthood are asked to do something they have not been expected to do previously. As a part of their development as unique people, they are expected to "pay back" society for the support it has given them. Most people in middle adulthood begin to realize that the collective society, through its institutions (families, schools, churches), has been generous in its support of their growth and development and that it is time to replenish these resources.[24,25] Younger and older people may have needs that middle-aged people can best meet. By meeting the needs of others, people in middle adulthood can fulfill their own needs to grow and develop. *Generativity* reflects this process of contributing to the collective good.

The process of repaying society for its support is structured around familiar types of activities. Developmentally speaking, people in middle adulthood are able to select the activities that best use their abilities to contribute to the good of society.

The most traditional way in which people in middle adulthood repay society is through parenting. Children, with their potential for becoming valuable members of the next generation, need the support of people who recognize the contribution they can make. By supporting children, either directly through quality parenting or through institutions that function on behalf of children, middle-aged people repay society for the support they have themselves received. As they extend themselves outward on behalf of the next generation, they ensure their own growth and development. In a similar fashion, their support of aging parents and institutions that serve older adults provides another means to express generativity.

For people who possess artistic talent, generativity may be accomplished through the pleasure brought to others. Artists, craftspeople, and musicians have unique opportunities to speak directly to others through their talents. Volunteer work serves as another avenue for generativity. Most people in middle adulthood also express generativity through their jobs by providing quality products or services and thus contribute to the well-being of those who desire or need these goods and services.

Reassessing the Plans of Young Adulthood

People in middle adulthood must also begin coming to terms with the finality of their death. In conjunction with doing this, they often feel compelled to take time to think about their goals for adulthood they formulated 25 or more years previously. Their dreams are thus revisited. This reassessment constitutes a second developmental task of people in middle adulthood.

By carefully reviewing the aspirations they had as young adults, middle-aged people can more clearly study their short- and long-term goals. Specifically, strengths and limitations that were unrecognizable when they were young adults are now more clearly seen. The inexperience of youth is replaced by the insights gained through experience. A commitment to quality often replaces the desire for quantity during the second half of the life cycle. Time is valued more highly because it is now seen in a more realistic perspective. The dream for the future is more sharply focused, and the successes and failures of the past are more fully understood as this developmental task of reassessing earlier plans of young adulthood is accomplished.

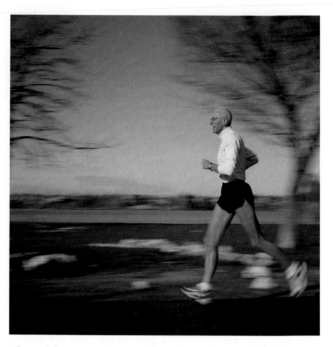

Physical fitness is important throughout all stages of the life span, including older adulthood.

Developmental Tasks of Older Adulthood

In this section, we focus on the developmental tasks confronted by older adults. Accepting the physical changes of aging, maintaining a high level of physical function, and establishing a sense of integrity are tasks of the older adulthood period.

Accepting the Changes of Aging

The general decline associated with the latter part of the life cycle is particularly serious between the 7th and 8th decades. Physically, emotionally, socially, intellectually, and occupationally, older adults must accept at least some decline. For example, a person may no longer be able to drive a car, which could in turn limit participation in social activities. Even a spiritual loss may be encountered at those times when life seems less humane. Clearly, a developmental task to be accomplished by the older adult is to accept the nature and extent of these changes.

Maintaining High Levels of Function

Because each segment of the life cycle should be approached with the fullest level of involvement possible, the second developmental task of the older adult is to maintain as much functionality in each segment as possible, particularly, those that support independence.

For areas of decline in which some measure of reversal is possible, older adults are afforded an opportunity to seek *rehabilitation.* Whether through a self-designed and individually implemented program or with the aid of a skilled professional, older adults can bring back some function to a previously high level.

The second approach, often used in combination with rehabilitation, is *remediation,* whereby an alternative to the area of loss is introduced. Examples of remediation include the use of hearing aids, audiocassettes, and caregivers or home health aids. By using alternative resources, function can often be returned.

For a growing number of older adults, rehabilitation and remediation are rarely necessary because of the high level of health that they enjoy. For most, only minor modifications are necessary to enjoy full independence.

Establishing a Sense of Integrity

The third major developmental task that awaits the older adult is to establish a sense of integrity, or a sense of wholeness, concerning the journey that may be nearly complete.[26] The elderly must look back over their lives to see the value in what they were able to accomplish. They must address the simple but critical questions, "Would I do it over again?" "Am I satisfied with what I managed to

The extra longevity of women in our society is well established. In fact, the difference in life expectancy for infants born today is projected to be 80 years for females and only 75 for males. This 5-year difference has commonly been attributed to genetic factors. However, new evidence demonstrates that this discrepancy may be affected more by male behavior rather than genetic traits.

Men outrank women in all of the top 15 causes of death except for Alzheimer's disease. Men's death rates are twice as high for suicide, homicide, and cirrhosis of the liver. In every age group, American males have poorer health and higher risk of mortality than do females. Common increased risks include:

- More men smoke than women.
- Men are twice as likely to be heavy drinkers and to engage in other risky behaviors such as abusing drugs and driving without a seatbelt.
- More men work in dangerous settings than women do, and men account for 90 percent of on-the-job fatalities.
- More men drive SUVs that are rollover prone and suffer fatalities in motorcycle accidents.

Perhaps some of these increased risks are associated with deep-seated cultural beliefs, which reward men for taking risks and facing danger head-on. This "macho" attitude seems to extend to the care that men take of their own physical and mental health. Women are twice as likely to visit their doctor on an annual basis and explore preventative medical treatments than are men. Men are more likely to ignore symptoms and less likely to schedule checkups or seek follow-up treatment. Psychologically, men tend to internalize their feelings or stressors, or even self-medicate to deal with stress, while women tend to seek psychological help. Almost all stress-related diseases are more common in men.

In the final analysis, men and women alike must be responsible for their own health and well-being. By making sound choices regarding diet, exercise, medical care, and high-risk behaviors, both genders can attempt to maximize the full potential of their life expectancy.

---

accomplish?" "Can I accept the fact that others will have experiences to which I can never return?"

If older adults can answer these questions positively, then they will feel a sense of wholeness, personal value, and worth. Having established this sense of integrity, they will believe that their lives have had meaning and that they have helped society.

Since they have already experienced so much, many older adults have no fear of death, even though they may fear the process of dying. Their ability to come to terms with death thus reinforces their sense of integrity.

Like all the other developmental tasks, this critical area of growth and development is a personal experience. Older adults must assume this last developmental task with the same sense of purpose they used for earlier tasks. When older adults can feel this sense of integrity, their reasons for having lived will be more fully understood.

The Multiple Dimensions of Health

In an earlier section of the chapter we promised to give you a new definition of health that would be less focused on morbidity (illness) and mortality (death) than most others are. However, before we present that new definition, we introduce here a *multidimensional concept of health* (**holistic health**)—a requirement for any definition of health that moves beyond the cure/prevention of illness and the postponement of death.

Although our modern health care community too frequently acts as if the structure and the function of the physical body are the sole basis of health, common experience supports the validity of a holistic nature to health. In this section we examine six components, or dimensions, of health, all interacting in a synergistic manner allowing us to engage in the wide array of activities of daily living (see Figure 1-2).

Physical Dimension

Most of us have a number of physiological and structural characteristics we can call on to aid us in accomplishing the wide array of activities that characterize a typical day and, on occasion, a not-so-typical day. Among these physical characteristics are our body weight, visual ability, strength, coordination, level of endurance, level of susceptibility to disease, and powers of recuperation. In certain situations the physical dimension of health may be the most important. This importance almost certainly is why traditional medicine for centuries has equated health with the design and operation of the body.

> **Key Terms**
>
> **holistic health** a view of health in terms of its physical, emotional, social, intellectual, spiritual, and occupational makeup

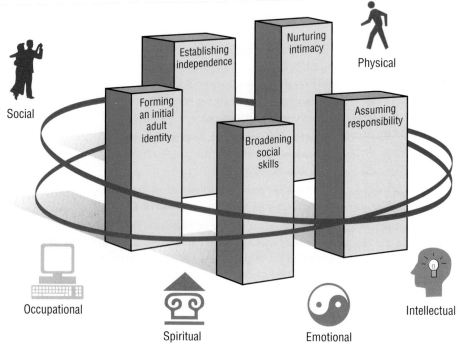

Figure 1-2 Mastery of the five developmental tasks of young adulthood through a balanced involvement of the six dimensions of health leads to the enjoyment of a more productive and satisfying life.

Emotional Dimension

We also possess certain emotional characteristics that can help us through the demands of daily living. The emotional dimension of health encompasses our ability to see the world in a realistic manner, cope with stress, remain flexible, and compromise to resolve conflict.

For young adults, growth and development often give rise to emotional vulnerability, which may lead to feelings of rejection and failure that can reduce productivity and satisfaction. To some extent we are all affected by feeling states, such as anger, happiness, fear, empathy, guilt, love, and hate. People who consistently try to improve their

Nurturing your spirituality is an integral part of holistic health.

emotional health appear to enjoy life to a much greater extent than do those who let feelings of vulnerability overwhelm them or block their creativity.

Social Dimension

A third dimension of health encompasses social skills and cultural sensitivity. Initially, family interactions, school experiences, and peer group interactions foster development in these areas, but future social interactions will demand additional skill development and refinement of already existing skills and insights. In adulthood, including young adulthood, the composition of the social world changes, principally because of our exposure to a wider array of people and the expanded roles associated with employment, parenting, and community involvement.

The social abilities of many nontraditional-age students may already be firmly established. Entering college may encourage them to develop new social skills that help them socialize with their traditional-age student colleagues. After being on campus for a while, nontraditional-age students are often able to interact comfortably with traditional-age students in such diverse places as the library, the student center, and the classroom. This interaction enhances the social dimension of health for both types of students.

Intellectual Dimension

The abilities to process and act on information, clarify values and beliefs, and exercise decision-making capacity rank among the most important aspects of total health. For many college-educated persons, the intellectual dimension of health may prove to be the most important and satisfying of the six. In fact, for all of us, at least on certain occasions, this holds true. Our ability to analyze, synthesize, hypothesize, and then act on new information enhances the quality of our lives in multiple ways.

Spiritual Dimension

The fifth dimension of health is the spiritual dimension. Although certainly it includes religious beliefs and practices, many young adults would expand it to encompass more diverse belief systems, including relationships with other living things, the nature of human behavior, and the need and willingness to serve others. All are important components of spiritual health.

Through nurturing the spiritual dimension of our health, we may develop an expanded perception of the universe and better define our relationship to all that it

Discovering Your Spirituality

How Does Spirituality Affect Your Life?

Spirituality or faith can include religious practice, but it can also be quite distinct from it. Spirituality is the most fundamental stage in the human quest for the meaning of life. It's a developing focus of the total person that gives purpose and meaning to life.

By the time people reach college age, their spirituality or faith may have already placed them in uncomfortable situations. Taking seriously their responsibility for their own commitments, lifestyles, beliefs, and attitudes, they've had to make some difficult personal decisions. This demands objectivity and a certain amount of independence. It requires finding a balance between personal aspirations and a developing sense of service to others. Finally, the symbols and doctrines of faith must be translated into personalized spiritual concepts that become part of everyday living.

- Have you had any experiences that show you're growing in your spirituality or faith?
- Do you consider yourself more spiritual or less spiritual than your friends or family members?
- What school-related experiences have affected the spiritual dimension of your health most powerfully?

contains, including other people. To achieve growth in the spiritual dimension of health, many people undertake a serious study of doctrine associated with established religious groups and assume membership in a community of faith, believed by some. For others, however, spiritual growth is believed to occur, in the absence of a theist-based belief system, as they open themselves to new experiences that involve nature, art, body movement, or stewarding of the environment.

Interestingly, the role of the spiritual dimension of health was recently given an increased measure of credence when studies published in the scientific literature, including a statistical review of 42 earlier studies, demonstrated a consistently longer life for persons who regularly participated in religious practices, particularly for women.[27,28] This was true even when factors such as smoking, alcohol use, and income were statistically eliminated.

Perhaps more relevant to college students than the spiritual dimension of health's relationship to life expectance is spirituality's positive influence during college. In the 2004 College Student Survey conducted by UCLA's Higher Education Research Institute, college students who defined themselves as spiritual seemed less stressed during school than did those reporting a less spiritually related focus.[31]

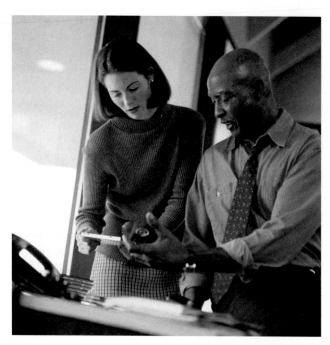

The occupational dimension of health is especially important to nontraditional-age students, who often have to balance school with work, parenting, and other responsibilities.

Occupational Dimension

A significant contribution made by the currently popular wellness movement is that it defines for many people the importance of the workplace to their sense of well-being. In today's world, employment and productive efforts play an increasingly important role in how we perceive ourselves and how we see the "goodness" of the world in which we live. In addition, the workplace serves as both a testing ground for and a source of life-enhancing skills. In our place of employment we gain not only the financial resources to meet our demands for both necessities and luxuries but also an array of useful skills such as conflict resolution, experiences in shared responsibility, and intellectual growth that can be used to facilitate a wide range of non-employment-related interactions. In turn, the workplace is enhanced by the healthfulness of the individuals who contribute to its endeavors.

Environmental Dimension

Some academics would add to the dimensions just discussed an *environmental dimension*. If this dimension is defined on the basis of land, air, and water, then it might be an additional dimension to consider. However,

should the environmental dimension be extended to include all that is material and metaphysical surrounding each individual, such a concept seems beyond the scope of this chapter. Thus, we have elected not to expand the number of holistic dimensions of health beyond those traditionally discussed. Contradictory to these findings, however, was a more recent report suggesting that the association between religious attendance and survival may be weaker than other studies have suggested. In this study certain specific health-related behavioral patterns, for both attenders and nonattenders, were statistically removed from the data; as a result, the influence of religious attendance fell by approximately one third.[30]

Wellness

Expanded perceptions of health are the basis for **wellness.** Recall that episodic health care, preventive medicine, and community health promotion are directly aligned with concerns about morbidity and mortality, whereas health promotion at the individual level is focused on aspects of appearance, weight management, body composition, and physical performance capabilities. Wellness differs from these kinds of health care concerns because it has virtually no interest in morbidity and mortality.

Practitioners describe wellness as a process of extending information, counseling, assessment, and lifestyle-modification strategies leading to a desirable change in the recipients' overall lifestyle, or the adoption of a wellness lifestyle. Once adopted, the wellness lifestyle produces a sense of well-being that in turn enables recipients to unlock their full potential.

This explanation of how wellness differs from episodic health care, preventive medicine, and health promotion does, on first hearing, seem progressive and clearly devoid of interest in morbidity and mortality concerns. But in practice, wellness programs are not all that different from other kinds of health care. We have consistently noted that wellness programs, as carried out on college campuses, in local hospital well centers,

---

Key Terms

wellness A process intended to aid individuals in unlocking their full potential through the development of an overall wellness lifestyle

Although not primarily interested in illness or premature death, wellness practitioners consider it essential to inform their clients about the role of elevated blood pressure in the development of cardiovascular disease.

and in corporate settings, routinely transmit familiar health-related information and engage in the same risk-reduction activities that characterize preventive medicine and health promotion. It is in the final aspect of wellness, the "unlocking of full potential," that wellness differs from other concepts of health. More than the absence of chronic illness, it involves achieving optimal health across all six of the dimensions of health discussed in the previous section.

A New Definition of Health

At the beginning of the chapter we hinted at a new way to view health—a view that would be far less centered in morbidity and mortality concerns than are traditional concepts of health and even of wellness. The definition that we propose takes into account the differences between *what health is for* (its role) and *what health is* (its composition).

The Role of Health

The role of health in our lives is similar to the role of a car. Much as a car (or other vehicle) takes us to the place we need or want to be at, good health enables us to accomplish the activities that transition us into and through developmental tasks associated with each stage of adulthood (pages 13–17). Recall that the process of moving through each stage of adulthood does not occur simply because of the passage of time but rather because we actively participate, on a day-to-day basis, in demands of life appropriate to our life stage, as defined by society and carried out by us as individuals in our own unique manner.

The Composition of Health

Now that you know what the role of health is, its composition can be seen as being more than simply having a body free of illness and apparently destined for a long life. Rather, the composition of health is that of a collection of resources, from each dimension of health (pages eighteen through twenty), determined to be necessary for the successful accomplishment of activities that you need or want to do. Some of these needed resources are already within you (intrinsic), whereas others need to come from outside (extrinsic). However, regardless of their origin, once they are accessed and applied to activities, small forward growth steps will occur. Obviously, to recognize what resources are needed, you must be a student of society's expectations for persons of your age, as well as your own highly personalized developmental aspirations.

Our Definition of Health

By combining the role of health with the composition of health, we offer a new definition of **health.** In light of this definition, do not be surprised when we ask whether you are resourceful (healthy) enough to attain the goals you wish to reach, whether you are healthy enough to sustain a particular behavioral pattern that you have adopted, or whether you are experiencing the sense of well-being to which you aspire.

Key Terms

health a reflection of one's ability to use the **intrinsic** and **extrinsic** resources related to each dimension of health to participate fully in the activities that contribute to growth and development, with the goal of feeling a sense of well-being as one evaluates one's progress through life

- Complete the Comprehensive Health Assessment on pages 25–34. Develop a plan to modify your behavior in the areas in which you need improvement.
- Take part in a new spiritual activity, such as meditating, creating art or music, or attending a religious service.

- To promote the social dimension of your health, try to meet one new person each week during the semester.
- Choose one developmental task you would like to focus on, such as assuming responsibility, and plan the steps you can follow to progress in this area.

- Volunteer to be an assistant in a community service program, such as a literacy project or a preschool program.

SUMMARY

- When used to define health, *morbidity* and *mortality* relate to the prevalence of particular diseases and illnesses and to death resulting from those diseases and illnesses.
- When we seek the services of health care practitioners because of symptoms of illness or disease, we are said to be seeking episodic health care.
- Preventive medical care attempts to minimize the incidence of illness and disease by identifying early indicators of risk to bring them under control.
- Individual health promotion involves risk-reduction activities similar to those used in preventive medical care, except that the techniques cannot be invasive and are directed by professionals who are not physicians. Its most visible emphasis tends to be on fitness and body composition.
- Community health promotion involves the empowerment of individuals so that they can organize and participate in their own health promotion activities.
- Healthy People 2010 is a federally funded program to improve the nation's health, increase life expectancy, and expand access to comprehensive health care.
- A decision to change a health behavior is often difficult to make because of the multiplicity of factors underlying the maintenace of the high-risk behavior.
- Health behavior change requires movement through a multistaged process, including precontemplation, contemplation, preparation, action, maintenance, and termination.
- A wide array of health problems (for example, cancer, cardiovascular disease, HIV/AIDS) persist despite today's highly sophisticated health care technology.
- Today's college campus is a dynamic blend of students of both traditional and nontraditional ages and of diverse backgrounds, cultures, and attributes.

- Complementary and integrative medicine involves the integration of alternative forms of care, such as acupuncture and therapeutic massage, into traditional medical practices. Today several forms of complementary care are under careful study by the Office of Complementary and Alternative Medicine of the National Institutes of Health.
- Young adulthood is characterized by five key developmental tasks: forming an initial adult identity, establishing independence, assuming responsibility, broadening social skills, and nurturing intimacy.
- Each phase of the life cycle involves a set of personal developmental tasks that are common to all people yet may be undertaken differently by each individual. Generativity and integrity are developmental tasks of midlife and older adulthood, respectively.
- Multidimensional definitions of health, including holistic health, have existed for decades—although the primary emphasis has always been on the physical dimension.
- Current multidimensionals definitions of health may include many or all of the following dimensions: physical, emotional, social, intellectual, spiritual, and occupational.
- Wellness contends a disinterest in morbidity and mortality, rather emphasizing living a wellness lifestyle that leads to a sense of well-being.
- Our new definition of health includes the role of health and the composition of health. The role of health is to enable individuals to participate in the activities that collectively constitute growth and development. The composition of health is the intrinsic and extrinsic resources on which individuals can draw to participate fully in their own growth and development.

REVIEW QUESTIONS

1. What are morbidity and mortality, and how are they involved in the more traditional definitions of health?
2. In preventive medical care, who determines a person's level of risk and decides what risk-reduction techniques should be implemented?

3. What does the term *empowerment* mean, and how would it appear as a component of a community-based health promotion program?
4. What factors could underlie the inability or unwillingness of persons to change their health behavior?

5. What are the six stages that persons pass through as they consider and then attempt to change their health behavior?

6. In what ways is the current U.S. college student population more diverse than any that came before?

7. What are the five developmental tasks of young adulthood, and how can the accomplishing of one influence the accomplishing of any of the remaining four?

8. What is implied by the statement, "growth and development are predictable yet unique"?

9. What is the most likely route that midlife adults will take in their quest for a sense of generativity?

10. What are the most frequently included dimensions of a holistically centered definition of health?

11. What is the main reason that proponents of wellness give for being uninterested in morbidity and mortality?

12. How does our definition of health differ from traditional definitions?

13. How does your textbook define the role of health? Composition of health?

14. Why is it necessary to understand developmental expectations before we can answer the question, "Are you healthy enough to . . . ?"

ENDNOTES

1. Woodwell DA and Cherry DK. *National Ambulatory Medical Care Survey: 2002 Summary.* Advance Data From Vital and Health Statistics. National Center for Health Statistics. Number 346. August 26, 2004.

2. Centers for Disease Control and Prevention. *National Ambulatory Medical Care Survey: 2000.* Atlanta, GA: July 2002.

3. Roper Center for Public Opinion Research (for Pfizer Women's Health), University of Connecticut. Adults know their family history. *USA Today.* May 30, 2000. p. 5D.

4. *U.S. Surgeon General's Family History Initiative.* Washington, DC: U.S. Department of Health and Human Services. 2004. www.hhs.gov/familyhistory/download.html.

5. Smith PC, et al. Missing information during primary care visits. 2005. *JAMA.* Feb 2; 293(5): 565–571.

6. Cottrell RR, Girvan JT, McKenzie JF. *Principles and Foundations of Health Promotion and Education* (3rd ed.). San Francisco: Benjamin Cummings. 2005.

7. Kreuter MW, Lezin NA, Kreuter MW, Green LW. *Community Health Promotion Ideas That Work: A Field-Book for Practitioners.* Sudbury, MA: Jones and Bartlett Publishers. 2003.

8. McKenzie JF, Neiger BL, Smeltzer JL. *Planning, Implementing, and Evaluating Health Promotion Programs* (4th ed.). San Francisco: Benjamin Cummings. 2005.

9. *Priority Areas for National Action: Transforming Health Care Quality.* Washington, DC: The National Academies Press. 2003.

10. *Healthy People 2000: National Health Promotion and Disease Prevention Objectives* (full report with commentary). Washington, DC: U.S. Department of Health and Human Services. Public Health Service. 1991.

11. *Healthy People 2000: Midcourse Review and 1995 Revisions.* Washington, DC: U.S. Department of Health and Human Services. Public Health Service. 1995.

12. *Healthy People 2010: Understanding and Improving Health.* Washington, DC: U.S. Department of Health and Human Services. Public Health Service. 2000.

13. *Healthy People 2010: Understanding and Improving Health* (2nd ed.). Washington, DC: U.S. Department of Health and Human Services. Public Health Service. 2000.

14. Visschedijk J, Simean TS. Targets for health for all in the 21st century. *World Health Stat Q,* 1998, 51(1), 560–567.

15. Prochaska JO, Velicer WF. The transtheoretical model of health behavior change. 1994. *Am J of Health Promotion.* 12:38–48.

16. Norcross JC, Prochaska JO. Using the stages of change. 2002. *Harv Ment Health Lett.* 18(11):507.

17. Prochaska JO, Norcross JC, Clemente CC. *Changing for Good.* New York: Willian Morrow and Company, 1994.

18. Diet and genes. *Newsweek* (with Harvard Medical School). January 17, 2005.

19. The quest for memory drugs. *Newsweek* (with Harvard Medical School). December 6, 2004.

20. College enrollment by sex, age, race, and hispanic origins: 1980 to 2001 (No. 280). Washington, DC: U.S. Census Bureau. *Statistical Abstract of the United States: 2003.*

21. Foreign (nonimmigrant) student enrollment in college: 1976 to 2002 (No. 281). Washington, DC: U.S. Census Bureau. *Statistical Abstract of the United States: 2003.*

22. Undergraduates reported disability status by selected characteristics: 1999–2000 (No. 285). Washington, DC: U.S. Census Bureau. *Statistical Abstract of the United States: 2003.*

23. U.S. National Center for Education Statistics, *Profile of Undergraduates in U.S. Postsecondary Education Institutions, 1999–2000.* Washington, DC: July, 2000.

24. McAdams DP, St. Aubin ED (Eds.) *Generativity and Adult Development: How and Why We Care for the Next Generation.* Washington, DC: American Psychological Association, 1998.

25. McAdams DP. Generativity in Midlife, in M. Lachman (Ed.), *Handbook of Midlife Development.* Hoboken, NJ: Wiley, 2001.

26. Erikson EH. *Childhood and Society* (reissues edition). New York: W.W. Norton, 1993.

27. Hummer RA, et al. Religious involvement and adult mortality in the United States: Review and perspective. *South Med J.* 2004. Dec: 97(12)1223–1230.

28. McCullough ME, et al. Religious involvement and U.S. adult mortality: A meta-analysis review. *Health Psychology,* 2000, 19(2): 211–222.

29. Musick MA, House JS, Williams, DR. Attendance at religious services and mortality in a national sample. *Journal of Health and Social Behavior.* 2004, 45(2): 198–213.

30. Bagiella W, Hong V, Sloan RP. Religious attendance as a predictor of survival in the EPESE cohorts. *Int J Epidemiol.* 2005, Jan 19 (34) 443–451.

31. *Spirituality in Higher Education: A National Search for Meaning and Purpose* (pilot survey 2003). Higher Education Research Institute, University of California, Los Angeles, www.spirituality.ucla.edu.

In 1996 the U.S. Preventive Services Task Force recommended that prenatal HIV testing need not be extended beyond those women determined to have come from high-risk backgrounds. When identified as HIV positive, these women were placed on a combination drug therapy, delivered by Caesarean section, and advised not to breast-feed their infants. For those compliant with this form of pregnancy management, the risk of infecting their infants dropped below 1 percent, from the otherwise expected 25 percent infant-infection rate. Five years later, in 2001, the Centers for Disease Control and Prevention (CDC) recommended that HIV testing become a routine part of prenatal care for all pregnant women.

In spite of CDC's recommendation for universal HIV prenatal testing, many pregnant women either were not offered testing by their prenatal care providers or declined the offer when it was extended. Accordingly, in the absence of knowing their HIV status, women who were unknowingly infected failed to receive treatment, and infant-infection rates remained unacceptably higher than necessary.

Recently, and in response to the continuing risks to both new mothers and their infants, a newer U.S. Preventive Services Task Force recommended that the emphasis on universal prenatal testing for HIV infection be significantly strengthened. In the opinion of this panel, should the health care community commit themselves to this task, women will feel increasingly more comfortable with the role of HIV testing as a part of prenatal care, and the risk of infection to newborns will fall accordingly. Recall that preventive medical care is, in the final analysis, more affordable than episodic care.

Source: U.S. Preventive Services Task Force. Screening for HIV: Recommendation statement. *Annals of Internal Medicine.* 2005 July; 143(1):32–37.

comprehensive health assessment

Now that you have read the first chapter, complete the following Comprehensive Health Assessment. We strongly suggest that you retake this assessment after you have completed your health course. Then compare your responses in each section of the assessment. Have your scores improved?

Social and Occupational Health

	Not true/ rarely	Somewhat true/ sometimes	Mostly true/ usually	Very true/ always
1. I feel loved and supported by my family.	1	2	3	4
2. I establish friendships with ease and enjoyment.	1	2	3	4
3. I establish friendships with people of both genders and all ages.	1	2	3	4
4. I sustain relationships by communicating with and caring about my family and friends.	1	2	3	4
5. I feel comfortable and confident when meeting people for the first time.	1	2	3	4
6. I practice social skills to facilitate the process of forming new relationships.	1	2	3	4
7. I seek opportunities to meet and interact with new people.	1	2	3	4
8. I talk with, rather than at, people.	1	2	3	4
9. I am open to developing or sustaining intimate relationships.	1	2	3	4
10. I appreciate the importance of parenting the next generation and am committed to supporting it in ways that reflect my own resources.	1	2	3	4
11. I recognize the strengths and weaknesses of my parents' childrearing skills and feel comfortable modifying them if I choose to become a parent.	1	2	3	4
12. I attempt to be tolerant of others whether or not I approve of their behavior or beliefs.	1	2	3	4
13. I understand and appreciate the contribution that cultural diversity makes to the quality of living.	1	2	3	4
14. I understand and appreciate the difference between being educated and being trained.	1	2	3	4
15. My work gives me a sense of self-sufficiency and an opportunity to contribute.	1	2	3	4
16. I have equal respect for the roles of leader and subordinate within the workplace.	1	2	3	4
17. I have chosen an occupation that suits my interests and temperament.	1	2	3	4
18. I have chosen an occupation that does not compromise my physical or psychological health.	1	2	3	4
19. I get along well with my coworkers most of the time.	1	2	3	4
20. When I have a disagreement with a coworker, I try to resolve it directly and constructively.	1	2	3	4

Points _____

Spiritual and Psychological Health

	Not true/ rarely	Somewhat true/ sometimes	Mostly true/ usually	Very true/ always
1. I have a deeply held belief system or personal theology.	1	2	3	4
2. I recognize the contribution that membership in a community of faith or spirituality can make to a person's overall quality of life.	1	2	3	4

	Not true/ rarely	Somewhat true/ sometimes	Mostly true/ usually	Very true/ always
3. I seek experiences with nature and reflect on nature's contribution to my quality of life.	1	2	3	4
4. My spirituality is a resource that helps me remain calm and strong during times of stress.	1	2	3	4
5. I have found appropriate ways to express my spirituality.	1	2	3	4
6. I respect the diversity of spiritual expression and am tolerant of those whose beliefs differ from my own.	1	2	3	4
7. I take adequate time to reflect on my own life and my relationships with others and the institutions of society.	1	2	3	4
8. I routinely undertake new experiences.	1	2	3	4
9. I receive adequate support from others.	1	2	3	4
10. I look for opportunities to support others, even occasionally at the expense of my own goals and aspirations.	1	2	3	4
11. I recognize that emotional and psychological health are as important as physical health.	1	2	3	4
12. I express my feelings and opinions comfortably, yet am capable of keeping them to myself when appropriate.	1	2	3	4
13. I see myself as a person of worth and feel comfortable with my own strengths and limitations.	1	2	3	4
14. I establish realistic goals and work to achieve them.	1	2	3	4
15. I understand the differences between the normal range of emotions and the signs of clinical depression.	1	2	3	4
16. I know how to recognize signs of suicidal thoughts and am willing to intervene.	1	2	3	4
17. I regularly assess my own behavior patterns and beliefs and would seek professional assistance for any emotional dysfunction.	1	2	3	4
18. I accept the reality of aging and view it as an opportunity for positive change.	1	2	3	4
19. I accept the reality of death and view it as a normal and inevitable part of life.	1	2	3	4
20. I have made decisions about my own death to ensure that I die with dignity when the time comes.	1	2	3	4

Points _____

Stress Management

	Not true/ rarely	Somewhat true/ sometimes	Mostly true/ usually	Very true/ always
1. I accept the reality of change while maintaining the necessary stability in my daily activities.	1	2	3	4
2. I seek change when it is necessary or desirable to do so.	1	2	3	4
3. I know what stress-management services are offered on campus, through my employer, or in my community.	1	2	3	4
4. When necessary, I use the stress-management services to which I have access.	1	2	3	4
5. I employ stress-reduction practices in anticipation of stressful events, such as job interviews and final examinations.	1	2	3	4
6. I reevaluate the way in which I handled stressful events so that I can better cope with similar events in the future.	1	2	3	4
7. I turn to relatives and friends during periods of disruption in my life.	1	2	3	4
8. I avoid using alcohol or other drugs during periods of stress.	1	2	3	4

	Not true/ rarely	Somewhat true/ sometimes	Mostly true/ usually	Very true/ always
9. I refrain from behaving aggressively or abusively during periods of stress.	1	2	3	4
10. I sleep enough to maintain a high level of health and cope successfully with daily challenges.	1	2	3	4
11. I avoid sleeping excessively as a response to stressful change.	1	2	3	4
12. My diet is conducive to good health and stress management.	1	2	3	4
13. I participate in physical activity to relieve stress.	1	2	3	4
14. I practice stress-management skills, such as diaphragmatic breathing and yoga.	1	2	3	4
15. I manage my time effectively.	1	2	3	4

Points _____

Fitness

	Not true/ rarely	Somewhat true/ sometimes	Mostly true/ usually	Very true/ always
1. I participate in recreational and fitness activities both to minimize stress and to improve or maintain my level of physical fitness.	1	2	3	4
2. I select some recreational activities that are strenuous rather than sedentary in nature.	1	2	3	4
3. I include various types of aerobic conditioning activities among the wider array of recreational and fitness activities in which I engage.	1	2	3	4
4. I engage in aerobic activities with appropriate frequency, intensity, and duration to provide a training effect for my heart and lungs.	1	2	3	4
5. I routinely include strength-training activities among the wider array of fitness activities in which I engage.	1	2	3	4
6. I routinely vary the types of strength-training activities in which I participate in order to minimize injury and strengthen all of the important muscle groups.	1	2	3	4
7. I do exercises specifically designed to maintain joint range of motion.	1	2	3	4
8. I believe that recreational and fitness activities can help me improve my physical health and my emotional and social well-being.	1	2	3	4
9. I include a variety of fitness activities in my overall plan for physical fitness.	1	2	3	4
10. I take appropriate steps to avoid injuries when participating in recreational and fitness activities.	1	2	3	4
11. I seek appropriate treatment for all injuries that result from fitness activities.	1	2	3	4
12. I believe that older adults should undertake appropriately chosen fitness activities.	1	2	3	4
13. My body composition is consistent with a high level of health.	1	2	3	4
14. I warm up before beginning vigorous activity, and I cool down afterward.	1	2	3	4
15. I select properly designed and well-maintained equipment and clothing for each activity.	1	2	3	4
16. I avoid using performance-enhancing substances that are known to be dangerous and those whose influence on the body is not fully understood.	1	2	3	4

	Not true/ rarely	Somewhat true/ sometimes	Mostly true/ usually	Very true/ always
17. I sleep seven to eight hours daily.	1	2	3	4
18. I refrain from using over-the-counter sleep-inducing aids.	1	2	3	4
19. I follow sound dietary practices as an important adjunct to a health-enhancing physical activity program.	1	2	3	4
20. My current level of fitness allows me to participate fully and effortlessly in my daily activities.	1	2	3	4

Points _____

Nutrition and Weight Management

	Not true/ rarely	Somewhat true/ sometimes	Mostly true/ usually	Very true/ always
1. I balance my caloric intake with my calorie expenditure.	1	2	3	4
2. I obtain the recommended number of servings from each of the food groups.	1	2	3	4
3. I select a wide variety of foods chosen from each of the food groups.	1	2	3	4
4. I understand the amount of a particular food that constitutes a single serving.	1	2	3	4
5. I often try new foods, particularly when I know them to be healthful.	1	2	3	4
6. I select breads, cereals, fresh fruits, and vegetables in preference to pastries, candies, sodas and fruits canned in heavy syrup.	1	2	3	4
7. I limit the amount of sugar that I add to foods during preparation and at the table.	1	2	3	4
8. I examine food labels to determine the presence of trans-fats (trans-fatty acids) and select foods free of these fats.	1	2	3	4
9. I select primarily nonmeat sources of protein, such as peas, beans, and peanut butter, while limiting my consumption of red meat and high-fat dairy products.	1	2	3	4
10. I consume an appropriate percentage of my total daily calories from protein.	1	2	3	4
11. I select foods prepared with unsaturated vegetable oils while reducing consumption of red meat, high-fat dairy products, and foods prepared with lard (animal fat) or butter.	1	2	3	4
12. I carefully limit the amount of fast food that I consume during a typical week.	1	2	3	4
13. I consume an appropriate percentage of my total daily calories from fat.	1	2	3	4
14. I select nutritious foods when I snack.	1	2	3	4
15. I limit my use of salt during food preparation and at the table.	1	2	3	4
16. I consume adequate amounts of fiber.	1	2	3	4
17. I routinely consider the nutrient density of individual food items when choosing foods.	1	2	3	4
18. I maintain my weight without reliance on over-the-counter or prescription diet pills.	1	2	3	4
19. I maintain my weight without reliance on fad diets or liquid weight loss beverages.	1	2	3	4
20. I exercise regularly to help maintain my weight.	1	2	3	4

Points _____

Alcohol, Tobacco, and Other Drug Use

	Not true/ rarely	Somewhat true/ sometimes	Mostly true/ usually	Very true/ always
1. I abstain or drink in moderation when offered alcoholic beverages.	1	2	3	4
2. I abstain from using illegal psychoactive (mind-altering) drugs.	1	2	3	4
3. I do not consume alcoholic beverages or psychoactive drugs rapidly or in large quantities.	1	2	3	4
4. I do not use alcohol or psychoactive drugs in a way that causes me to behave inappropriately.	1	2	3	4
5. My use of alcohol or other drugs does not compromise my academic performance.	1	2	3	4
6. I refrain from drinking alcoholic beverages or using psychoactive drugs when engaging in recreational activities that require strength, speed, or coordination.	1	2	3	4
7. I refrain from drinking alcoholic beverages while participating in occupational activities, regardless of the nature of those activities.	1	2	3	4
8. My use of alcohol or other drugs does not generate financial concerns for myself or for others.	1	2	3	4
9. I refrain from drinking alcohol or using psychoactive drugs when driving a motor vehicle or operating heavy equipment.	1	2	3	4
10. I do not drink alcohol or use psychoactive drugs when I am alone.	1	2	3	4
11. I avoid riding with people who have been drinking alcohol or using psychoactive drugs.	1	2	3	4
12. My use of alcohol or other drugs does not cause family dysfunction.	1	2	3	4
13. I do not use marijuana.	1	2	3	4
14. I do not use hallucinogens.	1	2	3	4
15. I do not use heroin or other illegal intravenous drugs.	1	2	3	4
16. I do not experience blackouts when I drink alcohol.	1	2	3	4
17. I do not become abusive or violent when I drink alcohol or use psychoactive drugs.	1	2	3	4
18. I use potentially addictive prescription medication in complete compliance with my physician's directions.	1	2	3	4
19. I do not smoke cigarettes.	1	2	3	4
20. I do not use tobacco products in any other form.	1	2	3	4
21. I minimize my exposure to secondhand smoke.	1	2	3	4
22. I am concerned about the effect that alcohol, tobacco, and other drug use is known to have on developing fetuses.	1	2	3	4
23. I am concerned about the effect that alcohol, tobacco, and other drug use is known to have on the health of other people.	1	2	3	4
24. I seek natural, health-enhancing highs rather than relying on alcohol, tobacco, and illegal drugs.	1	2	3	4
25. I take prescription medication only as instructed, and I use over-the-counter medication in accordance with directions.	1	2	3	4

Points _____

Disease Prevention

	Not true/ rarely	Somewhat true/ sometimes	Mostly true/ usually	Very true/ always
1. My diet includes foods rich in phytochemicals.	1	2	3	4
2. My diet includes foods rich in folic acid.	1	2	3	4
3. My diet includes foods that are good sources of dietary fiber.	1	2	3	4
4. My diet is low in dietary cholesterol.	1	2	3	4
5. I follow food preparation practices that minimize the risk of food-borne illness.	1	2	3	4
6. I engage in regular physical activity and am able to control my weight effectively.	1	2	3	4
7. I do not use tobacco products.	1	2	3	4
8. I abstain from alcohol or drink only in moderation.	1	2	3	4
9. I do not use intravenously administered illegal drugs.	1	2	3	4
10. I use safer sex practices intended to minimize my risk of exposure to sexually transmitted diseases, including HIV and HPV.	1	2	3	4
11. I take steps to limit my risk of exposure to the bacterium that causes Lyme disease and to the virus that causes hantavirus pulmonary syndrome.	1	2	3	4
12. I control my blood pressure with weight management and physical fitness activities.	1	2	3	4
13. I minimize my exposure to allergens, including those that trigger asthma attacks.	1	2	3	4
14. I wash my hands frequently and thoroughly.	1	2	3	4
15. I use preventive medical care services appropriately.	1	2	3	4
16. I use appropriate cancer self-screening practices, such as breast self-examination and testicular self-examination.	1	2	3	4
17. I know which chronic illnesses and diseases are part of my family history.	1	2	3	4
18. I know which inherited conditions are part of my family history and will seek preconceptional counseling regarding these conditions.	1	2	3	4
19. I am fully immunized against infectious diseases.	1	2	3	4
20. I take prescribed medications, particularly antibiotics, exactly as instructed by my physician.	1	2	3	4

Points _____

Sexual Health

	Not true/ rarely	Somewhat true/ sometimes	Mostly true/ usually	Very true/ always
1. I know how sexually transmitted diseases are spread.	1	2	3	4
2. I can recognize the symptoms of sexually transmitted diseases.	1	2	3	4
3. I know how sexually transmitted disease transmission can be prevented.	1	2	3	4
4. I know how safer sex practices reduce the risk of contracting sexually transmitted diseases.	1	2	3	4
5. I follow safer sex practices.	1	2	3	4
6. I recognize the symptoms of premenstrual syndrome and understand how it is prevented and treated.	1	2	3	4

	Not true/ rarely	Somewhat true/ sometimes	Mostly true/ usually	Very true/ always
7. I recognize the symptoms of endometriosis and understand the relationship of its symptoms to hormonal cycles.	1	2	3	4
8. I understand the physiological basis of menopause and recognize that it is a normal part of the aging process in women.	1	2	3	4
9. I understand and accept the range of human sexual orientations.	1	2	3	4
10. I encourage the development of flexible sex roles (androgyny) in children.	1	2	3	4
11. I take a mature approach to dating and mate selection.	1	2	3	4
12. I recognize that marriage and other types of long-term relationships can be satisfying.	1	2	3	4
13. I recognize that a celibate lifestyle is appropriate and satisfying for some people.	1	2	3	4
14. I affirm the sexuality of older adults and am comfortable with its expression.	1	2	3	4
15. I am familiar with the advantages and disadvantages of a wide range of birth control methods.	1	2	3	4
16. I understand how each birth control method works and how effective it is.	1	2	3	4
17. I use my birth control method consistently and appropriately.	1	2	3	4
18. I am familiar with the wide range of procedures now available to treat infertility.	1	2	3	4
19. I accept that others may disagree with my feelings about pregnancy termination.	1	2	3	4
20. I am familiar with alternatives available to infertile couples, including adoption.	1	2	3	4

Points _____

Safety Practices and Violence Prevention	Not true/ rarely	Somewhat true/ sometimes	Mostly true/ usually	Very true/ always
1. I attempt to identify sources of risk or danger in each new setting or activity.	1	2	3	4
2. I learn proper procedures and precautions before undertaking new recreational or occupational activities.	1	2	3	4
3. I select appropriate clothing and equipment for all activities and maintain equipment in good working order.	1	2	3	4
4. I curtail my participation in activities when I am not feeling well or am distracted by other demands.	1	2	3	4
5. I repair dangerous conditions or report them to those responsible for maintenance.	1	2	3	4
6. I use common sense and observe the laws governing nonmotorized vehicles when I ride a bicycle.	1	2	3	4
7. I operate all motor vehicles as safely as possible, including using seat belts and other safety equipment.	1	2	3	4
8. I refrain from driving an automobile or boat when I have been drinking alcohol or taking drugs or medications.	1	2	3	4
9. I try to anticipate the risk of falling and maintain my environment to minimize this risk.	1	2	3	4

		Not true/ rarely	Somewhat true/ sometimes	Mostly true/ usually	Very true/ always
10.	I maintain my environment to minimize the risk of fire, and I have a well-rehearsed plan to exit my residence in case of fire.	1	2	3	4
11.	I am a competent swimmer and could save myself or rescue someone who was drowning.	1	2	3	4
12.	I refrain from sexually aggressive behavior toward my partner or others.	1	2	3	4
13.	I would report an incident of sexual harassment or date rape whether or not I was the victim.	1	2	3	4
14.	I would seek help from others if I were the victim or perpetrator of domestic violence.	1	2	3	4
15.	I practice gun safety and encourage other gun owners to do so.	1	2	3	4
16.	I drive at all times in a way that will minimize my risk of being carjacked.	1	2	3	4
17.	I have taken steps to protect my home from intruders.	1	2	3	4
18.	I use campus security services as much as possible when they are available.	1	2	3	4
19.	I know what to do if I am being stalked.	1	2	3	4
20.	I have a well-rehearsed plan to protect myself from the aggressive behavior of other people in my place of residence.	1	2	3	4

Points _____

Health Care Consumerism

		Not true/ rarely	Somewhat true/ sometimes	Mostly true/ usually	Very true/ always
1.	I know how to obtain valid health information.	1	2	3	4
2.	I accept health information that has been deemed valid by the established scientific community.	1	2	3	4
3.	I am skeptical of claims that guarantee the effectiveness of a particular health care service or product.	1	2	3	4
4.	I am skeptical of practitioners or clinics who advertise or offer services at rates substantially lower than those charged by reputable providers.	1	2	3	4
5.	I am not swayed by advertisements that present unhealthy behavior in an attractive manner.	1	2	3	4
6.	I can afford proper medical care, including hospitalization.	1	2	3	4
7.	I can afford adequate health insurance.	1	2	3	4
8.	I understand the role of government health care plans in providing health care to people who qualify for coverage.	1	2	3	4
9.	I know how to select health care providers who are highly qualified and appropriate for my current health care needs.	1	2	3	4
10.	I seek a second or third opinion when surgery or other costly therapies are recommended.	1	2	3	4
11.	I have told my physician which hospital I would prefer to use should the need arise.	1	2	3	4
12.	I understand my rights and responsibilities as a patient when admitted to a hospital.	1	2	3	4
13.	I practice adequate self-care to reduce my health care expenditures and my reliance on health care providers.	1	2	3	4

	Not true/ rarely	Somewhat true/ sometimes	Mostly true/ usually	Very true/ always
14. I am open-minded about alternative health care practices and support current efforts to determine their appropriate role in effective health care.	1	2	3	4
15. I have a well-established relationship with a pharmacist and have transmitted all necessary information regarding medication use.	1	2	3	4
16. I carefully follow labels and directions when using health care products, such as over-the-counter medications.	1	2	3	4
17. I finish all prescription medications as directed, rather than stopping use when symptoms subside.	1	2	3	4
18. I report to the appropriate agencies any providers of health care services, information, or products that use deceptive advertising or fraudulent methods of operation.	1	2	3	4
19. I pursue my rights as fully as possible in matters of misrepresentation or consumer dissatisfaction.	1	2	3	4
20. I follow current health care issues in the news and voice my opinion to my elected representatives.	1	2	3	4

Points _____

Environmental Health

	Not true/ rarely	Somewhat true/ sometimes	Mostly true/ usually	Very true/ always
1. I avoid use of and exposure to pesticides as much as possible.	1	2	3	4
2. I avoid use of and exposure to herbicides as much as possible.	1	2	3	4
3. I am willing to spend the extra money and time required to obtain organically grown produce.	1	2	3	4
4. I reduce environmental pollutants by minimizing my use of the automobile.	1	2	3	4
5. I avoid the use of products that contribute to indoor air pollution.	1	2	3	4
6. I limit my exposure to ultraviolet radiation by avoiding excessive sun exposure.	1	2	3	4
7. I limit my exposure to radon gas by using a radon gas detector.	1	2	3	4
8. I limit my exposure to radiation by promptly eliminating radon gas within my home.	1	2	3	4
9. I limit my exposure to radiation by agreeing to undergo medical radiation procedures only when absolutely necessary for the diagnosis and treatment of an illness or disease.	1	2	3	4
10. I avoid the use of potentially unsafe water, particularly when traveling in a foreign country or when a municipal water supply or bottled water is unavailable.	1	2	3	4
11. I avoid noise pollution by limiting my exposure to loud noise or by using ear protection.	1	2	3	4
12. I avoid air pollution by carefully selecting the environments in which I live, work, and recreate.	1	2	3	4

13. I do not knowingly use or improperly dispose of personal care products that can harm the environment.	1	2	3	4
14. I reuse as many products as possible so that they can avoid the recycling bins for as long as possible.	1	2	3	4
15. I participate fully in my community's recycling efforts.	1	2	3	4
16. I encourage the increased use of recycled materials in the design and manufacturing of new products.	1	2	3	4
17. I dispose of residential toxic substances safely and properly.	1	2	3	4
18. I follow environmental issues in the news and voice my opinion to my elected representatives.	1	2	3	4
19. I am aware of and involved in environmental issues in my local area.	1	2	3	4
20. I perceive myself as a steward of the environment for the generations to come, rather than as a person with a right to use (and misuse) the environment to meet my immediate needs.	1	2	3	4

Points _____

YOUR TOTAL POINTS _____

Interpretation

770–880 points

Congratulations! Your health behavior is very supportive of high-level health. Continue to practice your positive health habits, and look for areas in which you can become even stronger. Encourage others to follow your example, and support their efforts in any way you can.

550–769 points

Good job! Your health behavior is relatively supportive of high-level health. You scored well in several areas; however, you can improve in some ways. Identify your weak areas and chart a plan for behavior change, as explained at the end of Chapter 1. Then pay close attention as you learn more about health in the weeks ahead.

330–549 points

Caution! Your relatively low score indicates that your behavior may be compromising your health. Review your responses to this assessment carefully, noting the areas in which you scored poorly. Then chart a detailed plan for behavior change, as outlined at the end of Chapter 1. Be sure to set realistic goals that you can work toward steadily as you complete this course.

Below 330 points

Red flag! Your low score suggests that your health behavior is destructive. Immediate changes in your behavior are needed to put you back on track. Review your responses to this assessment carefully. Then begin to make changes in the most critical areas, such as harmful alcohol or other drug use patterns. Seek help promptly for any difficulties that you are not prepared to deal with alone, such as domestic violence or suicidal thoughts. The information you read in this textbook and learn in this course could have a significant effect on your future health. Remember, it's not too late to improve your health!

To Carry This Further . . .

Most of us can improve our health behavior in a number of ways. We hope this assessment will help you identify areas in which you can make positive changes and serve as a motivator as you implement your plan for behavior change. If you scored well, give yourself a pat on the back. If your score was not as high as you would have liked, take heart. This textbook and your instructor can help you get started on the road to wellness. Good luck!

The Mind

Part One covers two topics that are closely linked to how we handle change in our lives. Chapter 2 discusses psychological health, and Chapter 3 deals with stress management. As explained below, your personal growth closely relates to each of the six health dimensions discussed in Chapter 1.

1. Physical Dimension

The physical dimension of health concerns the structure and the function of all body systems. Many of the experiences that shape your feelings about yourself are made possible by good physical health. In addition, effective coping skills often require us to draw on the physical dimension of health.

2. Psychological Dimension

Our responses to stress are primarily emotional. Feelings of uneasiness arising from the demands of college, relationships, parenting, or work are the hallmarks of stress. Fortunately, you can cope with change by using the resources of your psychological dimension of health. Your sense of humor, capacity for empathy, and attitude toward adversity will help you cope with demanding changes in your life.

3. Social Dimension

Growth and development are influenced by the people with whom you interact. When things go well with roommates, coworkers, or your spouse or children, you begin to feel capable as a social person. Occasional failures in social relationships can produce stress but can also remind you that emotional growth and coping skills take time to develop.

4. Intellectual Dimension

As you grow older, you will call on your intellectual resources with increasing frequency. These resources will help you enjoy life more fully and understand your emotional and spiritual growth. During difficult times, your mind may be your most dependable coping source. A book, a concert, or an art exhibit may be a refuge from the stress of the classroom, family, or office.

5. Spiritual Dimension

Many of today's students are searching for a deeper understanding of the meaning of life. Some students feel pressured to accept the spiritual beliefs of the majority. The uncertainties of exploring what to believe and how to express those beliefs can create stress. Your spirituality can be a valuable resource during periods of stress. Meditation, introspection, and prayer can free people from some of the stress of living in a fast-paced, sometimes uncaring world. To believe deeply in something and to act on that belief by serving others leads to personal growth.

6. Occupational Dimension

The vocation you choose will have a lasting effect on shaping the person you will become. Many people choose an occupation that allows them to serve others. However, work can be a primary source of life stress. Some of this stress is unwelcome and can be harmful. But occupational stress can also challenge you to perform at your peak, generating a sense of pride and accomplishment.

chapter two

Achieving Psychological Health

Eye on the Media

Television Advertisements for Psychological Medications: Informative or Misleading?

"Trouble sleeping? Difficulty concentrating? Crying most of the time? You might want to talk to your physician about taking Paxil." We are barraged by these types of media message on a daily basis. In fact, a recent study showed that drug advertising increased from $800 million in 1996 to $2.7 billion in 2001. Does it work? Well, for every dollar spent on drug advertising, $4.20 was made in sales. Viewers are typically encouraged to talk to their doctors about specific symptoms and problems and to ask for a particular medication. Physicians report that an increasing number of patients are making appointments because of something they saw on television. On the positive side, this trend results in finding and treating problems more quickly: before drug ads appeared on TV, patients erroneously believed that there was no treatment for, or were avoiding, the problems they were experiencing. When the possibility of a solution was brought to their attention by the commercials, people tended to feel less embarrassed, to be more hopeful, and to recognize problems sooner than they otherwise might have done. Research published in *Prevention Magazine* cited favorable responses to drug advertising on TV. It found that 84 percent of people felt better informed of new treatments. Seventy-eight percent said that the ads helped them to be more involved in their medical care, 34 percent reported talking to their physician about a drug they saw on TV, and 79 percent remembered hearing about risks and side effects. However, only 49 percent of these people said

they paid attention to side effects, with the majority of people believing that they would not experience them. Understanding all the side effects and risks when they are rattled off at breakneck speed or displayed in the smallest print possible at the bottom of the TV screen can be difficult. Of course, some people may be scared off by the side effects and risks and, as a result, won't even talk to their doctors about their concerns.

Sometimes it is difficult to know from watching TV advertisements what condition or problem a drug is designed to treat. And some physicians may disagree with an advertisement's promises or suggest a different drug. The drugs typically being advertised are the newest ones on the market and so are often more expensive and haven't been used for very long. Some physicians are hesitant to prescribe these medications until more evidence exists to show that they work better than the older medications do. There is also a concern that there hasn't been enough time to reveal all the potential side effects or the long-term effects of these drugs. Often it is only after people have been taking them for some time that certain side effects become apparent, such as those associated with the antidepressant Serzone, which has recently been linked to an increased risk of liver failure, jaundice, and hepatitis.

Sometimes the advertisements make misleading or even fraudulent claims. For example, the Food and Drug Administration (FDA)

Eye on the Media *continued*

recently sent a letter to GlaxoSmithKline requesting them to stop using a TV ad for Paxil. The letter stated that the ad was "false or misleading" because it suggested that the drug could be used by a broader range of patients than it was actually approved for and implied that it was safer than actually demonstrated. Pfizer Inc. was charged with illegal promotion of Neurontin, advertising it for use other than the one that the FDA approved. Also, the numbers of suicides and suicide attempts have increased with respect to individuals taking the drug. The FDA wanted the company to add suicide risk to its labeling, and Pfizer refused to do so, saying it remains "confident of the safety and effectiveness of this product."

A compromise might be to allow these ads to continue to air on television with more regulation. The FDA has announced a new proposal regarding consumer advertising and the health industry. The proposal would require ads for prescription drugs to contain language that consumers can better understand, to have possible adverse reactions displayed in larger type, and to include all warnings, contraindications, and major precautions. The FDA has further announced that it will begin a review of its direct-to-consumer ad policy to see if drug ads "confuse consumers and adversely affect the relationship between patients and their health-care providers." One hopes that having more guidelines in place will help educate the public, improve quality of care, and decrease the stigma and confusion surrounding the use of medications to alleviate psychological problems.

Sources:
"Plugged Into Prescription Drugs," *USA Today*, February 15, 2005.
"Prescription Drugs and the Cost of Advertising," www.therubins.com, Allan Rubin, February 27, 2005.
"Drug Advertising Skyrockets," CBS News, February 14, 2002.
"Group Urges Ban of Antidepressant Serzone," www.intelihealth.com, March 6, 2003.

Have you recently been frustrated, angry, fearful, content, excited, or happy? Have you occasionally felt anticipation or anxiety about doing something new? These feelings are all part of the psychological dimension of health. The terms *emotional wellness* and **psychological health** have been used interchangeably to describe how people function in the affective and cognitive realms of their lives. Such functioning includes how people express their emotions; cope with stress, adversity, and success; and adapt to changes in themselves and their environment. Psychological health also addresses cognitive functioning—the way people think and behave in conjunction with their emotions. There is some debate about whether thoughts influence feelings or feelings cause us to think and behave a certain way. However, the most accepted view is that the way we think can directly change how we feel about an event or situation. Thus you can change your feelings about something by changing your attitude and perspective about a situation. This ability has implications for how we can increase our self-esteem and confidence level, and enhance our interactions with others. You will learn more about psychological health in this chapter.

Psychological Health

How do you feel about yourself? When you apply resources from the multiple dimensions of health (Chapter 1) in ways that allow you to direct your growth, assess deeply held values, deal effectively with change, and have satisfying relationships with others, you are psychologically healthy.

Research in the area of health psychology has shown that there is a mind-body connection in which biological, psychological, and social factors interact to influence health or illness. This is referred to as the **biopsychological model.**[1] We know that one's psychological state has a significant effect on physical health; stress, depression, and anxiety have been associated with how the immune system responds and can impair physical health. Studies have shown that terminally ill cancer patients who had good psychological health lived longer lives and reported having higher quality of life than did other cancer patients.[2]

Key Terms

psychological health a broadly based concept pertaining to cognitive functioning in conjunction with the way people express their emotions; cope with stress, adversity, and success; and adapt to changes in themselves and their environment

biopsychological model a model that addresses how biological, psychological, and social factors interact and affect psychological health

Psychological health has also been associated with developing and maintaining a positive **self-concept,** positive **self-esteem,** and a higher level of **emotional intelligence.** However, as you will see, psychological health is much more than just the absence of mental illness.

Characteristics of Psychologically Healthy People

Some of the characteristics most people associate with being psychologically healthy are listed below. Psychologically healthy people:

- Accept themselves and others
- Like themselves
- Appropriately express the full range of human emotions, both positive and negative
- Give and receive care, love, and support
- Accept life's disappointments
- Accept their mistakes
- Express empathy and concern for others
- Take care of themselves
- Trust others as well as themselves
- Establish goals, both short and long term
- Can function both independently and interdependently
- Lead a health-enhancing lifestyle that includes regular exercise, good nutrition, and adequate sleep

The Changing for the Better box on this page suggests some activities that may enhance your current level of psychological health.

Self-Esteem

What is self-esteem? How do you know when someone is lacking in self-esteem? Most people answer this question by saying that they define positive self-esteem as:

- Having pride in yourself
- Treating yourself with respect
- Considering yourself valuable, important, worthy
- Feeling good about yourself
- Having self-confidence, being self-assured
- Accepting yourself

Key Terms

self-concept an individual's internal picture of himself or herself; the way one sees oneself

self-esteem an individual's sense of pride, self-respect, value, and worth

emotional intelligence the ability to understand others and act wisely in human relations and measure how well one knows one's emotions, manages one's emotions, motivates oneself, recognizes emotions in others, and handles relationships

People with low levels of self-esteem tend to allow others to mistreat them, don't take care of themselves, have difficulty being by themselves, and have little self-confidence. In addition, people with low self-esteem tend to take things personally and are sometimes seen as overly sensitive; they tend to be perfectionists who are highly critical of themselves and others. These individuals often have a pessimistic outlook on life and see themselves as undeserving of good fortune. We explore the concepts of optimism and pessimism as they relate to psychological health in a later section of this chapter.

Where do we get our self-esteem? Most people would say from their parents, teachers, peers, siblings, religious institutions, and the media. While these factors certainly can positively or negatively affect our self-concept and self-esteem, they are all *external* factors. Self-concept refers to our *internal* self-perception. People with low self-esteem tend to have a poor self-concept, meaning that their internal picture of themselves is very negative. Because of this poor self-concept, people with low self-esteem tend to allow others to mistreat or abuse them and fail to be assertive. Many psychological problems have their underpinnings in low self-esteem, including eating disorders, substance abuse problems, and depression.

People who suffer from low self-esteem tend to focus on outside factors. If our self-esteem and self-concept were based only on external factors, then we would need to change our environment and the people around us. Thus, many people believe that if they had more money, a nicer car, a better relationship, and so on they would feel better about themselves. This situation can become a vicious cycle, leaving the person always seeking more and being perpetually unsatisfied with himself/herself. This situation can also lead to perfectionism and not accepting yourself.

Although we don't have much control over other people, we do have control over what we internalize or accept as true and valid about ourselves. It is generally accepted that self-esteem comes from within and is ultimately within each individual's control. In addition, self-esteem is not an all-or-none commodity. Most people have varying degrees of self-esteem, depending on their stage of development, events in their lives, and their environment.[3]

Emotional Intelligence

A third aspect of psychological health is the degree of emotional intelligence you possess. Emotional intelligence refers to "the ability to understand others and act wisely in human relations."[4] Furthermore, emotional intelligence can be broken down into five primary domains:

- **Knowing your emotions.** This aspect of emotional intelligence is considered the cornerstone of emotional intelligence and relates to how much self-awareness and insight you have. How quickly you are able to recognize and label your feelings as you feel them determines the level of your emotional intelligence.

- **Managing your emotions.** How well can you express your feelings appropriately and cope with your emotions? People who have trouble coping with anxiety, distress, and failures tend to have lower levels of emotional intelligence.

- **Motivating yourself.** People who can motivate themselves tend to be more highly productive and independent than are those who rely on external sources for motivation. The more you can self-motivate and engage in goal-directed activities, the higher your emotional intelligence.

- **Recognizing emotions in others.** Another aspect of emotional intelligence is the degree of empathy you have or how sensitive you are to the feelings of others and how you come across to other people.

- **Handling relationships.** This refers to your level of social skills. The more interpersonally effective you are and able to negotiate conflict and build a social support network, the more emotional intelligence you possess.

Of course people have differing levels of emotional intelligence and may have higher levels in one domain than in another. People with overall high levels of emotional intelligence tend to take on leadership roles, are confident, assertive, express their feelings directly and appropriately, feel good about themselves, are outgoing, and adapt well to stress.[4]

Personality

What is meant when someone says, "She has a good personality"? Is it possible to have no personality? **Personality** is generally defined as a specific set of consistent patterns of behaviors and traits that help to identify and characterize an individual. Personality comprises thoughts, feelings, behaviors, motivation, instinct, and temperament.[5] Isn't it likely that you associate someone's "good" personality with the existence of psychological health?

Key Terms

personality a specific set of consistent patterns of behavior and traits that helps to identify and characterize an individual; personality comprises thoughts, feelings, behaviors, motivation, instinct, and temperament

How to Say You Are Sorry and Mean It!

Some people avoid relationships because they don't want to get hurt. Of course they are also avoiding feeling cared about and sharing their lives with others. While it is impossible not to hurt someone with whom you are in a relationship because you forgot something, inadvertently said the wrong thing, or you had a grouchy moment, it is possible to fix the damage you have done with little to no residual scarring, which is called "the art of effective apology."

There are some dos and don'ts that can make the difference between an effective, reparative apology and a lame, destructive one. In fact, an apology that is perceived as insincere, as blaming the other person, or as defensive, can do more harm than good. Here are some important things to keep in mind as you consider an apology.

Apologize . . .

1. As soon as you realize you have done something wrong. Don't wait for the "right time," because it will probably never come. Remember that the right time is as soon as you have realized your error.
2. When you have something truly to apologize for. Don't apologize for everything and everyone, including the bad weather. When you overapologize, it dilutes the apology's meaning.
3. By fully acknowledging what you did wrong. Don't sugarcoat or minimize the error. For example, don't say "I didn't understand what you said" when really you understood but didn't agree with what she said.
4. And include an explanation not an excuse for your actions. Take responsibility for your actions, don't blame other people or the situation. Help the person understand why you did what you did rather than making excuses or defending your behavior, which will only weaken your apology. Owning up to what you did and being willing to admit to it will increase trust in your relationship.
5. With remorse. Saying "I'm sorry you feel that way" versus "I'm sorry that I hurt you" will make or break how an apology is received. Saying "I'm sorry I hurt you but" also diminishes the sincerity of an apology, because "but" tends to negate whatever comes before it. However, this doesn't mean you have to beat yourself up to show how badly you feel about the situation, but you do need to acknowledge that you hurt the other person's feelings.
6. And fix what can be repaired. Saying "I'm sorry" but not offering to resolve or repair the damage can cause further hurt. Ask the person what you can do to make things right. Don't say "I said I'm sorry, what else do you want from me?" or "Get over it and move on. It wasn't that big a deal."
7. And learn from your mistakes. Saying you are sorry and then doing the same thing all over again destroys trust. You may be perceived as using an apology as a way of continuing the offensive behavior. The next time, do something different when that situation arises. Talk with the person about how you can handle that situation in a better way in the future.

With effective apologies can come forgiveness and rebuilding of trust and respect in relationships. An effective apology involves honesty, courage, humility, and a real commitment to the relationship. It means we admit to our imperfections and flaws, and it reinforces our commitment to improve ourselves and be acceptable as imperfect human beings.

Source: Martha Beck, "Love Means Never Having to Say You Are Sorry," *Oprah Magazine*, September 2004.

There is some debate about how personality is formed and where we acquire our personality traits. A general consensus is that two factors, **nature** and **nurture,** influence the shaping of personality. Nature refers to the innate factors we are born with that genetically determine our personality traits. Nurture is the effect that the environment, people, and external factors have on our personality.[6] While it is agreed that both nature and nurture influence personality development, there is some debate about how much of a role each one plays in its formation. We all know people who are introverted or quiet or shy "by nature" or "naturally outgoing." We seem to be born with a predisposition toward certain personality traits that often resemble our parents. "She is serious like her father" or "He is funny like his mother" are remarks people may make alluding to this genetic link. Environmental factors such as social relationships, family harmony, financial resources, job and academic concerns, and living situations, can influence your personality.

Often assumptions are made about an individual's personality based largely on his or her appearance. Studies have shown that physically attractive people are seen as warm, friendly, and intelligent, and unattractive people are viewed as cold, humorless, and not as bright.[7] First impressions also play a major role in how we perceive

Key Terms

nature the innate factors that genetically determine personality traits

nurture the effect that the environment, people, and external factors have on personality other people's personalities. Research shows that we tend to make a decision about someone's personality within four minutes of meeting them. Once an impression is formed, it is difficult to change, regardless of how the person behaves or of new information that you receive that might contradict what you initially perceived.[6] Thus, people can make errors in judgment because they have not taken the context into consideration or taken enough time to get to know someone over the course of several months and in a variety of settings.

The Normal Range of Emotions

You probably know people who seem to be cheerful all the time. Although some people like this may exist, they are truly the exceptions. For most people, emotions are more like a roller coaster ride. At times, they feel happy, confi-dent, and positive; other times, they feel sad, insecure, and negative. Once you know them better, these same people may show that they feel happy, sad, pleased, uncertain, confident, excited, and afraid all in the same day or week. To outsiders, they might even appear to be moody. To the mental health professional, however, these same people would probably seem to be normal, since the feeling states that they are demonstrating all fall within a normal range of emotions.

Everyone, not only college students, experiences a range of emotions. This is normal and healthy. You should not expect to remain calm and rational every minute of the day. You also should not expect to adjust effectively to every situation with which you are confronted. Life has its ups and downs, and the concept of the *normal range of emotions* reflects this. If one concept is important for you to understand about being psychologically healthy, it is this one.

Learning from Our Diversity
Diverse Personalities

When we think about diversity, we may think about differences in ethnicity, culture, religion, sexual orientation, and disabilities, but we don't often consider differences in personality as part of diversity. Diversity can refer to any difference or potentially separating factor between or within groups. With respect to psychological health, there certainly are differences in personality traits—for example, outgoing vs. shy, detail oriented vs. spontaneous, flexible vs. structured. Often people value certain personality characteristics over others—for instance, being extraverted, organized, responsible, humorous, and open minded. Other traits can seem positive in one situation but negative in another. For example, being sensitive can be seen as a positive quality when you are sensitive to the feelings of other people and can relate well to others. However, it can also be seen negatively if you are perceived as being overly sensitive in terms of taking things too personally or overreacting to situations or criticism.

A personality test called the Myers-Briggs Type Indicator (MBTI) examines individual personality traits on four different scales and gives a score for each: extraversion vs. introversion, sensing vs. intuitive, thinking vs. feeling, and judging vs. perception. Extraverts tend to get their energy from being with other people. They do their best thinking out loud and like to talk things through, whereas introverts tend to hang back and share their thoughts once they have them fully formed and put together in their own mind. Introverts tend to get their energy from solitary or one-on-one activities. Sensing people are good with facts and details, and they are practical, traditional, and down to earth. Intuitives tend to be nonconformist, creative, and divergent global thinkers. Thinking types are more analytical and logical, and they base their decisions on facts, rules, and policies. Feeling types base their decisions on how they will affect other people; they tend to be peacekeepers, conflict avoidant, and are sensitive to the feelings of others. Organized, good with time management, and structured are qualities of judging types, whereas spontaneous, adaptable, and flexible describe perceptives.

The MBTI maintains that there are no good or bad personality types, only important differences, and it uses the four scales to describe them. The MBTI talks about how you can play to your strengths and understand your weaknesses and how you can appreciate other people's personality types. In fact, the idea behind this instrument is that it is more helpful for opposites to work together or be in a relationship because each person can balance and complement the other. As a way to understand the diversity of people's personalities, the MBTI has been used in leadership styles, communication skills, conflict negotiation, career exploration, learning styles, and building work groups.

Psychological health entails finding a good balance between your own strengths and weaknesses as well as acknowledging and celebrating the differences among people. Knowing yourself, recognizing the impact you have on others, can help you to have more fulfilling interactions. Building relationships between diverse personality types and seeing these differences as strengthening, balancing, and enhancing is another way to celebrate diversity in our community.

Happiness and a Sense of Humor

Perhaps the most prized emotion to be experienced is a feeling of happiness about life—a feeling that is more likely to occur when day-to-day events are entered into with an underlying sense of humor.

Maintaining a sense of humor is now known to be a critically important component of the psychological dimension of health.[8] People who possess this resource understand that life is not meant to be one long, boring exercise. Life taken too seriously can be the most miserable life imaginable.

Recognizing the humor in daily situations and occasionally being able to laugh at yourself will make you feel better not only about others but also, more importantly, about yourself. Others will enjoy being associated with you, and your ability to perform physically and to recover from injuries and illnesses will also be enhanced.[9] In addition, laughter reduces stress,[10] boosts the immune system,[11] alleviates pain,[12] stabilizes mood,[13] decreases anxiety,[14] enhances communication,[15] and inspires creativity.[16] The research suggests that we need to laugh 30 minutes total in a 24-hour period in order to attain these benefits. This is an

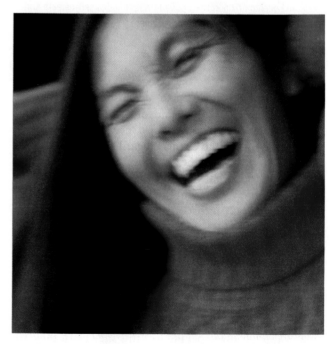

Laughing increases endorphin levels to help ease pain, decrease stress, and release tension from your body.

easy task for children who on average laugh 250 times a day but more challenging for adults who tend to only laugh 15 times a day.[17] Employers have been putting the benefits of laughter to good use to increase productivity in factories. Factories in India have created "laughing clubs" in which people laugh together for 20 minutes a day, resulting in less absenteeism and better performance among the workers.[18]

 TALKING POINTS How would you describe your personality? How do you think your friends or family would describe you? Do you think the descriptions would be the same or different?

Developing Communication Skills

When people find it difficult to initiate or even participate in conversations with others, it is likely, in part, that they have not developed some of the communication skills

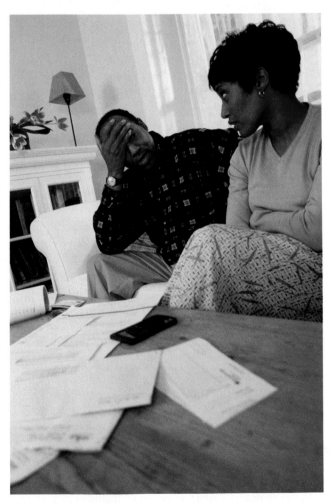

Nonverbal communication can be a powerful tool in sending messages to others through body language and posture as well as facial expressions.

with which others feel comfortable. In this section we investigate how speaking and listening can foster improved social relationships. We also look at the use of unspoken communication as an aid to social interaction. Remember that how people see themselves (their self-concept) influences how they feel about themselves (their self-esteem).

Verbal Communication

Communication between people can be viewed in terms of a particular person's role as sender or receiver. You can enhance your effectiveness as a sender of verbal information by implementing several important steps:[3]

- Take the time to think before speaking. Effective communication requires that you know what you want to say.
- Focus your words on your most important thoughts and ideas. Your main message may get lost in too many details or too long a story.
- Speak clearly and concisely. This will aid the listener, particularly when ideas are complex or new.
- Talk with, rather than at, the listener. Speaking with other people encourages listeners to share freely and comfortably with those speaking.
- Start on a positive note. Even when the message is negative, a more positive atmosphere is established when a conversation begins in this manner.
- Seek feedback from listeners. Provide frequent intervals between ideas to allow listeners to respond.
- Use other forms of communication to transmit important ideas when face-to-face conversation is not effective. Written communication or the use of a carefully selected third person is often highly effective.

Verbal communication requires that you function as skillfully as a listener, or receiver, as you do as a sender of spoken ideas. Certainly, there are skills for structuring the exchange of information. The following are a variety of listening approaches:

- Listen with attention. In many situations it will be important to hear and understand everything that is being said.
- Ask for clarification and summarize what you think you heard the speaker saying to ensure you have received the message accurately.
- On some occasions, it may be necessary to guide the speaker to ensure that excessive or confusing information is not being transferred. This is accomplished by asking carefully worded questions intended to stay on the topic and not get too far off on a tangent.

Nonverbal Communication

Nonverbal communication is what is communicated by your facial expressions, body posture, tone of voice, movements, and even the way you breathe, such as when you sigh or yawn. Nonverbal communication is a very powerful and sometimes more important aspect of the message than what is verbally communicated. Facial cues, particularly from the eyes, are attended to more than any other type of nonverbal communication, even when information from other sources, such as hand and body movements, may provide a more accurate picture of what the person is feeling. The following suggestions can enhance your nonverbal communication skills:

- *Facial expressions.* Facial expressions have been cited as one of the most important sources of nonverbal communication in terms of a person's emotional state.[19] When people speak with their eyebrows raised, they tend to be seen as more animated, excited, and happy. Flushing of one's face can indicate embarrassment, and crinkling one's nose can mean that you don't like something. Every part of your face can communicate some type of emotional reaction.

- *Eye contact.* Maintaining eye contact is an important component of positive nonverbal communication, while looking away or shifting your eyes can be read as seeming dishonest. But don't stare—5 to 7 seconds seems to be the maximum amount of time to look at someone's eyes before they begin to feel scrutinized.

- *Personal space.* There are cultural differences in how much personal space or distance is comfortable and accepted when sitting or standing next to another person. For example, Americans' personal space—about 3 to 4 feet for a casual conversation—tends to be much greater than that of Arabs or Italians but less than for Japanese or Britons. Gender and age and degree of familiarity are other factors that can determine the amount of personal space you are comfortable having between you and another person.

- *Body posture.* Assertiveness is equated with people who carry themselves with their heads up, shoulders back, and maintain eye contact. Folding your arms, crossing your legs, and turning your body away from the speaker can indicate defensiveness and rejection.

As with verbal communication, when nonverbal components are recognized and controlled, communication is more effective.

Managing Conflict

Communication can be especially challenging when there is a conflict or disagreement. Emotions such as anger, hurt, and fear might alter your ability to communicate as effectively as you would like. Some techniques for managing angry or upset people or conflictual situations are these:

- *Listen and acknowledge the other person's point of view, even if it differs from your own.* To ensure that you have heard the person accurately and to let that person know you are listening, repeat back or summarize what you heard and ask if you misunderstood something that was said.

- *Use assertive communication.* Using "I" statements rather than "You" helps to avoid putting people on the defensive and is especially helpful when negotiating conflict or disagreements. Rather than saying "You are inconsiderate," you can say "I feel upset when you're late and don't call to let me know."

- *Focus not just on what you say but how you say it.* Pay attention to your tone of voice and speak in a conversational tone. People tend to talk louder because they think they will be better heard that way. This can result in a shouting match in which neither person hears the other.

- *Acknowledge the others person's feelings.* Use statements like, "I can understand why this is so frustrating for you."

- *Watch your body posture.* Don't fold your arms in a closed, defensive posture, maintain eye contact, be aware of your facial expression so that you are not conveying hostility nonverbally. Make sure your nonverbal communication matches your verbal communication.

- *Accept valid criticism.* If you made a mistake, admit to it, apologize for whatever you think you did to contribute to the misunderstanding or conflict. This will open the door for the other person to take responsibility for his/her part in the conflict as well.

- *Focus on the problem at hand.* If you try to resolve every disagreement you have ever had with this person, you will become overwhelmed and won't accomplish much. Stay on track by talking about the present situation.

- *Take a team approach by engaging in mutual problem solving.* Avoid the winner versus loser paradigm, and look for areas of compromise. Find a middle ground you can both live with.

- *Agree to disagree.* There is probably more than one right answer, and you can agree that you will not persuade the other to change his or her point of view.

- *Agree to discuss this at a later time.* If the conversation becomes too volatile and heated, take some time to calm down and think about the situation. Some time and distance from the problem can be beneficial.

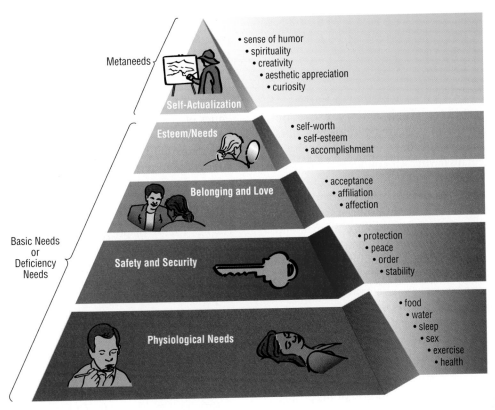

Figure 2-1 Maslow's hierarchy of needs.

Maslow's Hierarchy of Needs

Abraham Maslow has been among the significant contributors to the understanding of personality and emotional growth. Central to Maslow's contribution to 20th-century American psychological thought is his view of psychological health in terms of the individual's attempt to meet inner needs, what he called *the hierarchy of needs*[20] (see Figure 2-1).

Maslow's theory is a positive, optimistic theory of human behavior. He believed that people are motivated to grow and fulfill their potential, referring to this phenomenon as **self-actualization.** He described self-actualization as "the need to become more and more what one is, to become everything that one is capable of becoming."[21] Maslow differentiated between two different categories of needs: **basic needs** and **metaneeds.** Basic needs—physiological needs, belonging and love, and esteem needs—are the deficiency needs and are essential and urgent. Metaneeds come into play once the basic needs are met and include spirituality, creativity, curiosity, beauty, philosophy, and justice. Maslow's hierarchy of needs is arranged with the basic needs on the bottom, as they are the most fundamental and powerful needs. Lower level needs must be met before the next level of needs can be satisfied. Maslow believed that the fulfillment of metaneeds is needed to become a completely developed human being. Left unfulfilled, people can become cynical, apathetic, and lonely.[24]

Maslow arrived at this model by examining people whom he considered to be exceptionally healthy, people he defined as having developed to their fullest potentials. Self-actualized people whom Maslow identified included Albert Einstein, Albert Schweitzer, Eleanor Roosevelt, and Abraham Lincoln. He perceived these people to share

---

Key Terms

self-actualization the highest level of psychological health at which one reaches his or her highest potential and values truth, beauty, goodness, faith, love, humor, and ingenuity

basic needs deficiency needs that are viewed as essential and fundamental, including physiological needs, belonging and love, and esteem needs

metaneeds secondary concerns, such as spirituality, creativity, curiosity, beauty, philosophy, and justice, that can be addressed only after the basic needs are met similar personality characteristics, such as being self-assured, principled, innovative, compassionate, altruistic, goal-oriented, and internally motivated.[22]

Creative Expression

Another characteristic of people who have developed their psychological health is creativity. Allowing yourself to express your thoughts, feelings, and individuality in a creative manner entails having self-confidence, self-esteem, and flexibility. Confidence and self-esteem are essential so that you don't feel embarrassed by your creativity and feel free to share your creative side with others. Children can easily do this when they draw a picture or make up a dance and say, "Look at me; look at what I made." However, as we age, some of us become inhibited and don't allow ourselves to be creative or to share this part of ourselves. If you don't exercise your creative side, it can atrophy, just as unexercised muscles do.

What are some resources that you might need to develop to foster your creativity?

- *Nonconformity.* Creative individuals aren't terribly concerned about what other people think of them. They are willing to risk looking foolish or proposing ideas that are divergent from others or traditional ways of thinking.

- *Independence.* Highly creative people tend to work well alone and sometimes prefer this to working in a group. As children, they often were encouraged to solve problems on their own rather than having someone else to do so for them.

- *Motivation.* Creative people are motivated by intrinsic rather than external rewards, meaning they like to be creative for their own pleasure, not to please others or because it is expected of them. They don't fear failure, and success is not the main goal. They enjoy creativity for creativity's sake alone and not to reap rewards or praise from others.

- *Curiosity.* Creative people have a wide range of interests and a broad base of knowledge. They are open to new experiences and question things that other people ignore or take for granted.

- *Persistence.* This is seen as one of the most important traits of a creative person. As Thomas Edison said, "Genius is one-tenth inspiration and nine-tenths perspiration." Persistence requires not giving up when your first efforts are not successful and thinking of new ways of doing something, problem solving, or thinking "outside the box."[40]

Some people reviewing the preceding list may recognize many of these characteristics as being already well developed in their own personalities. Others may not have demonstrated some of the traits listed, and they may appear far beyond their reach. Nevertheless, most people can increase their creativity by giving themselves permission to be creative. Some people state, "I'm not a creative person," and yet they haven't explored that part of their personality, perhaps since childhood. There are many avenues of creativity, and the first step is to experiment, to be open and spontaneous. In this way, you can gain greater psychological health from accessing your inner strengths and resources.

Spiritual Health

Having a sense of purpose, direction, and awareness is a dimension of spiritual health. This aspect of psychological health also refers to how well we integrate our beliefs and values with our behavior. People with spiritual health

Discovering Your Spirituality

Mindfulness: Time to Pay Attention

Have you taken a moment today to be quiet and just be with yourself? Time alone can help you step away from a busy, fragmented world and draw inward for renewal. Having strengthened awareness of yourself in both mind and body allows you to experience the fullness of the moment, even to feel in sync with the universe. This is referred to as "mindfulness"—being aware of the present moment without judging or thinking.

Mindfulness can also help you establish your identity, clarify what's important to you, and strengthen your independence. Because most of our time is spent living with, caring for, or responding to others, it is only when we are observing the moment that we have the opportunity to fully emerge and become ourselves.

Any time you take for this meditation will be restorative. You may start with just five minutes every morning. You will need a place where you feel comfortable to be alone with your own thoughts, whether it be at the kitchen table, in bed, in the bath, at a coffee shop, in the library, or in the garden. Go for a walk, listen to music, weed the garden, write a letter to a friend, paint, read a poem, or just be still and concentrate on your breathing. All of these are ways to reconnect you to your life force. Pretty soon you may feel that your time of mindfulness is more energizing than sleep! When you are faced with a difficult project, a household disaster, or something more serious, such as sickness or death, these reflective moments will give you mental and spiritual renewal.

It's not selfish to carve out whatever time you need alone to refresh yourself. By paying attention to your thoughts and feelings, you're reconnecting to your inner self. This nourished spirit is what you can share with others, whether family, friends, coworkers, or strangers.

seek meaning and purpose in their lives and have a deep appreciation for a sense of unity and community. Spiritual health also includes one's morals, ethics, intrinsic values, and beliefs. It also refers to an awareness and appreciation of the vastness of the universe, and recognition of a dimension beyond the natural and rational, involving, perhaps, a belief in a force greater than oneself.[23] Spirituality has been found to increase psychological health; people who incorporate it into their lives reported better psychological coping, increased well-being, increased satisfaction with life, lower anxiety and fewer depressive symptoms, less hostility and anger, and greater happiness in general.[24] Similarly, spirituality has also been related to better physical health. Studies have shown that no matter how *spirituality* was defined or measured, it has a positive effect on reducing coronary heart disease, high blood pressure, stroke, cancer, and increasing life expectancy.[25]

As a resource in the spiritual dimension of health, the existence of spirituality provides a basis on which your belief system can mature and your expanding awareness of life's meaning can be fostered. In addition, the existence of spirituality gives meaning to your career and assists you in better understanding the consequences of your vocational efforts. Further, spirituality can influence many of the experiences that you will seek throughout life and can temper the emotional relationships that you have with these experiences. In virtually all cultures, spirituality provides individuals and groups with rituals and practices that foster the development of a sense of community. In turn, the community provides the authority and the guidance that nurtures the emotional stability, confidence, and sense of competence needed for living life fully.[26]

 TALKING POINTS How well do your actions reflect your beliefs and values? How can you better integrate your values, beliefs, and behavior? How much time and energy do you devote to what is most important to you?

Taking an Optimistic Approach to Life

Is your happiness within your control? Are people born naturally happy or sad? One important key to psychological health is the way that you think about and interpret events in your life. For example, if you say "hello" to someone and you don't get a response, do you begin to wonder if that person is angry with you? Or do you surmise that he or she didn't hear you or perhaps was distracted? Research shows that having a positive interpretation of life's events, particularly how you cope with adversity, can make a significant difference in terms of your health,

academic and work performance, as well as how long you will live.[27] Do you see the glass half empty, as pessimists do, or half full, as optimists do? Does it matter? Again studies overwhelmingly contend that your perspective makes a tremendous difference in your psychological health. Compared to pessimists, optimists tend to:

- Contract fewer infectious diseases
- Have better health habits
- Possess stronger immune systems
- Be more successful in their careers
- Perform better in sports, music, and academics

We do know that people can learn to be helpless and ultimately become depressed and even suicidal. Pavlov demonstrated the concept of **learned helplessness** in his classic study in which he administered an electric shock to dogs that were harnessed and couldn't escape the shock. When he moved the dogs to another room and delivered the shocks, the dogs lay down and whimpered and didn't try to avoid the shocks. This time the dogs were not harnessed and could have easily escaped the shocks by moving to another side of the room. This reaction has been referred to as learned helplessness. The dogs learned that there was nothing they could do to affect their situation, and they lost hope and felt trapped and powerless.[28] We have seen this same phenomenon with humans. College students volunteered for an experiment in which they were subjected to an earsplitting noise and their efforts to stop the noise were unsuccessful. Later, when they were placed in another situation in which they could have easily pulled a control lever to turn off the noise, they made no effort to do so and just suffered with the noise until the experimenter stopped it.[29] Battered women have demonstrated this same sense of powerlessness and helplessness in their inability to escape the abuse they are subjected to by their partners.

So, if people can learn to be helpless and pessimistic, can they also learn to feel more optimistic, powerful, and in control? Martin Seligman, a prominent psychologist, conducted studies to prove that this is possible, and he called this concept **learned optimism.** Learned optimism

> **Key Terms**
>
> **learned helplessness** a theory of motivation explaining how individuals can learn to feel powerless, trapped, and defeated
>
> **learned optimism** an attribution style comprising permanence, pervasiveness, and personalization; how people explain both positive and negative events in their lives, accounting for success and failure

refers to your explanatory style—in other words, if you describe the glass as being half full or half empty. Seligman identified three key factors that contribute to having an optimistic or pessimistic perspective. These crucial dimensions are **permanence, pervasiveness,** and **personalization.**

The first dimension is *permanence*. When something bad happens, pessimists tend to give up easily because they believe the causes of bad events are *permanent*. They say things like "Things never work out for me," "That won't ever work," or "He's always in a bad mood." They use permanent language—words like *never, always* and *forever*—which implies that this negative situation is not temporary but will continue indefinitely. Optimists tend to use temporary language—such words as *sometimes, frequently,* and *often*—and they blame bad events on transient conditions. Examples of optimistic language are "It didn't work out this time," "Doing it that way didn't work," and "He's in a bad mood today." Optimists see failure as a small, transitory setback and are able to pick themselves up, brush themselves off, and persevere toward their goals.

The second factor that affects our outlook is *pervasiveness*. It refers to whether you perceive negative events as universal and generalize them to everything in your life, or if you can compartmentalize and keep them defined to the specific situation. Pessimists tend to make universal explanations for their problems and when something goes wrong in one part of their lives, they give up on everything. While a pessimist would say that they are not good at math, an optimist would say that they didn't perform well in that particular class with that type of math: "I'm good at algebra but not as good with geometry."

The last aspect of an optimistic or pessimistic explanatory style is determined by whether you blame bad things on yourself or on other people or circumstances.

Pessimism and low self-esteem tend to come from personalizing events—blaming oneself and having an internal explanatory style for negative events. An optimist might say, "The professor wrote a very poor exam and that is the reason I received a lower score," whereas the pessimist would say, "I am stupid" or "I didn't study enough." This is different from not taking responsibility for one's actions and blaming other people for your problems or mistakes: the idea is to have a balanced perspective and outlook on life. Pessimists tend to give credit to other people or circumstances when good things happen and blame themselves when bad events occur. For example, a pessimist would say, "That was just dumb luck" rather than taking credit for a success. However, if pessimists fail, they readily blame themselves, saying, "I messed up." In contrast, optimists tend to give themselves credit for their accomplishments, saying, "I worked hard and did a good job," and they don't belittle themselves when things go wrong.

Seligman conducted many studies to test how an optimistic explanatory style might be useful in daily living. For example, he worked with a swimming team from the University of California, Berkeley, to see how optimism or pessimism might affect their performance. He had their coaches tell the athletes that their times were slower than they actually were. The swimmers were then asked to swim the event again as fast as they could. The performance of the pessimists deteriorated in their 100-yard event by 2 seconds, the difference between winning the event and finishing dead last. The optimists got faster by 2 to 5 seconds, again enough to be the difference between losing and winning the race.[27] So how you interpret events, your attribution style, can make a tremendous difference in the eventual success or failure in your endeavors.

How can you learn to be more optimistic? Albert Ellis developed a cognitive framework for positive thinking called the ABC method. When you encounter adversity, the "A" part of the formula, you try to make sense out of it and explain what has happened. For example, if you receive a notice from the bank that you have overdrawn your checking account, you start to think, "How did this happen?" These thoughts are associated with your beliefs, the "B" in ABC. Your beliefs affect your feelings, and so you can control your emotions by changing your beliefs and thoughts.[30] So if you think, "I'm irresponsible for letting this happen. I can't manage my money," then you will feel bad about yourself. But if you said, "The bank probably made a mistake" or "I might have added something incorrectly," you will most likely feel much better about yourself and the situation.

The "C" aspect is the consequence of the event, how you end up feeling about the situation. When someone feels depressed, he or she feels hopeless, trapped, and powerless. By adopting a more positive way of reframing or thinking about events, you create options, hope, and a strategy for solving problems rather than remaining stuck, like the whimpering dogs lying down and putting

---

Key Terms

permanence the first dimension of an individual's attribution style, related to whether certain events are perceived as temporary or long-lasting

pervasiveness the second dimension of an individual's attribution style, related to whether they perceive events as specific or general

personalization the final dimension of attribution style, related to whether an individual takes things personally or is more balanced in accepting responsibility for positive and negative events up with being shocked. In the previously described scenario with the overdraft, you can generate ideas such as "I need to check with the bank, go over my bank statement, be more careful in recording and calculating my balances, and request overdraft protection to prevent this from becoming a problem again."

Everyone encounters adversity sometime in his or her life. You can become discouraged by these events, blame yourself for these problems, and feel hopeless, worthless, and cynical about the world. Or you can be persistent and become stronger by overcoming these obstacles, by having positive beliefs, and by seeing these problems as short-lived, specific, and not as a flaw in your character. When you embrace an optimistic perspective, you will feel more hopeful, stronger, and confident. You will be able to accept new challenges and take risks in your life.

 TALKING POINTS Think about something bad that has happened in your life recently. What were your beliefs about this event? How did you feel? Using the concepts of permanence, pervasiveness, and personalization, how can you change your beliefs about this situation? How do you feel differently about the event?

Taking a Proactive Approach to Life

In addition to the approaches already discussed, the plan that follows is intended to give you other strategies for enhancing your psychological health. The following is a four-step process that continues throughout life: constructing perceptions of yourself, accepting these perceptions, undertaking new experiences, and reframing your perceptions based on new information.

Constructing Mental Pictures

Actively taking charge of your psychological health begins with constructing a mental picture of what you're like. Use the most recent and accurate information you have about yourself—what is important to you, your values, and your abilities. You may want to ask trusted friends and family members for their input.

To construct this mental picture, set aside a period of uninterrupted quiet time for reflection. Before proceeding to the second step, you also need to construct mental pictures about yourself in relation to *other people and material objects;* including your residence and college or work environment, to clarify these relationships.

Accepting Mental Pictures

The second step of the plan involves an *acceptance* of these perceptions. This implies a willingness to honor the truthfulness of the perceptions you have formed about yourself and other people.

Psychological development is an active process. You must be willing to be *introspective* (inwardly reflective) about yourself and the world around you and to apply these new perceptions.

Undertaking New Experiences

The next step of the plan is to test your newly formed perceptions. This *testing* is accomplished by *undertaking a new experience* or by reexperiencing something in a different way.

New experiences do not necessarily require high levels of risk, foreign travel, or money. They may be no more "new" than deciding to move from the dorm into an apartment, to change from one shift at work to another, or to pursue new friendships. The experience itself is not the goal; rather, it's a means of collecting information about yourself, others, and the objects that form your material world. The goal is to "try on" or test your perceptions to see what fits you.

Reframing Mental Pictures

When you have completed the first three steps in the plan, the new information about yourself, others, and objects becomes the most current source of information. Regardless of the type of new experience you have undertaken and its outcome, you are now in a position to modify the initial perceptions constructed during the first step. Then you will have new insights, knowledge, and perspectives. This is a continual process. As you grow and change, so will your perceptions.

Psychological Disorders

In the course of one year, an estimated 22 percent of Americans, about one in five, suffer from a diagnosable mental disorder.[31] This translates to 54 million people being diagnosed with a mental disorder each year, with many people suffering from more than one mental disorder at a given time.[32] In addition, four of the ten leading causes of disability in the United States and other developed countries are mental disorders.[33] However, two-thirds of these people do not receive treatment owing to the stigma and cost associated with mental health treatment.[34] Overall, minorities and Caucasians share the same prevalence rate of mental disorders; however, there are great disparities in the rate of mental health care for minorities as compared to the nonminority population.

How common are these disorders? Quite common, as the figures just mentioned suggest. In addition, the lives of millions of other people who work, live, and have relationships with people with mental illness also suffer the effect of these disorders. While there are over 300 different types of mental illness that can be diagnosed, we will cover three major categories of mental disorder: mood disorders, including depression and bipolar disorder; anxiety disorders, including panic disorder, obsessive-compulsive disorder, and posttraumatic stress disorder; and schizophrenia.[35] We will also briefly discuss attention deficit disorder. Over 450 million people worldwide are affected by mental disorders at any given time, and these numbers are expected to increase in the future.[36]

In the sections that follow, we will investigate selected disorders, identify professionals who are trained to treat these conditions, and take a look at the techniques they employ to help those who are afflicted.

Mood Disorders

Mood disorders, such as depression, seasonal affective disorder, and bipolar disorder, refer to psychological problems in which the primary symptom is a disturbance in mood.[35] You might perceive someone as moody, unable to predict if the person will be in a good or bad mood from one day to the next.

Depression

According to the World Health Organization (WHO), more than 340 million people worldwide, 18 million in the United States alone, are estimated to suffer from **clinical depression.**[36] WHO further contends that this will only worsen in the future, predicting that depression will become the second leading cause of disability worldwide by the year 2020, after heart disease, unless strides are made in prevention and treatment. We have already begun to see this trend, as the number of college students with depression has doubled over recent years.[37] About one in ten Americans suffers some form of depression, with women experiencing depression twice as often as men.[38] While depression can develop at any age, the average age of onset is the mid-20s.

How can you tell the difference between having the blues and clinical depression? The symptoms of depression are as follows:

- Depressed mood most of the day, nearly every day
- Frequent crying
- Withdrawing, isolating yourself from others
- Lack of interest in activities that are typically enjoyable
- Increase or decrease in appetite resulting in significant weight loss or weight gain
- Insomnia, disturbed or restless sleep, or sleeping more than usual

- Feeling tired most of the time, regardless of how much sleep you have had
- Low self-esteem, feelings of hopelessness and worthlessness
- Difficulty concentrating, remembering things, and focusing on a task, and indecisiveness
- Frequent thoughts of suicide

Most people have experienced some of these symptoms at one point or another in their lives; however, clinically depressed individuals experience most of these symptoms every day and have felt this way for at least two weeks. Most people can find ways of pulling themselves out of feeling down, but for those suffering from clinical depression, the normal methods used to cope with the blues don't work. Clinical depression can range from mild to severe depression and can result in significant impairment in functioning, for example, not being able to get out of bed to attend classes or go to work, lacking the energy or motivation to take care of basic needs for food, hygiene, and rest. Some people tend to become irritable, negative, and uncommunicative, which can cause greater stress and conflict in their relationships. Depression has been described as constantly having a black cloud over your head, not being able to get out from underneath it no matter what you do.

There are several causes or triggers for depression. Research suggests that if you have a family history of depression or any type of mood disorder, you are more prone to developing a depressive disorder. In fact, rates of depression for a child with a depressed parent are two to four times greater than for children without depressed parents.[39] While there is no single gene that causes depression, your genetic makeup can make you more vulnerable to depression. **Neurotransmitters** and hormone levels play a major role in the way your brain regulates your mood and emotions. Two neurotransmitters, serotonin and norepinephrine, are often found to be deficient in people with depression. (Chapter 7 includes a detailed discussion of neurotransmitters.)

However, biological processes are not the only explanation for depression. You may have a family history of depression and never develop depressive symptoms.

Key Terms

clinical depression a psychological disorder in which individuals experience a lack of motivation, decreased energy level, fatigue, social withdrawal, sleep disturbance, disturbance in appetite, diminished sex drive, feelings of worthlessness, and despair

neurotransmitters substances that transmit nerve signals; the chemical signals to activate or inhibit cell activity

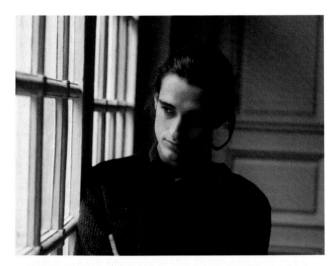

People who suffer from depression tend to feel hopeless and unmotivated and withdraw from others, which then increases their feelings of being trapped and stuck.

Conversely, you may have no genetic predisposition and still become clinically depressed. Depression can be caused by many psychological factors, such as:

- Loss of a significant relationship
- Death of a family member or friend
- Physical or sexual abuse or assault
- The response to a serious illness or health problems
- Experiencing numerous setbacks and problems simultaneously

Having a support system, effective coping strategies, and a positive attributional style can make the difference between succumbing to depression or being protected during stressful and adverse times in our lives.

There are many ways to treat depression, but the most effective treatment approach is a combination of counseling and medication. Counseling can help people develop healthy coping skills, learn stress management strategies, focus on developing an optimistic explanatory style, and improve relationships and social skills. Medication, such as antidepressants, can be helpful in the treatment of depression because they act to increase the serotonin or norepinephrine levels to a normal and functional range. Antidepressants include Prozac, Paxil, Zoloft, Celexa, Cymbalta, Remeron, Effexor, and Lexapro. It takes 4 to 6 weeks for an antidepressant to be fully effective, and there may be side effects such as dry mouth, decreased sexual drive, drowsiness, constipation, or diarrhea. Most of these side effects will disappear after 2 weeks of taking the medication. Interestingly, while the percentage of people with depression taking antidepressants has increased from 37 percent to 75 percent, those receiving psychotherapy has declined from 71 percent to 60 percent.[40] The use of antidepressants for youths 2 to 19 years of age has increased three to fivefold over recent years.[41] Most people take an antidepressant for 6 months to a year and then are able to taper off the medication without a reoccurrence of symptoms. If you have had three separate episodes of depression, recovering from each episode and then relapsing, this can be a sign that your depression has a biological basis and an indication that you may need to continue taking an antidepressant medication long term.

Herbal supplements, such as St. John's Wort, have also been touted as a treatment for depression, although there is some debate as to how effective they truly are. Most clinicians agree that St. John's Wort can be somewhat effective in alleviating mild depression but not moderate or severe types of depression. As is the case with all herbal supplements, St. John's Wort is not subject to FDA approval, and it has not been put through the clinical trials that prescription medications have undergone to establish therapeutic dose and efficacy. However, the National Institute of Mental Health, the National Center for Complementary and Alternative Medicine, and the Office of Dietary Supplements are currently conducting a $4 million collaborative four-year study to investigate the safety and the effectiveness of St. John's Wort, and so more definitive information will be available in the near future.

Exercise and activity level also play a significant role in alleviating and insulating people from depression. Again it seems that the endorphin levels and effects on brain chemistry and hormonal levels are part of the explanation for why this is a powerful antidote for depression.[42]

Electroconvulsive therapy (ECT) is another form of treatment for depression, with 100,000 Americans receiving this treatment each year. While ECT has fallen out of favor in recent years (owing in part to depictions of it in films such as *One Flew over the Cuckoo's Nest*), it has recently enjoyed a resurgence in popularity. This is due to improved technology. The procedure involves delivering a 90-volt burst of electricity, equal to the electricity in a 40-watt light bulb, for about a minute to the brain causing a grand mal seizure. The patient is under anesthesia and receives muscle relaxants before receiving the shock, and heart rate and oxygen level are constantly monitored during the treatment. Most patients receive three ECT treatments each week, for a total of six to twelve sessions. Proponents of ECT claim that it is an effective treatment for depression when no other antidepressant or treatment regime has worked. Critics of ECT say that it causes brain damage and memory loss and that the decrease in depressive symptoms are only temporary.[43] Although ECT has been used for more than 60 years, no one knows exactly how it works or why it alleviates depression.

TALKING POINTS Have you ever felt depressed? If so, what did you do to cope with these feelings? What did you do that worked and/or didn't help you to feel better?

Seasonal Affective Disorder

In addition to the types of depression just described, some people may be especially vulnerable to depression on a seasonal basis. **Seasonal affective disorder (SAD)** is a form of depression that develops in relation to the changes in the seasons. While most people with SAD begin to feel increasingly depressed in October and report their depression lifts in March or April, about one in six SAD sufferers experience Summer SAD, beginning in May or June and ending in the fall months. Twice as many women as men are affected with SAD.[47]

SAD seems to be related to environmental factors such as amount of light, temperature, and situational stressors. Weight gain, fatigue, increased sleep, diminished sex drive, and mood swings are some of the symptoms of Winter SAD; agitation, loss of appetite, insomnia, and increased suicidal thoughts are characteristic of Summer SAD. Seasonal depression in the winter seems linked to increases in the production of melatonin, a chemical that helps set the brain's daily rhythm, set off by the decrease in light. Antidepressants, counseling, and light therapy have been used to treat SAD. Light therapy for Winter SAD involves sitting in front of a white fluorescent bulb, housed in a plastic diffusing screen, for 20 to 90 minutes each day so that the light is falling on the eyes.[44] For Summer SAD, which tends to occur in hotter locales, individuals are instructed to travel to cooler climates, to swim in cool water, and to stay in darkened, air-conditioned rooms.

Postpartum Depression

Another unique form of depression is **postpartum depression,** a more severe kind of depression than is the commonly experienced "baby blues" that many women feel following childbirth. Postpartum depression occurs in one out of eight mothers who give birth and can last from a few days to over a year, but most commonly lasts for 2 weeks. Postpartum depression is characterized by fatigue, frequent crying, emotional withdrawal, anxiety, and other symptoms associated with depression. This should be differentiated from postpartum psychosis, which is marked by hallucinations and delusions. Sometimes people with postpartum depression have been associated with psychotic behavior, as was the situation with the much publicized case of Andrea Yates who in 2002 drowned her five children, ages 6 months to 7 years. Reportedly, Yates suffered from postpartum depression after the birth of her fourth child, and with the birth of her fifth child along with the death of her own father, became increasingly depressed and psychotic.

Suicide

Suicide is the third leading cause of death for young adults 15 to 24 years old and the 11th leading cause of all deaths in the United States. Men commit suicide four times more often than women do, and 72 percent of all suicides are committed by white men. Suicide occurs most often among Americans age 65 and older.[48] However, women are three times more likely than men to attempt suicide. Men tend to

Key Terms

seasonal affective disorder (SAD) a form of depression that develops in relation to the changes in the seasons

postpartum depression a form of depression that affects women in the weeks and months following childbirth employ more violent methods such as firearms, hanging, or jumping from high places, whereas women tend to use methods of suicide such as overdosing with pills or cutting their wrists, which are slower methods and allow more time for medical attention. Twice as many Caucasians complete suicide as African Americans, with Asian Americans being one of the lowest risk groups in terms of ethnicity. The suicide rate for the Hispanic population is lower than for Caucasians but higher than for African Americans.

Why do people attempt or commit suicide? The majority of suicidal people have depressive disorders and feel helpless and powerless over their lives. They say things like "I just want the pain to stop" and don't see any other options available to them. There are some risk factors associated with suicidal behavior such as:

- Little to no support system
- Previous suicide attempts
- Family history of mental illness, including substance abuse
- Family history of suicide
- Problems with drugs or alcohol
- Possession of a firearm
- Exposure to the suicidal behavior of others, including through the media

It is estimated that 300,000 suicide attempts occur each year in the United States, or one every 2 minutes.

Women tend to overdose on pills as a method of suicide, whereas men tend to use more lethal means, such as firearms, hanging, or jumping from high places.

Some people say that suicidal gestures or threats are a "cry for attention" or a "cry for help" and think it is better to ignore the person. But left ignored, the person may go ahead and take the next step to attempt suicide because no one seems to care. It is always best to take any threats or talk about suicide seriously and act accordingly. What should you do if a friend or family member talks to you about thoughts of suicide? See the Star Box on page 54 for the Dos and Don'ts of Suicide Intervention.

Bipolar Disorder

Another important mood disorder is **bipolar disorder,** a condition that was previously known as manic depression. The term *bipolar* refers to the extreme mood swings individuals with this disorder experience, from feeling euphoric, energetic, and reckless to feeling depressed, powerless, and listless. An estimated 2.3 million Americans suffer from bipolar disorder, with men and women equally likely to develop this condition. It is the least common of the mood disorders. The average age of onset for the first manic episode typically occurs in the early 20s. This change in mood or "mood swing" can last for hours, days, weeks, or months. Bipolar disorder is found across all ages, races, ethnic groups, and social classes. When one parent has bipolar disorder, the risk to each child is estimated to be 15 to 30 percent, when both parents have bipolar disorder, the risk increases to 50 to 75 percent.[35] A recent study contended that a flawed gene appears to promote bipolar disorder. Further research is needed to examine this particular variant of the gene to better identify people at risk and develop more effective medications to treat this disorder.

We have already described depression in the previous section. Bipolar disorder involves having both depressive periods and manic episodes. **Mania** is characterized by the following:

- Excessive energy, needing little sleep, being highly excitable
- Racing thoughts, feeling as though your mind is going 50 mph
- Rapid speech, changing from topic to topic quickly in conversation

> **Key Terms**
>
> **bipolar disorder** a mood disorder characterized by alternating episodes of depression and mania
>
> **mania** an extremely excitable state characterized by excessive energy, racing thoughts, impulsive and/or reckless behavior, irritability, and being prone to distraction

The Dos and Don'ts of Suicide Intervention

Do . . .

1. If possible, stay with the person until you can get further assistance.
2. Offer support and assistance. Tell them they are not alone.
3. Remain calm and talk about the person's feelings of sadness and helplessness.
4. Encourage problem solving and taking positive steps.
5. Emphasize the temporary nature of the problem. Suicide is a permanent solution to a temporary problem.
6. Seek help and don't try to handle this problem on your own. This might involve the person's family, religious advisor, friends, and teachers, or calling a mental health agency for consultation.

7. Ask the person to promise not to hurt or kill him/herself.

Don't . . .

1. Avoid talking about suicide or dancing around the topic. Talking about suicide doesn't upset people more. In fact, often people who are thinking about killing themselves say it is a relief to talk about it and it helps them to let go of this idea, not pursue it further.
2. Be judgmental or argumentative. Now is not the time to debate the morality of suicide—you will lose the debate and possibly the person.
3. Assume that the person is not serious. Saying "You're not serious" or "You don't

mean that" may inadvertently encourage the person to show you how serious she or he truly is.
4. Argue that things aren't that bad or that other people have it worse and the person should be happy about his or her life. This approach can make people feel worse about themselves and guilty about their feelings of unhappiness.
5. Don't promise not to tell anyone. If you keep this promise and something happens to this person, how will you feel?

- Easily irritated and distracted
- Impulsive and reckless in behavior: for example, spending sprees, increased involvement in sexual activity, and drug and alcohol use
- Trying to do too much, feeling as though you can accomplish a great deal

Many people with bipolar disorder will tell you that they enjoy the "highs" but dread the lows. However, manic behavior can become very destructive because when people are in a manic phase, they can create enormous credit card debt, abuse drugs and alcohol, drive recklessly, and often feel invincible. They stay up all night and feel very little need for rest or food, and eventually their bodies can't function and they collapse. Mood stabilizers such as Lithium, Lithobid, and anticonvulsant medications, such as Depakote, Neurontin, Topomax, and Lamictal, along with psychotherapy, have been used to treat bipolar disorder.

Anxiety Disorders

Bill, a very talented and bright 26-year-old, has a promising career as an executive in a large accounting firm. However, he is in jeopardy of losing his job because of his absenteeism and tardiness. It can take him hours to get to work even though he lives 15 minutes away, and sometimes he doesn't go to work even though he is in the car and ready to go. Bill has a routine in the morning that involves checking the windows, doors, iron, stove, and garage door five times to ensure that things are secure and safe. Sometimes he drives away and then returns to the house to check again. He feels a need to turn the handles on doors five times, and if he loses track, he starts all over again.

Susan has been having such severe panic attacks in the car while driving to work that she has needed to pull over. Her heart races, her breathing is labored, and she sometimes feels as though she is having a heart attack and might die. She is frightened of being in the car alone and having an attack and not being able to get help or having a car accident. She is beginning to be afraid to leave her house and feels safer at home. She has declined invitations to go out with her friends and on vacations and goes out only when absolutely necessary. She feels as though she is losing control of her life.

John worries constantly about what other people think of him. When he passes a group of people who are laughing, he assumes that they are laughing at him. He has trouble having conversations with people because he believes whatever he says will sound "stupid" and people will not like him. He also plays conversations over and over in his head when he is trying to go to sleep, thinking about what he should have said and worrying about how people are judging him.

Bill, Susan, and John are all suffering from *anxiety disorders*. While everyone tends to feel nervous or worry about something at some point in their lives, people with anxiety disorders feel anxious most, if not all, of the time. They also feel powerless to alleviate their anxiety, and tend to worry about becoming anxious, so their anxiety causes them even greater anxiety. Anxiety is related to fear and is part of daily life. Some anxiety can even be helpful and motivating at times. Anxiety is a physiological, adaptive response to danger or potential threat and can enhance performance and keep us out of harm's way. In Chapter 3, Managing Stress, we discuss the fight or flight response and how the stress response is related to anxiety. Anxiety disorders are differentiated from daily stress as being:

1. Intense, often debilitating, experiences during which people sometimes think they are going to die
2. Long lasting, persisting after the danger or stressful event has passed

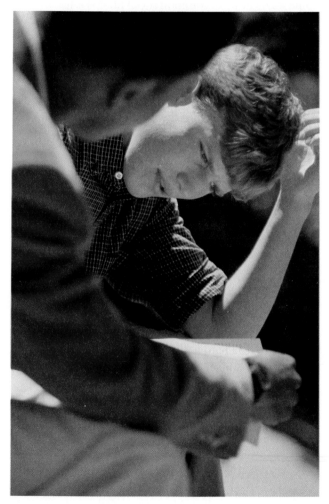

Anxiety is one of the three most frequent problems students report experiencing during college.

3. Dysfunctional, causing significant interference in daily functioning

Anxiety disorders include generalized anxiety disorder, obsessive-compulsive disorder (such as Bill's problem), posttraumatic stress disorder, panic disorder (which describes Susan's symptoms), and phobias such as the social phobia John suffered from in the example on page 54.[46] Approximately 19 million Americans have an anxiety disorder, and women are twice as likely as men to suffer from panic disorder, posttraumatic stress disorder, generalized anxiety disorder, agoraphobia, and specific phobias. There are no gender differences with obsessive-compulsive disorder or social phobia.[47]

Generalized Anxiety Disorder (GAD)

Generalized anxiety disorder (GAD) involves experiencing anxiety for at least 6 months in which the intensity and frequency of the worry is excessive and out of proportion to the situation. GAD can be distinguished from specific phobias in which people feel worried about a particular situation or stimulus. An individual with GAD appears to worry all the time about everything, thinks the worst, and overreacts to situations. Restlessness, fatigue, irritability, difficulty concentrating, muscle tension, and trouble sleeping are some of the symptoms associated with GAD. Physical symptoms include excessive sweating, nausea, diarrhea, being easily startled, shortness of breath, racing heart, and feeling shaky.[35] Because people with GAD are tense and anxious much of the time, they experience impairment in their relationships, work performance, and general functioning. Most people with GAD say that they are afraid of losing control, of failing, of rejection or abandonment, and death or disease. In addition, they feel unable to cope with their fears and thus out of control in managing their anxiety.

Panic Disorder

Shortness of breath, pounding heart, dizziness, trembling, sweating, nausea, tingling in hands and feet, hot and cold flashes, chest pain, and a feeling of choking are the

---

Key Terms

generalized anxiety disorder (GAD) an anxiety disorder that involves experiencing intense and nonspecific anxiety for at least 6 months, in which the intensity and frequency of worry is excessive and out of proportion to the situation symptoms of **panic disorder,** exemplified by Susan's situation. Many panic disorder sufferers feel as though they are going to die, are losing control or going crazy which of course makes them feel more anxious and panicked. Frequently, these individuals go to the emergency room thinking they are having a heart attack. This can seemingly occur out of the blue or because of some trigger, and can last for a few minutes or for hours. Because people become fearful of having a panic attack and don't know when the next attack might occur, they may develop **agoraphobia.** Agoraphobia is a fear of being in situations or places in which you can't escape or get help if you need it.[46]

Panic disorder can be treated with antidepressant medications such as imipramine and tranquilizers such as Xanax. Counseling can help individuals learn to recognize when a panic attack may be starting and to minimize and ward if off before it becomes a full blown attack, using relaxation and stress-management exercises, as well as positive self statements such as "I'm not going to die. I can get through this."

Obsessive-Compulsive Disorder (OCD)

Obsessive-compulsive disorder, or OCD, affects 3 million Americans and symptoms often begin during childhood or adolescence.[48] OCD involves more than just being neat and orderly: symptoms include having recurring thoughts and behaviors that seem irrational and out of control, and which can be extremely time consuming. Obsessions are intrusive thoughts, images, or impulses causing a great deal of distress. Most people recognize that their obsessions are ungrounded and senseless but can't seem to push them out of their minds. Obsessions may occur by themselves without being attached to compulsive behavior, but compulsions are associated with 25 percent of those with obsessive thoughts.[46] Compulsions refer to repetitive behaviors aimed at reducing anxiety and stress that are associated with the obsessive thoughts, such as checking that the iron is off, praying for your parent's good health, or washing your hands. Some compulsions seem relevant to a particular fear (such as handwashing out of a fear of germs), but others might seem unrelated—for example, having to do something an odd number of times so that your parents will not come to any harm. The most common compulsions are washing, checking, and counting.[35]

Even though the goal of compulsive behavior is to alleviate distress brought about by obsessions, it is in itself a source of shame and anxiety. Individuals with OCD, like Bill in the earlier example, realize that their behavior is excessive and unreasonable but are unable to resist engaging in this behavior. This can cause great distress in their relationships, problems completing their work, and getting to places on time. In addition, once they have performed the compulsive behavior, their anxiety is only temporarily alleviated; the obsessive thoughts return and the cycle continues.

Treatment for OCD can include antidepressant medication such as Prozac and also counseling. Counseling might involve response prevention strategies such as exposing the individual to the situations that trigger the obsessive thoughts and then preventing the person from engaging in the compulsive behaviors to break this vicious cycle. For example, the individual might be exposed to a dirty environment and then allowed to wash his or her hands only once.

Phobias

John is suffering from one of the most common anxiety disorders, **social phobia** previously called social anxiety disorder.[46] Social phobia refers to feelings of extreme dread and embarrassment in situations in which public speaking or social interaction is involved because the person worries she/he will be seen as stupid, clumsy, or lacking in some way. The most common social phobia is fear of public speaking. Commonly called stage fright, it is the most common of all phobias; many successful actors and performers suffer from this disorder, including actor Donny Osmond, gold medalist swimmer Susie O'Neill, and actresses Kim Basinger and Barbara Streisand.

Social phobia differs from another disorder called **specific phobia** in which the person has a strong fear and

---

Key Terms

panic disorder an anxiety disorder characterized by panic attacks, in which individuals experience severe physical symptoms; these episodes can seemingly occur "out of the blue" or because of some trigger and can last for a few minutes or for hours

agoraphobia a fear of being in situations from which there is no escape or in which help would be unavailable should an emergency arise; often associated with panic disorder

obsessive-compulsive disorder an anxiety disorder characterized by obsessions—intrusive thoughts, images, or impulses causing a great deal of distress—and compulsions—repetitive behaviors aimed at reducing anxiety or stress that is associated with the obsessive thoughts

social phobia a phobia characterized by feelings of extreme dread and embarrassment in situations in which public speaking or social interaction is involved

specific phobia an excessive and unreasonable fear about a particular situation or object that causes anxiety and distress and interferes with a person's functioning avoids one particular situation or object such as snakes, high places, or airplanes. Specific phobias affect 10 percent of the population and often begin as childhood fears that were never outgrown.[46] Sometimes a phobic reaction develops as a result of a traumatic event such as an accident, a particularly difficult visit to the doctor or dentist, or from an illness. Specific phobias tend to be easily treated with counseling in which the individual learns relaxation techniques and then is gradually exposed, first in imagery, then in real life situations, to the feared situation.

Posttraumatic Stress Disorder (PTSD)

The essential feature of **posttraumatic stress disorder** is the development of symptoms following exposure to an extreme stressor involving threat of death or serious injury. This threat may be directly experienced or be the result of witnessing an event that is life threatening and dangerous.[35] This disorder was first identified during World War I when soldiers were observed to be suffering from anxiety, flashbacks, and nightmares. Posttraumatic stress can be the result of not only combat but any trauma that produces intense fear, horror, and feelings of helplessness, such as sexual assault; natural disasters such as an earthquake or tornado; a car accident; life-threatening illness; or a mugging. The symptoms associated with PTSD are as follows:

- Recurrent and distressing thoughts about the event
- Nightmares about the event
- Flashbacks—feeling as though one is reliving the event
- Emotional numbness, feeling detached from oneself and one's feelings
- Avoidance of anything that reminds one of the event
- Detachment from others
- Difficulty expressing one's feelings
- Sleep disturbance
- Irritability, angry outbursts
- Being easily startled
- Difficulty concentrating
- Hypervigilence—extreme awareness of one's environment

People with PTSD tend to be highly anxious and depressed, to have problems with their relationships, and to have difficulty trusting people, and they may restrict their activities because of their fearfulness. It is also not uncommon to experience panic attacks when exposed to something that triggers a memory of the trauma. Again, counseling to express and resolve the feelings, losses, and negative thoughts associated with the trauma as well as antidepressant medications or tranquilizers may be beneficial in treating PTSD.

Attention Deficit Disorder (ADD)

Once thought to be only a childhood disorder, ADD is now being diagnosed in record numbers in adults. This increase might be the result of overlooking or misdiagnosing problems in childhood that later are accurately diagnosed in adults. With symptoms that include being fidgety, disorganized, overactive, and easily distracted, a child may be seen as simply misbehaving rather than having a diagnosable disorder. It is often the child with ADD who is seen as "disruptive" in the classroom and "lazy, stupid, a daydreamer" by friends and family. Actually the truth about these individuals is often the opposite: they tend to be highly intelligent, motivated, creative, and energetic individuals.

It is currently estimated that over 15 million Americans suffer from this disorder, affecting males more than females, 3:1. There is strong evidence to support a genetic cause for ADD, although environmental factors can certainly help or hinder the problem. One of the landmark studies in ADD was conducted on adults and showed that there is a difference at the cellular level in energy consumption, between the parts of the brain that regulate attention, emotion, and impulse control in people with ADD as compared to those without.[49]

Following are the symptoms often seen in adult ADD:

- A sense of underachievement, not meeting one's goals
- Difficulty getting organized
- Chronic procrastination or trouble getting started
- Trouble with follow-through and completing tasks
- Having many tasks going on simultaneously, switching from one to another
- Easily bored and a frequent search for high stimulation
- Easily distracted, trouble focusing and sustaining attention
- Creative, intuitive, highly intelligent
- Impulsive, doesn't stop to think things through
- Impatient, low frustration tolerance
- Tendency to worry needlessly and endlessly

> **Key Terms**
>
> **posttraumatic stress disorder** an anxiety disorder that sometimes develops following exposure to an extreme stressor involving threat of death or serious injury; symptoms include recurrent and distressing thoughts or nightmares about the event, emotional numbness, feelings of detachment, sleep disturbance, hypervigilance and irritability

- Insecure
- Moody
- Restless
- Tendency toward addictive behavior
- Low self-esteem
- Inaccurate self-concept, unaware of effect on others
- Childhood history of ADD or presence of symptoms since childhood

Psychological tests such as the Test of Variability of Attention (TOVA) and an IQ test can help substantiate a diagnosis of ADD. The TOVA tests the subject by flashing different shapes on a screen quantifying attention, distractibility, and impulsivity based on the subject's responses. The most effective treatment for ADD involves a multimodal approach: counseling and coaching the individual to provide strategies, techniques, and structure for daily life; education; tools such as daily planners and organizers; goal setting and time management; and medication such as Concerta, Strattera, Ritalin, and Adderall. (These medications are discussed in more detail in Chapter 7.)

Schizophrenia

Schizophrenia is one of the most severe mental disorders; it is characterized by profound distortions in one's thought processes, emotions, perceptions, and behavior. People with schizophrenia experience hallucinations (seeing things that are not there, hearing voices), delusions (believing that they are Jesus, the CIA is after them, or that radio waves are controlling their mind), and disorganized thinking (wearing multiple coats, scarves, and gloves on a warm day, shouting and swearing at passersby, maintaining a rigid posture and not moving for hours). The movie *A Beautiful Mind* gives a glimpse into the life of one schizophrenic, John Nash, and how he managed his symptoms.

There are several types of schizophrenia: paranoid, disorganized, catatonic, and undifferentiated. This disabling illness affects 1 percent of the U.S. population, and symptoms typically surface in people in their late teens and early 20s. Men and women are equally likely to develop schizophrenia, and it seems to run in families. Schizophrenia is often confused with multiple personality disorder, which is an entirely separate and distinct mental illness. While people with multiple personality disorder display two or more distinct identities or personalities that take control of the person's life, people with schizophrenia do not have multiple, separate, enduring personalities.

There are many theories to explain what causes schizophrenia. Some research suggests that heredity accounts for about 80 percent of the cause of schizophrenia and the other 20 percent is due to environmental stressors or situations. Researchers have also identified a number of abnormalities in the brains of diagnosed schizophrenics, including smaller temporal lobes, enlargement of the ventricles, and cerebral atrophy in the frontal lobes. Research is also being done on how the variations in chromosome-22 genes may be linked to schizophrenia. Individuals with schizophrenia also seem to have nearly double the number of dopamine receptors in their brains, leading to the theory that too much dopamine is being released into the brain pathways and causing schizophrenia symptoms. The antipsychotic medications act to block the receptors and prevent the transmission of dopamine, reducing the amount of dopamine in the system that is creating this chemical imbalance.[1]

Although there is no cure for schizophrenia, certain antipsychotic medications, such as Seroquel, Risperidone, Zyprexa, Geodon, and Abilify, can effectively treat this illness and enable people to live functional, satisfying lives. Psychotherapy can be helpful in developing problem-solving approaches, in addition to identifying stressors and triggers, and early detection of a psychotic episode. Unfortunately some people with schizophrenia are unable to recognize that they are delusional or irrational, and so do not get treatment or take their medications on a regular basis.

Health Providers Involved in the Treatment of Psychological Disorders

As in other areas of health care, a variety of practitioners, each of whom has unique training and uses specific therapies, treat and manage the mental health conditions just described.

Psychiatrists

A psychiatrist is a health care provider with a medical degree and has specialized in the field of psychiatry. Since

---

Key Terms

schizophrenia one of the most severe mental disorders, characterized by profound distortions in one's thought processes, emotions, perceptions, and behavior; symptoms may include hallucinations, delusions, disorganized thinking, and/or maintaining a rigid posture and not moving for hours

psychiatrist a medical doctor with specialized training in the diagnosis and treatment of psychological disorders through the use of biological and medical interventions psychiatrists are medical doctors, they may prescribe drugs and perform medical procedures such as electroshock therapy. Psychiatrists tend to treat psychological disorders through medical management and take a biological approach to addressing psychological disorders. They tend to give less focus to talking about one's problems and treat more severely and chronically ill patients.

Psychologists

A **psychologist** is a mental health care provider whose educational background includes a doctoral-level degree in the field of counseling or clinical psychology. Psychologists practice general psychology, and their clients range from those with severe pathology to those with more temporary problems of living. There is a variety of subspecialties such as children and adolescents, neurological disorders and assessments, psychological evaluations and assessments, forensic psychology, industrial psychology, health psychology, career counseling, and marriage counseling. Until recently, one difference between psychiatrists and psychologists was that psychologists did not have prescription privileges and so couldn't use drug therapies in their treatment interventions. However, the lines are beginning to blur, as there has been a push in many states for legislation that would allow psychologists to prescribe psychiatric medicines; such legislation exists in New Mexico already. In general, psychologists treat psychological disorders using behavior therapy, problem-solving approaches and talk therapy that focuses on changing the client's attitudes, behavior, affect, and cognitions. A psychologist must be licensed in the state in which he or she practices, and this typically requires passing a national certification examination and having a specific number of hours practicing psychology under the supervision of a licensed psychologist.

Counselors

Counselors typically have a master's degree in counseling or clinical psychology. Individuals with master's degrees usually work in group counseling practices, clinics, and schools and may specialize in areas such as substance abuse, divorce recovery, vocational rehabilitation, school counseling, marriage and family therapy, sexual assault, domestic violence, and employee assistance programs. In some states people with master's degrees must be supervised by a licensed doctoral level psychologist. However, there is a relatively new trend in licensure laws allowing masters level counselors to become licensed as professional mental health counselors. This has been passed in forty states to date. These licensing laws establish a standard of care and regulate the practice of counseling so that master's counselors can practice without being supervised by a psychologist.

Social Workers

Social workers have a master's degree in social work, and must be licensed to use the title social worker. Whereas psychologists, mental health counselors, and psychiatrists

> **Key Terms**
>
> **psychologist** a doctoral-level practitioner with specialized training in the diagnosis and treatment of psychological disorders through the use of psychotherapy
>
> **social worker** a professional with a master's degree in social work; social workers provide both mental health and social services to the community and are the largest group of professional to provide psychological services

A New Problem . . . Internet Addiction

The Internet has changed the way we work, socialize, and educate ourselves. While the Internet has provided connections that otherwise could not be made very easily with people all around the world, it has also created unique psychological problems for some individuals. There is some question about the psychological implications the Internet may be having on our society as we are moving from a world in which we used to know our neighbors and interact with people face to face to developing serious and deep relationships with people from a distance. Marriages have broken up, affairs have taken place, and teenagers have been kidnapped by people they met over the Internet. In fact, one teenager was encouraged to overdose on drugs by his Internet friends and died while communicating over the net to this group.

There is a feeling of anonymity that is created by talking on the Web. You can be who you want to be, reveal as much or as little as you want, and not be judged by your appearance. Of course, this also means people can be deceitful and dishonest about who they are and what they want from you. In addition, there is a blending of home and work and increased solitude. Studies show that greater use of the Internet is associated with less communication among family members, decreased socializing with local friends, and increased depression and loneliness.[51] One study showed that using the Internet more than 5 hours a week resulted in less time with friends, family, and social activities.[52]

In fact, there is such concern about the potential adverse effects of spending too much time on the Internet that some mental health professionals propose adding "Internet addiction" as a diagnosable mental disorder. How can you tell if you are addicted? Here are some warning signs:

1. Preoccupation with the Internet—planning and thinking about the next time you can get online.
2. Increased use of the Internet over time.
3. Repeatedly making unsuccessful attempts to curtail your use of the Internet.
4. Feeling irritable, restless, and moody when you attempt to cut down your use of the Internet or are prevented from getting online when you would like.
5. Unaware of how much time you are spending on the Internet, staying online longer than you originally intended.
6. Lying to family members and friends about your use of the Internet.
7. Jeopardizing your job or risking losing a relationship because of the time you are spending on the Web.
8. Using the Internet as a way of escaping from problems and coping with depression.
9. Declining invitations to spend time with family and friends because you would rather be online.

Of course, answering "yes" to one of these statements does not indicate a concern. However, if you can answer "yes" to more than half of them, then you may want to examine your use of the Internet. Here are some ways you can avoid being an Internet addict:

- Decide how much time you want to spend on the Internet before you get online and set an alarm for that time. Stick to that time allotment.
- Take frequent breaks. Spend at least 5 minutes out of every hour or 15 to 20 minutes of every 3 hours on unwired activity. Take a walk, stretch your body, eat a snack, or listen to music.
- Visit the net with a purpose and a strategy. Surfing the Web aimlessly can lead to being online for longer than you anticipated.
- Interact with people in a nonwired world. Make a commitment to socially interact at least once a day with someone who is not online.
- Don't let the Internet be the center of your existence or the most important, enjoyable part of your day. Remind yourself of your life goals, values, and interests. What are other ways to achieve these goals besides via the Web?[53]

tend to focus on the individual's problems, social workers look at the bigger picture and take into consideration the environment, community, and system the individual is living in. Social workers provide both mental health and social services to the community and are the largest group of professionals to provide psychological services.

Social workers typically consult and counsel clients and arrange for services that can help them. Often, they refer clients to specialists in services such as debt counseling, childcare or eldercare, public assistance, or alcohol or drug rehabilitation. Social workers then follow through with the client to assure that services are helpful and that clients make proper use of the services offered.

Social workers may review eligibility requirements, visit clients on a regular basis, and provide support during crises.[50]

Approaches in Treating Psychological Disorders

There are over 200 approaches to treating psychological disorders and new variations and models are continuing to develop. Most approaches have their foundations based on a few basic therapeutic models, which we will look at in the section that follows. These therapies can be utilized with individuals, families, or couples.

Dynamic Therapy

Dynamic therapy is based on the belief that effective treatment must focus on the psychological forces underlying the individual's problems. These forces begin in early childhood and have great significance on later behavior and personality development. Because this type of therapy focuses on the person's childhood years to uncover the source of the current problem, it usually is a long-term, intensive, and expensive form of therapy that many insurance companies refuse to cover.

Humanistic Therapy

Humanistic treatment approaches are based on the belief that people, left to their own devices, will naturally grow in positive and constructive ways. The job of the therapist is to help clients unearth their natural potential and gain greater self-awareness and self-acceptance. **Humanistic therapy** has its roots in Carl Rogers's "client-centered therapy" and in Abraham Maslow's hierarchy of needs. In client-centered therapy, the client, not the therapist, is responsible for behavior change. The task of the therapist is to facilitate in a nondirective manner the process of helping individuals resolve their problems.[7] Rogers further believed that when people accept themselves, they will also accept other people.

Behavior Therapy

Behavior therapy focuses not on one's thoughts or feelings but on behavior modification. Thus the goal of treatment is not to uncover the reasons underlying the problems an individual is having but to eliminate the symptoms and change behavior. Insight, awareness, and past history are unimportant in behavior therapy. The idea is that behavior has been learned and so can be unlearned, and different, more adaptive behavior can be taught. This can be especially effective for the treatment of anxiety such as phobias, panic disorder, and anxiety.

Cognitive-Behavioral Therapy

Cognitive-behavioral therapy focuses on changing an individual's thoughts or cognitive patterns in order to change his or her behavior and emotional state. Pioneered by psychologists Aaron Beck and Albert Ellis in the 1960s, cognitive therapy assumes that maladaptive behaviors and disturbed mood or emotions are the result of inappropriate or irrational thinking patterns. As with behavior therapy, cognitive-behavioral therapy does not explore why someone is thinking or behaving in a particular way, nor does it look at the client's past history. Instead, cognitive therapists attempt to make the client aware of distorted thought patterns and change them through strategies such as cognitive restructuring, cognitive reframing, challenging irrational beliefs, and thought stopping. This type of treatment has been especially effective in treating obsessive-compulsive disorder, eating disorders, anxiety disorders, and mood disorders. The learned optimism paradigm discussed earlier in this chapter was also based on cognitive-behavioral concepts.

Solution-Focused Therapy

Solution-focused therapy is a goal-oriented therapeutic approach that helps clients change by looking for solutions rather than dwelling on problems. Similar to cognitive-behavioral therapy, attention is directed to the present and the future, rather than to the past. Solution-focused therapists have confidence in the client and focus on the strength and resources within the individual. Clients are encouraged to envision a future in which their problems are no longer a dominant force in their lives, and in partnership with the therapist, treatment interventions are formulated in an effort to reach that goal.

Couples and Family Therapy

Couples counseling and family therapy includes premarital counseling, marital therapy, conflict mediation, and

---

Key Terms

dynamic therapy an intensive therapy based on the belief that effective treatment must focus on the psychological forces underlying the individual's problems

humanistic therapy a treatment approach based on the belief that people, left to their own devices, will naturally grow in positive and constructive ways

behavior therapy a behavior modification therapy based on the learning principles of reinforcement therapy, stimulus-response, and conditioning responses to change behavior

cognitive-behavioral therapy an action-oriented form of therapy that assumes that maladaptive, or faulty, thinking patterns cause maladaptive behavior and negative emotions; treatment focuses on changing an individual's thoughts or cognitive patterns in order to change his or her behavior and emotional state

solution-focused therapy a goal-oriented approach that helps clients change by looking for solutions rather than dwelling on problems divorce counseling. Communication skills, assertiveness skills, sexual disorders, intimacy and commitment, anger management, step-parenting, and blended families are some of the psychological issues that are typically addressed by these therapies.

Group Therapy

Group therapy usually comprises five to eight people who meet regularly with a therapist to focus on the psychological problems with which they are struggling. Often the group members share common problems such as eating disorders, childhood sexual abuse, substance abuse, or divorce recovery, and so they can support one another and understand one another's experiences. The group members can help and learn from one another and don't feel so alone in their problems. Group therapy is very beneficial in breaking your sense of isolation and challenging the belief that you are the only one having this type of problem. The idea behind group therapy is that you can learn new ways of behaving and practice these skills and behaviors in a safe, supportive atmosphere. In fact, the research strongly suggests that group therapy can be superior to individual therapy or at least a necessary next step for particular psychological problems, such as sexual abuse, eating disorders, substance abuse, and interpersonal relationship problems.

TALKING POINTS How do you think change occurs in people or yourself? What form of treatment described fits best with your perceptions of problems and behavior change?

Psychological Health: A Final Thought

As you can see, psychological health involves how your emotions, thoughts, and behavior interplay with one another and with the world around you. There is an important mind–body connection in terms of your psychological health having a significant effect on your physical health and vice versa. Psychological health is not just the absence of mental illness, and there is a range or continuum of psychological health. Possessing a positive self-concept, developing high self-esteem, and cultivating an optimistic attitude toward life can promote psychological health and enhance relationships with others. While heredity plays a role in the development of personality and psychological health, environmental factors and stressors seem to have an equally important role. As people age and encounter developmental milestones, they also encounter new challenges, obstacles, and resources in continuing to maintain their psychological health.

Taking Charge of Your Health

Assess how effective and healthy your style of communication is by considering the following questions:

- Do you know the difference between passive, aggressive, and assertive behavior?

- Do you use assertive language such as "I" statements rather than "you" statements?

- Do you have assertive body language such as making eye contact and keeping an open body posture without crossing your arms in front of you?

- Are you aware of your nonverbal communication?

- Are you aware of the volume and tone of your voice and the message you might be conveying?

- Do you acknowledge the other person's feelings and point of view before stating your own?

- Do you feel comfortable saying "no" to requests?

- Do you feel comfortable asking for someone's help, disagreeing with someone, or giving your opinion about something?

Having a positive and effective communication style is an important aspect of psychological health and can have a significant impact on your relationships, success at work, and your self-worth. Learn to be more optimistic in your attitude and communication by considering the characteristics of an optimist on page 47.

SUMMARY

- There is a mind–body connection in which biological, psychological, and social factors interact to influence health or illness. This is referred to as the biopsychological model.
- Psychological health has also been associated with developing and maintaining a positive self-concept, positive self-esteem, and emotional intelligence.

- Psychologically healthy people display a wide range of emotions.
- Personality is generally defined as a specific set of consistent patterns of behavior and traits that helps to identify and characterize an individual. Personality comprises thoughts, feelings, behaviors, motivation, instincts, and temperament.

- People with overall high levels of emotional intelligence tend to take on leadership roles, are confident and assertive, express their feelings directly and appropriately, feel good about themselves, are outgoing, and adapt well to stress.
- Two factors, nature and nurture, influence the shaping of personality. Nature refers to the innate factors we are born with that genetically determine our personality traits. Nurture is the effect that the environment, people, and external factors have on our personality.
- Nonverbal communication is what is communicated by your facial expression, body posture, tone of voice, and movements.
- Maslow's theory is a positive, optimistic theory of human behavior. He believed that people are motivated to grow and fulfill their potential, referring to this phenomenon as self-actualization.
- People with spiritual health seek meaning and purpose in their lives and have a deep appreciation for a sense of unity and community.
- Having a positive interpretation of life's events, particularly how you cope with adversity, can make a significant

difference in terms of your health and academic and work performance, as well as how long you will live.
- Clinical depression can range from mild to severe and can result in significant impairment in functioning.
- The majority of suicidal people have depressive disorders and feel helpless and powerless over their lives. It is always best to take any threats or talk about suicide seriously and act accordingly.
- Anxiety disorders include generalized anxiety disorder, obsessive-compulsive disorder, posttraumatic stress disorder, panic disorder, and phobias.
- Schizophrenia is one of the most severe mental disorders, characterized by profound distortions in one's thought processes, emotions, perceptions, and behavior.
- A number of different health care professionals are trained to treat mental disorders, including psychiatrists, psychologists, social workers, and counselors.
- Treatments for psychological illnesses include dynamic, humanistic, behavioral, cognitive-behavioral, and solution-focused therapies, as well as drug therapies.

REVIEW QUESTIONS

1. What are three factors that have been associated with psychological health?
2. What are the characteristics commonly demonstrated by psychologically healthy people?
3. What is the definition of self-esteem, and how can self-esteem be enhanced?
4. What is the definition of personality and what is it composed of?
5. What characterizes people with overall high levels of emotional intelligence?
6. What relationship is there between humor and psychological health?
7. What is nonverbal communication?
8. Describe Maslow's theory of the hierarchy of needs.
9. What traits are associated with people with spiritual health?
10. How can having a positive interpretation of life's events make a significant difference in people's health?
11. How is clinical depression different from having the "blues"?
12. How should you respond to someone threatening or talking about committing suicide?
13. List five different types of anxiety disorders.
14. How does a psychiatrist differ from a psychologist?
15. What are five different types of therapy approaches to treat psychological disorders?

ENDNOTES

1. Papalia D, Olds S. *Psychology* (2nd ed.). New York: McGraw-Hill, 1988.
2. Seligman M. *Learned Optimism.* New York: Simon & Schuster Inc., 1990.
3. McKay M, Fanning P. *Self-Esteem* (3rd ed.). Oakland, CA: New Harbinger Publications, 1992.
4. Goleman D. *Emotional Intelligence.* New York: Bantam Books, 1997.
5. Wade C, Tavris C. *Psychology.* New York: Harper & Row Publishers, 1987.
6. Spear P, Penrod S, Baker T. *Psychology: Perspectives on Behavior.* New York: John Wiley & Sons, 1988.
7. Kagan J, Segal J. *Psychology: An Introduction* (6th ed.). Orlando, FL: Harcourt Brace Jovanovich Inc., 1988.
8. Thorson JA, et al. Psychological health and sense of humor. *Journal of Clinical Psychology* 53(6), 605–619, 1997.
9. Yoshino S, Fujimori J, Kohda M. Effects of mirthful laughter on neuroendocrine and immune systems in patients with rheumatoid arthritis. *Journal Rheumatol* 23(4), 793–794, 1996.
10. Castro B, Eshleman J, Shearer R. Using humor to reduce stress and improve relationships. *Seminar Nurse Management* 7(2), 90–92, 1999.
11. Berk LS, et al. Immune System Changes During Humor Associated Laughter. *Clinical Research* 39, 124a, 1991.
12. Cogan R, et al. Effects of Laughter and Relaxation on Discomfort Thresholds. *Journal of Behavioral Medicine,* 139–144, 1987.
13. Martin RA, Lefcourt HM. Sense of Humor as a Moderator Between Stressors and Moods. *Journal of Personality and Social Psychology* 45, 1313–1324, 1983.
14. Nezu A, Nezu C, and Blissett S. Sense of humor as a moderator of the relationship between stressful events and psychological distress. *Journal of Personality and Social Psychology* 54, 520–525, 1988.
15. Miller J. Jokes and joking: A serious laughing matter, in Durant J and Miller J (Eds.) *Laughing Matters: A Serious*

Look at Humor. Essex England: Longman Scientific and Technical, 1988.

16. Lefcourt HM, Martin RA. *Humor and Life Stress: Antidote to Adversity.* New York: Springer-Verlag, 1986.

17. Kuhn C. *Humor Techniques for Health Care Professionals,* Presentation at Ball Memorial Hospital, April 22, 1998.

18. Nair M. A Documentary, *The Laughing Clubs of India,* 2001.

19. Collier G. *Emotional Expression.* Hillsdale, NJ: Lawrence Erlbaum Associates, 1985.

20. Maslow AH. *The Farthest Reaches of Human Nature.* Peter Smith, 1983.

21. Maslow AH. *Motivation and Personality* (2nd ed.). New York: Van Nostrand, 1970.

22. Lindzey G, Thompson R, and Spring B. *Psychology* (3rd ed.). New York: Worth Publishers, Inc. 1988.

23. May R. Values, myths, and symbols. *American Journal of Psychiatry,* 132, 703–706, 1975.

24. Hemenway JE, et al. *Assessing Spiritual Needs: A Guide for Caregivers.* Minneapolis: Augsburg Press, 1993.

25. Ayele H, Mulligan T, Gheorghiu S, Reyes-Ortiz C. Religious activity improves life satisfaction for some physicians and older patients. *Journal of the American Geriatrics Society* 43, 453–455, 1999.

26. Levin JS. Religion and health: Is there an association, is it valid and is it causal? *Social Science Medicine* 38(11), 1475–1482, 1994.

27. Seligman M. *Learned Optimism.* New York: Pocket Books, 1990.

28. Pavlov IP. *Conditioned Reflexes.* New York: Oxford University Press, 1927.

29. Hiroto D. Locus of control and learned helplessness. *Journal of Experiential Psychology* 102, 187–193, 1974.

30. Ellis A. *Reason and Emotion in Psychotherapy.* New York: Lyle Stuart, 1962.

31. *MHIC: Mental Illness and the Family,* National Mental Health Association and the Surgeon General's Report on Mental Health, 1999.

32. Narrow WE. *One-year prevalence of mental disorders, excluding substance use disorders, in the U.S.: NIMH ECA prospective data.* Population estimates based on U.S. Census estimated residential population age 18 and over on July 1, 1998, unpublished.

33. Murray CJL, Lopez AD (Eds.) *Summary: The Global Burden of Disease: A Comprehensive Assessment of Mortality and Disability from Diseases, Injuries, and Risk Factors in 1990 and Projected to 2020.* Cambridge, MA: Published by the Harvard School of Public Health on behalf of the World Health Organization and the World Bank, Harvard University, 2003.

34. Lehrer J. Transcript from On Line News Hour. *Living with Mental Illness,* December 13, 1999.

35. American Psychiatric Association. *Diagnostic and Statistical Manual on Mental Disorders, fourth edition (DSM-IV-TR).* Washington, DC: American Psychiatric Press, 2000.

36. World Health Organization. *Mental Health,* 2003.

37. Dramatic increases seen in college students' mental health problems over last 13 years. *Journal of Professional Psychology: Research and Practice,* February 2003.

38. National Institute of Mental Health, 2003.

39. Peterson K. Resilience, talking can help kids beat depression, *USA Today,* June 4, 2002.

40. Tanner L. With less stigma, more drugs, treatment for depression soars, *USA Today,* January 9, 2002.

41. Presentation of the *American Psychological Association* in New Orleans, 2001.

42. Exercise better than drugs for depression. *British Journal of Sports Medicine* 35, 114–117, April 2001.

43. Study puts spotlight on electroshock therapy, *USA Today,* March 13, 2001.

44. Rosenthal NE. *Winter Blues.* New York: The Guilford Press, 1998.

45. Understanding depression: A special health report from *Harvard Medical School,* 2003.

46. Bourne E. *The Anxiety and Phobia Workbook.* Oakland CA: New Harbinger Publications Inc., 1995.

47. Robins L, Regier D (Eds.). *Psychiatric Disorders in America: The Epidemiologic Catchment Area Study.* New York: The Free Press, 1991.

48. Narrow W, Raie D, Regier D. NIMH epidemiology note: prevalence of anxiety disorder. *One Year Prevalence Best Estimates Calculated from ECA and NCS Data.* Population estimates based on U.S. Census estimated residential population age 18 to 54 on July 1, 1998.

49. Hallowell, E, Ratey, J. *Driven to Distraction.* New York: Simon and Schuster, 1995.

50. *Occupational Outlook Handout,* U.S. Department of Labor Bureau of Labor Statistics, 2002–2003.

51. Kraut R, Patterson M, Lundmark V, Kiesler S, Mukopadyay T, Scherlis W. Internet paradox: A social technology that reduces social involvement and psychological well-being? *American Psychologist* 53(9), 1998.

52. Streitfeld D. Study finds heavy Internet users are isolated. *Washington Post,* February 16, 2000.

53. Goldstein D, Flory J. Best of the net, *Online Guide Book Series.* New York: McGraw-Hill, Irwin Professional Publishing Inc., 1996.

With suicide being the third leading cause of death for 10- to 20-year olds, there is reason to be concerned about how to provide effective treatment for depression in children and teenagers. The use of antidepressants to treat depression has significantly increased over the past few years. In 2004, over 1 million children were reported to take antidepressants. Thomas Insel, director of the National Institute of Mental Health stated "pediatricians write prescriptions for Prozac like it's penicillin." However, there has been mounting concern that antidepressants are increasing rather than decreasing suicidal behavior in children and adolescents. The FDA reports that "about 2 in 100 children taking antidepressants are more likely to think about or try suicide because they're on the pills." Because of recent government warnings and media coverage, there has been a sharp decline in the number of children and teens taking antidepressants.

Only Prozac has been approved by the FDA to treat children and teens with depression; however, physicians routinely prescribe other antidepressants such as Paxil, Zoloft, Celexa, Effexor, and Remeron for this population. In October 2004, the Food and Drug Administration ordered "black box" labels, the most severe warning, on all antidepressants. Researchers suggest that antidepressants may be triggering "akathisia," a rapid increase in impulsivity and energy level that might contribute to already depressed kids taking the next step and attempting suicide. Often people with depression are so lethargic, unmotivated, and tired that they don't have the energy to act on suicidal thoughts. However, when the medication starts to work, the individual's energy level increases. If the level of hopelessness has not decreased or has stayed the same, the risk of suicidal behavior increases. Also, more is known about how these medications work for adults, and medications can work differently in children and teens. The medication can change teens from lovable, friendly, bright students to hateful, angry, unmotivated kids who seem like strangers to their friends and families.

GlaxoSmithKline, maker of Paxil, has been accused of withholding information and misleading doctors about the safety of treating kids with Paxil. The company has been accused of reporting only positive results from their clinical trials and not releasing information about any negative results.

It is no wonder that physicians are becoming more reluctant to prescribe these medications for children and teens. However, this reluctance may be putting our youth at risk because they may not be receiving appropriate treatment and medication that could alleviate their depression. While some physicians perhaps were writing these prescriptions too freely, we may now have a situation that has gone to the opposite extreme in which children and adolescents are suffering needlessly, not having the quality of life they could have, which may result in losing them to depression and suicide. Work is currently underway to create national guidelines for physicians treating depression in 10- to 18-year-old patients to close the gap between over- and underprescribing antidepressants.

Sources: "Spitzer Says Glaxo Withheld Paxil Info," *USA Today,* June 3, 2004.

"Antidepressant Debate Takes a Delicate Turn," *USA Today,* October 18, 2004.

"Questions, Answers on "Black Box" Labels," *USA Today,* October 18, 2004.

"Warnings Slow Antidepressant Use," *USA Today,* February 1, 2005.

"Suicide Alert Has Parents Rethinking Antidepressants," *USA Today,* February 1, 2005.

"FDA Weighs Antidepressant Risk to Kids," www.intelihealth.com, January 27, 2004.

personal assessment

How does my self-concept compare with my idealized self?

Below is a list of fifteen personal attributes, each portrayed on a 9-point continuum. Mark with an X where you think you rank on each attribute. Try to be candid and accurate; these marks will collectively describe a portion of your sense of self-concept. When you are finished with the task, go back and circle where you wish you could be on each dimension. These marks describe your idealized self. Finally, in the spaces on the right, indicate the difference between your self-concept and your idealized self for each attribute.

Decisive				Indecisive				
9	8	7	6	5	4	3	2	1

Anxious				Relaxed				
9	8	7	6	5	4	3	2	1

Easily influenced				Independent thinker				
9	8	7	6	5	4	3	2	1

Very intelligent				Less intelligent				
9	8	7	6	5	4	3	2	1

In good physical shape				In poor physical shape				
9	8	7	6	5	4	3	2	1

Undependable				Dependable				
9	8	7	6	5	4	3	2	1

Deceitful				Honest				
9	8	7	6	5	4	3	2	1

A leader				A follower				
9	8	7	6	5	4	3	2	1

Unambitious				Ambitious				
9	8	7	6	5	4	3	2	1

Self-confident				Insecure				
9	8	7	6	5	4	3	2	1

Conservative				Adventurous				
9	8	7	6	5	4	3	2	1

Extroverted				Introverted				
9	8	7	6	5	4	3	2	1

Physically attractive				Physically unattractive				
9	8	7	6	5	4	3	2	1

Lazy				Hardworking				
9	8	7	6	5	4	3	2	1

Funny				Little sense of humor				
9	8	7	6	5	4	3	2	1

To Carry This Further . . .

1. Overall, how would you describe the difference between your self-concept and your self-ideal (large, moderate, small, large on a few dimensions)?

2. How do these differences for any of your attributes affect your sense of self-esteem?

3. How do you think someone who knows you well would rate you? Would they rate you in a similar way to how you see yourself? If not, why not?

4. Identify several attributes that you realistically believe can be changed to narrow the gap between your self-concept and your self-ideal and, thus, foster a well-developed sense of self-esteem.

chapter three

Managing Stress

Chapter Objectives

On completing this chapter, you will be able to:

▌ define stress, the stress response, and chronic stress.

▌ describe the fight or flight response.

▌ list at least ten physical responses to stress.

▌ discuss the general adaptation syndrome including three stages of stress: the alarm, resistance, and exhaustion stages.

▌ discuss at least five different types of student stress explored in this chapter.

▌ describe the differences between Type A and Type B personalities.

▌ describe the physical aspects of stress management.

▌ describe the social aspects of stress management.

▌ describe the environmental aspects of stress management.

▌ describe the psychological aspects of stress management.

▌ describe relaxation and deep breathing, progressive muscle relaxation, guided imagery and visualization, meditation and hypnosis, biofeedback, stress inoculation, and cognitive self-talk as tools for stress management.

Eye on the Media

Spit, Spam, Spim, and Phish—The Technological Stressors

We are learning to deal with a whole new type of stress—technological stress. Destructive computer viruses; hundreds of junk mail ads sent through e-mail, instant messages, cell phones, and voicemail; and increasing worry about identity theft have brought new meaning to stress management. With over 450 new viruses discovered each month and 82,000 hacking attacks made each year, it is no wonder that 500 or more professional hacking courses now instruct people how to think like and defend against computer intruders. Hacking costs companies over $17 billion dollars a year and creates paranoia, extreme stress, and frustration in victims of these attacks. Computer attacks have become increasingly wider in scope, automated, and harder to trace.

We are often overwhelmed by the amount of information we receive on a daily basis. If you are swamped by the catalogs, junk mail, and credit card applications you receive through the U.S. mail, your stress level will probably only intensify with the deluge of junk mail received via e-mail, voicemail, and instant messaging. And Internet telephony spam, called "spit," is predicted to become a bigger problem in the future as more people make phone calls over the Internet rather than use the regular phone lines. Marketers can program their computers to send 1,000 voice messages a minute over Internet telephony. "Spim" is spam sent out as an instant message, and it has increased to 2 billion messages in 2004, four times more than were sent in 2003.

Twenty percent of Americans reported receiving commercial messages and ads on their cell phones in 2004, an increase of 13 percent from the previous year. There were 75 million spam text messages received on cell phones in 2003, 150 million in 2004, and an estimated 450 million in 2005.

Even personal Web logs, or blogs, are not immune from these invasive advertisements. Spam messages masquerade as comments from readers, with some bloggers receiving 20 spam messages on their Web journals each day.

Phishing is the practice of sending e-mails and using fake Web sites to lure unsuspecting customers into sharing personal and financial data such as credit card account numbers, checking account numbers, and Paypal account numbers. Phishers create Web sites that look almost identical to the real ones, such as those of financial institutions like Citibank, and then ask their customers to verify their account information, which allows phishers easy access to people's financial data. An estimated 57 million people have received phish e-mails in 2004 alone. E-mails received from phishers are convincing because phishers copy the "from" line from the real company to make them look authentic. The incidence of phishing is growing at an alarming rate. In June 2004, the Anti-Phishing Working Group (APWG), an industry group, counted 1,422 phishing attacks—more than 12 times the number of attacks reported in December. Banks, eBay, and even some government agencies, including the IRS and the FBI, have been spoofed by phishers.

What Is Stress?

How do you know when you are stressed? You might experience headaches, stomachaches, or back and neck aches, or you might feel irritable, tired, anxious, and depressed. Some people eat more, while others find eating difficult when they are stressed. **Stress** refers to physiological and psychological responses to a significant or unexpected change or disruption in one's life. It can be brought on by real or imagined factors or events.

Stress was first described in the 1930s by Hans Selye. During his second year of medical school, Selye observed that, although his patients suffered from a variety of illnesses, they all showed common symptoms, such as fatigue, appetite disturbance, sleep problems, mood swings, gastrointestinal problems, and diminished concentration and recall. He began developing his now-famous theory of the influence of stress on people's ability to cope with and adapt to the pressures of injury and disease. He discovered that patients with a variety of ailments manifested many similar symptoms, which he ultimately attributed to their bodies' efforts to respond to the stresses of being ill. He called this collection of symptoms—this stress disease—stress syndrome, or the **general adaptation syndrome (GAS).** He also described this as "the syndrome of being ill."[1] We will discuss Selye's discovery further later in the chapter.

Selye defines stress as "the nonspecific response of the body to any demand whether it is caused by or results in pleasant or unpleasant conditions." Stress can be both positive or negative: again, it is our response to stress—how we manage stress—that makes a difference in terms of how it affects us. Stress resulting from unpleasant events or conditions is called **distress** (from the Greek *dys,* meaning bad, as in displeasure). Stress resulting from pleasant events or conditions is called **eustress** (from the Greek *eu,* meaning good, as in euphoria). Both eustress and distress elicit the same physiological responses in the body, as noted in Selye's general adaptation syndrome model.

While stress may not always be negative, our responses to it can be problematic or unhealthy. Both positive and negative stressful situations place extra demands on the body—your body reacts to an unexpected

Key Terms

stress the physiological and psychological state of disruption caused by the presence of an unanticipated, disruptive, or stimulating event

general adaptation syndrome (GAS) sequenced physiological responses to the presence of a stressor, involving the alarm, resistance, and exhaustion stages of the stress response

distress stress that diminishes the quality of life; commonly associated with disease, illness, and maladaptation

eustress stress that enhances the quality of life

Learning from Our Diversity

Different Stressors, Different Ways to Cope

While stressful situations can affect people differently, and we all have our unique ways of coping with stress, some important cultural differences exist in the types of stress and responses to stress that ethnic groups might experience. Clearly, being of minority status can cause a great deal of stress—for example, being the victim of hate crimes, having fewer opportunities for education and employment, earning less pay for the same work done by the majority population, experiencing higher mortality rates and illness and decreased access to health care, and suffering feelings of isolation and lack of support.

Latino/a Americans, for instance, are overrepresented among the poor, have a high unemployment rate, and often live in substandard housing. Many of those who do find employment hold semiskilled or unskilled jobs. Latino/a Americans also have disproportionately high rates of tuberculosis, AIDS, and obesity. Among Latino/a farm workers, infant mortality rates are reported to be as high as 25%, and infants are 50 times more likely than the general population to have parasitic infections. Nearly one-third of Latino/a students drop out of high school, which is more than double the rate for African Americans and three times higher than the rate for Caucasians.

The rate of alcoholism is higher among Native Americans, with deaths owing to alcoholism being more than four times higher than those reported for the general population. Fetal Alcohol Syndrome (FAS) is nearly 33 times higher in Native American infants than in Caucasians. The suicide rate among Native Americans is 77% higher than the national average. High school drop-out rates and unemployment rates are also higher for this group than for any other minority population.

Elderly Chinese immigrants report higher levels of stress and depression than do members of the majority population. Obesity, substance abuse, hypertension, and depression are significantly higher for African Americans than for others.

Because different ethnic groups experience different stressors, the ways that groups effectivley manage their stress are important to consider. For example, Native Americans incorporate story telling, spirituality, dreams, and visions into their stress-management strategies. A "talking circle" may be employed to help alleviate stress. This involves sitting in a circle, connecting with others by shaking hands around the circle, sharing one's innermost feelings without interruption or response from others, burning incense and passing it around the circle, and passing a sacred object such as an eagle feather to the person who is speaking. Asian Americans commonly use yoga, meditation, and acupuncture to manage stress. Transcendental meditation has been found to be twice as effective for African Americans than was progressive muscle relaxation.

Each of us needs to understand how we respond to stress and find strategies that work best to control stress levels. We should also consider issues of diversity in order to identify the unique stressors and stress-management techniques that might best fit us.

Sources:
Dolph L. Hatfield, "The Stereotyping of Native Americans," *Humanist,* September 2000.
"Native Americans of North America," *Microsoft® Encarta® Online Encyclopedia 2005,* http://encarta.msn.com © 1997–2005 Microsoft Corporation.
A. C. Mui, "Living Alone and Depression among Older Chinese Immigrants," *Journal of Gerontological Social Work,* 30, 147–166, 1998.
C. Alexander et al., "Trial of Stress Reduction for Hypertension in Older African Americans," *Hypertension,* 28, 228–237, 1996.

change or a highly emotional experience, regardless of whether this change is good or bad. If the duration of stress is relatively short, the overall effect is minimal and your body will rest, renew itself, and return to normal. But, as you will learn in this chapter, long-lasting stress, experiencing multiple stressors simultaneously, and not managing your stress effectively can take a toll on your body.

Stress is actually normal and healthy at a certain level. With functional, healthy levels of stress, overall physiological equilibrium is maintained at a balanced level. However, you really don't want to eliminate all stress because stress is adaptive, functional, and can be beneficial. You need to understand how you uniquely deal with stress and what works and doesn't work well for you in coping with day-to-day pressures and problems.

How We Respond to Stress

When we are stressed, we react in specific ways. The **stress response** is the result of learned and conditioned habits adopted early in life as a way of coping with problems, conflict, and disruptive events. But many of our responses to stress are innate, basic human survival

---

Key Terms

stress response the physiological and psychological responses to positive or negative events that are disruptive, unexpected, or stimulating mechanisms left over from our primordial roots. In pre-historic times, the best response to perceived danger, such as seeing a saber-toothed tiger about to attack, might be to either fight the animal or to run away. Stress in modern times remains the same except that we are responding to 21st-century threats and dangers rather than to saber-toothed tigers. Again, it is not the events that determine how stressed we feel but our response to these stressors. We next discuss the way that this innate stress response affects our modern lives.

Fight or Flight Response

Our response to stress involves many physiological changes that are collectively called the **fight or flight response.** In situations in which you must react immediately to danger, it is advisable to either fight off the danger or flee. For example, you are walking back from class at night, thinking about all the studying you need to do and you begin to cross the street. Suddenly, out of nowhere, a car's headlights are coming right at you. Since your best response is probably not to fight the car, you run as fast as you can to the other side of the road. In that split second when you see the car careening quickly toward you, your muscles tense, your heart beats faster, your adrenaline pumps faster and is released at increased levels into your bloodstream, your breathing becomes more shallow and rapid, and your pupils dilate to see the car better.

This is the fight or flight response. Receiving alert signals from the brain, the sympathetic nerves signal most of the organs of the body, and the adrenal glands are activated. Within the brain itself, neural pathways, involved in increased attention and focus, are activated. In this way, performance and learning can be heightened. Again, all these changes are adaptive and helpful to your survival in getting out of harm's way. In the preceding example, when you get to the other side of the road and realize that you are okay, your body begins to relax and return to its normal state. You take a large, deep breath, expressing a big sigh of relief. Your muscles may feel even weaker than usual, your breathing may become deeper and heavier than is typical, and you may feel shaky as your body goes from extreme arousal to relaxing very quickly. Figure 3-1a depicts the changes from the normal state to an arousal state to a very relaxed state then back to normal.

Accompanying this fight or flight reaction is a slower response. During stressful events, the pituitary gland secretes a peptide called adrenocorticotrophin, or ACTH, into the blood. ACTH travels through the blood to the adrenal gland, where it signals the production of a hormone called cortisol.[2] Cortisol aids the body in recovering from stressful experiences by freeing up energy stores. The logic behind the slower stress response is that the quick fight or flight response uses up a lot of the body's available energy.

The slower response helps to replenish that energy. The body usually has some small amount of cortisol circulating in the blood at all times. When the stress response lasts too long or is initiated too frequently, the cortisol level is increased. After enough of these small increases, the body soon resets its control mechanism to maintain a higher constant amount of cortisol in the body.

Chronic Stress

Now let's consider a different situation. You have a test in a week that you are very concerned about. It seems to be pre-occupying your every waking thought, and you have trouble sleeping as well. You are worried that you won't perform well on the test, and you really need to do better than you did on your last test. Your parents have been putting a great deal of pressure on you to do better in school in general. Because our bodies respond similarly to perceived or anticipated threat, you can have the same response to things that have and have not yet occurred. In other words, your heart races, breathing becomes labored, muscles are tense, the body sweats, and blood flow is constricted to the extremities and digestive organs and increases to the major muscles and brain. Your body is becoming ready to fight or flee the danger. However, you cannot take any action and make a fight or flight response, because nothing has happened yet. You haven't taken the test yet, and even once you have done so, you won't know your grade. So your body remains at this high level of arousal, as depicted in Figure 3-1b.

Remaining in a continued state of physiological arousal for an extended period of time is called **chronic stress.** This high level of arousal is similar to putting your foot on the accelerator of your car while it is in park and not letting up on the gas pedal. Since the fight or flight response is meant to be a very quick, short-acting response, your body begins to wear down if kept at this physiological state of arousal for too long; eventually, you will begin to feel exhausted. This is also the reason that people cope better with anxiety by taking some action, doing something about whatever they are worried about, rather than stewing about their problems. Thus the fight or flight response can be triggered inappropriately in

> ### Key Terms
>
> **fight or flight response** the physiological response to a stressor that prepares the body for confrontation or avoidance
>
> **chronic stress** refers to remaining at a high level of physiological arousal for an extended period of time; it can also occur when an individual is not able to immediately react to a real or a perceived threat

Adaptive Stress Response

3-1a

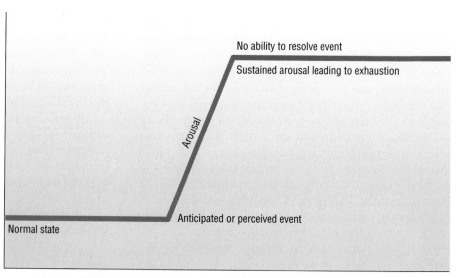

Chronic Stress Response

3-1b

Figure 3-1 Resolving Stress How quickly and effectively you act to resolve stress has a significant effect on how long your body remains at a high level of physiological arousal.
Source: H. Selye. "The Stress of Life," 1975.

response to phobias, irrational beliefs, an overactive imagination, or hallucinations or delusions.

The Three Stages of Stress

Once under the influence of a stressor, people's bodies respond in remarkably similar, predictable ways. For example, when asked to give a speech for a class, your heart rate may increase, your throat becomes dry, palms sweat, and you may feel lightheaded, dizzy, and nauseous. If an individual lost her or his job or discovered that her or his partner wanted to terminate their relationship, she or he might experience similar sensations. It is clear that different stressors are able to evoke common physical reactions.

Selye described the typical physical response to a stressor in his general adaptation syndrome model[3] discussed earlier in the chapter. Selye stated that the human body moves through three stages when confronted by stressors, as follows.

Stress and Psychoneuroimmunology

Can Stress Affect Our Immune System?
The newly emerging field of psychoneuroimmunology addresses the apparent interplay of the mind, the nervous system (the hypothalamus and the autonomic nervous system), and the immune system (see Chapter 13).

On the basis of clinical observation and laboratory studies, it is recognized that feelings associated with stress (depression and anxiety) and the disruption of social support systems relate to the weakening of the immune response and the development of some illnesses. For example, a study showed that happy, relaxed people are more resistant to illness than are those who tend to be unhappy and tense. In addition, work-related or personal stress experienced for at least one month increases a person's chances of catching a cold. In other words, the longer you live in a stressful state, the more likely you are to catch a cold. People in unhappy marriages, particularly wives, also have higher incidences

of colds. Extroverts are less likely to catch a cold, as are those with diverse social roles such as spouse, parent, worker, friend, community member, student. This situation makes sense, since we know that incorporating positive social interactions into our lives helps to alleviate stress, which in turn minimizes the risk of catching a cold. In another study, immunizations were less effective in producing an immune response in students stressed by upcoming examinations than in those not scheduled to take exams.

Stress triggers the release of inflammatory particles, cytokines and histamines, that fight off infection but can also cause cold symptoms. Researchers suspect that a sense of well-being decreases the release of cytokines and eases symptoms. This phenomenon may also explain why people can get through a state of acute stress and then become ill after the crisis is over, since stress produces adrenaline, which stimulates the immune system,

releasing cortisol. This is the hormone that battles inflammation but weakens immunity.

Our growing understanding of the relationship between our thoughts, the nervous system, and the functional status of the immune system enhances our insight into illnesses and their relationship to stress. As this understanding continues to mature, we will develop more effective coping strategies that enhance the connection between our feelings and their effect on nervous system and endocrine system function and the maintenance of immune system capabilities.

Sources:
Masek K et al. Past, present and future of psychoneuroimmunology. *Toxicology* 2000; 142(3): 179–188.
Marilyn Elias, "In the War on Colds Personality Counts," *USA Today*, December 1, 2003.
Cohen S et al. Types of stressors that increase susceptibility to the common cold in healthy adults. *Health Psychol* 1998; 17(3): 214–223.

Alarm Stage

Once exposed to any event that is perceived as threatening or dangerous, the body immediately prepares for difficulty, entering what Selye called the **alarm stage.** These involuntary changes, shown in Figure 3-2, are controlled by the hormonal and the nervous systems, and they trigger the fight or flight response. For example, you realize that the final exam you thought was today was actually scheduled for yesterday. You may begin to experience fear, panic, anxiety, anger, depression, and restlessness.[4]

Resistance Stage

The second stage of a response to a stressor is the **resistance stage,** during which the body attempts to reestablish its equilibrium or internal balance. The body is geared for survival, and because staying in the alarm stage for a prolonged amount of time is not conducive for the body's optimal functioning, it will resist the threat or attempt to resolve the problem and reduce the intensity of the response to a more manageable level. Specific organ systems, such as the cardiovascular and digestive systems, become the focus of the body's response.[5] During this phase, you might take steps to calm yourself down and relieve the stress on your body: You might deny the situation, withdraw and isolate yourself from others, and shut

down your emotions. Thus, in the example above, you may not tell anyone about missing the exam, may tell yourself that you don't care about that class anyway, and go back to bed.

Exhaustion Stage

Your ability to move from the alarm stage to a less damaging resistance stage determines the effect that the stressor has on your physical and psychological health. As you gain more control and balance is reestablished, you can begin to recover from the stress.

The length of time, the energy, and the effort required to accomplish recovery determines how exhausted your

Key Terms

alarm stage the first stage of the stress response involving physiological, involuntary changes that are controlled by the hormonal and the nervous systems; the fight or flight response is activated in this stage

resistance stage the second stage of a response to a stressor, during which the body attempts to reestablish its equilibrium or internal balance

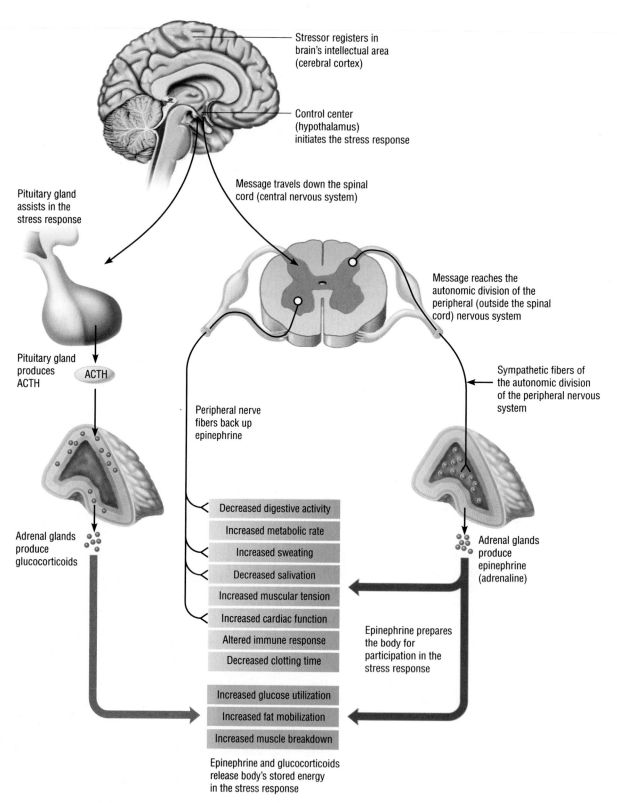

Stressor registers in brain's intellectual area (cerebral cortex)

Control center (hypothalamus) initiates the stress response

Message travels down the spinal cord (central nervous system)

Pituitary gland assists in the stress response

Message reaches the autonomic division of the peripheral (outside the spinal cord) nervous system

Pituitary gland produces ACTH

ACTH

Sympathetic fibers of the autonomic division of the peripheral nervous system

Peripheral nerve fibers back up epinephrine

Decreased digestive activity

Increased metabolic rate

Increased sweating

Decreased salivation

Increased muscular tension

Increased cardiac function

Altered immune response

Decreased clotting time

Adrenal glands produce epinephrine (adrenaline)

Epinephrine prepares the body for participation in the stress response

Adrenal glands produce glucocorticoids

Increased glucose utilization

Increased fat mobilization

Increased muscle breakdown

Epinephrine and glucocorticoids release body's stored energy in the stress response

Figure 3-2   The stress response: physiological reactions to a stressor.

body becomes as a result of the stressor. Of course, the longer the body is under stress and out of balance, the more negative the effect will be on your body. Long-term exposure to a stressor or coping with multiple stressors at the same time often results in overloading your system. Specific organs and body systems that were called on during the resistance stage may not be able to resist a stressor indefinitely. When all the psychological and physical resources we rely on to deal with stress are used up, an **exhaustion stage** results, and the stress-producing hormones such as adrenaline increase again. This is when chronic and serious illnesses can begin to develop, and the individual may even develop clinical depression.

The Sources of Stress

There are other causes of stress besides experiencing positive or negative events in life.[6] What events or situations trigger stress for you? For some it is financial worries, for others it might be relationship conflict, and for still others it is work-related stress. Even positive events, such as getting married, starting a new job, or moving to a new place, can be **stressors.** Going on vacation can be stressful as you get things done ahead of time to prepare for being away, pack your belongings, spend money on the trip, and completely change your routine. Any type of change in your life has the potential to trigger a stressful response.

Because stress involves a physiological response, it has a direct link to your physical and psychological health. The work of Thomas Holmes and Richard Rahe has found direct connections between changes in people's lives and physical illness. They developed a widely used inventory, called the Social Readjustment Rating Scale, to assess the degree of stress people experience in connection with particular life events. While one of these events alone might be tolerable, a combination of too many life changes within a short period of time may lead to illness.[7] To assess your level of stress and potential vulnerability to illness, complete the personal assessment inventory at the end of this chapter.

The Costs and Benefits of Stress

Stress can be costly, taking a toll on our physical and mental health as well as our finances.

Physical Toll of Stress

Constant arousal and increased levels of adrenaline in your system will eventually wear down your body's immunological system. As this occurs, you will be less able to cope with stress, and so it takes less and less to cause a stress reaction. When you are chronically stressed, it takes very little to frustrate you, and you can feel easily irritated and stressed at the littlest thing. Your body is both psychologically as well

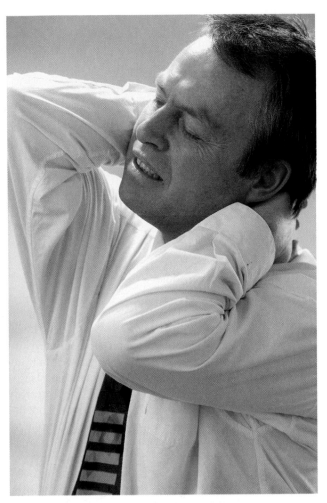

Tension and pain in the neck, shoulders, and back are common reactions to stress.

as physically less able to cope with stress. This can compromise your immune system, and you may become ill more easily. It may also take longer for you to recover from illness.

The following medical problems have been associated with stress[8] (to examine stress indicators for your personal stress, complete the rating scale at the end of this chapter):

- Cardiovascular problems (heart attacks, strokes, hypertension)
- Gastrointestinal problems (ulcers, irritable bowel syndrome, diarrhea, constipation, diverticulitis)

Key Terms

exhaustion stage the point at which the physical and the psychological resources used to deal with stress have been depleted

stressors factors or events, real or imagined, that elicit a state of stress

- Headaches and migraines
- Muscle spasms and cramps
- Sleep disorders
- Anxiety
- Jaw problems (temporomandibular joint [TMJ] syndrome)
- Allergies
- Cancer
- Back pain
- Asthma
- Kidney disease
- Sexual dysfunction
- Infertility
- Alcoholism and drug abuse

Other Costs of Stress

Stress can be very costly, not just in physical and psychological wellness but financially as well. While we can't put a price tag on quality of life, we do know that stress-related accidents, disease, early death, and absenteeism have been very costly. Stress-related symptoms and illnesses are costing industry a conservatively estimated $150 billion a year in absenteeism, company medical expenses, and lost productivity.[9] For example, researchers at the American Institute of Stress estimate that 75 to 90 percent of all visits to health-care providers result from stress-related disorders.[10] The American Heart Association says that more than 50 million workdays a year, totaling $8 billion, are lost annually to heart-related diseases.[11] The National Council on Compensation Insurance says that stress-related claims account for almost one-fifth of all occupational disease.[12] Researchers estimate that 60 to 80 percent of all industrial accidents are related to stress.[13]

Benefits of Stress

As we have said, while too much stress can have a negative effect and cause some serious health problems, a moderate level of stress is positive and beneficial. Stress can be motivating and energizing. Without some stress, many of us may not get much accomplished in our day or even get out of bed! Look at the diagram in Figure 3-3. What do you notice? Too little and too much stress are not helpful. When you are not stressed at all, you can be apathetic and lethargic. When you are too stressed, you are paralyzed with fear, like deer in the headlights. This is referred to as the **Yerkes-Dodson Law,** which uses a bell-shaped curve to demonstrate that there is an optimal level of stress for peak performance. This fact holds true for any type of performance, from academic or

Figure 3-3 The Yerkes-Dodson Law. Too little or too much stress is not helpful, but a moderate level of stress encourages peak performance.

Source: Hebb DO. Drive and the CNS (conceptual nervous system). *Psychological Review* 62(4), 243–254, 1955.

work activities to music or athletics.[14] Recognizing the appropriate level of stress for your ideal performance level is important in reaching your potential.

Student Stress

Going to college has been likened to "crossing into a new culture" where students face unique challenges and stressors.[6] Similar to going to live in another country, students must learn new customs and traditions, new ways of doing things, a new language, and must leave comfortable and familiar surroundings. This can cause a high level of stress for students, many of whom have left their support system behind to live in a place where they know few people. In the sections that follow, we cover some of the specific stressors college students face and offer ways to manage these situations.

> ### Key Terms
>
> **Yerkes-Dodson Law** a bell-shaped curve demonstrating that there is an optimal level of stress for peak performance; this law states that too little or too much stress is not helpful, whereas a moderate level of stress is positive and beneficial

Coping with Homesickness

Homesickness is one of the most common problems facing college students—which is understandable given that they are separated from friends and family and learning to live in an entirely new environment. When you are undergoing a great deal of change in your life, it is helpful to have the comfort and security of knowing that your home base remains stable and consistent. Moving from home to college can disrupt this sense of safety. While the college years can be an exciting and challenging time in your life, you may be missing your friends and family at home with whom you normally share these events. You may have also lost your sense of belonging while you struggle with finding a way to fit in with and navigate your new surroundings.

Often homesickness doesn't hit until a few weeks or maybe a month after you have moved, since the first few weeks are filled with meeting new people, social activities, and unpacking. After the dust settles, some people begin to feel lonely and alone. See Changing for the Better on page 80 for advice on how to deal with homesickness.

Relationship Problems

Along with homesickness, another very common stressor for students is relationship problems. Often students are separated by long distances from their best friends and romantic partners. While it can be difficult to maintain long-distance relationships, it is not impossible. Studies show that the key to effective long-distance relationships is communication. The quality of a long-distance relationship is improved if you both are committed to each other, you can talk openly about your concerns, feelings, and fears, and you can agree on the rules of the relationship, such as dating other people. In addition, there needs to be a strong level of trust between the partners, since trust is often tested in long-distance relationships. Both of you will change, and you must share these changes so that you can grow together, not apart. Agree on how often you will see each other, call or e-mail, and focus on spending high-quality time together.

It can be beneficial to have your friends visit you at college (rather than you going home) so that they can interact with you in your new environment and meet your new friends. Often students feel as though they live in two worlds, home and school, and it can be stressful to negotiate going from one to the other. The more you can connect these two worlds, the less stress you will experience. So it can be helpful to share what you are doing in your day— activities around campus, details of your classes, even who you ate lunch with—with your friends and family back home, and ask them what they have been doing.

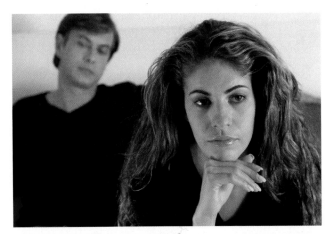

Stress caused by one aspect of your life can cause problems in other areas, such as your relationships.

Balancing Work, Home, and School

It is estimated that about three-quarters of students work while going to college, and more students are working full-time to pay for the costs of tuition (see Figure 3-4). In addition, it is estimated that between 5 and 10 percent of college students also have children. This, of course, adds stress to a student's life in balancing time for school, children, work, and household responsibilities. The increase in the number of students who have children is partly a result of a nationwide trend of more women in their mid-20s or older starting or returning to college. In fact, a national study by the University of Michigan showed that the number of full-time female students over 25 years old grew by 500 percent over recent years.[15]

While some campuses offer child care, many do not, which leaves students having to coordinate schedules and juggle responsibilities, causing even more stress. Also, the cost of child care can be exorbitant for some and can

Balancing Work and school
Almost two-thirds more then the nation's 1.8 million college students under age 25 worked at paying jobs in recent years.

4-year college	64%
2-year college	65.5%
All students	65%

Figure 3-4 Percentages of college students who also work at paying jobs
Source: Data from the U.S. Department of Labor, Bureau of Labor Statistics, March 25, 2005.

Yoga: The Union of Mind and Body

Yoga is often associated with Indian philosophy, such as Buddhism, but it has recently gained in popularity as a form of stress management. *Yoga* is a Sanskrit word meaning "union" of the individual soul with the universal soul. The practice of yoga directs and channels energy in a specific manner in the body. Individuals who practice yoga say they experience greater clarity in thinking and improved balance in their lives.

When individuals think of relaxation, they usually think of something that they like doing, that they find enjoyable or interesting. Such activities may include socializing, watching a movie or television, reading, going to a play or to a sporting event, or going to the beach or the mountains.

With yoga, relaxation involves slowing down the metabolism in order to let go of mental and physical tension. Many of the leisure activities mentioned above do not help us to slow down or to let go of mental and physical tension. It is purported that individuals who practice yoga experience better mental and physical health than those who do not, because of the conscious experience of slowing down the mind and the body. The idea behind yoga is that being consciously still each day for a set period of time is the best way to become more relaxed and develop and improve concentration and energy.

The reported benefits of regular yoga relaxation are numerous. They include:

- Better overall physical and mental health
- Less fatigue and a feeling of restfulness
- "Spiritual unfoldment," which refers to an improved mind-body integration and an increased sense of harmony and peacefulness
- Enhanced concentration and focus
- A greater ability to cope with anxiety and daily stressors

It is recommended to practice yoga relaxation techniques at least once a day. Suggested times are

- Before meals
- Before going to sleep at night
- After experiencing any stressful situation

Yoga has been shown to reduce heart rate and blood pressure, increase lung capacity, improve muscle relaxation, assist with weight management, and increase overall physical endurance. Yoga may affect levels of brain or blood chemicals, including monoamines, melatonin, dopamine, stress hormones (cortisol), and GABA (gamma-aminobutyric acid). Changes in mental functions, such as improved attention, cognition, processing of sensory information, and visual perception, have been described in some research studies in humans.

In yoga, poses are held for varying lengths of time using gravity, leverage, and tension. Breathing techniques are also used. Rapid breathing (*kapalabhati*) and slow breathing (*nadi suddhi*) may be practiced along with stretching exercises. The alignment of the head with the spine is important as is inhaling and exhaling through the nose only. Focus is on breathing and not allowing the mind to wander. One usually maintains a yoga position for 5 to 20 minutes.

To learn more about yoga, find a yoga class at your college or in the community.

Sources:
"Complementary & Alternative Medicine," *Alternative Modalities for Health and Well-Being,* www.inteliheath.com, July 8, 2005.
Kimbrough, J. *Yoga for Better Health and Living,* www.stress.about.com.

certainly add to financial worries. Managing time well and having a strong support system are essential for students with children, particularly single parents. Often there is little to no time available for relaxation, socializing, or exercising, and so employing stress relief strategies can be challenging.

Test Anxiety

You have studied for the test you are about to take and are well prepared. You look at the first test question and suddenly your mind goes blank. The harder you try to think, the more nervous and distressed you feel. You just can't think clearly and feel as though you have some type of mental block—what is happening? One-fifth of students experience these feelings, referred to as **test anxiety.** Exams are one of the greatest sources of stress for college students. The physical sensations associated with test anxiety are similar to those of general anxiety, such as fidgeting; having the feeling of butterflies in your stomach; rapid heart rate; difficulty breathing; nausea; tension in your neck, back, jaw, and shoulders; headaches; sweaty palms; and feeling shaky. People suffering from test anxiety make more mistakes on their tests, don't read the test accurately, and tend to make simple mistakes, such as spelling errors or adding something incorrectly. Many don't pace themselves well, and have a hard time finishing

Key Terms

test anxiety a form of performance anxiety that generates extreme feelings of distress in exam situations

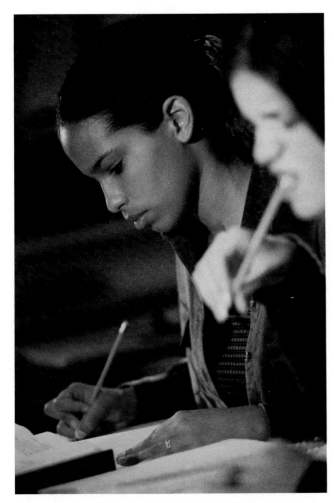

Test anxiety is related more to your confidence level than it is to how well you know the material.

exams. Test anxiety is a form of performance anxiety—people anticipate that they will perform poorly on the test.[16]

 TALKING POINTS What are some problems with stress described in this chapter that you have experienced?

Speech Anxiety

As we have mentioned, speech anxiety, or fear of public speaking, is one of the most common anxiety disorders. Since students are frequently required to give oral presentations, expected to engage in class discussion, and graded on class-participation points, this can present a problem for some.

In addition to the basic stress-management techniques outlined in this chapter, the following strategies can be used to cope with speech anxiety:

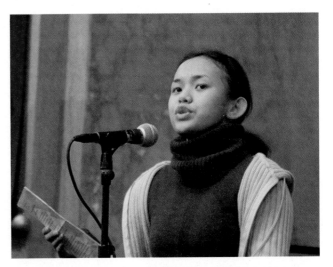

Effective behavioral and psychological interventions exist to treat speech anxiety.

- Volunteer to go first. Anxiety is dealt with best by taking action. Pressure and expectations tend to mount with each person who takes a turn so go first. Another advantage is that your performance is judged on its own merit without being compared to anyone else's.
- Practice in front of a mirror and for your friends. Solicit feedback: do you need to slow down or speak louder? Practice will also help you to remember your talk so that you don't read it word for word, which can seem less interesting to your audience.
- Engage in positive visualization. Take deep, comfortable breaths and imagine yourself giving your speech with confidence and receiving positive feedback and compliments about your performance.
- Vary your presentation style and format. Use visuals such as slides, and engage your audience in discussion so that they are an active not a passive part of your presentation. This takes some of the focus and pressure away from you.

Math Anxiety

Another common stressor for college students is math anxiety. Math anxiety is an intense emotional feeling of anxiety that some people have about their ability to understand mathematics. People who suffer from math anxiety feel that they are incapable of performing well in activities and classes that involve math. The incidence of math anxiety among college students has risen significantly over the last decade. Many students have even chosen their college major on the basis of how little math is required for the degree. Math anxiety has become so prevalent on college campuses

I just started college, and my family and friends are 5 hours away from me. I tend to be on the shy side and don't know anyone at my college. I miss my friends and family and don't feel like I belong here. I am thinking about withdrawing from school and going home. What should I do?

The following are some strategies to combat these feelings:

- Get involved! Become active in noncurricular, social activities such as special interest clubs, student government, religious clubs, fraternities, and sororities. Clubs associated with your major are a great way to meet people, further your academic and career interests, and keep you from feeling homesick.
- Call, e-mail, or write your family and friends regularly and let them know you would like to hear from them.
- Be open to meeting new people. Introduce yourself to people in your classes, and exchange e-mail addresses and phone numbers. This is also an excellent way to get a study partner or study group

together. Keep your door open when you are in your room, and spend time in public, common areas—not just hiding away in your room when you have spare time. Strike up a conversation while doing your laundry in the common laundry room area.

- Don't eat alone. Ask someone to join you to eat, or ask people at a table if you can eat with them.
- Don't go home on the weekends. Even though it may be tempting to visit your family and friends, the weekends are the best time to meet people and participate in the activities going on around campus.
- Be patient with yourself. Accept that loneliness and longing for home are normal, and it will take some time for you to adjust to all the changes you are experiencing. Don't decide to throw in the towel after the first few days! It may take a month or more before you begin to feel more comfortable in your new home. Give yourself some time to face this new challenge.

that many schools have designed classes and special counseling programs to help math-anxious students.

Typically, people with math anxiety have the potential to perform well in math; the anxiety is more of a psychological, rather than an intellectual, problem. However, since math anxiety interferes with a person's ability to learn math, it can create an intellectual problem. Often math anxiety is the result of a student's negative or embarrassing experience with math or a math teacher in previous years. Or perhaps the student was repeatedly told that he or she would not be able to perform well in math by a parent or a teacher. Such an experience can leave a student believing him- or herself deficient in math ability. This belief can actually result in poor performance, which serves as confirming evidence to the student. This phenomenon is known as *self-fulfilling prophecy*; it is described more fully later in this chapter.

Students who fear math often avoid asking questions to save embarrassment, sit in the back of the classroom, fail to seek help from the instructor, and usually put off studying math until the last moment. All these negative behaviors are intended to reduce the student's anxiety but actually result in more intense anxiety. However, there are a number of strategies to overcome math anxiety:

1. Be sure to have developed a solid arithmetic foundation. Since complex concepts build cumulatively on more simplistic ones, a remedial course or short course in arithmetic is often a significant first step in reducing the anxiety response to math.

2. Take an easier, slower math course as opposed to a faster-paced, more challenging one. It is better to

stack the odds in your favor than to risk reinforcing your negative experiences with math.

3. Be aware of thoughts, feelings, and actions as they are related to math. Develop a positive perspective toward math.

4. There is safety in numbers! Math anxiety is learned and reinforced over a long period of time and may take time to eliminate. You can reduce your anxiety with the help of a tutor, studying with a friend, and talking with your instructor.

5. Sit near the front of the class where you will experience fewer distractions and feel more a part of what is being discussed.

6. If you have questions or can't keep up with the instructor, ask for clarification and repetition of whatever you missed.[17]

7. Review the material. As with most things, skill in math comes from practice. Make sure you review the material covered in the class, and identify questions you need to ask the instructor as soon as possible after the class. Research shows that you will remember 50 percent of what you heard in class if you review it immediately after class, but only 20 percent is retained 24 hours later if you didn't review the material right away.[18]

Stress and Learning

How does stress affect learning? Research suggests that people who are highly anxious tend to perform better than others do at simple learning tasks but less well than others

Do You Suffer from Test Anxiety?

Test anxiety is a commonly experienced problem and can significantly impair your academic performance. Here are some questions you can ask yourself to help analyze if you might be suffering from test anxiety.

1. Are you aware of being really nervous on a test, maybe so nervous that you don't do your best and lose points, even though you know you've studied well and are prepared?
2. Does your stomach ever get tight or upset before or during a test? Hands cold and sweaty? Headaches? Do you have trouble sleeping the night before a test?
3. Do you ever find your mind racing or seeming dull or cloudy so that you can't think clearly while taking a test?
4. During a test, do you ever forget material you studied and learned, only to remember it again after the test is over?
5. Do you overanalyze questions, see too many possibilities, choose the complex answer, and overlook the simple, correct one?
6. Do you make many careless errors on a test?

7. Have you had some bad experiences with tests and made poor grades when you didn't expect them?
8. Do you spend a lot of time and energy studying and preparing for tests, yet fail to make grades that represent what you know?
9. Are tests and finals a particularly miserable time for you?

If you answered yes to more than half these questions, you might want to consider getting some help in managing the anxiety associated with test taking. College counseling centers frequently offer stress-management programs and can teach you techniques to manage your anxiety. Similar to managing other types of stress and anxiety, test anxiety can be coped with by using the following suggestions:

- Prepare well in advance. Don't cram at the last minute for the test. Rehearsal and repetition are the best ways of remembering information.
- Improve your odds by getting a good night's sleep before the test and eating a nutritious meal to give your brain needed energy.

- Have a positive attitude and watch your test talk. Don't talk about the test beforehand with friends, since this tends to increase anxiety. Go into the test with a confident attitude, reminding yourself that you are well prepared and have taken many tests and performed satisfactorily in the past.
- Activity reduces anxiety. If you stumble on a question, don't linger over it; go onto the next question and return to that one later.
- Ask for clarification if you don't understand a question or something on the test.
- Don't pay attention to the people around you. Focus on the test and don't allow yourself to get distracted.
- Take deep breaths, allow your breathing to help you to relax, and bring more oxygen to the brain so you can think more clearly.
- Look through the entire exam before starting to answer the questions. Pace yourself and be aware of your time. Know when you need to be halfway through the test according to the time allotted for the exam.

Source: Newman E. *No More Test Anxiety.* Los Angeles, CA: Learning Skills Publications, 1996.

---

do at difficult tasks, particularly those involving reasoning activities and time-limited tests. One interesting study showed that college students with average scholastic ability earned significantly better grades when they had low levels of anxiety as compared to highly anxious average students.[19] When you are more stressed or anxious, you have a diminished ability to concentrate, to recall information, and to master problem-solving activities. You may find yourself reading the same page in your textbook over and over again, not knowing what you read.[16]

Using Time Effectively

An overwhelming number of students identify time management as the reason for their academic success or failure. Setting priorities and goals, balancing academic life with your social life, and finding time for sleeping, eating, exercising, and working along with studying is an essential aspect of managing your stress effectively.

Time Management

Managing your time effectively can help you cope with your stress by feeling more in control, having a sense of accomplishment, and having a sense of purpose in your life. Establishing good time management habits can take two to three weeks. By using specific systems, even the most disorganized persons can make their lives less chaotic and stressful.

Assess Your Habits

The first step is to analyze how you are spending your time. What are your most productive and least productive times of day and night? Do you tend to underestimate how long something will take you to complete? Do you waste time or allow interruptions to take you off task? Carrying a notebook with you for a week and writing down how you spend your time might provide you with some insight into the answers to these questions and how you spend your time. You might find that you've been devoting most of your time to less important tasks. Perhaps it is tempting to do your laundry rather than to start writing that term paper, but this is probably not the best use of your time.

Use a Planner

Keeping a daily planner to schedule your time is the next step in managing your time more effectively. First block off all of the activities that are consistent, regular, weekly activities, such as attending classes, eating meals, sleeping, going to meetings, exercising, and working. Then look at the open, available time remaining. Schedule regular study time, relaxation time, and free time. Remember to schedule your study time during the more productive part of your waking hours. When you have a one-hour block of time, what can you realistically get done in that time? This could be a good time to review your notes from class, pay bills, or get some reading done.

Set Goals and Prioritize

Set goals for the week as well as for each day. If something unexpected interferes with your time schedule, modify your plans but don't throw out the entire schedule.

Managing your time well can greatly reduce your stress level.

Making a to-do list can be helpful, but it is only the first step. Breaking the large tasks into smaller, more manageable pieces and then prioritizing them is the key to effective time management. When you prioritize your tasks, try the ABC method of task management. The A tasks are those items that are most urgent and must be done today. Then the B tasks are those things that are important but, if need be, could wait 24 hours. The C tasks are activities that can easily wait a few days to a week. Don't fall into the C trap, which is when you do the less important tasks because they are quick and can be checked off your list with ease. This can lead to putting off the more important A activities, leaving them until you feel stressed and overwhelmed.[20] We discuss procrastination in the next section.

Procrastination

Procrastination means postponing something that is necessary to do to reach a goal.[21] Putting things off is a common problem that plagues students and can cause stress. A survey of college students found that approximately 23 percent of students said they procrastinated about half the time, and 27 percent of students said they procrastinated most of the time.[22] Procrastination has been viewed as a time-management problem, but it is really more than that, and so time-management strategies tend to be ineffective in resolving this problem. Procrastination is also different from indecision, because people can make a decision but still have trouble implementing it.

Typically there is a psychological aspect to procrastination because we tend to delay doing those things that we don't want to do. Emotions such as anxiety, guilt, and dread often accompany thinking about the task. By putting the dreaded activity off, you can temporarily alleviate your anxiety and discomfort, which is a reinforcing aspect of procrastination. In the short term, procrastination seems to be a good solution and helps you to feel better. However, in the long run, procrastination usually leads to bigger problems and more work. For example putting off paying your bills may feel good at the moment, but when your electricity is turned off and you have to pay late fees, and your roommates are upset with you because they thought you had paid the bill, your pleasurable feelings soon turn sour.

Men and women procrastinate equally often, but more people in the mid to late 20s and 60-year-olds procrastinate more than people in any other age group do.[23] Individuals who procrastinate are frequently referred to as

---

Key Terms

procrastination putting off completing tasks until some later time, sometimes resulting in increased stress "lazy" or "stupid," but actually there are no differences in levels of intelligence between procrastinators and non-procrastinators. However, students who procrastinate tend to perform less well and retain less than students who do not. You might want to take the survey at the end of this chapter to assess your risk for procrastination.

Many people who procrastinate report feeling overwhelmed and highly anxious. They have difficulty tuning out external stimulation and concentrating on the task at hand. They also worry about how their performance will be judged by others and have perfectionistic standards for themselves. We discuss perfectionism in the next section.

Some techniques for combating procrastination involve time management, stress management, assertiveness training, and increasing self-esteem and self-acceptance. Specifically with regard to time management, procrastinators tend to both over- and underestimate how much time a task will take. When they underestimate the time, they feel justified in procrastinating because they erroneously believe they have plenty of time to complete the task. When they overestimate the time needed, they feel intimidated by the magnitude of the job, feel anxious, and so have trouble getting started. Most students explain that their anxiety stems from a fear of failure or being evaluated. Sometimes their anxiety manifests itself because they don't understand the material or what the instructor is wanting but are afraid to ask for clarification.

People also report procrastinating when they feel forced or pressured to do something they don't want to do. Rather than communicating assertively, they rebel by agreeing to do something but constantly put it off, which can be a passive-aggressive way of behaving. They fear the consequences of saying no or not fulfilling their obligations but are also angry about what they perceive as unfair

expectations and demands on them. This is when some assertiveness training may be helpful. Finally, increasing self-esteem can solve problems with procrastination because feeling better about yourself relieves you of worrying about what others think of you and having constantly to prove yourself to them. Some people procrastinate because they think they need to do everything perfectly or not at all. With increased self-esteem, you are more accepting of mistakes and don't expect yourself to perform perfectly.

Perfectionism

Perfectionism leads to undue stress because perfection is an unattainable goal. By setting the standard at perfect, you will set yourself up to fail. Perfectionists tend to be their own worst critic; they are harder on themselves than anyone else is on them, and they are also critical of others. These individuals are described as neat and organized, seeming to "have it all together" and to be able to do more than most people and do it exceptionally well. Often people envy perfectionistic people because they seem very confident and competent; however, individuals who are perfectionistic never feel good enough and often feel out of control in their lives.[24] People who are perfectionists focus on what they

---

Key Terms

perfectionism a tendency to expect perfection in everything one does, with little tolerance for mistakes

---

My girlfriend is a perfectionist and she is driving me crazy. Nothing I do seems good enough for her as much as I try to please her. Her unrealistic expectations are causing a great deal of stress in our relationship and our friends are beginning to stay away from us because they don't like to hear us argue. What can I do?

Sometimes people who are perfectionist tend to blame others for their own sense of failure or rejection. Here are some ways to respond better to your girlfriend:

1. Communicate how you feel when she is critical of you or shows her disapproval. Suggest more positive ways that she can give you feedback or share her disappointments.
2. Give specific examples of how she may be expecting too much, and find a compromise between all or nothing.
3. Don't retaliate. It is tempting to point out her flaws when she is doing the same to you. Instead, reassure her that you think highly of her and point out her successes and accomplishments, since she is probably focusing on her failures.
4. Communicate your confidence in her abilities and ask her to have the same trust in you.
5. Model acceptance of imperfection in yourself and others. Show her that everybody is flawed, no one is perfect, and this makes us human.
6. Don't focus on her mistakes or tease her when she makes an error. Instead give positive reinforcement when she doesn't do something well.
7. Help her to relax and have fun even if all the work is not yet done.
8. Talk about how she is feeling rather than the content of her message, such as saying "You sound very stressed and overwhelmed."
9. Don't fall into the perfectionist trap yourself. It is easy to think, "If I just try harder, she will be happy with me." Perfectionism is an impossible goal to reach, and so you are setting yourself up for failure and rejection.
10. Help her to see the forest rather than the trees. It is easy for perfectionists to get lost in the details and lose sight of the overall goal. It may help to alleviate her stress if you can help her to refocus on what is really important and what the overall goal is such as having fun at the party you are throwing and not having the house perfectly clean.

---

haven't accomplished or haven't done right rather than on what they have completed or have done well. Making mistakes feels especially humiliating to persons who are perfectionistic, and they tend to feel a strong sense of shame and low self-esteem when someone catches them in error. They have difficulty with criticism or any negative feedback because much of their self-esteem is based on being accurate, competent, and being the best. While striving to do your best is an admirable quality, expecting to be perfect in everything you do and never making a mistake places a great deal of stress and pressure on yourself.

People with perfectionistic behavior tend to be rigid in their thinking, saying "I must be perfect or else I am a failure" and tend to put 100 percent of their effort into something or don't want to attempt it at all, which can lead to procrastination. In expecting perfection, there seems, to these individuals, to be a right and wrong way to do things. Thus, perfectionism can create a great deal of anxiety and distress.

Perfectionism is often associated with obsessive-compulsive disorder as well as with eating disorders. Having perfectionistic tendencies can also create stress and conflict in relationships because people who interact with perfectionists feel as though nothing they do is good enough or will please that person.

To help alleviate the stress of perfectionism, base your self-esteem on who you are rather than on what you do. This involves accepting yourself and others un-conditionally, including imperfections. Lowering your expectations of yourself and others and aiming for 80 percent rather than 100 percent is another strategy in battling perfectionism. Note what you are doing well and have accomplished rather than what is still left to do. Time-management strategies such as those outlined on pages 81–82 can be useful in managing your expectations of yourself. Push yourself to take risks and allow yourself to make mistakes. It can be useful to make mistakes on purpose in order to get accustomed to this experience and realize that people still like and accept you and nothing bad will happen. Relaxation and stress-management techniques such as the ones described at the end of this chapter can also help alleviate the stress that comes with perfectionism. You might want to take the survey at the end of this chapter to assess your level of perfectionism.

Type A and Type B Personalities

Cardiologists Meyer Friedman and Roy Rosenman identified two basic types of personalities when they interviewed individuals in order to identify people who may be susceptible to stress-related heart disease.[25] In the interview, they asked individuals the following questions:

1. Does your job carry heavy responsibility?
2. Is there any time when you feel particularly rushed or under pressure?

3. When you are under pressure, does it bother you?
4. Would you describe yourself as a hard-driving ambitious type of person in accomplishing the things you want, or would you describe yourself as a relatively relaxed and easy-going person?

From the responses to these questions, Friedman and Rosenman were able to distinguish two types of personalities with respect to stress: type A and type B personalities. **Type A** individuals often feel pressured, are ambitious, impatient, competitive, walk and talk rapidly, and can be easily annoyed by delays. **Type B** individuals tend to be calm, relaxed, easy-going, and patient. They also found that many cases of heart disease couldn't be attributed to other cardiac risk factors such as smoking or dietary habits but could be linked to stress. Type A personalities tend to share qualities of workaholism and perfectionism, such as having high expectations and feeling out of control, irritable and overwhelmed, stressed and pressured most of the time. There is a constant sense of needing to go faster and hurry through activities to get onto the next task. Thus type A people tend not to enjoy what they are doing because they are thinking about the next activity rather than enjoying the present.[26] This can of course cause tension in their relationships as well. Type A people tend to drive themselves to exhaustion and stop only when they collapse or become ill.

While Friedman and Rosenman didn't describe type A personalities as an illness but more as a personality type, they did find correlations with stress. As with perfectionism, type A people sometimes need to slow down, lower their expectations of themselves, delegate responsibilities to others, and prioritize their tasks. Type A individuals often complain that they have trouble relaxing and don't know how to relax. They also don't allow themselves to have fun until all of the work is done which rarely occurs. Scheduling social activities and time to relax is one important component in alleviating the stress that accompanies type A personalities. Exercising, meditation, massage, spiritual activities, and yoga are other ways to relax.

While some people are chronically stressed, which leads to exhaustion, other people seem to have a high stress tolerance. These "stress-hardy" individuals have a lower frequency of illness and absenteeism.[25] They view stressors as challenges and chances for new opportunities and seem to thrive with increased stress. They feel more in control of their lives and perceive themselves as having options and the power to make choices and influence situations. So it is not just the level of stress that an individual experiences that determines how he or she will respond but also the individual's ability to manage varying degrees of stress. Stress-hardy individuals who have a good social support system, exercise regularly, and maintain a healthy diet have fewer stress-related illnesses than do those who have less healthy lifestyles.

Managing Stress: Effective Coping Strategies

The research on how people cope with crisis and stress in their lives has shown that people tend to resolve problems within two weeks of experiencing a crisis. Because stress involves a disruption in equilibrium, and the body does not function well in a chronic state of unbalance, it is human nature to seek a way to alleviate the stress the body is experiencing and return to a steady state. As we discussed previously, our bodies cannot function for very long in a sustained fight or flight response without serious damage, and so a person will naturally strive to make changes to resolve the stress for survival. However, the way that people resolve their problems and alleviate stress may be positive or negative.

A number of negative ways of dealing with stress are quite common and often quite harmful. As indicated in Figure 3-5, some people turn to alcohol and drugs to avoid their problems and numb their feelings, and cigarettes are also cited as a way of relieving stress. Many people use food to comfort themselves. Putting off distasteful tasks and avoiding stressful situations is another negative way of coping with stress. Some people use sleep as a way of escaping their problems, and certainly depression has been associated with not having the ability to effectively manage stress. In the next section, we discuss ways of effectively managing stress.

What are some positive, effective methods to cope with stress? Different strategies and methods for stress management involve the physical, social, environmental, and psychological aspects of stress. We will review techniques and strategies within each of these dimensions, and you will need to practice and experiment to find the stress-management techniques that are right for you.

> ### Key Terms
>
> **type A personality** a personality type that tends to be competitive, ambitious, and impatient; often associated with heart attacks and other stress-related conditions
>
> **type B personality** a personality type that tends to be more relaxed and patient

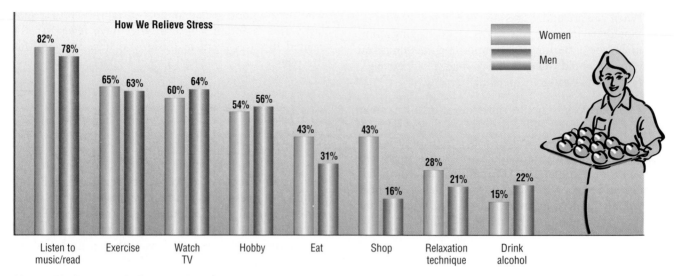

Figure 3-5 People have different ways of relaxing and relieving stress, such as cooking, reading a mystery novel, or swimming. How do you cope with stress?

The Physical Aspects of Stress Management

The physical aspects of stress management involve meeting your basic needs of nutrition, sleep, and exercise as was discussed in Chapter 2 under Maslow's Hierarchy of Needs.[27]

Nutrition

In Chapter 5 you will learn about the nutrients that provide the necessary fuel the body needs to function. When people are stressed, they often skip meals or eat on the run. Since the fight or flight response requires more energy during stressful times than is normally needed, you must eat a balanced, nutritious diet. Without proper nutrition, the body will begin to break down its own tissues in an effort to obtain the energy required to survive. The immune system can then become compromised, making the body more susceptible to disease. It is not a coincidence that many people who are under a great deal of stress for prolonged periods of time become ill and that regaining their health takes longer than it does for those who are managing their stress well.

As we previously mentioned, people often use food to cope with stress and can overeat, typically eating high-sugar and high-fat foods such as chips, candy, and cookies. One study showed that women who were exposed to a high level of noise, similar to that made by a jackhammer, ate 65 to 70 grams of fat when offered snacks as compared to women who were in a less stressful, quieter environment, who chose snacks with half as much fat. Eating too much or too little is not an effective way to manage stress and can eventually lead to serious health problems, such as obesity, eating disorders, diabetes, and hypertension.

Sleep

As with eating, too much sleep or too little is also an ineffective way of managing stress. Most adults require 7 to 8 hours of sleep a night.[28] Sometimes people get very little sleep during the week and try to "catch up" over the weekend, sleeping 14 hours at a time or taking naps during the day. Sleep is not like a bank account in which you can make deposits and withdrawals, and so getting an average of 7 to 8 hours a night over a week's time is not the same thing as sleeping this amount each night.

People also need uninterrupted sleep. Normal **circadian rhythms,** the biological processes related to the 24-hour light/dark cycle, are necessary for normal sleep and optimal daytime functioning. Our sleep patterns relate to these biological cycles, which also affect our patterns of hunger and eating, body temperature, and hormone release. These cycles must be in harmony for us to have a sense of well-being during our waking hours.[29] Sleep deprivation has been found to cause losses in higher cognitive processing tasks, decline in the performance of simple tasks, memory loss, and, with prolonged sleep deprivation, temporary psychosis, such as hallucinations and delirium.[25] Research also shows that sleeping too much

> **Key Terms**
>
> **circadian rhythms** the internal, biological processes that help coordinate physiological processes with the 24-hour light/dark cycle

Exercising is one of the best ways to manage your stress.

can result in increased depression and decreased energy levels. So getting the right amount of rest is an essential aspect of stress management.

Exercise

Exercise is another physical aspect of stress management. Exercising aerobically at least three times a week for 20 to 30 minutes has been found to manage stress effectively for several reasons. First, exercising requires you to focus on your breathing and to breath deeply, the key to stress management. By tensing and releasing the muscles through exercise, you are allowing your body to relax and unwind. Secondly, exercise can alleviate stress through the release of endorphins, naturally occurring chemicals in the brain. Endorphins help to counter stress, subdue pain, and increase pleasure, which is the reason people talk about the runner's high. Hitting a racquet ball against the wall or playing basketball can be a great way to release the frustrations of the day and let go of tension and stress. Aerobic exercise includes walking briskly, running, bicycling, skating, and dancing. The benefits of exercise are further discussed in Chapter 4.

The Social Aspects of Stress Management

To manage stress effectively, you must also make time for fun and play. Like exercise, laughter increases the release of endorphins and requires you to breath deeply,

and so having humor in your life is an essential part of stress management.[30] Research has shown that stress can be related to having inadequate social interactions.[31] Hugging and human contact have also been demonstrated as having a significant effect in reducing the harmful physical effects of stress.[32] Participating in social activities such as social organizations, sports, or just talking with friends can give you the break you need to rest your mind and focus on something other than work.

Actually you don't even have to have human contact to reduce stress—just owning a pet can make a difference. Studies have shown that just petting an animal produces calming effects such as lowered blood pressure and decreased heart rate. Cardiac patients who own pets tend to live much longer than those who have no pets.[33]

The Environmental Aspects of Stress Management

To effectively manage your stress, you need to take into consideration environmental stressors such as noise level, amount of light, and aesthetic quality of the space you inhabit. Stress has been linked to being exposed to prolonged, daily noise such as in a factory.[34] We know that depression can be related to the amount of light to which you are exposed, and this can also affect your circadian rhythms.[35] Natural light tends to elevate your mood, whereas prolonged exposure to artificial lighting can increase your stress level. Research also suggests that different colors can raise or lower your stress and energy level. Some people associate the color red with feelings of anger or hostility and blue with feeling depressed. Having plants or photos of friends and family around your living and workspace can also alleviate stress.

Smell can also play a significant role in managing stress. As the saying goes, "Stop and smell the roses." Studies have shown that aromatherapy, using different aromas or odors therapeutically, can lower stress levels. When you breathe in the oils, they send a direct message to your brain via your olfactory nerves, where they can then affect the endocrine and the hormonal systems via the hypothalamus. Odors have an amazing effect on our emotional states because they hook into the emotional or primitive parts of our brains. Aromatherapy has been used to relieve pain, enhance relaxation and stress relief, unknot tense muscles, soften dry skin, and enhance immunity. So it is wise to pay attention to your aromatic surroundings, because they may affect you much more than you may realize.

While social interaction has been shown to have positive results on lessening the effects of stress, this beneficial effect depends on the type of friends with whom you surround yourself. Spending time with negative, pessimistic people can increase your stress level rather than decrease it. It is obviously more advantageous to surround yourself with positive, optimistic friends.[36] Feeling crowded in a room and not having enough personal space can also lead to an increase in stress.[37] Interestingly, it is not being in crowds itself but how familiar you are with the people, the activity that is taking place, and how much control you feel over your personal space that makes the difference. In other words, being in a crowded room filled with your friends during a party feels subjectively different than feeling trapped in a crowded restaurant filled with strangers.

Other important aspects of managing stress in your environment include having meaningful work and challenging and interesting classes. Having work that is stimulating but not beyond your abilities helps to keep your stress response at a moderate, optimal level for performance.

The Psychological Aspects of Stress Management

Last, you can effectively cope with stress by using a variety of cognitive and psychological strategies. There are several different techniques, but as you will see, many are focused on deep breathing, which is the key to managing stress.

Relaxation and Deep Breathing

The relaxation response, developed by Herbert Benson, M.D., is an effective way to ensure that you do not remain in the stress response too long. It is effective because it entails the opposite of the stress response. Rather than taking shallow breaths, you are required to breathe deeply, inhaling to a count of four and exhaling to a count of four while sitting in a comfortable position. As you breathe deeply, your muscles unwind and relax, again the opposite of the stress response. It is generally advised not to cross your legs or arms so that your muscles can relax easily. Blood flows to the extremities, and your heart rate slows. In fact, experienced users of this technique can temporarily lower their breathing rate from a typical rate of 14 to 18 breaths per minute to as few as 4 breaths per minute. Body temperature decreases, and blood pressure is lowered as well. The entire nervous system is slowed, in direct opposition to its role in the stress response. You are instructed to focus on your breathing and inner experience and become less aware of your external environment. To help to tune out the outside world, you are instructed to close your eyes and let go of the worries and concerns of the day.[38]

To try this technique, take a moment to focus on your breathing and breathe in for a count of four and out for four. After doing so a few times, tighten your body, clench your hands, teeth, and jaw, close your eyes tightly, and pull your shoulders up while you are still breathing deeply. Are you able to do so? It is virtually impossible to tense your body and breathe deeply because they are mutually exclusive activities. Thus, the relaxation response is the foundation of most of the stress-management techniques described in this chapter. Deep breathing is the fundamental aspect of stress management.

Progressive Muscle Relaxation (PMR)

In 1929 Edmund Jacobson, M.D., published a book describing a simple procedure of deliberately tensing and releasing major muscle groups in sequence from head to toe to achieve total relaxation of the body. His technique, called Progressive Muscle Relaxation, still enjoys popularity.[39] By learning to recognize the difference between contracted and relaxed muscles, Jacobson believed that people would be able to have more of a sense of control over their bodies and the stress response. Progressive muscle relaxation enables you to intentionally put certain muscles into a controlled state of relaxation and reduce your overall stress level.

PMR is based on the use of positioning your body in a comfortable position, sitting or lying down, and concentrating on certain muscle groups. As you inhale, breathing in for a count of four, you contract your muscles starting with your forehead and count to four as you exhale and relax your muscles. Continue to clench and relax the muscles, using your breathing to help you to tighten and release, working your way down your body all the way to your feet and toes. Concentrate on the sensations of relaxation and how different they are from the feelings of tension and stress. Fifteen minutes, twice a day, is the recommended schedule. In one to two weeks, you will have mastered the basics and will be aware of which muscles need more attention in order to relax. You will also be more sensitive to the buildup of tension in your body so that you will be able to decrease your stress level before it becomes overwhelming.[40]

Guided Imagery and Visualization

In the early 1900s, Emil Coué, a French pharmacist, first suggested using human suggestibility to overcome the stress syndrome, to enhance recovery from illness, and to facilitate the accomplishment of positive goals.[41] By forming an image of a peaceful, serene place or seeing yourself being successful in accomplishing a task, you can use guided imagery or visualization to manage your stress. Guided imagery involves having someone describe a beautiful, relaxing scene while you focus on taking deep, comfortable breaths. While in a comfortable position, in an environment free from interruptions and distractions, you breathe deeply, relax your muscles, and imagine a pleasant scene. The imagery includes all the senses, not just what you see but pleasant smells, sounds, touch, and even taste. Guided imagery can be self-taught, or you can listen to recordings of narrated scripts.

Visualization is similar to guided imagery with the scene being more specifically focused on something you are about to do or want to accomplish, or on some performance or activity that may be causing you distress. Guided imagery and visualization techniques help you to consciously program change through positive mental images. For example, you might imagine yourself auditioning for a part in a play, seeing yourself go through your lines effortlessly and flawlessly, and feeling confident and proud of yourself. You are probably already skilled at visualization; unfortunately, we frequently engage in negative visualization and are unaware of doing so. For example, we imagine ourselves making fools of ourselves or making mistakes.

Athletes are trained in using positive visualization to improve their performance and visualize their goals.[40] Positive visualization has also been used in managing pain, especially in chronic pain management. This technique has also been effective in weight management, smoking cessation, insomnia, and for almost any type of behavior change. Some images commonly used to decrease stress are to visualize tightly twisted rope as uncoiling; hard, cold wax melting and softening; creaky hinges being oiled and becoming silent and gliding smoothly; or

the feeling of sandpaper turning into silk. Again, guided imagery and visualization exercises have optimal benefit when practiced at least once a day, every day for 15 to 20 minutes.

Meditation and Hypnosis

Meditation allows the mind to transcend thought effortlessly when the person concentrates on a focal point. In Transcendental Meditation, a widely recognized approach to meditation, people repeat a mantra, or a personal word, while using deep-breathing and relaxation techniques. In other meditation approaches, alternative focal points are used to establish the depth of concentration needed to free the mind from conscious thought. Physical objects, music, and relaxing environmental sounds or breathing can be used as focal points. Students who meditated twice a day for 15 minutes reported lowered blood pressure, better class attendance rates, and felt less stressed during their classes.

Hypnosis is an artificially induced state, resembling, but physiologically distinct from, sleep. It involves a heightened state of suggestibility that creates flexible and intensified attention and receptiveness, and an increased responsiveness to an idea or to a set of ideas. The focus is on the unconscious rather than on the conscious state of mind, using deep-breathing and relaxation techniques. Hypnosis is perhaps the oldest and most misunderstood type of relaxation technique. It has been given a bad reputation by stage entertainers who use hypnosis to have unsuspecting audience members engage in embarrassing behavior.

Hypnosis is a natural state of mind that occurs spontaneously in nearly every person. It is a trancelike state, similar to those that you experience upon awakening, before falling asleep, or when you are engrossed in thought while performing other tasks—such as driving down a highway—on autopilot. It is possible to learn self-hypnosis from a trained professional or participate in hypnosis sessions with a qualified hypnotherapist.

Similar to the other techniques described, meditation and hypnosis work best when you are in a comfortable, quiet environment and practice them at least once a day, every day, for 15 to 20 minutes.

Biofeedback

The word *biofeedback* was coined in 1969 to describe procedures to teach people to alter brain activity, blood pressure, muscle tension, heart rate, and other bodily functions that are not normally controlled voluntarily. Biofeedback is a training technique in which people are taught to improve their health and performance by using signals from their own bodies. It operates on the premise that individuals can alter their involuntary responses by being "fed back" information either visually or audibly about what was occurring

The Antidote for Anger . . . Relaxation

When we are angry, our muscles tense, we breathe shallowly, and our adrenaline level increases, similarly to how we feel when we are stressed. But expressing anger can reduce stress. As discussed earlier in the chapter, physiological arousal is associated with stress. Tension tends to build with the stress of increasing frustration, worry, discomfort, or unmet needs. The greater the stress, the more tension you feel. Expressing your anger can help to get rid of this tension, but only temporarily. You may have noticed that right after you get angry, maybe even blow up, you feel more relaxed and calm. Your muscles relax, the tension leaves your body, and you breathe more easily—but only briefly. Anger can create more anger because of the reinforcing effect that blowing up has in temporarily helping you feel better. Blowing up makes it easier to react the same way the next time, and the outbursts are usually stronger and harder to control each time.

As with the stress response, the key to managing anger is to change how we respond to events and express our anger. So, instead of blowing up, should you just keep your anger inside? No; this can eventually result in an explosion similar to that caused by pressure that builds in a pressure cooker or a shaken soda can. This is the "last straw" kind of anger response. To an observer, you may seem to be overreacting to a particular situation when you are really responding to a *multitude* of situations and frustrating events. You may take your anger out on an innocent bystander, or the dog.

Here are some tips on effective, respectful anger management:

1. Relax, take a deep breath, count to 10.
2. Take a time out if needed. Don't continue to engage in discussion if it is getting too heated.
3. Avoid name calling. Use "I" language, as was discussed in the previous chapter.
4. Stay connected to the individual with whom you are speaking. Don't withdraw physically or psychologically unless you need a time out, and then say this directly.
5. Ask yourself what underlies your anger. Hurt, guilt, feelings of rejection and shame, and fear of abandonment may be feelings that you need to express but that come out as anger. Especially for men, anger tends to be a more comfortable emotion to express.
6. Is there a hidden agenda to your anger? Are you using your anger to control, change, or punish someone? If so, use assertive language instead, and share your thoughts and feelings directly.
7. Speak in a quieter, calmer voice than you typically do. People tend to yell, speaking more loudly than normal in order to get the other person's attention. You may feel that you don't have power or people's attention unless you yell. While anger can be attention grabbing, this kind of attention is probably not what you want. People may tend to yell back, tune you out, or agree with you without meaning it, just to stop the yelling.
8. Choose your battles wisely. Don't argue every point. Ask yourself "Is this something that is really important to me and will be as meaningful tomorrow as it is right now?"
9. Express your anger in a timely fashion. Don't wait a week or a month to bring up issues when you have accumulated a bunch of things that have been bothering you over time. However, it may be more productive to wait until morning to express your anger if you are tired and irritable in the evenings. Another option is to wait and arrange a specific time to talk to avoid rushing through a conversation as you get ready to leave for work or class.
10. It might feel easier or safer to redirect the anger you feel toward your boss at your best friend or partner, but that doesn't solve your conflict with your boss and might create conflict with your friend or partner.

After you have respectfully expressed your anger, make sure you allow time and opportunity for the other person to express his or her feelings. Tell the person you appreciate how he or she listened to you and responded to you. Share other feelings besides the primary ones of hurt and anger, so that the person knows you can be angry with him or her and still care about him or her. Remember that your way of expressing anger and resolving conflict can either be destructive or be a way of connecting with people and improving relationships.

Sources: McKay, M., and Rogers, P. *The Anger Control Workbook*. Oakland: CA: New Harbinger Publications, Inc., 2000.
Paleg, K., and McKay, M. *When Anger Hurts Your Relationship*. Oakland: CA: New Harbinger Publications, Inc., 2001.

in their bodies. In addition, studies have shown that we have more control over so-called involuntary bodily functions than we once thought possible.

One commonly used device, for example, picks up electrical signals from the muscles and translates the signals into a form that people can detect. This device triggers a flashing light or activates a beeper every time muscles become more tense. To slow down the flashing or beeping, you need to relax tense muscles by breathing more slowly and deeply. People learn to associate sensations from the muscle with actual levels of tension and develop a new, healthy habit of keeping muscles only as tense as is necessary for as long as necessary. After treatment, individuals are then able to repeat this response at will without being attached to the sensors. Other biological functions that are commonly measured and used in a similar way to help people gain control are skin temperature, heart rate, sweat gland activity, and brainwave activity. People can manage stress by decreasing the physiological components of the stress response.

Melatonin is a natural hormone secreted by the pineal gland, a pea-size structure at the center of the brain. The production of melatonin goes hand in hand with the light-dark cycle. At night melatonin is produced to help our bodies regulate our sleep-wake cycles. As melatonin production rises, you begin to feel less alert. Body temperature starts to fall as well, and you begin to feel sleepier. Then melatonin levels drop quickly with the sunlight from the start of a new day. The amount of melatonin produced by our bodies seems to lessen as we get older. Scientists believe this may be why young people have fewer sleep problems than do older people.

Health food stores sell both synthetic and animal melatonin. Synthetic melatonin is made in factories where the manufacturing process is not controlled by the U.S. Food and Drug Administration (FDA). Melatonin is one of only two hormones not regulated by the FDA and sold over the counter without a prescription. (DHEA, or dehydroepiandrosterone, is the other.) Because melatonin does appear naturally in some foods, the U.S. Dietary Supplement and Health Education Act of 1994 allows it to be sold as a dietary supplement, and as such it does not need FDA approval.

Because melatonin has not undergone FDA approval or controlled laboratory studies, little is really known about its safety and efficacy. According to one report, "10% of the users said the hormone did nothing for them, and another 10% complained of side effects such as nightmares, headaches, morning grogginess, mild depression, and low sex drive." Information about reported side effects are not required to be listed on the product's packaging. Worsened fatigue and depression, constriction of the arteries to the heart, and possible negative effects on fertility have also been reported.

Without extensive research and testing, how much to take, when to take it, and the overall effectiveness of melatonin remains unclear. The doses listed on the bottles may not be accurate. In fact, one study found that a tested batch contained far more than the amount listed on the label.

As is true of all dietary supplements, melatonin must be taken with caution. Be aware of the risks of taking melatonin, given that so many questions remain unanswered about its safety and effectiveness.

Sources: American Academy of Family Physicians. *Melatonin: Frequently Asked Questions,* 1999; *Newsweek,* November 6, 1995, pp. 60–63.

Stress Inoculation

Working in a manner similar to a flu shot, stress inoculation involves exposing an individual to specific stressful situations, a little at a time, under controlled, safe conditions. Stress inoculation teaches individuals to relax using deep breathing and progressive muscle relaxation while they are being exposed to stressful situations.

The first step is to construct your personal list of stressful situations and arrange the list from the least to the most stressful items, and learn how to evoke each of these situations in your mind while at the same time focusing on your breathing and relaxing your muscles. The second step is to create an arsenal of stress-coping thoughts, such as "I'm going to be all right," "I've succeeded with this before," and "Getting started is the hardest part, then it will get easier for me." The third step is to practice this *in vivo,* meaning in real-life situations, while using the relaxation and cognitive techniques to minimize the stress response.[41] In addition to stress management, stress inoculation has also been helpful in anger management.

Cognitive Self-Talk

What we tell ourselves, our self-talk, has a tremendous effect on how well we manage our stress. Stress can be generated from faulty conclusions, misinterpretations, and expecting the worst. Some people claim that if they expect the worst, they won't feel disappointed or hurt, but in reality, they still feel the pain from their disappointment. We need to be careful about what we expect because we may inadvertently make it happen, a phenomenon referred to as **self-fulfilling prophecy.**[42] Self-fulfilling prophecies can work for you or against you. If you expect that work will be boring and uninteresting, you will tend to portray a negative, unmotivated attitude and will probably have a miserable time. However, if you expect to enjoy yourself at work, you are more likely to go looking for challenge and to have fun.

If we look more closely at how we make faulty conclusions and misinterpretations, we recognize a number

---

Key Terms

self-fulfilling prophecy the tendency to make something more likely to happen as a result of one's own expectations and attitudes of cognitive distortions that lead to a more stressed filled life, such as:

1. Filtering—Selectively paying attention to the negative and disregarding the positive.
2. Polarized Thinking—Putting things into absolute, all-or-nothing categories with no middle ground. For example, you have to be right or else you are wrong.
3. Overgeneralization—From one isolated event, you make a general, universal rule. For example, if you have failed once, you will always fail.
4. Mind Reading—Without people saying so, you believe you know what people are feeling and the reasons they behave the way they do. For example, if your friend seems tired, you think she doesn't really want to go out to the movies tonight as you had planned and so you cancel the plans thinking that is what she really wants.
5. Catastrophizing—Expecting disaster or the worst-case scenario.
6. Personalization—Thinking that things people do or say is in reaction to you and comparing yourself with others. For example, you walk past a group of people laughing and assume that they are laughing at you.
7. Control Fallacies—Feeling either that you have total control and responsibility for events or no control whatsoever over what is happening. You feel responsible for other people's happiness or pain.
8. Fallacy of Fairness—Feeling resentful when situations don't seem fair or just. Believing that good things happen to good people and bad things happen to bad people.
9. Blaming—Consistently blaming yourself or others for things that may not be entirely your or their fault.
10. Shoulds—Telling yourself what you are supposed to do, what is expected of you, or what you feel obligated to do rather than what you want to do. This is often something we don't want to do but think we should do and feel somewhat pressured or forced to do.
11. Emotional Reasoning—Believing that what you feel must be true and what you feel is what you are. For example, if you feel bad, then you are bad.
12. Fallacy of Change—Expecting that other people will change their behavior because you believe that your happiness is contingent upon it. For example, you tell yourself, "I would be happy if my parents showed more approval of me and my decisions."
13. Global Labeling—Applying stereotypes or labels to a whole group of people, behavior, or experiences, such as "Women are more emotional than men."
14. Being Right—Continually proving that your opinions and actions are correct. Being wrong is unacceptable and means you are inferior and less worthy.[41]

To change these cognitive distortions, you need to generate some rebuttals to your negative self-statements. This entails finding middle ground between all-or-nothing thinking by asking yourself what evidence proves that a statement is true and identifying some exceptions to this statement. Look for balance by asking yourself what is the opposite of this negative self-statement. Rather than telling yourself what you "should" do ask yourself what you "want" to do. Be specific instead of generalizing, and avoid labeling yourself and others. Instead of telling yourself "I'm lazy," you might say, "I wish I would have studied a few more hours for that test." Stick to the facts without blaming yourself or others. Question yourself as to how you know something is true and if you might be making an assumption or "mind reading." Be mindful of your self-fulfilling prophecies. It may be wiser to acknowledge that you don't know or consider many different possible outcomes rather than to expect the worst.

Changing negative self-talk requires time, practice, and patience. We develop these patterns of thinking over years, and they become almost automatic. It takes concentrated effort to be aware of and change negative thinking. Remember that your rebuttals need to be strong, nonjudgmental, and specific. Practice developing more flexible and balanced thinking about people, behavior, and situations.

As you can see, there are many different aspects to consider in managing stress, its physical, social, environmental, and psychological components. As you think about how you can more effectively manage your stress level, you will need to practice and experiment to find the stress-management techniques most beneficial for you.

 TALKING POINTS Think back to stressful times in your life. What were some positive ways you coped, and what were some negative things you did to cope?

A Realistic Perspective on Stress and Life

The development of a realistic approach to today's fast-paced demanding lifestyle may best be achieved by fostering many of the following perspectives:[43]

Anticipate problems and see yourself as a problem solver. Although each specific problem is unique, it is, most likely similar to past ones. Use these past experiences to quickly recognize ways of resolving new problems.

Search for solutions. Act on a partial solution, even when a complete solution seems distant. By resolving some aspects of a problem, you can gain time for more focused consideration of the remaining difficulties. In addition, some progress is a confidence builder that can help you remain committed to finding a complete solution.

Take control of your own future. Set out to accomplish your goals. Do not view yourself as a victim. Also, recall from Chapter 2 that being proactive and optimistic is an excellent way to take charge of your life and recognize capabilities that you were previously unaware of.

Be aware of self-fulfilling prophecies. Do not extend or generalize difficulties from one area into another. Further, negativity about yourself, in the form of self-doubt and self-blame, is certain to erode your feelings of success.

Visualize success. Focus on those things that are necessary and possible to ensure success. The very act of "imaging," seeing oneself performing skillfully, has proven beneficial in a variety of performance-oriented activities.

Accept the unchangeable. Focus on taking control of what you can and letting go of the rest. The direction your life takes is only in part the result of your own doing. Cope as effectively as possible with those events over which you have no direct control; beyond a certain point, however, you must let go of those things over which you have little control.

Live each day well. Combine activity, contemplation, and a positive attitude approaching the many things that must be done each day. Celebrate special occasions.

Undertake new experiences. Learn from your mistakes. Recognize your accomplishments. Most importantly, however, remember that the fabric of our lives is far more heavily influenced by day-to-day events than it is by the occasional milestones of life.

Act on your capacity for growth. Undertake new experiences and then extract from them new information about your own interests and capacities. The multiple dimensions of health identified in Chapter 1 will, over the course of your lifetime, provide a wide array of resources that will allow growth to occur throughout your entire life.

Allow for renewal. Make time for yourself, and take advantage of opportunities to pursue new and fulfilling relationships. Foster growth in each of the multiple dimensions of health—physical, psychological, social, intellectual, spiritual, and occupational. Initial renewal in one dimension may serve as a springboard for renewal in others.

Accept mistakes. Both you and others will make mistakes. Recognize that these can cause anger, and learn to avoid feelings of hostility. Mistakes, carefully evaluated, can serve as the basis for even greater knowledge and more likely success in those activities not yet undertaken.

Keep life simple. Keep the demands of life as orderly and manageable as you can. Just as adding too many appliances to an electrical circuit will quickly overload it and cause a power outage, excess demands and commitments added to our daily schedule can quickly burn out our psyches. Learning to prioritize and postpone activities is key to building a productive and enjoyable life.

Taking Charge of Your Health

- Analyze your past successes in resolving stressful situations, noting the resources that were helpful to you.
- Prioritize your daily goals in a list that you can accomplish, allowing time for recreational activities.
- Counteract a tendency to procrastinate by setting up imaginary (early) deadlines for assignments and rewarding yourself when you meet those dates.
- Add a new physical activity, such as an intramural team sport, to your daily schedule.
- Replace a negative coping technique that you currently use, such as smoking, with an effective alternative, such as deep breathing, relaxation exercises or yoga.
- List the positive aspects of your life, and make them the focus of your everyday thoughts.
- Explore the stress-reduction services that are available in your community, both on and off campus.

SUMMARY

- Stress refers to physiological changes and responses your body makes in response to a situation, a real or a perceived threat.
- The fight or flight response is a physiological response to perceived, anticipated, or real threat; it causes the heart to race, breathing becomes labored, muscles are tense, the body sweats, and blood flow is decreased to the extremities and digestive organs and increased to the major muscles and brain.
- Chronic stress refers to remaining at a high level of physiological arousal too long and not being able to take immediate, effective action to alleviate the perceived or real threat.
- While too much stress can have a negative effect and cause some serious health problems, a moderate level of stress is positive and beneficial.
- Constant arousal and increased levels of adrenaline in your system will eventually wear down your body's immunological system. You will be less able to cope with stress, and so it takes less and less stress to cause a stress reaction.
- General Adaptation Syndrome is a sequenced physiological response to the presence of a stressor, involving the alarm, resistance, and exhaustion stages of the stress response.
- When you are more stressed or anxious, you have a diminished ability to concentrate, recall information, and engage in problem-solving activities.
- An overwhelming number of students identify time management as the reason for their academic success or failure. Setting priorities and goals, balancing academic life with your social life, and finding time for sleeping, eating, exercising, and working along with studying is an essential aspect of managing your stress effectively.

- Procrastination means postponing something that is necessary to do to reach your goal. Typically, there is a psychological aspect to procrastination, since we tend to delay doing things we don't want to do.
- While striving to do your best is an admirable quality, expecting to be perfect in everything you do and never making a mistake places a great deal of stress and pressure on yourself.
- Type A individuals often feel pressured, are ambitious, impatient, competitive, walk and talk rapidly, and can be easily annoyed by delays. Type B individuals tend to be calm, relaxed, easy-going, and patient.
- To effectively manage your stress, you need to take into consideration environmental stressors such as the noise level, amount of light, and aesthetic quality of the space you inhabit. It is also important to get adequate amounts of rest, nutrition, and exercise.
- The relaxation response is effective because it entails the opposite of the stress response. Rather than taking shallow breaths, breathe deeply, inhaling to a count of four and exhaling to a count of four while sitting in a comfortable position.
- Effective psychological tools for stress management include progressive muscle relaxation, visualization, guided imagery, meditation, hypnosis, biofeedback, stress inoculation, and cognitive self-talk.
- Some of the ways people make cognitive distortions include filtering, polarized thinking, overgeneralization, mind reading, catastrophizing, personalization, control fallacies, fallacies of fairness, blaming, shoulds, emotional reasoning, fallacies of change, global labeling, and being right.

REVIEW QUESTIONS

1. What is stress?
2. How does stress relate to your physical and psychological health?
3. What is the fight or flight response?
4. What are some long-term physiological effects of chronic stress?
5. Describe the Yerkes-Dodson Law.
6. Explain the three stages of the General Adaptation Syndrome.
7. List at least five unique types of stress characteristics students can experience.
8. What are some common effects of test anxiety?
9. How does stress affect your ability to learn?
10. Define procrastination, and explain how it relates to stress.
11. How can being perfectionistic cause stress?
12. Describe type A and type B personality traits.
13. List some environmental stressors, and explain how high levels of stress have been linked to environmental factors.
14. Describe the relaxation response and how it is effective for stress management.
15. Name seven cognitive and psychological stress-management techniques, and explain how they work.

ENDNOTES

1. Selye H. *Stress Without Distress.* New York: New American Library, 1975.
2. Scott LV, Dinan T Vasopressin and the regulation of hypothalamic-pituitary-adrenal functions: Implications for the pathophysiology of depression. *Life Sci* 1998; 62(22): 1985–1998.
3. Selye, H. *The Stress of Life.* New York: McGraw-Hill, 1984.
4. Girdano DA, Everly GS, Dusek DE. *Controlling Stress and Tension.* Boston: Allyn & Bacon, 1996.
5. Raber M, Dyck G. *Managing Stress for Mental Fitness.* Menlo Park, CA: Crisp Publications, 1993.

6. Rowh M. *Coping with Stress in College.* New York: College Board Publications, 1989.

7. Holmes T, Rahe R. Social Readjustment Rating Scale. *Journal of Psychosomatic Research,* 11, 1967.

8. Kagan J, Segal J. *Psychology: An Introduction* (6th ed.). Orlando, FL: Harcourt Brace Jovanovich Inc., 1988.

9. Padus, E. *Positive Living and Health: The Complete Guide to Brain/Body Healing and Mental Empowerment.* Emmaus, PA: Rodale Press, 1990.

10. Kiev A. Managing stress to achieve success. *Executive Health,* 24(1): 1–4, 1987.

11. Lewen MK, Kennedy HL. The role of stress in heart disease. *Hospital Medicine,* 125–138, August 1986.

12. Byers SK. Organizational stress: Implications for health promotion managers. *American Journal of Health Promotion.* 21–26, Summer 1987.

13. O'Donnell MP, Ainsworth TH. *Health Promotion in the Workplace.* 185. New York: John Wiley & Sons, 1984,

14. Benson H, Allen R. How much stress is too much? *Harvard Business Review,* September/October, 1980.

15. Affordable care for kids squeezes college students. *The Detroit News,* November 23, 2001.

16. Newman E. *No More Test Anxiety.* Los Angeles, CA: Learning Skills Publications, 1996.

17. Arem C. *Conquering Math Anxiety: A Self-Help Workbook.* Pacific Grove: CA: Brooks/Cole Publishing Co., 1993.

18. Kahn N. *More Learning in Less Time.* Berkeley, CA. Ten Speed Press, 1992.

19. Lindzey G, Thompson R, Spring B. *Psychology* (3rd ed.). New York: Worth Publishers, Inc., 1988.

20. Lakein A. *How to Get Control of Your Time and Your Life.* New York: New American Library, 1973.

21. Hill MB, Hill DA, Chabot AE, Barrall JF. A survey of college faculty and student procrastination. *College Student Journal* 12, 256–262, 1978.

22. Roberts M. *Living Without Procrastination.* Oakland, CA: New Harbinger Publications, 1995.

23. Ferrari J, Johnson J, McGown W. *Procrastination and Task Avoidance: Theory, Research and Treatment.* New York: Plenum, 1995.

24. Basco M. *Never Good Enough.* New York: Simon & Schuster, 1999.

25. Davis M, Eshelmar E, McKay M. *The Relaxation and Stress Reduction Workbook.* Oakland, CA: New Harbinger, 2000.

26. Robinson B. *Overdoing It. How to Slow Down and Take Care of Yourself.* Deerfield Beach, FL: Health Communications Inc., 1992.

27. Maslow AH. *Motivation and Personality* (2nd ed.). NewYork: Van Nostrand, 1970.

28. Ferber R. *Solve Your Child's Sleep Problems.* New York: Simon & Schuster, 1985.

29. Saladin KS. *Anatomy & Physiology: The Unity of Form and Function.* New York: McGraw-Hill, 2001.

30. Lefcourt HM, Martin RA. *Humor and Life Stress: Antidote to Adversity.* New York: Spring-Verlag, 1986.

31. Asterita MF. *The Physiology of Stress.* 4–5. New York: Human Sciences Press, 1985.

32. Hugging warms the heart and also may protect it. *USA Today,* March 10, 2003.

33. Allen K, Shykoff BE, Izzo JL, Jr. Pet ownership but not ACE inhibitor therapy blunts home blood pressure responses to mental stress. *Hypertension 2001,* October, 38(4), 815–820.

34. Goliszek AG. *Breaking the Stress Habit.* Winston-Salem, NC: Carolina Press, 1987.

35. Rosenthal NE. *Winter Blues.* New York: The Guilford Press, 1998.

36. Seligman M. *Learned Optimism.* New York: Simon & Schuster Inc., 1990.

37. Wade C, Tavris C. *Psychology.* New York: Harper & Row, 1987.

38. Benson H. *The Relaxation Response.* New York: Avon, 1976.

39. Jacobson E. *Progressive Relaxation.* Chicago: University of Chicago Press, 1942.

40. Fanning P. *Visualization for Change.* Oakland, CA: New Harbinger Publications, Inc. 1988.

41. McKay M, Davis M, and Fanning P. *Thoughts and Feelings: The Art of Cognitive Stress Intervention.* Oakland, CA: New Harbinger Publications, 1981.

42. Jones RA. *Self-Fulfilling Prophecies.* Hillsdale, NJ: John Wiley & Sons, 1977.

43. McGinnis L. *The Power of Optimism.* New York: Harper & Row, 1990.

The aftermath of a natural disaster, such as Hurricane Katrina, which hit Louisiana, Alabama, and Mississippi in 2005, can have long-lasting effects. Hurricane Katrina cost over 1,000 people their lives as well as destroying homes, businesses, schools, churches, and personal belongings. The estimated cost from this disaster was over $100 billion, making Katrina the most costly storm in U.S. history. More than 400,000 people became jobless, and more than 150,000 properties were lost because of Katrina. People often experience feelings of vulnerability, confusion, loss, and helplessness when faced with such widespread devastation.

As we explained in Chapter 2, many people suffer from posttraumatic stress disorder after experiencing this type of natural disaster. Individuals are faced with rebuilding their lives, some starting completely from scratch with little or no resources. It can take years to recover from such trauma; people need positive, effective coping skills to get through an extended recovery period. Sights, sounds, and smells associated with hurricanes, such as rain, winds, and thunder, can create a great deal of distress in hurricane survivors. Seeing images of hurricanes on television or any similar reminders can bring back feelings of fear, powerlessness, and exposure. Merely hearing a loud noise, such as a pan dropping on the kitchen floor, can trigger a strong, negative emotional response. Survivors may also experience nightmares and flashbacks in addition to extreme startle responses to any kind of unexpected sound. People with posttraumatic stress disorder may experience clinical depression and severe anxiety for months and even years after the event.

Losing one's pets and significant places such as home, church, school, and work can leave people feeling lost and without their usual coping strategies. As you read in the stress management chapter, talking to friends and family members is a helpful way to express feelings associated with stress and to gain support. However, some people may be separated from their support group or have lost family and friends to the disaster. With the familiar, comfortable surroundings now gone, it may be extremely hard to connect to places and environments that help people to feel safe and secure. Some people may also experience survivor guilt—guilt associated with having escaped harm or one's home being untouched while others were destroyed.

Initially, many people respond to this type of disaster by feeling numb, as if the event didn't occur or couldn't have really happened. As the reality of what did occur sinks in, individuals may begin to feel a range of emotions—depression, anxiety, anger, and hopelessness. Helpers need to instill hope, the belief that people do survive these types of tragedies and can rebuild their lives again. They should encourage survivors to express their feelings and reassure them that these feelings are normal. This type of encouragement can bring a sense of stability and calmness to people's lives. Helpers should also remember that people have good days and bad days and remind survivors that soon the good days will outnumber the bad ones. Providing opportunities for survivors to share feelings appropriately with others who can understand and relate to how they are feeling is also helpful. Focusing on what one can control rather than what one cannot control is another positive coping strategy. Connecting with community resources and statewide efforts to assist survivors can also help. Knowing that people are there to help and that people don't have to rebuild their lives alone makes a tremendous difference in the recovery process.

Sometimes people are so focused on the logistics of what they need to do to get food, shelter, and clothing that they don't have time or energy to really process what has happened to them until after these basic needs are met. So it may be months later that the emotional toll becomes apparent. Often, assistance is plentiful when a disaster first hits, but later, when the psychological distress is worsening, the rescue efforts and relief efforts have dissipated and people are not getting the aid they need at that time. Having ongoing community support groups and mental health care services available is essential. It is also helpful to reestablish a routine as soon as possible. Returning to work, school, or just having a schedule can help people to feel safe, secure, and normal.

People also respond in individual ways to disaster, with some people being more resilient than others. Those who are experienced in coping with change, crisis, and adversity may recover more quickly than those who are unaccustomed to these problems. Most human beings are geared to survival, and so people eventually will rebuild their lives—one hopes to an equal or improved quality of living. Some people might find a "silver lining" and even find some positive outcomes in the aftermath of such disasters—for example, taking the chance to start over and reconsidering what is important to them in their lives.

personal assessment

How stressed are you?

A widely used life-stress scale called the Social Readjustment Rating Scale by Holmes and Rahe has been used to determine the degree of stress that you are experiencing because of life events over the past year. It also projects your chances of developing an illness- or stress-related health condition. Stress can lead to some serious health problems, and the more stress you have in your life, the more vulnerable you are to being susceptible to illness. Let's see how you score.

Life-Stress Scale

Check off the events that have happened to you **within the last year.** Then add up your total number of stress units for each life-stress event. The number on the right-hand side represents the amount, duration, and severity of change required to cope with each item. See the point scale at the end of the inventory to determine the health risk associated with your stress level.

Life Event	Value	Score
Death of a partner	100	_____
Divorce	73	_____
Relationship separation	65	_____
Jail term	63	_____
Death of a family member	63	_____
Personal injury/illness	53	_____
Marriage	50	_____
Fired from job	47	_____
Reconciliation with partner	45	_____
Retirement	45	_____
Illness—family member	44	_____
Pregnancy	40	_____
Sexual difficulties	39	_____
Addition of a family member	39	_____
Change in financial situation	38	_____
Death of a close friend	37	_____
Change in job	36	_____
Frequent arguments with partner	35	_____
Mortgage over $10,000	31	_____
Foreclosure of mortgage/loan	30	_____
Change in work responsibilities	29	_____
Child leaving home	29	_____
Trouble with in-laws	29	_____
Outstanding personal achievement	28	_____
Begin or end school	26	_____
Partner begins/stops working	26	_____
Change in living conditions	25	_____
Change in personal habits	24	_____
Trouble with supervisor	23	_____
Change in work hours	20	_____
Change in residence	20	_____
Change in schools	20	_____
Change in recreation	19	_____
Change in church activities	19	_____
Change in social activities	18	_____
Mortgage/loan less than $10,000	17	_____
Change in sleeping habits	16	_____
Change in family visits	15	_____
Change in eating habits	15	_____
Vacation	13	_____
Christmas	12	_____
Minor violations of the law	11	_____

TOTAL SCORE _____

What Is Your Health Risk?

Note that positive events such as outstanding personal achievements, vacations, and Christmas can be as stressful as negative ones. Think of events in your life that are not listed on this inventory. For example, where would you put running in a marathon or going on a diet?

⇒ If your score was 150 points or less . . .
You are on reasonably safe and healthy ground. You have about a one-in-three chance of a negative health change in the next 2 years.

⇒ If your score was between 150–300 points . . .
You have about a 50/50 chance of developing an illness related to stress in the next 2 years.

⇒ If your score was 300 points or more . . .
You have a 90 percent chance of developing a stress-related illness that could seriously affect your health. You need to be very watchful in how you manage your stress.

Based on Holmes and Rahe "Social Readjustment Scale".

personal assessment

Am I a perfectionist?

Below are some ideas that are held by perfectionists. Which of these do you see in yourself? To help you decide, rate how strongly you agree with each of the statements below on a scale from 0 to 4.

0	1	2	3	4
I do not agree		I agree somewhat		I agree completely

_____ 1. I have an eye for details that others can miss.

_____ 2. I can get lost in details and forget the real purpose of the task.

_____ 3. I can get overwhelmed by too many details.

_____ 4. It stresses me when people do not want to do things the right way.

_____ 5. There is a right way and a wrong way to do most things.

_____ 6. I do not like my routine to be interrupted.

_____ 7. I expect a great deal from myself.

_____ 8. I expect no less of others than I expect of myself.

_____ 9. People should always do their best.

_____ 10. I am neat in my appearance.

_____ 11. Good grooming is important to me.

_____ 12. I do not like being seen before I have showered and dressed.

_____ 13. I do not like making mistakes.

_____ 14. Receiving criticism is horrible.

_____ 15. It is embarrassing to make mistakes in front of others.

_____ 16. Sharing my new ideas with others makes me anxious.

_____ 17. I worry that my ideas are not good enough.

_____ 18. I do not have a great deal of confidence in myself.

_____ 19. I'm uncomfortable when my environment is untidy or disorganized.

_____ 20. When things are disorganized it is hard for me to concentrate.

_____ 21. What others think about my home is important to me.

_____ 22. I have trouble making difficult decisions.

_____ 23. I worry that I may make the wrong decision.

_____ 24. Making a bad decision can be disastrous.

_____ 25. I often do not trust others to do the job right.

_____ 26. I check the work of others to make certain it was done correctly.

_____ 27. If I can control the process it will turn out fine.

_____ 28. I am a perfectionist.

_____ 29. I care more about doing a quality job than others do

_____ 30. It's important to make a good impression.

_____ **TOTAL SCORE**

Scoring

Add all 30 items together to get total score. If your score was less than 30, then you are probably not a perfectionist, although you may have a few of the traits. Scores from 31 to 60 suggest mild perfectionism. When you are stressed your score may be higher. Scores of 61 to 90 suggest moderate perfectionism. This probably means that perfectionism is causing you trouble in some specific areas, but is not out of control. Scores higher than 91 suggest a level of perfectionism that could cause you serious problems.

Adapted from: _Never Good Enough_ by Monica Ramirez Basco.

The Body

Part Two comprises three chapters whose content is especially relevant to college students: fitness, nutrition, and weight management. This part will help you learn how to improve your health in these areas.

1. **Physical Dimension**
   Health experts believe that fitness, nutrition, and weight management are interrelated. How well our bodies work depends on what we eat and how we exercise. Healthy bodies allow us to participate in daily activities and recover more quickly from illness and injury.

2. **Psychological Dimension**
   When you start a fitness program or begin to pay attention to your diet, you learn about your level of motivation and commitment. You will be challenged, but the psychological rewards for your efforts, such as an improved self-concept and greater confidence, can be substantial.

3. **Social Dimension**
   The social dimension of health is closely related to fitness, nutrition, and weight management. Exercising with friends offers an opportunity for social interaction. Participation in most group fitness activities involves listening, sharing, and counseling. Food, like alcohol, can function as a "social lubricant" by bringing and holding people together. However, excessive food intake and lack of exercise can hinder social relationships when a person is significantly above his or her desirable weight.

4. **Intellectual Dimension**
   Some evidence suggests that people feel mentally sharper after they exercise. Many students report that they can study more efficiently after a workout. People deprived of adequate exercise and proper nutrition may suffer intellectual impairment. Regular physical activity, a sound diet, and effective weight management will allow you to enjoy a wide range of new experiences that can lead to improved intellectual functioning.

5. **Spiritual Dimension**
   Throughout this text we emphasize that an important part of your spiritual growth is serving others. Staying physically fit, following a healthful diet, and managing your weight can enhance your ability to serve others. You can express your own spirituality and help others find meaning in their lives when you take proper care of your health.

6. **Occupational Dimension**
   Just as you can better serve others when you feel your best, you can also pursue a career and carry out daily occupational tasks when you take care of your body. Some job functions, such as traveling and heavy lifting, require that you be in good physical condition. In addition, being fit can help you deal more effectively with the stress that inevitably accompanies employment. Taking care of your body can increase your self-esteem and improve your confidence—a definite plus when you are trying to land a job or earn a promotion.

chapter four

Becoming Physically Fit

Chapter Objectives

On completing this chapter, you will be able to:

▌ explain why cardiorespiratory fitness is more important to health than are other types of fitness, including muscular strength, muscular endurance, and flexibility.

▌ describe the effects that regular aerobic exercise has on the heart, lungs, and circulatory system.

▌ assess your own level of fitness in the areas of body composition, cardiorespiratory capacity, muscular strength, and flexibility.

▌ define aerobic energy production and anaerobic energy production.

▌ list and discuss the health concerns of midlife adults and of elderly adults.

▌ discuss the requirements of a suitable cardiorespiratory fitness program, including the mode of activity, frequency, intensity, duration, and resistance.

▌ explain the role of the warm-up, conditioning, and cooldown in an exercise session.

▌ explain the role exercise should play in pregnancy.

▌ discuss the role of fluid replacement in exercise, including when one should consume fluids and the best types of fluids one should consume.

▌ discuss the contribution of sleep to overall wellness.

▌ explain five principles for the prevention and care of sports injuries.

Eye on the Media

Infomercials for Fitness Equipment

As you channel surf with your TV's remote control, it's difficult to avoid seeing an infomercial for some type of fitness equipment. These paid commercials generally last from 15 to 30 minutes and often have an easily recognizable, healthy, attractive person as the spokesperson. The fitness equipment often has a catchy name. You've probably heard of most of them: BowFlex, Nordic Trac, Thigh-Master, Soloflex, and every imaginable name for equipment to improve the abdominal muscles.

The equipment advertisers frequently promise that by using their fitness device you will develop a beautiful, slim, strong, and well-toned body like that of the person "modeling" the equipment. And here is the best part: "You can achieve the body you want in just a few minutes each day . . . with very little effort on your part."

Is this possible? Probably not, say the fitness experts. There aren't many shortcuts to achieving overall fitness. The most lasting levels of fitness come from carefully designed programs that use a variety of activities and fitness equipment and encourage gradual increases in exertion and weight loss, if indicated.

TV's infomercials often try to sell equipment that tones just one part of the body. Also, the equipment sometimes comes with a "fitness and dietary plan" that includes a very low-calorie diet that may not be particularly safe for all individuals. You end up getting slimmer because you eat less and not because of the equipment's effectiveness.

Many of the less expensive fitness devices are poorly manufactured and break easily. Using just one piece of equipment can also become extremely monotonous, and you may find yourself avoiding exercise altogether.

So what should a consumer do? First, approach infomercials with a bit of skepticism. Try to find out if anyone you know has purchased the equipment and how well they liked it and how long they continued to use it. Ask fitness experts at your college or university about the equipment. If you are a member of a fitness club, ask the certified fitness experts on the staff about this equipment. You might also visit a local fitness equipment store and ask for the staff's input. Finally, if you should decide to purchase a piece of fitness equipment, try to use it as one part of your overall fitness program. Having "nice abs" is only marginally beneficial if the rest of your body remains out of shape and your cardiorespiratory fitness level remains low.

For many people, the day begins early in the morning; continues with classes, assignments, study, a job, and/or recreational activities; and does not end until after midnight. This kind of pace demands that one be physically fit. Even a highly motivated college student must have a conditioned, rested body to maintain such a schedule.

Of course, many college students do not look at physical fitness as a means to a more satisfying, exciting life. Instead, many students look for the cosmetic benefits of fitness. They want to look in the mirror and see the kind of body they see in the media: one with well-toned muscles, a trim waistline, and an absence of flabby tissue, especially on the arms, legs, abdomen, and hips. Thus, many students become motivated to start fitness programs because they hope that they can build a better body. Through their efforts to do so, students usually start to feel better, physically and mentally. They realize that physical fitness can improve every aspect of their lives, because they see it happening with each passing week.

Fortunately, you need not become a full-time athlete to enjoy the health benefits of fitness. Indeed, the Surgeon General has reported that significant health benefits can be achieved if you accumulate a moderate amount of physical activity on most, preferably all days of each week.[1]

Benefits of Fitness

Following a program of regular aerobic exercise improves the capacity of your cardiovascular and muscular systems. More specifically, regular aerobic exercise strengthens the muscles of your heart, enabling your heart to pump more blood with fewer strokes to meet the demands you place on it. As a result, your resting heart rate may become slower than in the past, indicating that you have become more physically fit. At the same time, your skeletal muscles develop improved metabolic machinery to allow them to use more oxygen and thus produce more energy. This cardiorespiratory endurance (also called cardiorespiratory fitness or aerobic fitness) enables you to deal more easily with the routine and extraordinary demands of your daily life.

Cardiorespiratory fitness is the foundation for whole-body fitness. It increases your capacity to sustain a given level of energy for a prolonged period. Thus your body can work longer and at greater levels of intensity.

As you will see, cardiorespiratory fitness has important benefits for everyone, including children (page 122), pregnant women (page 115), and older adults (page 113).

In addition, improving your cardiorespiratory (aerobic) fitness has a variety of benefits that can improve nearly all parts of your life. Aerobic fitness can help you gain the following physical benefits:

- Control of your weight
- Greater ability to perform a wide variety of activities throughout your life
- Ability to ward off infections
- Increased efficiency of your other body systems
- Reduced concentration of triglycerides and increased concentration of high-density lipoproteins ("good cholesterol") in your blood
- Reduced risk of heart disease and certain types of cancer
- Increased capillary network
- Prevention of hypertension and Type 2 diabetes
- Increased longevity
- Improved psychological health

Aerobic fitness also offers a variety of other benefits that, although not immediately obvious, are no less important. For example, the increased stamina that comes

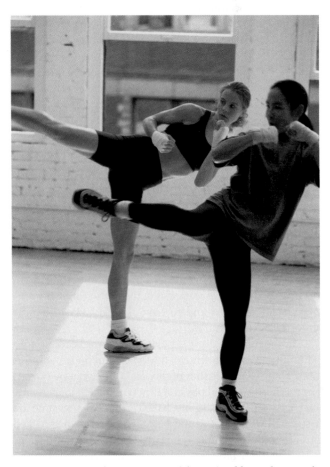

Cardiorespiratory fitness is essential for optimal heart, lung, and blood vessel function.

with cardiorespiratory fitness enables you to complete and better enjoy your daily activities. In addition, your improved fitness level may reduce the severity and shorten the duration of common illnesses. Likewise, you will find your ability to cope with stressors to be increased with your fitness level. As a result, you may find your sense of well-being and confidence to be improved.

Older adults will find that improving their cardiorespiratory fitness enables them to enjoy their later years to a greater extent, giving them the energy and ability to participate in activities that they might have delayed for many years, such as traveling, or even activities they might never have considered, such as joining a square dance club or learning how to line dance.

When you become aerobically fit, you may be able to achieve a long-held goal, such as hiking part of the Appalachian Trail, climbing Mt. Rainier, or bicycling through Europe. Others might find that becoming physically fit reduces their dependence on substances such as alcohol, cigarettes, or other drugs and that they sleep more soundly.

Finally, while you are pursuing your physical fitness activities, you probably will meet other healthy, active people and find that you are expanding your circle of friends. The Learning from Our Diversity box on page 103 takes a look at the physical and social benefits for persons with disabilities who participate in the Special Olympics.

 TALKING POINTS If your screening tests indicate that you cannot start a vigorous fitness program, are you prepared to ask your doctor about alternative activities?

Four Components of Physical Fitness

People who engage in regular **exercise** often choose **physical activities** that fit their lifestyles and individual preferences (Figure 4-1). These activities have the potential for helping them achieve a state of physical fitness. **Physical fitness** is characterized by the ability to perform occupational and recreational activities without becoming unduly fatigued and to have the capacity to handle unforeseen emergencies.

In the following sections, we discuss cardiorespiratory endurance, muscular fitness, flexibility, and body composition. These characteristics of physical fitness can be categorized as health-related physical fitness. Other characteristics, such as speed, power, agility, balance, and reaction time are associated with what would be called performance-related physical fitness. Although the latter type is most important for competitive athletes, it is the former type that has the most relevance to general population. Thus, this chapter focuses on health-related physical fitness.

Cardiorespiratory Endurance

If you were limited to improving only one area of your physical fitness, which would you choose—muscular strength, muscular endurance, or flexibility? Which would a dancer choose? Which would a marathon runner select? Which would an expert recommend?

The experts, exercise physiologists, would probably say that another fitness dimension is of even greater importance than those just listed. These research scientists regard improvement of heart, lung, and blood vessel function as the key focal point of a physical fitness program. **Cardiorespiratory endurance** forms the foundation for whole-body fitness. Cardiorespiratory endurance increases your capacity to sustain a given level of energy production for a prolonged period. Development of cardiorespiratory endurance helps your body to work longer and at greater levels of intensity.

Occasionally your body cannot produce the energy it needs for long-term activity. Certain activities require performance at a level of intensity that outstrips your cardiorespiratory system's ability to transport oxygen efficiently to contracting muscle fibers. When the oxygen demands of the muscles cannot be met, **oxygen debt** occurs. Any activity that continues beyond the point at

Key Terms

exercise a subcategory of physical activity; it is planned, structured, repetitive, and purposive in the sense that an improvement or maintenance of physical fitness is an objective[2]

physical activity any bodily movement produced by skeletal muscles that results in energy expenditure[2]

physical fitness a set of attributes that people have or achieve that relates to the ability to perform physical activity[2]

cardiorespiratory endurance the ability of the heart, lungs, and blood vessels to process and transport oxygen required by muscle cells so that they can contract over a period of time; cardiorespiratory endurance is produced by exercise that requires continuous, repetitive movements

oxygen debt a physical state in which one's activity exceeds the body's ability to produce energy aerobically, causing the body to switch to anaerobic energy production; this produces an excess buildup of by-products, especially lactic acid, and a feeling of inability to "catch one's breath"—respiration and heart rate remain increased until the excess by-products are cleared and the body can return to aerobic energy production

Learning from Our Diversity

A Different Kind of Fitness: Developmentally Disabled Athletes Are Always Winners in the Special Olympics

In America, as in many other countries around the world, physical fitness and athletic prowess carry a high degree of prestige, whereas lack of conditioning and poor sports performance often draw scorn and rejection. As anyone knows who's ever been picked last when sides were being chosen for a schoolyard game, few things are more damaging to youthful self-esteem than being the player nobody wants.

Some of these children blossom into accomplished athletes as they gain coordination or are inspired and guided by caring coaches. Others, lacking strong interest in sports, turn to less physical arenas in which they can excel—drama, debating, music, computers, science.

But what about people who want to be athletes at almost any cost but who have no realistic hope of attaining the standards of athletic accomplishment set for those in top physical condition? The Joseph P. Kennedy Foundation created an arena in which these athletes could compete when it established the Special Olympics in 1968. Joseph Kennedy was the father of President John F. Kennedy, whose older sister Rosemary was virtually shut away from the world when her family discovered she was mentally retarded. Many people at that time shared the Kennedys' view that the kindest way to treat family members who were developmentally disabled was to "protect" them from stares and whispers by keeping them at home or placing them in institutions or residential facilities. Spearheaded by President Kennedy's sister Eunice Kennedy Shriver, the Special Olympics was intended to

change the old attitudes toward developmentally disabled people by giving them an opportunity to compete at their own level and to celebrate their victories publicly.

Now, more than 30 years later, the Special Olympics holds both winter and summer games and boasts participation of more than 1 million developmentally disabled athletes in 140 countries around the world. The 2005 Special Olympics World Winter Games were held in Nagano, Japan.

The contests are open to athletes between the ages of 8 and 63, some of whom have proved wrong the specialists who claimed they would never walk, let alone compete internationally. "Mainstream" Olympic champions such as figure-skating silver medalist Brian Orser and a host of well-known entertainers have attended opening-day ceremonies to cheer and inspire the special athletes.

But medals aren't what the Special Olympics is all about. No matter where a Special Olympian finishes in a contest, he or she is applauded and celebrated for the accomplishment of playing the game and seeing it through. The oath taken by each participant in the Special Olympics aptly states the credo of this remarkable group of athletes: "Let me win. But if I cannot win, let me be brave in the attempt."

In what ways other than physical conditioning do you think a developmentally disabled person might benefit from participating in the Special Olympics? What can the rest of us learn from these athletes' courage and perseverance?

Physical Activity Preferences
Among adults who say they exercise regularly, here are the activities they prefer:

- 25% — At least 20 minutes aerobic exercise
- 21% — Work out on home equipment
- 19% — Participate in sports
- 16% — Strength training
- 14% — Jog/run
- 11% — Work out at club/gym
- 5% — Work out with exercise video

Figure 4-1 Running or working out in a gym is not for everyone. Which physical activities fit your preferences and lifestyle?

which oxygen debt begins requires a form of energy production that does not depend on oxygen.

This oxygen-deprived form of energy production is called **anaerobic** (without oxygen) **energy production,** the type that fuels many intense, short-duration activities. For example, rope climbing, weight lifting for strength, and sprinting are short-duration activities that quickly cause muscle fatigue; they are generally considered anaerobic activities. The key factor is if the energy demand of the activity exceeds the aerobic energy production capability. Thus, even activities that typically are considered to be aerobic (walking or cycling) can require anaerobic energy if the intensity is high.

If you usually work or play at low intensity but for a long duration, you have developed an ability to maintain **aerobic** (with oxygen) **energy production.** As long as your body can meet its energy demands in this oxygen-rich mode, it will not convert to anaerobic energy production. Thus fatigue will not be an important factor in determining whether you can continue to participate. Marathon runners, serious joggers, distance swimmers, bicyclists, and aerobic dancers can perform because of their highly developed aerobic fitness. The cardiorespiratory systems of these aerobically fit people have developed a large capacity to take in, transport, and use oxygen.

Besides allowing you to participate in activities such as those mentioned, aerobic conditioning (cardiorespiratory endurance conditioning) may also provide certain structural and functional benefits that affect other dimensions of your life (see the Discovering Your Spirituality box on page 105). These recognized benefits have received considerable documented support. It is now well accepted that regular physical activity that produces aerobic fitness will reduce the risk of heart disease, Type 2 diabetes, osteoporosis, obesity, depression, and cancer of the breast and colon.[3] For many women, exercise reduces the number and severity of symptoms that come with premenstrual syndrome (PMS). (See Chapter 14 for information regarding PMS.)

Muscular Fitness

Muscular fitness is the term used to represent the capabilities of the skeletal muscles to perform contractions. The capacity of the muscles have two distinct yet integrated characteristics: muscular strength and muscular endurance. The strength of the muscle is related to its ability to perform at or near its maximum for a short period of time. The endurance of the muscle is related to its ability to perform at submaximal levels for a long period of time.

Muscular fitness is essential for your body to accomplish work. Your ability to maintain good posture, walk, lift, push, and pull are familiar examples of the constant demands you make on your muscles to maintain or

Exercises for muscular fitness are important for both functional and health reasons. Functional reasons include the ability to perform daily tasks and recreational activities.

increase their level of contraction. The stronger you are, the greater your ability to contract muscles and maintain a level of contraction sufficient to complete tasks.

Key Terms

anaerobic energy production the body's alternative means of energy production, used when the available oxygen is insufficient for aerobic energy production; anaerobic energy production is a much less efficient use of stored energy

aerobic energy production the body's primary means of energy production, used when the respiratory and the circulatory systems can process and transport sufficient oxygen to muscle cells to convert fuel to energy

muscular fitness the ability of skeletal muscles to perform contractions; includes muscular strength and muscular endurance

Harnessing the Spirit: The Saga of Lance Armstrong

In the summer of 1999, American cyclist Lance Armstrong made one of the most amazing sports comebacks in history. Armstrong won the Tour de France, the most grueling cycling event in the world. In October 1996, Armstrong had been diagnosed with advanced testicular cancer and was given less than a 50% chance of survival. At the time of the diagnosis, the cancer had already spread to Armstrong's abdomen, lungs, and brain.

After being diagnosed with cancer, but before starting aggressive therapy, Armstrong declared himself "a cancer survivor, not a cancer victim." He convinced himself, his family, and his medical support team that he could beat the long odds facing him. He even established the Lance Armstrong Foundation (www.laf.org) before he had surgery and chemotherapy. He battled through his therapy without giving up the hope that the cancer would be defeated.

Miraculously, Armstrong's cancer disappeared. He then stunned the cycling world by returning to active training and planning a comeback that included competing for the 1999 Tour de France title. As Armstrong's physical condition improved and his training regimen became more demanding, cycling enthusiasts believed that Armstrong might be able to compete in—but certainly not win—the world's most famous bike race.

Armstrong proved his doubters wrong by winning the 1999 Tour de France. Perhaps even more amazingly, he has won the Tour de France *again* in the years 2000, 2001, 2002, 2003, 2004, and 2005, and he participated on the U.S. Olympic Cycling Team at the Sydney Olympics in 2000, winning a bronze medal in the Men's Individual Time Trial event. Armstrong chronicled his battle with testicular cancer in his best-selling book *It's Not About the Bike* (Putnam) and followed this with a cycling training book called *The Lance Armstrong Performance Program* (Rodale Press). Clearly, his powers of the mind and spirit worked to help him overcome his physical barriers. His success story has undoubtedly inspired others to take charge of their lives by doing their best to rise above mental and physical barriers to pursue the dreams that sometimes seem impossible.

Muscular strength can best be improved by training activities that use the **overload principle.** By overloading, or gradually increasing the resistance (load, object, or weight) your muscles must move, you can increase your muscular strength. The following three types of training exercises are based on the overload principle.

In **isometric** (meaning "same measure") **exercises,** the resistance is so great that the contracting muscles cannot move the resistant object at all. For example, you could contract your muscles against an immovable object such as a wall. Because of the difficulty of precisely evaluating the training effects, isometric exercises are not usually used as a primary means of developing muscular strength and can be dangerous for people with hypertension.

Isotonic resistance exercises, also called *same-tension exercises,* are currently the most popular type of strength-building exercises and include the use of traditional free weights (dumbbells and barbells), as well as many resistance exercise machines. People who perform progressive resistance exercises use various muscle groups to move (or lift) specific fixed resistances or weights. Although during a given repetitive exercise the weight remains the same, the muscular contraction effort required varies according to the joint angles in the range of motion.[4] The greatest effort is required at one angle (sticking point) in the range of motion of the movement.

Isokinetic (meaning "same motion") **exercises** use mechanical devices that provide resistances that consistently overload muscles throughout the entire range of motion. The resistance moves only at a preset speed regardless of the force applied to it. For the exercise to be effective, a user must apply maximal force. Isokinetic training requires elaborate, expensive equipment. Thus the use of isokinetic equipment may be limited to certain athletic teams, diagnostic centers, or rehabilitation clinics. The most common isokinetic machines are Cybex, Mini-Gym, ExerGenie, KinCom, and Biodex.

Which type of strength-building exercise (machines or free weights) is most effective? Take your choice, since all will help develop muscular strength. Some people

---

Key Terms

muscular strength the component of physical fitness that deals with the ability to contract skeletal muscles to a maximal level; the maximal force that a muscle can exert

overload principle the principle whereby a person gradually increases the resistance load that must be moved or lifted; this principle also applies to other types of fitness training

isometric exercises (eye so me trick) muscular strength-training exercises in which the resistance is so great that the object cannot be moved

isotonic resistance exercises muscular strength-training exercises in which traditional barbells and dumbbells with fixed resistances are used

isokinetic exercises (eye so kin e tick) muscular strength-training exercises in which machines are used to provide variable resistances throughout the full range of motion prefer machines because they are simple to use, do not require stacking the weights, and are already balanced and less likely to drop and cause injury. Other people prefer free weights because they encourage the user to work harder to maintain balance during the lift. In addition, free weights can be used in a greater variety of exercises than can weight machines.

Muscular endurance can be improved by performing repeated contractions of a less than maximal level. This aspect of muscular fitness is most related to common physical activities (leaf raking, pushing a lawn mower). Although it is not as glamorous as muscular strength, muscular endurance is an important part of muscular fitness.

Flexibility

The ability of your joints to move through their natural range of motion is a measure of your **flexibility.** This fitness trait, like so many other aspects of structure and function, differs from point to point within your body and among different people. Not every joint in your body is equally flexible (by design), and, over the course of time, use or disuse will alter the flexibility of a given joint. Certainly gender, age, genetically determined body build, and current level of physical fitness affect your flexibility.

One's inability to move easily during physical activity can be a constant reminder that aging and inactivity are the foes of flexibility. Failure to use joints regularly will quickly result in a loss of elasticity in the connective tissue and shortening of muscles associated with the joints. Benefits of flexibility include improved balance, posture, and athletic performance and reduced risk of low-back pain.

As seen in young gymnasts, flexibility can be highly developed and maintained with a program of activity that includes regular stretching. Stretching also helps reduce the risk of injury. Athletic trainers generally prefer **static stretching** to **ballistic stretching** for people who wish to improve their range of motion, since ballistic stretching carries a higher risk of soft-tissue tears. (See the Guidelines for Static Stretching on page 111.)

Body Composition

Body composition refers to what the body is made up of (muscle, bone, fat, water, minerals).[4] Of particular interest to fitness experts are percentages of body fat and fat-free weight. Health experts are especially concerned about the large number of people in American society who are overweight and obese. Cardiorespiratory fitness trainers increasingly are recognizing the importance of body composition and are including strength-training exercises to

Older Adults and Tai Chi Chuan

Continuing to follow a program of physical fitness is vital throughout midlife and older age. However, which types of exercise are most appropriate for older adults?

Many older adults choose gentle aerobic activities that put less stress and strain on joints, such as walking or water aerobics. Another option is the Chinese discipline tai chi chuan. Practitioners say that the slow, gentle movements of tai chi provide a variety of health benefits, such as improving physical strength and balance. At least one study[1] supports these beliefs, reporting that geriatric practitioners of tai chi enjoy greater flexibility, lower body fat, and greater peak oxygen uptake (an indication of cardiorespiratory fitness). The study concludes that tai chi may be prescribed as a suitable conditioning exercise for older adults.

[1] Lan C. et al: Cardiorespiratory function, flexibility, and body composition among geriatric tai chi chuan practitioners. *Arch Phys Med Rehabil* 1996 June; 77(6): 612–616.

help reduce body fat. (See Chapter 6 for further information about body composition, health effects of obesity, and weight management.)

Developing a Cardiorespiratory Endurance Program

For people of all ages, cardiorespiratory conditioning can be achieved through many activities. As long as the activity you choose places sufficient demand on the heart and lungs, improved fitness is possible. In addition to

Key Terms

muscular endurance the aspect of muscular fitness that deals with the ability of a muscle or muscle group to repeatedly contract over a long period of time

flexibility the ability of joints to function through an intended range of motion

static stretching the slow lengthening of a muscle group to an extended stretch, followed by a holding of the extended position for 10–30 seconds

ballistic stretching a "bouncing" form of stretching in which a muscle group is lengthened repetitively to produce multiple quick, forceful stretches engaging in the familiar activities of swimming, running, cycling, and aerobic dance, many people today participate in brisk walking, rollerblading, cross-country skiing, swimnastics, skating, rowing, and even weight training (often combined with some form of aerobic activity). Regardless of age or physical limitations, you can select from a variety of enjoyable activities that will condition the cardiorespiratory system. (Complete the Personal Assessment on pages 127–128 to determine your level of fitness.)

Many people think that any kind of physical activity will produce cardiorespiratory fitness. Many people consider golf, bowling, hunting, fishing, and archery to be forms of exercise. If performed regularly and for sufficient periods of time, they may enhance your health. However, they do not meet the requirements to be called exercise, and would not necessarily improve physical fitness. The American College of Sports Medicine (ACSM), the nation's premier professional organization of exercise physiologists and sport physicians,[7] has well-accepted guidelines for exercise training.

The ACSM's most recent recommendations for cardiorespiratory conditioning were published in 2005. The four major factors that are important for cardiorespiratory training are (1) mode of activity, (2) frequency, (3) intensity, and (4) duration. ACSM has also made recommendations for (5) muscular fitness and (6) flexibility training. We summarize these recommendations. You may wish to compare your existing fitness program with these standards.

Mode of Activity

The ACSM recommends that the mode of activity be any continuous physical activity that uses large muscle groups and can be rhythmic and aerobic in nature. Among the activities that generally meet this requirement are continuous swimming, cycling, aerobics, basketball, cross-country skiing, rollerblading, step training (bench aerobics), hiking, walking, rowing, stair climbing, dancing, and running. Water exercise (water or aqua aerobics) has become a popular fitness mode, because it is especially effective for pregnant women and older, injured, or disabled people.[8]

Endurance games and activities, such as tennis, basketball, racquetball, and handball, are fine as long as you and your partner are skilled enough to keep the ball in play; walking after the ball will do very little for you. Softball and football are generally less than sufficient continuous activities—especially the way they are played by weekend athletes. An old coaching adage applies here: You get in shape to play the game, you do not play the game to get in shape. In other words, using recreational sports is not an effective method to develop physical

fitness; however, it may be a useful (and enjoyable) way to maintain fitness.

Regardless of which continuous activity you select, it should also be enjoyable. Running, for example, is not for everyone—despite what some accomplished runners say! Find an activity you enjoy. If you need others around you to have a good time, corral a group of friends to join you. Vary your activities to keep from becoming bored. You might cycle in the summer, run in the fall, swim in the winter, and play racquetball in the spring. To help you maintain your fitness program, see the suggestions in the Changing for the Better box on page 108. In addition, the Star box on page 109 provides information on exercising in an urban environment.

Frequency of Training

Frequency of training refers to the number of times per week a person should exercise. The ACSM recommends three to five times per week. For most people, participation in fitness activities more than five times each week does not significantly further improve their level of conditioning. Likewise, an average of only two workouts each week does not seem to produce a measurable improvement in cardiorespiratory conditioning. Thus, although you may have a lot of fun cycling twice each week, do not expect to see a significant improvement in your cardiorespiratory fitness level.

Intensity of Training

How much effort should you put into an activity? Should you run quickly, jog slowly, or swim at a comfortable pace? Must a person sweat profusely to become fit? These questions all refer to **intensity** of effort.

The ACSM recommends that healthy adults exercise at an intensity level of between 65 percent and 90 percent of their maximum heart rate, which is estimated by subtracting one's age from 220. However, be aware that there could be a considerable difference between estimated maximal heart rate and actual maximal heart rate (measured during a maximal exercise test) Or, one should exercise at an intensity level between 50 percent and

---

Key Terms

frequency the number of exercise sessions per week; for aerobic fitness 3 to 5 days are recommended

intensity the level of effort put into an activity; for aerobic fitness 50 percent to 85 percent of heart rate range is recommended

85 percent of one's heart rate range. This level of intensity is called the **target heart rate (THR)** (see the Changing for the Better box on this page). This rate refers to the minimum number of times your heart needs to contract (beat) each minute to have a positive effect on your heart, muscles, and blood vessels. This intensity produces a *training effect*. Activity at an intensity below the THR will be insufficient to make a significant improvement in your fitness level. Although intensity below the THR will still help you expend calories and thus lose weight, it will probably do little to make you more aerobically fit. However, intensity that is significantly above your THR will probably cause you to become so fatigued that you will be forced to stop the activity before the training effect can be achieved.

Choosing a particular THR depends on your initial level of cardiorespiratory fitness. If you are already in relatively good physical shape, you might feel comfortable starting exercise at 70 percent of your heart rate range. A well-conditioned person needs to select a higher THR for his or her intensity level, whereas a person with a low cardiorespiratory fitness level will still be able to achieve a training effect at a lower THR of 50 percent of heart rate range.

In the example in the Changing for the Better box, the younger person would need to participate in a continuous activity for an extended period while working at a THR of 158 beats per minute. The older person would need to function at a THR of 150 beats per minute to achieve a positive training effect.

Changing for the Better

How to Calculate Your Target Heart Rate

The target heart rate (THR) is the recommended rate for increasing cardiorespiratory endurance. To maintain a training effect, you must sustain activity at your THR. To estimate your THR, subtract your age from 220 (the age-predicted maximum heart rate; note, the actual maximal heart rate may be as much as 30 beats per minute higher or lower than this estimate), then subtract your resting heart rate. This gives you your heart-rate range (HRR). Next, multiply your HRR by .70 (the desired training level), and then add this to your resting heart rate. Here are two examples:

For a 20-year-old person with a resting heart rate of 60 beats per minute (wanting a THR of 70% of heart-rate range)	For a 40-year-old person with a resting heart rate of 80 beats per minute (wanting a THR of 70% of heart-rate range)
Maximum heart rate:	Maximum heart rate:
$220 - 20 = 200$	$220 - 40 = 180$
$(200 - 60) \times .70 = 98$	$(180 - 80) \times .70 = 70$
$98 + 60 = 158$	$70 + 80 = 150$
THR = 158 beats per minute	THR = 150 beats per minute

InfoLinks

www.fitnesslink.com

Changing for the Better

Tips to Help You Stick to Your Exercise Program

Sometimes it seems difficult to continue an exercise program. Here are a few tips to keep you going:

- Fit your program into your daily lifestyle.
- Exercise with your friends.
- Incorporate music into your activity.
- Vary your activities frequently; cross-train.
- Reward yourself when you reach a fitness goal.
- Avoid a complicated exercise program; keep it simple.
- Measure your improvement by keeping a log or a diary.
- Take some time off to rest and recuperate.
- Keep in mind how important physical activity is to your life and health.

InfoLinks

http://primusweb.com/fitnesspartner

Determining your heart rate is not a complicated procedure. Find a location on your body where an artery passes near the surface of the skin. Pulse rates are difficult to determine by touching veins; the blood pressure is lower in veins than in arteries, making it more difficult to feel a pulse. Two easily accessible sites for determining heart rate are the carotid artery (one on each side of the windpipe at the front of your neck) and the radial artery (on the inside of your wrist, just above the base of the thumb).

Practice placing the front surface of your index and middle fingertips at one of these locations and feeling for a pulse. Once you have found a regular pulse, look at the second hand of a watch. Count the number of beats you

Key Terms

target heart rate (THR) the number of times per minute the heart must contract to produce a cardiorespiratory training effect

Exercising in an Urban Environment

People who live in large cities face special challenges as they pursue fitness activities. Some of these challenges are just annoying, but some challenges can be life-threatening. News reports occasionally tell of someone who was seriously injured or killed (accidentally or intentionally) while trying to exercise in an urban environment. Visitors to cities can also be confronted with these difficulties, and visitors may be less experienced adjusting to these challenges than those who live year-round in the city.

Among the obstacles are pollution, heavy vehicular and pedestrian traffic, and the possibility of criminal activity. These problems may also exist in small towns, but they likely exist to a lesser degree. Resist the temptation to use "the city" as an excuse not to exercise. Fortunately, you can tailor a fitness program to fit the urban environment in numerous ways. Consider these strategies as you plan your fitness activities in the city.

- If you are unfamiliar with the environment, exercise indoors. It can be dangerous to jog, rollerblade, or cycle in a place where you could become lost. Exercise inside your home or apartment, a local health club or YMCA, or in your hotel. Many indoor exercise machines provide a good cardiorespiratory and strength-training workout. Some facilities also have swimming pools, indoor tracks, handball courts, and special fitness classes.

- If you plan to exercise outdoors, always do so with a partner. There is, indeed, safety in numbers. Exercising with a friend or two (or jogging with a large, leashed dog) can provide a measure of protection. If you become injured, friends can help summon medical assistance.

- Try to avoid heavily congested areas. Cycling or jogging in heavy traffic is dangerous not only for you but also for other pedestrians and motorists. This is especially true during rush hours (7–9 A.M., noon, and 4–6 P.M.). Try to locate a relatively quiet place that also seems secure. If you are a visitor to an area, make certain you know whether a particular area is safe for walking, cycling, or jogging. Don't assume that every urban park is a safe haven for exercisers.

- Do not exercise outside at night. A city can take on an entirely different mood during the night. It is foolish to place yourself at risk by exercising outside when it is dark. Stick to the daylight hours.

- Be aware of pollution levels before you exercise. If there is a pollution warning, consider exercising indoors until the alert is over. If you are one who must exercise outside, you might wish to use a pollution mask; the mask will filter a significant amount of large particles. However, it may also serve to attract unnecessary attention.

- Consider carrying an alarm or protective spray device when exercising outdoors. This suggestion has both proponents and opponents. Carrying a protective spray device or alarm can be helpful, if you know how to use it in an emergency. Remember, some devices can be used against you, especially if an assailant surprises and overpowers you.

---

feel in a 15-second period. Multiply this number by 4. This number is your heart rate. With a little practice, you can become proficient at determining heart rate.

Duration of Training

The ACSM recommends that the **duration** of training be between 20 and 60 minutes of continuous aerobic activity. Generally speaking, the duration can be on the shorter end of this range for people whose activities use a high intensity of training (75 percent to 85 percent of heart-rate range). Those who choose activities with a low range of intensity (50 percent to 60 percent of heart-rate range) should maintain that activity for a longer time. Thus a fast jog and a moderate walk require different amounts of time to accomplish the training effect. The fast jog might be maintained for 25 minutes, whereas the brisk walk should be kept up longer—perhaps for 50 minutes. The bottom line is to achieve what ACSM calls an adequate volume (total amount) of exercise. ACSM recommends that individuals should expend between 1,000–2,000 kilocalories per week in aerobic exercises to obtain a cardiorespiratory training effect. This total volume can be achieved in a variety of ways. For example, some people may choose to exercise at a moderate intensity (50 percent to 60 percent of heart-rate range) for a longer duration (40 minutes per session) and higher frequency (5 days per week), whereas others can get similar benefits by choosing higher intensity (75 percent to 80 percent of heart-rate range) with a shorter duration (30 minutes per session) and lower frequency (4 days per week).

Resistance Training

Recognizing that overall body fitness includes muscular fitness, the ACSM now recommends resistance training in

Key Terms

duration the length of exercise time of each training session; for aerobic fitness 20–60 minutes per session are recommended its current standards. The ACSM suggests participation in resistance training two or three times a week. This training should help develop and maintain a healthy body composition—one with an emphasis on lean body mass. The goal of resistance training is not to improve cardiorespiratory endurance but to improve overall muscle strength and muscular endurance. For some people (individuals with hypertension or Type 2 diabetes), resistance training with heavy weights is not recommended because it can induce a sudden and dangerous increase in blood pressure.

The resistance training recommended by the ACSM includes one set of 8 to 12 repetitions (10 to 15 repetitions for individuals over age 50) of 8 to 10 different exercises. Although any weight that produces an overload will result in improvement, the greatest muscular fitness gains will be achieved if the weight lifting results in fatigue of the muscle (that is, more than 12 repetitions cannot be performed). These exercises should be geared to the body's major muscle groups (for example, legs, arms, shoulders, trunk, and back) and should not focus on just one or two

body areas. Isotonic (progressive resistance) or isokinetic exercises are recommended (see page 105). For the average person, resistance training activities should be done at a moderate-to-slow speed, use the full range of motion, and not impair normal breathing. With just one set recommended for each exercise, resistance training is not very time consuming.

Flexibility Training

To develop and maintain a healthy range of motion for the body's joints, the ACSM suggests that flexibility exercises be included in one's overall fitness program. Stretching can be done in conjunction with other (cardiorespiratory or muscular fitness) training or can be performed separately. Note that if flexibility training is done separately, a general warm-up should be performed before stretching. For most individuals, static stretching is the best type. Flexibility improvements can be obtained by training as little as two days per week; however, stretching is an activity that can be safely performed daily. ACSM recommends that a flexibility program should include all the major muscle and/or tendon groups. The intensity of each stretch should be at a position where you feel mild discomfort in the muscle. Each stretch should be held for between 10 to 30 seconds and should be repeated three to four times per training session. Stretching should be done according to safe and appropriate techniques. (See the Guidelines for Static Stretching that follow.)

Special Considerations

Warm-Up, Conditioning, Cooldown

Each training session consists of three basic parts: the warm-up, the conditioning, and the cooldown.[4] The warm-up should last 10 to 15 minutes. During this period, you should begin slow, gradual, comfortable movements related to the upcoming activity, such as walking or slow jogging. If the upcoming activity requires specific types of movement, some range of motion exercises mimicking those movements are beneficial. All body segments

Guidelines for Static Stretching

Take the following precautions to reduce the possibility of injury during stretching:

- Warm up using a slow jog or fast walk before stretching.

- Stretch only to the point at which you feel tightness or resistance to your stretching. Stretching should not be painful.

- Be sure to continue normal breathing during a stretch. Do *not* hold your breath.

- Use caution when stretching muscles that surround painful joints. Pain is an indication that something is wrong—it should not be ignored.

and muscle groups should be exercised as you gradually increase your heart rate. Near the end of the warm-up period, the major muscle groups should be stretched. This preparation helps protect you from muscle strains and joint sprains.

The warm-up is a fine time to socialize. Furthermore, you can mentally prepare yourself for your activity or think about the beauty of the morning sky, the changing colors of the leaves, or the friends you will meet later in the day. Mental warm-ups can be as beneficial for you psychologically as physical warm-ups are physiologically.

The second part of the training session is the conditioning phase, the part of the session that involves improving muscular fitness, cardiorespiratory endurance, and flexibility. Workouts can be tailor-made, but they should follow the ACSM guidelines discussed previously in this chapter.

The third important part of each fitness session is the cooldown. Ideally, one should not abruptly stop exercise as this could cause circulatory problems (insufficient blood returning to the heart). The cooldown consists of a 5- to 10-minute session of relaxing exercises, such as slow jogging, walking, and stretching. Note, this is the ideal time for flexibility training, since the muscles and joints are warmed from the conditioning phase. This activity allows your body to cool and return to a resting state. A cooldown period helps reduce muscle soreness.

Aging Physically

With aging, physical decline occurs and the components of physical fitness become more difficult to maintain. From the fourth decade onward, a gradual decline in vigor and resistance eventually gives way to various types of illnesses. In the opinion of many authorities, people do not die of old age. Rather, old age worsens specific conditions responsible for death. However, physical decline can be

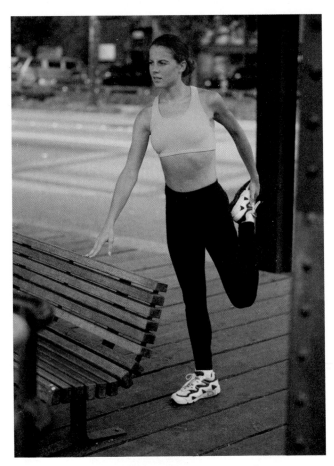

Flexibility exercises can be performed almost anywhere.

Have you received mixed messages about how much exercise is necessary? Some reports tout that all you need to do is more general types of activities (raking leaves, walking the dog.) Others suggest that you can get benefits with multiple short walks throughout the day. And of course, you can go to the gym and hear that you have to feel the burn to make it worthwhile. So which message is correct? Surprisingly, all of them! It just depends on what your goal is.

Prior to the 1990s, fitness professionals recommended that you needed to exercise above certain minimal (of time, intensity, and frequency) levels to obtain fitness benefits. Their message was correct; however, many people believed that if they could not meet the minimums, they were obtaining no benefits. Thus, it was viewed as an all-or-none proposition.

In 1995 the American College of Sports Medicine and the Centers for Disease Control and Prevention issued a public health statement on Physical Activity and Health. This report documented that there are clear benefits to 30 minutes a day of moderate-intensity physical activity and suggested that activities such as gardening and housework could be beneficial to health. Another important aspect of this report was that the health benefits could be obtained by accumulating activity throughout the day (for example: three 10-minute bouts of activity; one in the morning, one in the afternoon, and one in the evening). Unfortunately, many individuals misunderstood this message and started suggesting that more vigorous forms of activity (exercise) were not really necessary and the term *exercise* lite was born.

What got confused was the difference between health benefits and fitness benefits. The Surgeon General's Report on Physical Activity and Health was issued in 1996 and helped clarify the message from the ACSM/CDC report. Clearly there are numerous health benefits to regular physical activity. Among these benefits are control of body weight, blood pressure, blood sugar, and cholesterol. The Surgeon General also operationalized the amount of activity required to obtain health benefits as 150 kilocalories per day. The Report suggested that this could be achieved in a variety of ways (15 minutes of jogging, 30 minutes of walking, or 45 minutes of playing volleyball). Additionally, they clarified that doing more than this amount would result in additional benefits. In other words the more activity (dose), the greater the benefits (response).

Because exercise is a form of physical activity, when one exercises regularly, one gets the same (or greater) health benefits as those who choose to just maintain a regularly active lifestyle. Of course the bonus for those who exercise is that they will also derive physical fitness benefits from their program.

So, the choice is yours. If your principle goal is to maintain good health, accumulating a moderate amount of physical activity on most days will work. However, if your goal is health and physical fitness, then exercise is required.

slowed and the onset of illness delayed by staying physically active. The process of aging can be described on the basis of predictable occurrences,[5] as follows:

- Change is gradual. In aging, gradual changes occur in body structure or function before specific health problems are identified.

- Individual differences occur. When two people of the same age are compared for the type and the extent of change that has occurred with age, important differences can be noted. Even within the same person, different systems decline at differing rates and to varying extents.

- Greatest change is noted in areas of complex function. In physiological processes involving two or more major body systems, the most profound effects of physiological aging can be noted.

- Homeostatic decline occurs with age. Becoming older is associated with a growing difficulty in maintaining homeostasis (the dynamic balance among body systems). In the face of stressors, the older adult's system takes longer to respond, does not respond with the same magnitude, and may take longer to return to baseline.

Like growth and development, aging is predictable yet unique for each person.

Health Concerns for Midlife Adults

The period between 45 and 64 years of age brings with it a variety of subtle changes in the body's structure and function. When life is busy and the mind is active, these changes are generally not evident. Even when they become evident, they are not usually the source of profound concern. Nevertheless, older students in your class and people with whom you work could be experiencing these changes:[5]

- Decrease in bone mass and density
- Increase in vertebral compression
- Degenerative changes in joint cartilage
- Increase in adipose tissue—loss of lean body mass
- Decrease in capacity to engage in physical work
- Decrease in visual acuity
- Decrease in resting energy requirements
- Decrease in fertility
- Decrease in sexual function

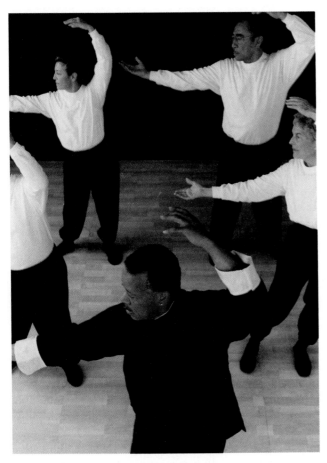

Exercising in a class can be fun and help you stick with your fitness program.

these are closely related to disease processes, but in most cases they reflect the gradual decline that is thought to be a result of the normal aging process. The most frequently seen changes include the following:

- Decrease in bone mass
- Changes in the structure of bone
- Decrease in muscle bulk and strength
- Decrease in oxygen uptake
- Loss of nonreproducing cells in the nervous system
- Decrease in hearing and vision abilities
- Decrease in all other sensory modalities, including the sense of body positioning
- Slower reaction time
- Gait and posture changes resulting from a weakening of the muscles of the trunk and legs

In addition to these changes, the most likely change seen in older adults is the increased sensitivity of the body's homeostatic mechanism. Because of this sensitivity, a minor infection or superficial injury can be traumatic enough to decrease the body's ability to maintain its internal balance. An illness that would be easily controlled in a young person could even prove fatal to a seemingly healthy 75-year-old person.

Continuing to follow a physical fitness plan throughout midlife and older adulthood is essential to minimizing age-related health problems. The plan should be modified as necessary to accommodate changes in physical functioning.

Exercise for Older Adults

An exercise program designed for younger adults may be inappropriate for older people, particularly those over age 50. Special attention must be paid to matching the program to the interests and abilities of the participants. Often, this is best achieved by having older individuals begin their exercise program under the supervision of a certified exercise professional. The goals of the program should include both social interaction and physical conditioning.

Older adults, especially those with a personal or family history of heart problems, should have a physical examination before starting a fitness program. This examination should include an evaluation of all the physiological systems of the body, especially the cardiovascular, respiratory, and musculoskeletal. Ideally, the evaluation should also include a maximal exercise test (a "stress" test). Participants should learn how to monitor their own cardiorespiratory status during exercise.

Well-designed fitness programs for older adults will include activities that begin slowly, are monitored frequently, and are geared to the enjoyment of the participants.[9] The

For some midlife adults these health concerns can be quite threatening, especially for those who view aging with apprehension and fear. Some middle-aged people reject these physical changes and convince themselves they are sick. Indeed, hypochondriasis is much more common among midlife people than among young people.

Health Concerns for Older Adults

In older people, it is frequently difficult to distinguish between changes caused by aging and those caused by disease. For virtually every body system, biomedical indexes for the old and young can overlap. In the respiratory system, for example, the cardiorespiratory endurance of a man of 70 may be no different from that of a man of 55 who has a history of heavy cigarette smoking. Is the level in the older man to be considered an indicator of a disease, or should it be considered a reflection of normal old age? In dealing with older adults, physicians frequently must make this kind of distinction.

In older people, as in midlife people, structural and physiological changes are routinely seen. In some cases, professional staff coordinating the program should be familiar with the signs of distress (excessively elevated heart rate, nausea, breathing difficulty, pallor, and pain) and must be able to perform CPR. Warm-up and cooldown periods should be included. Activities to increase flexibility are beneficial in the beginning and ending segments of the program. Participants should wear comfortable clothing and appropriate shoes, and they should be mentally prepared to enjoy the activities.

A program designed for older adults will largely conform to the ACSM criteria specified previously in this chapter, including both cardiorespiratory and muscular fitness training. Certainly, specific modifications or restrictions to the exercise program may be required due to health concerns of the individual. For example, because of possible joint, muscular, or skeletal problems, certain activities may have to be done in a sitting position. Pain or discomfort should be reported immediately to the fitness instructor.

Fortunately, properly screened older adults will rarely have health emergencies during a well-monitored fitness program. Many fit older adults can also safely exercise alone.

Low-Back Pain

A common occurrence among adults is the sudden onset of low-back pain. Four out of five adults develop this condition at least once in their lifetime, which can be so uncomfortable that they miss work, lose sleep, and generally feel incapable of engaging in daily activities. Many of the adults who have this condition will experience these effects two to three times per year.

Although low-back pain can reflect serious health problems, most low-back pain is caused by mechanical (postural) problems. As unpleasant as low-back pain is, the symptoms and functional limitations usually subside within a week or two. The services of a physician, physical therapist, or chiropractor are generally not required.

By engaging in regular exercise, such as swimming, walking, and bicycling, and by paying attention to your back during bending, lifting, and sitting, you can minimize the occurrence of this uncomfortable and incapacitating condition. Many commercial fitness centers and campus recreational programs are starting to offer specific exercises geared to muscular improvement in the lower back and abdominal areas.

Osteoporosis

Osteoporosis is a condition frequently seen in older middle-aged women. However, it is not fully understood why menopausal women are so susceptible to the increase in calcium loss that leads to fractures of the hip, wrist, and vertebral column. Approximately 80 percent of those with osteoporosis are women. Estimates from the National Osteoporosis Foundation are that half of women and one in eight men over age 50 will have an osteoporosis-related fracture in their lifetime.[6]

The endocrine system plays a large role in the development of osteoporosis. At the time of menopause, a woman's ovaries begin a rapid decrease in the production of estrogen, one of two main hormones associated with the menstrual cycle. This lower level of estrogen may decrease the conversion of the precursors of vitamin D into the active form of vitamin D, the form necessary for absorbing calcium from the digestive tract. As a result, calcium may be drawn from the bones for use elsewhere in the body.

Additional explanations of osteoporosis focus on two other possibilities—hyperparathyroidism (another endocrine dysfunction) and the below-average degree of muscle development seen in osteoporotic women. In the latter case the reduced muscle mass is associated with decreased activity, which in turn deprives the body of the mechanical stimulation needed to facilitate bone growth.

Premenopausal women have the opportunity to build and maintain a healthy skeleton through an appropriate intake of calcium. Current recommendations are for an intake of 1,200 mg of calcium per day. Three to four daily servings of low-fat dairy products should provide sufficient calcium. The diet also must contain adequate vitamin D because it aids in the absorption of calcium.

Many women do not consume an adequate amount of calcium. Calcium supplements, again in combination with vitamin D, can be used to achieve recommended calcium levels. It is now known that calcium carbonate, a much-advertised form of calcium, is no more easily absorbed by the body than are other forms of calcium salts. Consumers of calcium supplements should compare brands to determine which, if any, they should buy.

In premenopausal women, calcium deposition in bone is facilitated by exercise, particularly exercise that involves movement of the extremities. Today, women are encouraged to consume at least the recommended servings from the milk group and engage in regular physical activity that involves the weight-bearing muscles of the legs, such as aerobics, jogging, and walking.

Postmenopausal women who are not elderly can markedly slow the resorption of calcium from their bones

Key Terms

osteoporosis decrease in bone mass that leads to increased incidence of fractures, primarily in postmenopausal women through the use of estrogen-replacement therapy. When combined with a daily intake of 1,500 mg of calcium, vitamin D, and regular exercise, estrogen therapy almost eliminates calcium loss. Of course, women need to work closely with their physicians to monitor the use of estrogen because of continuing concern over the role of estrogen-replacement therapy in the development of breast cancer and the increased risk of coronary heart disease events and stroke.

Osteoarthritis

Arthritis is an umbrella term for more than 100 forms of joint inflammation. The most common form is **osteoarthritis.** It is likely that as we age, all of us will develop osteoarthritis to some degree. Often called "wear and tear" arthritis, osteoarthritis occurs primarily in the weight-bearing joints of the knee, hip, and spine. In this form of arthritis, joint damage can occur to bone ends, cartilaginous cushions, and related structures as the years of constant friction and stress accumulate.

The object of current management of osteoarthritis (and other forms) is not to cure the disease but rather to reduce discomfort, limit joint destruction, and maximize joint mobility. Aspirin and nonsteroidal anti-inflammatory agents are the drugs most frequently used to treat osteoarthritis.

It is now believed that osteoarthritis develops most commonly in people with a genetic predisposition for excessive damage to the weight-bearing joints. Thus the condition seems to run in families. Further, studies comparing the occurrence of osteoarthritis in those who exercise and those who do not demonstrate that regular movement may decrease the likelihood of developing this form of arthritis.

Fitness Questions and Answers

Along with the six areas to consider in your fitness program, you should think about many additional issues when you start a fitness program.

Should I See My Doctor Before I Get Started?

First of all, it is highly desirable to have regular checkups as part of your overall health plan. However, the Surgeon General has suggested that most adults can safely increase their activity level to a moderate amount without the need for a comprehensive medical evaluation. Individuals with chronic diseases should consult with their physician before increasing their activity level.

If vigorous forms of exercise are desired, then a medical exam is recommended for men over 40 and women over 50. It is also recommended for individuals with more than one risk factor for coronary artery disease or with any other notable health problems. The American College of Sports Medicine also recommends an exercise ("stress") test for these individuals.[10]

What Causes a "Runner's High"?

During or after exercise, a person occasionally experiences feelings of euphoria. Runners and joggers call these feelings the "runner's high." However, these positive feelings of relaxation, high self-esteem, and reduced stress are not limited to runners. Almost any fitness activity can leave participants with these intense positive feelings. Swimmers, aerobic exercisers, hikers, and cyclists all have reported exercise-induced highs.

Although these pleasurable feelings can be attributed in part to psychological causes, there is plenty of scientific evidence to suggest a physiological cause. During physical activity, the brain releases its own morphinelike (opiate-like) substances called *endorphins*. These chemicals are released by brain neurons and produce sensations that are pleasurable, and sometimes even numbing. Exercisers report that these episodes of euphoria are unpredictable. Sometimes they experience highs and sometimes they do not. However, endorphin highs are more likely to occur during or after a strenuous, challenging workout.

How Should "30-Somethings" Alter Their Exercise Programs?

People who are in their 30s need to make few if any significant adjustments in their fitness programs. Men and women can continue physical activities they have used since their 20s. If they feel mired in activities that now seem boring, "30-somethings" might try a new activity. However, any new activity (or increase in the intensity of a current activity) should be undertaken gradually.

Should Women Exercise during Pregnancy?

Pregnant women should continue to exercise.[11] During pregnancy a woman's entire body undergoes many physical changes. Muscles are stretched, joints are loosened,

---

> **Key Terms**
>
> **osteoarthritis** arthritis that develops with age; largely caused by weight bearing and deterioration of the joints

and tissues are subjected to stress. If a woman is in good physiological condition, she is more likely to handle these changes with few complications. The baby may also benefit. Studies have shown that women who exercise moderately during pregnancy tend to give birth to healthier babies.[12]

Some reports suggest that exercise during pregnancy can make delivery of the baby easier and faster. Exercise can also help control her weight gain and improve her balance during pregnancy, and make it easier to get back to normal weight after delivery.

The types of exercises a woman should perform during pregnancy depend on the individual and the stage of pregnancy.[11] Most pregnant women should perform general exercises that increase overall fitness and stamina, as well as exercises that strengthen specific muscle groups. Muscles of the pelvic floor, for example, should be exercised regularly, because these muscles will be supporting most of the extra weight of the baby.

A variety of exercises are appropriate, including walking, swimming, stretching, and strengthening exercises. Yoga and tai chi are also good forms of exercise for pregnant women. The muscles of the pelvic floor, abdomen, and back are especially subject to stress and strain during pregnancy and delivery, so certain exercises can also be performed to strengthen these muscles. Exercises can also be performed to speed up recovery after delivery. Such postpartum exercises can be started in some cases within 24 hours after delivery. Exercises can even be started before conception if a pregnancy is anticipated.

Some types of exercise can put the fetus at risk. A pregnant woman should avoid any activity in which she becomes overheated, because her elevated body temperature will warm up the fetal environment. Thus pregnant women should not use saunas or hot tubs, nor should they exercise in a hot, humid environment. During the last trimester of pregnancy, women should also avoid any strenuous or high-impact exercise that involves bouncing, jumping, or jarring motions. Obviously, pregnant women should first consult with their obstetricians to develop a safe, productive exercise routine.

How Beneficial Is Aerobic Dance Exercise?

One of the most popular fitness approaches is aerobic exercise, including aerobic dancing. Many organizations sponsor classes in this form of continuous dancing and movement. The rise in popularity of aerobic exercise video programs reflects the enthusiasm for this form of exercise. Because extravagant claims are often made about the value of these programs, the wise consumer should observe at least one session of the activity before enrolling. Discover for yourself whether the program meets the criteria outlined earlier in this chapter in terms of

mode of activity, frequency, intensity, duration, resistance training, and flexibility training.

Street dancing, swing dancing, and Latin dancing have become some of the most popular aerobic exercises. Popularized by rap music, hip-hop music, and the growth of vigorous dancing in music videos, these forms of dancing provide an excellent way of having fun and maintaining cardiorespiratory fitness. Have you experienced the exhilaration that results from an hour or two of dancing?

What Are Low-Impact Aerobic Activities?

Because long-term participation in some aerobic activities (for example, jogging, running, aerobic dancing, and rope skipping) may lead to injury of the hip, knee, and ankle joints, many fitness experts promote low-impact aerobic activities. Low-impact aerobic dancing, water aerobics, bench aerobics, and brisk walking are examples of this kind of fitness activity. Participants still conform to the principal components of a cardiorespiratory fitness program. THR levels are the same as in high-impact aerobic activities.

The main difference between low-impact and high-impact aerobic activities is the use of the legs. Low-impact aerobics require having one foot on the ground at all times. Thus, weight transfer does not occur with the forcefulness seen in traditional, high-impact aerobic activities. In addition, low-impact activities may include exaggerated arm movements and the use of hand or wrist weights. All these variations are designed to increase the heart rate to the THR without undue strain on the joints of the lower extremities. Low-impact aerobics are excellent for people of all ages, and they may be especially beneficial to older adults.

In-line skating (rollerblading) is one of the fastest-growing fitness activities. This low-impact activity has cardiorespiratory and muscular benefits similar to those of running without the pounding effect that running can produce. However, it should be recognized that it requires both skill and balance. Rollerblading requires important safety equipment: sturdy skates, knee and elbow pads, wrist supports, and a helmet. Obviously, the potential for falling makes this a higher-risk activity.

What Is the Most Effective Means of Fluid Replacement during Exercise?

Despite all the advertising hype associated with commercial fluid-replacement products, for an average person involved in typical fitness activities, water is still the best fluid replacement. The availability and cost are unbeatable. However, when activity is prolonged and intense, commercial sport drinks may be preferred over water because they contain electrolytes (which replace lost sodium and potassium) and carbohydrates (which replace depleted energy stores). However, the carbohydrates in sports drinks are actually simple forms of sugar. Thus, sports drinks tend to be high in calories just like regular soft drinks. Regardless of the drink you choose, exercise physiologists recommend that you drink fluids before and at frequent intervals throughout the activity, particularly in warm, humid environments.

What Effect Does Alcohol Have on Sport Performance?

It probably comes as no surprise that alcohol use is generally detrimental to sport performance. Alcohol consumption, especially excessive intake the evening before an activity, consistently decreases the level of performance. Many research studies have documented the negative effects of alcohol on activities involving speed, strength, power, and endurance.[13]

Lowered performance appears to be related to a variety of factors, including impaired judgment, reduced coordination, depressed heart function, liver interference, and dehydration. Understandably, sports federations within the International Olympic Committee have banned the use of alcohol in conjunction with sports competition.

Only in the sports of precision shooting (pistol shooting, riflery, and archery) have studies shown that low-level alcohol use may improve performance, by reducing the shooter's anxiety and permitting steady hand movements. However, alcohol use has also been banned from these sports.[13]

Why Has Bodybuilding Become So Popular?

The popularity of bodybuilding has increased significantly in recent years for many reasons. Bodybuilders often start lifting weights to get into better shape—to improve muscle tone. They may just want to look healthier and feel stronger. When they realize that they can alter the shape of their bodies, they find that bodybuilding offers challenges that, through hard work, are attainable. Bodybuilders also report enjoying the physical sensations (the "pump") that result from a good workout. The results of their efforts are clearly visible and measurable. Some bodybuilders become involved in competitive events to test their advancements.

Perhaps we should dispel a few myths about bodybuilding. Are bodybuilders strong? The answer is emphatically— yes! Will muscle cells turn into fat cells if weight-lifting programs are discontinued? No, muscle cells are physiologically incapable of turning into fat cells. Will women develop bulky muscles through weight training? No, they can improve muscle size, strength, and tone, but unless they take steroids, their muscle mass cannot increase to the same degree as men's muscle mass. Is bodybuilding socially acceptable? Yes, for many people. Just observe all the health clubs and campus exercise rooms that cater to weightlifters and bodybuilders.

Where Can I Find Out about Proper Equipment?

College students are generally in an excellent setting to locate people who have the resources to provide helpful information about sports equipment. Contacting physical education, exercise science, or health education faculty members who have an interest in your chosen activity might be a good start. Most colleges also have a number of clubs that specialize in fitness interests—cycling, hiking, and jogging clubs, for example. Attend one of their upcoming meetings.

Sporting goods and specialty stores (for runners, tennis and racquetball players, and cyclists) are convenient places to obtain information. Employees of these stores should be knowledgeable about sports and equipment; however, keep in mind their primary job is selling a product. So *caveat emptor*. Try to gather as much information as you can so that you can make an informed decision. The Star box on pages 118–119 provides tips for choosing an athletic shoe, and the Star box on pages 119–120 discusses various popular types of home fitness equipment.

How Worthwhile Are Commercial Health and Fitness Clubs?

The health and fitness club business is booming. Fitness clubs offer activities ranging from free weights to weight machines to step walking to general aerobics. Some clubs have saunas and whirlpools and lots of frills. Others have course offerings that include wellness, smoking cessation, stress management, time management, dance, and yoga. The atmosphere at most clubs is friendly, and people are encouraged to have a good time while working out.

If your purpose in joining a fitness club is to improve your cardiorespiratory fitness, measure the program offered by the club against the ACSM standards. If your primary purpose in joining is to meet people and have fun, request a trial membership for a month or so to see whether you like the environment.

Before signing a contract at a health club or spa, do some careful questioning. Find out when the business was established, ask about the qualifications of the employees, contact some members for their observations, and request a thorough tour of the facilities. You might even consult your local Better Business Bureau for additional information. Finally, make certain that you read and understand every word of the contract.

Proper-fitting sports shoes can enhance performance and prevent injuries. The American Academy of Orthopaedic Surgeons[1] provide the following advice for consumers of athletic or exercise shoes.

- Try on athletic shoes after a workout or run and at the end of the day. Your feet will be at their largest.
- Wear the same type of sock that you will wear for that sport.
- When the shoe is on your foot, you should be able to freely wiggle all your toes.
- The shoes should be comfortable as soon as you try them on. There is no break-in period.
- Walk or run a few steps in your shoes. They should be comfortable.
- Always re-lace the shoes you are trying on. You should begin at the farthest eyelets and apply even pressure as you crisscross a lacing pattern to the top of the shoe.
- There should be a firm grip of the shoe to your heel. Your heel should not slip as you walk or run.
- If you participate in a sport three or more times a week, you need a sports-specific shoe.

It can be hard to choose from the many different types of athletic shoes available. There are differences in design and variations in material and weight. These differences have been developed to protect the areas of the feet that encounter the most stress in a particular athletic activity. Specific recommendations for choosing selected types of shoes are presented below.

Aerobic Shoes

Flexibility: more at ball of foot than running shoes; less flexible than court shoes or running shoes; sole is firmer than running shoes. Uppers: most are leather or leather-reinforced nylon. Heel: little or no flare. Soles: rubber if you dance on wood floors; polyurethane for other surfaces. Cushioning: more than court shoes; less than running shoes. Tread: Should be fairly flat, especially on forefoot; may also have "dot" on the ball of the foot for pivoting.

Court Shoes (Basketball, Tennis, Volleyball)

Soles: can be made from rubber for durability, EVA for lightweight cushioning, or polyurethane, which is both lightweight and durable. Flexibility: should be most flexible in the forefoot, for making jump shots. Cushioning: should absorb shock in the ball of the foot, for landing from jump shots. Heel: a snug-fitting heel cup is essential to keep the ankle in place; the shoe can be high-, mid-, or low-cut, depending on the amount of ankle support desired. Tread: for playing outdoors, the sole should be harder and the tread deeper; a smoother tread works well for playing on a court. Uppers: can be made of leather for durability or nylon or other synthetics for breathability.

Running Shoes

Heel: flare gives foot broader, more stable base. Soles: usually carbon-based for longer wear. Cushioning: more than court shoes, especially at heel. Tread: "waffle" or other deep-cut tread for grip on many surfaces.

Walking Shoes

Cushioning: can be forefoot and heel, or primarily forefoot or heel. Heel: may have some flare, similar to running shoes. Soles: typically polyurethane for durability. Tread: some tread for traction, but slightly flatter than running shoes.

[1]http://orthoinfo.aaos.org/fact/thr_report.cfm?Thread_ID=32&topcategory=Foot

continued

Cross-Training Shoes
Cushioning: can be forefoot and heel, or primarily forefoot or heel.
Tread: can be moderate to aggressive.

Home Cardiorespiratory Fitness Equipment

In the past 10 years, there has been an explosion in the purchase and use of home fitness equipment. This equipment is especially helpful for those who do not have access to health/fitness clubs, who prefer to exercise alone and at home, and who must exercise at irregular hours. It is advisable to thoroughly test out the equipment before purchase. Unfortunately, many people purchase a machine and seldom use it. Most forms of equipment can provide a good cardiorespiratory workout. However, people looking for a complete workout may have to add some strength training, such as barbell work, to their fitness program. A discussion of current popular devices follows.

Stationary Bicycles
Many models of stationary bikes are available, ranging in price from about $150 to $3,500 or more for a computerized exercise bike. Some upright bikes have a "dual action" component, whereby the user can "pump" extended handlebars for an upper-body workout. Other bikes allow the user to sit back while pedaling. These recumbent bikes take pressure off the lower back and permit the rider to exercise the hamstring muscles to a greater degree than do upright bikes. Bike training stands that allow the user to convert a regular bicycle into a stationary bike are also available.

Treadmills
Treadmills are relatively simple devices that consist of a moving belt stretched over two rollers. Two basic forms of treadmills are commonly used. The less expensive is the variety that is driven manually by the walking or running action of the user. Motorized treadmills are much more expensive and driven, of course, by an electric motor. The cost of a treadmill can range from several hundred dollars to nearly $15,000 for top-of-the-line models. Most electric models allow the user to change speeds and also the incline angle of the platform. Changing the incline angle can increase the intensity of the workout. First-time users are cautioned to start slowly and gradually become familiar with the motion of the motorized models. Getting on and off a moving belt can be potentially dangerous.

Stair Climbers
These devices allow the user to simulate climbing up a series of stair steps. This form of movement is much preferred to the actual, repetitive climbing of stairs that some people undertake in high-rise buildings. Stair climbers take much of the pressure off the knee joint. These machines vary in price from around $200 for the simplest lever model to $5,000 for a programmable model that varies the speed and the amount of resistance. Some models come with an upper-body component that allows the user to pump the arms while climbing.

Rowing Machines
Users of these machines exercise by simulating the movements involved in rowing a boat. Most brands have a sliding seat and movable handles that are similar to oars. Users push their feet against footplates while pulling back on the handles. The simplest models may cost around $300, and prices range up to more than $3,000 for health club models.

Elliptical Machines
Elliptical machines provide a movement pattern whereby the feet describe an ellipse, with the longer action aligned roughly parallel to the ground. This is the same pattern that we move in when we walk or run. Recent studies have found that these types of machines actually can require more involvement of the gluteals (buttocks) and the thigh muscles than can be obtained from treadmill or stationary cycles. These machines are the fastest growing segment of all cardiovascular exercise equipment. Costs range from several hundred to several thousand dollars.

Which Machine Is Best for You?
The machine that is best for you is the one that you enjoy using. All too often, exercise machines are given as birthday or holiday gifts and used consistently for only a short time. (Note all the ads for used fitness equipment in the classified ads section of your local paper.) Remember that machines can be somewhat specific in their focus. You may wish to broaden your workout with

continued

additional exercises or strength-building activities.

In terms of which device produces the greatest level of energy expenditure, a recent *Journal of the American Medical Association* article indicated that treadmill users walking or running "somewhat hard" expended (burned) more calories per hour than users of five other common home exercise machines. In this study, exercisers using a dual-action stationary bike and a regular stationary bike expended the fewest calories per hour.[1]

[1]Zeni AL, et al. Energy expenditure with indoor exercise machines. *JAMA* 8 May 1996; 275(18).

Considering Complementary Care

Popular Ergogenic Aids

Androstendione ("andro") and creatine have recently received much attention for their use as possible **ergogenic aids.** Ergogenic aids are supplements taken to improve athletic performance.[1] These products presently can be purchased legally in health food stores. Andro is a steroidlike precursor to the male hormone testosterone. When taken into the body, andro stimulates the body to produce more of its natural testosterone. Increased levels of testosterone help a person build lean muscle mass and recover more quickly from injuries.

Andro's primary use as an ergogenic aid is to build muscle tissue, improve overall body strength, and boost performance, especially in anaerobic sports. Andro is banned by the National Football League, the National Collegiate Athletic Association, and the International Olympic Committee. The health concerns that most physicians attribute to andro are similar to those of anabolic steroids.

Perhaps the most famous user of andro was Mark McGwire, baseball player for the St. Louis Cardinals. In the summer of 1998, McGwire rocked the baseball world by surpassing Roger Maris's home run record (he hit 61 home runs in 1961) by hitting 70 home runs. It is interesting, though, that during the 1999 baseball season, McGwire opted to stop using andro but still managed to hit nearly 70 home runs.

Creatine is an amino acid found in meat, poultry, and fish. In a person's body, creatine is produced naturally in the liver, pancreas, and kidneys. Typically, people consume 1 to 2 grams of creatine each day from their food intake.[1] As an ergogenic aid, creatine performs its work in the muscles, where it helps restore the compound adenosine triphosphate (ATP). ATP provides quick energy for muscle contractions. It also helps to reduce the lactic acid buildup that occurs during physical exertion. This buildup causes a burning sensation that limits the amount of intense activity one can perform.

Early studies suggest that creatine can help athletes in anaerobic sports, which require short, explosive bursts of energy. However, the increase in performance has been small, the long-term health effects are unknown, studies have been restricted to highly trained subjects (not recreational athletes), and damage to the kidneys is possible with high dosages. Users are cautioned to consume ample amounts of water to prevent cramping and dehydration.

All in all, creatine is unlikely to prove as potentially dangerous as androstendione. If additional studies should indicate that creatine can consistently improve performance, this substance might be banned by many sports governing bodies. The safest, most prudent recommendation is for athletes to spend their time and energy improving their training programs rather than looking for a solution in a bottle.

[1]The creatine craze. *UC Berkeley Wellness Letter* 1998; 14(3):6.

What Is Cross-Training?

Cross-training is the use of more than one aerobic activity to achieve cardiorespiratory fitness. For example, runners may use swimming, cycling, or rowing periodically to replace running in their training routines. Cross-training allows certain muscle groups to rest and injuries to heal. In addition, cross-training provides a refreshing change of pace for the participant. You will probably enjoy your fitness program more if you vary the activities.

What Are Steroids, and Why Do Some Athletes Use Them?

Steroids are drugs that physicians can legally prescribe for a variety of health conditions, including certain forms of anemia, inadequate growth patterns, and chronic debilitating diseases. Steroids can also be prescribed to aid recovery from surgery or burns. **Anabolic steroids** are drugs that function like the male sex hormone testosterone. They can be taken orally or by injection (see the Considering Complementary Care box above).

> ### Key Terms
>
> **ergogenic aids** supplements that are taken to improve athletic performance
>
> **anabolic steroids** (ann uh **bol** ick) drugs that function like testosterone to produce increases in weight, strength, endurance, and aggressiveness

Figure 4-2 Effects of steroids on various parts of the body

Brain
Increased hostility can lead to tranquilizer use, hypertension, psychological dependence, and eating compulsions; increases aggression, which makes injuries more probable

Face
Facial hair growth, body hair growth, and baldness in women; acne in both men and women

Throat
Deepening of voice in women

Chest
Breast growth in men; breast cancer and decreased breast size in women

Heart
High blood pressure, clogging of arteries

Liver and prostate
Liver cancer in men and women; prostate cancer in men

Genitals
Sterility or atrophied testicles in men; menstrual irregularities, enlarged genitals in women

Arms, chest, and legs
Helps stimulate muscle growth, decreases recovery time needed between workouts

 TALKING POINTS If you suspected a young person you know was using steroids, what strategies would you use to encourage the person to change his or her behavior?

Anabolic steroids are used by athletes who hope to gain weight, muscular size and strength, power, endurance, and aggressiveness. Over the last few decades, many bodybuilders, weightlifters, track athletes, and football players have chosen to ignore the serious health risks posed by illegal steroid use. More recently, steroid use among high school and college campuses has reached epidemic levels. The mass media has begun to focus attention on the dangers of steroid use, but many young athletes choose to ignore these warnings.

The use of steroids is highly dangerous because of serious, life-threatening side effects and adverse reactions. These effects include heart problems, certain forms of cancer, liver complications, and even psychological disturbances. The side effects on female steroid users are as dangerous as those on men. Figure 4-2 shows the adverse effects of steroid use.

Steroid users have developed a terminology of their own. Anabolic steroids are called "roids" or "juice." "Roid rage" is an aggressive, psychotic response to chronic steroid use. "Stacking" is a term that describes the use of multiple steroids at the same time.

Many organizations that control athletic competition (such as the National Collegiate Athletic Association or the NCAA, The Athletics Congress, the National Football League, and the International Olympic Committee) have banned steroids and are testing athletes for illegal use. Fortunately, some athletes finally seem to be getting the message and are steering clear of steroids.

What Is the Female Athlete Triad?

In the early 1990s, the ACSM identified a three-part syndrome of disordered eating, **amenorrhea** (lack of menstruation), and osteoporosis as the female athlete triad.[14] The conditions of this syndrome appear independently in many women, but among female athletes they appear together. The female athlete triad is most likely to be found in athletes whose sport activities emphasize appearance (for example, diving, ice skating, or gymnastics) and can also be observed in women who become compulsive exercisers.

Key Terms
amenorrhea cessation of or lack of menstrual periods

Activities to Promote Sound Sleep

Can we work at being better sleepers? The answer is yes. Many activities, when done at the appropriate time, will aid in the quest for sound sleep.

Activities for the Day

Schedule. Maintain a consistent schedule of daily activities; a disrupted day makes sleeping difficult.

Physical activity. Regular vigorous activity promotes sleep; exercising too near bedtime, however, can make you too energized to sleep soundly.

Eating. A large meal taken late in the evening interferes with sleeping; avoid heavy late-night snacks as well.

Alcohol use. A single drink in the evening may be relaxing, but too many drinks during the day can make sleeping difficult.

Central nervous system (CNS) stimulants. Coffee, tea, soft drinks with caffeine, and some medications can disrupt normal sleeping patterns.

Worry. Problems and concerns should be put behind you by the time you retire for the night; practice leaving your concerns at the office or in the classroom.

Rituals. A ritualistic "winding down" over the course of the evening promotes sleep; watching television, listening to music, and reading during the evening are excellent ways to prepare the body for sleep.

Activities for the End of the Day

Bathing. For many people, a warm bath immediately before retiring promotes sleep.

Yoga. The quiet, relaxing exercises of yoga promote sleep by slowing the body's activity level.

Snack or nightcap. A light snack of foods high in l-tryptophan (for example, eggs, tuna, and turkey) and a glass of milk will help you fall asleep.

Muscular relaxation. Alternating contraction and relaxation of the large muscles of the extremities aids the body in falling asleep.

Imaging. Quieting images can distract the mind, thus allowing you to fall asleep more easily.

Fantasies. Escaping into fantasies slows the mind and encourages the onset of sleep.

Breathing. Slow, deep breaths set a restful rhythm the body can "ride" into sleep.

Thinking. By envisioning yourself as sleeping soundly, you may actually fall asleep quicker.

InfoLinks

www.sleepnet.com

Parents, coaches, athletic trainers, teammates, and friends should be watchful for signs of the female athlete triad. This syndrome has associated medical risks, including inadequate fuel supply for activities, inadequate iron intake, reduced cognitive function, altered hormone levels, reduced mental health, early onset of menopause, increased likelihood of skeletal trauma, altered blood fat profiles, and increased vulnerability to heart disease.[14] Vitally important is an early referral to a physician who is knowledgeable about the female athlete triad. The physician will likely coordinate efforts with a psychologist, a nutritionist, and an athletic trainer to improve the health of the athlete and prevent recurrences.

Are Today's Children Physically Fit?

Major research studies published during the last 10 years have indicated that U.S. children and teenagers lead very sedentary lives. Children ages 6 to 17 score extremely poorly in the areas of strength, flexibility, and cardiorespiratory endurance. In many cases, parents are in better shape than their children are. A major consequence of these sedentary habits in children is obesity.

The 1999–2000 National Health and Nutrition Examination Survey (NHANES) indicates that 15 percent of children and adolescents ages 6 to 19 years are overweight. Indeed, from NHANES II (1976–80) to NHANES III (1988–1994), the prevalence of overweight nearly doubled among children and adolescents and has continued to rise. The seriousness of these data is revealed by the fact that most obese children become obese adults.

This situation presents a challenge to educators and parents to emphasize the need for strenuous play activity. Television watching and parental inactivity were implicated as major factors in these studies.

How Does Sleep Contribute to Overall Fitness?

Sleep is an important adjunct to a well-planned exercise program (see the Changing for the Better box above). Sleep is so vital to health that people who are unable to sleep sufficiently (those with insomnia) or who are deprived of sleep experience deterioration in every dimension of their health. Fortunately, exercise is frequently associated with improvement in sleeping.

The value of sleep is apparent in a variety of positive changes in the body. Dreaming is thought to play an important role in supporting the emotional dimension of health. Problem-solving scenarios that occur during dreams seem to afford some carryover value in actual coping experiences. A variety of changes in physiological functioning, particularly a deceleration of the cardiovascular system, occur during sleep. The feeling of being well rested is an expression of the mental and physiological rejuvenation one feels after a good night's sleep.

The amount of sleep needed varies among people. In fact, for any person, sleep needs vary according to activity level and overall state of health. As we age, the need for sleep appears to decrease from the six to eight hours young adults require. Elderly people routinely sleep less than they did when they were younger. This decrease may be offset by the short naps older people often take during the day. For all people, however, periods of relaxation, daydreaming, and even an occasional afternoon nap promote electrical activity patterns that help regenerate the mind and body.

What Exercise Danger Signs Should I Watch For?

The human body is an amazing piece of equipment. It functions well regardless of whether you are conscious of its processes. It also delivers clear signals when something goes wrong.

You should monitor any sign that seems abnormal during or after your exercise. "Listen to your body" is a good rule for self-awareness. The Changing for the Better box lists some common warning signs to monitor.

However, such occurrences are extremely unusual. Fear of developing these difficulties should not deter you from starting a fitness program. These risks are minimal—and the benefits far outweigh the risks. Sports injuries are discussed further in the following section.

Sports Injuries

At any time during your participation in fitness or sport activities, it is possible that you will become injured, even if you carefully warm up before your exercise and cool down after your exercise. If you are lucky, the injury will be only a minor one and after a short period of rest you will be able to resume your fitness interests. Sometimes, however, an injury can be significant and require you to seek medical care and undergo extensive rehabilitation.

It is beyond the scope of this textbook to provide a comprehensive discussion of the prevention, care, and

Changing for the Better

Exercise Danger Signs

- A delay of more than one hour in your body's return to a fully relaxed, comfortable state after exercise.
- A change in sleep patterns.
- Any noticeable breathing difficulties or chest pains. Exercise at your THR should not initiate these problems, so you should consult a physician if you experience them.
- Persistent joint or muscle pain. Any lingering joint or muscle pain might signal a problem. Seek the help of an athletic trainer, a physical therapist, or your physician.
- Unusual changes in urine composition or output. Marked color change in your urine could signal possible kidney or bladder difficulties. Drink plenty of water before, during, and after you participate in your activity.
- Anything unusual that you notice after starting your fitness program. Examples are headaches, nosebleeds, fainting, numbness in an extremity, and hemorrhoids.

treatment of sports injuries. (You can find this information in an athletic training textbook, a fitness textbook, or a sports medicine book.) However, here we provide you with some general principles related to the prevention and care of sports injuries and a table that lists many common fitness injuries.[15] (See Table 4.1.)

1. *A well-planned fitness program starts at a low level and progresses gradually and consistently.* This principle supports the concept of starting at a level of activity that can be handled comfortably. If the activity is a walking program, an unfit person should not begin with walks of five or six miles a day but should start with a shorter distance and gradually add additional distance in a consistent manner to avoid muscle, skeletal, or joint injuries.
2. *If you stop exercising for an extended time, do not restart the activity at the level at which you stopped.* Do not plan on returning to a high level of activity if you have been inactive for an extended time. Rather, reduce your activity significantly and gradually return to your earlier levels of activity.
3. *"Listen to your body."* Always be aware of the nature of your body as you are exercising. If you sense that something is wrong, stop the activity and assess the situation. For example, if you think you might be hurting your back or that a joint or muscle is being strained, stop and evaluate the situation. If you think something is wrong, by all means don't test your

body by returning to the activity. (Have you ever seen a person with a suspected ankle injury "test" the ankle by hopping up and down on the injured leg? This makes no sense at all.) Pain indicates that something is wrong. If this is the case, seek a professional evaluation, perhaps from an athletic trainer or a physical therapist. A physician, especially one trained in sports medicine, can make an accurate diagnosis of the injury.

4. *Follow the rehabilitation instructions carefully.* Athletic trainers and physical therapists are trained to design effective rehabilitation programs. If you are injured, it is very important that you follow the advice of these professionals. This is especially true in cases where you start to feel better before the rehabilitation program is finished. Even though you feel better, your body may not be fully recovered. A return to activity too quickly may result in an even more serious injury than your original one. (This is especially true for adults over the age of 40.) The best advice is to resist the urge to return to your activity until you are given full clearance from your trainer or therapist.

5. *Develop a prevention approach.* After you recover from an injury, try to discover ways to prevent that injury from happening again. Learn about proper stretching exercises, effective strength-training activities,

Table 4.1 Common Injuries Associated with Physical Activity

Injury	Condition
Achilles tendinitis	A chronic tendinitis of the "heel cord" or muscle tendon, located on the back of the lower leg just above the heel. It may result from any activity that involves forcefully pushing off with the foot and ankle, such as in running and jumping. This inflammation involves swelling, warmth, tenderness to touch, and pain during walking and especially running.
Ankle sprains	Stretching or tearing of one or several ligaments that provide stability to the ankle joint. Ligaments on the outside or lateral side of the ankle are more commonly injured by rolling the sole of the foot downward and toward the inside. Pain is intense immediately after injury, followed by considerable swelling, tenderness, loss of joint motion, and some discoloration over a 24- to 48-hour period.
Groin pull	A muscle strain that occurs in the muscles located on the inside of the upper thigh just below the pubic area and that results from either an overstretch of the muscle or from a contraction of the muscle that meets excessive resistance. Pain will be produced by flexing the hip and leg across the body or by stretching the muscles in a groin-stretch position.
Hamstring pull	A strain of the muscles on the back of the upper thigh that most often occurs while sprinting. In most cases, severe pain is caused simply by walking or in any movement that involves knee flexion or stretch of the hamstring muscle. Some swelling, tenderness to touch, and possibly some discoloration extending down the back of the leg may occur in severe strains.
Patellofemoral knee pain	Nonspecific pain occurring around the knee, particularly the front part of the knee, or in the kneecap (patella). Pain can result from many causes, including improper movement of the kneecap in knee flexion and extension; tendinitis of the tendon just below the kneecap, which is caused by repetitive jumping; bursitis (swelling) either above or below the kneecap; and osteoarthritis (joint surface degeneration) between the kneecap and thigh bone. It may involve inflammation with swelling, tenderness, warmth, and pain associated with movement.
Quadriceps contusion "charley horse"	A deep bruise of the muscles in the front part of the thigh caused by a forceful impact or by some object that results in severe pain, swelling, discoloration, and difficulty flexing the knee or extending the hip. Without adequate rest and protection from additional trauma, small calcium deposits may develop in the muscle.
Shin splints	A catch-all term used to refer to any pain that occurs in the front part of the lower leg or shin, most often caused by excessive running on hard surfaces. Pain is usually caused by strain of the muscles that move the ankle and foot at their attachment points in the shin. It is usually worse during activity. In more severe cases it may be caused by stress fractures of the long bones in the lower leg, with the pain being worse after activity is stopped.
Shoulder impingement	Chronic irritation and inflammation of muscle tendons and a bursa underneath the tip of the shoulder, which results from repeated forceful overhead motions of the shoulder, such as in swimming, throwing, spiking a volleyball, or serving a tennis ball. Pain is felt when the arm is extended across the body above shoulder level.
Tennis elbow	Chronic irritation and inflammation of the lateral or outside surface of the arm just above the elbow at the attachment of the muscles that extend the wrist and fingers. It results from any activity that requires forceful extension of the wrist. Typically occurs in tennis players who are using faulty techniques hitting backhand ground strokes. Pain is felt above the elbow after forcefully extending the wrist against resistance or applying pressure over the muscle attachment above the elbow.

appropriate equipment, and the proper mechanics for your selected sports/fitness activities. Use this collective knowledge to prevent the injury from recurring.

For example, if you have injured your hamstring muscles while running, you will need to learn how to effectively stretch these muscles in the future. You will also need to learn how to strengthen these muscles

through resistance training. If your running shoes are old and worn, they may have to be replaced. Finally, don't run too fast before warming up; start slowly and gradually increase your speed after the muscles are fully warmed up. Preventive actions such as these will allow you to have a fitness program that is not regularly interrupted by a nagging injury.

Taking Charge of Your Health

- Assess your level of fitness by completing the National Fitness Test on pages 127–128.

- Start a daily stretching program based on the guidelines in this chapter.

- Implement or maintain a cardiorespiratory fitness program that uses the most recent American College of Sports Medicine recommendations.

- Examine your athletic shoes to determine their appropriateness for the fitness activities you do (see Choosing an Athletic Shoe on pages 118–119).

- Monitor your physical activities for potential danger signs indicating that you should consult an athletic trainer, physical therapist, or physician.

- For 2 weeks, keep track of the amount of sleep you are getting. Determine whether this is enough sleep, and make adjustments accordingly.

SUMMARY

- Physical fitness allows one to avoid illness, perform routine activities, and respond to emergencies.
- The health benefits of exercise can be achieved through regular, moderate exercise.
- Fitness comprises four components: cardiorespiratory endurance, muscular fitness, flexibility, and body composition.
- The American College of Sports Medicine's program for cardiorespiratory fitness has four components: (1) mode of activity, (2) frequency of training, (3) intensity of training, and (4) duration of training. Additionally, ACSM now recommends that everyone also include (5) resistance training and (6) flexibility training.
- The target heart rate (THR) refers to the number of times per minute the heart must contract to produce a training effect.

- Training sessions should take place in three phases: warm-up, workout, and cooldown.
- Static stretching is the recommended type of stretching.
- Fitness experts are concerned about the lack of fitness in today's youth.
- Street dancing, swing dancing, step aerobics, and rollerblading are currently popular aerobic activities.
- Low-impact aerobic activities have a lower risk of muscle and joint injuries than do high-impact activities.
- College students who are interested in fitness should be as knowledgeable as possible about the important topics of steroid use, cross-training, fluid replacement, bodybuilding, and proper sleep.
- Following a few simple principles can help prevent many common sports injuries.

REVIEW QUESTIONS

1. Identify the four components of fitness described in this chapter. How does each component relate to physical fitness?
2. What is the difference between anaerobic and aerobic energy production? What types of activities are associated with anaerobic energy production? With aerobic energy production?
3. List some of the benefits of aerobic fitness.
4. Describe the various methods used to promote muscular fitness.
5. What does the principle of overload mean in regard to fitness training programs?

6. Identify the ACSM's six components of an effective cardiorespiratory conditioning program. Explain the important aspects of each component.
7. Under what circumstances should you see a physician before starting a physical fitness program?
8. Identify and describe the three parts of a training session.
9. Describe some of the negative consequences of anabolic steroid use.
10. How can people improve their sleeping habits?
11. Describe the three-part female athlete triad.
12. Discuss the five basic principles important in avoiding sports injuries.

ENDNOTES

1. U.S. Department of Health and Human Services. *Physical Activity and Health: A Report of the Surgeon General.* Atlanta, GA: U.S. Department of Health and Human Services, Centers for Disease Control and Prevention, National Center for Chronic Disease Prevention and Health Promotion, 1996.

2. Casperson C, et al. *Public Health Reports* 100: 126, 1985.

3. American Heart Association, Councils on Clinical Cardiology and Nutrition, Physical Activity and Metabolism. *Exercise and Physical Activity in the Prevention and Treatment of Atherosclerotic Cardiovascular Disease.* Circulation; 107:3109, 2003.

4. Brubaker PH, Kaminksy LA, Whaley HM. Coronary artery disease. *Human Kinetics,* 2002.

5. Ferrini AF, Ferrini RL. *Health in Later Years* (2nd ed.). Guilford, CT: Brown & Benchmark, 1992.

6. Rubin R. Brittle bones: Promising strides against osteoporosis mean better, longer life for the elderly. *USA Today* 2000 March 28:1D.

7. American College of Sports Medicine. Position stand on the recommended quantity and quality of exercise for developing and maintaining cardiorespiratory and muscular fitness and flexibility in healthy adults. *Med Sci Sports Exerc* 1998; 30(6):975–991.

8. White MD. *Water Exercise.* Champaign, IL: Human Kinetics, 1995.

9. An exercise prescription for older people. *Harvard Health Letter* 1998; 8(10):1–4.

10. American College of Sports Medicine. *Guidelines for Exercise Testing and Prescription* (7th ed.). Philadelphia: Lippincott, Williams, and Wilkins, 2005.

11. Kaehler K, Tivers C. *Primetime pregnancy: The proven program for staying in shape before and after your baby is born.* Lincolnwood, IL: Contemporary Books, 1997.

12. Williams RD. Healthy pregnancy, healthy baby. *FDA Consumer* 1999; 33(2):18–23.

13. Williams MH. Alcohol and sports performance. *Sports Sci Exch* 1992; 4(40):1–4.

14. Stevens WC, Brey RA, Harris JE, Fowlkes-Godek S. The dangerous trio: A case study approach to the female athlete triad. *Athletic Therapy Today* 1997; 2(2):30–36.

15. Prentice WE. *Fitness for Wellness and Life* (6th ed.). New York: McGraw-Hill College Division, 1998.

personal assessment

What is your level of fitness?

You can determine your level of fitness in 30 minutes or less by completing this short group of tests based on the National Fitness Test developed by the President's Council on Physical Fitness and Sports. If you are over 40 years old or have chronic medical disorders such as diabetes or obesity, check with your physician before taking this or any other fitness test. You will need another person to monitor your test and keep time.

Three-Minute Step Test

Aerobic capacity. Equipment: 12-inch bench, crate, block, or step ladder; stopwatch. Procedure: face bench. Complete 24 full steps (both feet on the bench, both feet on the ground) per minute for 3 minutes. After finishing, sit down, have your partner find your pulse within 5 seconds, and take your pulse for 1 minute. Your score is your pulse rate for 1 full minute.

	Scoring standards (heart rate for 1 minute)									
Age	18–29		30–39		40–49		50–59		60+	
Gender	F	M	F	M	F	M	F	M	F	M
Excellent	<80	<75	<84	<78	<88	<80	<92	<85	<95	<90
Good	80–110	75–100	84–115	78–109	88–118	80–112	92–123	85–115	95–127	90–118
Average	>110	>100	>115	>109	>118	>112	>123	>115	>127	>118

Sit and Reach

Hamstring flexibility. Equipment: yardstick; tape. Positioned parallel to your legs and between them, tape a yardstick to the floor. Sit with legs straight and heels about 5 inches apart, heels even with the 15-inch mark on the yardstick. While in a sitting position, slowly stretch forward as far as possible. Your score is the number of inches reached.

	Scoring standards (inches)									
Age	18–29		30–39		40–49		50–59		60+	
Gender	F	M	F	M	F	M	F	M	F	M
Excellent	>22	>21	>22	>21	>21	>20	>20	>19	>20	>19
Good	17–22	13–21	17–22	13–21	15–21	13–20	14–20	12–19	14–20	12–19
Average	<17	<13	<17	<13	<15	<13	<14	<12	<14	<12

Arm Hang

Upper body strength. Equipment: horizontal bar (high enough to prevent your feet from touching the floor); stopwatch. Procedure: hang with straight arms, palms facing forward. Start watch when subject is in position. Stop when subject lets go. Your score is the number of minutes and seconds spent hanging.

Scoring standards (hanging time)

Age	18–29		30–39		40–49		50–59		60+	
Gender	F	M	F	M	F	M	F	M	F	M
Excellent	>1:30	>2:00	>1:20	>1:50	>1:10	>1:35	>1:00	>1:20	>:50	>1:10
Good	:46–1:30	1:00–2:00	:40–1:20	:50–1:50	:30–1:10	:45–1:35	:30–1:00	:35–1:20	:21–:50	:30–1:10
Average	<:46	<1:00	<:40	<:50	<:30	<:45	<:30	<:35	<:21	<:30

Curl-Ups

Abdominal and low back strength. Equipment: stopwatch. Procedure: Lie flat on upper back, knees bent, shoulders touching the floor, arms extended above your thighs or by your sides, palms down. Bend knees so that feet are flat and 12 inches from the buttocks. Curl up by lifting head and shoulders off the floor, sliding hands forward above your thighs or the floor. Curl down and repeat. Your score is the number of curl-ups in 1 minute.

Scoring standards (number in 1 minute)

Age	18–29		30–39		40–49		50–59		60+	
Gender	F	M	F	M	F	M	F	M	F	M
Excellent	>45	>50	>40	>45	>35	>40	>30	>35	>25	>30
Good	25–45	30–50	20–40	22–45	16–35	21–40	12–30	18–35	11–25	15–30
Average	<25	<30	<20	<22	<16	<21	<12	<18	<11	<15

Push-Ups (Men)

Upper body strength. Equipment: stopwatch. Assume a front-leaning position. Lower your body until chest touches the floor. Raise and repeat for 1 minute. Your score is the number of push-ups completed in 1 minute.

Scoring standards (number in 1 minute)

Age	18–29	30–39	40–49	50–59	60+
Excellent	>50	>45	>40	>35	>30
Good	25–50	22–45	19–40	15–35	10–30
Average	<25	<22	<19	<15	<10

Modified Push-Ups (Women)

Upper body strength. Equipment: stopwatch. Assume a front-leaning position with knees bent up, hands under shoulders. Lower your chest to the floor, raise, and repeat. Your score is the number of push-ups completed in 1 minute.

Scoring standards (number in 1 minute)

Age	18–29	30–39	40–49	50–59	60+
Excellent	>45	>40	>35	>30	>25
Good	17–45	12–40	8–35	6–30	5–25
Average	<17	<12	<8	<6	<5

To Carry This Further . . .

Note your areas of strengths and weaknesses. To improve your fitness, become involved in a fitness program that reflects the concepts discussed in this chapter. Talking with fitness experts on your campus might be a good first step.

chapter five

Understanding Nutrition and Your Diet

Chapter Objectives

On completing this chapter, you will be able to:

▌ name and describe the seven types of nutrients.

▌ describe saturated, monounsaturated, and polyunsaturated fats, and explain their effects on the human body.

▌ discuss the recent growth in fat-free foods and their possible advantages and disadvantages.

▌ define complete protein foods and incomplete protein foods, and give examples of each.

▌ describe three processes that vitamins help perform in the body.

▌ discuss the roles of minerals and water in the body.

▌ describe the benefits of soluble and insoluble fiber.

▌ describe the new Food Guide Pyramids and the USDA's dietary recommendations.

▌ describe foodborne illnesses and strategies for preventing them.

▌ name three types of vegetarian diets and describe the advantages and disadvantages of each.

Eye on the Media

How Low Is Low Carb?

We see advertising for "low carbs" on candy bars, chips, peanut butter, and even on beer. Restaurants have jumped on the low-carb bandwagon by putting low-carb choices on their menus. But what does "low carb" mean? Well, if you ask 10 different people, you may get 10 different answers, because there is no one answer. Currently there is no standard definition as to how few carbohydrates a product must contain to qualify as low carb. With the recent low-carb craze, the FDA has been subject to increased pressure to issue guidelines for what can be called "low carb." We saw a similar phenomenon with the low-fat and low-calorie craze; these terms were not defined by the FDA until foodmakers started using them on packaging, creating confusion and misinformation. The FDA eventually standardized the use of "low-fat" for advertising and packaging.

Many gimmicks are used to advertise and portray foods as having few carbohydrates, including phrases such as carb smart, carb aware, carb sense, low-carb lifestyles, carb free, carb conscious, and carb wise. Note the words linked with a low carbohydrate level—wise, smart, free, intelligent. Does this make a difference to the consumer or the manufacturer? Absolutely; sales have tripled for products that remain unchanged except for adding something on their packaging that suggests low carbs.

Actually, this type of advertising is illegal, because the FDA prohibits any nutrient claim that it hasn't defined. However, this fact doesn't seem to have stopped the tidal wave of low-carb advertising. "Net carb" is another phrase commonly being tossed around that has not been standardized or defined by the FDA. This term has been used to refer to the net effect that carbs have after one subtracts from the product the sugar, alcohol, fiber, and other carbohydrates that supposedly have a minimal effect on blood sugar. This approach is misleading and confusing to the consumer as well as being illegal, because it has not been approved by the FDA.

For now, the FDA is sending warnings to companies such as Russell Stover Candies and Peak Performance about mislabeling their products as low carb. Many companies are becoming more creative in the way they package their foods, using terms such as "good for a low-carb lifestyle" or "great for low-carb diets." Foodmakers are also limiting how much they are packaging so that they can be ready to change their advertising quickly, with little loss in revenue, in anticipation of the FDA's ruling. It's probably only a matter of time before the FDA defines what can be called "low carb"; in the meantime, in the absence of FDA regulation, it would be prudent for consumers to be wary of anything that claims to be low carb.

Sources:
"What Does It Mean to Be Low Carb?" *USA Today,* May 25, 2004.
"Cashing In on the Low-Carb Craze," *Nutrition Action,* March 2004.
"FDA Recommends Changes to Food Labels," *USA Today,* March 12, 2004.

Healthy eating is important from the prenatal period throughout life, in order to prevent malnourishment and minimize the development of illnesses. Food supports growth and development by providing the body with the nutrients needed for energy, repair of damaged tissue, growth of new tissue, and regulation of physiological processes, all of which support full participation in the activities that constitute our days, weeks, months, and years of living. But our diets are more than that. Our food selections reflect personal, familial, and cultural traditions. The preparation and serving of food at regular mealtimes and during holiday gatherings and other special occasions enhance all of the dimensions of health. For example, sharing a meal with fellow parishioners after a religious service supports the spiritual dimension of health; sharing popcorn at the movies with your friends can enhance the social dimension of health; and learning about the cuisine of another culture develops the cultural dimension of health. As you read this chapter, keep in mind this balanced view of food as sustenance and food as a resource for the dimensions of health.

Types and Sources of Nutrients

Your body relies on seven **nutrients** to carry out its physiological functions: carbohydrates, fats, protein, vitamins, minerals, dietary fiber, and water.* The first three—carbohydrates, fats, and protein—will be discussed together because they provide **calories.** [†] These calories are either used quickly by our bodies in energy metabolism or are stored in the form of glycogen or fat for delayed use as energy sources. The other nutrients—vitamins, minerals, dietary fiber, and water—are not sources of calories for the body. However, regardless of their relationship to calories, all nutrients are essential to human health. The function of each is discussed later in the chapter.

Carbohydrates

Carbohydrates are various combinations of sugar units, or saccharides, and are the major energy source for the body. Each gram of carbohydrate contains 4 calories. Since the average person requires approximately 2,000 calories per day and about 45–65 percent of our calories come from carbohydrates, it is recommended that

---

*Since most of our water intake comes from beverages rather than from food, some nutritionists do not consider water a nutrient, even though it is essential for life.

†The term *calorie* is used here to refer to a *kilocalorie* (1,000 calories), which is the accepted scientific expression of the energy value of a food.

Table 5.1 Find Your Calorie Count

The number of calories your body needs daily is based on age, gender, and lifestyle. While many people structure their diets around a 2,000-calorie plan, the actual number of calories an individual needs to maintain energy and health could be more or less than that amount. Look for your daily calorie requirements on the chart below.

| Gender | Age | ACTIVITY LEVEL | | |
		Sedentary	Moderately active	Active
Child	2–3	1,000	1,000–1,400	1,000–1,400
Female	4–8	1,200	1,400–1,600	1,400–1,800
	9–13	1,600	1,600–2,000	1,800–2,200
	14–18	1,800	2,000	2,400
	19–30	2,000	2,000–2,200	2,400
	31–50	1,800	2,000	2,200
	51+	1,600	1,800	2,000–2,200
Male	4–8	1,400	1,400–1,600	1,600–2,000
	9–13	1,800	1,800–2,200	2,000–2,600
	14–18	2,200	2,400–2,800	2,800–3,200
	19–30	2,400	2,600–2,800	3,000
	31–50	2,200	2,400–2,600	2,800–3,000
	51+	2,000	2,200–2,400	2,400–2,800

Sedentary means a lifestyle that includes only the light physical activity associated with typical day-to-day life.
Moderately active means a lifestyle that includes physical activity equivalent to walking about 1.5 to 3 miles per day at 3 to 4 miles per hour, in addition to the light physical activity associated with typical day-to-day life.
Active means a lifestyle that includes physical activity equivalent to walking more than 3 miles per day at 3 to 4 miles per hour, in addition to the light physical activity associated with typical day-to-day life.

Source: Dietary Guidelines for Americans 2005.

approximately 1,200 of our daily caloric intake come from carbohydrates.[1] However, age, gender, and activity level affect the number of calories an individual requires each day (see Table 5.1).

Key Terms

nutrients elements in foods that are required for the growth, repair, and regulation of body processes

calories units of heat (energy); specifically, 1 calorie is the amount of energy needed to raise the temperature of 1 gram of water by 1°C

carbohydrates the body's primary source of energy for all body functioning; carbohydrates are chemical compounds including sugar, starches, and dietary fibers

Mealtime—A Chance to Share and Bond

Food is important to your physical well-being—for energy, growth, repair, and regulation of your body and its functions. But it's also important to the well-being of your spirit. The sharing of food nourishes our spiritual sense of community. This happens through the type of foods selected, the method of preparation, the uniqueness of presentation, and the people involved. From a spiritual perspective, the sharing of food can be a highly satisfying activity.

When food is shared in the company of those who care about us in the deepest and most personal ways, we experience a sense of community and well-being. The simple act of being together and engaged in a familiar and comfortable practice is reassuring. Meals that involve family or friends, especially dinners for special occasions or important holidays, can be particularly rewarding.

Food is often at the center of the celebration of special occasions. Weddings, birthdays, anniversaries, graduations, promotions, retirements, and funerals take on a special meaning when people come together to share food and drink. From the first birthday cake through the retirement dinner to the lunch provided by neighbors after the funeral of a loved one, food can help to symbolize and acknowledge these events in our lives.

Food has been part of many religious practices and customs for centuries. Some foods have symbolic meanings related to major life experiences, and ceremonies and religious rites. Food can take on symbolic and spiritual meaning, such as bread representing the body of Christ in the Christian religion. The use of food in spirituality helps to bring groups together to build a stronger sense of community. For example, Ramadan, the ninth month of the Islamic Calendar, is considered one of the holiest months of the year in Islam, and from dawn to sunset Muslims abstain from food. The fast is broken at sunset when families and friends come together and enjoy traditional dishes such as fattoushi, a salad. For Jews, the Seder is the most important event in the Passover celebration. Gathering family and friends together, the Seder maintains long-held traditions and customs involving food. The home is cleaned and cleared of all leavened food (foods containing yeast) and grains, and only foods that are kosher are consumed. In the Christian religion, family and friends celebrate Easter by having a meal together on Easter Sunday, usually including lamb, which represents Christ and is seen as a good omen.

Finally, food connects people on a spiritual level by allowing them to share traditions, religious practices, and beliefs. These customs help people build a sense of fellowship and can unify them in times of joy and sorrow.

Carbohydrates occur in three forms, depending on the number of saccharide (sugar) units that make up the molecule:

- *Monosaccharides—carbohydrates with one saccharide unit.* These are the primary source of the body's energy. Examples include glucose, found in vegetables, honey, fruits, and syrup; and fructose, found in fruits and berries.

- *Disaccharides—carbohydrates with two saccharide units, one of which is always a glucose unit.* Examples include sucrose, or table sugar; maltose, which is derived from germinating cereals; and lactose, found in human and animal milk.

- *Polysaccharides—carbohydrates with more than two saccharide units.* Polysaccharides are referred to as starches.

Starches are found primarily in vegetables, fruits, and grains. Starches provide much overall nutrition benefit since most starch sources also contain significant amounts of vitamins, minerals, protein, and water. Dietary fiber is also a polysaccharide. Starches play an important role in all the dietary recommendations discussed later in the chapter.

The average adult American consumes approximately 150 pounds of sweeteners (sugar, corn sweetener, syrup, and honey) each year,[2] usually in colas, candies, and pastries, which offer few additional nutritional benefits. For years the consumption of sweeteners (particularly table sugar) was implicated in a number of major health concerns, including obesity, nutrient deficiencies, behavioral disorders, cavities, diabetes, and cardiovascular disease. With the exception of dental cavities, current scientific data fail to confirm that sugar directly causes any of these health problems. However, the inability of some people to digest milk sugar (lactose) is well documented. Lactose intolerance can be effectively managed.

Much of the sugar we consume is hidden; that is, sugar is a principal product we may overlook in a large number of food items. Foods such as ketchup, salad dressings, cured meat products, and canned vegetables and fruits can contain much hidden sugar. Corn syrup, frequently found in these items, is a highly concentrated sucrose solution. Whether the sugar is overt or hidden, the USDA has suggested a limit of 8 teaspoons of sugar per day for a 2,000 calorie diet.

For a number of years, sugar substitutes have been used in a wide array of beverages, candy, baked goods, chewing gum, frozen desserts, gelatins and puddings, jams, toppings, and syrups. Among the most familiar of these are saccharin and aspartame (Nutrasweet®), both of which are several hundred times sweeter than sucrose. Some of the newer artificial sweeteners are acesulfame potassium (ace K), used in Pepsi One®, and xylitol, found in some brands of chewing gum, as well as neotame found in candy and soft drinks, sucralose (Splenda®), and tagatose. These sweeteners can be more than 600 times sweeter than sugar; neotame is 7,000 to 13,000 times sweeter than sugar.

Fats

Fats (lipids, fatty acids) are an important nutrient in our diets. Fats provide a concentrated form of energy (over double that of carbohydrates—there are 9 calories per gram consumed versus 4 for carbohydrates and protein) Fats provide a sense of **satiety** and keep us from feeling hungry. Because fats take longer to leave the stomach than either carbohydrates or proteins do, our stomachs feel full for a longer period of time, decreasing our appetite. Fats also help to give our food its pleasing taste, and they serve as carriers of fat-soluble vitamins A, D, E, and K. Without fat, these vitamins would quickly pass through the body. Fat insulates the body and helps it retain heat. The new dietary guidelines recommend that no more than 20–35 percent of our calories come from fat. In addition it is suggested that people:

- Consume less than 10 percent of calories from saturated fatty acids and less than 300 mg/day of cholesterol, and keep trans-fatty acid consumption as low as possible.

- Get most fats from sources of polyunsaturated and monounsaturated fatty acids, such as fish, nuts, and vegetable oils.

- Make choices that are lean, low fat, or fat free when selecting and preparing meat, poultry, dry beans, and milk or milk products,

Dietary sources of fat are often difficult to identify. The visible fats in our diet, such as butter, salad oils, and the layer of fat on some cuts of meat, represent only about 40 percent of the fat we consume. Most of the fat we eat is "hidden" in food because it is incorporated into the food during preparation or used to fry the food, or it is in food that we have not learned to recognize as being high in fat, such as a candy bar.

When shopping, we often notice that the fat content of some foods is reported by its percentage of the product's weight. In selecting the type of milk we drink, for example, we see that milk ranges from skim milk (no fat) to low-fat milk (½ percent) through reduced-fat milk (1–2 percent) to whole milk (3–4 percent). The labeling term *reduced fat* for 1 percent and 2 percent milk was introduced to reflect that these types of milk are no longer considered low fat.

Parents of infants and toddlers need to know that current medical opinion advises strongly against any limiting of fats in the diets of children younger than two years of age.[3] This recommendation is, of course, based on the demands for energy and the nutritional requirements that accompany the rapid growth that occurs during this formative stage of life.

Every type of dietary fat is made up of a combination of three forms of fat (saturated, monounsaturated, and polyunsaturated), based on its chemical composition. In each of the three forms of fat, the absence of double bonds (saturated fats) or the presence of double bonds (nonunsaturated and polyunsaturated fats) and the location of the double bonds within the molecule determine the nature and degree of restructuring that the body can do in changing dietary fat into physiology-friendly forms. Today, consumers need to pay attention to the amount of each type of fat in dietary fat because of the role that each form plays in heart disease (see Chapter 10).

Not all fats are created equal. **Saturated fats,** including those found in animal sources and in vegetable oils to which hydrogen has been added (hydrogenated), becoming **trans-fatty acids,** need to be carefully limited in a modern healthy diet. The presence of trans-fatty acids (an altered form of normal vegetable oil molecule or from meat and dairy products, having formed naturally by fermentation in the intestinal tract of animals)[4] is associated with changes in the cell membrane, including those cells lining the artery wall. This possibly prevents these vessel wall cells from freeing cholesterol from their surfaces.[5] Processing can change the structure of fat, making it more saturated. As a result, the oils become semisolid and more stable at room temperature. The term *trans* describes the chemical makeup of a fatty acid. Most trans-fatty acids come from hydrogenated oil, which is found in foods such as stick margarine, peanut butter, and crackers. They are popular in food manufacturing because they can extend the shelf life of the food: the oil stays mixed in the food and doesn't rise to the top, and the food doesn't become too soft at room temperature. The fast-food industry uses

Key Terms

satiety (suh **tie** uh tee) the feeling of no longer being hungry; a diminished desire to eat

saturated fats fats in solid form at room temperature; primarily animal fats

trans-fatty acids an altered form of an unsaturated fat molecule in which the hydrogen atoms on each side of the double bond(s) are on opposite sides

Table 5.2 **Comparison of Dietary Fats***

Oil	Mono.	Poly.	Sat.	Chol.
Canola oil	62	32	06	00
Safflower oil	13	77	10	00
Corn oil	25	62	13	00
Olive oil	77	09	14	00
Peanut oil	49	33	18	00
Vegetable shortening	44	28	28	00
Beef fat	44	04	52	14
Palm oil	38	09	53	00
Butter	30	04	66	33
Coconut oil	06	02	92	00

*Comparisons of the percentages of monosaturated fat (Mono), polyunsaturated fat (Poly), and saturated fat (Sat) constituting selected dietary fats, in addition to their cholesterol (Chol) content

these fats to fry many foods.[6] Additionally, trans-fatty acids are associated with increases in low-density lipoprotein (LDL) the "bad" cholesterol, without corresponding increases in high-density lipoprotein (HDL), the "good" cholesterol[4] (see Chapter 10). The amount of trans-fatty acids in the diet should be limited. This can be accomplished in part by reducing the use of stick margarine and shortening.[7]

Fortunately, the replacement of saturated fats with monounsaturated and polyunsaturated fats and oils appears to lower blood cholesterol levels and reduce the risk of heart disease. Vegetable oils tend to be low in saturated fats, with the exception of the tropical oils (coconut, palm, and palm kernel oils). Monounsaturated fats are found in high quantities in olive oil, peanut oil, and sesame oil. Polyunsaturated fats are especially prevalent in safflower oil and corn oil (Table 5.2).

Tropical Oils

Although all cooking oils (and fats such as butter, lard, margarine, and shortening) have the same number of calories by weight (9 calories per gram), some oils contain high percentages of saturated fats. All oils and fats contain varying percentages of saturated, monounsaturated, and polyunsaturated fats. The tropical oils—coconut, palm, and palm kernel—contain much higher percentages of saturated fats than do other cooking oils. Coconut oil is 92 percent saturated fat. Tropical oils can still be found in some brands of snack foods, crackers, cookies, nondairy creamers, and breakfast cereals, although they have been removed from most national brands. Do you check for tropical oils on the ingredients labels of the food you select?

How Much Fat Is Enough?

How advisable is a diet in which fat intake is restricted to less than 20–35 percent of total calories? Controversy over this question was examined in a leading medical journal.[8] In the article cited, researchers reported that when fat intake was significantly restricted in men who had high cholesterol levels, a known risk factor for cardiovascular disease, the men showed an unexpected decline in levels of HDL cholesterol, the so-called "good" cholesterol thought to favor heart health (see Chapter 10).

Critics of the report contend that the researchers failed to consider the improved appearance of the arteries of people who restricted fat intake to as little as 10 percent of total calories. Resolution of the controversy will require studies in which both HDL levels and artery wall changes are considered in association with dietary modifications.

Cholesterol

There has been a great deal of focus and concern over cholesterol levels. **Cholesterol** is a white, fatlike substance found in cells of animal origin. It is not found in any vegetable product, so products such as peanut butter and margarine that claim they are cholesterol free never had it in the first place. Cholesterol is used to synthesize cell membranes and also serves as the starting material for the synthesis of bile acids and sex hormones. Although we consume cholesterol in our diet—in such foods as shrimp and other shellfish, animal fat, and milk—we don't need to obtain cholesterol from external sources—the human liver can synthesize enough of the substance to meet the body's needs. Note that some foods high in cholesterol may provide other important nutrients and could remain in a healthy diet on a modest basis. A high level of cholesterol has been reported to be a risk factor in the development of cardiovascular disease (see Chapter 10).

A number of medical conditions can give rise to high blood cholesterol, such as liver disease, kidney failure, hypothyroidism, and diabetes. Certain medications, (some diuretics, for example) can also raise blood cholesterol, irrespective of diet. Considerable evidence suggests that increased intake of saturated fats may increase serum (blood) cholesterol levels. Nutritionists recommend that people restrict their dietary intake of cholesterol to 300 mg or less per day. In other words, no more than 20–35 percent of your total caloric intake should come from fat, with most fats being monounsaturated and polyunsaturated. Trans fat should be limited as much as possible.

Trans fats can act like saturated fat, potentially raising LDL blood cholesterol levels and decreasing HDL cholesterol. This is the reason nutritionists encourage us to use butter rather than stick margarine. To reduce your intake of trans fat, make sure you check the labels on foods to see if they list "partially hydrogenated vegetable oil" as one of the ingredients. Foods such as cakes, cookies, crackers, snack foods, stick margarine, vegetable shortening, and fried foods are most likely to have hydrogenated vegetable oil as one of the ingredients.

Low-Fat Foods

Low fat and *low calorie* do not mean the same thing, but often people confuse the two. Fat-free, low-fat, and reduced-fat foods have been popular for many years, with people thinking they can eat as much as they want of these foods. This is far from true; a fat-free or reduced-fat product may have as many if not more calories per serving than regular products do. For example, 2 tablespoons of fat-free caramel topping have 103 calories, the same amount as homemade-with-butter caramel topping; 2 tablespoons of Skippy peanut butter have the same as 2 tablespoons Skippy reduced-fat peanut butter, 190 calories; and 2 tablespoons of Cool Whip are equal to lite Cool Whip, 25 calories.[9] Fatty foods make people feel fuller longer than do fat-free foods; thus people tend to eat more of the fat-free foods and so consume more calories. In general, the lower the fat, the higher the price tag, because the food industry recognizes that Americans are willing to pay more for reduced-fat and fat-free labels. However, this situation may be changing, since people have realized that lower fat with potentially higher calories doesn't equal weight loss or healthy weight management. With Subway trading in cookies for a fruit roll and soda for a 100 percent juice carton in its kids-pak meals and McDonald's offering fresh fruit in lieu of French fries for its Happy Meals and touting salads for adult fare, the fast-food tide seems to be turning from supersized and superfat toward healthier choices.

Fat-Free Substitutes

Newly developed fat-free products containing fat substitutes (Simplesse, Simple Pleasures, Olestra, and Trailblazer) are available or soon to be available in the marketplace. These products contain no cholesterol and have 80 percent fewer calories than do similar products made with fat. Although fat-free substitutes first appeared only in snack foods, today they are found in ice cream, salad dressing, cheese spreads, yogurt, cakes, pies, and French fries.

The development of Olestra (marketed as Olean) as an example, required more than 25 years and $200 million on the part of Procter & Gamble, as an array of new technologies were required. In general, fat-free substitutes are made through processes called *microparticulation*, in which several fatty acids are bonded to a sugar molecule to create a triglyceride-like molecule that imparts all the characteristics of fats but is incapable of being enzymatically broken down by the body as are the triglycerides.

In spite of the apparent desirability of the fat-free technology, concerns have been voiced regarding the inability of these "nouveau fats" to carry fat-soluble vitamins (vitamins A, D, E, and K). Additional concern was raised over side effects in some people, such as abdominal cramping, loose stools, anal leakage, and an unpleasant aftertaste.[10]

 TALKING POINTS What would you say to a friend who is following a low-carbohydrate, high-fat weight loss diet to help that person see the potential pitfalls of the diet?

Key Terms

cholesterol a primary form of fat found in the blood; lipid material manufactured within the body, as well as derived from dietary sources

---

Proteins

The word *protein* derives from the ancient Greek word *proteios*, meaning "first importance." **Proteins** are manufactured in every living cell; they are composed of chains of amino acids. **Amino acids** are the "bricks" from which the body constructs its own protein. Twenty amino acids are used in various combinations to build the protein required for physiological processes to continue in a healthy manner.

The human body obtains amino acids from two sources—by breaking down protein from food (as if to take a brick wall apart for its bricks) or by manufacturing its own bricks (amino acids) within its cells. The latter process is less than fully successful because only 11 of the necessary 20 amino acids can be built by the body. The 9 amino acids that *cannot* be built by the body are called *essential amino acids* (indispensable amino acids), because they must be obtained from outside the body through the protein in food. The 11 amino acids that the body itself can make are called *nonessential amino acids* (dispensable amino acids), because the body does not have to rely solely on food protein to obtain these bricks.[11]

In terms of food sources of amino acids, foods can be classified into one of two types, depending on whether they can supply the body with the essential amino acids or not. Complete protein foods contain all nine essential amino acids and are of animal origin (milk, meat, cheese, and eggs). The incomplete protein foods do not contain all the essential amino acids and are of plant origin (vegetables, grains, and legumes [peas or beans, including chickpeas, butter beans, and tofu]). Vegan vegetarians (see page 164), people with limited access to animal-based food sources, and those who have significantly limited their meat, egg, and dairy product consumption, need to understand how essential amino acids can be obtained from incomplete protein sources. Fortunately, various sources of incomplete protein foods can be combined to achieve complete sources. This requires the careful selection of plant foods in combinations that provide all the essential amino acids. The list below shows many usable combinations that include legumes and grains:

> Sunflower seeds/green peas
>
> Navy beans/barley
>
> Green peas/corn
>
> Red beans/rice
>
> Sesame seeds/soybeans
>
> Black-eyed peas/rice and peanuts
>
> Green peas/rice
>
> Corn/pinto beans

When even one essential amino acid is missing from the diet, deficiency can develop.

Protein serves primarily to promote growth and maintenance of body tissue. However, when calorie intake falls, protein is broken down for glucose. This loss of protein can impede growth and repair of tissue. From this, it can be seen that adequate carbohydrate intake prevents protein from serving as an energy source.[11] Protein also is a primary component of enzyme and hormone structure; it helps maintain the *acid-base balance* of our bodies and serves as a source of energy (4 calories per gram consumed). Nutritionists recommend that 12–15 percent of our caloric intake be from protein. The RDA for adults is 58 grams of dietary protein for men and 46 grams for women each day. Malnutrition in the world's underdeveloped countries is often seen in the protein deficiency disease called *kwashiorkor*. This disease is rarely seen in countries that have an abundant supply of protein.

The specific protein currently gaining the attention of the American public is *soy protein*. Nutritionists currently recommend that the daily diet include 25 grams of soy protein. This can be obtained from soy milk, soy nuts (as snack foods), or from a wide array of products made with soy flour. Soybeans provide the same high-quality protein equal to that of animal protein.[12] Furthermore, soybeans contain no cholesterol or saturated fat and can actually lower blood lipid levels, reducing the risk of heart disease.[13]

Vitamins

Vitamins are organic compounds that are required in small amounts for normal growth, reproduction, and maintenance of health. Vitamins differ from carbohydrates, fats, and proteins because they do not provide calories or serve as structural elements for our bodies. Vitamins serve as *coenzymes*. By facilitating the action of **enzymes,** vitamins help initiate a wide variety of body responses, including energy production, use of minerals, and growth of healthy tissue.

Key Terms

proteins compounds composed of chains of amino acids; primary components of muscle and connective tissue

amino acids the building blocks of protein; manufactured by the body or obtained from dietary sources

vitamins organic compounds that facilitate the action of enzymes

enzymes organic substances that control the rate of physiological reactions but are not altered in the process

Table 5.3 Adult Recommended Dietary Allowances (RDAs) for Four Different Caloric Levels

Food Groups	1,600 Calories	2,000 Calories	2,600 Calories	3,100 Calories	Serving Sizes
Grains	6 servings	7–8 servings	10–11 servings	12–13 servings	1 slice bread, 1 oz dry cereal, ½ cup cooked rice, pasta, or cereal
Vegetables	3–4 servings	4–5 servings	5–6 servings	6 servings	1 cup raw leafy vegetable ½ cup cooked vegetable 6 oz vegetable juice
Fruits	4 servings	4–5 servings	5–6 servings	6 servings	6 oz fruit juice 1 medium fruit ¼ cup dried fruit ½ cup fresh, frozen, or canned fruit
Low-fat or fat-free dairy foods	2–3 servings	2–3 servings	3 servings	3–4 servings	8 oz milk 1 cup yogurt 1½ oz cheese
Meat, poultry, fish	1–2 servings	2 or less servings	2 servings	2–3 servings	3 oz cooked meats, poultry, or fish
Nuts, seeds, legumes	3–4 servings	4–5 servings	1 serving	1 serving	⅓ cup or 1½ oz nuts 2 Tbsp or ½ oz seeds ½ cup cooked dry beans or peas
Fat and oils	2 servings/ week	2–3 servings/ week	3 servings	4 servings	1 tsp soft margarine 1 Tbsp low-fat mayonnaise 2 Tbsp light salad dressing 1 tsp vegetable oil
Sweets	0 servings	5 servings/week	2 servings	2 servings	1 Tbsp sugar 1 Tbsp jelly or jam ½ oz jelly beans 8 oz lemonade

Discovered just after the turn of the 20th century, the 13 essential vitamins can be classified as *water soluble* (capable of being dissolved in water) or *fat soluble* (capable of being dissolved in fat or lipid tissue). Water-soluble vitamins include the B-complex vitamins and vitamin C. Most of the excess of these water-soluble vitamins is eliminated from the body during urination. The fat-soluble vitamins are A, D, E, and K. These vitamins are stored in the body in the adipose tissue or fat with excessive intake. It is therefore possible to consume and retain too many of these vitamins, particularly A and D. All the fat-soluble vitamins, however, hold the potential for toxicity if taken in amounts that far exceed recommended dietary allowances (RDAs) (see Table 5.3). Most toxicity results from the use of supplements by adults or through excessive food intake of particular sources in very small children. When toxicity develops, the condition is referred to as **hypervitaminosis.**

People often think taking megadoses of vitamins such as vitamin C can be health-enhancing, but the reverse is true. Taking large doses of vitamin C from a dietary supplement can put a strain on your kidneys, causing kidney stones and diarrhea. Too much niacin, vitamin B6, and folate can also be harmful.[6]

Because water-soluble vitamins dissolve rather quickly in water, you should be cautious in the preparation of fresh fruits and vegetables. One precaution is to avoid overcooking fresh vegetables. The longer fresh vegetables are steamed or boiled, the more water-soluble vitamins will be lost. More vitamins are retained with

> **Key Terms**
>
> **hypervitaminosis** excessive accumulation of vitamins within the body; associated with the fat-soluble vitamins

microwave cooking than with stove-top cooking. Even soaking sliced fresh fruit or vegetables can result in the loss of vitamin C and B-complex vitamins.

To ensure an adequate vitamin intake, do not rely on bottled vitamins sold in grocery stores or health food stores. The best way is really the simplest and least expensive way: eat a variety of foods. Unless there are special circumstances, such as pregnancy, infancy, or an existing health problem, virtually everyone in our society who eats a reasonably well-rounded diet consumes appropriate levels of all vitamins. The validity of this was recently substantiated by a study of 42,000 women in which it was demonstrated that those women with a sustained history of eating a balanced diet were significantly less likely to die prematurely from a variety of chronic conditions than were those women who ate less balanced diets.[14]

In spite of the availability of vitamin-rich foods, not all people eat a balanced diet based on a variety of foods. Most likely a large percentage of these persons, as well as many who also eat nutritionally, use vitamin supplements. Some proportion of these supplement users believe that additional vitamin intake will prevent or delay the onset of chronic health conditions such as cancer and cardiovascular disease. To date there seems to be no absolute consensus regarding the effectiveness of most supplements in chronic disease prevention. This said, there is at least one well-established success story regarding vitamin supplementation. That success story is the effectiveness of folic acid supplementation (found in vitamin B) in assuring the appropriate closure of the neural tube during embryonic development, thus preventing the development of spina bifida.[15] In spite of widespread awareness of the necessity for folic acid, however, nearly one-third of women of childbearing age do not take this B vitamin on a daily basis.

Who else might benefit from vitamin supplementation? In the opinion of nutritionists, this group might include vegans, people with limited milk intake and limited exposure to sunlight, people with lactose intolerance, and people on a severely restricted weight loss diet. Children and adolescents are another group that may benefit from vitamin D supplements. Physicians have been increasingly concerned about vitamin D deficiency owing to reduced outdoor activity and decreased milk consumption among children and adolescents. Preteens and teens need 1,200 to 1,500 mg of calcium per day, while adults require 1,200 mg per day. Stress, as well as soft drinks, fiber, and iron in foods, can decrease calcium absorption, and calcium is best absorbed when taken in frequent, small amounts and with meals. Vitamin C improves the absorption of calcium, as does the presence of estrogen. So women after menopause are at increased risk of calcium deficiency.

Except for the people identified above, most Americans could go without supplementation. How would this occur? Today it is known that few Americans obtain 100 percent of the 14 RDAs on a daily basis, although the majority of people regularly obtain most (77 percent) of the RDAs every day. In fact, experts are confident that virtually all Americans would achieve the recommended RDAs on a daily basis by increasing their fruit and vegetable consumption to the recommended 4½ cups daily. Therefore, in light of current eating patterns and the increase in fruit and vegetable consumption needed to achieve desired nutritional intake, the American Dietetic Association does not recommend the wide-scale use of vitamin and mineral supplements, particularly in amounts exceeding 100 percent of the current RDAs.[16] Physicians, however, routinely recommend supplementation to individual patients because of pregnancy, lactation, smoking, or recovery from specific conditions. Some recommend that supplements be taken with food, since they're really components of food and help the body metabolize other food components. The fat-soluble nutrients should be taken with a little oil or fat to enhance absorption. The water-soluble nutrients are easily absorbed without food but may work better when taken with meals. In addition, some people complain of stomach upset when they take vitamins on an empty stomach.

Phytochemicals

Certain physiologically active components are believed to deactivate carcinogens or function as antioxidants. Among these are the carotenoids (from green vegetables), polyphenols (from onions and garlic), indoles (from cruciferous vegetables), and the allyl sulfides (from garlic, chives, and onions). These **phytochemicals** may play an important role in sparking the body to fight and slow the development of some diseases, such as cancer. At this time, however, the exact mechanisms through which the various phytochemicals reduce the formation of cancer cells is not understood. Although it is generally agreed that these foods are important in planning food selections, no precise recommendations regarding the amounts of various phytochemical-rich plants have been made.

Minerals

Nearly 5 percent of the body is composed of inorganic materials, the *minerals.* Minerals function primarily as structural elements (in teeth, muscles, hemoglobin, and

---

Key Terms

phytochemicals physiologically active components believed to deactivate carcinogens and to function as antioxidants thyroid hormones). They are also critical in the regulation of a number of body processes, including fluid balance, nerve impulses, muscle contraction, heart function, blood clotting, protein synthesis, and red blood cell synthesis. Approximately 21 minerals have been recognized as being essential for human health.[1] Unlike vitamins, minerals are inorganic and can't be destroyed by heat or food processing.

Macronutrients (major minerals) are those minerals that are seen in relatively high amounts in our body tissues. The RDAs include 250 mg of each one daily. Examples of macronutrients are calcium, phosphorus, sodium, potassium, and magnesium. Examples of *micronutrients,* minerals seen in relatively small amounts in body tissues, include zinc, iron, copper, selenium, and iodine. Although micronutrients (trace elements) are required only in small quantities, fewer than 20 mg daily of each, they are still essential. Active, menstruating women need at least 18 milligrams of iron daily; however, a well-balanced diet supplies around 12 mg of iron for 2,000 calories. Eating a food rich in vitamin C along with iron-rich foods will help your body efficiently utilize iron. Examples of this might be eating spaghetti with meat and tomato sauce, meat and potatoes, hamburger and coleslaw, fruit and iron-fortified cereal or fruit with raisins.

Water

Water may well be our most essential nutrient, since without water most people would die from **dehydration** effects in less than a week. People could survive for weeks and even years without some of the essential minerals and vitamins. More than half the body's weight comes from water. Water provides the medium for nutrient and waste transport and temperature control and plays a key role in nearly all of the body's biochemical reactions. A common indication of inadequate fluid intake is strained, uncomfortable bowel movements.

Most people seldom think about the importance of an adequate intake of water and fluids. The average adult loses about 10 cups of water daily through perspiration, urination, bowel movements, and breathing. Adults require about 6 to 10 glasses a day, depending on their exercise level and environment. However, because of the dehydrating effects of coffee, tea, and alcohol, the average American consumes the equivalent of only 4.6 glasses per day.[17] To see if you're drinking enough fluid, check your urine. A small amount of dark-colored urine can be an indication that you are not consuming enough fluid and need to drink more. Urine that is pale or almost colorless means you are most likely taking in enough fluids. Of course, people also obtain needed fluids from fruits, vegetables, fruit and vegetable juices, milk, and noncaf-feinated soft drinks. However, excessive water consumption by persons of any age, including forced consumption by infants, can lead to fatal brain edema (swelling) and aspiration pneumonia.[18, 19]

Fiber

Although not considered a nutrient by definition, **fiber** is an important component of sound nutrition. Fiber consists of plant material that is not digested but rather moves through the digestive tract and out of the body. Cereal, fruits, and vegetables all provide us with dietary fiber.

Fiber can be classified into two large groups on the basis of water solubility. *Insoluble* fibers are those that can absorb water from the intestinal tract. By absorbing water, the insoluble fibers give the stool bulk and decrease the time it takes the stool to move through the digestive tract. In contrast, *soluble* fiber turns to a "gel" within the intestinal tract and in so doing binds to liver bile, which has cholesterol attached. Thus, soluble fiber is valuable in removing (or lowering) blood cholesterol levels. Also, since foods high in soluble fiber are generally low in sugar and saturated fats, fiber may indirectly contribute to keeping blood sugar low[20] and reduce the risk of colon cancer associated with diets high in saturated fats, although today this latter contention is being seriously challenged.[21] How much fiber do you need? Adults should eat from 25 to 35 g of fiber each day; however, most American adults eat only 11 g per day. Fiber has many benefits, including helping to curb your appetite and prevent overeating because it is filling, requires more chewing, stays in the stomach longer, and absorbs water, adding to the feeling of fullness. Fiber also helps to slow the absorption of sugar from the intestines, thus steadying the blood sugar and slowing down the absorption of fat from the foods you eat. Consuming adequate amounts of fiber has an important effect on reducing serious medical problems because soluble fiber lowers LDL cholesterol and protects against cardiovascular disease, whereas insoluble fiber protects against developing colon cancer.[22]

In recent years attention has been directed toward three forms of soluble fiber—oat bran, psyllium (from the weed

---

> **Key Terms**
>
> **trace elements** minerals whose presence in the body occurs in very small amounts; micronutrient elements
>
> **dehydration** abnormal depletion of fluids from the body; severe dehydration can lead to death
>
> **fiber** cellulose-based plant material that cannot be digested; found in cereal, fruits, and vegetables

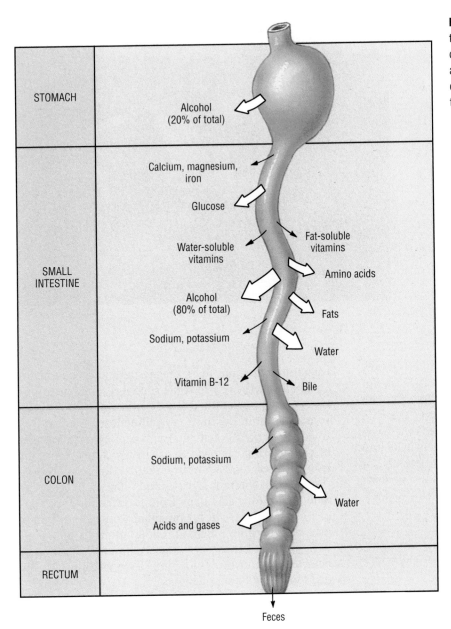

Figure 5-1 Important sites of nutrient absorption along the gastrointestinal (GI) tract. The size of the arrow indicates the relative amount of absorption at that site. (Note that this drawing depicts the GI tract as being "uncoiled" to simplify the presentation of its absorption sites.)

STOMACH

Alcohol
(20% of total)

SMALL
INTESTINE

Calcium, magnesium,
iron

Glucose

Fat-soluble
vitamins

Water-soluble
vitamins

Amino acids

Alcohol
(80% of total)

Fats

Sodium, potassium

Water

Vitamin B-12

Bile

COLON

Sodium, potassium

Water

Acids and gases

RECTUM

Feces

plantain), and rice bran—for their ability to lower blood cholesterol levels and prevent heart disease.[23] To accomplish a five- to six-point lowering in cholesterol, a daily consumption of oat bran equaling a large bowl of oat bran cold cereal or three or more packs of instant oatmeal would be necessary. One serving of bran plus one serving of beans each day will also give you more than half your total daily fiber needs. It is recommended to eat fiber from a variety of sources to obtain a good balance of soluble and insoluble fibers.

The Absorption of Nutrients

In a very real sense, food (as nutrients) is not "in the body" until it is digested and then absorbed into and through the walls of the gastrointestinal (GI) tract, into the bloodstream, and is distributed to the cell sites at which it will be used for energy, growth, repair, and regulation. Figure 5-1 depicts a highly diagrammatic representation of the GI tract showing specific absorption sites for several important nutrients. The first 18 inches of the small intestine make up the most active site for absorption, surpassing the level of activity in the remainder of the small intestine, the large intestine, and the stomach. Some portion of the alcohol contained in alcoholic drinks enters the body through the stomach wall (more in women than in men), although most is absorbed in the small intestine. Water and salts are principally regulated by the walls of the large intestine.

Eating a healthy diet including fruits and vegetables is the best way to get the necessary vitamins and minerals.

In light of the importance of the small intestine, any injury or disease in this location could seriously harm nutritional status by impairing the body's ability to obtain nutrients. In fact, in extreme cases of obesity (morbid obesity) a portion of small intestine is resected (cut away) in an attempt to restrict the movement of nutrients into the body. This drastic approach to weight loss is, of course, a double-edged sword in that many nutrients needed for overall health must then be supplemented, often for the rest of the person's life.

The New Dietary Guidelines for Americans 2005

The Dietary Guidelines for Americans is science-based and summarizes the analysis of new scientific information regarding nutrition, health, physical activity, and food safety. The goal of these guidelines is to lower the risk of chronic disease and promote health through diet and physical activity.

The United States Department of Agriculture (USDA) releases a revision of their dietary guidelines for Americans every five years. However, the food pyramid had not undergone a revision since it was created in 1992. A recent revision, announced in 2005, has some significant changes. These changes are based on evidence that found that Americans are consuming too many calories and yet are not meeting the recommended intake for some nutrients. It was determined that Americans have too much saturated and trans fats, cholesterol, and added sugar and salt in their diets and not enough

calcium, potassium, fiber, magnesium, and vitamins A, C, and E. There are also some special recommendations for specific population groups. For people over 50, consuming vitamin B_{12} in its crystalline form (such as fortified foods or supplements) is recommended. Women of childbearing age need to eat iron-rich plant food or iron-fortified food with an enhancer for iron absorption, such as vitamin-C-rich foods. Taking in adequate amounts of folic acid daily from fortified foods or supplements is important for pregnant women and women who may become pregnant. Older adults, people with dark skin, and those not exposed to enough sunlight need to consume extra vitamin D from vitamin-D-fortified foods and/or supplements.

These findings were used to formulate the new USDA Food Guide for Americans (Table 5.4), which focuses on overall caloric intake rather than on one particular food group, such as fats or carbohydrates. Portion sizes are emphasized, and the recommendations are made in cups rather than in serving sizes, to help people have better portion control. There is also increased emphasis on consuming **nutrient-dense foods,** which provide substantial amounts of vitamins and minerals and comparatively few calories. Junk foods typically are not nutrient-dense, since

Key Terms

nutrient-dense foods foods that provide substantial amounts of vitamins and minerals and comparatively few calories

Table 5.4 USDA Food Guide

The suggested amounts of food to consume from the basic food groups, subgroups, and oils to meet recommended nutrient intakes at 12 different calorie levels.

Daily Amount of Food from Each Group (vegetable subgroup amounts are per week)

Calorie Level	1,000	1,200	1,400	1,600	1,800	2,000	2,200	2,400	2,600	2,800	3,000	3,200
Food Group	Food group amounts shown in cup (c) or ounce-equivalents (oz-eq), with number of servings (srv) in parentheses when it differs from the other units. See note for quantity equivalents for foods in each group. Oils are shown in grams (g).											
Fruits	1 c (2 srv)	1 c (2 srv)	1.5 c (3 srv)	1.5 c (3 srv)	1.5 c (3 srv)	2 c (4 srv)	2 c (4 srv)	2c (4 srv)	2c (4 srv)	2.5c (5 srv)	2.5c (5 srv)	2.5c (5 srv)
Vegetables	1 c (2 srv)	1.5 c (3 srv)	1.5 c (3 srv)	2 c (4 srv)	2.5 c (5 srv)	2.5 c (5 srv)	3 c (6 srv)	3 c (6 srv)	3.5 c (7 srv)	3.5 c (7 srv)	4 c (8 srv)	4 c (8 srv)
Dark green veg.	1 c/wk	1.5 c/wk	1.5 c/wk	2 c/wk	3 c/wk	3 c/wk	3 c/wk	3 c/wk	3 c/wk	3 c/wk	3 c/wk	3 c/wk
Orange veg.	.5 c/wk	1 c/wk	1 c/wk	1.5 c/wk	2 c/wk	2 c/wk	2 c/wk	2 c/wk	2.5 c/wk	2.5 c/wk	2.5 c/wk	2.5 c/wk
Legumes	.5 c/wk	1 c/wk	1 c/wk	2.5 c/wk	3 c/wk	3 c/wk	3 c/wk	3 c/wk	3.5 c/wk	3.5 c/wk	3.5 c/wk	3.5 c/wk
Starchy veg.	1.5 c/wk	2.5 c/wk	2.5 c/wk	2.5 c/wk	3 c/wk	3 c/wk	6 c/wk	6 c/wk	7 c/wk	7 c/wk	9 c/wk	9 c/wk
Other veg.	4 c/wk	4.5 c/wk	4.5 c/wk	5.5 c/wk	6.5 c/wk	6.5 c/wk	7 c/wk	7 c/wk	8.5 c/wk	8.5 c/wk	10 c/wk	10 c/wk
Grains	3 oz-eq	4 oz-eq	5 oz-eq	5 oz-eq	6 oz-eq	6 oz-eq	7 oz-eq	8 oz-eq	9 oz-eq	10 oz-eq	10 oz-eq	10 oz-eq
Whole grains	1.5	2	2.5	3	3	3	3.5	4	4.5	5	5	5
Other grains	1.5	2	2.5	2	3	3	3.5	4	4.5	5	5	5
Lean meat and beans	2 oz-eq	3 oz-eq	4 oz-eq	5 oz-eq	5 oz-eq	5.5 oz-eq	6 oz-eq	6.5 oz-eq	6.5 oz-eq	7 oz-eq	7 oz-eq	7 oz-eq
Milk	2 c	2 c	2 c	3 c	3 c	3 c	3 c	3 c	3 c	3 c	3 c	3 c
Oils	15 g	17 g	17 g	22 g	24 g	27 g	29 g	31 g	34 g	36 g	44 g	51 g
Discretionary calorie allowance	165	171	171	132	195	267	290	362	410	426	512	648

they are high in sugar and saturated and trans fat, high in calories, and low in vitamins and minerals.

Americans are advised to consume more whole grains, milk products, fruits, and vegetables as well. Another key aspect is the focus on daily exercise, with 60 to 90 minutes of moderate exercise as the recommended amount. Restricting salt, alcohol, and trans fats are other important aspects of the dietary guidelines.

The new food pyramid, referred to as *MyPyramid*, takes a more personalized approach to healthy eating (see Figure 5-2). The pyramid has been tipped onto its side, and the colors and size of the bands reflect the proportion of each food group that people generally need to consume each day. The steps signify the importance of daily exercise. The food pyramid acknowledges that people have different dietary needs based on age, gender, and physical activity level. There are 12 different recommendations based on these factors, and you can find the one that best fits you through the USDA's Web site at www.mypyramid.gov. People can also assess their activity level and food intake through www.mypyramid-tracker.gov.

Some of the specific key recommendations for a healthy pattern of eating, physical activity, and handling food on a daily basis that have been suggested by these new guidelines include:[26]

1. Choose a variety of fruits and vegetables. Select from all five vegetable subgroups (dark green, orange, legumes, starchy vegetables, and other vegetables).
2. Eat 2 cups of fruit and 2½ cups of vegetables.
3. Consume 3 1-ounce equivalents of whole-grain products per day, with at least half of the grains coming from whole grains.
4. Drink 3 cups of fat-free or low-fat milk or the equivalent.
5. Engage in at least 30 minutes of moderate intensity physical activity on most days of the week to reduce the risk of chronic disease. Engage in 60 to 90 minutes of physical activity for weight management.
6. Those who choose to drink alcoholic beverages should consume no more than 1 drink per day for women and 2 drinks per day for men.
7. Consume less than 10 percent of calories from saturated fats and less than 300 mg/day of cholesterol. Keep trans fats at a minimum.

MyPyramid
STEPS TO A HEALTHIER YOU
MyPyramid.gov

1% MILK

Yogurt

GRAINS	VEGETABLES	FRUITS	MILK	MEAT & BEANS
Make half your grains whole	Vary your veggies	Focus on fruits	Get your calcium-rich foods	Go lean with protein
Eat at least 3 oz. of whole-grain cereals, breads, crackers, rice, or pasta every day 1 oz. is about 1 slice of bread, about 1 cup of breakfast cereal, or ½ cup of cooked rice, cereal, or pasta	Eat more dark-green veggies like broccoli, spinach, and other dark leafy greens Eat more orange vegetables like carrots and sweet potatoes Eat more dry beans and peas like pinto beans, kidney beans, and lentils	Eat a variety of fruit Choose fresh, frozen, canned, or dried fruit Go easy on fruit juices	Go low-fat or fat-free when you choose milk, yogurt, and other milk products If you don't or can't consume milk, choose lactose-free products or other calcium sources such as fortified foods and beverages	Choose low-fat or lean meats and poultry Bake it, broil it, or grill it Vary your protein routine — choose more fish, beans, peas, nuts, and seeds

For a 2,000-calorie diet, you need the amounts below from each food group. To find the amounts that are right for you, go to MyPyramid.gov.

Eat 6 oz. every day	Eat 2½ cups every day	Eat 2 cups every day	Get 3 cups every day; for kids aged 2 to 8, it's 2	Eat 5½ oz. every day

Find your balance between food and physical activity
- Be sure to stay within your daily calorie needs.
- Be physically active for at least 30 minutes most days of the week.
- About 60 minutes a day of physical activity may be needed to prevent weight gain.
- For sustaining weight loss, at least 60 to 90 minutes a day of physical activity may be required.
- Children and teenagers should be physically active for 60 minutes every day, or most days.

Know the limits on fats, sugars, and salt (sodium)
- Make most of your fat sources from fish, nuts, and vegetable oils.
- Limit solid fats like butter, stick margarine, shortening, and lard, as well as foods that contain these.
- Check the Nutrition Facts label to keep saturated fats, *trans* fats, and sodium low.
- Choose food and beverages low in added sugars. Added sugars contribute calories with few, if any, nutrients.

MyPyramid.gov
STEPS TO A HEALTHIER YOU

U.S. Department of Agriculture
Center for Nutrition Policy and Promotion
April 2005
CNPP-15

Anatomy of MyPyramid

One size doesn't fit all

USDA's new MyPyramid symbolizes a personalized approach to healthy eating and physical activity. The symbol has been designed to be simple. It has been developed to remind consumers to make healthy food choices and to be active every day. The different parts of the symbol are described below.

Activity

Activity is represented by the steps and the person climbing them, as a reminder of the importance of daily physical activity.

Moderation

Moderation is represented by the narrowing of each food group from bottom to top. The wider base stands for foods with little or no solid fats or added sugars. These should be selected more often. The narrower top area stands for foods containing more added sugars and solid fats. The more active you are, the more of these foods can fit into your diet.

Personalization

Personalization is shown by the person on the steps, the slogan, and the URL. Find the kinds and amounts of food to eat each day at MyPyramid.gov.

Proportionality

Proportionality is shown by the different widths of the food group bands. The widths suggest how much food a person should choose from each group. The widths are just a general guide, not exact proportions. Check the Web site for how much is right for you.

Variety

Variety is symbolized by the 6 color bands representing the 5 food groups of the Pyramid and oils. This illustrates that foods from all groups are needed each day for good health.

Gradual Improvement

Gradual improvement is encouraged by the slogan. It suggests that individuals can benefit from taking small steps to improve their diet and lifestyle each day.

U.S. Department of Agriculture
Center for Nutrition Policy
and Promotion
April 2005 CNPP-16

USDA is an equal opportunity provider and employer.

| GRAINS | VEGETABLES | FRUITS | OILS | MILK | MEAT & BEANS |

Figure 5-2 The new look for the food pyramid takes a personal approach to healthy eating.

8. Keep total fat intake between 20–35 percent of calories, with most fats coming from polyunsaturated and monounsaturated fats.

9. Choose low-fat, fat-free, or lean meat, poultry, milk, and bean products.

10. Consume less than 2,300 mg (approximately 1 teaspoon) of sodium daily.

11. Clean hands, food-contact surfaces, and fruits and vegetables. Meat and poultry shouldn't be washed or rinsed.

12. Separate raw, cooked, and ready-to-eat foods while shopping, preparing, and storing foods.

13. Cook foods to a safe temperature, and chill perishable food promptly.

14. Avoid unpasteurized milk and milk products, raw or partially cooked eggs, and foods containing raw eggs or undercooked meat and poultry, unpasteurized juices, and raw sprouts.

The most effective way to take in adequate amounts of nutrients is to eat a balanced diet as outlined by the USDA's most current guidelines. The USDA particularly focuses on meeting these dietary needs by consuming food, not dietary supplements. In addition, the USDA advises consuming a variety of nutrient-dense foods and beverages (discussed later in the chapter). To determine whether you are eating a healthful diet balanced with choices from each food group, complete the personal assessment entitled "Rate Your Plate" on page 171.

Fruits

As previously mentioned, the new guidelines suggest eating 2 cups of fruits per day for a 2,000 calorie/day adult diet. One medium-sized fruit, ¼ cup dried fruit, or 1 cup of fresh, frozen, or canned fruit is equivalent to 1 serving or 1 cup. Orange fruits such mango, cantaloupe, apricots, and red or pink grapefruit provide sources of vitamin A. Kiwi, strawberries, guava, papaya, and cantaloupe and citrus fruits are good sources of vitamin C. Oranges and orange juice also provide folate. Some good sources for potassium are bananas, plantains, dried fruits, oranges and orange juice, cantaloupe and honeydew melons, and tomato products. For the majority of your fruit intake, it is generally recommended to consume whole fruits and avoid fruit juices to ensure adequate fiber and to avoid the high sugar content associated with fruit juices. The American Cancer Society indicates that this food group may play an important role in the prevention of certain forms of cancer.

Vegetables

Two and one-half cups of vegetables per day is the new recommendation for adults following a 2,000 calorie diet. As with the fruit group, the important function of this group is to provide vitamin A, vitamin C, complex carbohydrates, and fiber. Because Americans tend to eat only a few vegetables, such as potatoes, corn, and carrots, the new guidelines give specific recommendations about the types of vegetable. One general rule is to "eat your colors," meaning you should consume a variety of vegetables over the course of a week. The USDA recommends:

- Dark green vegetables—3 cups/week
- Orange vegetables—2 cups/week
- Legumes (dry beans)—3 cups/week
- Starchy vegetables—3 cups/week
- Other vegetables—6½ cups /week

Again, avoid drinking vegetable juices as a way of meeting these requirements because they can be high in salt and sugar and don't provide the fiber intake that whole vegetables do. **Cruciferous vegetables,** such as broccoli, cabbage, brussels sprouts, and cauliflower, may be particularly helpful in the prevention of certain forms of cancer.[24] It has also been determined that antioxidants in vegetables and fruits may slow the age-related changes in cognitive function.[25] Decreased risk of heart disease has also been associated with the consumption of fruits and vegetables.

Milk and Milk Products

The new dietary guidelines recommend increasing the consumption of milk to 3 cups of fat-free or low-fat milk each day, or its equivalent in another milk product. Milk consumption has been associated with higher bone den-

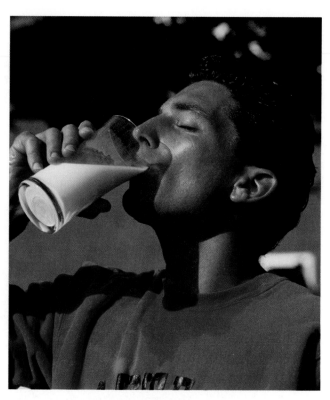

Three cups of milk or the equivalent from this group is the recommended daily amount for adults.

sity and can help fight osteoporosis. Calcium and high-quality protein, required for bone and tooth development, are two primary nutritional benefits provided by this food group. The guidelines further suggest that children 2 to 8 years old should consume 2 cups per day of fat-free or low-fat milk, or equivalent milk products, whereas children 9 years of age and older should consume 3 cups per day of fat-free or low-fat milk, or equivalent milk products. Milk, cheese, yogurt, and ice cream are included in this food group.

Meat, Poultry, Fish, Eggs, Dry Beans, and Nuts

Our need for selections from this protein-rich group is based on our daily need for protein, iron, and the

---

Key Terms

cruciferous vegetables group of vegetables that includes broccoli, cabbage, brussels sprouts, and cauliflower

To get an idea of portion sizes—a stacked deck of cards is equivalent to 3 ounces.

B vitamins. Meats include all red meat (beef, pork, and game), fish, and poultry. It is strongly recommended that we choose lean meats and low-fat or fat-free foods in this group. Meat substitutes include dry beans, eggs, tofu, peanut butter, nuts, and seeds. For individuals who are lactose intolerant (lactose upsets their intestines) or are vegan (vegetarians who don't consume any animal products, including dairy products), soybeans, tofu, spinach, kale, okra, beet greens, and oatmeal are good alternative sources of calcium. The 2005 USDA guidelines recommend that adults eat 5½ ounces of meat or protein foods each day. One ounce is equivalent to:

- 1 ounce cooked lean meat, poultry, or fish
- 1 egg
- ¼ cup cooked dry beans
- ¼ cup tofu
- 1 tablespoon peanut butter
- ½ ounce nuts or seeds

The fat content of meat varies considerably. Some forms of meat yield only 1 percent fat, whereas others may be as high as 40 percent fat. Poultry and fish are generally significantly lower in overall fat than are red meats. Interestingly, the higher the grade of red meat, the more fat is marbled throughout the muscle fiber. Indeed, people usually find that higher-grade steak usually tastes better, but that is because of its higher fat content.

Meats are generally excellent sources of iron. Iron is present in much greater amounts in red meats and organ meats (liver, kidney, and heart) than in poultry and fish. Iron plays a critically important role in hemoglobin synthesis on red blood cells and thus is an important contributor to physical fitness (see Chapter 4) and overall cardiovascular health (see Chapter 10). However, meat and fish should be fresh, stored appropriately, and cooked adequately to reduce the likelihood of serious foodborne illnesses.

Breads, Cereals, Rice, and Pasta

The nutritional benefit from the breads, cereals, rice, and pasta group lies in its contribution of B-complex vitamins and energy from complex carbohydrates. Some nutritionists believe that foods from this group promote protein intake, since many of them are prepared as complete-protein foods—for example, macaroni and cheese, cereal and milk, and bread and meat sandwiches.

This group is referred to as the "grain group" by the USDA, and there is a particular emphasis on consuming at least 3 of the 6 ounces of this group from whole grains. Whole grains can reduce the risk of chronic disease and help with weight maintenance.

Whole grains consist of the entire grain seed, or the kernel, and can't be identified by the color of the food. The FDA requires that food contain 51 percent or more whole-grain ingredients by weight and be low fat in order to be called "whole grain." On food labels, "whole grain" should be the first ingredient listed. Avoid refined grains, because the grain-refining process typically removes most of the bran and some of the germ, resulting in the loss of dietary fiber, minerals, vitamins, and other important nutrients. Wheat flour, enriched flour, and degerminated cornmeal are *not* whole grains.

Some products are labeled **enriched,** meaning that some of nutritional elements that were removed during processing are returned to the food; however, only three B vitamins (thiamine, niacin, riboflavin) and iron are replaced.

The USDA recommends 6 ounces of grains daily, with at least 3 ounces coming from whole grains. One ounce is equivalent to:

- 1 slice bread
- 1 cup dry cereal
- ½ cup cooked rice, pasta, cereal

The food industry has risen to the challenge of providing nutritious whole-grain foods with improved taste and texture. For example, ConAgra has spent millions of dollars over the past five years to develop "white wheat"

Key Terms

enriched the process of returning to foods some of the nutritional elements (B vitamins and iron) removed during processing made from a naturally occurring albino variety of flour. It has 3½ times more dietary fiber, 11 times more vitamin E, 5 times more magnesium, and 4 times more niacin than does refined, unenriched wheat flour. It also tastes milder and sweeter than most whole grains do. It combines the best of both worlds—the nutrition of whole wheat with the taste of white flour.[27]

Fats, Oils, and Sweets

Where do such items such as beer, butter, candy, colas, cookies, corn chips, and pastries fit into your diet? Most of these items contribute relatively little to healthful nutrition; they provide additional calories, generally from sucrose and significant amounts of salt and fat. The new dietary guidelines make specific recommendations about fats, salt, sugar, and alcohol intake.

The USDA refers to the fats and oils group as the "oil group" on the MyPyramid. The recommended total daily fat intake should be 20–35 percent of total calories, with most fats coming from sources of polyunsaturated and monounsaturated fatty acids, such as fish, nuts, and vegetable oils. Canola oil and olive oil are preferred over other types of oils. Less than 10 percent of total calories should be from saturated fats, and less than 300 mg/day should come from cholesterol. Trans-fatty acid consumption is to be kept "as low as possible." A limit of 24 grams, or 6 teaspoons of oils, is the daily recommendation. One teaspoon is equivalent to:

- 1 teaspoon soft margarine
- 1 tablespoon low-fat mayonnaise
- 2 tablespoons light salad dressing
- 1 teaspoon vegetable oil

The USDA also suggests that we choose and prepare foods and beverages with little added sugars or caloric sweeteners. The new food guide recommends no more than 8 teaspoons of added sugars per day, which is equivalent to ½ ounce of jelly beans or an 8-ounce glass of lemonade. Eating too much sugar has been thought to be a major contributor to the increase in obesity in Americans.

Something new to the USDA guidelines is the limitation on salt intake. They advise consuming less than 2,300 mg, or 1 teaspoon, of sodium each day and to choose and prepare foods with little salt. Most of our salt intake comes from processed or prepared foods. Many people are unaware of the high sodium content in prepared foods, sauces, soups, and canned foods, and so reading the labels for ingredients is extremely important. You might be surprised by some of the foods that contain salt—cookies, minute rice, canned green beans, soft drinks, and cereal. It is also difficult to know how to

make healthy choices when eating out if you don't know the sodium content in the menu items. Too much sodium is linked to hypertension, and about 30 percent of Americans have sodium-sensitive high blood pressure, which can lead to heart attack or stroke. It is estimated that about 150,000 deaths each year are caused by too much salt.

Another difference in the new dietary guidelines is the recommendation concerning alcohol consumption. The USDA states that "those who choose to drink alcoholic beverages should do so sensibly and in moderation." *Moderation* is defined as the consumption of up to 1 drink per day for women and up to 2 drinks per day for men. One drink is defined as either 12 fluid ounces of regular beer, 5 fluid ounces of wine, or 1½ fluid ounces of 80-proof distilled spirits. Since alcoholic beverages tend to contribute calories but little nutrition, they are counterproductive to taking in sufficient nutrients while not going over the daily caloric allotment. However, there are some indications that moderate alcohol consumption, such as having a glass of red wine each day, assists in decreasing the risk of coronary heart disease.

Table 5.5 provides a sample 2,000-calorie menu based on the new USDA dietary guidelines.

Table 5.5 Sample 2,000-Calorie Menu Based on the New USDA Dietary Guidelines for Americans, 2005

Breakfast
1 cup oatmeal
1 cup low-fat vanilla yogurt
½ cup blackberries

Snack
1 medium banana

Lunch
2 whole wheat tortillas each filled with 1 ounce of cooked chicken breast, ¼ cup refried beans, ¼ cup onion and tomato, 2 tablespoons shredded light cheese, and ¼ cup shredded romaine lettuce
16 ounces water

Snack
¼ cup unsalted peanuts
1 medium apple

Dinner
1½ cups cooked whole wheat pasta topped with ½ cup low-fat pasta sauce, ½ cup cooked mushrooms, ¼ cup cooked onions, and 2 ounces cooked extra-lean ground turkey breast
1 cup skim milk

Snack
6 ounces fat-free yogurt
1 cup grapes

Fast Foods

Fast foods are convenience foods usually prepared in walk-in or drive-through restaurants. The nutritional values of fast foods can vary considerably (see Table 5.6), and **fat density** remains a serious limitation of fast foods. In comparison to the recommended standard (20–35 percent of total calories from fat), 40–70 percent of the calories in fast foods are obtained from fats. A conversion some years ago from animal fat to vegetable oil for frying (to reduce cholesterol levels) did not alter the fat-dense nature of these food items. In fact, the vegetable oil formula now used by the major fast-food companies is hydrogenated vegetable shortening and not liquid vegetable oil as advertised. This shortening contributes fat in the form of trans-fatty acids, which, as we have discussed, are suspected contributors to arterial wall damage. Table 5.6 shows how many fast foods are high in sodium and saturated and trans fat.

Although many fast-food restaurants have broadened their menus to include whole-wheat breads and rolls, salad bars, fruit, and low-fat milk, a recent study showed that those who said they ate out at fast-food restaurants at least twice a week or more gained 10 pounds more than those who did not. Also, sit-down chain restaurants such as Applebees, Outback Steakhouse, Chili's, Cracker Barrel, Denny's, Olive Garden, and Red Lobster offer children's meals that are adult sized in calories and fat content. For example, the boomerang cheeseburger with fries at Outback Steakhouse has 840 calories and 31 grams of saturated-plus-trans fat. Applebee's grilled cheese sandwich with fries has 900 calories and 14 grams of saturated fat in the grilled cheese alone.

Some fast-food restaurants seem to be turning away from their healthy food offerings and reinstating high-fat and high-calorie meals. For example, Burger King recently introduced its Enormous Omelet Sandwich, which comprises one sausage patty, two eggs, two American cheese slices, and three strips of bacon on a bun. This adds up to a whopping 730 calories and 47 grams of fat. It has a suggested retail price of $2.99, or $3.49 for the value meal, which comes with fried potatoes and coffee or juice. The hash browns add 230 calories and 15 grams of fat to the meal.

Hardee's has also bucked the "health trend" in fast-food restaurants by offering a burger it dubbed the "Monster Thickburger," with 1,400 calories and 107 grams of fat. The Grand Slam breakfast at Denny's, which comes with two pancakes, two eggs, two strips of bacon, and two sausage links, has 665 calories and 49 grams of fat, according to the Denny's Web site. The Fabulous French Toast Platter—with three slices of French toast, two bacon strips, and two sausage links—contains 1,261 calories and 79 grams of fat. Many of the "meal deals" offered by restaurants, such as Burger King's King Value Meal (a Double Whopper with Cheese) and Wendy's Classic Triple with Cheese plus Great Biggie Fries and a Biggie Cola, supply more than a day's worth of calories and sodium and two days of saturated and trans fat.

Who are these restaurants appealing to with these menu items? Research shows that men ages 18 to 24 make fast-food choices based on getting the most for the least amount of money, not on nutritional value. And don't be fooled by thinking that if it's salad it's healthy; that can be far from the truth. Wendy's Garden Sensations Salads, for example, have half the daily fat allowance and one third of the day's sodium. Burger King's TenderCrisp salads have 500 calories and 11 grams of fat, and McDonald's salads have 500 calories, 19 grams of fat, and half the day's allotment of sodium.

On the other side of the coin, some healthy fast-food choices are Burger King's veggie burger with 380 calories (although it contains 930 mg of sodium), Wendy's Ultimate Chicken Grill (360 calories), McDonald's Chicken McGrill (400 calories), McDonald's Hamburger (260 calories,) and McDonald's fruit and yogurt (160 calories).

Table 5.7 shows some other healthy food choices you can make at several fast-food restaurants.

Functional Foods

At the forefront of healthful nutrition is the identification and development of foods intended to affect a particular health problem or to improve the functional capability of the body. **Functional foods** contain not only recognized nutrients but also new or enhanced elements that impart medicinelike properties to the food. Alternative labels also exist for various subclasses of functional foods, such as *nutraceutics,* or food elements that may be packaged in forms appearing more like medications (for example, pills or capsules), and *probiotics.*[31] **Probiotics** are living bacteria (good bugs) that are thought to help prevent disease and boost the immune system. They make the environment in the digestive

---

Key Terms

fat density the percentage of a food's total calories that are derived from fat; above 35 percent reflects high fat density

functional foods foods capable of contributing to the improvement/prevention of specific health problems

probiotics living bacteria (good bugs) that help to prevent disease and strengthen the immune system

Table 5.6 The Fast Lane

Within each section, foods are ranked from least to most bad fat (saturated + trans), then calories.

Burgers, etc.

	Calories	Total Fat (grams)	Saturated + Trans Fat (grams)	Sodium (milligrams)
Burger King BK Veggie	380	16	3	930
McDonald's Hamburger	260	9	4	530
Wendy's Jr. Hamburger	280	9	4	600
McDonald's McVeggie*	350	8	4	1,200
Burger King Hamburger	310	13	6	550
McDonald's Cheeseburger	310	12	7	740
Burger King Whopper Jr.	390	22	8	550
McDonald's Quarter Pounder	420	18	8	730
Wendy's Classic Single	430	20	8	890
Burger King The Angus Steak Burger	570	22	9	1,270
McDonald's Big N' Tasty	520	29	11	730
McDonald's Big Mac	560	30	12	1,010
McDonald's Quarter Pounder with Cheese	510	25	14	1,150
Wendy's Big Bacon Classic	580	29	14	1,390
Burger King Whopper	700	42	14	1,020
Wendy's Classic Double with Cheese	700	39	19	1,470
Burger King Whopper with Cheese	800	49	20	1,450
McDonald's Double Quarter Pounder with Cheese	730	40	22	1,330
Burger King Double Whopper	970	61	24	1,110
Wendy's Classic Triple with Cheese	970	59	29	2,060
Burger King Double Whopper with Cheese	1,060	69	30	1,540

Chicken & Fish Sandwiches

	Calories	Total Fat (grams)	Saturated + Trans Fat (grams)	Sodium (milligrams)
Wendy's Ultimate Chicken Grill	360	7	2	1,090
McDonald's Chicken McGrill	400	16	3	1,010
McDonald's Filet-O-Fish	400	18	5	640
Wendy's Spicy Chicken Fillet	510	19	5	1,480
Burger King Chicken Whopper	570	25	5	1,410
McDonald's McChicken	420	22	6	760
McDonald's Crispy Chicken	500	23	6	1,090
Wendy's Homestyle Chicken Fillet	540	22	6	1,320
Burger King Chicken	560	28	8	1,270
Burger King TenderCrisp Chicken	780	45	11	1,730
Burger King BK Fish Filet	520	30	NA	840

French Fries

	Calories	Total Fat (grams)	Saturated + Trans Fat (grams)	Sodium (milligrams)
McDonald's, small (2½ oz)	230	11	5	140
Burger King, small (2½ oz)	230	11	6	410
Wendy's, small (3 oz)	280	14	6	270
McDonald's, medium (4 oz)	350	16	7	220
Wendy's, medium (5 oz)	440	21	9	430
Burger King, medium (4 oz)	360	18	10	640
Wendy's, Biggie (5½ oz)	490	24	10	480
McDonald's, large (6 oz)	520	25	11	330
Wendy's, Great Biggie (6½ oz)	590	29	12	570
Burger King, large (5½ oz)	500	25	13	880
Burger King, king (7 oz)	600	30	16	1,070

Chicken Nuggets (no. pieces–weight)

	Calories	Total Fat (grams)	Saturated + Trans Fat (grams)	Sodium (milligrams)
McDonald's McNuggets (6–3½ oz)	250	15	5	670
Burger King Tenders (5–2½ oz)	210	12	6	530
McDonald's Selects (3–4½ oz)	380	20	6	930
Wendy's Homestyle Strips (3–5½ oz)	410	18	7	1,470
McDonald's McNuggets (10–5½ oz)	420	24	8	1,120
Burger King Tenders (8–4½ oz)	340	19	9	840
McDonald's Selects (5–8 oz)	630	33	11	1,550
McDonald's McNuggets (20–11½ oz)	840	49	16	2,240
McDonald's Selects (10–15½ oz)	1,270	66	21	3,100

Entrée Salads

	Calories	Total Fat (grams)	Saturated + Trans Fat (grams)	Sodium (milligrams)
Burger King Fire-Grilled Chicken or Shrimp Garden Salad, Vinaigrette[1]	310	18	4	1,770
Wendy's Mandarin Chicken Salad, Oriental Sesame dressing	550	26	4	1,210
Burger King Fire-Grilled Chicken or Shrimp Caesar Salad, Caesar dressing[1]	320	20	5	1,600
McDonald's California Cobb Salad with Grilled Chicken, Cobb dressing	380	20	7	1,500
McDonald's Caesar Salad with Grilled Chicken, Caesar dressing	390	24	7	1,330
McDonald's Bacon Ranch Salad with Grilled Chicken, Ranch dressing	410	24	7	1,470
Wendy's Spring Mix Salad, Low Fat Honey Mustard dressing	420	27	8	630
McDonald's California Cobb Salad with Crispy Chicken, Cobb dressing	480	27	9	1,580
McDonald's Bacon Ranch Salad with Crispy Chicken, Ranch dressing	510	31	9	1,560

Table 5.6—*continued*

	Calories	Total Fat (grams)	Saturated + Trans Fat (grams)	Sodium (milligrams)
McDonald's Caesar Salad with Crispy Chicken, Caesar dressing	490	32	10	1,410
Burger King TenderCrisp Garden Salad, Ranch dressing	530	32	10	1,780
Wendy's Spring Mix Salad, House Vinaigrette	500	42	11	1,040
Burger King TenderCrisp Caesar Salad, Caesar dressing	520	33	11	1,870
Wendy's Chicken BLT Salad, Honey Mustard dressing	680	47	13	1,320
Wendy's Homestyle Chicken Strips Salad, Ranch dressing	670	45	15	1,760
Wendy's Taco Supremo Salad	680	31	17	1,700
Baked Potatoes & Chili				
Burger King Chili (7½ oz)	190	8	3	1,040
Wendy's Chili, small (8 oz)	220	6	3	780
Wendy's Broccoli & Cheese Potato	440	15	3	540
Wendy's Chili, large (12 oz)	330	9	4	1,170
Wendy's Sour Cream & Chives Potato	340	6	4	40
Wendy's Bacon & Cheese Potato	560	25	7	850
Desserts & Shakes				
Wendy's Fresh Fruit Bowl with Yogurt	220	1	0	90
McDonald's Apple Dippers with Dip (3 oz)	100	1	1	40
McDonald's Fruit 'n Yogurt Parfait (5½ oz)	160	2	1	90
McDonald's Ice Cream Cone (3 oz)	150	4	2	60
Wendy's Frosty, small (12 oz)	330	8	5	150
Burger King Dutch Apple Pie (4 oz)	340	14	6	470
McDonald's Triple Thick Shake (12 oz)[2]	430	10	7	150
McDonald's Baked Apple Pie (3 oz)	250	11	8	150
Burger King Shake, small (9 oz)[2]	410	14	8	250
Wendy's Frosty, large (20 oz)	540	13	9	250
Burger King Shake, medium (13 oz)[2]	580	18	12	360
McDonald's McFlurry (12 oz)[2]	590	18	12	220
McDonald's Triple Thick Shake (21 oz)[2]	750	18	12	270
Burger King Shake, large (19 oz)[2]	830	27	18	520
McDonald's Triple Thick Shake (32 oz)[2]	1,130	26	18	410

	Calories	Total Fat (grams)	Saturated + Trans Fat (grams)	Sodium (milligrams)
McDonald's Extra Value Meals (includes medium fries and medium Coke, unless noted)				
Chicken McGrill Sandwich	960	32	10	1,250
Filet-O-Fish Sandwich	960	34	12	880
Crispy Chicken Sandwich	1,060	39	13	1,330
Chicken McNuggets (10 pieces)	980	40	15	1,360
Big N' Tasty	1,080	45	18	970
Chicken Selects (5 pieces)	1,190	49	18	1,790
Big Mac	1,120	46	19	1,250
Quarter Pounder with Cheese	1,070	41	21	1,390
Double Quarter Pounder with Cheese, large fries, large Coke	1,560	65	33	1,680
Burger King Value Meals (includes medium fries and medium Coke, unless noted)				
Chicken Whopper	1,130	43	14	2,050
Chicken Tenders (8 pieces)	900	37	18	1,480
Chicken Sandwich	1,120	46	18	1,910
TenderCrisp Chicken Sandwich	1,340	63	21	2,370
Whopper	1,260	60	24	1,660
Whopper, king fries, king Coke	1,690	72	30	2,090
Whopper with Cheese, large fries, large Coke	1,590	74	33	2,330
Double Whopper with Cheese, king fries, king Coke	2,050	99	46	2,610
Wendy's Combo Meals (includes Biggie fries and medium cola, unless noted)				
Ultimate Chicken Grill Sandwich, Salad with Low Fat Honey Mustard, Iced Tea	510	10	2	1,450
Homestyle Chicken Fillet Sandwich	1,150	46	16	1,800
Homestyle Chicken Strips (3 pieces)	1,020	42	17	1,950
Classic Single	1,040	44	18	1,370
Big Bacon Classic	1,190	53	24	1,870
Classic Double with Cheese, Great Biggie fries, Biggie cola	1,480	68	31	2,040
Classic Triple with Cheese, Great Biggie fries, Biggie cola	1,750	88	41	2,630

*Limited availability. [1]Average of the items listed. [2]Average of all flavors. NA Number not available.

Daily Values (daily limits for a 2,000-calorie diet): **Total Fat:** 65 grams. **Saturated + Trans Fat:** 20 grams. **Sodium:** 2,400 milligrams.

Source: Nutrition Action Letter, "Fast Food in '05," March, 2005.

Table 5.7 Making Better Fast-Food Choices

Fast-food meals can be high in calories, fat, cholesterol, and sodium. But it is still possible to eat fast food occasionally and follow a sensible diet. Take a look at how a few sample meals stack up against one another, and against the recommended daily intake for calories (2,000–2,700 per day), fat (no more than 50–80 g), cholesterol (no more than 300 mg), and sodium (no more than 1,100–3,300 mg).

	Poor Choice	Sensible Choice
Burger (McDonald's)	Double quarter-pound burger with cheese, large fries, 16 oz soda *1,560 calories* *65 g fat* *98 mg cholesterol* *1,680 mg sodium*	Hamburger, small fries, 16 oz diet soda *490 calories* *20 g fat* *30 mg cholesterol* *670 mg sodium*
Pizza (Domino's)	4 slices sausage and mushroom pizza, 16 oz soda *1,000 calories* *28 g fat* *62 mg cholesterol* *2,302 mg sodium*	3 slices cheese pizza, 16 oz diet soda *516 calories* *15 g fat* *29 mg cholesterol* *1,470 mg sodium*
Chicken (KFC)	2 pieces fried chicken (breast and wing), buttermilk biscuit, mashed potatoes with gravy, corn-on-the-cob, 15 oz soda *1,232 calories* *57 g fat* *157 mg cholesterol* *2,276 mg sodium*	1 piece fried chicken (wing), mashed potatoes with gravy, cole slaw, 15 oz diet soda *373 calories* *19 g fat* *46 mg cholesterol* *943 mg sodium*
Taco (Taco Bell)	Taco salad, 16 oz soda *1,057 calories* *55 g fat* *80 mg cholesterol* *1,620 mg sodium*	3 light tacos, 16 oz diet soda *420 calories* *15 g fat* *60 mg cholesterol* *840 mg sodium*

Source: Adapted from "Fast Food Facts" from the office of the Minnesota Attorney General, www.olen.com/food/book.html.

Changing for the Better

Eating on the Run

I am always in a hurry and don't have time to cook, and so a lot of my meals end up being fast food. Are there better choices I can make when eating on the run?

The typical American eats about three hamburgers and four orders of French fries each week so you aren't alone. With over 300,000 fast-food restaurants in the United States, fast food is definitely part of the American lifestyle. Here are some things to consider when eating at fast food restaurants:

- Don't supersize! Go for the "small" or "regular" size.
- Don't wait until you are starving because that leads to overeating and supersizing!
- Decide what you want to order ahead of time, and don't be swayed by "value meal" or what "looks good."
- Ask for a nutritional guide for the menu. Look at the calories, fat grams, and sodium when making your selection.

- Order grilled instead of fried chicken or fish.
- Look for the "light" choices.
- Limit your condiments. Mustard, ketchup, salsa, or low-fat or fat-free condiments and dressing are preferable to regular mayonnaise or high-fat dressings.
- For breakfast, choose cereal and milk or pancakes rather than a breakfast sandwich (which can have about 475 calories, 30 grams of fat, and 1,260 mg of sodium).
- Bring fast food from home! Buy portable foods at the grocery store to take with you that can be eaten quickly and easily such as portable yogurt, banana, apple, low-fat granola bar, or breakfast bar.
- Order low-fat or skim milk or water instead of soda.
- Go to a variety of different kinds of fast-food restaurants so you aren't eating hamburgers every day, and set a limit on how many meals you are going to eat out each week.

system inhospitable for harmful bacteria (the bad bugs). More than 400 types of bacteria reside in and on our bodies and outnumber human cells 10 to 1. Yogurt is one example of a food that gives you a dose of these good bugs—lactobacillus bulgaris.

Examples of functional foods include garlic (believed to lower cholesterol), olive oil (thought to prevent heart disease), foods high in fiber (which prevent constipation and lower cholesterol), and foods rich in calcium (which help prevent osteoporosis). In addition, foods that contain high levels of vitamins A, C, and E—primarily fruits and vegetables—and provide the body with natural sources of antioxidants are functional foods.

 TALKING POINTS What fast-food restaurants are your favorites? Are you surprised at any of the information in this chapter regarding your favorite meals? Will you change your order next time you visit a fast-food restaurant?

Other functional foods are those that contain or are enriched with folic acid. These vitamin B family foods aid in the prevention of spina bifida and other neural tube defects (see Chapter 12) and the prevention of heart disease. Foods that are rich in selenium are sometimes categorized as functional foods because of selenium's potential as an agent in cancer prevention. Most recently, the FDA approved a "heart healthy" label for foods that are rich in soy protein.[32] All the functional foods discussed here are approved to carry **health claims** on the basis of current FDA criteria.[33]

One category of functional foods being researched is vegetables that are genetically engineered to produce a specific biological element that is important to human health. An example is tomatoes that are high in lycopene. Another example is a new type of margarine that can lower the level of and change the properties of blood cholesterol. Food technologists are interested in expanding the functional food family to include a greater array of health-enhancing food items.

Dietary Supplements

In 2004 it was estimated that Americans spent 19 billion dollars on a wide array of over-the-counter (OTC) products

---

Key Terms

health claims statements authorized by the FDA as having scientific proof of claims that a food, nutrient, or dietary supplement has an effect on a health-related condition known collectively as *dietary supplements.* These nonprescription products are legally described as:

- Products (other than tobacco) that are intended to supplement the diet, including vitamins, amino acids, minerals, glandular extracts, herbs, and other plant products such as fungi.
- Products that are intended for use by people to supplement the total daily intake of nutrients in the diet.
- Products that are intended to be ingested in tablet, capsule, softgel, gelcap, and liquid form.
- Products that are not in themselves to be used as conventional foods or as the only items of a meal or diet.

Unlike prescription medications, dietary supplements have been available in the marketplace for years almost without restriction. However, dietary supplements now must be deemed safe for human use on the basis of information supplied to the Food and Drug Administration (FDA) by the manufacturers. In addition, the labels on these products cannot make a direct claim, with the exception of calcium and folic acid supplements, that they can cure or prevent illnesses. However, other materials with such claims may be displayed close to the dietary supplements themselves. Further, the labels on dietary supplements must remind consumers that the FDA has not required these products to undergo the rigorous research required of prescription medications, and so the FDA cannot attest to their effectiveness. Beyond this, consumers are left to themselves to decide whether to purchase and use dietary supplements.

As we mentioned, probiotic products, dietary supplements with live bacteria, are gaining in popularity. The U.S. sales of probiotic supplements have increased 19 percent since 2003, with total sales of $714 million in 2005. Actimel is one of the biggest sellers, claiming to "help to strengthen your body's natural defenses" and enhance your immune system.[34]

Easily accessible to anyone, over 15,000 different dietary supplements can be purchased in grocery stores, drugstores, and discount stores, through mail-order catalogs, and over the Internet. Because of the great demand for these products, major pharmaceutical companies are now entering the dietary supplement field. Whether this trend leads to the development of more effective products, or to a greater effort on the part of the FDA to demand proof of effectiveness, remains to be seen. By definition, supplements are not foods but simply "supplements." Therefore, they remain free from requirements to substantiate their claims of effectiveness (as now required for functional foods).

 TALKING POINTS A friend asks you about the advantages and disadvantages of taking a dietary supplement. What would you point out to your friend?

Food Allergies

Foods enjoyed by the vast majority of people may be harmful and even deadly to others because of their unique food allergies. For some people, peanuts, the familiar snacks once served on many plane flights, are such a food. Today, U.S. airlines are replacing peanuts with pretzels in order to provide "peanut-free" flights and to protect people known to be allergic to peanuts and peanut-based products. Many schools have already established peanut-free tables in their lunchrooms for the same purpose.

Being intolerant to certain foods is not the same as being allergic to particular foods. **Food intolerance** means that a food upsets your intestines, usually because of an enzyme deficiency. A lactase deficiency, for example, causes lactose intolerance. Lactose intolerance affects 20 percent of Caucasian Americans, 75 percent of African Americans, and 50 percent of Hispanic Americans. Intolerance of gluten (found in wheat, rye, barley, and perhaps oats) affects 1 of every 150 Americans and can cause malnutrition, premature osteoporosis, colon cancer, thyroid disease, diabetes, arthritis, miscarriage, and birth defects.

A **food allergy** mistakenly calls the body's disease-fighting immune system into action, creating unpleasant and sometimes life-threatening symptoms. Peanuts, milk, eggs, shellfish, tree nuts, fish, soy, and wheat account for 90 percent of food allergies. Eight percent of children and 2 percent of adults have food allergies. For some members of this group, food-based allergies may be serious or even life threatening.

Because food allergies generally develop slowly, initial symptoms may not be fully recognized or even associated with the food. It takes three exposures to the allergic food

Key Terms

food intolerance an adverse reaction to a specific food that does not involve the immune system; usually caused by an enzyme deficiency

food allergy a reaction in which the immune system attacks an otherwise harmless food or ingredient; allergic reactions can range from mildly unpleasant to life threatening to obtain a significant food allergy reaction. The first time a person eats a food she is allergic to, she may have little or no reaction. The second time she eats this food, she will most likely have a more observable reaction, such as breaking out in hives, itching, runny nose, burning in the mouth, and wheezing. The third exposure can bring on a full-blown reaction, which, for peanut allergies among others, can result in death within minutes. There is no cure for food allergies, and the treatment is for the food-allergic person to avoid these foods and carry an epi-pen (epinephrine) at all times.

For the first time, an experimental drug has proven highly effective against potentially deadly peanut allergies. The once-a-month shots don't cure peanut allergy, which affects about 1.5 million Americans and kills 50 to 100 people each year. Xolair, a drug currently patented for patients with asthma, may hold promise in preventing or reducing the severity of reactions for people who suffer from peanut allergy. Xolair, an anti-IgE therapy, blocks a protein called *immunoglobulin E* from causing an asthmatic reaction. Genentech and Novartis Pharmaceuticals are currently conducting clinical trials for use with people who suffer from peanut allergy in hope that anti-IgE therapy can be used to diminish or eliminate the reaction caused by peanut allergy in the same way it treats asthma. However, Xolair is not a cure or a vaccine. It just adds protection against a fatal reaction in case of accidental ingestion of peanut-containing food. Scientists also are working on treatments that could suppress peanut allergy permanently, but those developments are probably 5 to 10 years in the future.

Organic foods tend to be safer and healthier.

Food Labels

Since 1973, food manufacturers have been required by the FDA to provide nutritional information (labels) on products to which one or more nutrients have been added or for which some nutritional claim has been made. Despite the presence of these labels, there was concern about whether the public could understand the labels as they appeared and whether additional information was required. Accordingly, the FDA, in consultation with individual states and public interest groups, developed new labeling regulations. Revised labels began appearing on food packages in 1993. The currently used label is shown in Figure 5-3. Specific types of information contained on the new label are highlighted. Additionally, newly developed definitions for nutrition-related terms are shown in the Star box on page 157.

Proposals for the labeling of raw foods, including fresh produce, meat, and seafood, are now being studied. Concern for consumer protection stems from recent disclosures regarding inadequate meat inspection, undercooking of hamburgers, and the risk of contaminated seafood.

Processed meat, fish, and poultry products, such as hot dogs, fish sticks, and chicken patties, must be labeled. Produce, such as vegetables and fruit, is not required to be labeled. Currently, single-ingredient meat, fish, and poultry products are not required to have a label. However, in conjunction with the National Nutrition Summit meetings held in the spring of 2000, it was announced that food labels for meats, including information on fat, saturated fat, cholesterol, and other nutrients, would be forthcoming.

Beginning January 1, 2006, foodmakers have been required by the FDA to put the amount of trans fat on food labels, sparking some companies such as Frito-Lay and Kraft to start reducing and even eliminating trans fat from its products. The FDA has further recommended that food labels list calories in larger type print, list the percentage of the consumer's daily allotment of calories, and list the total amount of calories in the container, not just the calories per serving. For example, pretzels might be listed as having 100 calories per serving and approximately 15 servings per bag and so it is up to you to compute how

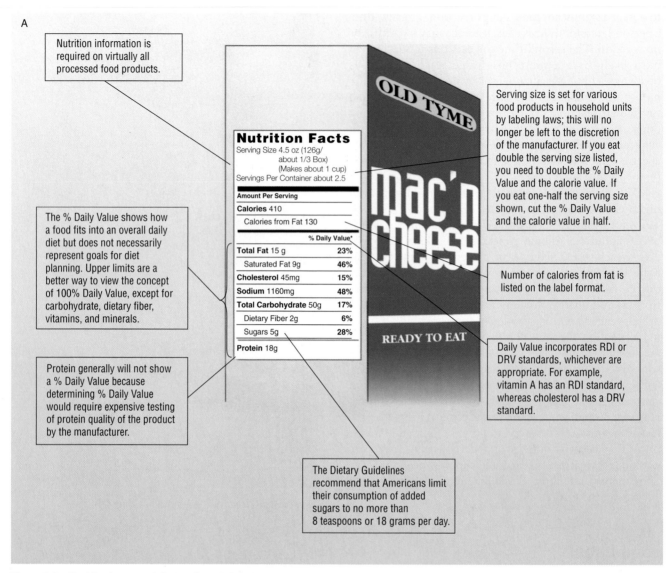

A

Nutrition information is required on virtually all processed food products.

Nutrition Facts
Serving Size 4.5 oz (126g/ about 1/3 Box) (Makes about 1 cup) Servings Per Container about 2.5

Amount Per Serving	
Calories 410	
Calories from Fat 130	
	% Daily Value*
Total Fat 15 g	23%
Saturated Fat 9g	46%
Cholesterol 45mg	15%
Sodium 1160mg	48%
Total Carbohydrate 50g	17%
Dietary Fiber 2g	6%
Sugars 5g	28%
Protein 18g	

Serving size is set for various food products in household units by labeling laws; this will no longer be left to the discretion of the manufacturer. If you eat double the serving size listed, you need to double the % Daily Value and the calorie value. If you eat one-half the serving size shown, cut the % Daily Value and the calorie value in half.

Number of calories from fat is listed on the label format.

Daily Value incorporates RDI or DRV standards, whichever are appropriate. For example, vitamin A has an RDI standard, whereas cholesterol has a DRV standard.

The % Daily Value shows how a food fits into an overall daily diet but does not necessarily represent goals for diet planning. Upper limits are a better way to view the concept of 100% Daily Value, except for carbohydrate, dietary fiber, vitamins, and minerals.

Protein generally will not show a % Daily Value because determining % Daily Value would require expensive testing of protein quality of the product by the manufacturer.

The Dietary Guidelines recommend that Americans limit their consumption of added sugars to no more than 8 teaspoons or 18 grams per day.

OLD TYME
mac'n cheese
READY TO EAT

Figure 5-3 Nutrition facts panel. **A:** top of panel; **B:** bottom of panel

many servings and calories you have consumed. The FDA is also urging restaurants to list calories on their menus. The FDA prohibits any nutrient claim that it has not defined. For example, the FDA recently defined *low fat* as containing 3 grams or less of fat per serving (see the Star Box on page 157 for more on this). The FDA has not yet defined what can be considered to be low carb even though many foodmakers and restaurants use this term in their advertising. Consumers need to know what is meant by claims such as *low calorie, low fat,* and *low carb*; having a standard definition makes it much easier to make healthy and informed nutritional choices.

There is also a push for the FDA to make food labels clearer, more understandable to children as well as to adults, and uniform. This is especially important for peo-

ple with food allergies, whose health may depend on the clarity of a food label. For example "whey, casein, and lactoglobulin" can be used to indicate the presence of milk in a product, but some people who are lactose intolerant may not realize that they are consuming a milk product.

The new USDA organic food labels went into effect in October 2002 to standardize regulations for foods grown without synthetic pesticides or other chemicals. Under the new USDA rules, organic means:

- Meat, poultry, and eggs are from animals given no growth hormones or antibiotics. Vitamin and mineral supplements are allowed. Livestock are given organic feed and live in conditions that allow for "exercise, freedom of movement and reduction of stress."

B

Many vitamin and mineral amounts no longer need to be listed on the nutrition label. Only vitamin A, vitamin C, calcium, and iron remain. The interest in or risk of deficiencies of the other vitamins and minerals is deemed too low to warrant inclusion.

Vitamin A 10%•Vitamin C 0%

Calcium 30% •Iron 15%

Percent Daily Values are based on a 2,000 calorie diet. Your daily values may be higher or lower depending on your calorie needs:

		Calories:	2,000	2,500
Total Fat	Less than		65g	80g
Sat Fat	Less than		20g	25g
Cholest	Less than		300mg	300mg
Sodium	Less than		2,400mg	2,400mg
Total Carb			300g	375g
Fiber			25g	30g

Some Daily Value standards, such as grams of total fat, increase as energy intake increases. The % Daily Values on the label are based on a 2,000 kcal diet.

**Calories per gram:
Fat 9 • Carbohydrate 4
• Protein 4**

GOOD SOURCE OF CALCIUM SEE SIDE PANEL FOR NUTRITION INFORMATION

Absolute and comparative claims, as well as health claims, can appear on the front panel or on the sides of the package. All must follow legal definitions.

Labels on larger packages may list the number of calories per gram of fat, carbohydrate, and protein.

INGREDIENTS: WATER, ENRICHED MACARONI (ENRICHED FLOUR [NIACIN, FERROUS SULFATE (IRON), THIAMINE MONONITRATE AND RIBOFLAVIN], EGG WHITE), FLOUR, CHEDDAR CHEESE (MILK, CHEESE CULTURE, SALT, ENZYME), SPICES, MARGARINE (PARTIALLY HYDROGENATED SOYBEAN OIL, WATER, SOY LECITHIN, MONO- AND DIGLYCERIDES, BETA CAROTENE FOR COLOR, VITAMIN A PALMITATE), AND MALTODEXTRIN.

Ingredients, listed in descending order by weight, appear here or in another place on the package. The sources of some ingredients, such as certain flavorings, will be stated by name to help people better identify ingredients that they avoid for health, religious, or other reasons.

- Products are not genetically engineered or irradiated to kill germs.
- Crops are grown on land that has not been fertilized with sewage sludge or chemical fertilizers.
- Pests and plant disease are treated primarily with insect predators, traps, natural repellants, and other nonchemical methods.

- Weeds are controlled by mulching, mowing, hand weeding, or mechanical cultivation, not chemical herbicides.

There are different types of organic foods: "100 percent organic," meaning the food contains all organic ingredients; "organic," which means at least 95 percent of the product is organic; and "made with organic ingredients," which means at least 70 percent of the food is organic as previously defined.[35]

Organic foods have enjoyed a 20 percent annual growth rate over the past several years. One-hundred and twenty new organic snacks were introduced to meet the needs of people trying to find healthier snacks. It is projected that the now 10.4-billion-dollar organic food industry will increase to 32 billion dollars by 2009, owing to its increasing popularity.

Food Safety

Technological advances in food manufacturing and processing have done much to assure that the food we eat is fresh and safe. Yet concern is growing that certain recent developments may also produce harmful effects on humans. For example, the preparation, handling and storage of food, irradiation of foods, and genetic engineering of foods all contribute to the safety of our food in terms of contamination.

Foodborne Illness

Foodborne illness or food poisoning is the result of eating contaminated food. The symptoms of food poisoning can be easily mistaken for the flu—fatigue, chills, mild fever, dizziness, headaches, upset stomach, diarrhea, and severe cramps. Illness develops within 1 to 6 hours following ingestion of the contaminated food, and recovery is fairly rapid.[36] Bacteria are the culprits in most cases of food poisoning, which can be the result of food not being cooked thoroughly to destroy bacteria or not keeping food cool enough to slow their growth. In addition, nearly half of all cases of food poisoning can be prevented with proper hand washing so as to not contaminate food by viruses, parasites, or toxic chemicals. Food safety is such an important issue that the USDA incorporated it into the new dietary guidelines. (Some of the guidelines are included in the Star Box on page 160.) Food should be refrigerated below 40° Fahrenheit or kept warm above 140° Fahrenheit. Between 40° and 140° Fahrenheit, bacteria can double in number in as little as 20 minutes, so it is important to keep food at safe temperatures. (See Figure 5-4 on temperature rules for safe cooking and handling of foods.)

Most of us know that we must wash our hands before handling food; however, do you use the USDA's recommended protocol for hand washing? They recommend washing your hands often during food preparation, wetting your hands, applying soap, rubbing your hands for 29 seconds, rinsing hands thoroughly under clean, warm, running water and drying your hands completely using a clean disposable or cloth towel.

It is estimated that 76 million Americans are the victims of food poisoning each year, and about 5,000 of these people die.

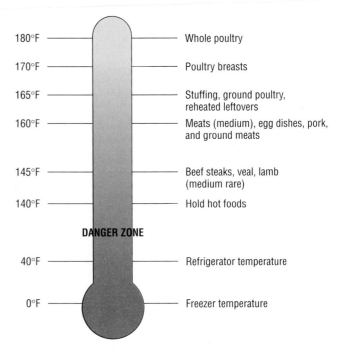

Figure 5-4 Temperature rules for cooking and safe handling of food

Salmonella is the most common foodborne illness and is found mostly in raw or undercooked poultry, meat, eggs, fish, and unpasteurized milk. Clostridium perfringens, also called the "buffet germ," grows where there is little to no oxygen and grows fastest in large portions held at low or room temperatures. For this reason, buffet table servings should be replaced often and leftovers should be refrigerated quickly. Refrigerated leftovers may become harmful to eat after 3 days. The old adage "if in doubt, throw it out" applies to any questionable leftovers. A third type of food poisoning is botulism, which is rare but often fatal. It is caused by home-canned or commercially canned food that hasn't been processed or stored properly. Some warning signs are swollen or dented cans or lids, cracked jars, loose lids, and clear liquids turned milky.

The Center for Science in the Public Interest found that fruits and vegetables account for the majority of foodborne illnesses. Salads are by far the biggest culprit. The reason for this seems to be because some of the water used to irrigate and wash produce is contaminated with human and animal feces. This problem can be difficult to regulate or correct, because produce comes from all over the world, not just from the United States.

What do you do if you suspect food poisoning?

1. Contact a medical professional immediately. Don't wait to see if you feel better.
2. Report the incident to your local health department as soon as possible if the suspected food came from a public place.

Speaking Label-ese

Food labels constitute a language all their own, defined by government regulation. You need to learn this language and understand its terms. Here are some translations of what is meant by the labels you read:

- Calorie-free = contains less than 5 calories per serving

- Low calorie = contains 40 calories or less per serving

- Reduced calorie = contains at least 25 percent fewer calories than regular versions of the food do

- Lite or light = contains ⅓ fewer calories than do regular versions of the product or no more than half the fat of the regular version of the product

- Fat free = contains less than 0.5 g of fat per serving

- Free = contains none or trivial amounts of a substance such as sodium, fat, cholesterol, calories, or sugars

- Low fat = contains 3 g or less per serving

- Reduced fat = at least 25 percent or less fat than regular versions of the food

- Cholesterol free = contains no more than 2 mg of cholesterol and 2 g or less of saturated fat per serving

- Low saturated fat = contains 1 g or less of saturated fat per serving

- Lean = contains fewer than 10 g of fat, 4 g of saturated fat, and 95 mg of cholesterol per serving or per 100 g of food

- Fresh = unprocessed, uncooked, unfrozen

- Healthy = contains no more than 3 g of fat, including 1 g of saturated fat and 60 mg of

cholesterol per serving and must also contain at least 10 percent of RDA of one of these: vitamin A, vitamin C, calcium, iron, protein, fiber. Must contain no more than 300 mg of sodium, but there is no limit on sugar content

- Good source = serving must contain 10 to 19 percent of RDA of a particular nutrient

- High = serving contains 20 percent or more of the RDA of a particular nutrient

- More = serving contains 10 percent or more of the RDA of a particular nutrient than does the regular food to which it is being compared

- Less = contains at least 25 percent less of the nutrient to which it is being compared

- Energy = refers to any product that contains calories; so any drink, except water, can meet this definition

3. Preserve the suspected food including any packaging to give to the health department for investigation and possible prevention of further poisoning.

Safe Handling of Food

Handle food properly to avoid food poisoning. Frequent hand washing is at the top of the list of food safety tips. Bacteria live and multiply on warm, moist hands, and hands can inadvertently transport germs from one surface to another. It is also important to clean work surfaces with hot, soapy water and keep nonfood items such as the mail, newspapers, and purses, off the countertops. Some people advocate the use of antibacterial products, whereas others maintain that if they are overused, these products can lose their effectiveness, and bacteria then become resistant to them. Utensils, dishes, cutting boards, cookware, and towels and sponges need to be washed in hot, soapy water and rinsed well.

Irradiation of Food

Because of the increasing concern about contaminated meat and meat products, the first irradiated meat, ground beef, arrived in American supermarkets in early 2000. Irradiated frozen chicken was introduced more recently. Irradiation is a process that causes damage to the DNA of disease-causing bacteria such as salmonella and E. coli as well as of insects, parasites, and other organisms so that they can't reproduce.

While irradiated meat has much lower bacteria levels than regular meat does, irradiation doesn't destroy all bacteria in meat. In fact, irradiation actually destroys fewer bacteria than does proper cooking.[36] There is also some concern that irradiation will lull consumers into a false sense of security so that they erroneously believe that they don't have to take the usual precautions in food handling and preparation. For example, undercooking, unclean work surfaces or cooking utensils, and improper storage can still contaminate meat. Some also claim that irradiated meat has a distinct off-taste and a smell like "singed hair."

Safe Farming Techniques

In recent decades, there has been an increased push toward ensuring better treatment of animals raised for slaughter and for dairy production in the United States. As a result of recent reforms, more than half of beef cattle in North America meet their end at slaughterhouses based on innovative designs that consider the fears and inclinations of herd animals. The cages of laying hens are nearly one third larger than the old ones were, and the practice of starving hens for weeks at a time to stimulate egg production is beginning to be phased out. These reforms are important to ensure more humane treatment of these animals, but they are also proving beneficial to human health and food quality. It has been suggested that there is an increase in the quality of meat when animals are

Learning from Our Diversity

Diverse Food Pyramids

Besides the new food pyramid discussed earlier in this chapter, other food pyramids exist. The Mediterranean food pyramid (Figure 5-5) emphasizes fruits, beans, legumes, nuts, vegetables, whole grains, and breads. In fact, the new food pyramid recommended by the USDA looks similar to the existing Mediterranean food pyramid. Many of the changes from the old to the new USDA food pyramid are in keeping with what had already been suggested by the Mediterranean food pyramid—for example, using more olive oil, limiting consumption of alcohol, eating more whole grains, fruits, and vegetables, choosing lean meat, and exercising daily.

The Asian food pyramid (Figure 5-6) limits meat consumption even more by recommending consumption of meat on a monthly basis and daily consumption of fish, shellfish, and dairy products. The Asian diet, like the Mediterranean diet, encourages daily intake of fruit, legumes, vegetables, and whole grains. In addition, the Asian diet includes rice and noodles and suggests eating poultry, eggs, and sweets only once a week.

The Latin American food pyramid (Figure 5-7) also advises consumption of meat, sweets, and eggs only once a week. Like the Asian diet, it encourages eating fish and shellfish on a daily basis, and, unlike the Mediterranean and Asian diets, it advises consumption of poultry on a daily basis. As in the other food pyramids, fruit, vegetables, beans, and whole grains are to be consumed every day, and physical exercise is emphasized by all three food pyramids.

The changes the USDA made to its new dietary guidelines appear to have some similarities to the Mediterranean, Asian, and Latin American pyramids in the emphasis on fruit, vegetables, whole grains, limited alcohol consumption, and increased physical activity.

Source: Nowack, D., & Sarnoff, J. (2003). *Food for Thought*, National Multiple Sclerosis Society, www.nationalmssociety.org/pdf/brochures/Food.pdf.

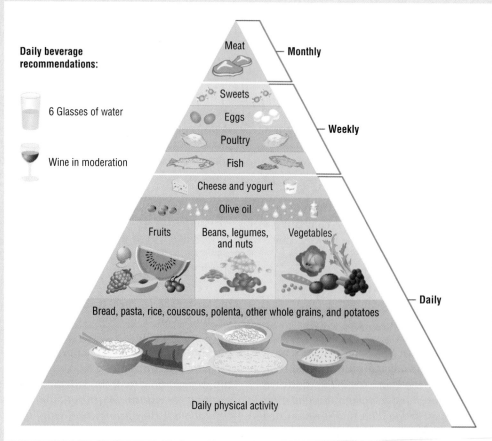

Figure 5-5   The Mediterranean Diet Pyramid

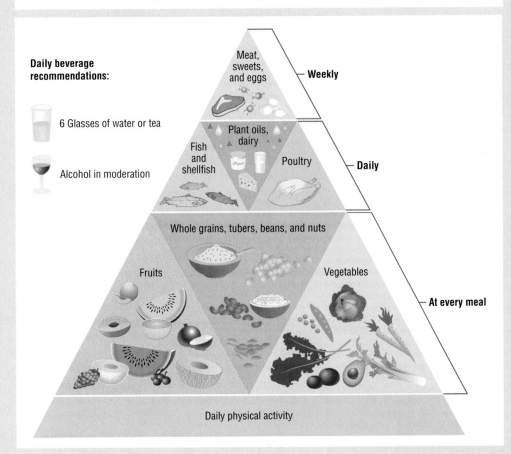

Figure 5-6 The Asian Diet Pyramid

Daily beverage recommendations:

6 Glasses of water or tea

Sake, wine, or beer in moderation

Monthly — Meat

Weekly — Sweets / Eggs and poultry

Optional daily — Fish and shellfish or dairy

Daily — Vegetable oils / Fruits / Legumes, seeds and nuts / Vegetables / Rice, noodles, breads, millet, corn, and other whole grains

Physical activity

Figure 5-7 The Latin American Diet Pyramid

Daily beverage recommendations:

6 Glasses of water or tea

Alcohol in moderation

Weekly — Meat, sweets, and eggs

Daily — Fish and shellfish / Plant oils, dairy / Poultry

At every meal — Whole grains, tubers, beans, and nuts / Fruits / Vegetables

Daily physical activity

More humane treatment of animals has contributed to increased quality, taste, and safety in food production.

treated humanely, with less bruising, improved tenderness, lower incidence of dark-cutting beef, and lessened occurrence of pale, soft, and dry pork. Furthermore, the taste of eggs is said to be significantly better if they come from humanely treated hens.

One important component in these reforms—some of which have been government mandated and others voluntarily adopted by the agricultural industry—relates to the feed given to beef cattle. The spread of bovine spongiform encephalopathy, more commonly known as Mad Cow Disease, has largely been attributed to the use of animal feed containing the protein-rich by-products of slaughtered cows, including nerve tissue, the tissue most likely to harbor the disease. Such feed—which is believed to be the primary, if not the only, way the disease can be transmitted—was banned in the United States and Canada in August 1997.[37] While the disease had been restricted to European cows, a number of cases of Mad Cow detected in American cattle in late 2003 encouraged the U.S. government to impose even stricter rules to protect the nation's beef supply from the disease, including banning the butchering of sick or injured cows, banning certain animal parts from the food supply, and increased testing on suspect animals.[38]

Eliminating animal products from feed has also proven beneficial in hens. Many consumers choose only to eat poultry and eggs from free-range, vegetarian-fed chickens, for health and safety reasons. Several companies (such as Eggland's Best) claim that their vegetarian-fed hens produce eggs that have seven times more vitamin E, are lower in cholesterol, have a higher unsaturated/saturated fat ratio, and contain more omega-3 fatty acids than do factory-farmed eggs.[39]

Interestingly, McDonald's Corporation has been one of the champions for animal welfare reform. Since 1997, the fast-food leader has required all of its meat producers to undergo animal welfare audits; in 1999 they conducted 100 audits in the United States, and in 2002, they did 500

I have heard that incorporating fish into my diet is a good source of protein and part of healthy eating. However, I recently learned that fish may be toxic. Should I limit my intake of fish?

While it is true that fish is a good source of protein and other nutritional benefits, there has been some compelling research to suggest that the big fish, swordfish, halibut, tuna, red snapper, flounder, freshwater bass, grouper, trout, marlin, king mackerel, tilefish, shark, and freshwater bass, have been associated with toxic levels of mercury in the people who consume them regularly, some of whom had more than double the amount the EPA deemed safe. Memory lapses, hair loss, stomach cramps, headaches, muscle and joint aches, nausea, and dizziness are the symptoms people reported who had toxic levels of mercury from eating these fish. Physicians claim that, within 6 months of avoiding eating fish, their patients' mercury levels decreased significantly, their hair stopped falling out, and their other symptoms subsided. Recent studies also suggest that mercury may raise the risk of heart attack. Some experts are even drawing links between mercury levels and autism in children and Alzheimer's disease in adults. Pregnant women and infants are at even greater risk, since mercury excreted through breast milk has been found to lower IQ level and may cause learning disorders and other developmental problems.

So should you swear off fish forever? No, not necessarily. It is suggested that women of childbearing age, pregnant women, nursing mothers, and children under 8 years old select a variety of cooked fish and eat a maximum of 12 ounces a week. Women and children should also avoid the fish associated with high mercury levels and eat fish such as salmon, sole, catfish, shrimp, clams, scallops, and oysters. Orange roughy and sea bass should be limited to once a month for women and children.

Source: Jetter A. How safe is your food? *Reader's Digest,* August 2003, pp. 53–63.

worldwide. Because McDonald's makes up such a formidable part of the meat industry, few companies could afford to lose its business by not complying with its animal welfare standards. Thus McDonald's has been instrumental in pushing the entire industry to change its production techniques.[40] The state of Florida has also been a forerunner in pushing for animal welfare in its recent passage of a measure outlawing slow stalls, where pregnant pigs are confined in stalls 2 feet wide and 7 feet long, unable to turn around or walk for much of their 115-day pregnancy.

Food Additives

Food additives refers to substances added to food to provide color or flavor, replace sugar or fat, or improve nutritional content, texture or shelf life. Food additives must undergo FDA testing and approval to ensure that the benefits outweigh any risks associated with these additives. For example, emulsifiers help to give peanut butter a more consistent texture and prevent separation while stabilizers and thickeners can give ice cream a smooth, uniform texture. Preservatives such as antioxidants prevent apples from turning brown from exposure to air and fats and oils in baked goods from spoiling. The three most common additives are sugar, salt, and corn syrup.[41]

Genetically Modified Foods

Biotech crops increased 20 percent in 2004, with the United States, Argentina, and Canada being the front-runners.[43] The success of American agriculture, in terms of food quality and marketability, has been based on the ability to genetically alter food sources to improve yield, reduce production costs, and introduce new food characteristics. Today, however, genetic technology is so sophisticated that changes are being introduced faster than scientists can fully evaluate their effects. For example, the genetic makeup of plant seeds and animals is being modified while scientists are still trying to determine whether human consumption of these products will be safe over extended periods. Concerned individuals and agencies in the United States and abroad are calling for more extensive longitudinal research* into safety issues and stricter labeling requirements for genetically altered foods. The label *GM* (for genetically modified) is appearing on some food items. Some food manufacturers have announced that they will discontinue the use of genetically modified ingredients in their products. The American public appears about equally divided in believing that genetically modified foods are safe (44%) or unsafe (20%) or that they are uncertain (36%) about the safety of such foods.[42]

Guidelines for Dietary Health

Vegetarian Diets

For some, vegetarianism is a way of eating, and for others, it is a way of life. In the sections that follow, various forms of vegetarianism will be addressed. Figure 5-8 shows a

---

*Longitudinal research is repeated observation of subjects to see if there is a long-term effect over time.

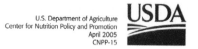

Figure 5-8 The new food pyramid for ovolactovegetarians

vegetarian food guide pyramid modeled after the USDA Food Guide Pyramid.

A *vegetarian diet* relies on plant sources for most of the nutrients the body needs. Studies show that vegetarians who eat a balanced diet don't seem to have any more iron-deficiency problems than do meat eaters. Although the iron in plant food is not as well absorbed as the iron in animal food is, vegetarians tend to eat more of iron-containing foods and more vitamin C foods, which help with the absorption of the iron.[22] In addition, vegetarians tend to get enough calcium from dairy foods, tofu, beans, soybeans, calcium-fortified cereals, and vegetables such as broccoli. There has been some concern about a vitamin B_{12} deficiency, because animal foods are the best source for B_{12} and plant foods don't naturally contain this vitamin. However, soy foods such as tempeh may contain vitamin B_{12}, although it is not as biologically active as the source in animal foods. Many soy products are fortified with vitamin B_{12} as well. Note also that the liver stores so much B_{12} that it would take years to become deficient in this vitamin.[22] Vegetarian diets encompass a continuum from diets that allow some animal sources of nutrients to those that exclude all animal sources. We briefly describe three vegetarian diets, beginning with the least restrictive in terms of food sources.

Ovolactovegetarian Diet

Depending on the particular pattern of consuming eggs (*ovo*) and milk (*lacto*) or using one but not the other, ovolactovegetarianism can be an extremely sound approach to healthful eating during the entire course of the adult years. An **ovolactovegetarian diet** provides the body with the essential amino acids while limiting the high intake of fats seen in more conventional diets. The exclusion of meat as a protein source lowers the total fat intake, while the consumption of milk or eggs allows for an adequate amount of saturated fat to remain in the diet. The consistent use of vegetable products as the primary source of nutrients supports the current dietary recommendations for an increase in overall carbohydrates, an increase in complex carbohydrates, and an increase in fiber. Most vegetarians in the United States fit into this category.

Meatlike products composed of textured vegetable protein are available in supermarkets. Nonmeat bacon strips, hamburger and chicken patties, and link sausage can be used by people who want to restrict their meat intake but still want a meatlike product. Soybeans are a primary source of this textured vegetable protein.

Vegetarians who do consume dairy products face challenges when making food choices if they wish to avoid other animal products in their food. Because most cheese is made with rennet, a coagulating agent that usually

Over 12 million Americans are vegetarian.

comes from stomachs of slaughtered newly born calves, many vegetarians eliminate cheese from their diet or opt for rennetless cheese. Vegetarian cheeses are manufactured using rennet from either fungal or bacterial sources. Similarly, yogurt is often made with gelatin derived from animal ligaments, skins, tendon, and bones (gelatin is also found in marshmallows, candy such as jelly beans, and candy corn, poptarts, and a variety of other foods).

It has become easier to follow a vegetarian diet since stores have begun offering organic vegetarian items that do not contain these animal products. However, it can be difficult to avoid all animal products without being an avid and knowledgeable label reader. For example, McDonald's recently acknowledged it failed to disclose its use of beef flavoring in its French fries and hashbrowns.

> ### Key Terms
>
> **ovolactovegetarian diet** (oh voe **lack** toe veg a **ter** ee in)
> a diet that excludes all meat but does allow the consumption of eggs and dairy products

Good nutrition can make a tremendous difference in increasing your endurance, preventing dehydration, avoiding injury, and enhancing performance. Even small losses of 1%–2% of your body weight can diminish your physical performance significantly. While water is generally the drink of choice, research shows that sports drinks may offer some performance benefits for high-intensity activity lasting 30 minutes or more. Temperature, intensity, body size, duration of activity, and fitness level all play a role in determining the appropriate fluid intake.

An increase in carbohydrate intake is generally appropriate for the majority of endurance athletes. In comparison to the non-athlete who most likely is well served by a carbohydrate intake of 5 g/kg of body weight, the endurance athlete may require 8–10 g/kg of body weight. This higher carbohydrate intake should be obtained through foods high in complex carbohydrates rather than foods characterized by a high carbohydrate/high fat composition. Carbohydrates should generally supply 60% to 70% of daily caloric intake.

Protein intake for athletes may exceed that of non-athletes by a factor of two (1.2–1.6 g/kg of body weight for athletes versus 0.8 g/kg for non-athletes). This increase in protein intake can, in most cases, be achieved without supplementation. For athletes in the early phase of weight training, when increased muscle mass is the focus, a threefold increase in protein intake can be justified on a relatively short-term basis.

Athletes may also increase their intake of vitamin E and vitamin C above that seen in the general population. The antioxidant/free radical scavenger contribution of these two vitamins is thought by some to contribute to more sustainable health during periods of intense training and competition. Intakes greater than 150% of daily values are not, however, recommended.

In addition to vitamins, an increased intake of iron and calcium is often noted among endurance athletes, particularly among women athletes. Increased iron can assist in red blood cell replacement and increase oxygen transportation, thus offsetting to some degree the loss of iron through menstruation and high-impact training (foot pounding) that physically damages red blood cells. In terms of increased calcium, an intake of 1,500 mg per day will help sustain acceptable levels of bone density in women athletes who menstruate, but the supplement alone will not sustain bone health in athletes whose menstrual periods are suppressed by the rigors of training. In this latter group of women athletes, osteoporosis-like changes, including stress fractures, are common.

The dietary changes noted above are only a few of the adjustments commonly seen among serious athletes. Additional changes are likely to be even more highly personalized and based on careful laboratory and performance-based testing.

Lactovegetarian and Ovovegetarian Diets

People who include dairy products in their diet but no other animal products, such as eggs and meat, are *lactovegetarians*. In contrast, people who exclude dairy products such as milk and cheese, yet consume eggs, are *ovovegetarians*. Both diets carry the advantages of ovolactovegetarianism.

Vegan Vegetarian Diet

A **vegan vegetarian diet** is one in which not only meat but also other animal products, including milk, cheese, and eggs, are excluded from the diet. When compared with the ovolactovegetarian diet, the vegan diet requires a higher level of nutritional understanding to avoid nutritional inadequacies.

One potential difficulty is that of obtaining all the essential amino acids. Since a single plant source does not contain all the essential amino acids, the vegan must learn to consistently employ a complementary diet. By carefully combining various grains, seeds, and legumes, amino acid deficiency can be prevented.

In addition to the potential amino acid deficiency, the vegan could have some difficulty in maintaining the necessary intake of vitamin B_{12}. Possible ramifications of inadequate B_{12} intake include depression, anemia, back pain, and menstrual irregularity. Vegans often have difficulty maintaining adequate intakes of iron, zinc, and calcium.[1] Calcium intake must be monitored closely by the vegan. In addition, vitamin D deficiencies can occur. Supplements and daily exposure to sunshine will aid in maintaining adequate levels of this vitamin.

A final area of potential difficulty for the vegan is that of an insufficient caloric intake because of the satiation resulting from the nature of the diet. Early satiation caused by a large amount of fiber may lower carbohydrate intake to the point that protein stores (muscle mass) are used for energy.

When practiced knowledgeably, vegan vegetarianism is sound for virtually all people, including pregnant and

---

Key Terms

vegan vegetarian diet (**vee** gun *or* **vay** gun) a vegetarian diet that excludes the consumption of all animal products, including eggs and dairy products

Antioxidant Supplementation: Chocolate Can Be Good for You!

Chocolate may actually be good for you. Dutch researchers indicate that dark chocolate contains four times the amount of catechin antioxidants than does black tea, which is suspected of having a protective effect against heart disease and possibly cancer, owing to its antioxidant properties. Milk chocolate was slightly higher in catechin antioxidants than was black tea.

Following multiple vitamins and multiple vitamins with herbs, antioxidants are the most frequently purchased dietary supplements. This lofty sales position within the massive dietary supplement industry likely reflects the public's belief and confidence in the ability of antioxidants to improve health by removing *free radicals,* which are highly excited and highly damaging organic molecules produced in cells during periods of incomplete oxidation. Eliminating free radicals is considered by many people to be important in reducing the chances of developing cardiovascular disease, cancer, Alzheimer's disease, and Parkinson's disease. Additionally, some people believe that free-radical damage is the basis of many of the age-related changes seen in humans.

Currently, five antioxidants have reached the attention of the American public and are available as dietary supplements. These include *vitamin C,* the most frequently taken antioxidant, which may be beneficial to heart health, and *vitamin E,* the "anti-aging vitamin,"

which may provide protection to the cardio-vascular system as well as being beneficial in preventing or slowing the development of Alzheimer's and Parkinson's diseases. Additionally, *vitamin A* and *beta carotene* (a precursor to vitamin A) are frequently taken and were once thought to provide protection against the development of cardiovascular disease and lung cancer. Recent studies have, however, failed to demonstrate a positive role for either. Two additional antioxidants, *selenium* (a mineral) and *coenzyme Q10,* both found naturally in seafoods, are taken as supplements. Selenium may be a preventative against the development of cancer, particularly prostate cancer, while coenzyme Q10 may be helpful in reducing the onset of congestive heart failure.

Perhaps it is most appropriate to suggest that the "jury is still out" in regard to the effectiveness of supplemental antioxidants. That said, however, their use at recommended levels may provide some benefit without producing serious detriment to the normal structure and function of the body. Long-term and excessively heavy use may, however, eventually be found to be detrimental to human health. For example, recent studies showed that some antioxidants may interfere with cholesterol drugs taken by heart patients.

---

breastfeeding women, infants and children, older adults, and athletes.

Semivegetarian Diets

People become vegetarians for many reasons. Some shun meat and animal products for ethical or spiritual reasons. Others choose vegetarianism for health or environmental reasons. In recent years, however, some people have found a middle ground between the two eating styles. These so-called **semivegetarians** are increasing their intake of vegetables and cutting back greatly on meat consumption but not necessarily eliminating meat entirely. Semivegetarians add occasional servings of fish and poultry to the ovolactovegetarian diet, and some even eat red meat on occasion. **Pesco-vegetarians** eat fish, dairy products, and eggs along with plant foods.

A semivegetarian diet is much healthier than the typical meat-laden Western diet. The American Cancer Society, the American Heart Association, and the National Academy of Science all recommend dietary changes that are closely related to the typical semivegetarian diet. The health benefits of such a diet are well documented.

The semivegetarian diet may be desirable to some people because the limited consumption of meat products may help ward off some nutrient deficiencies, and

such a diet can be healthier than that of the typical American.

 TALKING POINTS What do you think about vegetarian diets? If you were to follow a vegetarian diet, which one would you be likely to choose?

Nutrition and the Older Adult

Nutritional needs change as adults age. Age-related alterations to the structure and function of the body are primarily responsible for this. Included among the changes that alter nutritional requirements and practices are changes in the teeth, salivary glands, taste buds, oral

---

Key Terms

semivegetarianism a diet that significantly reduces but does not eliminate meat consumption and allows consumption of dairy products and eggs

pesco-vegetarian diet a vegetarian diet that includes fish, dairy products, and eggs along with plant foods muscles, gastric acid production, and peristaltic action (movement of food through the gastrointestinal tract). Older adults can find food less tasteful and harder to chew. Chronic constipation resulting from changes in gastrointestinal tract function can also decrease interest in eating.

The progressive lowering of the body's basal metabolism is another factor that eventually influences dietary patterns of older adults. As energy requirements fall, the body gradually senses the need for less food. This gradual recognition of lower energy needs results in a lessened food intake and loss of appetite in many older adults. Because of this decreased need for calories, nutrient density—the nutritional value of a food relative to the number of calories supplied—is an important factor for older adults. The new USDA dietary guidelines make some specific suggestions for people over 50. They include consuming more vitamin B_{12}, because older people tend to have difficulty absorbing this vitamin. Older adults are also encouraged to consume extra vitamin D-fortified foods, since this vitamin may be lacking in this group.

Besides the physiological factors that influence dietary patterns among the elderly, several psychosocial factors alter the role of food in the lives of many older adults. Social isolation, depression, chronic alcohol consumption, loss of income, transportation limitations, and housing restrictions are factors in lifestyle patterns that can alter the ease and enjoyment associated with the preparation and consumption of food.

International Nutritional Concerns

Whereas nutritional concerns in this country are centered on overnutrition, including fat density and excessive caloric intake, the main concern in many areas of the world is the limited quantity and quality of food. Reasons for these problems are many, including the limitations imposed by weather, the availability of arable land, religious practices, political unrest, war, social infrastructure, and material and technical shortages. Underlying nearly all of these factors, however, is unabated population growth.

To increase the availability of food to the 82 countries and 840 million people whose demand for food outweighs their ability to produce it, a number of steps have been suggested, including the following:

Increase the yield of land currently under cultivation.

Increase the amount of land under cultivation.

Increase animal production on land not suitable for cultivation.

Use water (seas, lakes, and ponds) more efficiently for the production of food.

Develop unconventional foods through the application of technology.

Improve nutritional practices through education.

In these countries, little progress is being made despite impressive technological breakthroughs in agriculture and food technology (such as "miracle" rice, disease-resistant high-yield corn, and soybean-enhanced infant foods), the efforts of governmental programs, and the support of the Food and Agricultural Organization of the United Nations and the USDA. In developing countries, where fertility rates are two to four times higher than those of the United States, annual food production would have to increase between 2.7 percent and 3.9 percent. If population growth and food production are not altered in these countries, basic needs will continue to be unmet.

Smart Supermarket Shopping

- Make a shopping list before you go and stick to it!
- Don't go grocery shopping when you are hungry.
- Shop just once a week, don't make special trips.
- Read the food labels and check for the percentage of fat, sodium, sugar, and so on.
- Take note of the "sell by" or expiration date. The items stocked toward the back are usually the newest.
- For the single shopper, look for foods sold in single servings: juice, yogurt, frozen meals, soup, and pudding, for example.
- Buy fresh fruits and vegetables over canned and frozen. If buying canned or frozen fruits and vegetables, look for ones without added sugar, fats, salt, and sodium.
- Choose brown rice over white, whole-wheat over white bread.
- Skip the ramen noodle soups; the noodles are usually flash-cooked in oil and high in fat and sodium.
- Avoid giant muffins, bagels, and donuts, and select the smaller ones.
- Meat labeled "select" is leaner than meat graded "choice."
- Leaner cuts of beef are flank, sirloin, and tenderloin. The leanest pork is fresh, canned, cured, or boiled ham, Canadian bacon, pork tenderloin, rib chops, and roast.
- Ground turkey and chicken can contain the skin, which makes it higher in fat and calories. For a lower-fat option, look for ground turkey or chicken meat. Ground turkey breast is lower still.
- Buy water-packed tuna and sardines rather than those packed in oil.
- Buy low-fat or fat-free milk rather than 2% or whole milk.
- Look for low-fat cheeses, sour cream, mayonnaise, and cream cheese that are labeled "part skim," "reduced fat," or "fat free."
- Buy canola or olive oil rather than corn oil, or use nonstick cooking spray.
- Consider buying cholesterol-free or reduced-cholesterol egg substitutes, especially if you don't use eggs very often, because they tend to last longer than fresh eggs do.

Source: Kirby J. *Dieting for Dummies.* New York: Wiley, 1998.

SUMMARY

- Carbohydrates, fats, and protein supply the body with calories.
- The molecular complexity of carbohydrates differs, with sugars being the least complex and starches the most complex.
- Fat plays an important role in nutritional health beyond serving as the body's primary site for the storage of excess calories.
- Dietary fats can be classified on the basis of their molecular makeup. Alteration of a fat's chemical bonding through hydrogenation may result in the formation of potentially harmful trans-fatty acids.
- Cholesterol-free and low-fat foods play important roles in today's dietary practices.
- Protein supplies the body with amino acids that subsequently provide the material needed by the body to construct its own protein.
- Vitamins serve as catalysts for the body and are found in either water-soluble or fat-soluble forms.
- Minerals are incorporated into various tissues of the body and also participate in regulatory functions within the body.
- Adequate water and fluids are required by the body on a daily basis and are obtained from a variety of food sources, including beverages.
- Fiber is undigestible plant material and can be found in two forms, water-soluble and water-insoluble. Soluble fiber contributes to the removal of cholesterol from the blood, while insoluble fiber contributes to stool formation.
- To follow a food group-based dietary plan, it is important to be able to classify each food, know the number of recommended servings from each food group, and recognize the amount of food that constitutes a single serving.
- Fast foods should play a limited role in daily food intake because of their high fat density, as well as their high levels of sugar and sodium.
- Food allergies such as peanut allergies may be life threatening.
- Preventive strategies such as hand washing and proper preparation, cooking, and storage of food can help to decrease foodborne illnesses.
- The *USDA Dietary Guidelines for Americans* focus on the role of trans fat, saturated fat, sugar, sodium, alcohol, and weight management in health and disease. The current *Dietary Guidelines for Americans* address the importance of daily physical activity.

REVIEW QUESTIONS

1. What unique contributions do carbohydrates, fats, and protein each make to overall nutrition that are not made by other nutrients?
2. Of the two forms of carbohydrate, which form has the most complex molecular structure and which has the simplest?
3. What concern is being voiced over the role of tropical oils in sound dietary practices?
4. What is the principal role of protein in the body?
5. What are the important nutritional differences between plant and animal sources of protein? Which food source supplies complete protein and which supplies incomplete protein?
6. Which vitamins are water soluble and which are fat soluble? What is the most current perception regarding the need for vitamin supplementation?
7. What roles do minerals play in the body? What is a trace element?
8. What is the current recommendation regarding daily fluid intake? Why is water considered an essential nutrient?
9. What are the two principal forms of fiber, and how does each of them contribute to health?
10. Identify each of the five food groups. What makes up the additional sixth group? Explain the nutritional benefit of each food group and the recommended daily adult allotments.
11. What is the principal concern regarding excessive fast-food consumption? How can food selection at a fast-food restaurant be made nutritionally healthier?
12. In the most general sense, what are phytochemicals, and in which foods are they most abundant?
13. What are functional foods, and what contribution do they make to health beyond supplying various nutrients as do all foods?
14. Describe food allergies and how they can be managed effectively.
15. What are the specific areas of nutritional concern addressed by the current *Dietary Guidelines for Americans?*
16. Define a vegetarian diet. Explain the differences among ovolactovegetarian, lactovegetarian, pescovegetarian, vegan vegetarian, and semivegetarian diets. Which one poses more potential nutritional problems? In what ways?
17. What is nutrient density?

ENDNOTES

1. Wardlaw GM. *Perspectives in Nutrition* (5th ed.). New York: McGraw-Hill, 2002.
2. *USDA Agricultural Outlook.* Washington, DC: U.S. Department of Agriculture, April 2000.
3. U.S. Department of Health and Human Services. *Report of the Expert Panel on Population Strategies for Blood Cholesterol Reduction.* NIH Pub No 9-3049. Washington, DC: Author, 1990.
4. Lichtenstein AH. Dietary trans fatty acid. *J Cardiopulm Rehabil;* 20(3):143–146, 2000.
5. Willet WC, Ascherio A. Trans fatty acids: Are the effects only marginal? *Am J Public Health;* 84:722, 1994.
6. Duyff R. *American Dietetic Association Complete Food and Nutrition Guide* (2nd ed.). Hoboken, NJ: Wiley, 2002.
7. Katan MB. Trans fatty acids and plasma lipoproteins. *Nutr Rev;* 58(6):188–191, 2000.
8. Noop RH, et al. Long-term cholesterol-lowering effects of 4 fat-restricted diets in hypercholesterolemic and combined hyperlipidemic men: The dietary alternatives study. *JAMA;* 278(18): 1509–1525, 1997.
9. National Institutes of Health. *Practical Guide to the Identification, Evaluation and Treatment of Overweight and Obesity in Adults,* 2001.
10. Cheskin LJ, et al. Gastrointestinal symptoms following consumption of Olestra or regular triglyceride potato chips score. *JAMA;* 279(2): 150–152, 1998.
11. Wardlaw GM. *Contemporary Nutrition: Issues and Insights.* New York: McGraw-Hill, 1999.
12. Young VR. Soy protein in relation to human protein and amino acid nutrition. *J Am Diet Assoc.* 91, 828–835, 1991.
13. Anderson J, Johnstone R, Cook-Newell M. Meta-analysis of the effects of soy protein intake on serum lipids. *N Engl J Med* 333, 276–282, 1995.
14. Kant AK. A prospective study of diet quality and mortality in women. *JAMA;* 283(16): 2109–2115, 2000.
15. Czeizel AE, Dudaz I. Prevention of the first occurrence of neural-tube defects by periconceptional vitamin supplementation. *N Engl J Med;* 327(26): 1832–1835, 1992.
16. Position of the American Dietetic Association. *Vitamin and mineral supplementation,* 1998. www. eatright.org/ asupple.html.
17. In Yankelovich, *Partners for the Nutrition Information Center at The New York Hospital and the Bottled Water Association.* April, 1998. www.bottledwater.org/public/ PressRel1.htm.
18. Garigan TP, Ristedt DE. Death from hyponatremia as a result of acute water intoxication in an Army basic trainee. *Mil Med;* 164(3):234–238, 1999.
19. Arieff AI, Kronlund BA. Fatal child abuse by forced water intoxication. *Pediatrics;* 103(6 Pt 1): 1292–1295, 1999.
20. Chandalia M, et al. Beneficial effects of high dietary fiber intake in patients with type 2 diabetes mellitus. *N Engl J Med;* 342(19):1392–1398, 2000.

21. Schatzkin A, et al. Lack of effect of a low-fat, high-fiber diet on the recurrence of colorectal adenomas. Polyp Prevention Trial Study Group. *N Engl J Med;* 342(16): 1149–1115, 2000.

22. Sears W, Sears M. *The Family Nutrition Book.* New York: Little, Brown and Co., 1999.

23. FDA allows whole oat foods to make health claim on reducing the risk of heart disease. *FDA Talk Paper,* January 1998.

24. American Cancer Society. *Cancer Facts and Figures—2000.* The Association, 2000.

25. Joseph JA, et al. Long-term dietary strawberry, spinach, or vitamin E supplementation retards the onset of age-related neuronal signal-transduction and cognitive behavioral deficits. *J Neurosci;* 18(19):8047–8055, 1998.

26. www.health.gov/dietaryguidelines/dga, 2005.

27. Flour power: A slice of multigrain can taste like bread, *USA Today,* August 9, 2004.

28. U.S. Department of Agriculture. *The Healthy Eating Index* (executive summary). July 2000. http://Warp.nal.usda.gov/fnic/HEI/execsum.html.

29. Willett W. *Eat, Drink and Be Healthy.* New York: Free Press, 2001.

30. Waladkhani AR, Clemens MR. Effect of dietary phytochemicals on cancer. *Int J Mol Med;* 1(4):747–753, 1998.

31. Fransworth ER. What we are trying to do? *Medicinal Food News;* 1(1):1–6, 1999. www.medicinalfoodnews.com/vol01/issue1.html.

32. U.S. Food and Drug Administration Center for Food Safety and Applied Nutrition. *FDA Approves New Health Claim for Soy Protein and Coronary Heart Disease* [FDA talk paper]. October 1999. www.fda.gov/fdac/bbs/topics/ANSWERS/ANSoo980.html.

33. Kurtzweil P. Staking a claim to good health. *FDA Consumer,* November–December 1998. www.fda/gov/fdac/features/1998,689-labl.html.

34. A bug for what's bugging you. *USA Today,* July 9, 2003, D-1.

35. USDA gives bite to organic label. *USA Today,* October 16, 2002.

36. The truth about irradiated meat. *Consumer Reports,* 34–37, August 2003.

37. Oppel RA, Jr. Infected cow old enough to have eaten now-banned feed. *The New York Times,* December 30, 2003.

38. Grady D. U.S. imposes stricter safety rules for preventing mad cow disease. *The New York Times,* December 31, 2003.

39. Corporate Web Site, www.eggland.com.

40. Food sellers push animal welfare, *USA Today,* August 13, 2003.

41. Insel P, Turner E, Ross D. *Nutrition.* Sudbury, MA: Jones and Barlett, 2002.

42. Americans are iffy on genetically modified foods, *USA Today,* September 18, 2003.

43. Biotech crops gained ground across globe. *USA Today,* January 13, 2005.

44. Williams S, Schlenker E. *Essentials of Nutrients and Diet Therapy* (8th ed.). St. Louis, MO: Mosby, 2003.

Is Cookie Monster Going on a Diet?

"C" is not for cookie anymore. C is for carrots. With the increase in childhood obesity, the ever-popular children's television show, *Sesame Street,* has decided to focus on teaching children about healthy foods and physical activity. According to Sesame Street's spokesperson, each show will open with a health tip for kids about nutrition, exercise, hygiene, and rest. There will be talking eggplants and carrots and new songs about the importance of physical activity. The Cookie Monster's new song is "A Cookie Is a Sometimes Food," as he learns the difference between sometimes foods (sweets) and anytime foods (fruits and vegetables). Senator Hillary Clinton teaches him about the various textures and tastes of food, and Elmo learns to exercise with the help of Senate Majority Leader Bill Frist.

Of course, sitting in front of the television is probably not conducive to children increasing their activity level. Sixty percent of children reported that they don't participate in sports, and 25 percent say that they engage in no physical activity outside school. Researchers from the Harvard School of Health suggested that the more television children watch, the fewer fruits and vegetables they eat. This study found that, over the course of a year, children lack 13 percent of recommended nutrition from fruits and vegetables, owing to increased television viewing.

However, we can't hold the Cookie Monster solely responsible for the rising obesity rates in children. Surely Ronald McDonald, Burger King's Burgermeister, and that larger-than-life mouse Chuck E. Cheese have to shoulder some of the responsibility for children eating burgers, fries, pizza, and soft drinks. Junk food accounts for one-third of all calories consumed by Americans, so adults are not necessarily good role models for children regarding healthy eating. Most school vending machines are filled with junk food such as sodas, chips, and candy bars. Sixty-seven percent of adolescents say they buy junk food from vending machines at school on a regular basis.

Legislation is being considered on a national level to regulate food sales in schools in order to restrict the types of foods and drinks sold there. School cafeterias are also under scrutiny as to how healthy the choices are for students. Some schools have eliminated the sale of soft drinks entirely and may eliminate other junk foods as well.

It is increasingly apparent that a number of factors contribute to the rising obesity rates among children. It will be interesting to see what kind of effect the Sometimes Cookie Monster and the All-the-Time Carrot Monster will have on children's eating habits.

Sources: "Cookie Monster Eating Less Cookies," *USA Today,* April 7, 2005. "School Vending Rated as Junk," *USA Today,* May 12, 2004.

personal assessment

Rate your plate

Take a closer look at yourself—your current food decisions and your lifestyle. Think about your typical eating pattern and food decisions.

Do You . . .

	Usually	Sometimes	Never
Consider nutrition when you make food choices?	❑	❑	❑
Try to eat regular meals (including breakfast), rather than skip or skimp on some?	❑	❑	❑
Choose nutritious snacks?	❑	❑	❑
Try to eat a variety of foods?	❑	❑	❑
Include new-to-you foods in meals and snacks?	❑	❑	❑
Try to balance your energy (calorie) intake with your physical activity?	❑	❑	❑

Now for the Details

Do You . . .

Eat at least 6 ounces of grain products daily?	❑	❑	❑
Eat at least 2½ cups of vegetables daily?	❑	❑	❑
Eat at least 2 cups of fruits daily?	❑	❑	❑
Consume at least 3 cups of milk, yogurt, or cheese daily?	❑	❑	❑
Go easy on higher-fat foods?	❑	❑	❑

Go easy on sweets?	❑	❑	❑
Drink 8 or more cups of fluids daily?	❑	❑	❑
Limit alcoholic beverages (no more than 1 daily for a woman or 2 for a man)?	❑	❑	❑

Score Yourself

Usually = 2 points
Sometimes = 1 point
Never = 0 points

If you scored . . .

24 or more points—Healthful eating seems to be your fitness habit already. Still, look for ways to stick to a healthful eating plan—and to make a "good thing" even better.

16 to 23 points—You're on track. A few easy changes could help you make your overall eating plan healthier.

9 to 15 points—Sometimes you eat smart—but not often enough to be your "fitness best."

0 to 8 points—For your good health, you're wise to rethink your overall eating style. Take it gradually—step by step!

Whatever your score, make moves for healthful eating. Gradually turn your "nevers" into "sometimes" and your "sometimes" into "usually."

Adapted from *The American Dietetic Association's Monthly Nutrition Companion: 31 Days to a Healthier Lifestyle*, Chronimed Publishing, 1997.

personal assessment

Are you feeding your feelings?

Sometimes people use food as a way of coping with their emotions and problems. To identify how you might be using food as a coping strategy and what feelings you tend to associate with eating, complete the following inventory.

1 = Never

2 = Rarely

3 = Occasionally

4 = Often

5 = Always

1. _____ Do you eat when you are angry?
2. _____ When you feel annoyed, do you turn to food?
3. _____ If someone lets you down, do you eat to comfort yourself?
4. _____ When you are having a bad day, do you notice that you eat more?
5. _____ Do you eat to cheer yourself up?
6. _____ Do you use food as a way of avoiding tasks you don't want to do?
7. _____ Do you view food as your friend when you are feeling lonely?
8. _____ Is food a way for you to comfort yourself when your life seems empty?
9. _____ When you are feeling upset, do you turn to food to calm yourself down?
10. _____ Do you eat more when you are anxious, worried, or stressed?
11. _____ Does eating help you to cope with feeling overwhelmed?
12. _____ Do you eat more when you are going through big changes or transitions in your life?
13. _____ Do you reward yourself with food?
14. _____ When you think you have done something wrong, do you punish yourself by eating?
15. _____ When you are feeling badly about yourself, do you eat more?
16. _____ When you feel discouraged about your efforts to improve yourself, do you eat more, thinking "what's the use of trying"?

_____ **TOTAL SCORE**

Interpretation

If you scored between . . .

0–13 You don't eat to cope with your emotions. Your eating may not be related to your emotional state. However, you may avoid eating when you are upset or having trouble coping with your feelings. You may run away from food rather than running to food to cope.

14–66 Although you fall in the average range, you may use food to deal with specific situations or feelings such as anger, loneliness, or boredom. See the breakdown of scores below to identify how you may be using food to cope with particular feelings.

67 and above You run to food to cope with your emotions, and you may want to consider developing other ways of appropriately expressing your feelings.

If you answered "4" or "5" to most of questions #1–#4, this can be indicative of eating when you are angry.

If you answered "4" or "5" to most of questions #5–#8, this can be indicative of eating when you are lonely or bored.

If you answered "4" or "5" to most of questions #9–#12, this can be an indication that you are a stress eater.

If you answered "4" or "5" to most of questions #13–#16, this can be an indication that you are using food to cope with feelings of low self-esteem and self-worth.

chapter six

Maintaining a Healthy Weight

Chapter Objectives

On completing this chapter, you will be able to:

▌ describe the role of the media and entertainment industry in defining the ideal body image.

▌ define overweight and obesity.

▌ discuss how effective body mass index, electrical impedance, skin fold measurements, hydrostatic weighing, and appearance are as methods of assessing body weight.

▌ discuss the causes of obesity, including genetics, metabolism, physiological and hormonal changes, environmental factors, dietary practices, sociocultural factors, and psychological factors.

▌ describe the body's use of food in activity requirements, in basal metabolism, and in the thermic effect.

▌ discuss the primary types of weight-management techniques, including dietary alterations, surgical interventions, medications, weight loss programs, and physical activity.

▌ provide evidence supporting physical exercise as the most important component of a weight-loss program.

▌ define anorexia nervosa, bulimia nervosa, binge eating disorder, chewing and spitting food syndrome, night-time eating syndrome, body dysmorphic disorder, and bigorexia.

▌ discuss the at-risk groups for eating disorders and factors to consider for males with eating disorders.

▌ discuss ways of treating eating disorders.

Eye on the Media

Weight Loss and Reality

The Biggest Loser, The Swan, and *America's Next Top Model*—we are bombarded by television programs that tell us how we should be focused on our appearance, particularly on losing weight. Since the majority of adult Americans are overweight, weight loss would seem appealing to most television viewers. However, this preoccupation with appearance and weight sends a perilous message—that to feel good about yourself, you must be thin and beautiful. The shows also create an expectation of achieving the perfect body, which is an impossible goal.

The Biggest Loser is described as a "weight-loss drama" in which contestants follow comprehensive diet and exercise plans, supervised by physicians and personal trainers. They compete to see which team can lose the most weight. There are temptations and physical challenges along the way to make the endeavor even more difficult and perhaps more like real life. All the contestants from the first season continued to lose weight after the show ended, by continuing to exercise regularly and monitoring their caloric intake. Most of the contestants also refer to the support of their families and friends as another key factor in continuing to manage their weight. Some of the more positive components of the show are

- *Realization*—You must realize where you are so that you can figure out where you want to be. As Kirstie Alley from the show *Fat Actress* stated, "I didn't really realize I was fat until I saw the first show."

- *Coaching*—Many of the contestants continued to work with a personal trainer or exercised with a friend.

- *Accountability*—With millions of television viewers watching, along with family and friends, contestants feel some accountability. It is important to broadcast your weekly progress toward your goals. This is the reason many people find keeping a food diary to be helpful.

- *Rewards*—A healthier body, a grand prize of $250,000, book and television offers, tours, interviews, and notoriety are some of the obvious rewards mentioned by the contestants. They also talk of additional rewards, such as increased sense of self-esteem and self-worth, taking new risks, having more energy, and experiencing less stress.

- *Goals*—The contestants set weight goals during the show and continued to set weight management goals after the show ended. They also set goals such as helping others to manage their weight, wearing a swimsuit, or developing relationships.

- *Support*—Team members supported one another during the show, which seems to be a significant factor in continued success in managing their weight. Support from friends, family, and fans also helped to inspire and motivate these individuals to stay on course.

Of course you don't have to be on a television show to incorporate these factors into your own life. *USA Today* conducted a "Weight Loss Challenge" in 2004 and looked at what it takes to be a successful loser. They reported that according to 126 registered dieticians, the key factors are being honest with yourself, setting goals and priorities, having a positive attitude, and being organized. These factors sound remarkably similar to the weight-loss components identified in *The Biggest Loser* and *The Swan*.

On *The Swan,* a nine-episode series, 18 women get plastic surgery and a full makeover over a three-month time. The premise of the show is that women are transformed from "ugly ducklings" to "beautiful swans." The contestants are not permitted to see their new look until the end of their three-month makeover. The final episode consists of a two-hour beauty pageant with all the episodes' "winners." Their transformations include exercising with a personal trainer, following a commercial diet plan, having therapy sessions, and undergoing extensive cosmetic surgery such as brow-lift, chin implant, lower-eye-lift, face-lift, fat transfer to lips and cheek folds, tummy tuck, breast-lift, rhinoplasty, hair implants, dental surgery, and liposuction. The winners of the beauty pageants have been awarded such prizes as a contract as a spokesperson for NutriSystem, continued educational opportunities, a $100,000 neck-lace, a new car, a mink coat, and vacations to Las Vegas, Hawaii, and Thailand. As with *The Biggest Loser*, this program utilizes the important positive components of realization, accountability, coaching, rewards, and support. However, this show also presents a dangerous message in linking self-esteem to beauty and setting some unrealistic goals (discussed later in this section).

America's Next Top Model shows the transformation of everyday young women who train to become supermodels. With supermodel Tyra Banks as their mentor, the participants learn how to model on catwalks, engage in intense physical-fitness exercises, and do fashion photo shoots and publicity skills. The Grand Prize package includes the opportunity to receive a Revlon modeling contract and to be managed by Wilhelmina Models, in addition to a guaranteed appearance in *Marie Claire* magazine.

Consider the goals of these contestants: Most of the people on these shows are not just looking to lose weight and change their appearance; they believe that, by focusing on their appearance and weight, they will save their marriages, increase their self-esteem and self-confidence, become better mothers, have more successful careers—in essence become different people. For example, one of the contestants on *The Swan* beauty pageant said that one of the reasons she applied to be on the show was to save her marriage (which ended before the show did). Another contestant said she wanted to reinvent herself by changing her appearance so that she could stand up to her abusive husband. How realistic are these goals? Tiffany, a contestant on *Top Model* said that it was "one of the most humiliating experiences of my life."

What is the message to viewers? One of the contestants on *The Biggest Loser* said, "When you feel good, you look good," but these programs are sending the opposite message—that you need to look good to feel good, and looking good means being thin and fitting the cultural ideal of beauty.

The other component of these reality television makeover shows is the extensive use of plastic surgery costing tens of thousands of dollars for each contestant. How many of us have the money or the desire to undergo extensive plastic and reconstructive dental surgery? Actually, the numbers are rising to epidemic proportions. From 1996 to 2001, the number of Americans undergoing cosmetic surgery increased 1,125 percent. According to the American Society for Aesthetic Plastic Surgery, nearly 6.9 million cosmetic procedures occurred in the United States in one year, with women undergoing 88 percent of them. In this quick-fix society, some Americans are no longer willing to wait for the results they want. However, these fixes come with costs of their own, such as complications from surgeries and having to have repeated surgeries.

In addition, medical problems such as hypertension, heart attacks, gastrointestinal problems, osteoporosis, and kidney problems can result from unhealthy diets and taking diet supplements. These dangers would seem to outweigh the benefits of trying to reach the unrealistic goal of having the perfect body.

Rather than undergoing a series of diet programs, surgeries, and pills to manage your weight, you will be much healthier if you follow a balanced diet and engage in regular exercise. Shows like *The Swan, The Biggest Loser,* and *America's Next Top Model* prey on people's low self-esteem and exploit their fears about appearance. As was discussed in Chapter 2, there is much more to self-esteem than external factors such as how people see us and our outer appearance. In addition, the research shows that physical attractiveness does not predict self-esteem. In other words, some people who didn't think they were physically attractive had higher self-esteem than those who did see themselves as attractive.

Sources:
Attansai, K. "Anti-Aging Options Require Balanced Approach to Health, Beauty," *Today's Pentecostal Evangel*, August 10, 2003.
www.realitytvcalendar.com, 2005.
www.nbc.com/The Biggest Loser.

Weight management has become an obsession in American culture as well as a significant health problem. In the United States, obesity has risen at an epidemic rate during the past 20 years. One of the national health objectives for the year 2010 is to reduce the prevalence of obesity among adults to less than 15 percent.[1] Research indicates that the situation is worsening rather than improving. According to the National Center for Chronic Disease Prevention and Health Promotion, an estimated 65 percent of adult Americans are either overweight or obese.[2] Currently 30 percent, or 60 million, adult Americans are obese with more women (33 percent) than men (28 percent) meeting the criteria for obesity. Up 74 percent since 1991, the number of overweight children and adolescents has

Table 6.1 Health Problems Associated with Excess Body Fat

Health Problems	Partially Attributed to:
Surgical risk	Increased anesthesia needs and greater risk of wound infections
Pulmonary disease	Excess weight over lungs
Type 2 diabetes mellitus (NIDDM)	Enlarged fat cells, which then poorly bind insulin and also poorly respond to the message insulin sends to the cell
Hypertension	Increased miles of blood vessels found in the fat tissue; however, no validated cause is yet known
Coronary heart disease	Increases in serum cholesterol and triglyceride levels, as well as a decrease in physical activity
Bone and joint disorders	Excess pressure put on knee, ankle, and hip joints
Gallbladder stones	An increase in the cholesterol content of bile
Skin disorders	The trapping of moisture and microbes in fat folds
Various cancers	Estrogen production by fat cells; animal studies suggest excess energy intake encourages tumor development
Shorter stature (in some forms of obesity)	An earlier onset of puberty
Pregnancy risk	More difficult delivery and increased anesthesia needs (if used)
Early death	A variety of risk factors for diseases listed above

The greater the degree of obesity, the more likely and the more serious these health problems generally become. They are much more likely to appear in people who are greater than twice their desirable body weight.

tripled in the past 20 years.[3] These people face an increased risk of developing serious health problems, independent of other risk factors not directly related to weight.

What accounts for the high percentage of Americans defined as overweight or obese? Experts point to two salient factors: greater daily caloric consumption and a relatively low level of consistent physical activity. Women eat 335 more calories and men eat 168 more calories per day than they did 30 years ago. Meanwhile, nearly two-thirds of Americans are not physically active on a regular basis, and 25 percent are completely sedentary[4] (see Chapter 4).

The increase in weight occurs, of course, when the body is supplied with more energy than it can use and the excess energy is stored in the form of **adipose tissue,** or fat. This is called a positive caloric balance. The continuous buildup of adipose tissue leads to excess weight and can eventually result in obesity. Obesity may account for as many as 400,000 deaths annually.[5]

Among the health problems caused by or complicated by excess body fat are increased surgical risk, hypertension, various forms of heart disease, stroke, type 2 diabetes, several forms of cancer, deterioration of joints, complications during pregnancy, gallbladder disease, and an overall increased risk of mortality (see the Star box on page 177 and Table 6.1). So closely is obesity associated with chronic conditions, that medical experts now recommend that obesity itself be defined and treated as a chronic disease. In fact, the combination of type 2 diabetes, hypertension, and atherosclerosis along with

obesity is so common that it is now referred to as *Syndrome X.*[6]

Body Image and Self-Concept

Although clinicians now have specific guidelines for the diagnosis and treatment of obesity, the general public has its own set of definitions and concerns regarding body weight. Principal among these is the issue of perceived physical attractiveness. This concern is caused (or reinforced) by the media, which tells people that being overweight does not conform to certain ideal **body images** (such as being tall, thin, and "cut" with muscular definition). The average actress or model, for example, is thinner than 95 percent of the female population and weighs 23 percent less than the average woman.[7] The average American woman is 5'4", 143 pounds, and wears a size 10–12, but the average model is 5'10" and 110 pounds.[8]

Key Terms

adipose tissue tissue made up of fibrous strands around which specialized cells designed to store liquefied fat are arranged

body image our subjective perception of how our body appears

Health Risks of Obesity

Each of the diseases listed below is followed by the percentage of cases that are caused by obesity:

Colon cancer	10%
Breast cancer	11%
Hypertension	33%
Heart disease	70%
Diabetes (type 2, non-insulin-dependent)	90%

As these statistics show, being obese greatly increases your risk of many serious and even life-threatening diseases.

Today's lean but muscular version of perfection is a very demanding standard for both women and men to meet. Men, in fact, make up approximately 10 percent of those with eating disorders, for which body image concerns is an important component. For both men and women, the demands of athletics seems to be a significant factor in the development of body image-related concerns, particularly in sports such as gymnastics, boxing, wrestling, dancing, track, swimming, and rowing, in which "making weight" is an important component.[9]

In light of this challenge, people may become dissatisfied and concerned about their inability to resemble ideal images. The scope of this dissatisfaction is evident in a study of more than 800 women, which revealed that nearly half were unhappy with their weight, muscle tone, hips, thighs, buttocks, and legs.[10] Not surprisingly, when this dissatisfaction exists, people can question their own attractiveness, and eventually their self-concept and self-esteem declines.

In the body image that seems to be popular for today's women, the hips, waist, and shoulders line up in a vertical line. The once-popular emphasis on an "hourglass" figure has given way to a more angular, athletic appearance, somewhat similar to the body build of many young men. As is true for women, most men do not achieve their ideal weight and body composition. Men tend toward wanting a V-shaped body with a full chest, muscular legs, well-defined abdominal muscles, and a thin waist. However, men with eating disorders prefer the lean, toned, thin shape.[11]

Whether the body image desired can realistically be achieved seems unimportant to many people. Some spend hours each week in weight rooms and reduce or increase their food intake dramatically in a quest to attain the desired body image. For those who are ultimately unsuccessful, disappointment, frustration, and serious medical problems can result.

Overall, men report feeling more comfortable with their weight and perceive less pressure to be thin than women do. A national survey showed that 41 percent of men were dissatisfied with their weight, with many of these men wanting to gain weight and increase muscle mass. While the average American woman wants to lose 11 pounds, the average American man wants to lose 1 pound or is happy with his weight.[11]

However, men do tend to have the desire to be more muscular, more "cut," bigger, and stronger. An increasing number of men have become obsessed with being bigger and more muscular, referred to as the "Adonis Complex."[12] This term comes from Greek mythology, which depicted Adonis as half man and half god, considered to be the ultimate in masculine beauty. Men with this preoccupation obsessively lift weights for hours a day, sometimes sacrificing important social relationships, jobs, or physical health.

In many cases, these men take anabolic steroids or diet supplements to get bigger. They manifest a sort of "reverse anorexia nervosa", also referred to as **bigorexia.** The main characteristic of bigorexia is the thought that no matter how hard you try, your body is never muscular enough.[12] Some men with the Adonis complex become preoccupied with fat as opposed to muscle and, hence, may develop eating disorders (discussed later in this chapter).

Research suggests that 2 to 3 million American men have used steroids or other supplements to increase muscle mass, often starting as teenagers. Steroid use can result in side effects such as psychiatric symptoms, including manic and aggressive symptoms while using steroids and depressive symptoms from withdrawal. Remarkably, parents, teachers, and even trained clinicians often remain unaware of steroid use despite these obvious physical and personality changes.

Dietary supplements such as creatine, glutamine, and androstenedione products have been advertised as "muscle and strength builders," as aids in recovering from workouts more quickly, and as immunity boosters. Baseball player Mark McGuire came under fire for his use of androstenedione, called *andro,* and brought increased attention of the use of these supplements among athletes and body builders. McGuire publicly discouraged young people from taking andro and discontinued taking it himself. As with all dietary supplements, there is no regulation or standardization among these drugs, so the safe and

Key Terms

bigorexia the obsession with getting bigger and more muscular, and thinking that your body is never muscular enough

Studies show that mirrors can make us more self-conscious, critical, and conforming.

a person's weight is 20 percent or more above normal weight. *Morbid obesity* refers to being 50–100 percent above normal weight, more than 100 pounds over normal weight, or sufficiently overweight to interfere with health or normal functioning.[12] Of course, an exception to this relationship between overweight and obesity is excessive weight caused by extreme muscularity, such as that seen in many athletes.

Being most familiar with the weight guidelines used in the past, most clinicians and the general public continue to use standard height/weight tables to determine the extent to which scale weight exceeds **desirable weight** and, thus, the existence of mild, moderate, or severe obesity. However, other techniques are now available that can be used to determine body composition. The next section describes several of these techniques, including waist/hip ratio (*healthy body weight*), body mass index, hydrostatic weighing, "BOD POD" assessment, skinfold measurements, and electrical impedance.

Most recently the scientific community has issued guidelines for determining obesity for purposes of medical intervention. People with a **body mass index (BMI)** over 25 are considered overweight. Individuals are considered obese when BMI is 30.0 or above. Severe or morbid obesity is when the BMI is greater than 40.[13] Aggressive medical intervention is necessary for people who, in addition to being obese, have a waist circumference of 40 or more inches (males) or 35 or more inches (females) and two or more of the following risk factors: diabetes, high blood pressure, high blood cholesterol, and **sleep apnea.**[14] For obese

effective dosage is not known. There is no research proving that these supplements actually do enhance athletic performance or increase muscle mass. What is known is that the side effects associated with taking these dietary supplements include shrinkage of testicles, growth of breast tissue, and impotence for men. Side effects for all youth include acne, early start of puberty, and stunted growth. For this reason, the FDA has announced a crackdown on products containing androstenedione and is requesting companies to stop distributing dietary supplements containing androstenedione. The FDA is also encouraging Congress to consider legislation to classify these products as a controlled substance.

Defining Overweight and Obesity

How can people tell the difference between overweight and obesity? Doctors usually define **overweight** as a condition in which a person's weight is 1–19 percent higher than normal, as defined by a standard height/weight chart. **Obesity** is usually defined as a condition in which

Key Terms

overweight a condition in which a person's excess fat accumulation results in a body weight that exceeds desirable weight by 1–19 percent

obesity a condition in which a person's body weight is 20 percent or more above desirable weight as determined by standard height/weight charts

desirable weight the weight range deemed appropriate for people, taking into consideration gender, age, and frame size

body mass index (BMI) a mathematical calculation based on weight and height; used to determine desirable body weight

sleep apnea a condition in which abnormalities in the structure of the airways lead to periods of greatly restricted air flow during sleep, resulting in reduced levels of blood oxygen and placing greater strain on the heart to maintain adequate tissue oxygenation

Childhood obesity, a condition that is increasing in incidence, is viewed as a precursor to the development of type 2 diabetes mellitus.

people who demonstrate fewer risk factors, less aggressive treatment may suffice.

Obesity, although perhaps genetically and behaviorally determined early in life, often takes many years to develop fully. A daily caloric surplus of only 10 calories yields 10 unwanted pounds of fat in 10 years; 20 or 30 years of consistent excess food intake or gradually declining activity can easily result in a **positive caloric balance** and, eventually, being overweight and even obese. Accordingly, to maintain a specific weight people must balance their energy intake with their energy expenditure. The key to losing weight and keeping it off is regular, aerobic exercise and a balanced diet that is consistent with the current nutritional recommendations described in Chapter 5; in other words, eat healthfully and exercise regularly.

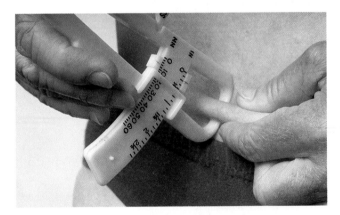

Body fat determination using skinfold calipers. Skinfold measurements are used in equations that calculate body fat density and percentage of body fat.

Determining Weight and Body Composition

A wide array of techniques exist to determine weight and body composition. Some techniques are, of course, much more accurate and more expensive than others. The following section describes a variety of these techniques.

Body Mass Index

As we mentioned in the previous section, one means of assessing healthy body weight is the body mass index (BMI). The BMI indicates the relationship of body weight (expressed in kilograms) to height (expressed in meters) for both men and women. The BMI does not reflect body composition (fat versus lean tissue) or consider the degree of fat accumulated within the central body cavity. It is, nevertheless, widely used in determining obesity (see Table 6.2). BMI is calculated metrically as weight divided by height squared (kg/m^2).

An alternative method of determining the BMI is to use a **nomogram** such as that in Figure 6-1. Like the BMI, the nomogram requires information about both weight and height. Once you have determined your BMI,

> ### Key Terms
>
> **positive caloric balance** caloric intake greater than caloric expenditure
>
> **nomogram** a graphic means of finding an unknown value

Table 6.2 Charting Weight

Body Mass Index Table

Height (inches) / BMI	Normal 19	20	21	22	23	24	Overweight 25	26	27	28	29	Obese 30	31	32	33	34	35	36	37	38	39	Extreme Obesity 40	41	42	43	44	45	46	47	48	49	50	51	52	53	54
												Body Weight (pounds)																								
58	91	96	100	105	110	115	119	124	129	134	138	143	148	153	158	162	167	172	177	181	186	191	196	201	205	210	215	220	224	229	234	239	244	248	253	258
59	94	99	104	109	114	119	124	128	133	138	143	148	153	158	163	168	173	178	183	188	193	198	203	208	212	217	222	227	232	237	242	247	252	257	262	267
60	97	102	107	112	118	123	128	133	138	143	148	153	158	163	168	174	179	184	189	194	199	204	209	215	220	225	230	235	240	245	250	255	261	266	271	276
61	100	106	111	116	122	127	132	137	143	148	153	158	164	169	174	180	185	190	195	201	206	211	217	222	227	232	238	243	248	254	259	264	269	275	280	285
62	104	109	115	120	126	131	136	142	147	153	158	164	169	175	180	186	191	196	202	207	213	218	224	229	235	240	246	251	256	262	267	273	278	284	289	295
63	107	113	118	124	130	135	141	146	152	158	163	169	175	180	186	191	197	203	208	214	220	225	231	237	242	248	254	259	265	270	278	282	287	293	299	304
64	110	116	122	128	134	140	145	151	157	163	169	174	180	186	192	197	204	209	215	221	227	232	238	244	250	256	262	267	273	279	285	291	296	302	308	314
65	114	120	126	132	138	144	150	156	162	168	174	180	186	192	198	204	210	216	222	228	234	240	246	252	258	264	270	276	282	288	294	300	306	312	318	324
66	118	124	130	136	142	148	155	161	167	173	179	186	192	198	204	210	216	223	229	235	241	247	253	260	266	272	278	284	291	297	303	309	315	322	328	334
67	121	127	134	140	146	153	159	166	172	178	185	191	198	204	211	217	223	230	236	242	249	255	261	268	274	280	287	293	299	306	312	319	325	331	338	344
68	125	131	138	144	151	158	164	171	177	184	190	197	203	210	216	223	230	236	243	249	256	262	269	276	282	289	295	302	308	315	322	328	335	341	348	354
69	128	135	142	149	155	162	169	176	182	189	196	203	209	216	223	230	236	243	250	257	263	270	277	284	291	297	304	311	318	324	331	338	345	351	358	365
70	132	139	146	153	160	167	174	181	188	195	202	209	216	222	229	236	243	250	257	264	271	278	285	292	299	306	313	320	327	334	341	348	355	362	369	376
71	136	143	150	157	165	172	179	186	193	200	208	215	222	229	236	243	250	257	265	272	279	286	293	301	308	315	322	329	338	343	351	358	365	372	379	386
72	140	147	154	162	169	177	184	191	199	206	213	221	228	235	242	250	258	265	272	279	287	294	302	309	316	324	331	338	346	353	361	368	375	383	390	397
73	144	151	159	166	174	182	189	197	204	212	219	227	235	242	250	257	265	272	280	288	295	302	310	318	325	333	340	348	355	363	371	378	386	393	401	408
74	148	155	163	171	179	186	194	202	210	218	225	233	241	249	256	264	272	280	287	295	303	311	319	326	334	342	350	358	365	373	381	389	396	404	412	420
75	152	160	168	176	184	192	200	208	216	224	232	240	248	256	264	272	279	287	295	303	311	319	327	335	343	351	359	367	375	383	391	399	407	415	423	431
76	156	164	172	180	189	197	205	213	221	230	238	246	254	263	271	279	287	295	304	312	320	328	336	344	353	361	369	377	385	394	402	410	418	426	435	443

Source: Adapted from *Clinical Guidelines on the Identification, Evaluation, and Treatment of Overweight and Obesity in Adults: The Evidence Report*, National Institute of Health.

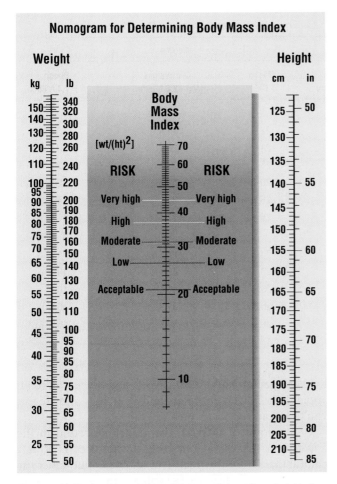

Nomogram for Determining Body Mass Index

Figure 6-1 To use this nomogram, place a ruler or other straightedge between the body weight in kilograms or pounds (without clothes) located on the left-hand column and the height in centimeters or in inches (without shoes) located on the right-hand column. The BMI is read from the middle of the scale and is in metric units.

Table 6.3 Healthy and Unhealthy BMIs

BMI	Weight Status
Below 18.5	Underweight
18.5–24.9	Normal
25.0–29.9	Overweight
30.0 and Above	Obese

information on this newly released BMI chart can be obtained at www.cdc.gov/growthcharts.

Height/Weight Tables

Traditionally the 1983 Metropolitan Life Insurance Height and Weight Table has been the basis for determining the desirable or ideal weight for your gender, height, and frame size. However, the use of this table and others like it is no longer considered the best way to determine whether body weight is acceptable. It is now recognized that this table excludes uninsurable people, disregards the influence of age, fails to consider other causes of mortality (such as smoking), and relies on subjective determinations of frame size to express the influence of body composition on weight. In addition, people have failed to take into consideration that the Metropolitan Life Insurance Height and Weight Tables were based on height that included 1-inch heel shoes and allowed 3 pounds of clothing. The tables were also designed for adults aged 25–59 years of age and were not intended for use with children.[15] Fortunately, the newer tables are intended for use with the guidelines describing healthy body weight and body mass index (BMI) (Table 6.2).

Healthy Body Weight

You can determine your healthy body weight by using the weight guidelines found in the 2005 *Dietary Guidelines for Americans.*[16] This assessment involves converting two body measurements, the waist and the hip circumferences, into a waist-to-hip ratio (WHR) that can then be applied to weight ranges found in Table 6.2 for people of particular ages and heights. The size of your waist is a surprisingly accurate measure of your abdominal fat. Among people who have an acceptable WHR, female "healthy weight" is near the lower end of each weight range, whereas male "healthy weight" is at the higher end of each weight range.

To use these new weight ranges, the following procedure must be performed:

you can determine whether it falls within a healthy range (see Table 6.3). Note that with aging, generally higher BMI values are found.[13] This reflects the gradual weight gain (and indirectly the changing body composition) seen in adults as they age. Table 6.4 on page 182 presents data on BMI related to age, gender, and ethnicity.

The newest BMI chart to appear is the recently released BMI chart for children and adolescents. The importance of having a BMI chart appropriate for age 2 years through 20 years was stimulated by the increasing percentage of children and adolescents who are now classified as being overweight (20 percent). Because of the availability of this chart, pediatricians and parents now have the ability to more quickly and more accurately determine the risk of potential obesity in children and take appropriate action to minimize its occurrence. Additional

Table 6.4 Mean Body Mass Index and Percentage of Overweight and Obese U.S. Adults

	Men			Women		
	Mean BMI	Overweight (N = 15.4 Million)	Obese (N = 5.1 Million)	Mean BMI	Overweight (N = 18.6 Million)	Obese (N = 7.4 Million)
AGE						
20–24	23.5	12.1	4.2	22.6	11.4	3.5
25–34	25.2	20.4	6.7	24.1	20	8.8
35–44	26	28.9	8.9	25.3	27	12.1
45–54	26.3	31	10.7	26.1	32.5	12.9
55–64	26.1	28.1	9.2	26.5	37	14.2
All ages	25.3	24.2	8	25	27.1	10.6
ETHNICITY						
White	25.4	24.4	7.8	24.8	24.6	9.6
Black	25.3	26.3	10.4	27.1	45.1	19.7
Mexican	25.9	31.2	10.8	26.6	41.5	16.7
Cuban	26	28.5	10.3	25.8	31.9	6.9
Puerto Rican	25.5	25.7	7.9	26.1	39.8	15.2

1. Measure around your waist near your navel while you stand relaxed, not pulling in your stomach.
2. Measure around your hips, over the buttocks where your hips are the largest.
3. Divide the waist measurement by the hip measurement.

Women with a WHR of .80 or less generally have a body weight that falls within the healthy range for their age and height as depicted in Table 6.2; men with a WHR of .90 or less will also probably fall within the range that is considered healthy for their age and height.

This assessment procedure was developed in response to the growing concern over the relationship between the amount of fat in the central abdominal cavity (upper body obesity) and the development of several serious health problems. As we mentioned earlier, the risk of health problems such as heart disease and diabetes increases at a waist measurement of 35 inches for women and 40 inches for men, regardless of height.[16]

In comparison with the "spare tire" pattern of fat distribution seen in men, women more often demonstrate an excessive accumulation of fat in the hips, thighs, and buttocks. This lower body obesity is less closely associated with chronic health problems.

Research shows that women who have more fat concentrated around the waist, as opposed to their hips, have a greater risk of cardiovascular disease and diabetes. This has been referred to as the "apple versus pear shape" phenomenon. Whether you're an apple or pear depends on where your body stores its excess fat. If fat tends to gather high around your abdomen, you're an apple. If it collects more around your hips and thighs, you're a pear.

As a point of interest, the guidelines found in the *Dietary Guidelines for Americans* do not use WHR as a clinical marker for the treatment of obesity but rather use only waist circumference, believing it to be a better predictor of risk. Only time will tell about the continued use of healthy body weight in assessing risk for cardiovascular disease and other chronic conditions.

The *Dietary Guidelines for Americans* assessment procedure recognizes increasing age as a factor that influences body weight.[16] For people older than 35 years of age, this alleviates some of the pressure to maintain an unrealistic weight. Some nutritionists, however, believe that the same weight standards should apply to both older adults and younger adults.

Electrical Impedance

Electrical impedance is a relatively new method to determine body composition. This assessment procedure measures the electrical impedance or resistance to a weak electrical flow directed through the body. Because adipose

---

Key Terms

electrical impedance a method used to measure the percentage of body fat using a harmless electrical current tissue resists the passage of the electrical current more than muscle tissue does, electrical impedance can be used to calculate the percentage of body fat. However, in addition to high cost and limited availability, psychological variables, such as fear or discomfort associated with the electrical current flow, can reduce the practicality of electrical impedance.

BOD POD (Body Composition System)

The newest method of determining body composition involves the use of the BOD POD, an egg-shaped chamber that uses computerized pressure sensors to determine the amount of air displaced by the person's body (larger people displace more air than smaller people). The person is allowed to breath normally during the test, and the amount of air in the lungs can either be measured directly in the BOD POD or is estimated. A complete test, with printed results, can be achieved in less than 4.5 minutes.[18] Body density can itself be used to determine the percentage of the subject's body that is comprised of fat. Upon knowing the percent body fat, the percent of lean body mass can be calculated, again using a mathematical formula.[19] The BOD POD is highly accurate and much more comfortable for subjects than is hydrostatic weighing.

Skinfold Measurements

A **skinfold measurement** provides another way to measure body fat percentage. Skinfold measurements rely on constant-pressure **calipers** to measure the thickness of the layer of fat beneath the skin's surface. Skinfold measurements of subcutaneous fat are taken at several key places on the body. Measurements of skinfold thickness can then be used to calculate the percentage of body fat, and then a relatively simple conversion can be made to determine desired body weight. There are some drawbacks to this type of measure: First, a second person may be required to perform the test, because it is sometimes difficult to get an accurate measurement on yourself. Second, skinfolds are notoriously hard to locate precisely, and being just a few millimeters off can make a significant difference. Research recommends that 50–100 tests are needed before an examiner can be classified as "competent" with body fat calipers. Body fat calipers used correctly are accurate to within 4 percent at best.[13]

Young adult men normally have a body fat percentage of 10–15 percent. The normal range for young adult women is 22–25 percent. When a man's body fat percentage exceeds 25 percent and a woman's body fat percentage exceeds 30 percent, these people are classified as obese.

The relatively higher percentage of fat found in women compared to men is related to the female's capacity for pregnancy and lactation. Women require a sufficient amount of body fat in order to ovulate, menstruate, and become pregnant. In fact, some experts suggest that lack of sex drive can be related to the adverse changes in hormonal level owing to insufficient body fat. The danger zone begins when a woman's BMI is about 18 or below. Women tend to store fat in their pelvic region, around their hips and thighs. Not only does this fat help to protect vital reproductive organs, it also acts as a source of stored energy for pregnancy and breast-feeding. As women enter menopause, they produce less estrogen. This leads to a change in body shape and fat distribution. During a woman's fertile years, the female hormones estrogen and progesterone are responsible for maintaining the female shape of a narrow waist and rounded hips. During and after menopause, the female waist thickens and fat is deposited around the stomach area similar to the male's pattern of fat distribution. In addition, as in men, the metabolic rate slows and fewer calories are required. So if a woman continues to eat the same amount of food as she has throughout her fertile years, without increasing her exercise, weight and fat gain are likely to occur.[20]

Hydrostatic Weighing

Hydrostatic weighing (underwater weighing) is a precise method for determining the relative amounts of fat and lean body mass that make up body weight. A person's percentage of body fat is determined by comparing the underwater body weight with the body weight out of the water and dry. The necessity for expensive equipment and trained technicians makes the use of this method impractical for the average person. Traditionally hydrostatic weighing has been considered the most accurate or sensitive means of determining body composition, with a 97 percent accuracy rate. The BOD POD appears to be just as accurate and certainly more comfortable to use than underwater weighing.

Additional techniques used to determine body composition include computerized axial tomography (CAT) scans, magnetic resonance imaging (MRI), infrared light transmission, and neutron activation. These techniques have limited application because of cost and availability.

Key Terms

skinfold measurement a measurement to determine the thickness of the fat layer that lies immediately beneath the skin; used to calculate body composition

caliper a device used to measure the thickness of a skinfold from which percentage of body fat can be calculated

hydrostatic weighing weighing the body while it is submerged in water

Appearance

While it may seem as though the simplest method of determining one's body size is to look in the mirror, for most people this is not an accurate measure. Research shows that most women are dissatisfied with their appearance or body image and perceive themselves as needing to lose an average of 10–15 pounds when in actuality they are in a healthy weight range. Body dissatisfaction is endemic to young women in Western culture as evidenced by the rate of dieting in the United States, starting at a young age. In fact, on any given day, 50 percent of 10-year-olds are on a diet, and two-thirds of high school women and a third of all adult women are dieting.[21] There is also an important difference between one's internal concept of one's body and actual body perception, and this is particularly problematic for people with eating disorders.

Home Scale

Most people use scales at home or in a gym to determine their weight, but scales can be highly inaccurate, as evidenced by weighing yourself on a variety of scales and weighing different amounts. Also, you will probably weigh less in the morning when you first wake up and more in the evening, after having eaten during the day. So, if you are using a scale to monitor your weight, you need to do so on the same scale, at the same time of day, and with approximately the same weight of clothing. Also, remember that muscle weighs more than fat, which explains why some toned and muscular athletes can weigh as much as someone who is sedentary and overweight. In general, risk of disease increases with a higher percentage of body fat, not weight.

For many people, it is important to appear physically attractive. This desired body image may or may not be compatible with their inherited body type or their ability to gain or lose weight. Nevertheless, they try to achieve the look that they have in mind.

Causes of Obesity

Debate continues as to the causes of obesity. Genetic, physiological, metabolic, environmental, psychological, and other factors may all play a part. In the past decade, the overall prevalence of obesity has increased so that currently one-third of all Americans are obese. Moreover, in the last 20 years, the number of overweight children in the United States has tripled to one in five children.[22] Genetics, dietary practice, and activity level seem to all play a role in this dramatic increase.

Four additional factors seem to play a significant role in the prevalence of obesity: sex, age, socioeconomic status, and race. Biology accounts for only 33 percent of the variation in body weight, so the environment can also exert an enormous influence. According to the Centers for Disease Control, prevalence rates for obesity in women is 35 percent and 31 percent among men and is found mainly in the 20–55 age group. Among women, obesity is strongly associated with socioeconomic status, being twice as common among those with lower socioeconomic status as it is among those with higher status.[23] Although prevalence among black and white men does not differ significantly, obesity is far more common among black than among white women, affecting 66 percent of black women compared with 49 percent of white women.

While the precise cause of obesity remains unclear, we do know that obesity is a complex condition caused by a variety of factors. Until we are sure what causes obesity, it will remain difficult to develop effective ways of managing weight.

Genetic Factors

Through years of research, we do know that heredity plays a major role in the development of body size and obesity.[24] Based on studies comparing both identical and fraternal (nonidentical) twins raised together and separately, it's evident that both environment and genetics influence obesity. In fact, it is estimated that heredity accounts for 25 percent to 40 percent of the development of obesity.[12] Women have a higher percentage of body fat than do men, and this seems stable across cultures and dietary habits.[24] While some scientific research has explored whether the X chromosome may be linked to fat distribution, no conclusive evidence has substantiated this link.

There is also some speculation about population differences and prevalence of obesity suggesting that some groups possess a "thrifty genotype."[25] For example, the differences in diabetes and obesity rates in Native Americans compared with European Americans prompted some researchers to consider that some groups of people have survived periods of feast and famine by increased efficiency in energy storage and expenditure through a particular genotype. However, no specific thrifty gene or genotype has been identified.

A complex interplay of genetic factors very likely influence the development of obesity, since more than 250 genes may play a role in obesity. Promising research has explored how the leptin gene influences obesity. Discovered in the mid 1990s, the leptin gene, referred to as the "fat gene," was thought to influence satiety or the feeling of fullness in mice.[26] When the leptin gene was faulty in mice, it produced lower leptin levels, and the mice experienced excessive weight gain. However, when the leptin gene was normal, the leptin levels were higher and the mice were able to maintain normal weight. It has been theorized that leptin resistance may be involved in weight

Dieting and Religion

As was discussed in Chapter 5, spirituality guides some of our eating habits and traditions. Many stories from medieval times tell of female saints who ate almost nothing or fasted as a way of purifying the body. Catherine of Siena is said to have eaten a handful of herbs each day and occasionally shoved twigs down her throat to bring up any other food she was forced to eat. Fasting was a way of demonstrating female holiness; it was thought that prayer provided sustenance.[1] Fasting is part of other religions besides Christianity—for example, the Islamic celebration of Ramadan (Chapter 5).

Some modern diets promote spiritual components, and some food has been referred to as sinful. *The Weigh Down Diet* by Gwen Shamblin approaches weight loss from a religious perspective, advising people to feed the human soul with a relationship with God rather than with food. Holding meetings in local churches, Shamblin teaches you "God's rules for eating." She advocates allowing your stomach to become empty before eating and to give your appetite to God to control. In fact, she suggests waiting to eat until your stomach is growling and to focus on making the desire for eating go away. This is counter to what many nutritionists, physicians, and psychologists suggest in terms of healthy eating. She states that exercise is not important for weight management, writing in her book that "the only exercises we insist on are getting down on your knees to pray and getting the muscle of your will to surrender some of the extra food you have been eating."[2] Again, this advice is not consistent with the USDA's guidelines of engaging in daily physical exercise for 30–90 minutes.

There are a number of other religious or spiritually based approaches to weight loss. For example, the *Hallelujah Diet* by Rev. George Malkmus suggests that we eat a vegan diet. He states, "the Lord gave us everything we need in the Garden of Eden; fruits, vegetables, nuts, and seeds." He calls this the "Hallelujah diet" to "celebrate its true creater." Dr. Don Colbert wrote a book based on a similar philosophy called *What Would Jesus Eat?*, which encourages the consumption of non-animal-derived living foods rather than dead or processed foods. One of the newest Christian weight-management books is *The Maker's Diet* by Jordan S. Rubin. He warns against a vegan diet and suggests eating meat and dairy products instead. He further recommends eating foods in their most organic and least-processed states and consuming food in the form the body was designed by God to eat them. For example, he doesn't think milk should be pasteurized nor should the fat be removed to make skim or low-fat milk.[3]

While Shamblin is a registered dietician and has a master's degree in food and nutrition, most of the diet ministries are led by people without these types of degrees and credentials. There has been some concern raised about food safety issues with unprocessed dairy products, meat, and other foods as well as how these diets contradict the new dietary guidelines released by the USDA, particularly those concerning exercising daily and eating a balanced diet. Some critics say that God is being used as a gimmick to get in on the $50 billion dollar diet industry, while others view giving dietary advice as part of God's ministry.

[1]Brumberg, J. *Fasting Girls.* Cambridge, MA: Harvard University Press, 1989.

[2]Shamblin, G. *The Weigh Down Diet.* New York: Bantam Doubleday Dell Publishing Group, 1997.

[3]"What Would Jesus Eat? Diets Grapple with God's Gastronomic Will," *Muncie Star Press,* Volume 105, No. 364, June 2004.

---

gain and the maintenance of excessive weight, but much more research needs to be conducted in this area.[27] While we know that leptin helps to regulate fat storage and energy efficiency in humans, it still remains unclear as to how this research can be utilized in the treatment of obesity.

Physiological and Hormonal Factors

Building on the new information about the genetic and neuropsychological basis of obesity, researchers have identified centers for the control of eating within the hypothalamus of the central nervous system (CNS). These centers—the feeding center for hunger and the satiety center for fullness—tell the body when it should begin consuming food and when food consumption should stop. It takes 20 minutes on average for these signals to go from the stomach to the brain to relay the message "stop eating." These centers are thought to continuously monitor a variety of factors regarding food intake including smell, taste, visual cues, glucose levels, amino acids, the degree of stomach distention, and information regarding basal metabolic rate, gastrointestinal hormone level, orexin A, and orexin B that influence hunger in rats.[27]

Hormonal factors also influence obesity. Obesity can be caused by a condition called **hypothyroidism,** in

Key Terms

hypothyroidism a condition in which the thyroid gland produces an insufficient amount of the hormone thyroxin which the thyroid gland produces an insufficient amount of thyroxin, a hormone that regulates metabolism. Over five million Americans have this common medical condition, and as many as 10 percent of women may have some degree of thyroid hormone deficiency. In such individuals, the underactive thyroid makes burning up food difficult, and so weight gain is common. As we acquire greater understanding of the hormones and neurotransmitters that influence hunger and satiety, drugs designed to influence their actions will be developed. Some of these drugs already exist and will be described later in this chapter.

The effects of hormonal changes on eating can be seen each month just before a woman's menstrual cycle; many women say that they crave salty and sugary foods during this time. Pregnancy brings about another host of hormonal and metabolic changes. During a normal pregnancy, a woman requires an extra 300 calories a day to support the developing fetus and supportive tissues, and to fuel her elevated maternal metabolic rate. In addition, pregnant women will develop approximately 9 extra pounds of adipose tissue that will be used as an energy source during lactation. The average woman is expected to gain 25–35 pounds during pregnancy.[12] Many women express concern about their ability to lose this weight following the birth of the child, and some women do gain much more than the recommended amount of weight. However, the majority of women lose their pregnancy weight within 6 months to a year after having a baby. Nevertheless, obesity is one of the most frequent causes for complications in pregnancy. Women who are obese during pregnancy have a much higher risk of hypertension and gestational diabetes. Obesity has also been associated with infertility, poor pregnancy outcomes, and miscarriage.[28]

Typically, breast-feeding can help women to burn more calories and return to their prepregnancy weight, although extra fat may linger, since nature intended this to be a store of energy for breast-feeding. Breast-feeding requires an additional 500 calories a day.[29] Mothers who breast-feed tend to lose more weight when their babies are 3 to 6 months old than do formula-feeding mothers who consume fewer calories. One study of mothers at 1 month postpartum found that mothers who breast-fed had slimmer hips and weighed less than did women whose babies received formula.[29] Infants who are breast-fed also have a lower chance of developing obesity and asthma in childhood and adolescence.[30, 31, 32]

Metabolic Factors

Traditional theory has suggested that the energy expenditure and energy storage centers of the body possess a genetically programmed awareness of the body's most physiologically desirable weight, called **set point.**[33] However, the term *set point* is somewhat misleading in that it does not refer to a certain number or point but a weight range that the body is genetically programmed to maintain. When the body falls below its natural set point, one's metabolism reacts by slowing down the body's functioning in order to conserve energy. In other words, the body senses that it is not receiving enough calories to maintain healthy functioning and so it sends calories to essential areas of the body and uses the energy as efficiently as possible. Alternatively, when someone consumes more calories than are needed, the body begins to increase the rate of metabolism in an effort not to gain weight above the set point. The process of storing or burning more energy to maintain the body's "best" weight is called **adaptive thermogenesis.** This process also explains the reason that 90 percent of people who go on any diet gain all the weight back plus more within a year of going off the diet. When dieting, people reduce their caloric intake, which in turn lowers their metabolism. When they discontinue the diet, they typically eat more calories and foods with higher fat content on a lowered metabolism. This is a good formula for weight gain. In addition, dieters tend to lose muscle and regain their weight as fat.

There is a great deal of debate on how an individual's set point can be altered. The number of fat cells in the body, the blood level of insulin, and regions of the brain such as the hypothalamus all seem to play a role in determining set point. Certain drugs such as amphetamines and other diet pills and herbal supplements can act on the brain to temporarily lower the set point. However, once these drugs are discontinued, the set point returns to the previous level or perhaps an even higher level and weight increases as a result. Healthier and more permanent methods of changing one's set point are through regular exercise and healthy eating patterns. In fact, a recent study of 8,000 successful dieters found that the majority of them used "my own diet and exercise regimen" and did not follow any formal weight reduction program.[34]

The body's requirement for energy to maintain basic physiological processes decreases progressively with age. This change reflects the loss of muscle tissue as both men and women age. This loss of muscle mass eventually alters the ratio of lean body tissue to fat. As the proportion of fat

---

Key Terms

set point a genetically programmed range of body weight, beyond which a person finds it difficult to gain or lose additional weight

adaptive thermogenesis the physiological response of the body to adjust its metabolic rate to the presence of food increases, the energy needs of the body are more strongly influenced by the lower metabolic needs of the fat cells.[35] This excess energy is then stored in the fat cells of the body. A gradual decrease in caloric intake and a conscious effort to expend more calories can effectively prevent this gradual increase in weight leading to obesity.

Social and Cultural Factors

Ethnic and cultural differences also relate to the incidence of obesity and what is considered to be a healthy weight. African American, American Indian, and Hispanic American women have the highest risk of becoming overweight, according to the Centers for Disease Control. In fact, the results of a national study showed that more than half of all African American and Hispanic women in the United States are above what is considered a healthy body weight. The statistics are startling: 66 percent of African American women are overweight, with 33 percent of these being obese. For Caucasian women, 49 percent are considered overweight with 24 percent of these being obese. Only one minority group, Asian Americans, has a lower rate of obesity than does the general population.

Obesity is second only to tobacco as the leading cause of premature deaths and disproportionately affects women of color and women of lower socioeconomic classes. On the positive side, African American women report less pressure to be thin than do their white counterparts and tend to be less self-conscious about their weight.[36] Acculturation also has a significant effect on the rates of obesity—the more an ethnic group has adapted to and absorbed Western culture, the higher the rate of obesity within that group.[37]

Socioeconomic status is also an important influence on obesity, particularly in women. Upper socioeconomic women tend to be thinner than lower socioeconomic women, while among men there is not such a pattern.[38] Limited access to health care, lower education levels, lower income levels, and increased stress are some of the reasons cited for this disparity. Interestingly, higher obesity levels are also related to marriage, parenthood, and geographical location; married men, parents, and people living in rural areas tend to have a higher incidence of obesity.[39]

Environmental Factors

Certainly environmental factors such as the smell or sight of freshly made cookies, or an advertisement for a candy bar, can affect your eating habits. Even the clock signaling it is "time to eat" can encourage us to eat even when we aren't hungry. While this may seem adaptive and helpful in regulating our food intake, Dr. Kelly D. Brownell, a professor of psychology at Yale and an expert on eating disor-

ders, has gone so far as to label American society a "toxic environment" when it comes to food. Researchers contend that the local environment has a powerful effect on eating. Factors such as portion size, price, advertising, the availability of food, and the number of food choices presented all can influence the amount the average person consumes. For example, moviegoers will eat 50 percent more popcorn if given an extra-large tub of popcorn instead of a container one size smaller, even if the popcorn is stale. If a tabletop in the office is stocked with cookies and candy, coworkers tend to nibble their way through the workday, even if they are not hungry. One study showed that when the candy was in plain sight on workers' desks, they ate an average of nine pieces each. Storing the candy in a desk drawer reduced consumption to six pieces, as compared to putting the candy a couple of yards from the desk, cutting the number to three pieces per person.[40] In response to these and other findings, many public schools have begun offering only healthy foods in their cafeterias, replacing soft drinks, candy, and chips with juice, milk, fruit, and granola bars.

Packaging and price can also influence the amount people consume, a concept of which advertisers, restaurants, and grocery stores are well aware. Dropping the price of the low-fat snacks by even a nickel resulted in dramatically increased sales. In contrast, stickers signaling low-fat content or cartoons promoting the low-fat alternatives had little influence over which snacks were more popular. This is true not only of food but also of beverages: people tend to drink *more* from short, wide glasses than from thin, tall ones, thinking they are drinking less.[40]

Having more choices also appears to make people eat more. In one study, people ate more when offered sandwiches with four different fillings than they did when they were given sandwiches with their single favorite filling. In another study, participants who were served a four-course meal with meat, fruit, bread, and a pudding ate 60 percent more food than did those served an equivalent meal of only their favorite course. Even the cup holders in automobiles have grown larger to make room for giant drinks. Note that these findings apply to people of all body sizes not just people who are overweight or obese, as is often the misconception. However, one difference seems to relate to the age of the individuals studied. One study found that 3-year-olds who were served three different portion sizes of macaroni and cheese for lunch on three different days ate the same amount each time. Five-year-olds, however, ate more when more was put in front of them.[40]

 TALKING POINTS Do you think there should be more regulation of the food industry? If so, what recommendations would you make? What food would you include for regulation and how should this be determined?

The South Beach diet, the Atkins' diet—many of these fad diets make the same promises and offer consistent misinformation:

1. *It's not a diet but a way of life.* While this is true of healthy eating habits, it is not true of most popular diets, because it is very difficult and not healthy to remain on them for the rest of your life. Eating a healthy, balanced diet along with exercising regularly is more realistic on a long-term basis.

2. *The food is delicious, and you won't be hungry.* Again, because most diets severely cut calories, people are hungry and end up falling off the diet and eating high-fat and high-sugar foods. This is another reason that these diets can't be a way of life—people feel too deprived.

3. *You're overweight because you eat the wrong food.* This means you didn't buy the food advertised by that weight loss company. What the "wrong food" is changes depending on whom you are listening to. It might be too many carbohydrates, too much fat, too many fruits and vegetables, or too few fruits and vegetables! The truth is that you are overweight because you eat too much food period!

4. *The diet will prevent diseases.* Actually the truth is the opposite. Many of these diets are dangerous and have been associated with cancer, kidney failure, heart disease, hypertension, and other problems.

Perhaps the most startling evidence that these diets aren't effective and are unhealthy can be gained from learning about their creators. For example, Robert Atkins, the originator of *Dr. Atkins' New Diet Revolution,* was reported by *The Wall Street Journal* to have weighed 258 pounds at 6 feet at the time of his death. He went into cardiac arrest after falling on the ice and died. Dr. Phil, of *The Ultimate Weight Solution,* is said to weigh 240 pounds at 6'4"—again, clearly overweight.

These diets do have a kernel of truth in that they propose that to effectively manage your weight you need to make a lifestyle change, not just change your diet for a brief time; eat foods you enjoy to avoid feeling deprived; reduce portion sizes and cut your calories; and follow the new USDA dietary guidelines to help you to prevent the development of chronic diseases.

Psychological Factors

Psychological factors related to overeating concern the reasons people eat other than physiological hunger. Individuals with eating disorders often report that they don't know when they are hungry and often eat when they are not hungry and don't eat when they have a biological reason for doing so. Why do people eat if not in response to hunger? Frequently people eat in response to their emotions—for example, to comfort themselves or when bored, tired, stressed, or depressed. Some people say they use food as a way of coping with hurt, sadness, and anger, "swallowing" their feelings and putting food on top of them. Others eat out of habit and associate food with certain activities, such as eating popcorn at a movie, eating chips in front of the television, and having dessert after dinner. Certainly many people think of chocolate when they want to cheer themselves up. Food is also part of celebrations, holidays, and family bonding, as well as a mainstay of socialization. It is difficult to think about social activities we engage in that don't involve food in some way.

Some people develop relationships with food that substitute for real human relationships. Comments such as "Food is my best friend" and "A great meal is better than sex" are indicative to the degree to which many people rely on food to fill their needs. As we'll learn in our discussion of eating disorders later in the chapter, psychological issues with food can become serious, even life-threatening problems.

Dietary Practices

Many researchers believe that the number of fat cells a person has is initially determined during the first two years of life. Babies who are overfed will develop a greater number of fat cells than will babies who receive a balanced diet of appropriate, infant-sized portions. Overfed babies, especially those with a family history of obesity, tend to develop **hypercellular obesity.** When these children reach adulthood, they will have more fat cells. An increase in fat cells during infancy and childhood can increase the chances of developing obesity. This increase can result in five times as many fat cells in obese people as in people of normal weight. Dieting reduces only the size of fat cells not the number of fat cells. People who have hypercellular obesity have an abnormally high number of fat cells and are biologically limited in their ability to lose weight.[41]

Hypercellular obesity in adulthood can also result from excessive weight gain in late childhood and adolescence. If an individual's weight is 75 percent above the desirable weight, this can stimulate an increase in the number of fat cells, resulting in eventual obesity.

> ### Key Terms
>
> **hypercellular obesity** a form of obesity that results from having an abnormally high number of fat cells

Hypertrophic obesity is the result of a pattern of overeating for a long period of time. Over a period of years, the existing fat cells increase in size to accommodate excess fat intake. Note that, after puberty, as your body stores more fat, the number of fat cells remains the same but each fat cell can get bigger. Hypertrophic obesity is generally associated with excessive fat around the waist and is thought to contribute to conditions such as type 2 diabetes, high levels of fat in the blood, high blood pressure, and heart disease. Hypertrophic obesity generally appears during middle age when physical activity tends to decline, whereas caloric intake remains the same.[41]

The information, values, traditions, and messages you receive from your family also have a significant impact on your dietary habits. If an infant's cries for food are immediately responded to, that child will likely learn what the sensation of hunger is and what the appropriate response is. If crying unrelated to hunger is responded to by the offer of a cookie or candy, the child will learn to soothe himself or herself with food. Studies show that children become confused about what hunger is and how to satisfy it if their hunger needs are neglected or overindulged in infancy.[42]

Some of the first power struggles between parents and their children revolve around issues of food. A child who has little power in her life can exert some power and control through refusing to eat certain foods and demanding other foods and determining when she wants to eat. Parents who use food as a reward for good behavior ("If you get an 'A' on your test, I will treat you to ice cream"); as punishment ("You weren't behaving so you can't have dessert"); or as a guilt trip ("Don't waste food. Clean your plate. Children are starving in the world") may inadvertently be creating negative dietary practices that will continue throughout the child's life. Interestingly, research has shown that children are extraordinarily adept at meeting their nutritional needs when left to their own devices. One study allowed children to eat whatever they wanted for a week. Did they always pick high-fat, high-sugar foods? No. Actually, when we look at each day's intake, they didn't eat a balanced diet. However, when one takes the full week into consideration, they met their nutritional needs perfectly.

What your parents say to you not only has a tremendous influence on your eating behavior; what they do, their own eating practices, can have even a greater impact. Children are exposed to different foods and model what their parents eat. If a parent makes comments such as "I shouldn't eat that because I will get fat" or doesn't eat fruits or vegetables, or sits down with a bag of chips in front of the television every night, the child will probably do the same. In the same vein, when parents exercise regularly, eat a balanced diet, and make positive comments about their weight, children tend to mimic this behavior.

Inactivity

When weight management experts are asked to identify the single most important reason that obesity is so high in today's society, they are most certain to point to inactivity. People of all ages tend to be less active and burn fewer calories than did their ancestors only a few generations ago. (See the Star box on page 196.) Both adults and children spend less time devoted to exercise as a result of longer work hours at sedentary jobs, a decline in physical education programs in school, and increased participation in sedentary recreational activities, such as browsing the Internet, playing video games, and watching television. In addition, many of the laborsaving devices and increased automation in the home and workplace have contributed to increased inactivity. According to some studies, nearly two-thirds of Americans are not physically active on a regular basis, and 25 percent are completely sedentary.[44] It is not surprising that as inactivity becomes the norm so does overweight.

 TALKING POINTS What were the messages you received in childhood regarding food? What positive and negative eating habits have you learned from your family?

Caloric Balance

As previously mentioned, any calories consumed beyond those that are used by the body are converted to fat stores. People gain weight when their energy input exceeds their energy output. Consuming about 3,500 calories a week more than is needed results in a weight gain of 1 pound of fat.[43] Conversely, they lose weight when their energy output exceeds their energy input (Figure 6-2). The basic formula is quite simple and can be analogous to a seesaw. Weight remains constant when caloric input and caloric output are equal. In such a situation, our bodies are said to be in *caloric balance*.

Energy Needs of the Body

What are our energy needs? How many calories should we consume (or expend) to achieve a healthy weight? There is no single answer for everyone. The new USDA dietary guidelines are based on consuming 2,000 calories a day.[44]

Key Terms

hypertrophic obesity a form of obesity in which there are a normal number of fat cells, but the individual fat cells are enlarged

---

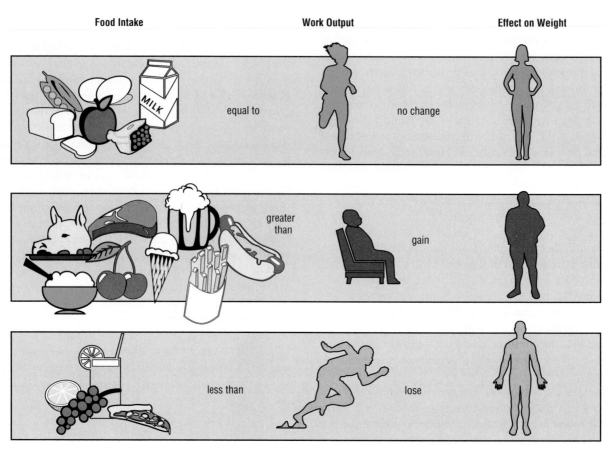

Food Intake	Work Output	Effect on Weight
equal to		no change
greater than		gain
less than		lose

Figure 6-2 Caloric balance: energy input equals energy output, some of which comes from physical activity.

(See Chapter 5.) Age and gender both affect the amount of calories people need. In addition, they need fewer or more than the USDA recommendation depending on these three factors: (1) basal metabolism, (2) activity requirements, and (3) the thermic effect of food. Of these factors, basal metabolism is the most important determinant of the total calories required by an individual.

Basal Metabolic Rate

Basal Metabolic Rate (BMR) is a measure of resting energy expenditure that is taken upon awakening, 10–12 hours after eating, or 12–18 hours after significant physical activity. A closely related construct, resting metabolic rate (RMR), is often used interchangeably with BMR. In comparison with the BMR, the RMR is measured at rest, without the stringent controls on physical activity required as with measuring BMR. RMR measures the calories needed for functioning such as blood circulation, respiration, brain activity, muscle function, body temperature, and heart beat.[45]

Basal metabolism changes as people age. For both males and females, the BMR is relatively high at birth and continues to increase until the age of 2. Except for a slight rise at puberty, the BMR gradually declines throughout the remainder of life. A variety of other variables also affect BMR, including body composition (muscular bodies are associated with higher BMRs), physical condition (fit people have higher BMRs), sex (males have 5 percent higher BMRs), hormone secretions (people with excessively active thyroid and adrenal glands have higher BMRs), sleep (BMRs are about 10 percent lower during sleep), pregnancy (a 20 percent increase in BMR is typical, especially in the last trimester), body temperature (a 1° rise in body temperature increases BMR about 7 percent), and environmental temperature (deviations above and below 78° F result in increased BMRs).[46]

> **Key Terms**
>
> **basal metabolic rate (BMR)** the amount of energy, expressed in calories, that the body requires to maintain basic functions

The most important variables related to BMR are age, body composition, activity level, and caloric intake. For example, if people fail to recognize that BMR declines with aging, they might fail to adjust food intake accordingly, and weight gain will occur. Also, for those who are thinner, the presence of lean tissue favors a higher basal metabolic rate with greater resistance to weight gain. Finally, an increase in physical activity fosters a faster BMR, which contributes to weight loss. In contrast, in those people with above-average levels of body fat, BMR rates are lower, thus providing the body with excess calories that will be stored as fat. Use the formula in the Star box [on this page] to determine your BMR and the approximate number of calories you require.

Activity Requirements

Each person's caloric *activity requirements* vary directly according to the amount of daily physical work completed. For example, sedentary office workers require a smaller daily caloric intake than do construction workers, letter carriers, and farm workers. Even within a given general job type, the amount of caloric expenditure varies according to the physical effort required. A police officer who walks a neighborhood beat usually expends many more calories than does the typical police dispatcher, equestrian, or motorcycle officer.

Physical activity that occurs outside the occupational setting also adds to caloric needs. Sedentary office workers may be quite active in their recreational pursuits, or active employees may spend their off-hours lounging in front of the television. You must closely examine the total amount of work or activity you perform to accurately estimate your caloric requirements. Physical activity uses between 20–40 percent of caloric intake. See Table 6.5 for a breakdown of caloric expenditures for various activities.

Thermic Effect of Food

Thermic effect of food (TEF) refers to the amount of energy our bodies require for the digestion, absorption, and transportation of food. This energy breaks down the bonds that hold complex food molecules together, resulting in smaller nutritional units that can be distributed throughout the body. The amount of TEF burned varies for different types of food, with some food such as fat requiring less energy to convert to energy stores and others such as protein and carbohydrates requiring more. The TEF peaks in about 1 hour after eating and accounts for approximately 10 percent of total energy expenditure.[46]

Weight-Management Techniques

Weight loss occurs when the calories consumed are fewer than required by the body for physiological maintenance and activity. This may sound overly simplified, and certainly the $50 billion-a-year weight loss industry would like us to think it is much more complicated than this.

Weight loss followed by weight gain may be less healthy and certainly more frustrating than maintaining body weight, even at weight above the desirable levels. When a diet or weight loss strategy fails, the person, not the diet, is blamed. This causes people to jump to another weight loss method and then another, and a vicious cycle has begun. However, a commitment to a lifestyle change of eating in healthy ways and engaging in regular exercise seems to be the most effective strategy for weight loss and weight maintenance. Set a goal to lose not more than 2 pounds a week, because the body tends to lose muscle rather than fat if the weight loss occurs too rapidly.[43] Many people also complain of "hanging skin" after a rapid, drastic weight loss, which can then require cosmetic surgery to rectify.

A number of approaches to weight loss can be pursued. How do dieters know when they have succeeded?

Calculating Basal Metabolic Rate

The basal metabolic rate (BMR) reflects the amount of energy in calories (C) that your body requires to sustain basic functions. The formula below can be used to calculate your approximate basal metabolic rate.

$$\text{BMR per day} = 1\,C \times \frac{\text{body weight (lb)}}{2.2} \times 24$$

Example: 150-lb person

$$\text{BMR per day} = 1\,C \times \frac{150}{2.2} \times 24$$
$$= 1\,C \times 6.82 \times 24$$
$$= 1636.8\,C$$

This person would need approximately 1,637 calories to sustain the body at rest for an entire day. Activity of any kind, of course, elevates the requirement for calories.

Note: A woman's BMR would be approximately 5% lower than that of a man of the same age.

Key Terms

thermic effect of food (TEF) the amount of energy our bodies require for the digestion, absorption, and transportation of food

Table 6.5 Calories Expended during Physical Activity

To determine the number of calories you have spent in an hour of activity, simply multiply the *calories per hour per pound* column by your weight (in pounds). For example, after an hour of archery, a 120-pound person will have expended 209 calories; a 160-pound person, 278 calories; and a 220-pound person, 383 calories.

Activity	Calories/Hour/Pound	Activity	Calories/Hour/Pound
Archery	1.74	Marching (rapid)	3.84
Baseball	1.86	Painting (outside)	2.10
Basketball	3.78	Playing music (sitting)	1.08
Boxing (sparring)	3.78	Racquetball	3.90
Canoeing (leisure)	1.20	Running (cross-country)	4.44
Cleaning	1.62	Running	
Climbing hills (no load)	3.30	11 min 30 sec per mile	3.66
Cooking	1.20	9 min per mile	5.28
Cycling		8 min per mile	5.64
5.5 mph	1.74	7 min per mile	6.24
9.4 mph	2.70	6 min per mile	6.84
Racing	4.62	5 min 30 sec per mile	7.86
Dance (modern)	2.28	Scrubbing floors	3.00
Eating (sitting)	0.60	Sailing	1.20
Field hockey	3.66	Skiing	
Fishing	1.68	Cross-country	4.43
Football	3.60	Snow, downhill	3.84
Gardening		Water	3.12
Digging	3.42	Skating (moderate)	2.28
Mowing	3.06	Soccer	3.54
Raking	1.44	Squash	5.76
Golf	2.34	Swimming	
Gymnastics	1.80	Backstroke	4.62
Handball	3.78	Breaststroke	4.44
Hiking	2.52	Free, fast	4.26
Horseback riding		Free, slow	3.48
Galloping	3.72	Butterfly	4.68
Trotting	3.00	Table tennis	1.86
Walking	1.14	Tennis	3.00
Ice hockey	5.70	Volleyball	1.32
Jogging	4.15	Walking (normal pace)	2.16
Judo	5.34	Weight training	1.90
Knitting (sewing)	0.60	Wrestling	5.10
Lacrosse	5.70	Writing (sitting)	0.78

Figure 6-3 shows how Americans measure their progress at losing weight.

Dietary Alterations

A diet that reduces caloric intake is the most common approach to what seems to be a national obsession with weight loss. The choice of foods included in the diet and the amount of food that can be consumed are the two factors that distinguish the wide range of diets currently available. Unfortunately, dieting alone usually does not result in long-term weight loss. Effective and lasting weight loss requires a lifestyle change, not just going on a diet for a specific time period only to return to your old patterns of eating. This is the problem many people face when they go on strict diets and overly restrict their calories. Because the diet is so restrictive and demanding, they are unable to continue to follow it for very long and return to their previous eating patterns. In addition, people tend to overeat the foods they denied themselves while dieting, because they feel deprived and the forbidden food seems even more alluring. This can also lead to binge eating. Thus diets tend not to work in the long run. The Changing for the Better box on page 197 provides suggestions for changing your eating patterns to increase your chances for long-term success.

Balanced Diets Supported by Portion Control

For nutritional health, a logical approach to weight loss and subsequent management of that loss is to establish a nutritionally sound balanced diet (see Chapter 5) that

Dropping a
clothing size

Don't know, 1.1%

Other,
2.8%

48.8%

34.1%

Feeling
more
energetic

Being able to
avoid fattening
foods, 6.5%

Getting
compliments,
9.7%

Figure 6-3 How do Americans measure success when it comes to losing weight? Most say dropping a clothing size is the best indicator that their diet is working.

controls portions. This approach is best undertaken with nutritionists and physicians who are knowledgeable in diet management. After a study of your day-to-day energy needs, they can establish a diet designed to produce a gradual loss. Food scales or food models can assist in gaining an understanding of portion sizes.

The new food pyramid outlines the breakdown of daily caloric intake for each food group. You can get a personalized dietary guideline by inputting your gender, age, and activity level at www.mypyramid.gov. One study showed that people cut 256 calories a day just by trimming their portion sizes by 25 percent.

Maintaining a balanced diet and watching your portion sizes is especially important on the weekends. Many people throw their good eating habits out the window on the weekends, as evidenced by a recent study that found that Americans eat an average of 115 extra calories per day from Friday to Sunday as compared to the rest of the week. Most of these calories came from alcohol and increased fat consumption. These extra calories can result in a gain of 5 pounds over the course of a year.

TALKING POINTS Have you ever tried to lose weight? What methods were effective for you? What is the longest time you have stuck to a particular weight management strategy?

A balanced diet-portion control approach to weight loss reflects a nutritionally sound program that offers some probability of success without the negative feature of forcing people to adapt to a restrictive approach to eating. People have extreme difficulty adjusting to a diet that presents them with uncommon foods. To people who need to lose weight, dieting is often bad enough without feeling that they must be deprived of foods that satisfy their emotional needs. Figure 6-4 depicts favorite foods that are the biggest hazards to a healthy diet.

Fad Diets

People use a variety of fad diets in an attempt to achieve rapid weight loss. Currently there are over 150 popular diets, often promoted by celebrities or people who claim to be nutrition experts. With few exceptions, these approaches are both ineffective and potentially dangerous. In addition, some require far greater expense than would be associated with weight loss or management techniques using portion control and regular physical activity. The pros and cons of a variety of popular diet plans are presented in Table 6.6.

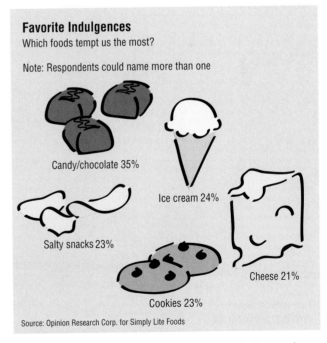

Favorite Indulgences
Which foods tempt us the most?

Note: Respondents could name more than one

Candy/chocolate 35%

Ice cream 24%

Salty snacks 23%

Cheese 21%

Cookies 23%

Source: Opinion Research Corp. for Simply Lite Foods

Figure 6-4 Late-night kitchen raids and too many daytime snacks can compromise a healthy diet. Which foods are the most difficult for you to resist?

Table 6.6 Advantages and Disadvantages of Selected Diets

Type of Diet	Advantages	Disadvantages	Examples
Limited food choice diets	Reduce the number of food choices made by the users Limited opportunity to make mistakes Almost certainly low in calories after the first few days	Deficient in many nutrients, depending on the foods allowed Monotonous—difficult to adhere to Eating out and eating socially are difficult Do not retrain dieters in acceptable eating habits Low long-term success rates No scientific basis for these diets	Good Carbs, Bad Carbs Banana and milk diet Fitonics for Life diet Kempner rice diet The New Beverly Hills Diet Fit for Life Sommersizing
Restricted-calorie, balanced food plans	Sufficiently low in calories to permit steady weight loss Nutritionally balanced Palatable Include readily available foods Reasonable in cost Can be adapted from family meals Permit eating out and social eating Promote a new set of eating habits May employ a point system	Do not appeal to people who want a "unique diet" Do not produce immediate and large weight losses	Eat Right for Your Type Weight Watchers Diet Prudent Diet (American Heart Association) Eating Thin for Life Take Off Pounds Sensibly (TOPS) Overeaters Anonymous Jenny Craig
Fasting starvation diet	Rapid initial loss	Nutrient deficient Danger of ketosis >60% loss is muscle <40% loss is fat Low long-term success rate	ZIP Diet 5-Day Miracle Diet Hollywood Diet
High-carbohydrate diet	Emphasizes grains, fruits, and vegetables High in bulk Low in cholesterol	Limits milk, meat Nutritionally very inadequate for calcium, iron, and protein	Eat More, Weigh Less Quick Weight Loss Diet Pritikin Diet Hilton Head Metabolism Diet
High-protein, low-carbohydrate diets	Rapid initial weight loss because of diuretic effect Very little hunger Usually include all the meat, fish, poultry, and eggs you can eat Occasionally permit milk and cheese in limited amounts Limits fruits, vegetables, and bread or cereal products	Too low in carbohydrates Deficient in many nutrients—vitamin C, vitamin A (unless eggs are included), calcium, and several trace elements High in saturated fat, cholesterol, and total fat Extreme diets of this type could cause death Impossible to adhere to these diets long enough to lose any appreciable amount of weight Dangerous for people with kidney disease Weight lost, which is largely water, is rapidly regained Expensive Unpalatable after first few days Difficult for dieter to eat out Unattractive side effects (e.g., bad breath) May require potassium and calcium supplements	Dr. Phil's Ultimate Weight Solution The New Glucose Revolution The Fat Flush Plan Dr. Stillman's Quick Weight Loss Diet Dr. Atkins' New Diet Revolution The Zone Diet The Carbohydrate Addict's Diet Sugar Busters Protein Power South Beach Diet
Low-calorie, high-protein supplement diets	Usually a premeasured powder to be reconstituted with water or a prepared liquid formula	Usually prescribed at dangerously low calorie intake of 300 to 500 cal Overpriced Low in fiber and bulk—constipating in short amount of time	Metracal Diet Cambridge Diet Liquid Protein Diet Last Chance Diet Oxford Diet

continued

Table 6.6 Advantages and Disadvantages of Selected Diets—*Continued*

Type of Diet	Advantages	Disadvantages	Examples
	Rapid initial weight loss Easy to prepare—already measured Palatable for first few days Usually fortified to provide recommended amount of micronutrients Must be labeled if > 50% protein		Genesis New Direction
High-fiber, low-calorie diets	High satiety value Provide bulk	Irritating to the lower colon Decreases absorption of trace elements, especially iron Nutritionally deficient Low in protein	Pritikin Diet F Diet Zen Macrobiotic Diet
Protein-sparing modified fast < 50% protein: 400 cal	Safe under supervision High-quality protein Minimize loss of lean body mass	Decreases BMR Monotonous Expensive	Optifast Medifast
Premeasured food plans	Provide prescribed portion sizes—little chance of too small or too large a portion Total food programs Some provide adequate calories (1,200) Nutritionally balanced or supplemented	Expensive Do not retrain dieters in acceptable eating habits Preclude eating out or social eating Often low in bulk Monotonous Low long-term success rates	Nutri-System Carnation Plan

Currently, the most popular of the faddish diets are those that reduce carbohydrate intake to an extremely low level while permitting an almost unlimited consumption of animal protein (meat), with its accompanying high fat content. As indicated in Table 6.6, these diets, such as *Dr. Atkins' New Diet Revolution, The South Beach Diet; Good Carbs, Bad Carbs; The Zone;* and *Dr. Phil's Ultimate Weight Solution,* involve potential problems, particularly if followed for long periods. (See the Star Box on page 197.)

The restriction of calories is the basis of all diets. Some suggest limiting the consumption of fat, others sugar, or the caloric intake is dangerously low for all food groups. Many diet plans, such as the South Beach diet and the Atkins' diet, advocate the restriction of carbohydrates, which can cause ketosis. When the carbohydrate calories are limited, intake of fat usually increases. This high-fat diet can cause an increase in blood ketones from fat breakdown and too few carbohydrates. Ketosis can cause the blood to become too acidic, and dehydration can occur. The body requires a minimum of 50–100 grams of carbohydrate per day to avoid ketosis.[46] Low-carbohydrate diets are characterized by initial rapid weight loss, which is appealing to most people, but this loss is primarily due to water and not fat loss.

Complications associated with low-carbohydrate, high-protein diets include dehydration, hypertension, heart disease, cancer, electrolyte loss, calcium depletion, weakness due to inadequate dietary carbohydrates, nausea due to ketosis, vitamin and mineral deficiencies, and possible kidney problems. Gout (painful inflamation of the joints) and kidney failure are potential side effects. The risk of coronary heart disease may be higher in those who stay on the diet a long time, owing to the increased consumption of foods high in saturated fat and cholesterol.

Low-Calorie Foods and Controlled Serving Sizes

Recently, a variety of familiar foods have been developed in a reduced-calorie form. By lowering the carbohydrate content with the use of nonnutritive sweeteners, reducing the portion size, reducing the fat content of the original formulations, or removing fat entirely (see the discussion of Olestra in Chapter 5), manufacturers have produced "lite" versions of many food products. For example, many frozen entrees, such as Healthy Choice Oriental Beef with Vegetables (290 calories), Weight Watchers Lasagna Florentine (210 calories), and Healthy Choice Fettucine with

The Growing Problem of Obesity

Children are 9 pounds heavier today, and teens are 12–16 pounds heavier than they were in the early 1960s. This can lead to greater chances of developing type 2 diabetes, high cholesterol, and a host of other health problems. The trend doesn't stop with the adolescent years. Obesity doubles from the teen years to the mid-20s. Though college students fear "the Freshman 15," the rumored tendency for first-year college students to gain 15 pounds, researchers have found that freshmen women gained an average of 4 pounds, and men gained 6 pounds.

One of the reasons American children and adolescents gain weight over the generations is that children expend significantly less energy on a daily basis than their parents or grandparents did at their age. Today's youth spend endless hours engaged in sedentary play—watching television and playing computer and handheld electronic games. Schools have not helped the situation by cutting back on physical education classes and recess.

In our fast-paced society, we are eating more and more fast food and vending machine food than we have in the past. Again, schools have come under attack for providing high-sugar and high-fat foods, as well as sodas, in the cafeterias and vending machines. College students frequently complain about the food at the college dining hall being loaded with fat and sugar; however, it is often the midnight delivery of pizza or study breaks to the vending machines that lead to weight gain. College students also say that they have trouble finding time to exercise regularly and rely on walking to and from classes and on physical education classes to provide their exercise. Unfortunately

this does not typically add up to at least 30 minutes of daily physical activity as suggested by the new USDA dietary guidelines.

Americans are working more hours than they have in the past, usually well beyond the 40-hour work week, leaving little to no time for daily exercise. Many adults perceive themselves as working hard at their jobs and have no energy reserves left for exercise when they come home. They also mistakenly believe that they have already expended enough energy on the job to count toward fulfilling the daily requirement for physical activity. For some, this is an accurate assumption, but the vast majority of Americans' jobs are sedentary and don't involve manual labor or have great physical demands.

So, what can we do to curb the growing trend toward obesity? One of the most important steps to take is to get parents to role-model healthy eating to their children and to reward behavior with activities, not food. When a child's parents maintain a healthy weight, this increases the likelihood that the child will do the same. Other factors that seem important are to

1. *Go outside and play!* Parents need to encourage their children to play outside. Play with them! Go for a bike ride, play ball, take a walk.

2. *Limit screen time.* Decrease television, computer, and electronic game time to one to two hours a day maximum. Don't hit the couch or the computer as soon as you get home, because it is likely you will spend the evening there. Plan to do something active when you first get home from work or school.

3. *Avoid vending machines and fast food restaurants.* Pack nutritious snacks such as apples, carrots, nuts, and yogurt.

4. *Downsize your dishes.* Studies have repeatedly shown that we eat more when we are offered more food. Use narrower glasses, and smaller bowls and plates.

5. *Quit the clean plate club!* Researchers have also shown that we tend not to feel more full even if we eat more. In one study, a bowl automatically refilled itself with soup, unbeknownst to the subjects, and they ate almost double the amount as the group with normal bowls, and yet they didn't report feeling more full.

6. *Eat weighty food.* We tend to eat the same amount or weight in food each day. Eating food that is high in fiber and water, such as fruits and vegetables, helps us to consume fewer calories. Nutrient-dense food fills you up faster, so you eat fewer calories but get more nutrition compared to eating foods that are less nutrient dense.

7. *Water yourself.* Drink water instead of juice and sodas.

If we look at the lifestyles Americans led 40 years ago, we can see why they didn't struggle with overweight and obesity in the way we do today. Perhaps a lesson to learn from the past is to not take advantage of every convenient way to accomplish our daily living but to make choices based on a healthy lifestyle.

Turkey and Vegetables (350 calories), are low in calories. Because fat helps us to feel satiated or not hungry, these low-fat, low-calorie meals tend not to satisfy our hunger for very long, and we may find ourselves wanting to snack or binge by late afternoon.

TALKING POINTS Your best friend is trying to follow a low-fat, low-calorie diet in order to lose weight but is finding herself constantly hungry. What can you tell her about the diet plan she's chosen? What changes might she make to increase her chances of success?

Controlled Fasting

In cases of extreme obesity, some patients are placed on a complete fast in a hospital setting. The patient consumes only water, electrolytes, and vitamins. Weight loss is substantial because the body is forced to begin **catabolizing**

> **Key Terms**
>
> **catabolizing** the metabolic process of breaking down tissue for the purpose of converting it to energy

its fat and muscle tissue. Complete fasting is such an extreme approach to weight loss that it must be done in an institutional setting so that the patient can be closely monitored. Inadequate protein and sodium and potassium loss are particular health concerns.

Today some people regularly practice short periods of modified fasting. Solid foods are removed from the diet for a number of days. Fruit juices, water, supplements, and vitamins are used to minimize the risks associated with total fasting. However, unsupervised short-term fasting can be dangerous and is not recommended.

In addition to the controlled fasting just discussed, a somewhat different version of this practice is appearing with the long-term use of readily available, low-calorie, nutrient-dense food supplementation products

such as Ensure, Boost, SlimFast, and Sustical. Regardless of whether they are marketed as nutrient-dense supplements for older adults or as adjuncts to weight loss diets, these drinks should not be viewed, or used, as meal replacements. Because these products contain no more than 400 calories (and the lite versions contain as few as 200 calories), their routine use as meal replacements could move even a young, healthy adult dangerously close to caloric inadequacy in a short time. Perhaps if used in place of a high-calorie snack or as a very occasional substitute for breakfast, these supplements may not present the dangers that their routine use does.

Weight Reduction Programs

In virtually every area of the country, at least one version of the popular weight reduction programs, such as TOPS (Take Off Pounds Sensibly), Jenny Craig, and Nutri-System Weight Loss Centers, can be found. Pioneered by Weight Watchers, these programs generally feature a format consisting of (1) a well-balanced diet emphasizing portion control and low-fat, low-saturated fat, and high-complex carbohydrate foods, (2) specific weight loss goals to be attained over a set period of time, (3) encouragement from supportive leaders and fellow group members, (4) emphasis on regular physical activity, and (5) a maintenance program (follow-up program). The Changing for the Better box on page 198 presents some guidelines for choosing a weight loss program.

Although in theory these programs offer an opportunity to lose weight for people who cannot or will not participate in a physical activity program, their effectiveness is very limited. The minimal success of these programs and the difficulty that working adults have in attending meetings has resulted in falling enrollment and the development of home-based programs, such as those developed by hospital-based wellness programs, many YMCAs and YWCAs, and even Weight Watchers. Further, these programs can be costly when compared with self-directed approaches, especially when the program markets its own food products.

The Weight Loss Industry

In response to our nation's near obsession with thinness, a thriving weight loss industry exists to assist us in our attempts to lose weight. Americans are spending in excess of $50 billion each year in an attempt to achieve and maintain weight loss (see Table 6.7).

The weight loss industry has capitalized and profited on the meaning that thinness has in the American culture, including a bias against large people. These programs are promising not just weight loss but happiness and success in life as well. Thinness is associated

Table 6.7 The Real Cost of Dieting

Plan	Annual Cost
Weight Watchers	$709
Over-the-counter diet pills	$500
Nutritional counseling	$450–$1200
Physician-supervised weight loss program	$2,000–$3,5000
Prescription diet pills	$1,090–$1,343
Gastric bypass surgery	$20,000–$25,000

Source: Chatzky JS. The real costs of diets, *USA Weekend*, December 2002.

not only with beauty but also with one's ability to have successful relationships, careers, and self-worth. A study was conducted asking 32,000 women what they would choose: a successful career, a satisfying romantic relationship, or a loss of 10–15 pounds. The majority of these women chose to lose weight, believing that they would also have a successful career and relationship if they lost 10–15 pounds.[7] Another study showed that the

winner of the Miss America Pageant, five years consecutively, was always the thinnest contestant, looking at height proportional to weight. Another study showed children pictures of a minority child, a disabled child, and an overweight child and asked them to choose who they would like to be their friend. Overwhelmingly, the overweight child was their last choice. The American Association of University Women conducted a study to examine the changing attitudes children and adolescents have of themselves in terms of their body image. While 60 percent of elementary school girls said "I am always happy with the way I am," only 29 percent of high school girls said the same thing. For boys, 67 percent of elementary school boys liked how they looked, and 46 percent of high school boys continued to feel this way. It is these attitudes that play into the measures to which individuals will go and the price they will pay to achieve the cultural ideal.

The financial success of the weight loss industry in this country has in part been because of its effective television advertising. Skillfully produced commercials featuring successful program members suggest likely success for the viewer willing to sign on. Before 1994, these commercials were regular fare on daytime television. Today, however, commercials for diet programs such as Jenny Craig, Nutri-System, Weight Watchers, and others are considerably more restrained in their messages about success. Under directives issued by the Federal Trade Commission (FTC), today's advertisements cannot misrepresent program performance. They must disclose that most weight loss is temporary, and they now inform the viewer that their loss will most likely not approximate that of the successful subjects featured in their commercials.

Most recently some nationally franchised weight loss programs have added a "medical" component to their format that involves prescribing medications. Consumers should find out if medical supervision will be a regular component of the program or a brief, one-time physician visit involving little more than basic screening.

Physical Intervention

A second approach to weight loss involves techniques and products designed to change basic eating patterns.

Hunger- and Satiety-Influencing Products

Many overweight people want to lessen their desire to eat or develop a stronger sense of when they have eaten enough. Today, many dieters are confused about the safety of pharmaceutical approaches to weight loss, including both over-the-counter (OTC) and prescription drugs.

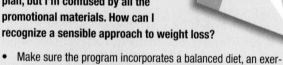

Changing for the Better

Choosing a Diet Plan

I've been trying to find a good diet plan, but I'm confused by all the promotional materials. How can I recognize a sensible approach to weight loss?

- Make sure the program incorporates a balanced diet, an exercise program, and behavior modification.
- Beware of inflexible plans, such as those that require you to eat certain foods on certain days.
- Avoid plans that allow fewer than 1,200 calories a day, which is the minimum needed to get essential nutrients.
- Make sure the recommended rate of weight loss does not exceed 2 pounds per week.
- Avoid programs that promote vitamins, pills, shots, gimmicks, gadgets, or brand-name diet foods.
- Look for a statement of approval by a reputable nutrition expert or institution.
- Beware of diets that promise fast, easy, or effortless weight loss or "a new secret formula."
- Choose a plan that teaches you how to keep the weight off once you've lost it.

InfoLinks

www.shapeup.org

Learning from Our Diversity

You are in London, England, and decide to buy some of the latest English fashions. You find a pair of pants you like and try them on. They don't fit. In fact nothing in your size fits. Why not? Because not all sizes are the same for women.

As you can see from Table 6.8, if you wear a size 12 in American stores, you will need to find a size 14 in the British stores or an 11 in Japanese stores or a 40 in the Parisian boutiques.[1] Is this true for men's clothing? No, you will find that a waist size of 38 is the same in American, British, and Japanese clothing. Why is this? Well, it is the same reason that you will find that not all women's size-12 clothing is the same even in the same country! What you will find is that the more expensive the clothing, the smaller the size compared to its true size. In other words, you can compare a pair of jeans from a discount store to the identical pair of pants in an expensive department store and find that the expensive pants are labeled one to two sizes smaller than the pants in the discount store. You will also discover that the smaller-size pants have a much larger-size price tag. Again, does this hold true for men's clothing? No, it doesn't. The reason is that women will pay more for a smaller size, a lot more, while most men will not. There is not a market for smaller-size clothing for men the way there is for women.

Women feel much more pressure to comform to the popular size. The popular size can vary from generation to generation and between different cultures. Whereas a size 6 was the desired size for women in the 1980s, size 4 in the early 1990s, and size 2 in the late 1990s, now size 0 is the size to be for American women. When size 4 was popular in the United States, size 6 was the British size to strive for, whereas in Japan it was size 3. This situation reflects the changing cultural ideal for female beauty, which can lead to unhealthy eating, dangerous dieting, and the development of eating disorders in order to fit into the current fad size. Women are increasingly succumbing to this pressure and going to greater lengths to achieve perfection. This includes undergoing plastic surgery because they can't achieve the perfect body naturally and so turn to unnatural methods to try to meet the perception of perfection.

Men, however, are not immune to the trend of rising obesity around the world. In Cyprus, the Czech Republic, Finland, Germany, Greece, Malta, and Slovakia, more men are overweight or obese than American men are. Although the Mediterranean diet has been touted as a healthy diet, obesity is also higher in the Mediterranean countries.[2]

Eating disorders and distorted eating are more prevalent in cultures adopting Westernized values. One startling example of how quickly and significantly Western ideals of beauty can influence others was seen when television first came to the island of Fiji in 1995. Before the introduction of television, a common compliment given to someone was "you've gained weight," and dieting was almost nonexistent. Telling someone that he or she looked thin was a way of saying that the person didn't look well. Within three years of having television, the number of teenagers at risk for eating disorders more than doubled; 74 percent of teens said they felt too big or too fat, and 62 percent reported that they had been dieting in the past month.[3]

In the United States and other Westernized societies, the cultural ideal for beauty is becoming thinner and thinner. A generation ago, a model weighed 8 percent less than the average woman did, but she now weighs 23 percent less. With the ideal dress size for women now at a size 0, there is a message for women to aspire to nothingness. What can be done about this alarming trend? Women can refuse to buy more expensive clothing just because they are labeled with smaller sizes, as men have done for years. We can glorify all sizes and shapes of women. As Angel, a 17-year-old high school basketball player from West Los Angeles stated, "I'm 5'8" and 165 pounds. I'm not a size 4. I'm tall. I'm muscular. I'm a thick girl. I accept that."[4]

Table 6.8 Size Comparisons

Women's Clothing

UK	6	8	10	12	14	16	18	20	22
USA	4	6	8	10	12	14	16	18	20
Russia	40	42	44	46	48	50	52	54	56
Spain/France	34	36	38	40	42	44	46	48	50
Italy	38	40	42	44	46	48	50	52	54
Germany	32	34	36	38	40	42	44	46	48
Japan	3	5	7	9	11	13	15	17	19
Dominican Republic	10	12	14	16	18	20	22	24	26

Men's Clothing

Suits, Sweaters, Jackets, and Pants

UK	34	36	38	40	42	44	46	48
USA	34	36	38	40	42	44	46	48
Europe	44	46	48	50	52	54	56	58
Japan	S	–	M	–	–	L	–	–

Shirt Collars

UK	14	14½	15	15½	16	16½	17	17½
USA	14	14½	15	15½	16	16½	17	17½
Europe	36	37	38	39	40	41	42	43
Japan	36	37	38	39	40	41	42	43

Source: www.hostelscentral.com/hostels-article-34.html.

[1] "International Clothes Sizes Compared," www.hostelscentral.com.

[2] "Some European Countries More Obese Than in U.S.," *USA Today,* March 28, 2005.

[3] Kilbourne, J. *Can't Buy My Love.* New York: Simon & Schuster Inc., 1999.

[4] "The New Girls," *Oprah Magazine,* May 2004.

Ma Huang: A Deadly Way to Lose Weight

Advertised as a "natural" herbal version of "phenfen," ma huang is a powerful, amphetaminelike drug that has been used for years for weight loss until recently. In late 2003, the FDA placed a ban on any products containing ephedra, such as ma huang. This is the first time U.S. officials have blocked the sale of an over-the-counter nutritional supplement, as dietary supplements don't have to be proven safe before going on the market. In fact, it is difficult to stop the sale of dietary supplements that appear dangerous because there must be enough proof to substantiate the health risks.

About 1% of dietary supplements contain ephedra, and yet 64% of reports about adverse effects from supplements have been related to ephedra. More focus was put on the dangers of ephedra after the well-publicized deaths of Baltimore Orioles pitcher Steve Bechler and semiprofessional football player Christopher Mills, both of whose deaths have been linked to ephedra use. Ephedra has been associated with at least 155 deaths and dozens of heart attacks and strokes, and it can cause high blood pressure, seizures, heart irregularities, insomnia, anxiety, and tremors.

The FDA issued a statement to the 62 companies that made or sold ephedra to "stop selling these products" owing to their health risk. Before the FDA ruling, New York, Illinois, and California passed their own bans at a state level owing to the complaints and allegations of the health risks.

So, what will replace ephedra in the herbal supplement industry, and will this replacement be a healthier option? Although there had been longstanding concerns about the safety of ephedra, it took years to gather enough evidence and the deaths of innocent people before ephedra was removed from the market. Thus it is recommended that you take extreme caution when using any type of herbal supplement, since these supplements do not have to prove that they are safe in order to be sold over the counter.

Sources: "Ephedra Ban Puts Herb Industry on Notice," *New York Times*, December 31, 2003.
"Government Announces Ban on Ephedra," CNN, December 31, 2003.
U.S. Health Chief: Evidence Strong for Ephedra Ban, December 30, 2003.

Some OTC appetite suppressants containing **phenylpropanolamine (PPA)** may still be sold in drugstores and supermarkets. PPA can also be found in OTC and prescription cough and cold medications. The FDA recommends that consumers not use any products with PPA because of its association with higher risk for stroke.

The FDA also continues to advise against using OTC weight loss products containing the recently banned ephedrine (*ma huang* and Chinese ephedra) (see Considering Complementary Care above).

In 1994 Congress passed the Dietary Supplement and Education Act (DSHEA), which regulated herbal agents to the category of "dietary supplements." Thus the FDA can't regulate these products to ensure that they meet certain standards or are safe and effective. Many people see these supplements as safe because they are "natural," and yet they can be more dangerous and deadly than prescription medications because they are not inspected as to the purity and accuracy of the contents or the potency of the ingredients. Recently, more than $5 billion was spent on herbal supplements with one of every three Americans reporting using them.

Ephedrine, found in most herbal diet pills, has been linked to heart attacks, strokes, hepatitis, headache, tremors, anxiety, extreme irritability, and insomnia in consumers of all ages. Metabolife, an herbal diet supplement that contains ephedra, has sold more than 50 million bottles over the past few years, about 225,000 pills an hour. In 2003 the death of 23-year-old Baltimore Orioles pitcher Steve Bechler was linked to an ephedra supplement, prompting the FDA to reexamine the supplement. Ephedra was banned by the FDA in late 2003.[47]

Another herb, Aristolochia fangchi, was used as a weight loss supplement until many people developed kidney damage or complete renal failure, as well as precancerous and cancerous lesions in the kidneys. There is also a danger in the potential interactions between prescription medications and herbal agents that people can be unaware of and physicians may overlook because 70 percent of patients do not disclose the use of herbal medicines to their physicians. Research shows that the

Key Terms

phenylpropanolamine (PPA) (fen ill pro pan **ol** ah meen) the active chemical compound still found in some over-the-counter diet products average person taking a combination of ephedra and caffeine lost 8.8 pounds over 6 months compared to 1.8 pounds among those who took a placebo pill. This translates into one-third of a pound a week that the ephedra subjects lost over the control group, roughly the same a person might lose cutting out 146 calories a day.[48]

Some prescription medications have also been shown to produce serious side effects. Two such medications, *phentermine* and *fenfluramine,* have been prescribed for patients who wanted to lose weight. Both drugs affect levels of serotonin, the neurotransmitter associated with satiety. This popular combination, referred to as *phenfen,* gradually raised concern among health experts because of the side effects it produced in people with angina, glaucoma, and high blood pressure. In addition, reports began to surface that some patients had developed a rare but lethal condition called *pulmonary hypertension.*

During the mid-1990s, a new serotonin-specific weight loss drug, *dexfenfluramine* (Redux), was approved for use in the United States. Results among patients who used the drug, in combination with dietary modification and exercise, seemed impressive during the initial months of its widespread use. However, some patients began to take dexfenfluramine with fenfluramine in an attempt to find a new combination that would be even more effective than phenfen or Redux used alone, and death resulted in some cases.

Thus, two combinations of three serotonin-specific drugs were in vogue in early 1997. However, by May of 1997, there were reports of weight loss patients with newly diagnosed heart valve damage who had been using these drug combinations. In some cases, damage was correctable only by valve-replacement surgery. Accordingly, in September 1997, the FDA requested voluntary withdrawal of fenfluramine and dexfenfluramine from the market.[49] Manufacturers responded by ceasing all distribution of the drugs. In October 1999, a $4.8 billion class-action settlement was proposed, through which patients whose use of the drugs resulted in heart valve damage would receive monetary compensation and continuing medical care. Phentermine remains on the market and is used in combination with various antidepressants, such as Prozac, Zoloft, and Paxil. For those people whose use of the diet drug combinations led to heart valve damage, a study reported at the end of 1999 indicated that once medication use ceased, damage did not progress, and some indication of improvement was noted.[50]

At the same time of the initial concern over the use of phentermine and fenfluramine, the FDA approved yet another obesity drug, *sibutramine* (brand name Meridia), even though an advisory committee within the FDA recommended against approving it. Meridia acts on serotonin in the body similarly to how phenfen and Redux functioned and, like its predecessors, has been linked to heart attacks, high blood pressure, strokes, and death; however, it still remains on the market in the United States. Italy recently pulled Meridia from the market following reports of death linked to this drug.

Nonhunger/Nonsatiety-Influencing Drugs

Currently a third approved medication, *orlistat* (brand name Xenical), is available for use in treating obesity. Unlike phentermine and sibutramine, which influence the neurotransmitter serotonin, orlistate reduces fat absorption in the small intestine by about 30 percent. The drug is intended for use among people who are 20 percent or more over their ideal weight. In persons who tolerate the drug's side effects, a 10 percent reduction of weight without significant dietary restriction is possible.

Some concerns related to the use of orlistat include anal leakage, severe abdominal cramping, excessive flatulence, and inhibition of the absorption of vitamins and minerals in the body. Olestra has been used in fat-free chips such as "Wow!" potato chips and there have been complaints of stomach discomfort among people who ate them. In addition, people erroneously believe that they can eat as much as they want since it is fat free, but it is not calorie free and so they may end up gaining weight as a result.

Surgical Interventions

It used to be that surgical measures were undertaken only if the person's weight was severely endangering his or her health and other less invasive methods had been unsuccessful. Now surgeries such as liposuction, tummy tucks, gastric bypass surgery, and gastric band surgeries are becoming increasingly popular and commonplace, especially among teenagers. Insurance companies are approving these expensive surgeries because the cost of obesity and its related medical problems are even more costly. Gastric bypass surgery, vertical banded gastroplasty, and laparoscopic adjustable gastric banding all involve major surgery. All three operations limit the amount of food a person can eat at one time, because overeating results in vomiting or severe diarrhea. Because the stomach is made smaller, individuals who have undergone these procedures must limit their food intake to half a cup to a cup of food at each "meal." However, it is possible to regain weight by eating small portions of high-calorie foods on a consistent basis. Individuals lose weight because this type

Three types of obesity surgery

The success depends on how good a candidate the patient is, how skilled the surgeon is, and how much support follows the operation. Risks range from death, to a hernia or ulcer, to surgical failures such as internal leaks. Although the surgery limits the amount of food the patient can eat in one sitting, it's possible to gain the weight back by eating small but continuous portions of high-calorie junk food. the following techniques are becoming increasingly popular for treating severely obese patients:

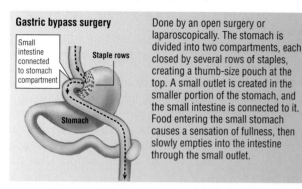

Gastric bypass surgery

Done by an open surgery or laparoscopically. The stomach is divided into two compartments, each closed by several rows of staples, creating a thumb-size pouch at the top. A small outlet is created in the smaller portion of the stomach, and the small intestine is connected to it. Food entering the small stomach causes a sensation of fullness, then slowly empties into the intestine through the small outlet.

Vertical banded gastroplasty

Four rows of staples are placed vertically in the upper part of the stomach. The outlet at the lower end of the pouch created by these staples is restricted by a ring that limits the passage of food into the rest of the stomach. The person feels full after a few bites of food.

Laparoscopic adjustable gastric banding

An inflatable band is placed around the outside of the upper stomach to create a small pouch with a narrow outlet to the rest of the digestive tract.

Sources: USA TODAY research; the American Society for Bariatric Surgery, May 5, 2004

Figure 6-5 Three types of obesity surgery

of surgery limits the amount of food that can be digested, therefore decreasing the amount of calories that they can eat at one time.

Gastric Bypass Surgery

This is the most common type of weight loss surgery, and it has gained interest since celebrities such as singer Carnie Wilson, American Idol judge Randy Jackson, and weatherman Al Roker have gone public about their experiences with this surgery. It is a major operation and involves dividing the stomach into two compartments to create a pouch, the size of a thumb, for food to enter. The small intestine is cut below the stomach and connected to a smaller portion of the stomach, bypassing the larger stomach and a section of the intestine, which are no longer used (see Figure 6-5). In 2003, 103,200 gastric bypass surgeries (also referred to as *bariatric surgery*) were performed, compared to 16,800 in 1993. The average cost per surgery is $25,000, and the average death rate is 1 in 200. Candidates for this surgery typically have a BMI above 40 or are 100 pounds or more (men) or at least 80 pounds (women) overweight. People with a BMI between 35 and 40 who suffer from type 2 diabetes or life-threatening cardiopulmonary problems may also be candidates for surgery.

Gastric bypass surgery tends to result in greater weight loss (93.3 pounds on average) than does gastroplasty (67 pounds on average) after one year. Over two years, gastric bypass surgery patients have been shown to lose two-thirds of excess weight. These surgeries are not without their risks: hernias, ulcers, liver damage, infection, internal leaks, and even death. These surgeries are not a cure-all for weight management; individuals who have these operations must continue to exercise regularly, take nutritional supplements, eat small portions very slowly, and decrease intake of high-sugar foods in order to maintain their weight loss.

Gastric Band Surgery

There are two types of gastric band surgery: vertical banded gastroplasty and laparoscopic adjustable gastric banding. Vertical banded gastroplasty uses both a band and staples to create a small stomach pouch, limiting the passage of food into the rest of the stomach. This results in a feeling of fullness after only a few mouthfuls of food. This used to be the most common weight loss surgery, but it has decreased in popularity with the rise of gastric bypass surgery. Laparoscopic adjustable gastric banding, a less invasive procedure, involves an inflatable band being placed around the upper end of the stomach, again creating a small pouch. A narrow passage is also made into the rest of the stomach. The band is inflated with a salt solution through a tube that connects the band to an access port positioned under the skin. In this way, the band can be tightened or loosened over time to change the size of the passageway into the stomach.

Liposuction and Abdominoplasty

Liposuction is the most frequent cosmetic operation in the United States in which fat tissue is removed. Liposuction involves removing unwanted fat from specific areas, such as the abdomen, hips, buttocks, thighs, knees, upper arms, chin, cheeks, and neck. A small tube is inserted through the skin, and adipose tissue is vacuumed out. This is more of a sculpting or contouring operation than a weight loss surgery, because little weight is lost. Potential risks and outcomes include infection; the formation of fat clots or blood clots, which may travel to the lungs and cause death; excessive fluid loss, which can lead to shock or fluid accumulation that must be drained; friction burns or other damage to the skin or nerves; numbness; skin discoloration; irregular body contours; and sagging skin.

Abdominoplasty, known more commonly as a tummy tuck, is a major surgical procedure to remove excess skin and fat from the middle and lower abdomen and to tighten the muscles of the abdominal wall. It leaves a permanent scar, which can extend from hip to hip. Infection and blood clots are some of the potential risks. A balanced diet and regular exercise are required to maintain the results from this surgery.

People considering these procedures should carefully investigate all aspects, including the training and experience of the surgeon, to determine whether they are appropriate for them.

There exists a growing concern regarding the safety of liposuction based on a comparison of surgery-related deaths during liposuction and the death rates for all surgery, including trauma-based cases. In the case of all types of surgery, the mortality rate is reported to be between 1 death for every 100,000 cases and 1 death for every 300,000 surgical cases, whereas for liposuction the rate may be 20 to 60 times higher (1 death per 5,000 cases between 1995 and 1998).[51] In spite of these figures, the Society of Plastic and Reconstructive Surgeons believes the procedure is still acceptably safe, explaining that an office-based procedure often carries a higher mortality rate than do procedures conducted in hospitals.

Body Wrapping

Although not a surgical procedure or weight loss technique, *body wrapping* is another form of body contouring. In this procedure, various areas of the body are tightly wrapped with 6-inch strips of material soaked in a solution of amino acids that are claimed to draw toxins out of the underlying tissue, shrink fatty deposits, diminish **cellulite,** lighten stretch marks, and eliminate inches of fat. Once the wrapping is removed, the newly contoured body area may remain this way for 4 to 10 weeks. Although the secret to the success of a particular spa's body wrapping approach is supposed to lie in its uniquely formulated soaking solution, the contouring effect probably results from dehydration of the underlying tissue and

redistribution of extracellular fluids through pressure from the wrapping.

Regarding cellulite, note that no product or noninvasive procedure currently in the marketplace has been shown to be effective in removing or reducing this tissue. Thus, the dimpled appearance of the buttocks, back of the arm, and upper leg seems destined to remain, despite cosmetic companies' advertisements of lotions and creams that claim to eliminate cellulite.

Underweight

For some young adults, the lack of adequate body weight, called **underweight,** can be a serious concern, particularly for those who have inherited a tendency toward thinness (see Changing for the Better on page 204). Males tend to be particularly concerned with too thin a body type, preferring a lean, muscular V-shape appearance.

Nutritionists believe that the healthiest way to gain weight is to increase the intake of "calorie-dense" food. These foods are characterized by high fat density resulting from high levels of vegetable fats (polyunsaturated fats). Particularly good foods in this regard are dried fruits, bananas, nuts, granola, and cheeses made from low-fat milk. The current recommendation is to eat three calorie-dense meals of moderate size per day, interspersed with two or three substantial snacks. Using the Food Guide Pyramid shown on page 143, one should eat the higher number of recommended amounts for each group.[52]

A second component of weight gain for those who are underweight is an exercise program that uses weight training activities intended to increase muscle mass. For all the reasons detailed in Chapter 4, the use of anabolic drugs in the absence of highly competent medical supervision has no role in healthful weight gain. In addition, carefully monitored aerobic activity should be undertaken in sessions adequate to maintain heart-lung health, while at the same time one should restrict unnecessary activity that expends calories.

For those who cannot gain weight in spite of having tried the preceding approaches, a medical evaluation

> ### Key Terms
>
> **cellulite** tissue comprised of fat cells intertwined around strands of fibrous connective tissue
>
> **underweight** a condition in which the body is below the desirable weight

could supply an explanation for being underweight. If no medical explanation can be found, the person must begin to accept the reality of his or her unique body type.

Behavior Change Strategies

Several approaches designed to change learned eating patterns, such as *behavior modification,* aversive conditioning, and hypnosis, have been used by people who want to lose weight. Because of the relatively small number of people involved in many of these approaches and the limited extent to which they have been scientifically studied, it is difficult to assess their long-term effectiveness. Nevertheless, they remain as alternatives to the approaches already described.

Lifetime Weight Control

Obesity and frequent fluctuation in weight are clearly associated with higher levels of morbidity and mortality. Therefore, maintenance of weight and body composition at or near optimum levels is highly desirable. Although you may believe that this is a difficult goal to achieve, it is not unrealistic when practiced on a consistent basis. You will need to draw on resources from each dimension of your health to maintain a lifestyle that fosters the maintenance of optimum weight and body composition. Keys to your success will include:

- **Exercise** Caloric expenditure through regular exercise, including cardiovascular exercise and strength training, is a key to maintaining a healthy weight and body composition. The weight loss resulting from dieting alone, in comparison to dieting in combination with exercise, tends to be less effective and temporary at best.

- **Dietary modification** Plan your meals around foods low in total fat and saturated fat and high in complex carbohydrates. Choose fresh fruits, vegetables, pastas, and, occasionally, lean meat such as skinless chicken and baked fish (see the discussion of semivegetarianism in Chapter 5).

- **Lifestyle support** Not only do you need to be committed to a lifestyle of regular physical activity and healthy food choices, but you also need to build a support group that will encourage you in these endeavors. Inform family, friends, classmates, and coworkers about your intent to rely on them for support and encouragement. Perhaps you will eventually serve as a role model for their involvement in a similar process.

- **Problem solving** Reevaluate your current approach to dealing with stressors. Replace any reliance on food as a coping mechanism with nonfood options, such as exercise or talking with friends or family members. Additionally, your personal reward system may need to be reviewed to decrease the use of food as a reward for a job well done.

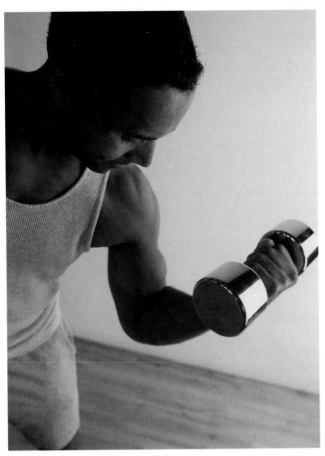

The most important component of weight management is regular exercise.

- **Redefinition of health** Set your personal goals for your health and wellness in a manner that reinforces the importance of prevention and self-care (see Chapter 2) rather than waiting to become sick or incapacitated before attending to your diet and exercise.

The lifestyle choices just suggested will make a significant contribution to lessening the chances of developing a weight problem or weight-related health problems during your remaining adult years. Aging will exert its effects to some degree on weight and body composition, but you will avoid the damaging influences that poor dietary practices and a sedentary lifestyle present.

Physical Activity

The emphasis placed on physical activity in the model just described reflects our support of the many experts who now believe that the most important component of a weight-loss program is regular physical activity. Physical activity contributes to weight loss and the maintenance of weight loss because activity burns calories. Remember, the need for calories decreases with age and with decreased activity.

An additional benefit derived from physical activity is that proportionately more fat is lost than is lost through dieting alone. Studies suggest that the weight loss achieved through physical activity is 95 percent fat and 5 percent lean tissue, such as muscle, in comparison with a loss of 75 percent fat and 25 percent lean tissue when dieting alone is used. Exercise also offers the benefits of increased heart and lung endurance, muscular strength, and flexibility.

How much exercise is enough? The new USDA dietary guidelines (see Chapter 5) advise American adults to engage in at least 30 minutes of moderately intense aerobic exercise almost every day for weight maintenance and 60–90 minutes of this type of exercise for weight loss. Weight training has become a more important factor in weight management. As with most things, too much or too little exercise is not beneficial. As will be discussed in the next chapter, some people with eating disorders tend to overexercise which results in diminishing returns.

The importance of regular physical activity along with sound nutrition in the prevention of obesity is especially important for children. Today Americans are in the throes of an "epidemic" of diabetes type 2 (glucose intolerance) that begins in childhood, in comparison to the disease's traditional onset during adulthood.[53] When this form of diabetes develops and then cannot be adequately managed, the risks of heart attack, stroke, blindness, kidney failure, and inadequate wound healing leading to amputation increase significantly. Parents, educators, and society in general must place a greater emphasis on physical activity for children in order to lessen the likelihood of the obesity that fosters the development of this condition.

Eating Disorders

Perhaps it is not surprising that some people have medically identifiable, potentially serious difficulties with body image, body weight, and food selection. Among these disorders are two that are frequently seen among college students, anorexia nervosa and bulimia nervosa. In addition, binge eating and disordered eating are also found in college populations. We have included these topics in the chapter on weight management because most eating disorders begin with dieting. However, most eating disorders also involve inappropriate food choices, as well as psychological issues. Those issues are discussed in Chapters 2 and 5.

A recent survey showed that dieting has become the norm for females starting at an early age. Fifty percent of

9-year-olds and 80 percent of 10-year-olds have reported dieting.[4] While eating disorders involve a preoccupation with food and weight, much deeper psychological issues underly these conditions.

In the United States, conservative estimates indicate that after puberty 5 to 10 million females and 1 million males struggle with eating disorders such as anorexia, bulimia, or binge eating disorder. It is estimated that approximately 8 percent of college women will develop an eating disorder, and the population most at risk for developing bulimia is college freshmen women. Ninety to 95 percent of people with eating disorders are women, although the prevalence of eating disorders in men is on the rise. Athletes such as dancers, gymnasts, swimmers, runners, and wrestlers are at risk for developing eating disorders because of the focus on weight and appearance for successful performance. In fact, any group in which success in influenced by weight or attractiveness is at risk for the development of an eating disorder, such as those involved in the performance arts, theatre, television, and modeling.

Anorexia Nervosa

Anorexia nervosa is an eating disorder in which a person denies his or her own feelings of hunger and avoids food, with marked weight loss occurring. Anorexics tend to run from food in the relentless pursuit of thinness, although they never perceive themselves as thin enough. To meet the diagnostic criteria for anorexia nervosa, the individual has an intense fear of gaining weight, even though he or she weighs less than 85 percent of the expected weight for his/her age, gender, and height, and, in females, menstruation ceases for at least 3 consecutive months.[54] In addition, people with anorexia perceive themselves as overweight and much larger than they really are. Anorexics lose their ability to recognize when they are hungry and have difficulty eating even if they want to do so. Depression, irritability, withdrawal, perfectionism, and low self-esteem are some of the psychological problems associated with anorexia. In addition, anorexics tend to feel cold most of the time because they have very little body fat (2–10 percent) and also suffer from lightheadedness, dizziness, insomnia, hair loss, muscle cramps, stress fractures, fatigue, decreased memory and concentration, and gastrointestinal problems. More serious complications include heart and kidney failure, hypothermia, osteoporosis, infertility, and, in 25 percent of cases, death.

As with other eating disorders, anorexia nervosa also involves a sense of feeling out of control in one's life and attempting to find control through food and weight loss. It is not a coincidence that anorexia nervosa typically begins around puberty: most individuals with anorexia have a fear of growing up and all that goes with being an adult,

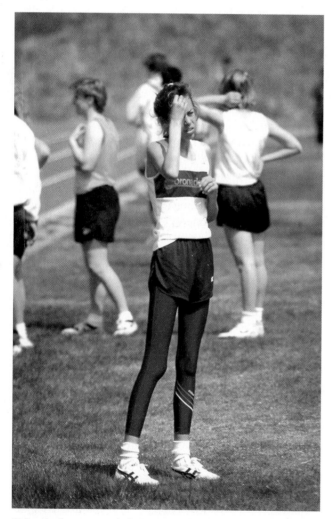

Using food to cope with feeling stressed, out of control, lonely, upset, or bored can lead to the development of an eating disorder.

Key Terms

anorexia nervosa an eating disorder in which the individual weighs less than 85 percent of the expected weight for his or her age, gender, and height, has an intense fear of gaining weight, and, in females, ceases to menstruate for at least 3 consecutive months. People with anorexia perceive themselves as overweight, even though they are underweight.

such as financial responsibility, sexual relationships, leaving one's family, and becoming more autonomous and independent.

Anorexia often begins with dieting but may also begin as a result of an illness such as the stomach flu, a relationship that breaks up, or after dental surgery, when it might be expected that one would temporarily eat less. However, anorexics will tell you that the disorder begins to take on a life of its own after what started as wanting to lose a few pounds turns into losing 15 percent or more of body weight and still not feeling satisfied with one's appearance. Friends and family might initially encourage the person on his or her weight loss and say complimentary things about his or her appearance but soon become concerned when the person's weight continues to dramatically decrease.

Anorexia has become more common as changing cultural ideals for beauty have changed. Our standards have gone from Marilyn Monroe who was a voluptuous 5'5", 128-pound woman to Kate Moss who has been reported to be 5'7" and 105 pounds.[7] Now the "lollipop look" is considered the "in look" in Hollywood, with actresses and models having stick-thin bodies, making their heads seem huge. More attention has been drawn to this disorder since Mary-Kate Olsen went public with her battle with anorexia in the summer of 2004. She is not alone; other stars have admitted to having anorexia—for example, Tracey Gold (*Growing Pains* sitcom), fashion model Carrie Otis, Spice Girl Victoria Beckem, singer Whitney Houston, Courtney Thorne-Smith (from *Alley McBeal*), and actress Christina Ricci. Because many of these stars are seen as the standard for the American body ideal, they may be inadvertently increasing the number of women with eating disorders.

Denial of problems plays a major role in eating disorders in that the individual refuses to acknowledge that there is anything wrong, even though she is becoming thinner and wasting away, and family and friends are expressing great concern. Anorexia nervosa is considered a serious medical and psychological disorder; however, some anorexics argue that "Anorexia is a lifestyle not a disorder." Heated debates and discussions often occur on pro-anorexia Web sites. With names like "Thinspiration," "Stick Figures," and "Anorexic and Proud," these pro-anorexia forums have become very popular and deadly in the past few years. These Web sites show computer-enhanced pictures of models and actresses such as Calista Flockhart and Lara Flynn Boyle, making them appear thinner and more skeletal than they really are.[55] Messages on these Web sites include tips on how to starve, how to purge, and ways of hiding one's disorder, as well as encouragement to lose more weight. There has been a push among health providers, educators, and health organizations to eliminate these types of Web sites, and they have been somewhat successful. However, these sites still do exist, although somewhat disguised and underground.[56]

Three groups that have traditionally been overlooked in the incidence of anorexia are women of color, female athletes (see the Female Athlete Triad in Chapter 4), and men. The research shows a significant increase in the incidence of anorexia among these three groups. More focus has been given to anorexia among women of color, and it has been proposed that this group might be more vulnerable to developing eating disorders than Caucasian women are because of ethnocultural identity issues. It has been suggested that the more pressure women of color feel to fit into the dominant culture's standards of beauty and thinness, the more likely they are to develop eating disorders.

Often female athletes are not diagnosed with eating disorders because the symptoms of anorexia—absence of menses, low body fat and weight, and osteoporosis—are referred to as the female athletic triad and are not uncommon among athletes, and so they don't necessarily signify the presence of an eating disorder.

The incidence of anorexia nervosa (as well as bulimia nervosa, which we'll cover later) has traditionally been much lower in men than in women. Today, however, the incidence of both conditions is increasing in men as they begin to feel some of the same pressures that women feel to conform to the weight and body composition standards imposed by others. The "lean look" of young male models serves as a standard for more and more young men, whereas the requirements to "make weight" for various sports drives others. Runners, jockeys, swimmers, and gymnasts frequently must lose weight quickly to meet particular standards for competition or the expectations of coaches and trainers. Researchers report that men are less inclined than women are to admit that they may have an eating disorder, thinking it is a "woman's illness." Thus they are less likely to seek treatment. In addition, physicians tend not to suspect men of having eating disorders, and so they go untreated.

Fortunately, psychological treatment in combination with medical and dietary interventions can return the person with anorexia nervosa to a more life-sustaining pattern of eating. The person with anorexia needs to receive the care of professionals experienced in the treatment of this disorder. It is not uncommon for this treatment to take 3 to 5 years. If others, including friends, coworkers, roommates, and parents, observe this condition, they should consult a health care provider for assistance.

Recognizing Anorexia Nervosa and Bulimia Nervosa

The American Psychological Association uses the following diagnostic criteria to identify anorexia nervosa and bulimia

Anorexia	Bulimia
• Body weight is 15 percent or more below desirable weight • Fear of weight gain • Distorted body image • In women, the absence of three or more menstrual periods (young girls may not start menstruating at the appropriate age); In men, sex hormones decrease	• Binge eating two or more times a week for at least 3 months • A lack of control over bingeing • Engaging in inappropriate compensatory behavior purging two or more times a week for at least 3 months to prevent weight gain • Overly concerned about body image

Characteristic symptoms include the following. Note that it is unlikely that all the symptoms will be evident in any one individual.

Anorexia	Bulimia
• Looks thin and keeps getting thinner • Skips meals, cuts food into small pieces, moves food around plate to appear to have eaten • Loss of menstrual periods and possible infertility • Wears baggy clothes in an attempt to disguise weight loss and to keep warm • Significant hair loss • Extreme sensitivity to cold • Dizziness, lightheadedness, headaches • Withdrawn, irritable, depressed • Insomnia • Decreased sex drive • Dehydration, kidney dysfunction • Fatigue, loss of energy • Decreased concentration • Lanugo (fine downy body hair) • Heart irregularities, heart failure	• Bathroom use immediately after eating • Eating in secret • Excessive time (and money) spent food shopping • Shopping for food at several stores instead of one store • Menstrual irregularities and possible fertility problems • Excessive constipation • Swollen and/or infected salivary glands, sore throat • Bursting blood vessels in the eyes • Dental erosion in teeth and gums • Dehydration and kidney dysfunction • Significant hair loss; dry, brittle hair and nails • Increased acne and skin problems • Heart irregularities, heart failure

 TALKING POINTS What would you do if you suspected that a friend of yours had an eating disorder? Would you share your concern with him or her? If so, what would you say?

Bulimia Nervosa

Whereas anorexics are underweight, people with **bulimia nervosa** often are of a normal weight. These

Resources for Anorexia and Bulimia Treatment

Local Resources

- College or university health centers
- College or university counseling centers
- Comprehensive mental health centers
- Crisis intervention centers
- Mental health associations

Organizations and Self-Help Groups

National Association of Anorexia Nervosa and Associated Disorders (ANAD)

ANAD is the oldest national nonprofit organization helping eating disorder victims and their families. In addition to its free hotline counseling, ANAD operates an international network of support groups for sufferers and their families, and it offers referrals to health care professionals who treat eating disorders across the U.S. and in 15 other countries.

PO Box 7 E-mail: *anad20@aol.com*
Highland Park, IL 60035
Hotline: 847-831-3438
www:anad.org

American Psychological Association (APA) HelpCenter

The American Psychological Association is the largest professional organization comprised of health care professionals whose practices are limited to the diagnosis, treatment, and management of psychological health problems. The APA HelpCenter provides information concerning eating disorders and the treatment options that are available for both patients and their families. Links are provided to assist in finding psychological services in your local area.

www.helping.apa.org

Academy for Eating Disorders (AED)

The Academy for Eating Disorders' membership comprises academics and clinical professionals with demonstrated interest and expertise in the field of eating disorders. In addition to providing information to both professionals and the public regarding eating disorders, the AED also advocates on behalf of patients and the general public. The AED can provide guidelines to assist in the selection of a competent healthcare provider.

60 Revere Dr., #500 E-mail: *info@aedweb.org*
Northbrook, IL 60062-1577
Telephone: 847-498-4274
www.aedweb.org/index.cfm

Anorexia Nervosa and Related Eating Disorders, Inc. (ANRED)

ANRED is a nonprofit organization that provides information about anorexia, bulimia nervosa, compulsive eating, and other less well-known food and weight disorders. Printed and Web-based information regarding treatment, recovery, and prevention are available to the general public.

PO Box 5102 E-mail: *jarinor@rio.com*
Eugene, OR 97405
541-344-1144
www.anred.com

American Anorexia/Bulimia Association, Inc. (AABA)

AABA is a national, nonprofit organization of concerned members of the public and health care industry dedicated to the prevention and treatment of eating disorders. General information related to eating disorders is provided to the general public, as well as more focused specific information for patients, families, and professionals. A list of upcoming events in various areas of the country is also provided.

418 East 76th Street, New York, NY 10021
212-501-8351
www.aabainc.org

National Eating Disorder Association

The National Eating Disorders Association is the largest nonprofit organization in the United States dedicated to the elimination of eating disorders and body dissatisfaction. It disseminates information, offers prevention programs, publishes and distributes educational materials, and operates the nation's first toll-free eating disorders information and referral line. It states as part of its mission to "continually work to change the cultural, familial, and interpersonal factors which contribute to the development of eating disorders and body dissatisfaction."

603 Stewart St., #803 E-mail: *info@NationalEatingDisorders.org*
Seattle, WA 98101
206-382-3587
www.NationalEatingDisorders.org

Additional Resources

Bulimia Anorexia Nervosa Association (BANA)
2109 Ottowa St.
Windsor, Ontario (Canada) N8Y 1R8 E-mail: *info@bana.ca*
(519) 969-2112

National Eating Disorders Association (NEDO) at Laureatte Psychiatric Hospital
6655 S. Yale
Tulsa, OK 74136
918-491-5600

This organization publishes a quarterly newsletter appropriate for professional and personal use.

individuals use food and weight as a way of coping with stress, boredom, conflict in relationships, and low self-esteem. It is not uncommon in our society to comfort ourselves with food, to have social activities based on food, and to eat as a way of procrastinating a dreaded activity. However, people with bulimia take this to the extreme, engaging in recurrent bingeing, consuming unusually large amounts of food, and feeling out of control with their eating.[54]

While anorexics run away from food, bulimics run to food to cope with their emotions, problems, and stress. Because they feel so guilty, ashamed, and anxious about the food they have consumed, people with bulimia **purge** by self-induced vomiting, taking an excessive number of laxatives and diuretics, excessively exercising or fasting. There is a strong preoccupation with weight, calories, and food among sufferers of bulimia. Most people with bulimia constantly count calories, weigh themselves throughout the day, and frequently make negative statements concerning different parts of their bodies, primarily focusing on the thighs, stomach, and waist. As with anorexia, bulimia is associated with depression, isolation, anxiety, perfectionism, and low self-esteem. Dental erosion, hair loss, esophageal lesions, blood in the vomit and stools, loss of voluntary gag reflex, kidney damage, heart failure, gastrointestinal problems, ketosis, edema, infertility, parotid gland swelling, depression, and insomnia are just some of the medical problems associated with bulimia nervosa.

The recent publicity surrounding Terri Schiavo's death highlights the lethality of this disorder—she entered a persistent vegetative state following a heart attack possibly caused by bulimia. She had developed a potassium deficiency that was reportedly caused by bulimia nervosa. Many public figures have acknowledged struggling with this disorder, including Jane Fonda, Paula Abdul, Sally Field, Justine Bateman, Joan Rivers, and the late Princess Diana. All these individuals have talked about the pressures to be thin in order to be successful in their careers and how they succumbed to this pressure by developing an eating disorder.

As mentioned previously, bulimia often begins around age 17 to 18 years of age when young adults are separating from their families and are forging lives of their own; some conflict arises around issues of independence, autonomy, and relationships with family. There is a higher incidence of bulimia than anorexia, although some bulimics may have had anorexia in the past. There is also a higher rate of bulimia among female college students as compared to their peers who are not attending college. Treatment for bulimia nervosa involves nutritional counseling, psychological counseling, and consultation with a physician. Often people with bulimia recover from this disorder within a year of beginning treatment.

Binge Eating Disorder

Binge eating disorder is the newest term for what was previously referred to as compulsive overeating. Binge eaters use food to cope in the same way that bulimics do and also feel out of control and unable to stop eating during binges. People with this disorder report eating rapidly and in secret or may snack all day. They tend to eat until they feel uncomfortably full, sometimes hoarding food and eating when they aren't physically hungry.[54] Like people with bulimia, they feel guilty and ashamed of their eating habits and have a great deal of self-loathing and body hatred. People who have binge eating disorder do not engage in purging behavior, which differentiates it from bulimia nervosa. Typically, binge eaters have a long history of diet failures, feel anxious, are socially withdrawn from others, and are overweight. Heart problems, high blood pressure, joint problems, abnormal blood sugar levels, fatigue, depression, and anxiety are associated with binge eating. The treatment of this eating disorder involves interventions similar to those described for treating bulimia nervosa.

Chewing and Spitting Out Food Syndrome

Chewing and spitting out one's food without swallowing it has also been used as a method for weight loss or weight management. This is a common eating disorder and falls within the "Eating Disorder Not Otherwise Specified" diagnosis. It differs from bulimia nervosa, and researchers contend that chewing and spitting out food without swallowing may indicate a more severe eating disorder.[57]

Night Eating Syndrome

Night eating syndrome has not yet been formally defined as an eating disorder. The signs and symptoms of this syndrome include eating more than half of one's daily food intake after dinner and before breakfast; feeling tense, anxious, and guilty while eating; difficulty falling or staying asleep at night; and having little to no appetite in the morning. Unlike binge eating, night eating involves eating

---

Key Terms

purging using vomiting, laxatives, diuretics, enemas, or other medications, or means such as excessive exercise or fasting, to eliminate food

binge eating disorder an eating disorder formerly referred to as compulsive overeating disorder; binge eaters use food to cope in the same way that bulimics do and also feel out of control, but do not engage in compensatory purging behavior throughout the evening hours rather than in short episodes. There is a strong preference for carbohydrates among night eaters. Some researchers speculate that night eating may be an unconscious attempt to self-medicate mood problems, because eating carbohydrates can trigger the brain to produce so-called "feel good" neurochemicals. Research is underway in examining the underlying causes of this syndrome and developing subsequent treatment interventions. It seems likely that a combination of biological, genetic, and psychological factors contribute to this problem.

Body Dysmorphic Disorder

Body dysmorphic disorder (BDD) is a secret preoccupation with an imagined or slight flaw in one's appearance. Sometimes, people become almost completely fixated on concerns regarding body image, leading to repeatedly weighing themselves and checking mirrors throughout the day, compulsively dieting, exercising, and undergoing cosmetic surgery.[58] Perceptions of an imperfect body may lead to psychological dysfunction, such as not wanting to leave the house because of imagined defects.

Treating Eating Disorders

The treatment for eating disorders is multimodal and multidimensional involving nutritionists, psychologists, physicians, family, and friends. There are different treatment modalities, such as individual, group, and family counseling. Sometimes treatment requires inpatient hospitalization to medically stabilize the individual. In extreme cases, a feeding tube may be inserted to treat starvation, especially if the person refuses to eat. Behavioral modification and cognitive therapy are utilized in counseling people with eating problems. Medications such as antidepressants are often used to decrease

obsessive-compulsive behavior, reduce anxiety, alleviate depression, and improve mood. Some medications can stimulate or reduce appetite as well. There is some debate over the efficacy of using an addictions model, similar to the 12-step Alcoholics Anonymous philosophy, with eating disorders. Overeaters Anonymous utilizes this model in helping people with eating problems, and many hospital programs employ this model in their treatment programs. While there seems to be some overlap of eating disorders with substance abuse problems, such as denial of problems, feeling out of control of one's behavior, and using food or drugs or alcohol to cope with problems, this is where the similarities end—obviously one needs food to live, which is not the case with drugs and alcohol.

A Final Thought about Health and Weight Management

Recognizing the attention placed on physical attractiveness and its relationship to thinness, ask yourself if you are healthy enough to accept your unique body even if it does not match the cultural ideal. As you recall from Chapter 1, it is important to develop every dimension of health, not simply the physical dimension. We hope that focusing on all dimensions of health, including the psychological aspects outlined in Chapter 2, will balance the pressure most of us feel to strive for a body image that is unrealistic and obtainable by only a few.

Key Terms
body dysmorphic disorder a secret preoccupation with an imagined or slight flaw in one's appearance

---

Taking Charge of Your Health

- Investigate the resources available on your campus that you could use to determine your healthy weight and body composition profile.

- Evaluate your eating behaviors to find out if you are using food to cope with stress. If you are, develop a plan to use nonfood options, such as exercise or interaction with friends or family members, to deal with stress.

- Formulate a realistic set of goals for changing your weight and body composition in a time frame that allows you to do so in a healthful way.

- Establish a daily schedule that lets you make any necessary dietary and physical activity adjustments.

- Keep a daily journal of your weight-management efforts.

- Monitor your progress toward meeting your weight-management goals.

- Design a reward system for reaching each goal.

- Learn to accept your body including the imperfections.

- Focus on other aspects of yourself that you like that are not related to appearance.

SUMMARY

- Weight management has become an obsession in American culture as well as a significant health problem; an estimated 65 percent of U.S. adults are either overweight or obese.
- Doctors usually define "overweight" as a condition in which a person's weight is 1 percent to 19 percent higher than "normal," as defined by a standard height/weight chart. Obesity is usually defined as a condition in which a person's weight is 20 percent or more above normal weight. "Morbid obesity" refers to being 50 percent to 100 percent over normal weight, more than 100 pounds over normal weight, or sufficiently overweight to interfere with health or normal functioning.
- Some of the methods for assessing one's weight are: Body Mass Index, current height and weight tables, waist to hip ratios, electrical impedance, BOD POD, skinfold measurements, hydrostatic weighing, and home scales.
- Basal Metabolic Rate (BMR) is a measure of resting energy expenditure that is taken upon awakening, 10–12 hours after eating, or 12–18 hours after significant physical activity.
- Thermic effect of food (TEF) refers to the amount of energy our bodies require for the digestion, absorption, and transportation of food.
- Four factors seem to play a significant role in the prevalence of obesity: sex, age, socioeconomic status, and race.
- The energy expenditure and energy storage centers of the body possess a genetically programmed awareness of the body's most physiologically desirable weight, called *set point*.
- Environmental factors such as portion size, price, advertising, the availability of food, and the number of food choices presented all influence the amount the average person consumes.
- Psychological reasons for eating refer to eating not out of hunger but as a way of coping with feelings, as a way of socializing and celebrating with others, and by associating certain activities with eating.
- Weight loss occurs when the calories consumed are fewer than the energy the body needs for physiological maintenance and activity.
- The primary types of weight-management technique include dietary alterations, surgical interventions, medications, weight loss programs, and physical activity.
- A commitment to a lifestyle change of eating in healthy ways and engaging in regular aerobic exercise seem to be the most effective strategy for weight loss and weight maintenance.
- Anorexia nervosa is a psychological condition in which the individual weighs less than 85 percent of his/her expected weight for his/her age, gender, and height.
- People with bulimia nervosa use food and weight as a way of coping with stress, boredom, conflict in relationships, and low self-esteem. They engage in recurrent bingeing and purging to eliminate the food from their bodies.
- Binge eaters use food to cope in the same way that bulimics do and also feel out of control and unable to stop eating during binges, but they do not engage in purging behaviors.

REVIEW QUESTIONS

1. What percentage of U.S. adults are either overweight or obese?
2. How has the average caloric intake and physical activity level for Americans changed over the past two decades?
3. Define *overweight, obesity,* and *morbid obesity.*
4. List at least four of the methods used for assessing weight.
5. Define Basal Metabolic Rate (BMR).
6. Describe the thermic effect of food (TEF) and how it relates to the BMR.
7. What are four factors that seem to play a significant role in the prevalence of obesity?
8. Define *set point.*
9. The process of storing or burning more energy to maintain the body's "best" weight is called what?
10. Give four examples of how environmental factors can influence the amount the average person consumes.
11. Describe at least two psychological reasons for eating.
12. Give examples of four different types of weight-management techniques.
13. What is the most effective strategy for weight loss and weight maintenance?
14. Describe the symptoms of anorexia nervosa, bulimia nervosa, and binge eating disorder.

ENDNOTES

1. National Center for Chronic Disease Prevention and Health Promotion. *Defining Overweight and Obesity,* April 2005.
2. National Research Council, *Healthy People 2010.* www.healthypeople.gov.
3. National Center for Health Statistics. Center for Disease Control. *Obesity Still a Major Problem, New Data Show.* October 6, 2004.
4. Harvard Women's Health Watch: Panel issues new guidelines for healthy eating. *Harvard Medical School,* November 2002, Volume 10(3).
5. www.usda.gov. *USDA Revamps Food Pyramid to Unveil New Symbol.* April 18, 2005.
6. Heart and Stroke Facts. *American Heart Association,* 2003.
7. Poulton T. *No Fat Chicks.* Secaucus, NJ: Carol Publishing Group, 1997.
8. Maine M. *Body Wars.* Carlsbad, CA: Gurze Books, 2000.
9. Andersen A, Cohn L, Holbrook T. *Making Weight: Men's Conflicts with Food, Weight, Shape and Appearance.* Carlsbad, CA: Gurze Books, 2000.
10. Cash T, Henry P. Women's body images: The results of a national survey in the U.S.A. *Sex Role Res* 33(1), 19–29, 1995.

11. Andersen A. *Males with Eating Disorders*. Philadelphia, PA: Brunner/Mazel Inc., 1990.

12. Pope, M, Phillips, K, Olivardia, R. *The Adonis Complex*. New York: Simon and Schuster, 2000.

13. Brownell KD, Fairburn CG. *Eating Disorders and Obesity: A Comprehensive Handbook*. New York: Guilford Press, 1995.

14. National Institute of Health. Clinical guidelines on the identification, evaluation, and treatment of overweight and obesity in adults. As reported in *First Federal Obesity Clinical Guidelines* (NIH News Advisory). The National Institutes of Health, 17 June, 1998.

15. Gaesser G. *Big Fat Lies*. Carlsbad, CA: Gurze Books, 2002.

16. U.S. Department of Agriculture/U.S. Department of Health and Human Services. Nutrition and your health: Dietary guidelines for Americans. *Home and Garden Bulletin,* 232, 2000.

17. Waist Management, Gauging Your Risk. *Consumer Reports,* p. 48, August 2003.

18. International Health Racquet and Sportsclub Association. BOD POD Body Composition System to Descend on San Francisco's *IHRSA CONVENTION,* as reported in the 29th Anniversary Exhibition in San Francisco's Moscone Convention Center, March 22–24, 2001.

19. Dempster P, Aitkens S. A new air displacement method for the determination of human body composition. *Medical Science Sports Exercise* 27(2), 1692–1697, 1995.

20. Lindzey G, Thompson R, Spring B. *Psychology* (3rd ed.). New York: Worth Publishers, Inc., 1988.

21. Thelen MH, Powell AL, Lawrence C, Kuhnent ME. Eating and body image concerns among children. *Journal of Consulting and Clinical Psychology* 21, 41, 46, 1992.

22. U.S. Department of Health and Human Services. *The Surgeon General's Call to Action to Prevent and Decrease Overweight and Obesity*. Rockville, MD: U.S. Department of Health and Human Services, Public Health Service, Office of the Surgeon General, 2001. Available from U.S. GPO, Washington www.surgeongeneral.gov/topics/obesity/calltoaction/CalltoAction.pdf.

23. Sobal J. Obesity and socioeconomic status: A framework for examining relationships between physical and social variables. *Medical Anthropology* 13, 231–247, 1991.

24. Wadden TA, Stunkard AJ. *Handbook of Obesity Treatment*. New York: Guilford Press, 2002.

25. Halaas J, et al. Weight-reducing effects on the plasma protein encoded by the obese gene. *Science* 269(5223), 543–546, 1995.

26. Folsom AR, Jensen MD, Jacobs DR, Hilner JE, Tsai AW, Schreiner PJ. Serum leptin and weight gain over eight years in African American and Caucasian young adults. *Obesity Research* 7(1), 1–8, 1999.

27. Sakurai T, et al. Orexins and orexin receptors: A family of hypothalamic neuropeptides and G protein-coupled receptors that regulate feeding behavior. *Cell* 92(4), 573–585, 1998.

28. Pettigrew R, Hamilton FD. Obesity and female reproductive function. *Br Med Bull* 53:2, 341–358, 1997.

29. La Leche League International. *The Womanly Art of Breastfeeding*. 1997.

30. Dell S, To T. Breastfeeding and asthma in young children. *Archives of Pediatric and Adolescent Medicine* 155: 1261–1265, 2001.

31. Hediger ML, et al. Association between infant breast-feeding and overweight in young children. *JAMA* 285(19): 2453–2460, 2001.

32. Gillman MW, et al. Risk of overweight among adolescents who were breastfed as infants. *JAMA* 285(19): 2461–2467, 2001.

33. Set Point: What your body is trying to tell you. *National Eating Disorders Information Centre Bulletin,* 7(2), June, 1992.

34. The truth about dieting. *Consumer Reports,* 26–31 June, 2002.

35. Saladin KS. *Anatomy & Physiology: The Unity of Form and Function*. Dubuque, IA: William C. Brown/McGraw-Hill, 1998.

36. Sorbara M, Geliebter A. Body image disturbance in obese outpatients before and after weight loss in relation to race, gender and age of onset of obesity. *Internal Journal of Eating Disorders,* 416–423, May, 2002.

37. Sobal J, Stunkard AJ. Socioeconomic status and obesity: A review of the literature. *Psychological Bulletin* 105, 260–275, 1989.

38. Stunkard AJ, Wadden TA. *Obesity: Theory and Therapy*. New York: Raven Press, 1993

39. Sobal J, Rauschenbach B, Frongillo E. Marital status, fatness and obesity. *Social Science and Medicine* 35, 915–923, 1992.

40. Obesity in America: The gorge yourself environment. *The New York Times,* August 19, 2003.

41. Shils, M, Olson, J. Shike, Ross, A. *Modern Nutrition in Health and Disease* (9th ed.). Philadelphia: Lippincott, Williams, and Wilkins, 1999.

42. Weight Watchers. *Stop Stuffing Yourself: 7 Steps to Conquering Overeating*. New York: Wiley Publishing Inc., 1988.

43. Kirby, J. *Dieting for Dummies*. New York: Wiley Publishing Inc., 1998.

44. *Dietary Guidelines for Americans*. www.health.gov/dietaryguidelines. 2005.

45. Insel P, Turner RE, Ross D. *Nutrition*. Sudbury, MA: Jones and Bartlett Publishers, 2002.

46. Wardlaw, GM. *Perspectives in Nutrition* (4th ed.). New York: McGraw-Hill, 1999.

47. Ephedra ban puts herb industry on notice. *The New York Times,* December 31, 2003.

48. Roering JL. Herbal agents used by eating disorder patients. *Eating Disorders Review,* 13(4), July/August 2002.

49. Center for Drug Evaluation and Research, U.S. Food and Drug Administration. FDA announces withdrawal of fenfluramine and dexfenfluramine. *News Release #97-32,* September 15, 1997.

50. Hensrud DD, et al. Echocardiographic improvement over time after cessation of use of fenfluramine and phentermine. *May Clin Pro* 74(12), 1191–1197, 1999.

51. Grazer FM, de Jong RH. Fatal outcomes from liposuction: Census survey of cosmetic surgeons. *Plastic Reconstructive Surgery* 105(1) 436–446, 2000.

52. The American Dietetic Association. Gaining weight: A healthy plan for adding pounds. *Hot Topics,* www.eatright.org/nfs10html, 1998.

53. Young TK, et al. Childhood obesity in a population at high risk for type 2 diabetes. *Journal of Pediatrics* 136(3), 365–369, 2000.

54. *Diagnostic and Statistical Manual of Mental Disorders IV TR.* Washington, D.C., American Psychiatric Association, 2000.

55. Gotthelf M. The new anorexia outrage. *Self Magazine,* 82–84. August 2001.

56. Lilenfeld L. Academy members debate over pro-anorexia websites. *Academy of Eating Disorders Newsletter,* June 2001.

57. Update: Chewing and Spitting Out Food. *Eating Disorders Review,* July/August, 2002.

58. A dangerous duo: Body dysmorphic disorder with anorexia nervosa. *Eating Disorders Review,* November/December, 4–5, 2002.

As We Go to Press...

Want to Lose Weight? Get More Sleep!

Research has recently discovered that not getting enough sleep doesn't just make you grumpy and sluggish—it can make you gain weight as well! People who sleep 2 to 4 hours a night have been found to be 73 percent more likely to be obese than those who sleep 7 to 9 hours. Sleeping 5 hours a night results in a 50 percent chance of being obese compared to those consistently sleeping 7 to 9 hours. Twenty-three percent of people who sleep 6 hours tend to be obese. In other words, the higher the BMI, the less sleep the person got.

Why does less sleep equal more weight? We used to think that sleeping too much made us gain weight and staying up meant we were more active and so burned calories, but this has been disproved. People tend to watch television, read, or be online late at night, and so they are not active. In addition, people tend to eat high-fat, high-sugar foods while they are engaging in these activities. Some people say that they eat sugary foods in order to give themselves more energy to stay up late to study or to get work done.

Two hormones, ghrelin and leptin, have been found to regulate both sleep and hunger. A sleep study at the University of Chicago found that leptin levels were 18 percent lower and ghrelin levels 28 percent higher after subjects slept 4 hours. Sleep-deprived subjects reported feeling the most hungry and craved carbohydrates, the energy food. Ghrelin has been referred to as the accelerator for eating. When ghrelin levels are up, people feel hungrier. Leptin is the brake for eating; higher levels are associated with feeling full and decreased appetite.

These sleep studies seem to indicate that a hormonal relationship exists between sleep and hunger. The ghrelin level in people who routinely slept 5 hours a night was 15 percent higher, compared to 15 percent lower leptin levels in people who slept 8 hours a night. The first group had higher BMIs than did individuals sleeping 8 hours at night. Studies have also found that children are not getting the 10 to 11 hours of sleep a night they require, which may also help explain the increase in childhood obesity.

So, one way for us to manage our weight is to manage our sleep better. This means managing our time better—prioritizing our commitments and activities and not overloading our schedules, so that we can get the rest we need.

Sources: "Sleep Loss May Equal Weight Gain," *USA Today,* December 7, 2004. "One More Reason to Get Enough Sleep," *Harvard Women's Health Watch,* May 2005.

personal assessment

How many calories do you need?

Resting Energy Requirement (RER)

Women

3–10 years 22.5 × weight (kg) + 499
10–18 years 12.2 × weight (kg) + 746
18–30 years 14.7 × weight (kg) + 496
30–60 years 08.7 × weight (kg) + 829
>60 years 10.5 × weight (kg) + 596

Men

3–10 years 22.7 × weight (kg) + 495
10–18 years 17.5 × weight (kg) + 651
18–30 years 15.3 × weight (kg) + 679
30–60 years 11.6 × weight (kg) + 879
>60 years 13.5 × weight (kg) + 487

Activity Energy Requirement (AER)

At bed rest: 1.20
Low activity (walking): 1.30
Average activity: 1.50–1.75
High activity: 2.0

Instructions: Calculate your resting energy requirement based on your sex, age, and weight. Then multiply your RER by your AER to determine how many calories you need each day to maintain your weight.

Example: Woman
    24 years
    120 lbs = 54.5 kg
    High activity
    (RER) × (AER) = Total Energy Requirement
    14.7 × 54.5 (kg) + 496 × 2.0 = 2594 calories/day

Note: 1 kg = 2.2 lbs.

Data from *Energy and protein requirements: report of a joint FAO/WHO/UNU expert consultation.* Technical Report Series 724. World Health Organization, 1985; Zeam FJ: *Clinical nutrition and dietetics,* Macmillan, 1991.

personal assessment

Body love or body hate?

When you catch a glimpse of yourself in a mirror, do you smile at what you see or grimace? The following quiz will help you to assess your body self-esteem associated with your appearance. Please answer using the following rating scale:

1 = Rarely or never

2 = Sometimes

3 = Almost always or always

Add up your scores to determine your total score, and look at the summary below for an interpretation of your scores.

_____ 1. I worry about my weight and weighing "too much."

_____ 2. I prefer to eat by myself and not with other people.

_____ 3. My mood is determined by the scale and how I feel about my appearance.

_____ 4. I make negative comments about my appearance to myself and others.

_____ 5. I think I look less attractive on days that I haven't exercised.

_____ 6. I have a difficult time accepting compliments about my appearance from others.

_____ 7. I compare myself to other women and find myself lacking.

_____ 8. I ask other people how I look.

_____ 9. I avoid social situations, activities, and events involving food.

_____ 10. I feel more anxious about my body in the summertime because of the need to wear bathing suits and clothing suitable for warmer temperatures.

_____ **TOTAL SCORE**

Interpretation

If you scored between 10 and 15, you have positive body self-esteem and are accepting of yourself and your appearance.

If you scored between 16 and 23, you scored in the average range. While you are in good company, feeling about your body the way most people do, you may want to reframe your body image and develop more of an appreciation for your body and appearance.

If your score was between 24 and 30, you have poor or low body self-esteem. Your self-esteem in general is probably driven by how you see yourself, and you may be putting too much emphasis on your appearance and are too self-critical. You may feel as though you never are thin enough or look good enough and can always find a flaw when looking in the mirror. To improve your body self-esteem, focus on other aspects of yourself, focus on the positive aspects of your body, and be more accepting of yourself and less perfectionistic.

Preventing Drug Abuse and Dependence

Health educators have no doubt that the use, misuse, and abuse of many drugs can impair health. These substances not only alter the functioning of the body and mind but also affect the other dimensions of health. In Part Three, we take a look at addictive substances and their effects on the user.

1. **Physical Dimension**
   The effects of substance use, especially the long-term use of tobacco and alcohol, are well understood. These substances cause illness and death. Alcohol abuse can destroy the structure and function of many body systems. Tobacco use damages the cardiovascular system and the tissues of the respiratory tract and can cause cancer in many sites throughout the body. Chronic abuse of psychoactive drugs impairs many central nervous system functions. Even the experimental use of these drugs carries the danger of toxic overdose.

2. **Emotional Dimension**
   Because psychoactive drugs alter nervous system functioning, many users experience depression and mood swings. For people who are predisposed to enter dependent relationships, drug use can become an unhealthy way of relieving stress. When psychological dependence combines with physical dependence, the addict may begin to lose touch with reality.

3. **Social Dimension**
   Psychoactive drug use often takes place in social settings. For many people, drinking or using other drugs is a necessary first step toward enjoying the company of others. However, most people have little tolerance for inappropriate substance use, such as use of illegal drugs, excessive alcohol intake, and smoking in public places where tobacco use is banned.

4. **Intellectual Dimension**
   Intellectual impairment is one consequence of chemical abuse. People cannot perform well intellectually when they are feeling high or low or when their senses are dulled. Some people prefer to disregard information about the dangers of substance abuse, a choice that could prove extremely harmful to their health.

5. **Spiritual Dimension**
   Although drug use has long played a role in the religious practices of people throughout the world, the nonceremonial use of drugs conflicts with the principles of service to others. Substance abuse can hinder spiritual growth by turning a person's focus inward, making it impossible to develop the other-directedness that is essential to a rich spiritual life.

6. **Occupational Dimension**
   Use of both legal and illegal drugs clearly stands in the way of occupational health. Most workplaces are smoke-free, forcing smokers to stand outside or walk to the smoker's lounge to have a cigarette. These continual interruptions lower a worker's productivity. Illegal drug use can keep a job candidate from being hired, and use of illegal drugs or alcohol on the job can be dangerous and will certainly lower a worker's level of performance.

chapter seven

Making Decisions about Drug Use

Eye on the Media

Do Media Scare Tactics Keep People from Using Drugs?

The media has tried to frighten people in many ways to keep them away from unhealthy behaviors. Bloody films showing the aftermath of a prom night car crash have been used to scare teenagers about dangerous drinking and driving behaviors. Television ads and public service announcements have featured celebrities speaking out against drug use. More recently, antidrug campaigns stated that buying illegal drugs helped finance anti-American terrorists.

Advertisements for drug and alcohol rehabilitation facilities have shown alcoholics drowning in a sea of alcohol, drug users being confronted by their families, and employees caught by a drug screening test. The message is that miserable life situations can be changed if people are willing to get help.

It's difficult to measure the effectiveness of these approaches to drug prevention. Many people recall these media presentations, so they do make an impression. But, given the variables involved in drug-taking behavior—family influence, inherited predispositions, life events and situations, drug availability, and peer influence—it's impossible to pinpoint the influence of a single media event. These scare tactics seem to be especially effective among people who have already made the decision not to use drugs. They remind these people how dangerous it is to use drugs. For people who are thinking about starting drug use, these messages may be beneficial, since they portray drug use in a negative light.

For hard-core drug users, though, it's unlikely that scare tactics will be effective. These people tend to lead chaotic lives, may never see the ads, and often remain in denial about their addiction. Despite the fact that these ad campaigns are highly visible and costly, they seem to have only limited influence in drug prevention.

The use of psychoactive drugs can be tremendously disruptive in many people's lives, from causing tragic deaths or the loss of employment opportunities (most Fortune 500 companies use preemployment drug testing) to causing personal relationships to deteriorate and babies to be born with profound birth defects. Perhaps realizing this, college students have generally moved away from using the most dangerous illegal drugs.

However, it is safe to say that drug use remains a significant problem for both college students and the general population. Alcohol is the most important problem drug for most college students (see Chapter 8), but other drugs pose risks for certain students (Table 7.1). Additionally, many nontraditional-age students see the destructive effects of drug use on their neighborhoods and worry about their children being exploited by drug dealers.

Table 7.1 Annual Prevalence among College Students: Alcohol and Other Drugs

Drug	% Students Using Drug 1 or More Times
Tobacco	30.8
Alcohol	74.7
Marijuana	20.3
Cocaine	2.4
Amphetamines	4.6
Sedatives	2.2
Hallucinogens	1.6
Opiates	.8
Inhalants	.8
Designer drugs	1.3
Steroids	.6
Other	1.0

Note: Statistics were drawn from a sample of 38,857 college students from 89 two- and four-year colleges in the United States in 2003.
Source: CORE Institute: Center for Alcohol and Other Drug Studies. *American Campuses: 2001 Statistics on Alcohol and Other Drug Use.* Southern Illinois University at Carbondale (online). www.siu.edu/departments/coreinst/public_html/2003.htm, accessed February 11, 2005.

Prevention: The Best Solution

We combat the drug problem in the United States on two fronts: the demand side and the supply side. The United States government attempts to reduce the supply of illegal (illicit) drugs through drug interdiction efforts at our borders, through joint efforts with countries such as Mexico and Colombia, and through law-enforcement measures within our own borders.

However, the best way to avoid the immense costs of drug abuse is simply to reduce the demand. We do this by helping people develop the tools needed to avoid the use of illegal drugs (see Changing for the Better below). Experts are currently mounting prevention efforts on three levels: primary, secondary, and tertiary. Take a look at each of these three levels. Which level is most familiar to you?

Changing for the Better

Improving Your Mood without Drugs

It's tempting to reach for a pill when I feel down, but I don't want to get into that habit. What can I do to improve my mood without using drugs?

Talk with a trusted friend. Confide your feelings to a close, trusted friend or family member. By opening up to another person, you'll gain insights into how you can get beyond your negative feelings without resorting to drug use.

Get moving. Go for a walk, ride your bike, or swim a few laps. Physical activity is a natural way to enhance your mood. Nearly every college provides recreation programs such as aerobics, swimming, dancing, or weight lifting.

Give yourself a break. If you're tired, take a quick power nap. If you're overworked, set aside some personal time—just for yourself. Read, watch TV, surf the net, or phone an old friend. Decide what you like to do, and then do it. You'll return to your responsibilities with renewed enthusiasm.

Do volunteer work. One way to feel good is to help others. Teach reading to adults, become a Big Brother or Big Sister, work in a soup kitchen, or drive a van for the elderly in your community.

Reexamine your spiritual health. Many people find comfort by making connections to their spiritual life. Through activities such as meditation, spiritual reflection, and renewal of faith, people often gain reassurance and a sense of calmness.

Restructure your daily activities. If you have one hectic day after another but feel as though you're not accomplishing anything, try reorganizing your daily activities. Experiment with new patterns. Plan to get sufficient sleep, eat regular meals, and set aside specific times for work, family activities, and pleasure. Find out what works best for you.

Seek professional guidance. If you've tried these strategies but your mood still isn't improving, consider seeking professional help. This important first step is up to you. Visit your college health center or counseling center, and talk with people who are trained to help you learn how to become a happier person.

Primary Prevention

Primary prevention means reaching people who have not yet used drugs and reducing their desire to try drugs. Primary prevention programs can target individuals, families, peer groups, neighborhoods, schools, workplaces, colleges, and the community. The key to primary prevention is to keep potential users from starting to use drugs.[1]

Secondary Prevention

Secondary prevention targets those who are beginning to experiment with drugs and uses detection, screening, intervention, and treatment of early drug abuse to help avoid further drug use. These programs do not prevent initial drug use but instead involve detection and early treatment of drug problems before they become severe. Popular methods include crisis telephone hotlines, peer counseling, individual and family counseling, school and worksite drug screening programs, and student and employee assistance programs.[1]

Tertiary Prevention

Tertiary prevention (third-level prevention) targets drug-dependent people, such as cocaine abusers, heroin addicts, or alcoholics. These individuals require specialized, intensive help that includes rehabilitation and maintenance. Such intensive treatments may require temporary hospitalization. Additional treatment methods include intensive outpatient care, support groups, and after-care programs. Relapse prevention is designed to help people recovering from drug abuse maintain their drug-free lifestyles.[1]

Effects of Drugs on the Central Nervous System

To better understand the disruption caused by the actions of psychoactive drugs, a general knowledge of the normal functioning of the nervous system's basic unit, the **neuron,** is required.

First, stimuli from the internal or external environment are received by the appropriate sensory receptor, perhaps an organ such as an eye or an ear. Once sensed, these stimuli are converted into electrical impulses. These impulses are then directed along the neuron's **dendrite,** through the cell body, and along the **axon** toward the synaptic junction near an adjacent neuron.[2] On arrival at the **synapse,** the electrical impulses stimulate the production and release of chemical messengers called **neurotransmitters.** These neurotransmitters transmit the electrical impulses from one neuron to the dendrites of adjoining neurons. Thus neurons function in a coordinated fashion to send information to the brain for interpretation and to relay appropriate response commands outward to the tissues of the body.

The role of neurotransmitters is critically important to the relay of information within the system. A substance that has the ability to alter some aspect of neurotransmitter function has the potential to seriously disrupt the otherwise normally functioning system. Psychoactive drugs are capable of exerting these disruptive influences on the neurotransmitters. Drugs "work" by changing the way neurotransmitters work, often by blocking the production of a neurotransmitter or forcing the continued release of a neurotransmitter (see Figure 7-1).

Addictive Behavior

This chapter explores the health consequences of drug use, misuse, and abuse. Before we talk about specific drugs, however, we need to put drug use in the broader context of addictive behavior. Experts in human behavior view drug use and abuse as just one of the many forms of

---

Key Terms

primary prevention measures intended to deter first-time drug use

secondary prevention measures aimed at early detection, intervention, and treatment of drug abuse before severe physical, psychological, emotional, or social consequences can occur

tertiary prevention treatment and rehabilitation of drug-dependent people to limit physical, psychological, emotional, and social deterioration or prevent death

neuron a nerve cell

dendrite the portion of a neuron that receives electrical stimuli from adjacent neurons; neurons typically have several such branches or extensions

axon the portion of a neuron that conducts electrical impulses to the dendrites of adjacent neurons; neurons typically have one axon

synapse (**sinn** aps) the location at which an electrical impulse from one neuron is transmitted to an adjacent neuron; also referred to as a *synaptic junction*

neurotransmitters chemical messengers that transfer electrical impulses across the synapses between nerve cells

---

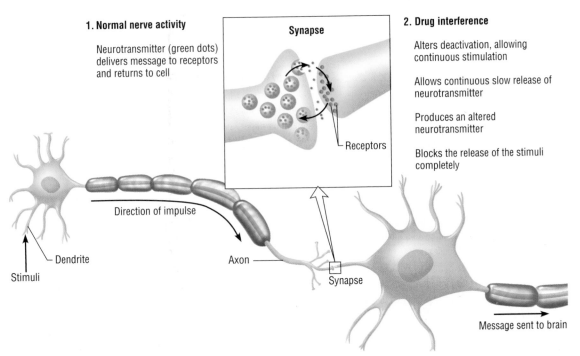

1. Normal nerve activity

Neurotransmitter (green dots) delivers message to receptors and returns to cell

Synapse

Receptors

2. Drug interference

Alters deactivation, allowing continuous stimulation

Allows continuous slow release of neurotransmitter

Produces an altered neurotransmitter

Blocks the release of the stimuli completely

Direction of impulse

Dendrite

Axon

Stimuli

Synapse

Message sent to brain

Figure 7–1   This illustration depicts the disruption caused by the action of psychoactive drugs on the central nervous system. Neurotransmitters are chemical messengers that transfer electrical impulses across the synapses between nerve cells. Psychoactive drugs interrupt this process, thus disrupting the normal functioning of the nervous system.

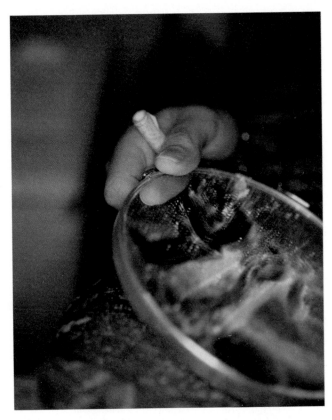

Drug use of all types remains a significant problem in our society.

addictive behavior. Addictive behavior includes addictions to shopping, eating, gambling, sex, television, video games, Internet use, or work, as well as addictions to alcohol or other drugs.

TALKING POINTS How would you approach a friend and tell him he has a gambling addiction that needs to be controlled?

The Process of Addiction

The process of developing an addiction has been a much-studied topic. Addictive behavior seems to have three common aspects: exposure, compulsion, and loss of control.

Exposure

An addiction can begin after a person is exposed to a drug (such as alcohol) or a behavior (such as gambling) that he or she finds pleasurable. Perhaps this drug or behavior temporarily replaces an unpleasant feeling or sensation. This initial pleasure gradually (or in some cases quickly) becomes a focal point in the person's life.

Compulsion

Increasingly more energy, time, and money are spent pursuing the drug use or behavior. At this point in the addictive process, the person can be said to have a compulsion

According to many college and university drug counselors, students who undergo drug counseling often say that they started (or continued) to use drugs because they felt inadequate in social situations. These students believed that they were not attractive, talented, wealthy, or socially skilled enough to start and maintain relationships. In a dating situation, the drug allowed them to be more relaxed and less conscious of their perceived shortcomings. Then, if they did something foolish while socializing, they had an instant excuse—the drug made them act inappropriately.

What are some drug-free strategies you can use to enhance your social relationships? Start by finding people and activities that are free of drug use. Contrary to popular opinion, most college students do not use illegal drugs. More students than ever are supportive of a drug-free lifestyle, so it shouldn't be difficult to find individuals and groups who will be a good match for you. Be aware of all the people around you. Don't get locked into one group too quickly. Keep your options open.

As you explore your inner self and try to connect with people at a deeper level, also consider these approaches:

Be true to yourself. Most people like someone who is genuine, so try to be the person you know yourself to be. Don't present a false image of yourself to others.

Be a good listener. One sure way to discourage a growing relationship is to talk more than you listen. Show others that you're interested in them by hearing what they have to say. Let the other person be the center of attention, at least early in the relationship. By listening carefully, you can evaluate the person or group better and see if you're a good fit.

Be open to new people and ideas. It's good to have firm opinions and ideas, but it's also important to be open to new people and ideas. Take the attitude that the next person you meet or the next group you interact with may change your life forever. Don't limit yourself to a particular group of people or friends. Flexibility can be a real asset to your social life.

Be willing to laugh at yourself. Most surveys indicate that people rate humor as an important quality in people they want to date. Try to find humor in everyday situations. Focusing on the lighter side will make things easier for you and the people around you. Most important—be willing to laugh at yourself sometimes.

Be prepared for setbacks. One sign of social maturity is to recognize that setbacks can happen. Don't be defeated by them. Sometimes it's best for everyone involved when things don't work out. You'll always have another opportunity. Focus on the attitude that things will get better. Don't give in to the idea that drugs will make up for an unsatisfying social life. Seek professional help if things do not improve after a reasonable time.

---

for the drug or behavior. Frequently, repeated exposure to the drug or behavior continues despite negative consequences, such as the gradual loss of family and friends, unpleasant physical symptoms after taking the drug, and problems at work.

During the compulsion phase of the addictive behavior, a person's "normal" life often degenerates while she or he searches for increased pleasures from the drug or the behavior. An addicted person's family life, circle of friends, work, or study patterns become less important than does the search for more and better "highs." The development of tolerance and withdrawal are distinct possibilities. (These terms are discussed later in the chapter.)

Why some people develop compulsions and others do not is difficult to pinpoint, but addiction might be influenced by genetic makeup, family dynamics, physiological processes, personality type, peer groups, and available resources for help.

Loss of Control

Over time, the search for highs changes to a desire to avoid the effects of withdrawal from the drug or behavior. Addicted people lose their ability to control their behavior. Despite overwhelming negative consequences (for example, deterioration of health, alienation of family and friends, or loss of all financial resources), addicted people continue to behave in ways that make their lives worse. The person addicted to alcohol continues to drink heavily, the person addicted to shopping continues to run up heavy debts, and the person addicted to food continues to eat indiscriminately. This behavior reflects a loss of control over one's life. Frequently, a person has addictions to more than one drug or behavior.

Intervention and Treatment

The good news for people with addictions is that help is available. Within the last two decades, much attention has been focused on intervention and treatment for addictive behavior. Many people can be helped through programs such as those described at the end of this chapter. These programs often include inpatient or outpatient treatment, family counseling, and long-term aftercare counseling.

It is common for people in aftercare treatment for addictive behavior to belong to a self-help support group, such as Alcoholics Anonymous, Gamblers Anonymous, or Sex Addicts Anonymous. These groups are often listed in the phone book or in the classified ads section of the newspaper.

Codependence

With all the focus placed on the person with a drug problem, often the families and loved ones of the addict do not receive the attention and help they need. You may already be familiar with the term *codependent,* but you might have assumed that this term applies only to those close to an alcoholic. In fact, this term can apply to anyone who is close to an individual addicted to any type of behavior, including addiction to drugs, sex, gambling, or other behaviors.

Codependent people typically become unaware of their own feelings, needs, and boundaries in their preoccupation with the addicted individual. They become focused on protecting or coping with the addict and often lose their own sense of identity. This stress often results in chaotic behaviors, addictions, and physical illnesses in the codependent person.

Private and public programs are also available to help the codependent person learn new behaviors. (See Chapter 8 for more information about codependent behavior and resources.)

Drug Terminology

Before examining drug actions or drug behavior, you must first be familiar with some basic terminology. Much of this terminology originates in the field of pharmacology, or the study of the interaction of chemical agents with living material.

What does the word **drug** mean? Each of us may have different ideas about what a drug is. Although a number of definitions are available, we consider a drug to be "any substance, natural or artificial, other than food, that by its chemical or physical nature alters structure or function in the living organism."[3] Included in this broad definition is a variety of psychoactive drugs, medicines, and substances that many people do not usually consider to be drugs.

Psychoactive drugs alter the user's feelings, behavior, perceptions, or moods when using stimulants, depressants, hallucinogens, opiates, or inhalants. Prescribed medications function to heal unhealthy tissue as well as ease pain, prevent illness, and diagnose health conditions. Although some psychoactive drugs are used for medical reasons, as in the case of tranquilizers and some narcotics, the most commonly prescribed medicines are antibiotics, hormone replacement drugs, sulfa drugs, diuretics, oral contraceptives, and cardiovascular drugs. Legal substances not usually considered to be drugs (which certainly are drugs) include caffeine, tobacco, alcohol, aspirin, and other over-the-counter (OTC) drugs. These common substances are used so frequently in our society that they are rarely perceived as true drugs.

For organizational reasons, this chapter primarily deals with psychoactive drugs. Alcohol is covered in Chapter 8. The effects of tobacco are delineated in Chapter 9. Prescription and OTC drugs and medicines are discussed at length in Chapter 18. Anabolic steroids, drugs used primarily for increasing muscle growth, are discussed in Chapter 4.

Dependence

Psychoactive drugs have a strong potential for the development of **dependence.** In this chapter the term **addiction** is used interchangeably with physical dependence. When users take a psychoactive drug, the patterns of nervous system function are altered. If these altered functions provide perceived benefits for the user, drug use may continue, perhaps at increasingly larger dosages. If persistent use continues, the user can develop a dependence on the drug. Pharmacologists have identified two types of dependencies—physical and psychological.

A person can be said to have developed a *physical dependence* when the body cells have become reliant on a drug. Continued use of the drug is then required because body tissues have adapted to its presence.[4] The person's body needs the drug to maintain homeostasis, or dynamic balance. If the drug is not taken or is suddenly withdrawn, the user develops a characteristic **withdrawal illness.** The symptoms of withdrawal reflect the attempt by the body's cells to regain normality without the drug. Withdrawal symptoms are always unpleasant (ranging from mild to severe irritability, depression, nervousness, digestive difficulties, and abdominal pain) and can be life threatening, as in the case of abrupt withdrawal from barbiturates or alcohol.

> ### Key Terms
>
> **drug** any substance, natural or artificial, other than food, that by its chemical or physical nature alters structure or function in the living organism
>
> **psychoactive drug** any substance capable of altering feelings, moods, or perceptions
>
> **dependence** a general term that refers to the need to continue using a drug for psychological or physical reasons or both
>
> **addiction** compulsive, uncontrollable dependence on a substance, habit, or practice to such a degree that cessation causes severe emotional or physiological reactions
>
> **withdrawal illness** an uncomfortable, perhaps toxic response of the body as it attempts to maintain homeostasis in the absence of a drug; also called *abstinence syndrome*

Continued use of most drugs can lead to **tolerance.** Tolerance is an acquired reaction to a drug in which continued intake of the same dose has diminishing effects.[4] The user needs larger doses of the drug to receive previously felt sensations. The continued use of depressants, including alcohol, and opiates can cause users to quickly develop a tolerance to the drug.

 TALKING POINTS You're out with your friends and they decide to compete to see who can drink the most beer. How would you tell them that what they are doing is dangerous without sounding like a parent?

Tolerance developed for one drug may carry over to another drug within the same general category. This phenomenon is known as **cross-tolerance.** The heavy abuser of alcohol, for example, might require a larger dose of a preoperative sedative to become relaxed before surgery than the average person would. The tolerance to alcohol "crosses over" to the other depressant drugs.

A person who possesses a strong desire to continue using a particular drug is said to have developed *psychological dependence.* People who are psychologically dependent on a drug believe that they need to consume the drug to maintain a sense of well-being (see Discovering Your Spirituality on page 224). They crave the drug for emotional reasons despite having persistent or recurrent physical, social, psychological, or occupational problems that are caused or worsened by the drug use. Abrupt withdrawal from a drug by such a person would not trigger the fully expressed withdrawal illness, although some unpleasant symptoms of withdrawal might be felt. The term *habituation* is often used interchangeably with the term *psychological dependence.*

Drugs whose continued use can quickly lead to both physical and psychological dependence are depressants (barbiturates, tranquilizers, and alcohol), narcotics (the opiates, which are derivatives of the Oriental poppy: heroin, morphine, and codeine), and synthetic narcotics (Demerol and methadone). Drugs whose continued use can lead to various degrees of psychological dependence and occasionally to significant (but not life-threatening) physical dependence in some users are the stimulants (amphetamines, caffeine, and cocaine), hallucinogens (LSD, peyote, mescaline, and marijuana), and inhalants (glues, gases, and petroleum products).

Drug Misuse and Abuse

So far in this chapter we have used the term *use* (or *user*) in association with the taking of psychoactive drugs. At this point, however, it is important to define *use* and to introduce the terms *misuse* and *abuse.*[3] By doing so, we can more accurately describe how drugs are used.

The term use is all-encompassing and describes drug-taking in the most general way. For example, Americans use drugs of many types. The term use can also refer more narrowly to misuse and abuse. We often use the word in this latter regard.

The term **misuse** refers to the inappropriate use of legal drugs intended to be medications. Misuse may occur when a patient misunderstands the directions for use of a prescription or OTC drug or when a patient shares a prescription with a friend or family member for whom the drug was not prescribed. Misuse also occurs when a patient takes the prescription or OTC drug for a purpose or condition other than that for which it was intended or at a dosage other than that recommended.

The term **abuse** applies to any use of an illegal drug or any use of a legal drug when it is detrimental to health and well-being. The costs of drug abuse to the individual are extensive and include absenteeism and underachievement, loss of job, marital instability, loss of self-esteem, serious illnesses, and even death. (Complete the Personal Assessment on page 247 to test your drug awareness.)

Dynamics of Drug Abuse

Many factors influence drug-taking behavior, including individual factors, immediate environmental factors, and societal factors. Specific aspects of each are discussed in the following sections.

Individual Factors

Genetic predisposition, personality traits, attitudes and beliefs, interpersonal skills, and unmet developmental needs can lead to drug use.

Genetic Predisposition

The importance of genetic predisposition (inherited vulnerability) to drug use has not been fully determined.

Key Terms

tolerance an acquired reaction to a drug in which the continued intake of the same dose has diminished effects

cross-tolerance transfer of tolerance from one drug to another within the same general category

misuse the inappropriate use of legal drugs intended to be medications

abuse any use of a legal or illegal drug in a way that is detrimental to health or well-being

Family Impact on Children's Drug Use

The family has undeniably one of the most important environmental influences on drug-taking behavior. Adolescents who are likely to abuse drugs tend to come from families who foster the abuse of drugs. While all children can be considered vulnerable to drug use and abuse to some degree, those who are at greatest risk are children whose parents exhibit poor management skills, antisocial behavior, or criminality. These children live in disorganized families in which the roles for children and adults are poorly defined. The lack of family closeness and low educational goals seem to correlate with an early onset of drug-taking behavior among children.

The National Center on Addiction and Substance Abuse (CASA) at Columbia University published the results of a study that examined the attributes and attitudes of the parent and the household that increased the risk of drug abuse among teens. The parental risk factors include these:

- No specified curfew for the teen
- Parental disapproval of the teen's friends
- Parental expectation that their teen will try drugs
- The teen's family rarely has dinner together
- The parents do not attend religious services and do not take the teen with them if they do
- A parent smoked or smokes marijuana, and the teen knows it
- The parents think that marijuana is benign.
- The parents feel powerless, blame drug use on others, or do not assume responsibility.

It is very important that parents believe that their attitudes and actions will make a difference in the lives of their children. According to the CASA report, parents who think that they have little influence on their children's decision to use illegal drugs are probably correct. This negative attitude alone will likely become a self-fulfilling prophesy. CASA indicates that the most important thing that parents can do is to accept the responsibility to keep their kids off drugs. The parents' activism, diligence, and confidence are vitally important characteristics to develop in themselves. Parents can make a difference.

Sources:
Pinger RR, Payne WA, Hahn DB, Hahn EJ. *Drugs: Issues for Today.* 3rd ed. New York: McGraw-Hill, 1998. The National Center on Addiction and Substance Abuse at Columbia University. *Family Relationships: CASA's 1999 Teen and Parent Survey,* www.casacolumbia.org accessed February 24, 2005.

However, studies of alcoholics have demonstrated that genetic factors do play some role in the development of alcoholism. Research on genetic predisposition to the abuse of other drugs is much farther behind than for alcohol abuse.

Personality Traits, Attitudes, and Beliefs

Although drug-taking behavior cannot be predicted strictly on the basis of personality type, correlations have been noted with certain aspects of personality (or temperament). For example, children who are easily bored and need continual activity and challenge are more likely to take drugs when they are older. A similar tendency is seen in children who are driven to avoid negative consequences for their actions and who crave immediate external reward for their efforts. Clusters of traits (as measured by personality inventories), including rebelliousness, rejection of behavioral norms, resistance to authority, and high tolerance for deviance, are also reported in drug abusers.

However, a cause-and-effect relationship between personality profile and drug abuse is difficult to prove. Perhaps the abuse of drugs actually creates the personality traits, rather than the other way around.

Interpersonal Skills and Self-Esteem

Drug abusers are usually deficient in interpersonal skills. They are likely to score lower on tests that measure well-being, tolerance of others, and achievement. They also often have lower self-esteem than do those who do not abuse drugs. Again, the question of cause and effect must be raised.

Personal development results from success in daily living. When people lack positive experiences in school, employment, parenting, and varied aspects of community involvement, they may attempt to compensate through chronic heavy drug use. Of course, drug abuse removes them further from productive and satisfying growth and development, thus increasing the desire for the compensatory use of drugs.

Environmental Factors

Drug use can be fostered by factors within the immediate environment, which includes home and family, school, peers, and the community.

Home and Family

Drug abuse that begins in childhood is often associated with the home and family.[4] Children seem to be at greater risk when parents exhibit poor management skills, antisocial behavior, and even criminality. These families are often disorganized and have poorly defined roles for parenting and being a productive member of society. In many cases, adult family members abuse drugs themselves or tolerate those who do. As with tobacco use, parents can be the best or worst models children can have. The Star box above explores the family environment in greater detail.

School

Children from disorganized or socially maladjusted families often have difficulty adjusting to the organized environment of the school. The following chain of events has been suggested to explain the relationship of a poor home environment and weak academic performance to drug abuse: An undesirable home environment contributes to poor school performance and poor social development; failure at school leads to loss of self-esteem, aggressive behavior, and loss of interest in school; these factors in turn may foster truancy and drug experimentation.

Peers

A clear relationship exists between peer group drug abuse and drug abuse among individual members. It is unusual for a student to remain an active member of a peer group and abstain from drug use while other members abuse drugs. The pressure to "join in" is just too powerful to resist.

Community

Drug availability, drug education, and drug treatment and rehabilitation vary among communities. As a result, drug abuse rates differ from one community to another. Students who are parents may be interested in the degree to which their communities foster or deter drug abuse.

Societal Factors

Factors such as the existence of a youth subculture, modeling and advertising, and the self-care movement affect drug use.

Youth Subculture

For many reasons, a distinctive youth subculture exists in the United States. It comprises people from 12 to 17 years of age. This subculture has its own expectations, roles, and standards, and its own language, dress code, and behaviors.

Many people assume that the rate of drug abuse is higher in this group than in any other segment of American society. However, this belief is not supported by research. A recent study indicates that a higher rate of drug abuse occurs among 18- to 25-year-olds.[5] Nevertheless, the drug abuse that does occur among those in the younger age group is of concern because patterns that are established at an early age can carry over into later life. In fact, during this period, experimentation with a gateway drug (alcohol, nicotine, or marijuana) often begins, which may lead to heavier drug use later.[3]

Modeling and Advertising

Modeling of drug use within the peer group and family has already been presented. However, movie stars, musi-cians, and athletes also serve as models of behavior. Their example exerts a powerful influence on children and adolescents.

When models are employed by the media to sell products, advertising becomes an important factor in fostering drug use. The marketing of tobacco and alcohol products is perhaps the best example. "Beautiful people" are depicted enjoying a social drug, such as alcohol, coffee, tea, or tobacco, in opulent surroundings that most viewers can only dream of being in. Celebrities participate in events sponsored by alcohol or tobacco companies.

The Self-Care Movement

People's ability to engage in medical self-care makes drug use easier and more socially acceptable than in the past. In a society conditioned by the effectiveness and availability of OTC and prescription medications, the use of other drugs, both legal and illegal, to make ourselves feel better seems more reasonable than ever before. This attitude fosters drug misuse and, for some, drug abuse.

Combination Drug Effects

Drugs taken in various combinations and dosages can alter and perhaps intensify effects.

A **synergistic effect** is a dangerous consequence of taking different drugs in the same general category at the same time. The combination exaggerates each individual drug's effects. For example, the combined use of alcohol and tranquilizers produces a synergistic effect greater than the total effect of each of the two drugs taken separately. In this instance, a much-amplified, perhaps fatal sedation will occur. In a simplistic sense, "one plus one equals four or five."

When taken at or near the same time, drug combinations produce a variety of effects. Drug combinations have additive, potentiating, or antagonistic effects. When

---

Key Terms

gateway drug an easily obtainable legal or illegal drug that represents a user's first experience with a mind-altering drug; this drug can serve as the "gateway" to the use of other drugs

modeling the influence others have on us by example of their own behavior

synergistic effect a heightened, exaggerated effect produced by the concurrent use of two or more drugs two or more drugs are taken and the result is merely a combined total effect of each drug, the result is an **additive effect.** The sum of the effects is not exaggerated. In a sense, "one plus one plus one equals three."

When one drug intensifies the action of a second drug, the first drug is said to have a **potentiated effect** on the second drug. One popular drug-taking practice during the 1970s was the consumption of Quaaludes and beer. Quaaludes potentiated the inhibition-releasing, sedative effects of alcohol. This particular drug combination produced an inexpensive but potentially fatal drunklike euphoria in the user. More recently, the combined use of various "**club drugs**" results in unpredictable potentiated drug effects (see the Star box above).

An **antagonistic effect,** on the other hand, is a drug's action in reducing another drug's effects. Knowledge of this principle has been useful in the medical treatment of certain drug overdoses, as in the use of tranquilizers to relieve the effects of LSD or other hallucinogenic drugs.

Because of these possible synergistic drug effects, patients should always inform their doctors and dentists of any illegal drugs they have taken.

Drug Classifications

Drugs can be categorized according to the nature of their physiological effects. Most psychoactive drugs fall into one of six general categories: stimulants, depressants, hallucinogens, cannabis, narcotics, and inhalants (Table 7.2).

Key Terms

additive effect the combined (but not exaggerated) effect produced by the concurrent use of two or more drugs

potentiated effect a phenomenon whereby the use of one drug intensifies the effect of a second drug

club drug one of a variety of psychoactive drugs typically used at raves, bars, and dance clubs

antagonistic effect the effect produced when one drug reduces or offsets the effects of a second drug

Table 7.2 Psychoactive Drug Categories

Drugs	Trade or Common Names	Medical Uses	Possible Effects
STIMULANTS			
Cocaine*	Coke, crack, gin, girlfriend, girl, double bubble, California cornflakes, caballo, bouncing powder, flake, snow	Local anesthetic	Increased alertness, excitation, euphoria, increased pulse rate and blood pressure, insomnia, loss of appetite
Amphetamines	Biphetamine, Delcobese, Desoxyn, Dexedrine, mediatric, black Mollies, aimies, amps, bam, beans, benz	Hyperactivity, narcolepsy,	
Methamphetamine	Speed, ice, chalk, meth, crystal, crank, fire, glass	Weight control	Memory loss, violence, psychotic behavior, cardiac and neurological damage
Phendimetrazine	Prelu-2		
Methylphenidate	Ritalin, Methidate		
Other stimulants	Adipex, Bacarate, Cylert, Didrex, Ionamin, Plegine, PreSate, Sanorex, Tenuate, Tepanil, Voranil, ephedra		
DEPRESSANTS			
Chloral hydrate	Noctec, Somnos	Hypnotic	Slurred speech, disorientation, drunken behavior without odor of alcohol
Barbiturates	Amobarbital, Butisol, phenobarbital, phenoxbarbital, secobarbital, Tuinal, blockbusters, black bombers, blue devils, blue dogs, blue tips, tombica	Anesthetic, anticonvulsant, sedative, hypnotic	
Glutethimide	Doriden	Sedative, hypnotic	
Methaqualone	Optimil, Parest, Quaalude, Somnafec, Sopor	Sedative, hypnotic	
Benzodiazepines	Ativan, Azene, Clonopin, Dalmane, diazepam, Librium, Serax, Tranxene, Valium, Verstran	Antianxiety, anticonvulsant, sedative, hypnotic	
GHB	Gamma-hydroxybutyrate (G, Liquid ecstacy, Georgia Home Boy)	None	Unconsciousness, seizures, amnesia, vomiting, coma
Other depressants	Equanil, Miltown, Noludar, Placidyl, Valmid	Antianxiety, sedative, hypnotic	
HALLUCINOGENS			
LSD	Acid, microdot, brown dot, cap, California sunshine, brown bomber	None	Delusions and hallucinations, poor perception of time and distance
Mescaline and peyote	Mesc, buttons, cactus, chief	None	
Amphetamine variants (designer drugs)	2,5-DMA, DOM, DOP, MDA, MDMA, PMA, STP, TMA, clarity, chocolate chips, booty juice	None	
Phencyclidine	Angel dust, hog, PCP, AD, boat, black whack, amoeba, angel hair, angel smoke	Veterinary anesthetic	
Phencyclidine analogs	PCE, PCPy, TCP	None	Euphoria, relaxed inhibitions, increased appetite, disorientation
Other hallucinogens	Bufotenin, DMT, DET, ibogaine, psilocybin, psilocyn	None	
CANNABIS			
Marijuana	Acapulco gold, black Bart, black mote, blue sage, bobo, butterflowers, cannabis-T, cess, cheeba, grass, pot, sinsemilla, Thai sticks	Under investigation	Euphoria, relaxed inhibitions, increased appetite, disoriented behavior
Tetrahydrocannabinol	THC	Under investigation	
Hashish	Hash	None	
Hashish oil	Hash oil	None	
NARCOTICS			
Opium	Dover's powder, paregoric, Parapectolin, cruz, Chinese tobacco, China	Analgesic, antidiarrheal	Euphoria, drowsiness, respiratory depression, constricted pupils, nausea
Morphine	Morphine, Pectoal syrup, emsel, first line	Analgesic, antitussive	
Codeine	Codeine, Empirin compound with codeine, Robitussin A–C	Analgesic, antitussive	
Heroin	Diacetylmorphine, horse, smack, courage pills, dead on arrival (DOA)	Under investigation	

Table 7.2—*continued*

Hydromorphone	Dilaudid	Analgesic	Intoxication, excitation, disorientation, aggression, hallucination
Meperidine (pethidine)	Demerol, Pethadol	Analgesic	
Methadone	Dolophine, Methadone, Methadose	Analgesic, heroin substitute	
Other narcotics	Darvon,[†] Dromoran, Fentanyl, LAAM, Leitine, Levo-Dromoran, Percodan, Tussionex, Talwin,[†] Lomotil	Analgesic, antidiarrheal, antitussive	
INHALANTS			
Anesthetic gases	Aerosols, petroleum products, solvents	Surgical anesthetic	Intoxication, excitation, disorientation, aggression, hallucination, variable effects
Vasodilators (amyl nitrile, butyl nitrite)	Aerosols, petroleum products, solvents	None	

*Designated a narcotic under the Controlled Substances Act.
[†]Not designated a narcotic under the Controlled Substances Act.

Stimulants

In general, **stimulants** excite or increase the activity of the CNS. Also called "uppers," stimulants alert the CNS by increasing heart rate, blood pressure, and the rate of brain function. Users feel uplifted and less fatigued. Examples of stimulant drugs include caffeine, amphetamines, and cocaine. Most stimulants produce psychological dependence and tolerance relatively quickly, but they are unlikely to produce significant physical dependence when judged by life-threatening withdrawal symptoms. The important exception is cocaine, which seems to be capable of producing psychological dependence and withdrawal so powerful that continued use of the drug is inevitable in some users.

Caffeine

The methylxanthines are a family of chemicals that includes three compounds: caffeine, theophylline, and theobromine. Of these, caffeine is the most heavily consumed.

Caffeine is a tasteless drug found in coffee, tea, chocolate, many soft drinks, energy drinks, and several groups of over-the-counter drugs. It is a relatively harmless CNS stimulant when consumed in moderate amounts. Many coffee drinkers believe that they cannot start the day successfully without the benefit of a cup or two of coffee.

The chronic effects of long-term caffeine use are less clear. Chronic users show evidence of tolerance and withdrawal, indicating that they are physically dependent. Researchers have attempted to link caffeine to coronary heart disease, pancreatic cancer, and fibrocystic breast disease. So far, the results have been inconclusive, or, in some cases, inconsistent with those of other studies.

For the average healthy adult, moderate consumption of caffeine is unlikely to pose any serious health threat. However, excessive consumption (equivalent to eight or

Energy Drinks

Energy drinks have risen in popularity owing to the increased effect in alertness it gives consumers. Energy drinks contain caffeine, sugar, vitamins, amino acids, and a mixture of herbs. Students and athletes consume energy drinks to pull all-nighters or to boost performance, while party-goers mix them with alcohol. Health experts strongly advise consumers not to mix alcohol and energy drinks because of the dangerous effect it can have on the heart. Caffeine, like alcohol, is also diuretic and can cause dehydration.

Sources:
Cohen, E. "Energy Drinks Pack a Punch, but Is It Too Much?," *CNN.com*, May 29, 2001.
Associated Press. "'Energy Drinks' Stir Health Debate," *USA Today*, December 21, 2001.

more cups of coffee daily) could lead to anxiety, diarrhea, restlessness, delayed onset of sleep or frequent awakening, headache, and heart palpitations. Pregnant women are advised to avoid caffeine consumption.

Ephedra

Health professionals are warning people about the dangers of using any over-the-counter herbal supplement containing ephedra. Also known as *ma huang*, ephedra (Chapter 5) is an amphetaminelike drug that provides

> **Key Terms**
>
> **stimulants** psychoactive drugs that stimulate the function of the central nervous system

benefits to consumers who need to lose weight but[6] can be especially dangerous for people with hypertension or other cardiovascular disease. Presently, ephedra has been used in many over-the-counter decongestants and asthma drugs; warning labels indicate possible harmful side effects and drug interactions. The FDA announced its ban on ephedra in dietary supplements in April 2004.

Amphetamines

Amphetamines produce increased activity and mood elevation in almost all users. The amphetamines include several closely related compounds: amphetamine, dextroamphetamine, and methamphetamine. These compounds do not have any natural sources and are completely manufactured in the laboratory. Medical use of amphetamines is limited primarily to the treatment of obesity, narcolepsy, and attention deficit hyperactivity disorder (ADHD).

Amphetamines can be ingested, injected, or snorted (inhaled). At low-to-moderate doses, amphetamines elevate mood and increase alertness and feelings of energy by stimulating receptor sites for two naturally occurring neurotransmitters. They also slow the activity of the stomach and intestine and decrease hunger. In the 1960s and 1970s, amphetamines were commonly prescribed for dieters, but when it was discovered that the appetite suppression effect of amphetamines lasted only a few weeks, most physicians stopped prescribing them. At high doses, amphetamines can increase heart rate and blood pressure to dangerous levels. As amphetamines are eliminated from the body, the user becomes tired.

When chronically abused, amphetamines produce rapid tolerance and strong psychological dependence. Other effects of chronic use include impotence and episodes of psychosis. When use is discontinued, periods of depression may develop.

Methamphetamine

Today the abuse of amphetamines is a more pressing concern than it has been in the recent past because of the sharp increase in the abuse of methamphetamine. Known by a variety of names and forms, including "crank," "ice," "crystal," "meth," "speed," "crystal meth," "chalk," "fire," "glass," and "Zip," methamphetamine has a high potential for abuse and is produced in illegal home laboratories with over-the-counter ingredients.[8]

Methamphetamines can be smoked, ingested orally, snorted, or injected.

Crystal methamphetamine, glass or ice, is among the most dangerous forms of methamphetamine. Ice is a very pure form of methamphetamine that looks like rock candy.[9] When smoked or injected, the effects of ice are felt in about seven seconds as a wave of intense physical and psychological exhilaration. This effect lasts for several

Meth Lab Warning Signs

- Strong chemical odors (ammonia, ether, cat urine)
- Blocked out windows in the residence
- Renters who pay rent in cash
- A high-traffic area, especially at night
- Significant amount of trash (containers, fuel cans, coffee filters, duct tape)
- Clear glass containers being brought into the residence
- Items including but not limited to batteries, house cleaners, gasoline, automobile chemicals, hot plates, alcohol, ether, rock salts, and diet aids

If you suspect a meth lab in your neighborhood, please contact your local police department.

Source: KCI The Anti-Meth Site. *Is There a Meth Lab Cookin' in Your Neighborhood?* www.kci.org/meth_info/neighborhood_lab.htm, March 7, 2005.

hours (much longer than the effects of crack), until the user becomes physically exhausted. The user experiences a rush of pleasure that is the result of the drug telling the brain to release large amounts of dopamine.[10] When ingested orally or snorted, methamphetamine induces euphoria, which may result in quick addiction for the user.

Abuse can lead to memory loss, violence, anxiety, paranoia, euphoria, hyperthermia, convulsions, increased wakefulness and physical activity, and cardiac and neurological damage. Chronic use can result in Parkinsonlike symptoms, rotten teeth ("meth mouth"), stroke, anorexia, increased heart rate and blood pressure, death,[11] nutritional difficulties, weight loss, reduced resistance to infection, and damage to the liver, lungs, and kidneys. Psychological dependence is quickly established. Withdrawal causes acute depression and fatigue but not significant physical discomfort.

Key Terms

narcolepsy a sleep-related disorder in which a person has a recurrent, overwhelming, and uncontrollable desire to sleep, often at inappropriate times

attention deficit hyperactivity disorder (ADHD) an above-normal rate of physical movement; often accompanied by an inability to concentrate well on a specified task; also called *hyperactivity*

crystal methamphetamine a dangerous form of methamphetamine that quickly produces intense physical and psychological exhilaration when smoked

① **The nose:** as cocaine is snorted, nasal vessels immediately constrict and prohibit about 40% of the drug from entering the body. The remaining 60% enters the bloodstream.

② **The heart:** electrical impulses that regulate rhythmic pumping are impaired. Beating becomes irregular (arrhythmia). The heart can no longer supply itself with enough oxygenated blood.

③ **The brain:** dopamine and norepinephrine are released into the brain, producing a feeling of euphoria and confidence. Electrical signals to the heart are distorted, heart rate and pulse increase. A seizure may occur, causing coma and breathing stoppage.

④ **The heart:** blood circulation is out of control. The heart may simply flutter and stop, or it can be pumping so little oxygenated blood to the brain that the brain dies and the heart stops beating.

Figure 7-2   Cocaine's effects on the body

Ritalin

Although Ritalin has not historically been considered a significant drug of abuse, the recent surge in the prescribing of Ritalin for children and teens has become a subject of debate. In a recent year, 8 million prescriptions were written for children and adolescents.

Ritalin is typically prescribed to children to help focus attention if they are hyperactive or cannot concentrate. Critics argue that the drug is being prescribed to treat a variety of problems. Studies suggest that access to health care may influence a diagnosis of ADHD, when the better course of treatment would be to identify and treat the root cause of the problems.[12] Supporters respond that Ritalin enables their children to succeed in school (see the Star box on page 234).

Cocaine

Cocaine, perhaps the strongest of the stimulant drugs, has received much media attention. Cocaine is the primary psychoactive substance found in the leaves of the South American coca plant.[13] The effects of cocaine last only briefly—from 5 to 30 minutes (Figure 7-2). Regardless of the form in which it is consumed, cocaine produces an immediate, near-orgasmic "rush," or feeling of exhilaration. This euphoria is quickly followed by a period of marked depression. Used only occasionally as a topical anesthetic, cocaine is usually inhaled (snorted), injected, or smoked (typically as crack). There is overwhelming scientific evidence that users quickly develop a strong psychological dependence on cocaine. Considerable evidence suggests that physical dependence also rapidly develops. Cocaine users risk a weakened immune system making them "more susceptible to infections, including HIV."[14]

However, physical dependence on cocaine does not lead to death on withdrawal.

The status of cocaine as a substitute for amphetamines (during the 1960s), as a recreational drug for the wealthy (during the 1970s), and as a widely abused drug by many segments of society (during the 1980s) is well documented. During the 1990s, overall cocaine use decreased, although heavy use increased. In addition, the proportion of high school seniors who used cocaine at least once decreased from 9.8 percent in 1999 to 5 percent in 2000 and to 4.8 percent in 2001, about where it remained in 2003 according to the annual *Monitoring the*

Intravenous injection of cocaine results in an almost immediate high for the user.

Ritalin and Adderall Abuse on College Campuses

Ritalin and Adderall abuse on college campuses continue to rise. Studies have shown that one in every five college students has used Ritalin illegally. Adderall is a fairly new drug similar to Ritalin, and it is being abused like Ritalin. Students who take Ritalin or Adderall without a prescription are using these drugs to help enhance concentration during late-night study sessions, to obtain a cocaine-like high, or to suppress their appetites. However, students may not realize the serious side effects they can experience from taking these drugs illegally.

Side effects of Ritalin can include nervousness, insomnia, loss of appetite, headaches, increased heart and respiratory rates, dilated pupils, dry mouth, perspiration, and feelings of superiority. Higher doses can result in tremors, convulsions, paranoia, and/or a sensation of bugs crawling under the skin. These health risks are considerably higher if Ritalin is snorted. Death can occur from abusing Ritalin.

Side effects of Adderall are similar to those of Ritalin. These effects include loss of appetite, weight loss, insomnia, headache, and dizziness. Owing to a longer-lasting dose, Adderall has been growing in popularity. In comparison to Ritalin users, Adderall patients have experienced softer side effects, withdrawal symptoms, stomach discomfort, and mood changes. Adderall abuse can also result in death.

Sources:
The Johns Hopkins News-Letter. *Ritalin Abuse Is Increasing,* www.jhunewsletter.com/vnews/display.v/ART/2002/11/22/3ddd766faebeb, February 21, 2005.
The Johns Hopkins News-Letter. *Hopkins Students Turning to Drugs to Keep Grades Up,* www.jhunewsletter.com/vnews/display.v/ART/2004/04/02/406cd1793dfb2?in_archive=1, February 21, 2005.
Attention Deficit Disorder Help Center. *Adderall Side Effects,* www.add-adhd-help-center.com/adderall_side_effects.htm, February 21, 2005.

Future Study of drug use.[15] Studies have shown that the mean age of first cocaine use has declined from 22 years in the early 1980s to 21 years in the late 1990s to about 20.3 years in 2002.[13]

Crack Cocaine   Crack is made by combining cocaine hydrochloride with common baking soda. When this paste-like mixture is allowed to dry, a small rocklike crystalline material remains. This crack is heated in the bowl of a small pipe, and the vapors are inhaled into the lungs.[13] Some crack users spend hundreds of dollars a day to maintain their habit.

The effect of crack is almost instantaneous. Within ten seconds after inhalation, cocaine reaches the CNS and influences the action of several neurotransmitters at specific sites in the brain. As with the use of other forms of cocaine, convulsions, seizures, respiratory distress, and cardiac failure have been reported with this sudden, extensive stimulation of the nervous system.

Within about 6 minutes, the stimulating effect of crack has been completely expended, and users frequently become depressed. Dependence develops within a few weeks, because users consume more crack in response to the short duration of stimulation and rapid onset of depression.

Intravenous administration has been the preferred route for cocaine users who are also regular users of heroin and other injectable drugs. Intravenous injection results in an almost immediate high, which lasts about 10 minutes. A "smoother ride" is said to be obtained from a "speedball," the injectable mixture of heroin and cocaine (or methamphetamine).[4] However, such a mixture can be volatile and even fatal.

Freebasing   As inhaling crack did, freebasing developed as a technique for maximizing the psychoactive effects of cocaine. Freebasing first requires that the common form of powdered cocaine (cocaine hydrochloride) be chemically altered (alkalized). This altered form is then dissolved in a solvent such as ether or benzene. This liquid solution is heated to evaporate the solvent. The heating process leaves the freebase cocaine in a powder form that can then be smoked, often through a water pipe. Because of the large surface area of the lungs, smoking cocaine facilitates fast absorption into the bloodstream.

One danger of freebasing cocaine is the risk related to the solvents used. Ether is a highly volatile solvent capable of exploding and causing serious burns. Benzene is a known carcinogen associated with the development of leukemia. Clearly, neither solvent can be used without increasing the level of risk normally associated with cocaine use.

Depressants

Depressants (or sedatives) sedate the user, slowing down CNS function. Drugs included in this category are alcohol (see Chapter 8), barbiturates, and tranquilizers. Depressants produce tolerance in abusers, as well as strong psychological and physical dependence.

> **Key Terms**
>
> **depressants** a category of drugs that sedate the user by slowing CNS function; they produce tolerance and strong psychological and physical addiction in users

Barbiturates

Barbiturates are the so-called sleeping compounds that function by enhancing the effect of inhibitory neuro-transmitters. They depress the CNS to the point where the user drops off to sleep or, as is the case with surgical anesthetics, the patient becomes anesthetized. Medically, barbiturates are used in widely varied dosages as anesthetics and for treatment of anxiety, insomnia, and epilepsy.[3] Regular use of a barbiturate quickly produces tolerance—eventually such a high dose is required that the user still feels the effects of the drug throughout the next morning. Some abusers then begin to alternate barbiturates with stimulants, producing a vicious circle of dependence. Other misusers combine alcohol and barbiturates or tranquilizers, inadvertently producing toxic or even lethal results. Abrupt withdrawal from barbiturate use frequently produces a withdrawal syndrome that can involve seizures, delusions, hallucinations, and even death.

Methaqualone (Quaalude, "ludes," Sopor) was developed as a sedative that would not have the dependence properties of other barbiturates.[3] Quaaludes were occasionally prescribed for anxious patients. Today, compounds resembling Quaaludes are manufactured in home laboratories and sold illegally so that they can be combined with small amounts of alcohol for an inexpensive, drunklike effect.

Tranquilizers

Tranquilizers are depressants that are intended to reduce anxiety and to relax people who are having problems managing stress. They are not specifically designed to produce sleep but rather to help people cope with stress during their waking hours. Such tranquilizers are termed *minor tranquilizers,* of which alprazolam (Xanax),

diazepam (Valium), and chlordiazepoxide (Librium) may be the most commonly prescribed examples. Unfortunately, some people become addicted to these and other prescription drugs.[16]

Some tranquilizers are further designed to control hospitalized psychotic patients who may be suicidal or who are potential threats to others. These major *tranquilizers* subdue people physically but permit them to remain conscious. Their use is generally limited to institutional settings. All tranquilizers can produce physical and psychological dependence and tolerance.

"Date Rape" Depressants "Date rape" drugs or club drugs are commonly used on college campuses. These drugs are usually slipped into the drink of an unsuspecting woman or man and can result in a coma or even death.

Common "date rape" drugs include GHB (gamma-hydroxybutyrate), also known as G, liquid esctasy, Easy Lay, and Georgia Home Boy, and Rohypnol ("roophies"). When these drugs are consumed they cause a drunklike or sleepy state that can last for hours. During this time is when unsuspecting individuals are taken advantage of, against their will and sometimes against their knowledge. (For additional information see the Club Drugs Star box on page 229.)

High school and college students should not accept drinks from people they do not know. This recommendation extends to all parties where drinkers do not know what has been added to the punch or other drinks.[17]

Hallucinogens

As the name suggests, hallucinogenic drugs produce hallucinations—perceived distortions of reality. Also known as *psychedelic drugs,* or *phantasticants,* **hallucinogens** reached their height of popularity during the 1960s (see Learning from Our Diversity on page 235). At that time, young people were encouraged to use hallucinogenic drugs to "expand the mind," "reach an altered state," or "discover reality." Not all the reality distortions, or "trips," were pleasant. Many users reported "bummers," or trips during which they perceived negative, frightening distortions.

Hallucinogenic drugs include laboratory-produced lysergic acid diethylamide (LSD), mescaline (from the peyote cactus plant), and psilocybin (from a particular genus of mushroom). Consumption of hallucinogens seems to produce not physical dependence but mild levels of psychological dependence. The development of tolerance is questionable. **Synesthesia,** a sensation in which users report hearing a color, smelling music, or touching a taste, is sometimes produced with hallucinogen use.

The long-term effects of hallucinogenic drug use are not fully understood. Questions about genetic abnormalities in offspring, fertility, sex drive and performance, and the development of personality disorders have not been fully answered. One phenomenon that has been identified and documented is the development of flashbacks—the unpredictable return to a psychedelic trip that occurred months or even years earlier. Flashbacks are thought to result from the accumulation of a drug within body cells.

LSD

The most well-known and powerful hallucinogen is lysergic acid diethylamide (LSD). LSD was first isolated in 1938 by Albert Hoffmann, who was studying a group of chemicals that were extracted from a fungus that infects rye and other cereal grains. Five years later, he accidentally discovered its hallucinogenic effects. Dr. Timothy Leary helped to spread the popularity of LSD in the 1960s by promoting the use of LSD in mind expansion and experimentation. LSD helped define the counterculture movement of the 1960s. During the 1970s and the 1980s, this drug lost considerable popularity. LSD use peaked in 1996, with an annual prevalence of 8.8 percent. The 2003 *Monitoring the Future* reported a sharp decrease in LSD use among high school seniors, at 1.9 percent. The researchers suggest that this sharp decline may be due to an increase in Ecstasy use or a drop in LSD availability.[18]

LSD is manufactured in home laboratories and frequently distributed in absorbant blotter paper decorated with cartoon characters.[19] Users place the paper on their tongue or chew the paper to ingest the drug. LSD is similar in structure to the neurotransmitter serotonin and produces psychedelic effects by interfering with the normal activity of this neurotransmitter. The effects can include altered perception of shapes, images, time, sound, and body form. Synesthesia is common to LSD users. LSD

is metabolized in the liver and excreted. Its effects last an average of six to nine hours.

Users may describe LSD experiences as positive and "mind-expanding," or negative and "mind-constricting," depending on the user's mood and the social setting in which the drug is taken. Positive sensations include feelings of creativity, deep understanding of oneself and the universe, and feelings of grandeur. Although LSD users report feelings of increased insight and creativity, a real increase in these skills has not been demonstrated. At the same time, some reports of bad trips on LSD are thought to have been caused by other substances, such as PCP, that were sold to the user as LSD. Deaths resulting from bizarre behavior after taking LSD have been reported. Dangerous side effects include panic attacks, flashbacks, and occasional prolonged psychosis.

Although the typical doses ("hits") today are about half as powerful as those in the 1960s, users still tend to develop high tolerance to LSD. Physical dependence does not occur.

Designer Drugs

In recent years, chemists who produce many of the illicit drugs in home laboratories have designed versions of drugs listed on **FDA Schedule 1.** Under the Controlled Substances Act, substances regulated by the Food and Drug Administration are placed in one of five schedules. Schedule 1 contains the most dangerous drugs that have no medical use.[20] Designer drugs are similar to the controlled drugs on the FDA Schedule 1 but are sufficiently different so that they escape governmental control. The designer drugs are either newly synthesized products that are similar to already outlawed drugs but against which no law yet exists, or they are reconstituted or renamed illegal substances. Designer drugs are said to produce effects similar to their controlled drug counterparts.

People who use designer drugs do so at great risk because the manufacturing of these drugs is unregulated. The neurophysiological effect of these homemade drugs can be quite dangerous. So far, a synthetic heroin product

> ### Key Terms
>
> **hallucinogens** psychoactive drugs capable of producing hallucinations (distortions of reality)
>
> **synesthesia** a sensation of combining of the senses, such as perceiving color by hearing it or perceiving taste by touching it
>
> **FDA Schedule 1** a list of drugs that have a high potential for abuse but no medical use

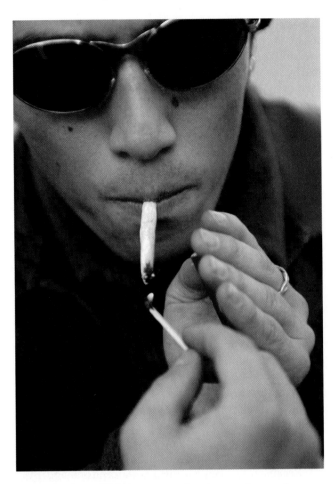

Marijuana is considered a gateway drug because its use often leads the user to heavier drug use.

(MPPP) and several amphetamine derivatives with hallucinogenic properties have been designed for the unwary drug consumer.

DOM (STP), MDA (the "love drug"), and ecstacy ("MDMA" or "XTC") are examples of amphetamine-derivative, hallucinogenic designer drugs. These drugs produce mild LSD-like hallucinogenic experiences, positive feelings, and enhanced alertness. They also have a number of potentially dangerous effects. These dangers include increased heart rate and blood pressure, muscle tension, involuntary teeth clenching, nausea, blurred vision, faintness, and chills or sweating. MDMA use can also cause hyperthermia from a sharp increase in body temperature, which can result in kidney, liver, and cardiovascular system failure.[21] Experts are particularly concerned that MDMA can produce strong psychological dependence and can deplete serotonin, an important excitatory neurotransmitter associated with a state of alertness. Permanent brain damage is possible.[3] On a positive note, one recent major survey indicates that MDMA use is declining among teens. In 2001, 9.2 percent of high school seniors reported using MDMA. In 2002, 7.4 percent reported using MDMA, and in 2003 the percentage declined to 4.5 percent.[22]

Phencyclidine

Phencyclidine (PCP, "angel dust") is unique because it not only produces hallucinogenic effects but also acts as an analgesic, a depressant, a stimulant, and an anesthetic. This makes the typical PCP experience impossible to predict or describe. The physical effects of PCP begin a few minutes after consumption and continue for four to six hours. PCP was studied for years during the 1950s and 1960s and was found to be an unsuitable animal and human anesthetic.[23]

Manufactured in tablet or powder form, PCP can be injected, inhaled, taken orally, or smoked. Some users report mild euphoria, although most report bizarre perceptions, paranoid feelings, and aggressive behavior. PCP overdose may cause convulsions, cardiovascular collapse, and damage to the brain's respiratory center.

In a number of cases the aggressive behavior caused by PCP has led users to commit brutal crimes against both friends and innocent strangers. PCP accumulates in cells and may stimulate bizarre behavior months after initial use.

PCP is an extremely unpredictable drug. Although PCP has been blamed in many reports of bizarre, even homicidal, behavior, it continues to be abused. Because PCP is easily and cheaply manufactured in home laboratories, authorities have difficulty limiting its availability.

Cannabis

Cannabis (marijuana) has been labeled a mild hallucinogen for a number of years. However, most experts now consider it to be a drug category in itself. Marijuana produces mild effects like those of stimulants and

Thai sticks are a potent form of marijuana.

depressants. The recent implication of marijuana in a large number of traffic fatalities makes this drug one whose consumption should be carefully considered. Marijuana is actually a wild plant (*Cannabis sativa*) whose fibers were once used in the manufacture of hemp rope. When the leafy material and small stems are dried and crushed, users can smoke the mixture in rolled cigarettes ("joints"), cigars ("blunts"), or pipes. The resins collected from scraping the flowering tops of the plant yield a marijuana product called hashish, or hash, commonly smoked in a pipe.[24]

The potency of marijuana's hallucinogenic effect is determined by the percentage of the active ingredient, tetrahydrocannabinol (THC), present in the product. The concentration of THC averages about 3.5 percent for regular grade marijuana, 7–9 percent for higher-quality marijuana (sinsemilla), 8–14 percent for hashish, and as high as 50 percent for hash oil.[3] Today's marijuana has THC levels that are higher than in past decades.

THC is a fat-soluble substance and thus is absorbed and retained in fat tissues within the body. Before being excreted, THC can remain in the body for up to a month. With the sophistication of today's drug tests, trace metabolites of THC can be detected for up to 30 days after consumption.[3] It is possible that the THC that comes from passive inhalation of high doses (for example, during an indoor rock concert) can also be detected for a short time after exposure.

Once marijuana is consumed, its effects vary from person to person (see Table 7.3). Being "high" or "stoned" means different things to different people. Many people report heightened sensitivity to music, cravings for particular foods, and a relaxed mood. There is widespread consensus that marijuana's behavioral effects include four probabilities: (1) Users must learn to recognize what a marijuana high is like, (2) marijuana impairs short-term memory, (3) users overestimate the passage of time, and (4) users lose the ability to maintain attention to a task.[3]

The long-term effects of marijuana use are still being studied. Chronic abuse may lead to an amotivational syndrome in some people. Heavy marijuana users have trouble paying attention and retaining new information for at least a day after last using the drug, according to a recent study.

The irritating effects of marijuana smoke on lung tissue are more pronounced than those of cigarette smoke, and some of the more than 400 chemicals in marijuana are now linked to lung cancer development. In fact, one of the most potent carcinogens, benzopyrene, is found in higher levels in marijuana smoke than in tobacco smoke. Marijuana smokers tend to inhale deeply and hold the smoke in the lungs for long periods. It is likely that at some point the lungs of chronic marijuana smokers will be damaged.

Long-term marijuana use is also associated with damage to the immune system and to the male and female reproductive systems and with an increase in birth defects in babies born to mothers who smoke marijuana. Chronic marijuana use lowers testosterone levels in men, but the effect of this change is not known. The effect of long-term marijuana use on a variety of types of sexual behavior is also not fully understood.

Because the drug can distort perceptions and thus perceptual ability (especially when combined with alcohol), its use by automobile drivers clearly jeopardizes the lives of many innocent people.

Table 7.3 Effects of Marijuana

Short-Term Effects	Long-Term Effects
• Increased heart rate and blood pressure • Feeling of elation • Drowsiness and sedation • Increased appetite • Red eyes • Food cravings • Slow reaction time • Feelings of depression, excitement, paranoia, panic, and euphoria • Problems with attention span, memory, learning, problem-solving, and coordination • Sleeplessness[1]	• Lung damage • Increased risk of bronchitis • Emphysema • Lung cancer • Heart attack[2] • Loss of motivation and short-term memory • Increased panic or anxiety • May become tolerant to marijuana • Damage to lungs, immune system, and reproductive organs • Can remain in the body for up to a month • Can cause birth defects • Five times more damaging to the lungs than tobacco products[1]

[1]National Institute on Drug Abuse. National Institutes of Health, *NIDA Research Report-Marijuana Abuse,* www.nida.nih.gov/ResearchReports/Marijuana/default.html, February 15, 2005.
[2]"Stronger Marijuana Is Major Health Risk," *The Independent,* February 1, 2001.

Medical Marijuana Ruling

In May of 2001, the United States Supreme Court ruled that the distribution of marijuana for medicinal purposes to people in California must be stopped. The court decided in an 8–0 decision that there is no medical necessity exception to the federal laws prohibiting the manufacturing and distribution of marijuana. This Supreme Court ruling does not overturn similar state laws in Alaska, Arizona, Hawaii, Maine, Nevada, Oregon, and Washington where these laws have made it possible for seriously ill patients to grow (or purchase) marijuana for pain relief, when recommended by a physician. This ruling allows the federal government to prosecute individuals for the manufacturing and distribution of marijuana even though some state laws might have decriminalized medical marijuana use.[1] In June 2005, the U.S. Supreme Court ruled in a 6–3 decision that the federal government can continue to ban the use of medicinal marijuana. Individuals who use marijuana for medicinal purposes risk federal legal action with state laws providing no defense. The government's position is that marijuana is not a safe product, has no medical purpose, and cannot be administered safely under medical supervision, and conflicts with the Controlled Substance Act.

Proponents of medical marijuana argue that marijuana can act as an appetite stimulant, muscle relaxant, and pain reliever, and that it can treat the following conditions:

- Nausea resulting from cancer treatment

- Appetite loss in persons with AIDS

- Pain from diseases such as multiple sclerosis

- Eye pressure and pain resulting from glaucoma

In 1985, the FDA approved the drug dronabinol (Marinol) for use by cancer chemotherapy patients who were experiencing nausea. Marinol is a capsule that contains a controlled amount of marijuana's active ingredient, THC. In 1993, the FDA approved Marinol for use as an appetite stimulant in persons with AIDS. Proponents of medical marijuana, however, believe that the THC dose is better controlled and more effective (and thus safer) when taken by smoking the raw plant material.

[1] *The United States* v. *Oakland Cannabis Buyer's Co-op.*, (2001), 121 S. Ct. 1711.

The only medical uses for marijuana are to relieve the nausea caused by chemotherapy, to improve appetite in AIDS patients, and to ease the pressure that builds up in the eyes of glaucoma patients. However, a variety of other drugs, many of which are nearly as effective, are also used for these purposes. The U.S. Supreme Court recently struck a blow to the proponents of the medical use of marijuana (see the Star box above).

Narcotics

The **narcotics** are among the strongest dependence-producing drugs. Medically, narcotics are used to relieve pain and induce sleep. On the basis of origin, narcotics can be subgrouped into the natural, quasisynthetic, and synthetic narcotics.

Natural Narcotics

Naturally occurring substances derived from the Oriental poppy plant include opium (the primary psychoactive substance extracted from the Oriental poppy), morphine (the primary active ingredient in opium), and thebaine (a compound not used as a drug). Morphine and related compounds have medical use as analgesics in the treatment of mild to severe pain.

Quasisynthetic Narcotics

Quasisynthetic narcotics are compounds created by chemically altering morphine. These laboratory-produced drugs are intended to be used as analgesics, but their benefits are largely outweighed by a high dependence rate and a great risk of toxicity. The best known of the quasisynthetic narcotics is heroin. Although heroin is a fast-acting and very effective analgesic, it is extremely addictive. Heroin can be inhaled ("snorted"), smoked, injected into a vein, or "skin-popped" (injected beneath the skin surface). Heroin produces dreamlike euphoria and, like all narcotics, strong physical and psychological dependence and tolerance.

Most new heroin users are smoking or snorting heroin, rather than injecting the drug. Many new heroin users are also young, with one-quarter of the new users of heroin being under age 18, while nearly half are age 18 to 25.[25]

Heroin users who inject the drug face an additional risk. As with the use of all other injectable illegal drugs, the practice of sharing needles increases the likelihood of transmission of various communicable diseases, including hepatitis C and HIV (see Chapter 13). Abrupt withdrawal from heroin use is rarely fatal, but the discomfort during **cold turkey** withdrawal is reported to be overwhelming.

Key Terms

narcotics opiates; psychoactive drugs derived from the Oriental poppy plant; narcotics relieve pain and induce sleep

cold turkey immediate, total discontinuation of use of a drug; associated withdrawal discomfort

Synthetic Narcotics

Meperidine (Demerol) and propoxyphene (Darvon), common postsurgical painkillers, and methadone, the drug prescribed during the rehabilitation of heroin addicts, are synthetic narcotics. These opiatelike drugs are manufactured in medical laboratories. They are not natural narcotics or quasisynthetic narcotics because they do not originate from the Oriental poppy plant. Like true narcotics, however, these drugs can rapidly induce physical dependence. One important criticism of methadone rehabilitation programs is that they merely shift the addiction from heroin to methadone. (See the Star Box on OxyContin above.)

Inhalants

Inhalants constitute a class of drugs that includes a variety of volatile (quickly evaporating) compounds that generally produce unpredictable, drunklike effects in users and feelings of euphoria.[26] Users of inhalants may also have some delusions and hallucinations. Some users may become quite aggressive. Drugs in this category include anesthetic gases (chloroform, nitrous oxide, and ether), vasodilators (amyl nitrite and butyl nitrite), petroleum products and commercial solvents (gasoline, kerosene, plastic cement, glue, typewriter correction fluid, paint, and paint thinner), and certain aerosols (found in some propelled spray products, fertilizers, and insecticides).

Most of the danger in using inhalants lies in the damaging, sometimes fatal effects on the respiratory and cardiovascular systems.[26] Furthermore, users may unknowingly place themselves in dangerous situations because of the drunklike hallucinogenic effects. Aggressive behavior might also make users a threat to themselves and others.

For more information about inhalants, contact the National Inhalant Prevention Coalition at www.inhalants.org.

Society's Response to Drug Use

During the last 25 years, society has responded to illegal drug use with growing concern. Most adults see drug abuse as a clear danger to society. This position has been supported by the development of community, school, state, and national organizations interested in the reduction of illegal drug use. These organizations have included such diverse groups as Parents Against Drugs, Parents for a Drug-Free Youth, Drug Abuse Resistance Education (DARE), Mothers Against Drunk Driving (MADD), Narcotics Anonymous, and the federal Drug Enforcement Administration. Certain groups have concentrated their efforts on education, others on enforcement, and still others on the development of laws and public policy.

The personal and social issues related to drug abuse are very complex. Innovative solutions continue to be devised. Some believe that only through early childhood education will people learn alternatives to drug use. Starting drug education in the preschool years may have a more positive effect than waiting until the upper elementary or junior high school years. The focus on reducing young people's exposure to gateway drugs (especially tobacco, alcohol, and marijuana) may help slow down the move to other addictive drugs. Some people advocate much harsher penalties for drug use and drug trafficking, including extreme measures such as public executions.

Key Terms

inhalants psychoactive drugs that enter the body through inhalation

Preemployment Drug Testing: An Invasion of Privacy?

Drug abuse in the workplace is a growing concern. In factories, stores, and offices, employee drug use is suspected to be the cause of one-third to one-half of all absenteeism, accidents, medical claims, insubordination, thefts, and loss of productivity.

In response, more than half of Fortune 500 companies have instituted mandatory preemployment drug screening. Prospective employees of these firms are required to pass one or more drug tests to be considered for employment. Preemployment screening is also becoming more popular in the public employment sector. Such drug testing is controversial in several ways.

Supporters of mandatory preemployment drug screening argue that employers have an obligation to provide a safe and healthy work environment. They also contend that drug abuse is driving the cost of health care to ever-higher levels. Workers' compensation costs are also high, perhaps in part because of an increase in drug-related accidents and the chronic nature of drug-related illnesses. Employers also say that those who have taken drugs and have failed a drug screening have already broken the law and thus have forfeited their right to be considered for employment.

Opponents of preemployment screening express two concerns. First, they argue that the validity and reliability of screening tests are too low. If 1 million tests are performed in a year, a conservative estimate, and .05 percent of those tests yield false positives, also a conservative estimate, then 500 people may be fired from their jobs or not offered jobs for which they are qualified, according to the American Civil Liberties Union (ACLU).

The second concern is that employers invade the privacy of applicants by assuming them guilty until proved innocent by the testing laboratory. Privacy is invaded in two ways, says the ACLU. First, the specimen-collection process itself often involves direct or indirect observation to prevent tampering by the employee. Even indirect observation can be degrading. Typically, employees must remove all outer garments and urinate in a bathroom in which the water supply has been cut off. A second search takes place in the lab. Urinalysis can reveal not only the presence of illegal drugs, but also many other physical and medical conditions, such as medication for epilepsy, hypertension, or diabetes; a genetic predisposition to heart disease or cancer; and pregnancy. Employees are usually required to fill out forms listing all the medications they currently are taking, a clear invasion of privacy, says the ACLU.

Do you feel that mandatory preemployment drug screening is justified? Do you feel that it is an invasion of privacy? Would you agree to take a preemployment drug test as a condition of employment?

Others support legalizing all drugs and making governmental agencies responsible for drug regulation and control, as is the case with alcohol. Advocates of this position believe that drug-related crime and violence would virtually cease once the demand for illegal products is reduced. Sound arguments can be made on both sides of this issue. What is your opinion?

Unless significant changes in society's response to drug use take place soon, the disastrous effects of virtually uncontrolled drug abuse will continue to be felt. Families and communities will continue to be plagued by drug-related tragedies. Law enforcement officials will be pressed to the limits of their resources in their attempts to reduce drug flow. Our judicial system will be heavily burdened by thousands of court cases. Health care facilities could face overwhelming numbers of patients.

In comparison with other federally funded programs, the "war on drugs" is less expensive than farm support, food stamps, Medicare, and national defense. However, it remains to be seen whether any amount of money spent on enforcement, without adequate support for education, treatment, and poverty reduction, can reduce the illegal drug demand and supply. Currently, approximately $19.2 billion is spent to fight the drug war in the United States—$13 billion on law enforcement (supply reduction) and $6.2 billion on education, prevention, and treatment (demand reduction).[27]

Drug Testing

Drug testing is one of society's responses to drug use and is becoming an increasingly popular prevention tool. In 1986 the federal government instituted drug-testing policies for federal employees in safety-sensitive jobs. In 1988 the Drug Free Workplace Act extended the drug-free federal policy to include all federal grantees (including universities) and most federal contractors. Although this act did not mandate drug testing, it encouraged tougher approaches to prevent and deal with drug problems at the work site.

Private companies have developed drug-testing procedures similar to those used with federal agencies. Most Fortune 500 companies use drug testing to screen applicants or monitor employee drug use.

Drug tests commonly search for amphetamines, barbiturates, benzodiazepines (the chemical bases for prescription tranquilizers such as Valium and Librium), cannabinoids (THC, hashish, and marijuana), methaqualone, opiates (heroin, codeine, and morphine), and PCP. With the exception of marijuana, most traces of these drugs are eliminated by the body within a few days after use. Marijuana can remain detectable for up to 30 days after use.

How accurate are the results of drug testing? At typical cutoff standards, drug tests are likely to identify 90 percent of recent drug users. This means that about 10 percent of recent users will pass undetected. (These 10 percent are

Acupuncture involves the insertion of very fine needles on the body's surface to help influence the body's physiological functioning. Although many people in the Western world think of acupuncture as a new alternative type of medicine, the practice has been a part of Chinese medicine for thousands of years.

Acupuncture theory holds that there is an energy force that runs throughout the body on special pathways called *meridians*. When the meridians become unbalanced, perhaps through various obstructions, deficiencies, or excesses, the body can become sick. Acupuncture restores the balance in the energy forces and helps return the body to good health.

Acupuncture has been used to treat a number of health conditions. Among these are low back pain, headaches, arthritis, and relief of muscle spasms. According to the National Institutes of Health (NIH) 1997 Consensus Statement,[1] acupuncture may be helpful in treating musculoskeletal conditions, such as fibromyalgia, myofacial pain, and tennis elbow. Additionally, postoperative pain and low back pain seem to respond well to acupuncture. The NIH Consensus Panel reported that there is clear evidence that needle acupuncture reduces adult postoperative nausea and chemotherapy nausea and vomiting, and it may reduce the nausea of pregnancy.

However, the Consensus Statement indicated that there was insufficient evidence to demonstrate that acupuncture was significantly helpful in promoting the cessation of smoking and some other conditions. Studies suggest that acupuncture can help reduce drug cravings.[2] Certainly, interest in the practice of Eastern medicine is increasing in the United States, and studies are underway to examine the benefits of acupuncture in treating addictions. However, because there are so many factors that impact on a person's ability to be successfully treated, it will be difficult to isolate acupuncture as the sole reason for treatment success.

It is likely that acupuncture will eventually be viewed as one of a number of beneficial approaches used in a comprehensive drug treatment program. Acupuncture will probably be helpful to some people and not so helpful to others.

If you had a drug addiction, would you be willing to try acupuncture? Why or why not?

[1] *Acupuncture,* National Institutes of Health Consensus Statement Online, 3–5 November 1997; 15(5): 1–34.
[2] Leinwand D. "Study: Acupuncture Cuts Cocaine Cravings: Counseling, Recovery Programs Also Advised," *USA Today,* August 14, 2000.

considered *false negatives.*) Nonusers whose drug tests indicate drug use (*false positives*) are quite rare. (Follow-up tests on these false positives would nearly always show negative results.) Human errors are probably more responsible than technical errors for inaccuracies in drug tests.

Recently, scientists have been refining procedures that use hair samples to detect the presence of drugs. These procedures seem to hold much promise, although certain technical obstacles remain. Watch for refinements in hair-sample drug testing in the near future.

Do you think that the possibility of having to take a drug test would have any effect on college students' use of drugs? Do you think that drug testing is an acceptable method of prevention? See the Star box on page 241 for differing viewpoints.

College and Community Support Services for Drug Dependence

Students who have drug problems and realize they need assistance might select assistance based on the services available on campus or in the surrounding community and the costs they are willing to pay for treatment services.

One recently developed approach to convince drug-dependent people to enter treatment programs is the use of *confrontation.* People who live or work with chemically dependent people are being encouraged to confront them directly about their addiction. Direct confrontation helps chemically dependent people realize the effect their behavior has on others. Once chemically dependent people realize that others will no longer tolerate their behavior, the likelihood of their entering treatment programs is increased significantly. Although effective, this approach is very stressful for family members and friends and requires the assistance of professionals in the field of chemical dependence. These professionals can be contacted at a drug treatment center in your area.

Treatment

Comprehensive drug treatment programs are available in very few college or university health centers. College settings for drug dependence programs are more commonly found in the university counseling center. At such a center the emphasis will probably be not on the medical management of dependence but on the behavioral dimensions of drug abuse. Trained counselors and psychologists who specialize in chemical dependence counseling will work with students to (1) analyze their particular concerns, (2) establish constructive ways to cope with stress, and (3) search for alternative ways to achieve new "highs" (see the Personal Assessment on page 247).

Medical treatment for the management of drug problems may need to be obtained through the services of a community treatment facility administered by a local health department, community mental health center, private clinic, or local hospital. Treatment may be on an inpatient or outpatient basis. Medical management might include detoxification, treatment of secondary health complications and nutritional deficiencies, and therapeutic counseling related to chemical dependence (see the Considering Complementary Care box on page 242).

Some communities have voluntary health agencies that deliver services and treatment programs for drug-dependent people. Check your telephone book for listings of drug treatment facilities. Some communities have drug hot lines that offer advice for people with questions about drugs. (See Changing for the Better above for a list of antidrug abuse organizations and hot line numbers.)

 TALKING POINTS Do you think that confronting a friend about her regular marijuana use will prompt her to seek treatment?

Costs of Treatment for Dependence

Drug treatment programs that are administered by colleges and universities for faculty and students usually require no fees. Local agencies may provide either free services or services based on a **sliding scale.** Private hospitals, physicians, and clinics are the most expensive forms of treatment. Inpatient treatment at a private facility may cost as much as $1,000 per day. Since the length of inpatient treatment averages three to four weeks, a patient can quickly accumulate a very large bill. However, with many types of health insurance policies now providing coverage for alcohol addiction and other types of drug dependence, even these services may not require additional out-of-pocket expenses.

Key Terms

sliding scale a method of payment by which patient fees are scaled according to income

- Assess your knowledge of drug use by completing the Personal Assessment on page 247–249.
- Calculate the amount of caffeine you consume daily. If you're drinking more than three cups of caffeinated beverages per day, develop a plan to reduce your overall intake.

- Prepare a plan of action to use if someone you know needs professional assistance with a drug problem.
- Identify five activities that can provide you with a drug-free high.
- Analyze your drug use patterns (if any), and assess the likelihood that you might fail a pre-employment drug test.

- Assess your lifestyle for addictive behaviors that do not involve drugs, such as over-exercising or watching too much TV. Develop a plan to moderate these activities and achieve more balance in your life.

SUMMARY

- Abuse of drugs takes a tremendous toll on human lives and has a devastating effect on society.
- Primary prevention of drug abuse targets individuals and groups to reach people who have not used illegal drugs and reduce their desire to try drugs.
- Secondary prevention targets people who are beginning to use drugs.
- Tertiary prevention (third-level prevention) targets people who are drug dependent, such as crack or heroin addicts, and their families.
- Drugs affect the CNS by altering neurotransmitter activity on neurons.
- The addiction process has three components: exposure, compulsion, and loss of control.
- A drug is any substance, natural or artificial, other than food, that by its chemical nature alters structure or function in the living organism.
- Psychoactive drugs alter the user's feelings, behavior, perceptions, or moods.
- Physical drug dependence occurs when body cells become reliant on a drug, causing withdrawal illness if the drug is not taken.

- Tolerance to a drug has developed when continued intake of the same dose has diminishing effects.
- Psychological drug dependence occurs when a user has a strong desire to continue using a particular drug and believes that he or she must use the drug to maintain a sense of well-being.
- Drug misuse is the inappropriate use of legal drugs intended to be medications.
- Drug abuse is any use of an illegal drug or use of a legal drug in a way that is detrimental to health and well-being.
- Individual, environmental, and societal factors influence drug taking behavior.
- Combination drug effects include synergistic, additive, potentiated, and antagonistic effects.
- Psychoactive drugs are classified as stimulants, depressants, hallucinogens, cannabis, narcotics, or inhalants.
- Society has responded to drug use with educational programs, law enforcement efforts, and legislation and public policy.
- Drug testing can be used as a means of primary, secondary, or tertiary prevention.

REVIEW QUESTIONS

1. Explain the terms *primary prevention, secondary prevention,* and *tertiary prevention,* and give examples of each.
2. Describe how neurotransmitters work.
3. Identify and explain the three steps in the process of addiction.
4. How is the term *drug* defined in this chapter? What are psychoactive drugs? How do medicines differ from drugs?
5. Explain what *dependence* means. Identify and explain the two types of dependence.
6. Define the word *tolerance.* What does *cross-tolerance* mean? Give an example of cross-tolerance.
7. Differentiate between drug misuse and drug abuse.
8. Identify some individual, environmental, and societal factors that affect drug abuse.
9. Explain the terms *synergistic effect, additive effect, potentiated effect,* and *antagonistic effect.*

10. List the six general categories of drugs. For each category, give several examples of drugs and explain the effects they would have on the user. What are designer drugs?
11. What are the side effects and health risks of abusing Ritalin.
12. What is the active ingredient in marijuana? What are its common effects on the user? What are the long-term effects of marijuana use?
13. Identify three or four so-called "club-drugs" and describe how they can cause serious medical problems.
14. How accurate is drug testing?
15. Describe several drug treatment services that are available. Who administers these services and how do their approaches differ?

ENDNOTES

1. Tricker, R. *Preventing Substance Use in Young Athletes,* www.tpronline.org, February 11, 2005.

2. Shier D, Butler J, Lewis R. *Hole's Essentials of Human Anatomy and Physiology* (9th ed.). New York: McGraw-Hill, 2002.

3. Ray O, Ksir C. *Drugs, Society, and Human Behavior* (10th ed.). New York: McGraw-Hill, 2004.

4. Pinger RR, Payne WA, Hahn DB, Hahn EJ. *Drugs: Issues for Today* (3rd ed.). New York: McGraw-Hill, 1998.

5. Substance Abuse and Mental Health Services Administration (SAMHSA). *Overview of Findings from the 2003 National Survey on Drug Use and Health,* http://oas.samhsa.gov/nhsda/2k3nsduh/2k3overview.htm, February 12, 2005.

6. Ephedra Education Council. *Ephedra Supported by Science—A Ban Is Not, Industry Tells FDA,* April 8, 2003.

7. U.S. Food and Drug Administration. FDA Statement. *FDA Announces Rule Prohibiting Sale of Dietary Supplements Containing Ephedrine Alkaloids Effective April 12,* www.fda.gov/bbs/topics/NEWS/2004/NEW01050.html, April 12, 2004.

8. National Institute on Drug Abuse. National Institutes of Health. *NIDA Research Report-Methamphetamine Abuse and Addiction,* www.nida.nih.gov/ResearchReports/Methamph/Methamph.html. NIH Publication, No. 02-4210, January 2002.

9. U.S. Department of Justice. Drug Enforcement Administration. *Methemphetamine,* www.usdoj.gov/dea/concern/meth.htm, December 31, 2001.

10. Frackelmann, K. Breaking bonds of addiction: Compulsion traced to part of the brain, *USA Today,* April 18, 2002.

11. National Institute on Drug Abuse. National Institutes of Health. NIDA InfoFacts *Methamphetamine,* www.nida.nih.gov/Infofax/methamphetamine.html, March 7, 2005.

12. Attention deficit rate tops estimates, *Cox News Service,* May 22, 2002.

13. U.S. Department of Justice. Drug Enforcement Administration. *Drugs of Abuse,* www.dea.gov/pubs/abuse/5-stim.htm, 2005 Edition.

14. Cocaine weakens immune system, *Boston Herald,* March 7, 2003.

15. Johnston LD, O'Malley PM, Bachman JG, Schulenberg, JE. *Monitoring the Future: National Results on Adolescent Drug Use: Overview of Key Findings, 2003.* University of Michigan Institute for Social Research, www.monitoringthefuture.org/pubs/monographs/overview2003.pdf, NIH Publication No. 04-5506. Bethesda, MD: 2004.

16. National Institute on Drug Abuse. National Institutes of Health. *NIDA Research Report-Prescription Drugs Abuse and Addiction,* www.drugabuse.gov/ResearchReports/Prescription/Prescription.html, NIH Publication No. 01-4881, July 2001.

17. National Institute on Drug Abuse. *NIDA InfoFacts—Rohypnol and GHB,* www.nida.nih.gov/Infofax/RohypnolGHB.html, February 14, 2004.

18. Johnston LD, O'Malley PM, Bachman JG, Schulenberg, JE. *Monitoring the Future: National Survey Results on Drug Use: 1975–2003. Volume I: Secondary School Students,* www.monitoringthefuture.org/ pubs/monographs/voll_2003.pdf. NIH Publication No. 04-5507. Bethesda, MD: 2004.

19. National Institute on Drug Abuse. *NIDA InfoFacts—LSD,* www.nida.nih.gov/Infofax/lsd.html, February 15, 2005.

20. U.S. Drug Enforcement Administration. Controlled Substances Act, www.usdoj.gov/dea/agency/csa.htm, Feburary 16, 2005.

21. National Institute on Drug Abuse. National Institutes of Health. *NIDA InfoFacts—MDMA (Ecstasy),* www.nida.nih.gov/Infofax/ecstasy.html, February 16, 2005.

22. Johnston LD, O'Malley PM, Bachman JG, Schulenberg, JE National Press Release, *Overall Teen Drug Use Continues Gradual Decline; but Use of Inhalants Rises.* University of Michigan News and Information Services, Ann Arbor, MI: December 21, 2004.

23. National Institute on Drug Abuse. National Institutes of Health, *NIDA InfoFacts—PCP (Phencyclidine),* www.nida.nih.gov/Infofax/pcp.html, February 15, 2005.

24. National Institute on Drug Abuse. National Institutes of Health, *NIDA InfoFacts—Marijuana,* www.nida.nih.gov/Infofax/marijuana.html, February 16, 2005.

25. Leinwand, D. Heroin's resurgence closes drug's traditional gender gap: Teenage girls are increasingly falling prey to narcotic in purer, 'more mainstream,' sniffable form, *USA Today,* May 9, 2000.

26. Frackelmann, K. Inhalants' hidden treat: Access makes huffing popular but kids can recover with help, *USA Today,* June 25, 2002.

27. www.whitehousedrugpolicy.gov/publications/policy/04budget/exec_sum.pdf, May 21, 2003.

An anti-methamphetamine bill has been advancing in Congress to restrict the sales of over-the-counter cold medicines that contain pseudoephedrine, such as Sudafed, NyQuil, and Tylenol Cold, which are used in home laboratories to make methamphetamine. This bill will require consumers to present a photo identification card, sign a log, and be limited to a particular number of grams of pseudoephedrine bought in a 30-day period. Computer tracking would also prevent consumers from purchasing pseudoephedrine in other stores. Walgreen Company announced that they would move all pseudoephedrine products behind the pharmacy counter nationwide in October 2005. Other retailers are restricting sales of pseudoephedrine to help curb methamphetamine production.

personal assessment

Test your drug awareness

1. What is the most commonly used drug in the United States?
   a. heroin
   b. cocaine
   c. alcohol
   d. marijuana

2. Name the three drugs most commonly used by children.
   a. alcohol, tobacco, and marijuana
   b. cocaine, crack, alcohol
   c. heroin, inhalants, marijuana

3. Which drug is associated with the most teenage deaths?
   a. heroin
   b. cocaine
   c. alcohol
   d. marijuana

4. By the 8th grade, how many kids have tried at least one inhalant?
   a. 1 in 100
   b. 1 in 50
   c. 1 in 25
   d. 1 in 5
   e. 1 in 2

5. "Crack" is a particularly dangerous drug because it is
   a. cheap.
   b. readily available.
   c. highly addictive.
   d. all of the above.

6. Fumes from which of the following can be inhaled to produce a high?
   a. spray paint
   b. model glue
   c. nail polish remover
   d. whipped cream canisters
   e. all of the above

7. People who have not used alcohol and other drugs before their 20th birthday:
   a. have no risk of becoming chemically dependent.
   b. are less likely to develop a drinking problem or use illicit drugs.
   c. have an increased risk of becoming chemically dependent.

8. A speedball is a combination of which two drugs?
   a. cocaine and heroin
   b. PCP and LSD
   c. valium and alcohol
   d. amphetamines and barbiturates

9. Methamphetamines are dangerous because their use can cause
   a. anxiety/nervousness/irritability.
   b. paranoia/psychosis.
   c. loss of appetite/malnutrition/anorexia.
   d. hallucinations.
   e. aggressive behavior.
   f. all of the above.

10. How is marijuana harmful?
    a. It hinders the user's short-term memory.
    b. Students may find it hard to study and learn while under the influence of marijuana.
    c. It affects timing and coordination.
    d. All of the above.

Answers to Personal Assessment

1. c
2. a
3. c
4. d
5. d
6. e
7. b
8. a
9. f
10. d

Source: *A Parent's Guide to Prevention*, U.S. Department of Education.

personal assessment

Getting a drug-free high

Experts agree that drug use provides only short-term, ineffective, and often destructive solutions to problems. We hope that you have found (or will find) innovative, invigorating drug-free experiences that make your life more exciting. Circle the number for each activity that reflects your intention to try that activity. Use the following guide:

1 No intention of trying this activity
2 Intend to try this within 2 years
3 Intend to try this within 6 months
4 Already tried this activity
5 Regularly engage in this activity

1. Learn to juggle	1	2	3	4	5
2. Go backpacking	1	2	3	4	5
3. Complete a marathon race	1	2	3	4	5
4. Start a vegetable garden	1	2	3	4	5
5. Ride in a hot air balloon	1	2	3	4	5
6. Snow ski or water ski	1	2	3	4	5
7. Donate blood	1	2	3	4	5
8. Go river rafting	1	2	3	4	5
9. Learn to play a musical instrument	1	2	3	4	5
10. Cycle 100 miles	1	2	3	4	5
11. Go skydiving	1	2	3	4	5
12. Go rockclimbing	1	2	3	4	5
13. Play a role in a theater production	1	2	3	4	5
14. Build a piece of furniture	1	2	3	4	5
15. Solicit funds for a worthy cause	1	2	3	4	5
16. Learn to swim	1	2	3	4	5
17. Overhaul a car engine	1	2	3	4	5
18. Compose a song	1	2	3	4	5
19. Travel to a foreign country	1	2	3	4	5
20. Write the first chapter of a book	1	2	3	4	5

TOTAL POINTS _____

Interpretation

61–100 You participate in many challenging experiences
41–60   You are willing to try some challenging new experiences
20–40   You take few of the challenging risks described here

To Carry This Further . . .

Looking at your point total, were you surprised at the degree to which you are aware of alternative activities? What are the top five activities, and can you understand their importance? What activities would you add to this list?

chapter eight

Taking Control of Alcohol Use

Chapter Objectives

On completing this chapter, you will be able to:

▪ describe the prevalence of drinking on college campuses.

▪ discuss the dysfunctional behaviors of an alcoholic's family.

▪ describe the physiological effects of alcohol and how these effects differ by gender.

▪ list the symptoms and first aid procedures for acute alcohol intoxication.

▪ explain how alcohol use plays a role in accidents, crime, and suicide.

▪ list the major organizations that support responsible drinking.

▪ describe problem drinking and alcoholism.

▪ explain how denial and enabling can prolong problem drinking.

▪ define codependence and describe how it damages the alcoholic and codependent.

▪ list the common traits of adult children of alcoholics.

Eye on the Media

TV Ads Target Drunk Driving

The first successful national campaign against drunk driving, "Designated Driver," began in 1998. Besides targeting specific audiences and using well-timed and strategically placed public service announcements, its developers convinced TV producers and writers to work references to the designated driver into the dialogue of their shows. Gradually, the message got through to young people. It does make sense to plan to have someone else drive if you're not going to be up to it. The designated-driver approach is still considered a good idea on college campuses today.

In contrast, the "Campaign for Alcohol Free Kids," relied heavily on dramatic graphics, such as grisly photos of car crash scenes on prom night.[1] Although the overall visual impact was powerful, the campaign lacked a practical element. Worse, the ads seemed to be preaching.

The Ad Council's "Friends Don't Let Friends Drive Drunk" is based on the idea that we all have responsibility for one another. If someone is your friend, you want to take care of that person. So don't let your friend do something dangerous.[2] Here the message is practical, not preachy.

The "You Drink & Drive, You Lose" campaign, a part of the National Public Education Campaign, targets two high-risk groups, 21- to 34-year-olds and repeat offenders. The message is simple: Make the right choice—don't drink and drive. The "Don't Lose It!" TV spot focuses on the fact that it's inconvenient to be stopped but the time spent at the checkpoint is for your own safety. It seems to be saying: "Sure, you're in a hurry, but this is important. So be patient." The graphics range from a serious-looking police officer talking to a motorist to hands locked in handcuffs.

What the successful campaigns have in common is a message that is simple, believable, and acceptable. Rather than scolding or preaching, the ads emphasize the fact that you have a choice and ask you to make the right choice.

"Road Predators," an American Public Television special that aired in December 1999, touched off strong controversy. Funded by the Century Council, a corporation backed by a group of U.S. distillers, the program used tragic accounts of alcohol-related accidents to dramatize the fact that innocent people lose their lives, families are shattered, and billions of dollars are spent because of drunk drivers.

What is the motivation for an alcohol industry group to fund a campaign to discourage drunk driving? How do such campaigns compare with the tobacco industry's efforts to discourage smoking among teenagers? How effective do you think each kind of ad campaign is?

Campaign for Alcohol Free Kids: Who We Are, www.alcoholfreekids.com/au_who_ we_are.html, March 8, 2005. Web site Information: Ad Council, www.adcouncil.org/, March 8, 2005.

The push for zero tolerance laws, the tightening of standards for determining legal intoxication, and the growing influence of national groups concerned with alcohol misuse show that our society is more sensitive than ever to the misuse of alcohol.

People are concerned about the consequences of drunk driving, alcohol-related crime, and lowered job productivity. Alcohol use remains quite high among young people in the United States and national data indicate that per capita, alcohol consumption has slowly decreased in the United States since the 1980s.[1] Alcohol use remains the preferred form of drug use for most adults (including college students), but as a society, we are increasingly uncomfortable with the ease with which alcohol can be misused.

Choosing to Drink

Clearly, people drink for many different reasons. Most people drink because alcohol is an effective, affordable, and legal substance for altering the brain's chemistry. As **inhibitions** are removed by the influence of alcohol, behavior that is generally held in check is expressed (Figure 8-1). At least temporarily, drinkers become a different version of themselves—more outgoing, relaxed, and adventuresome.

TALKING POINTS If alcohol did not make people more outgoing, relaxed, and adventuresome, then do you think they would consume as much?

Alcohol Use Patterns

From magazines to billboards to television, alcohol is one of the most heavily advertised consumer products in the country.[2] You cannot watch television, listen to the radio, or read a newspaper without being encouraged to buy a particular brand of beer, wine, or liquor. The advertisements create a warm aura about the nature of alcohol use. The implications are clear: alcohol use will bring you good times, handsome men or seductive women, exotic settings, and a chance to forget the hassles of hard work and study.

Given the many pressures to drink, it is not surprising that most adults drink alcoholic beverages. Two-thirds of all American adults are classified as drinkers. Yet one in three adults does not drink. In the college environment, where surveys indicate that 85–90 percent of all students drink, it is difficult for many students to imagine that every third adult is an abstainer. (Complete the Personal Assessment on page 275 to rate your own alcohol use.)

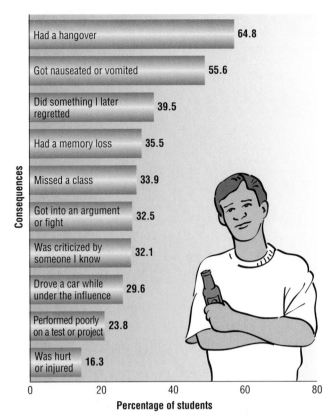

Figure 8-1 Negative consequences of alcohol and drug use as reported by college students. (Occurred at least once in the past year.)

Source: Core Institute. *2003 The Core Alcohol and Drug Survey*, www.siu.edu/departments/coreinst/public_ html/, February 27, 2005.

Alcohol consumption figures are reported in many different ways, depending on the researchers' criteria. Figures from various sources support the contention that about one-third of adults eighteen years of age and older are abstainers, about one-third are light drinkers, and one-third are moderate-to-heavy drinkers (see the Star box on page 253). As a single category, heavy drinkers make up about 10 percent of the adult drinking population.

Drinking on Campus

Students who drink in college tend to classify themselves as light-to-moderate drinkers. It comes as a shock to

---

Key Terms

inhibitions inner controls that prevent a person from engaging in certain types of behavior

Two-thirds of American adults are classified as drinkers. Only one-third choose to abstain from using alcohol.

students, though, when they read the criteria for each drinking classification. Many students will find that they fall into the category of heavy drinkers. The criteria are based on a combination of quantity of alcohol consumed per occasion and the frequency of drinking, as shown in Table 8.1.

 TALKING POINTS How would you tell a friend you think she has a drinking problem?

Binge Drinking

Alcohol abuse by college students usually takes the form of a drinking pattern called **binge drinking.** Binge drinking refers to the consumption of five drinks in one

---

Key Terms

binge drinking the consumption of five drinks or more on one drinking occasion

---

Table 8.1 Criteria for Drinking Classifications

Classification	Alcohol-Related Behavior
Abstainers	Do not drink or drink less often than once a year
Infrequent drinkers	Drink once a month at most and drink small amounts per typical drinking occasion
Light drinkers	Drink once a month at most and drink medium amounts per typical drinking occasion, or drink no more than three to four times a month and drink small amounts per typical drinking occasion
Moderate drinkers	Drink at least once a week and small amounts per typical drinking occasion or three to four times a month and medium amounts per typical drinking occasion or no more than once a month and large amounts per typical drinking occasion
Moderate/heavy drinkers	Drink at least once a week and medium amounts per typical drinking occasion or three to four times a month and large amounts per typical drinking occasion
Heavy drinkers	Drink at least once a week and large amounts per typical drinking occasion

Note: Small amounts = One drink or less per drinking occasion
Medium amounts = Two to four drinks per drinking occasion
Large amounts = Five or more drinks per drinking occasion (binge drinking)
Drink = 12 fluid oz of beer, 5 fluid oz of wine, or 1.5 fluid oz of 80 proof distilled spirits
[1]U.S. Department of Health and Human Services: *Fourth Special Report to the U.S. Congress, Washington, D.C.,* 1981, DHHS Pub No. ADM 81-1080.
[2]Dufour M. (1999). "What Is Moderate Drinking? Defining 'Drinks' and Drinking Levels," *Alcohol Research and Health,* 23(1), 5–14.

Moderate Drinking Redefined

Alcohol Research and Health defines moderate drinking as no more than two drinks each day for most men and one drink each day for women. A drink is defined as one 12-ounce regular beer, a 5-ounce glass of wine, or 1.5 ounces of 80 proof distilled spirits.[1] These cutoff levels are based on the amount of alcohol that can be consumed without causing problems, either for the drinker or society. (The gender difference is due primarily to the higher percentage of body fat in women and to the lower amount of an essential stomach enzyme in women.) Elderly people are limited to no more than one drink each day, again due to a higher percentage of body fat.

These consumption levels are applicable to most people. Indeed, people who plan to drive, women who are pregnant, people recovering from alcohol addiction, people under age 21, people taking medications, and those with existing medical concerns should not consume alcohol at all. In addition, although some studies have shown that low levels of alcohol consumption may have minor psychological and cardiovascular benefits, nondrinkers are not advised to start drinking.

[1]Dufour M. "What Is Moderate Drinking? Defining 'Drinks' and Drinking Levels," *Alcohol Research and Health* 23(1), 5–14, 1999.

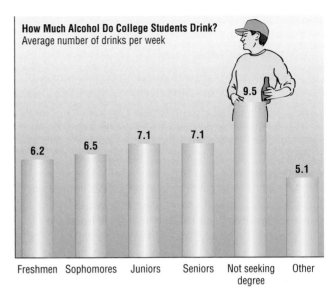

How Much Alcohol Do College Students Drink?
Average number of drinks per week

- Freshmen: 6.2
- Sophomores: 6.5
- Juniors: 7.1
- Seniors: 7.1
- Not seeking degree: 9.5
- Other: 5.1

Figure 8-2   Research shows that 20- to 24-year-olds drink more alcohol than does any other age group. How many servings a month do you have?

Source: Core Institute. *2003 The Core Alcohol and Drug Survey,* www.siu.edu/departments/coreinst/public_html, March 8, 2005.

sitting at least once during the previous 2-week period. One large study of more than 17,000 students on 89 campuses found that 49.7 percent of students binged.[3] The strongest predictors for bingeing were living in a fraternity or sorority, adopting a party-centered lifestyle, and engaging in other risky behavior. The study also suggested that many college students began binge drinking in high school. Individuals may experience peer pressure to participate in a drinking game. Drinking games are a form of binge drinking in which individuals consume large amounts of alcohol in a small period of time.

By its very nature, binge drinking can be dangerous. Drunk driving, physical violence, property destruction, date rape, police arrest, and lowered academic performance are all highly associated with binge drinking. Besides the role that heavy drinking may play in the aggressor in date rape, a recent study found that more than half the victims in sexual assaults also were at least somewhat drunk.

The direct correlation between the amount of alcohol consumed and lowered academic performance results in impaired memory, verbal skill deficiencies, and altered perceptions.[4] Frequently, the social costs of binge drinking can be very high, especially when intoxicated people demonstrate their level of immaturity. How common is binge drinking on your campus?

For large numbers of students who drink, the college years are a time when they drink more heavily than at any other period during their lifetime (Figure 8-2). Some will

suffer serious consequences as a result. These years will also mark the entry into a lifetime of problem drinking for some.

Drinking Games

Drinking games are one form of binge drinking that seeks to make binge drinking socially acceptable.

Drinking games are especially risky for inexperienced drinkers who are unfamiliar with changes associated with heavy alcohol consumption. They place themselves at increased risk for drinking-related problems, such as alcohol poisoning, injuries, property destruction, legal problems, and sexual assaults.

Declining Alcohol Use

As you learned in Chapter 7, "Making Decisions about Drug Use," being able to decline drugs and alcohol when others around are using these substances is a challenge that you can learn to meet. For example, participating in a long bicycle ride or run can leave you with an excellent sense of well-being produced by endorphins, natural painkillers produced by the brain. Such a "high" is enhanced by the knowledge that you have earned the good feeling through your efforts (see Discovering Your Spirituality on page 254). Consider some additional techniques for avoiding alcohol:

- Avoid parties where you can expect heavy drinking.
- Avoid people who are drinking heavily or becoming erratic or threatening.

What's a Social Life without Alcohol?

When was the last time you went to a get-together where alcoholic drinks weren't served? It's probably been years. Socializing and drinking are connected in our consciousness in many ways. For instance, it's Friday night after a hard week and your friends ask you to join them for a beer. Why not? It'll be fun. Or you're invited to a party and want to bring something. How about a bottle of wine? That's easy and always appreciated.

Associating drinking with fun is something that many people, including college students, do. For various reasons, though, some college students are choosing to plan their fun around activities that don't involve drinking. Instead of going to a bar for a beer, they find a coffee shop and have a latte. Or they order soda with their pizza (not bad!). Others have discovered that they can get something that tastes great and is actually healthy at a juice bar.

What happens, though, when you go to a party and everyone else seems to be drinking? Choose something nonalcoholic—club soda, juice, soda, or water. (You probably won't be the only one doing this.) If someone gives you trouble about your choice, be firm. Just say that's what you want. You don't need to explain. And you don't have to say "yes" to be nice.

But maybe you want to drink at a party because it loosens you up and makes it easier to talk to people. How will you start a conversation without a drink to relax you? Think about how you talk easily and naturally with the people in your drama group or one of your favorite classes. You've got things in common, so it's easier to do. When you meet someone new at a party, look for common interests. You may feel self-conscious at first. But soon you'll forget about the fact that he or she is a stranger because you'll be involved in what you're talking about. Without that drink, you'll actually be more yourself.

Some students are making the commitment to be active instead of sitting around and drinking. They're going backpacking, joining a cycling group, taking an exercise class, or playing a team sport. What they're discovering is that it feels good—physically and mentally. They're socializing, doing something they enjoy, and getting in better shape. Think about something you've always wanted to try, and get going on it.

Making the choice to have fun without alcohol doesn't mean cutting yourself off from your friends. (If they're real friends, they'll respect your choice.) It's all about deciding what's right for you and making a commitment to that choice.

- Request a nonalcoholic beer, soft drink, or glass of water instead of alcohol.
- Participate in activities that can provide a nonchemical high. See the Personal Assessment on page 248 of Chapter 7 for a variety of suggestions.
- Cultivate friends who find their highs through natural, positive activities in which you share an interest.

Alcohol and the Family

The alcohol abuser hurts more than just himself or herself. Everyone around the addicted person suffers. Alcoholism is a family disease, and a family can be defined as a person, a family, a fraternity, a sorority, a dormitory floor, even a therapy group or a 12-step group. Many family members deny there is an alcohol problem in their family. They may feel embarrassed; have suffered from physical, sexual, or mental abuse; and may not want to deal with or think about their personal family situation.

Following are some of the behaviors that the dysfunctional family typically experiences.[5] The family:

- Lives in fear and fears others different from them in race, religion, color, nationality, appearance, and so forth.

- Depends on family members to the exclusion of the outside world. An exception can be made for outsiders who are very like the family members.
- Believes that, to be successful, you must have money, make money, or marry into money.
- Believes that the authority figures in the family are always right.
- Teaches every member of the family to adapt to the emotional sickness present and feels threatened when a member attempts to recover.
- Teaches conditional love.
- Teaches that to have a worthwhile identity you must gain the approval of the outside world, and especially of the family itself.
- Feels threatened and abandoned at the death or departure of a member of the group.
- Tries to maintain the group through guilt and pity, which it calls "love."
- Expects all members to like the same things and people.
- Thrives on excitement and teaches that if you are not excited you are not alive.

As a result of these constant dysfunctional behaviors, the person living with an alcoholic can develop many of the following problems:

- Become isolated and afraid of people and authority figures.
- Become an approval-seeker and lose his or her identity in the process.
- Become frightened by angry people and any criticism.
- Become an alcoholic, marry one, or find another compulsive personality such as a workaholic to continue the sickness.
- Develop a victim mentality and be attracted by weakness in potential friends or loved ones.
- Have an extreme sense of responsibility and focus on others to the detriment of himself or herself.
- Feel guilty when being assertive or saying no.
- Become addicted to excitement.
- Confuse pity with love.
- Lose the ability to feel or express feelings.
- Be terrified of abandonment and be willing to tolerate abuse to hold on to a relationship.
- Develop all the symptoms of an alcoholic without actually drinking.

The good news is that many resources, such as recovery and support groups, are now available for both the alcoholic and those who live with the alcoholic. (See the sections on alcohol self-assessment, codependence, rehabilitation and recovery, and adult children of alcoholic parents beginning on page 265.)

Those who have lived with an alcoholic will face their own issues as they work through their own recovery. They may find that they learned compulsions from the alcoholic, or they may transfer the compulsions to other behaviors, such as excessive eating, gambling, house cleaning, or taking up lost causes or people. Those who know, or are still living with, an active alcoholic also can consider intervention to urge the alcoholic to seek help.

The Nature of Alcoholic Beverages

Alcohol (also known as *ethyl alcohol* or *ethanol*) is the principal product of **fermentation.** In this process, yeast cells act on the sugar content of fruits and grains to produce alcohol and carbon dioxide.[6]

The alcohol concentration in beverages such as whiskey, gin, rum, and vodka is determined through a process called **distillation.** These distilled beverages are expressed by the term *proof,* a number that is twice the percentage of alcohol by volume in a beverage. Thus 70 percent of the fluid in a bottle of 140 proof gin is pure alcohol. Most proofs in distilled beverages range from 80 to 160. The pure grain alcohol that is often added to fruit punches and similar beverages has a proof of almost 200.

The nutritional value of alcohol is extremely limited. Alcoholic beverages produced today through modern processing methods contain nothing but empty calories—about 100 calories per fluid ounce of 100-proof distilled spirits and about 150 calories per each 12-ounce bottle or can of beer. Alcohol consumption is a significant contributor to the additional pounds that many college students accumulate. Pure alcohol contains only simple carbohydrates; it has no vitamins and minerals, and no fats or protein.

Recently, researchers have suggested that moderate consumption of alcoholic beverages can reduce the risk of coronary heart disease.[7] Alcohol appears to increase levels of HDL cholesterol (the good cholesterol) in the bloodstream and, perhaps, reduce LDL cholesterol levels. However, there are various other ways to alter a person's cholesterol profile. Doctors caution anyone against drinking merely because of this one possible health benefit.

"Light" beer and low-calorie wines have been introduced in response to concerns about the number of calories in alcoholic beverages. These light beverages are not low-alcohol beverages but merely low-calorie beverages. Only beverages marked "low alcohol" contain a lower concentration of alcohol than do the usual beverages of that type. Recently, manufacturers have introduced a new form of beer called low carbohydrate beer. For the diet-conscious consumer, low-carb beer contains a lower carbohydrate content but the same alcohol and calorie contents that other beers have.

Ice beers actually contain a higher percentage of alcohol than do other types of beer. The term *ice* refers to the way in which this beer is processed. After brewing and fermentation, it is deep-chilled at 24 to 28 degrees Fahrenheit, which causes ice crystals to form in the mixture. When these ice crystals are removed, the remaining liquid contains a higher percentage of alcohol. Most regular and light beers contain less than 5 percent

> ### Key Terms
>
> **fermentation** a chemical process whereby plant products are converted into alcohol by the action of yeast cells on carbohydrate materials
>
> **distillation** the process of heating an alcohol solution and collecting its vapors into a more concentrated solution

alcohol, whereas ice beer generally contains 5–6 percent alcohol. Do you think beer drinkers are choosing this beer for its reportedly rich flavor or simply because it contains more alcohol?

The Physiological Effects of Alcohol

First and foremost, alcohol is classified as a drug—a very strong CNS depressant. The primary depressant effect of alcohol occurs in the brain and spinal cord. Many people think of alcohol as a stimulant because of the way most users feel after consuming a serving or two of their favorite drink. Any temporary sensations of jubilation, boldness, or relief are attributable to alcohol's ability as a depressant drug to release personal inhibitions and provide temporary relief from tension.

Factors That Influence the Absorption of Alcohol

The **absorption** of alcohol is influenced by several factors, most of which can be controlled by the individual. These factors include the following:

Strength of the Beverage

The stronger the beverage, the greater the amount of alcohol that accumulates within the digestive tract.

Number of Drinks Consumed

As more drinks are consumed, more alcohol is absorbed.

Speed of Consumption

If consumed rapidly, even relatively few drinks will result in a large concentration gradient that leads to high blood alcohol concentration.

Presence of Food

Food can compete with alcohol for absorption into the bloodstream, thus slowing the absorption of alcohol. When you slow your alcohol absorption, your body can remove alcohol already in the bloodstream. Serving food at a party is a healthy idea.

Body Chemistry

Each person has an individual pattern of physiological functioning that may affect the ability to process alcohol. For example, in some conditions, such as that marked by "dumping syndrome," the stomach empties more rapidly than is normal, and alcohol seems to be absorbed more quickly. The emptying time may be either slowed or quickened by anger, fear, stress, nausea, and the condition of the stomach tissues.

Race/Ethnicity

Research suggests that alcohol tolerance levels may range from weak to strong based on an individual's race/ethnic origin.

Gender

Women produce much less alcohol dehydrogenase than do men.[8] This enzyme is responsible for breaking down alcohol in the stomach. With less alcohol dehydrogenase action, women absorb about 30 percent more alcohol into the bloodstream than men do, despite an identical number of drinks and equal body weight.

Three other reasons help explain why women tend to absorb alcohol more quickly than do men of the same body weight: (1) Women have proportionately more body fat than men do. Since alcohol is not stored easily in fat, it enters the bloodstream relatively quickly. (2) Women's bodies have proportionately less water than do men's bodies of equal weight. Thus consumed alcohol does not become as diluted as it does in men. (3) Alcohol absorption is influenced by a woman's menstrual cycle. Alcohol is more quickly absorbed during the premenstrual phase of a woman's cycle. Also, there is evidence that women using birth control pills absorb alcohol more quickly than usual.[8]

With the exception of a person's body chemistry, race/ethnicity, and gender, all factors that influence absorption can be moderated by the alcohol user.

Blood Alcohol Concentration

A person's **blood alcohol concentration (BAC)** rises when alcohol is consumed faster than it can be removed (oxidized) by the liver.[9] As outlined in Figure 8-3, a fairly predictable sequence of events takes place when a person drinks alcohol at a rate faster than one drink every hour. When the BAC reaches 0.05 percent, initial measurable changes in mood and behavior take place. Inhibitions and everyday tensions appear to be released, while judgment and critical thinking are somewhat impaired. This BAC would be achieved by a 160-pound person drinking

---

Key Terms

absorption the passage of nutrients or alcohol through the walls of the stomach or the intestinal tract into the bloodstream

blood alcohol concentration (BAC) the percentage of alcohol in a measured quantity of blood; BAC can be determined directly, through the analysis of a blood sample, or indirectly, through the analysis of exhaled air

Table 8.2 Blood Alcohol Concentration and the Effects of Alcohol

Blood Alcohol Concentration	Sporadic Drinker	Chronic Drinker	Hours for Alcohol to be Metabolized
.05%	Congenial euphoria; decreased tension	No observable effect	2–3
.075%	Talkative	Often no effect	
.10%	Uncoordinated; legally drunk (as in drunk driving) in most states; a level of 0.08% is legal drunkenness in 18 states	Minimal signs	4–6
.125%–.150%	Unrestrained behavior; episodic uncontrolled behavior	Pleasurable euphoria or beginning of uncoordination	6–10
.20%–.25%	Alertness lost; sluggish	Effort required to maintain emotional and motor control	10–24
.30%–.35%	Stupor to coma; death is possible	Drowsy and slow	
.40%–.50%	Death is likely	Coma; some will die	>24

about two drinks in an hour (see Table 8.2 above and Figure 8-3).

At a level of 0.10 percent (one part alcohol to 1,000 parts blood), the drinker typically loses significant motor coordination. Voluntary motor function becomes quite clumsy. At this BAC, most states consider a drinker legally intoxicated and thus incapable of safely operating a vehicle. Although physiological changes associated with this BAC do occur, certain users do not feel drunk or appear impaired.

As a person continues to elevate the BAC from 0.20–0.50 percent, the health risk of **acute alcohol intoxication** increases rapidly. A BAC of 0.20 percent is characterized by the loud, boisterous, obnoxious drunk person who staggers. A 0.30 percent BAC produces further depression and stuporous behavior, during which time the drinker becomes so confused that he or she may not be capable of understanding anything. The 0.40 percent or 0.50 percent BAC produces unconsciousness. At this BAC a person can die, because brain centers that control body temperature, heartbeat, and respiration may virtually shut down.

An important factor influencing the BAC is the individual's blood volume. The larger the person, the greater the amount of blood into which alcohol can be distributed. Conversely, the smaller person has less blood into which alcohol can be distributed, and as a result, a higher BAC will develop.

Sobering Up

Alcohol is removed from the bloodstream principally through the process of **oxidation.** Oxidation occurs at a constant rate (about ¼ to ⅓ ounce of pure alcohol per hour) that cannot be appreciably altered. Because each

typical drink of beer, wine, or distilled spirits contains about ½ ounce of pure alcohol, it takes about 2 hours for the body to fully oxidize one typical alcoholic drink.[10]

After a night of drinking alcohol, the next morning people may experience uncomfortable symptoms such as headache, nausea, fatigue, diarrhea, loss of appetite, or an overall feeling of being sick. These symptoms are commonly known as a *hangover* and are the result of the body reacting to too much alcohol in its system. These symptoms may be intensified by dehydration, poor nutrition, an empty stomach, lack of sleep, poor health, or increased physical activity while drinking.

Although people have attempted to sober up by drinking hot coffee, taking cold showers, or exercising, the oxidation rate of alcohol is unaffected. Thus far the FDA has not approved any commercial product that can help people achieve sobriety. Since alcohol causes dehydration, rehydration and the passage of time remain the only effective way to sober up.

First Aid for Acute Alcohol Intoxication

Not everyone who goes to sleep, passes out, or even becomes unconscious after drinking has a high BAC. People who are

> **Key Terms**
>
> **acute alcohol intoxication** a potentially fatal elevation of BAC, often resulting from heavy, rapid consumption of alcohol
>
> **oxidation** the process that removes alcohol from the bloodstream

Number of drinks consumed in two hours	Alcohol in blood (percentage)	Typical effects
2	0.05	Judgment, thought, and restraint weakened; tension released, giving carefree sensation
3	0.08	Tensions of everyday life lessened; cheerfulness
4	0.10	Voluntary motor action affected, making hand and arm movements, walk, and speech clumsy
7	0.20	Severe impairment—staggering, loud, incoherent, emotionally unstable, 100 times greater traffic risk; exuberance and aggressive inclinations magnified
9	0.30	Deeper areas of brain affected, with stimulus-response and understanding confused; stuporous; blurred vision
12	0.40	Incapable of voluntary action; sleepy, difficult to arouse; equivalent of surgical anesthesia
15	0.50	Comatose; centers controlling breathing and heartbeat anesthetized; death increasingly probable

Note: A drink refers to a typical 12-ounce bottle of beer, a 1.5-ounce shot of hard liquor, or a 5-ounce glass of wine.

Figure 8-3 Effects of alcohol by number of drinks

already sleepy, have not eaten well, are sick, or are bored may drink a little alcohol and quickly fall asleep. However, people who drink heavily in a rather short time may be setting themselves up for an extremely unpleasant, toxic, potentially life-threatening experience because of their high BAC.

Although responsible drinking would prevent acute alcohol intoxication (poisoning), such responsible drinking will never be a reality for everyone. As caring adults, what should we know about this health emergency that may help us save a life?

The first real danger sign we need to recognize is **shock** and its typical signs. By the time these signs are evident, a drinker will already have become unconscious. He or she cannot be aroused from a deep stupor. The person will probably have a weak, rapid pulse (over 100 beats per minute). The skin will be cool and damp, and breathing

Key Terms

shock profound collapse of many vital body functions; evident during acute alcohol intoxication and other serious health emergencies will be increased to once every three or four seconds. These breaths may be shallow or deep but will certainly occur in an irregular pattern. The skin will be pale or bluish. (In a person with dark skin, these color changes will be more evident in the fingernail beds or in the mucous membranes inside the mouth or under the eyelids.) Whenever any of these signs are present, seek emergency medical help immediately. (See Changing for the Better above for a summary of these signs.)

Involuntary regurgitation (vomiting) can be another potentially life-threatening emergency for a person who has drunk too much alcohol. When a drinker has consumed more alcohol than the liver can oxidize, the pyloric valve at the base of the stomach tends to close. Additional alcohol remains in the stomach. This alcohol irritates the lining of the stomach so much that involuntary muscle contractions force the stomach contents to flow back through the esophagus. By removing alcohol from the stomach, vomiting may be a life-saving mechanism for conscious drinkers.

An unconscious drinker who vomits, however, may be lying in such a position that the airway becomes obstructed with the vomitus from the stomach. This person is in great risk of dying from **asphyxiation.** As a first-aid measure, unconscious drinkers should always be rolled onto their sides to minimize the chance of airway obstruction. If you are with a person who is vomiting, make certain that his or her head is positioned lower than the rest of the body. This position minimizes the chance that vomitus will obstruct the air passages.

Also keep a close watch on anyone who passes out from heavy drinking. Unfortunately, partygoers sometimes make the mistake of carrying these people to bed and then forgetting about them. You should do your best to monitor the physical condition of anyone who becomes unconscious from heavy drinking because of the risk of death. If you really care about these people, you will observe them at regular intervals until they appear to be clearly out of danger. Although this may mean an evening of interrupted sleep for you, you might save a friend's life.

Alcohol-Related Health Problems

The relationship of chronic alcohol use to the structure and function of the body is reasonably well understood. Heavy alcohol use causes a variety of changes in the body that lead to an increase in morbidity and mortality. Figure 8-4 describes these changes.

Research shows that chronic alcohol use also damages the immune system and the nervous system. Thus chronic users are at high risk for a variety of infections and neurological complications.

Fetal Alcohol Syndrome and Fetal Alcohol Effects

A growing body of scientific evidence shows that alcohol use by pregnant women can cause birth defects in unborn children. When alcohol crosses the **placenta,** it enters the fetal bloodstream in a concentration equal to that in the mother's bloodstream. Because the fetal liver is underdeveloped, it oxidizes this alcohol much more slowly than the alcohol in the mother. During this time of slow detoxification, the developing fetus is certain to be overexposed to the toxic effects of alcohol. Mental retardation frequently develops.

This exposure has additional disastrous consequences for the developing fetus. Low birth weight, facial abnormalities, such as a small head and widely spaced eyes, and heart problems are often seen in such

> **Key Terms**
>
> **asphyxiation** death resulting from lack of oxygen to the brain
>
> **placenta** the structure through which nutrients, metabolic wastes, and drugs (including alcohol) pass from the bloodstream of the mother into the bloodstream of the developing fetus

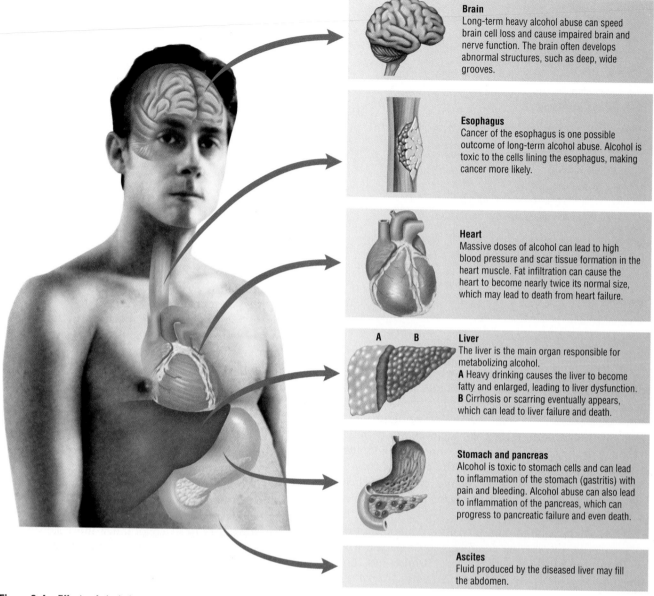

Brain
Long-term heavy alcohol abuse can speed brain cell loss and cause impaired brain and nerve function. The brain often develops abnormal structures, such as deep, wide grooves.

Esophagus
Cancer of the esophagus is one possible outcome of long-term alcohol abuse. Alcohol is toxic to the cells lining the esophagus, making cancer more likely.

Heart
Massive doses of alcohol can lead to high blood pressure and scar tissue formation in the heart muscle. Fat infiltration can cause the heart to become nearly twice its normal size, which may lead to death from heart failure.

Liver
The liver is the main organ responsible for metabolizing alcohol.
A Heavy drinking causes the liver to become fatty and enlarged, leading to liver dysfunction.
B Cirrhosis or scarring eventually appears, which can lead to liver failure and death.

Stomach and pancreas
Alcohol is toxic to stomach cells and can lead to inflammation of the stomach (gastritis) with pain and bleeding. Alcohol abuse can also lead to inflammation of the pancreas, which can progress to pancreatic failure and even death.

Ascites
Fluid produced by the diseased liver may fill the abdomen.

Figure 8-4 Effects of alcohol use on the body. The mind-altering effects of alcohol begin soon after it enters the bloodstream. Within minutes, alcohol numbs nerve cells in the brain. The heart muscle strains to cope with alcohol's depressive action. If drinking continues, the rising BAC causes impaired speech, vision, balance, and judgment. With an extremely high BAC, respiratory failure is possible. Over time, alcohol abuse increases the risk for certain forms of heart disease and cancer and makes liver and pancreas failure more likely.

infants (Figure 8-5). This combination of effects is called **fetal alcohol syndrome (FAS).** Recent studies estimate that the full expression of this syndrome occurs at a rate of 1 to 3 per 1,000 births. Partial expression (*fetal alcohol effects, [FAE]*) can be seen in 3 to 9 per 1,000 live births. In addition, it is likely that many cases of FAE go undetected.[11]

Is there a safe limit to the number of drinks a woman can consume during pregnancy? Because no one can accurately predict the effect of drinking even small amounts of alcohol during pregnancy, the wisest plan is to avoid alcohol altogether.

> **Key Terms**
>
> **fetal alcohol syndrome (FAS)** characteristic birth defects noted in the children of some women who consume alcohol during their pregnancies

Figure 8-5 Fetal alcohol syndrome. The facial features shown are characteristic of affected children. Additional abnormalities in the brain and other internal organs accompany fetal alcohol syndrome but are not obvious in the child's appearance.

Labels (left illustration):
- Small head circumference
- Low nasal bridge
- Short eyelid tissues
- Short nose
- Small midface
- Indistinct depression under nose
- Thin upper lip

Because of the critical growth and development that occur during the first months of fetal life, women who have any reason to suspect they are pregnant should stop all alcohol consumption. Furthermore, women who are planning to become pregnant and women who are not practicing effective contraception should also keep their alcohol use to a minimum.

Alcohol-Related Social Problems

Alcohol abuse is related to a variety of social problems. These problems affect the quality of interpersonal relationships, employment stability, and the financial security of both the individual and the family. Clearly, alcohol's negative social consequences lower our quality of life. In financial terms the annual cost of alcohol abuse and dependence has been estimated at more than $185 billion.[12]

Accidents

The four leading causes of accidental deaths in the United States (motor vehicle collisions, falls, drownings, and fires and burns) have significant statistical connections to alcohol use.

Motor Vehicle Collisions

Data from the National Highway Traffic Safety Administration (NHTSA) indicate that in 2004 over 17,000 alcohol-related vehicular crash deaths occurred. This figure represented 40 percent of the total traffic fatalities for 2003. Although 17,000 remains an unacceptably high

On August 4, 2000, 23-year-old Casey Ray Beaver was driving with two friends along U.S. Highway 71 near Goodman, Missouri, when an oncoming vehicle crossed the center line and collided with his car. Casey, a recent graduate of the University of Kansas, was pronounced dead at the scene, as was the driver of the other vehicle. The offender, who had seven prior convictions of driving under the influence and whose driver's license had been revoked seven years earlier, had a BAC above 10 percent. Casey was due to begin classes at the Illinois College of Optometry 10 days after the accident occurred.

Figure 8-6 A BAC of .08% constitutes legal intoxication. However, a BAC as low as 0.05% can impair functioning enough to cause a serious accident.

Number of drinks in a 2-hour period
(1½ oz 86-proof liquor or 12 oz beer)

Body weight (lbs)									
100	1	2	3	4	5	6	7	8	9
120	1	2	3	4	5	6	7	8	9
140	1	2	3	4	5	6	7	8	9
160	1	2	3	4	5	6	7	8	9
180	1	2	3	4	5	6	7	8	9
200	1	2	3	4	5	6	7	8	9

Could impair driving (BAC to .05%)

Driving significantly impaired (BAC .05% to .09%)

Driving seriously impaired (BAC .10% and up)

figure represented 40 percent of the total traffic fatalities for 2003. Although 17,000 remains an unacceptably high figure, this total represented a 12 percent reduction from the 20,000 alcohol-related fatalities reported in 1991.[13]

Presently in the United States, an alcohol-related car crash fatality occurs every 31 minutes. Every 2 minutes, an alcohol-related car crash injury happens. More than 275,000 people were injured in such crashes in 2001. In 2002, the NHTSA reported that approximately 1.5 million drivers were arrested for drunk driving, reflecting an arrest rate of 1 for every 130 licensed drivers in the United States.[13] (To find out what happens to people after they are arrested, read the Star box on page 263.)

One response to drunk driving has been for all states to raise the minimum legal drinking age to 21 years. This was accomplished in the mid-1980s. In October 2000, President Clinton signed into law a federal bill that requires all states to lower the legal BAC to .08 percent by the year 2003 or risk losing federal highway funds. All states have lowered the driving standard to .08 percent BAC. You can search the MADD website at www.madd.org to find out current .08 percent BAC law information (see Figure 8-6).

Other programs and policies are being implemented that are designed to prevent intoxicated people from driving. Many states have enacted **zero-tolerance laws** to help prevent underage drinking and driving. Also included have been efforts to educate bartenders to recognize intoxicated customers, to use off-duty police officers as observers in bars, to place police roadblocks, to develop mechanical devices that prevent intoxicated drivers from starting their cars, and to encourage people to use designated drivers.

Falls

Many people are surprised to learn that falls are the second leading cause of accidental death in the United States.

Alcohol use increases the risk for falls. Various studies suggest that alcohol is involved in 21–77 percent of deadly falls and 18–53 percent of nonfatal falls.[15]

Drownings

Drownings are the third leading cause of accidental death in the United States. Studies have shown that alcohol use is implicated in 21–47 percent of these deaths.[15] High percentages of recreational boaters have been found to drink alcohol while boating. Alcohol can impair judgment and swimming ability and reduce body temperature.[16]

Fires and Burns

Fires and burns are responsible for an estimated 5,000 deaths each year in the United States, the fourth leading cause of accidental death. This cause is also connected to alcohol use: studies indicate that half of burn victims have BACs above the legal limit.[15]

Crime and Violence

Have you noticed that most of the violent behavior and vandalism on your campus is related to alcohol use? The connection of alcohol to crime has a long history. Prison

---

Key Terms

zero-tolerance laws laws that severely restrict the right to operate motor vehicles for underage drinkers who have been convicted of driving under the influence of alcohol or any other drug

Getting Arrested for Drinking and Driving: The Aftermath

Many college students admit to having driven a car after drinking alcohol. Some even admit that they have left a party after drinking and then driven to another location, but could not remember actually driving the car. This behavior reflects an alcoholic blackout. These dangerous activities are serious enough for the driver, the passengers, and anyone else on (or near) the road. For people who get arrested, another drama will unfold—the aftermath of an arrest for drinking and driving.

Although laws vary from state to state, here is the general sequence of events: If you are driving a car and are stopped by a police officer who suspects you may have been driving under the influence of alcohol, you will first be asked to show your driver's license and proof of your car's registration. You may be asked to get out of your car and undergo a field test for sobriety. This test could include tests of motor coordination, such as walking in a line in a heel-to-toe fashion. You may even be given an alcohol breath test on the spot.

If you appear to fail the field test, you could be arrested and frisked, read your Miranda rights, and taken to the local jail. There you will likely be fingerprinted and photographed. A more precise blood alcohol test may be given. Depending on local or state law, you will either spend some hours in jail (until your BAC is lowered) or be immediately eligible for bail (if you, a family member, or a friend can come up with the cash to get you released).

A date for your court appearance will be set. You will be required to face a judge and answer the charges against you. By this time, you probably will have hired an attorney to help you in this process. If you are convicted or decide to plead guilty to misdemeanor charges of driving while intoxicated (DWI) and this is your first offense, a typical scenario will follow. You will receive a fine (perhaps $200–$500) and be required to pay court costs (perhaps $125). You will probably be required to attend alcohol education classes and be placed on probation (for a year). Many states also require a person convicted of DWI to pay a probationer's fee of $50 plus $10 each month during the probation period. You will generally be required to see your probation officer once a month, and you may be required to take random drug tests.

Some communities require people convicted of DWI to pay a fee (perhaps $200) that goes to local drug prevention programs. Finally, some jurisdictions require judges to impose a term of community service hours that you must serve. You will likely lose points on your driver's license and have an official police and court record. The total cost for a simple, first-time conviction can easily reach $1,000 or more, depending on fines and legal fees.

For first-time offenders in jurisdictions in which the courts and jails are overcrowded, "pretrial diversionary programs" may exist. In these programs, lawyers work with local prosecutors to help first-time offenders avoid facing a judge and having a court record. Those arrested agree to pay a set community drug program fine (perhaps $300-$500) and attend alcohol education classes. They typically must perform community service and meet with a probation office each month. (They must also pay the probationer's fees.) At the end of a year, after a positive probationary experience, the arrest record is removed from the police files. Again, the total cost can amount to over $1,000.

The preceding discussion applies to misdemeanor charges. However, if you are arrested and charged with a felony (such as operating a vehicle while intoxicated and you kill or injure someone), the whole ball game changes radically. You will be arrested and put in jail. You may not be able to be bailed out of jail. Almost certainly, you will need an attorney to assist you through a lengthy court process. If you are ultimately convicted of a felony, you are likely to pay a heavy fine and spend time in jail or prison. After a criminal trial, injured people can also pursue a civil suit against you. A civil suit can be quite expensive and time consuming. Indeed, the repercussions of a criminal DWI felony conviction will last for years and will have a significant impact on you, your family, and the lives of others.

Unfortunately, people who drink and drive fail to consider the aftermath of their behavior before it is too late.

populations have large percentages of alcohol abusers and alcoholics: people who commit crimes are more likely to have alcohol problems than are people in the general population. This is especially true for young criminals. Furthermore, alcohol use has been reported in 53–66 percent of all homicides, with the victim, the perpetrator, or both found to have been drinking. In rape situations, rapists are intoxicated 50 percent of the time and victims 30 percent of the time.[17]

Because of research methodological problems, pinpointing alcohol's connection to family violence is difficult.[18] However, it seems clear that among a large number of families, alcohol is associated with violence and other harmful behavior, including physical abuse, child abuse, psychological abuse, and abandonment.[17]

The difficult question that arises when discussing the relationship between alcohol use and violence is whether a cause-effect link can be proven. Obviously, not everyone who drinks becomes violent, but in many violent crimes, at least one person involved has been drinking. The answer perhaps is that alcohol use by itself is not enough to cause violence, but use of alcohol may be one of several factors that act in combination to cause violent behavior in some instances.

Suicide

Alcohol use has been related to large percentages of suicides. Alcoholism plays a large role in 30 percent of completed suicides.[19] Also, alcohol use is associated with

Partying 101: How to Party Responsibly

My friends and I are planning a big holiday party. We want to have fun, but we also want to be responsible about alcohol. What guidelines should we follow?

- Provide other social activities as a primary focus when alcohol is served.
- Respect an individual's decision about alcohol if that decision is either to abstain or to drink responsibly.
- Recognize the decision not to drink and the respect it warrants by providing equally attractive and accessible nonalcohol drinks when alcohol is served.
- Recognize that drunkenness is neither healthy nor safe. One should not excuse otherwise unacceptable behavior solely because of "too much to drink."
- Provide food when alcohol is served.
- Serve diluted drinks, and do not urge that glasses be constantly full.

- Keep the cocktail hour before dinner to a reasonable time and consumption limit.
- Recognize your responsibility for the health, safety, and pleasure of both the drinker and the nondrinker by avoiding intoxication and helping others do the same.
- Make contingency plans for intoxication. If it occurs in spite of efforts to prevent it, assume responsibility for the health and safety of guests—for example, by providing transportation home or overnight accommodations.
- Serve or use alcohol only in environments conducive to pleasant and relaxing behavior.
- Discard unattended drinks immediately. This reduces the possibility of someone consuming a drink containing Rohypnol, GHB, Ketamine (see Chapter 7), or other powerful intoxicants.

impulsive suicides rather than with premeditated ones. Drinking is also connected with more violent and lethal means of suicide, such as the use of firearms.[17]

For many of these social problems, alcohol use impairs critical judgment and allows a person's behavior to quickly become reckless, antisocial, and deadly. Because most of us wish to minimize problems associated with alcohol use, acting responsibly when we host a party is a first step in this direction.

Hosting a Party Responsibly

Some people might say that no party is totally safe when alcohol is served. These people are probably right, considering the possibility of unexpected **drug synergism,** overconsumption, and the consequences of released inhibitions. Fortunately, an increasing awareness of the value of responsible party hosting seems to be spreading among college communities. The impetus for this awareness has come from various sources, including respect for an individual's right to choose not to drink alcohol, the growing recognition that many automobile crashes are alcohol related, and the legal threats posed by **host negligence.**

For whatever reasons, responsibly hosting parties at which alcohol is served is becoming a trend, especially among college-educated young adults. The Education Commission of the States' Task Force on Responsible Decisions about Alcohol has generated a list of guidelines for hosting a social event at which alcoholic beverages are served. The list includes the recommendations shown in Changing for the Better above.

In addition to these suggestions, the use of a **designated driver** is an important component of responsible alcohol use. By planning to abstain from alcohol or to carefully limit their own alcohol consumption, designated drivers are able to safely transport friends who have been drinking.

Designated drivers have indisputably saved many lives. However, there may be a down side. Some health professionals are concerned that the use of designated drivers allows the nondrivers to drink more heavily than they might otherwise. In effect, designated drivers "enable" drinkers to be less responsible for their own behavior. This freedom from responsibility might eventually lead to further problems for the drinkers.

Key Terms

drug synergism (**sin** er jism) enhancement of a drug's effect as a result of the presence of additional drugs within the system

host negligence a legal term that reflects the failure of a host to provide reasonable care and safety for people visiting the host's residence or business

designated driver a person who abstains from or carefully limits alcohol consumption to be able to safely transport other people who have been drinking

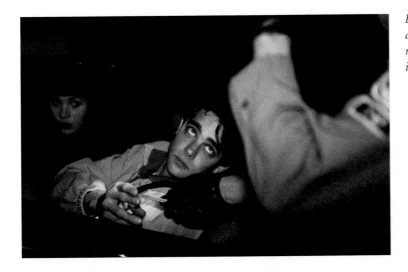

Police have stepped up their efforts to keep drunk drivers off the road by using sobriety checkpoints and roadside sobriety tests for people suspected of being intoxicated.

 TALKING POINTS Have you noticed an increased use of designated drivers in your community? Would you be willing to be a designated driver?

Organizations That Support Responsible Drinking

The serious consequences of the irresponsible use of alcohol have led to the formation of a number of concerned-citizen groups. Although each organization has a unique approach, all attempt to deal objectively with two indisputable facts: Alcohol use is part of our society, and irresponsible alcohol use can be deadly.

Mothers Against Drunk Driving

Mothers Against Drunk Driving (MADD) is a national network of over 600 local chapters in the United States and Canada. This organization attempts to educate people about alcohol's effects on driving and to influence legislation and enforcement of laws related to drunk drivers. For more information about MADD, visit its Web site at www.madd.org.[14]

Students Against Destructive Decisions

Many students have known the acronym *SADD* to stand for the youth group Students Against Driving Drunk or Students Against Destructive Decisions. Recently, the group has restructured itself to expand beyond drunk driving to include other high-risk activities that are detrimental to youth, such as underage drinking, drug use, drugged driving, and failure to use seat belts. Founded in 1981, this organization now has millions of members in thousands of chapters throughout the country. Remaining central to the drunk driving aspect of SADD is the "Contract for Life," a pact that encourages students and parents to provide safe transportation for each other if either is unable to drive safely after consuming alcohol. This contract also stipulates that no discussions about the incident are to be started until both can talk in a calm and caring manner. For more information about SADD, visit its Web site at www.saddonline.com.[20]

BACCHUS and GAMMA Peer Education Network

BACCHUS (Boost Alcohol Consciousness Concerning the Health of University Students) began in 1975 as an alcohol-awareness organization at the University of Florida. Run by student volunteers, this organization promoted responsible drinking among college students who chose to drink. It was not an anti-alcohol group, but a "harm reduction" group. Over the years, hundreds of chapters were formed on campuses across the country.

When supporters of BACCHUS realized that many students interested in alcohol awareness were from fraternities and sororities, they developed GAMMA (Greeks Advocating Mature Management of Alcohol) to join BACCHUS to form a peer education network. Campuses are now able to choose BACCHUS, GAMMA, or any other acronym or name of their groups.

With the broadening of the original BACCHUS organization has come an expansion of the health issues this group addresses. Originally, the focus was on alcohol abuse and prevention. Now the BACCHUS and GAMMA Peer Education Network confronts a variety of student health and safety issues. For additional information about this organization, check out its Web site at www.bacchusgamma.org.[21]

Other Approaches

Other responsible approaches to alcohol use are surfacing nearly every day. Even among college fraternity organizations, attitudes toward the indiscriminate use of alcohol are changing. Most fraternity rush functions are now conducted without the use of alcohol, and growing numbers of fraternities are alcohol-free.

Another encouraging sign on college campuses is the increasing number of alcohol use task forces. Although each of these groups has its own focus and title, many are meeting to discuss alcohol-related concerns on their particular campus. These task forces often try to formulate detailed, comprehensive policies for alcohol use across the entire campus community. Membership on these committees often includes students (on-campus and off-campus, graduate and undergraduate), faculty and staff members, academic administrators, residence hall advisors, university police, health center personnel, alumni, and local citizens. Does your college have such a committee?

Problem Drinking and Alcoholism

Problem Drinking

At times the line separating problem drinking from alcoholism is difficult to distinguish (see the Star box). There may be no true line, with the exception that an alcoholic is unable to stop drinking. **Problem drinking** is a pattern of alcohol use in which a drinker's behavior creates personal difficulties or difficulties for other people. What are some of these behaviors? Examples might be drinking to avoid life stressors, going to work intoxicated, drinking and driving, becoming injured or injuring others while drinking, solitary drinking, morning drinking, an occasional **blackout,** high-risk sexual activity, and being told by others that you drink too much. For college students, two clear indications of problem drinking are missing classes and lowered academic performance caused by alcohol involvement. (Changing for the Better on page 267 offers suggestions that can help you keep drinking under control.)

Problem drinkers are not always heavy drinkers; they might not be daily or even weekly drinkers. Unlike alcoholics, problem drinkers do not need to drink to maintain "normal" body functions. However, when they do drink, they (and others around them) experience problems . . . sometimes with tragic consequences. It is not surprising that problem drinkers are more likely than other drinkers to eventually develop alcoholism.

 TALKING POINTS Do you know people who show signs of problem drinking?

Progressive Stages of Alcohol Dependence

Early
- Escape drinking
- Binge drinking
- Guilt feelings
- Sneaking drinks
- Difficulty stopping after beginning to drink
- Increased tolerance
- Preoccupation with drinking
- Occasional blackouts

Middle
- Loss of control
- Self-hate
- Impaired social relationships
- Changes in drinking patterns (more frequent binge drinking)
- Temporary sobriety
- Morning drinking
- Dietary neglect
- Increased blackouts

Late
- Prolonged binges
- Alcohol used to control withdrawal symptoms
- Alcohol psychosis
- Nutritional disease
- Frequent blackouts

Alcoholism

In the early 1990s, a revised definition of **alcoholism** was established by a joint committee of experts on alcohol dependence.[22] This committee defined alcoholism as follows: *Alcoholism is a primary, chronic disease with genetic, psychosocial, and environmental factors influencing its*

Key Terms

problem drinking an alcohol use pattern in which a drinker's behavior creates personal difficulties or difficulties for other people

blackout a temporary state of amnesia experienced by an alcoholic; an inability to remember events that occurred during a period of alcohol use

alcoholism a primary, chronic disease with genetic, psychosocial, and environmental factors influencing its development and manifestations *development and manifestations. The disease is often progressive and fatal. It is characterized by impaired control over drinking, preoccupation with the drug alcohol, use of alcohol despite adverse consequences, and distortions in thinking, most notably denial. Each of these symptoms may be continuous or periodic.*

This definition incorporates much of the knowledge gained from addiction research during the last two decades. It is well recognized that alcoholics do not drink for the pleasurable effects of alcohol but to escape being sober. For alcoholics, being sober is stressful.

Unlike problem drinking, alcoholism involves a physical addiction to alcohol. For the true alcoholic, when the body is deprived of alcohol, physical and mental withdrawal symptoms become evident. These withdrawal symptoms can be life threatening. **Delirium tremens (DTs)** can progress to nausea, vomiting, hallucinations, shock, and cardiac and pulmonary arrest. Delirium tremens are an occasional manifestation of alcohol withdrawal.[23]

The complex reasons for the physical and emotional dependence of alcoholism have not been fully explained. Why, when more than 100 million adults use alcohol without becoming dependent on it, do 10 million or more others become unable to control its use?

Could alcoholism be an inherited disease? Studies in humans and animals have provided strong evidence that genetics plays a role in some cases of alcoholism.

Two forms of alcoholism are thought to be inherited: type 1 and type 2. Type 1 is thought to take years to develop and may not surface until midlife. Type 2 is a more severe form and appears to be passed primarily from fathers to sons. This form of alcoholism frequently begins earlier in a person's life and may even start in adolescence.

Genetics may also help protect some Asians from developing alcoholism. About half of all Far East Asians produce low levels of an important enzyme that helps metabolize alcohol. These people cannot tolerate even small amounts of alcohol. In addition, genetic factors influencing the absorption rates of alcohol in the intestinal tract have been hypothesized to predispose some Native Americans to alcoholism. More research is needed about the role of genetic factors in all forms of chemical dependence.

The role of personality traits as conditioning factors in the development of alcoholism has received considerable attention. Factors ranging from unusually low self-esteem to an antisocial personality have been implicated. Additional factors making people susceptible to alcoholism may include excessive reliance on denial, hypervigilance, compulsiveness, and chronic levels of anxiety. Always complicating the study of personality traits is the uncertainty of whether the personality profile is a predisposing factor (perhaps from inheritance) or is caused by alcoholism.

Denial and Enabling

Problem drinkers and alcoholics frequently use the psychological defense mechanism of *denial* to maintain their drinking behavior. By convincing themselves that their lives are not affected by their drinking, problem drinkers and alcoholics are able to maintain their drinking patterns. A person's denial is an unconscious process that is apparent only to rational observers.

Formerly, alcoholics were required to admit that their denial was no longer effective before they could be admitted to a treatment program. This is not the case today. Currently, family members, friends, and coworkers of alcohol-dependent people are encouraged to intervene (with the help and supervision of a professional) and force an alcohol-dependent person into treatment.

During treatment, chemically dependent people must break through the security of denial and admit that

Key Terms

delirium tremens (DTs) uncontrollable shaking combined with irrational hallucinations alcohol controls their lives. This process is demanding and often time consuming, but there is no alternative path to recovery.

For family and friends of chemically dependent people, denial is part of a process known as *enabling.* In this process, people close to the problem drinker or alcoholic inadvertently support drinking behavior by denying that a problem really exists. Enablers unconsciously make excuses for the drinker, try to keep the drinker's work and family life intact, and in effect make the continued abuse of alcohol possible. For example, college students enable problem drinkers when they clean up a drinker's messy room, lie to professors about a student's class absences, and provide class notes or other assistance to a drinker who cannot perform academically. Even the use of designated drivers has been criticized as enabling behavior.

Alcohol counselors contend that enablers can significantly delay the onset of effective therapy. Do you know of a situation in which you or others have enabled a person with alcohol problems?

Codependence

A new term was coined in the 1980s to describe the relationship between drug-dependent people and those around them—*codependence.* This term implies a kind of dual addiction. The alcoholic and the person close to the alcoholic are both addicted, one to alcohol and the other to the alcoholic. People who are codependent often find themselves denying the addiction and enabling the alcohol-dependent person.

Unfortunately, this kind of behavior damages both the alcoholic and the codependent. The alcoholic's intervention and treatment may be delayed for a considerable time. Codependent people often pay a heavy price as well. They often become drug or alcohol dependent themselves, or they may suffer a variety of psychological consequences related to guilt, loss of self-esteem, depression, and anxiety. Codependents may be at increased risk for physical and sexual abuse.

Fortunately, researchers continue to explore this dimension of alcoholism. Many students have found some of the sources listed at the end of this chapter to be especially helpful. (To determine whether you could benefit from a support program such as Al-Anon or Alateen, answer the questions in the Personal Assessment on page 277.)

Helping the Alcoholic: Rehabilitation and Recovery

When an alcoholic realizes that alcoholism is not a form of moral weakness but rather a clearly defined illness, the chances for recovery are remarkably good. It is estimated that as many as two-thirds of alcoholics can recover. Recovery is especially improved when the addicted person has a good emotional support system, including concerned family members, friends, and employer. When this support system is not well established, the alcoholic's chances for recovery are considerably lower. (See the Star box on page 269 concerning older adults and alcohol.)

Alcoholics Anonymous (AA) is a voluntary support group of recovering alcoholics who meet regularly to help each other get and stay sober. There are over 100,000 groups in 150 countries worldwide.[24] AA encourages alcoholics to admit their lack of power over alcohol and to turn their lives over to a higher power (although the organization is nonsectarian). Members of AA are encouraged not to be judgmental about the behavior of other members. They support anyone with a problem caused by alcohol.

Al-Anon and Alateen are parallel organizations that give support to people who live with alcoholics. Al-Anon is geared toward spouses and other relatives, whereas Alateen focuses on children of alcoholics. Both organizations help members realize that they are not alone and that successful adjustments can be made to nearly every situation. AA, Al-Anon, and Alateen chapter organizations are usually listed in the telephone book or in the classified sections of local newspapers. You can locate Al-Anon and Alateen on the web at www.al-anon.alateen.org.[25]

For people who feel uncomfortable with the concept that their lives are controlled by a higher power, secular recovery programs are becoming popular. These programs maintain that sobriety comes from within the alcoholic. Secular programs strongly emphasize self-reliance, self-determination, and rational thinking about one's drinking. Secular Organizations for Sobriety (SOS) and Rational Recovery are examples of secular recovery programs.

Medical Treatment for Alcoholism

Could there be a medical cure for alcoholism? For nearly fifty years, the only prescription drug physicians could use to help drinkers stop drinking was antabuse. Antabuse would cause drinkers to become extremely nauseated whenever they used alcohol.

In 1995 the Food and Drug Administration approved a drug called naltrexone that works by reducing the craving for alcohol and the pleasurable sensations felt when drinking. Combining naltrexone with conventional behavior modification has been shown to reduce alcohol relapse significantly. For a nontraditional approach to treatment of alcoholism, see Considering Complementary Care on page 270.

Alcohol and Older Adults: A Hidden Problem

We know that children, adolescents, and adults all can succumb to the risks of alcohol abuse. Unfortunately, we should not assume that the risk goes away as we age.

As the body ages, everyone experiences the effects of alcohol differently. In older adults, the body becomes more sensitive to alcohol, and the effects of alcohol can become greatly exaggerated. Alcohol levels can rise 30 percent to 40 percent higher than that of younger drinkers who consume the same amount.

About 3 million people over the age of 60 are alcoholics. Alcohol abuse by widowers and older men is higher than for widows and older women. Twenty-one percent of hospitalized people 50 and older are alcoholics. Alcohol-related hospital care in the elderly costs over $60 billion per year.

As the number of older adults is expected to grow over the next few decades as baby boomers begin retiring, we will see an increase in the number of older problem drinkers. Likewise, we can expect alcohol to continue to contribute to motor vehicle accidents involving older adults, because alcohol already appears at a relatively high frequency in crashes involving older adults, especially men.

Health care professionals need to be aware of this growing problem and offer help to older people facing the risks of alcohol abuse. In particular, we need to realize that older adults have special needs:

- Older adults may experience problems even at lower levels of alcohol consumption.

- Signs and symptoms of alcohol problems in older adults may differ from those of younger problem drinkers.

- Those most at risk are men, especially those men in transition from work to retirement.

- Older alcoholics tend to do well in alcohol treatment.

Sources:
Alcohol Use and Abuse. National Institute on Aging: Age Page, www.niapublications.org/engagepages/alcohol.asp, March 10, 2005.
Brody JE. "Hidden Plague of Alcohol Abuse by the Elderly," *New York Times,* April 2, 2002.
Campbell B. *Elderly Drug and Alcohol Abuse Often Undetected,* www.csindy.com/csindy/2000-02-02/news.html, February 2, 2000.
About Men's Health. Illinois Department on Aging. www.state.il.us/aging/1news_pubs/onage05.htm, May 15, 1999.

Current Alcohol Concerns

Adult Children of Alcoholic Parents

In recent years a new dimension of alcoholism has been identified—the unusually high prevalence of alcoholism among adult children of alcoholics (ACOAs). It is estimated that these people are about four times more likely to develop alcoholism than are persons whose parents are not alcoholics. Even the ACOAs who do not become alcoholics may have a difficult time adjusting to everyday living. Janet Geringer Woititz, author of the best-selling book *Adult Children of Alcoholics,*[26] describes 13 traits that, to some degree, most ACOAs exhibit. (See the Star box on page 271).

In response to this concern, support groups have been formed to prevent the adult sons and daughters of alcoholics from developing the condition that afflicted their parents. If a stronger link for an inherited genetic predisposition to alcoholism is found, these groups may play an even greater role in the prevention of alcoholism.

Women and Alcohol

For decades, women have consumed less alcohol and had fewer alcohol-related problems than men. Evidence is mounting that a greater percentage of women are choosing to drink and that some subgroups of women, especially young women, are drinking more heavily. A greater number of admissions of women to treatment centers may also reflect that alcohol consumption among women is on the rise. Special approaches for women to use for staying sober are discussed in Learning from Our Diversity on page 271.

Studies show that there are now almost as many female as male alcoholics. However, differences appear to exist between men and women when it comes to alcohol abuse.[17] Some of the more pronounced differences are (1) More women than men can point to a specific triggering event, such as a divorce, death of a spouse, a career change, or children leaving home, that started them drinking heavily. (2) Alcoholism among women often starts later and progresses more quickly than alcoholism among men. (3) Women tend to be prescribed more mood-altering drugs than men are. Thus women face a greater risk of drug interaction or cross-tolerance. (4) Nonalcoholic men tend to divorce their alcoholic spouses nine times more often than nonalcoholic women divorce their alcoholic spouses. Thus alcoholic women are not as likely to have a family support system to aid them in their recovery attempts. (5) Female alcoholics do not tend to receive as much social support as men in their treatment and recovery. (6) Although men outnumber women entering treatment programs by almost 4 to 1, women alcoholics tend to come into treatment earlier than men. (7) Women alcoholics are more likely than male alcholics to have medical complications. This may result from the differences in the metabolism of alcohol between men and women. Women are particularly susceptible to diseases of the liver. (8) Unmarried or divorced single-parent women often have economic problems that make entry into treatment programs especially difficult. In light of the generally recognized educational, occupational, and social gains made by women during the last two decades, it will be interesting to see whether these male-female differences continue. What's your best guess?

Alcohol Advertising

Every few years, careful observers can see subtle changes in the ways the alcoholic beverage industry markets its products. Recently, the marketing push appears to be directed toward minorities (through advertisements for malt liquor and fortified wines), women (through wine and wine cooler ads), and youth (through trendy, young adult-oriented commercials).

On the college campus, aggressive alcohol campaigns have used rock stars, beach party scenes, athletic event sponsorships, and colorful newspaper supplements to encourage the purchase of alcohol. Critics claim that most of the collegiate advertising is directed at minors and that the prevention messages are not strong enough to offset the potential health damage to this population. As a college student, how do you feel about alcohol advertising on your campus? If you are a nontraditional-age student, do you find the advertising campaigns amusing or potentially dangerous?

Some beer and liquor companies have begun using websites on the Internet to promote their products. Critics contend that the colorful graphics, hip language, games, chat rooms, and "virtual bars" are designed to recruit underage drinkers.

Alcohol Advertising in Ethnic Communities

A literature review by the Trauma Foundation at San Francisco General Hospital[27] reports some interesting facts concerning alcohol availability and alcohol advertising in ethnic communities. In the United States, low-income Latino and African American communities have a disproportionate number of alcohol outlets compared to white communities. This concentration of alcohol outlets seems to be related to an increase in traffic injuries and assaults. Additionally, as the number of alcohol outlets increases, the likelihood of increased crime and violence rises. Crime and violence drive out existing business establishments and discourage new businesses from locating in the area. Economic development can become thwarted.

Learning from Our Diversity

Staying Sober: New Pathways for Women

Since 1935, when it was founded by two white American male alcoholics, Alcoholics Anonymous has expanded to encompass millions of members in virtually every region of the world who strive to achieve and maintain sobriety by adhering to AA's well-known 12-step program of recovery. With its strong spiritual orientation emphasizing the acknowledgment of a "higher power," AA offers safety, comfort, and structure to people of all ages and backgrounds, and both sexes. For decades, women as well as men have made AA the cornerstone of their efforts to get sober and stay sober.

Not all women, however, are comfortable with AA's focus on Christian spirituality and the perceived masculine orientation of its chief text, Alcoholics Anonymous (familiarly known as the "Big Book"), and other program literature. These women place an equally high value on sober living as do AA adherents, but they prefer to pursue that goal in other settings. In recent years, alternatives to AA have emerged that offer peer group acceptance and support for recovering alcoholic women but do so in a nonspiritual, nonsexist context.

One such group, Women for Sobriety, is a mutual aid organization for women with alcohol problems that was founded in 1975 by Dr. Jean Kirkpatrick. The WFS program focuses on improving self-esteem; members achieve sobriety by taking responsibility for their actions and by learning not to dwell on negative thoughts. Another alternative, Rational

Recovery, is open to both men and women. RR, which is based on the theories of psychologist Albert Ellis's Rational Emotive Therapy, also uses a cognitive, nonspiritual approach that fosters cohesiveness and provides the emotional support sought by people who seek to gain and maintain sobriety.

Particularly for "marginalized" alcoholic women such as lesbians, members of racial and ethnic minorities, and those of non-Christian religious backgrounds, alcoholism treatment professionals increasingly are being encouraged to present the full range of support-group options, including but not emphasizing the approach of Alcoholics Anonymous.

If you were seeking help to achieve and maintain sobriety, would you be more inclined to attend a program based on spirituality, or one that offers a rational, cognitive approach? Why?

Sources:
Galanter M, et al. Rational recovery: Alternative to AA for addiction? *American Journal of Drug and Alcohol Abuse,* 1993, vol. 19, p. 499.
Hall J. Lesbians' participation in Alcoholics Anonymous: Experience of social, personal, and political tensions. *Contemporary Drug Problems,* Spring 1996, vol. 23, no. 1, p. 113.
Kaskutas L. A road less traveled: Choosing the "Women for Sobriety" program. *Journal of Drug Issues.* Winter 1996, vol. 26, no. 1, p. 77.
Women for Sobriety, Inc. www.womenforsobriety.org/, March 10, 2005.

Common Traits of Adult Children of Alcoholics

Adult children of alcoholics may:

- Have difficulty identifying normal behavior
- Have difficulty following a project from beginning to end
- Lie when it would be just as easy to tell the truth
- Judge themselves without mercy
- Have difficulty having fun
- Take themselves very seriously
- Have difficulty with intimate relationships

- Overreact to changes over which they have no control
- Constantly seek approval and affirmation
- Feel that they are different from other people
- Be super-responsible or super-irresponsible
- Be extremely loyal, even in the face of evidence that the loyalty is undeserved
- Tend to lock themselves into a course of action without considering the consequences

Experts agree that adult children of alcoholics who believe they have come to terms with their feelings can sometimes face lingering problems. Support groups to contact include Al-Anon (www.al-anon.alateen.org). Adult Children of Alcoholics (www.adultchildren.org), and Children of Alcoholics Foundation (www.coaf.org).

Woititz JG. *Adult Children of Alcoholics.* Health Communications, Inc., 1990.

The Trauma Foundation also reports that alcohol is more heavily advertised in low-income African American and Latino communities than in other neighborhoods. The advertisements are found on billboards as well as the displays inside and around the alcohol outlets. Advertising frequently exploits important cultural symbols, and promotions are targeted toward specific ethnic groups. For example, malt liquor is marketed especially to African Americans. Thus, rap singers are frequently featured in promotions and advertisements for malt liquor.

- Determine whether you are affected by someone's drinking by doing the Personal Assessment on page 277.

- Prepare for a possible alcohol-related emergency by reviewing the signs listed in Changing for the Better on page 259.

- Assess your level of social responsibility by using Changing for the Better on page 264.

- If you think that you are a problem drinker or an alcoholic, join a support group to get help.

- Enter into a "Contract for Life" with your parents or closest friends, a pact that says that you will provide safe transportation for one another if any of you is/are unable to drive safely after consuming alcohol.

- Make a commitment to responsible alcohol use by joining a campus group that works toward this goal.

SUMMARY

- Most people drink because alcohol is an effective, affordable, legal substance for altering the brain's chemistry.
- People are categorized as abstainers, light drinkers, moderate drinkers, or heavy drinkers, according to their alcohol use patterns.
- Binge drinking is dangerous and can lead to drunk driving, violence, lowered academic performance, and social problems.
- As BAC rises, predictable depressant effects take place, and the risk of acute alcohol intoxication increases; people with this condition are in danger and must receive first aid immediately.
- Federal legislation has pushed all states to lower the legal BAC standard to .08 percent.
- Alcohol is removed from the bloodstream through the process of oxidation.
- Chronic alcohol use causes a variety of serious health problems for the drinker and can cause fetal alcohol syndrome in infants when a woman drinks during pregnancy.
- Alcohol-related social problems include accidents (motor vehicle crashes, falls, drownings, and fires and burns), crime and violence, and suicide.
- People who host events at which alcohol is served should follow certain guidelines, such as providing nonalcoholic alternative beverages, to help ensure the safety of their guests.

- Several groups of concerned citizens, such as MADD, SADD, BACCHUS, and GAMMA promote responsible alcohol use.
- Problem drinking is an alcohol use pattern in which a drinker's behavior creates personal difficulties or problems for others.
- Alcoholism is a primary, chronic disease characterized by addiction to alcohol; it has a variety of possible causes and manifestations.
- Enabling is a behavior pattern in which people close to the problem drinker or alcoholic make the continued use of alcohol possible by keeping the drinker's work and family life intact.
- An alcoholic's family members may unintentionally delay the alcoholic's intervention and treatment by becoming codependent.
- Alcoholics Anonymous and other support groups may help an alcoholic recover from the disease.
- The drugs antabuse and naltrexone are sometimes prescribed to discourage alcohol use.
- Alcohol advertising is often targeted at minorities, women, and youth.

REVIEW QUESTIONS

1. What percentage of American adults consume alcohol? Approximately what percentage of adults are classified as abstainers? What percentage of college students drink?
2. What is binge drinking?
3. What is meant by the term *proof*?
4. What is the nutritional value of alcohol? How do "light" and low-alcohol beverages compare?
5. Identify and explain the various factors that influence the absorption of alcohol. Why is it important to be aware of these factors?
6. What is BAC? Describe the general sequence of physiological events that takes place when a person drinks alcohol at a rate faster than the liver can oxidize it.
7. What are the signs and symptoms of acute alcohol intoxication? What are the first-aid steps you should take to help a person with this problem?

8. Describe the characteristics of fetal alcohol syndrome and fetal alcohol effects.
9. Explain the differences between problem drinking and alcoholism.
10. What roles do denial and enabling play in alcoholism? What is codependence?
11. What are some common traits of ACOAs?
12. What unique alcohol-related problems do women face?
13. Describe the activities undertaken by SADD, MADD, BACCHUS, and GAMMA, and by AA, Al-Anon, and Alateen.
14. Describe the progressive stages of alcohol dependence.
15. List some ways you can keep alcohol consumption under control.

ENDNOTES

1. U.S. Department of Health and Human Services. *Alcohol and Health: Tenth Special Report to the U.S. Congress,* NIH Publication No 00-1583. Washington, DC: U.S. Government Printing Office, 2000.
2. U.S. Bureau of the Census. *Statistical Abstract of the United States, 1999* (199th ed.). Washington, DC: U.S. Government Printing Office, 1999.
3. Core Institute. *The Core Alcohol and Drug Survey 2003,* www.siu.edu/departments/coreinst/public_html/, March 9, 2005.
4. Brown SA, Tapert SF, Granholm E, et al. Neurocognitive functioning of adolescents: Effects of protracted alcohol use, *Alcoholism, Clinical and Experimental Research,* 24(2), 2000, 164–171.
5. Adult Children Educational Foundation Computer Bulletin Board. *Sick Families,* www.recovery.org/acoa/families.html, December 24, 1997.
6. Zest for Life. *Alcohol and Ethanol Information Page,* www.anyvitamins.com/alcohol-ethanol-info.htm, March 9, 2005.
7. Gaziano, JM, et al. Light-to-moderate alcohol consumption and mortality in the Physicians' Health Study enrollment cohort. *Journal of the American College of Cardiology,* 35(1), 2000, 96–105.
8. Be Responsible About Drinking. *Women and Alcohol,* www.brad21.org/alcohol_and_women.html, March 9, 2005.
9. Pinger RR, et al. *Drugs: Issues for Today* (3rd ed.). New York: McGraw-Hill, 1998.
10. Ray O, Ksir C. *Drugs, Society, and Human Behavior* (8th ed.). New York: McGraw-Hill, 1999.
11. ADA: Division of Drug and Alcohol Abuse. *As a Matter of Fact . . . Fetal Alcohol Syndrome,* www.well.com/user/woa/fsfas.htm, March 9, 2005.
12. National Institute on Alcohol Abuse and Alcoholism. *Tenth Special Report to the U.S. Congress on Alcohol and Health,* Chapter 6. NIH Publication No. 00-1583. Rockville, MD: U.S. Department of Health and Human Services, 2000.
13. Traffic Safety Facts 2003: *Alcohol.* U.S. Department of Transportation National Highway Traffic Safety Administration.
14. Mothers Against Drunk Driving. *About Us,* www.madd.org, March 9, 2005.
15. The Trauma Foundation. *Alcohol and Unintentional Injury: A Brief Review of the Literature,* www.tf.org/tf/alcohol/ariv/reviews/injurev5.html, June 16, 2003.
16. USLA Lifeguards for Life. *Training Guide for USLA Safety Tips: General Information on Drowning,* www.usla.org/PublicInfo/Safety_guide.shtml, June 16, 2003.
17. Kinney J. *Loosening the Grip: A Handbook of Alcohol Information* (7th ed.). New York: McGraw-Hill, 2003.
18. Vaughn, C. *Children of Alcoholics: At Risk for Family Violence.* U.S. Department of Health and Human Services and SAMHSA's National Clearinghouse for Alcohol and Drug Information, February 10, 2003.
19. *Facts about Suicide.* CDC Prevention, National Center for Health Statistics, 1998.
20. SADD History. *Students Against Drunk Driving,* www.saddonline.com, March 1, 2005.
21. Organization History and Mission. The Bacchus and Gamma Peer Education Network, www.bacchusgamma.org/, March 1, 2005.
22. Morse RM, et al. The definition of alcoholism, *JAMA* 1992; 268(8): 1012–1014.
23. Burns, M. *Delirium Tremens,* emedicine.com, Inc., November 8, 2004.
24. Alcoholics Anonymous. *AA At a Glance,* www.alcoholics-anonymous.org, March 1, 2005.
25. Al-Anon/Alateen Web Site Information, www.al-anon.alateen.org/, March 1, 2005.
26. Woititz JG. *Adult Children of Alcoholics.* Health Communications, Inc., 1990.
27. Trauma Foundation at San Francisco General Hospital. *The Effects of Alcohol on Different Ethnic Communities: Fact Sheet,* www.tf.org/tf/alcohol/ariv/facts/ethfct25.html, June 20, 2003.

As We Go to Press

To help enforce underage drinking laws, the Justice Department announced in August 2005 that all 50 states and the District of Columbia would each be awarded $350,000. This $20 million federal initiative consists of block grants to be used for media outreach programs stressing the dangers of binge drinking, underage drinking, drinking and driving, and a zero-tolerance policy for offenders. This funding would also support alcohol-free programming for minors.

personal assessment

How do you use alcoholic beverages?

Answer the following questions about your own alcohol use. Record your number of "yes" and "no" responses at the end of the questionnaire.

Do you: **Yes**   **No**

1. Drink more often than you did a year ago? _____ _____

2. Drink more heavily than you did a year ago? _____ _____

3. Plan to drink, sometimes days in advance? _____ _____

4. Gulp or "chug" your drinks, perhaps in a contest? _____ _____

5. Set personal limits on the amount you plan to drink but then consistently disregard these limits? _____ _____

6. Drink at a rate greater than two drinks per hour? _____ _____

7. Encourage or even pressure others to drink with you? _____ _____

8. Frequently want a nonalcoholic beverage but then end up drinking an alcoholic drink? _____ _____

9. Drive your car while under the influence of alcohol or ride with another person who has been drinking? _____ _____

10. Use alcoholic beverages while taking prescription or OTC medications? _____ _____

11. Forget what happened while you were drinking? _____ _____

12. Have a tendency to disregard information about the effects of drinking? _____ _____

13. Find your reputation fading because of alcohol use? _____ _____

        TOTAL _____ _____

Interpretation

If you answered yes to any of these questions, you may be using alcohol irresponsibly. Two or more yes responses indicate an unacceptable pattern of alcohol use and may reflect problem drinking behavior.

To Carry This Further . . .

Ask your friends or roommates to take this assessment. Are they willing to take this assessment and then talk about their results with you? Be prepared to discuss any follow-up questions they might have about their (or your) alcohol consumption patterns. Your willingness to talk about drinking behavior might help someone realize that this topic can and should be discussed openly. Finally, be aware of how people in your area can get professional help with drinking or other drug concerns.

Use the space below to write down important phone numbers where you can find alcohol-related assistance for you or your friends and relatives.

_____

_____

_____

_____

_____

_____

_____

_____

personal assessment

Does someone's drinking trouble you?

The following questions are designed to help you decide whether you are affected by someone's drinking and could benefit from a program such as Al-Anon. Record your number of yes and no responses in the boxes at the end of the questionnaire.

	Yes	No
1. Do you worry about how much someone else drinks?	_____	_____
2. Do you have money problems because of someone else's drinking?	_____	_____
3. Do you tell lies to cover up for someone else's drinking?	_____	_____
4. Do you feel that if the drinker loved you, he or she would stop drinking to please you?	_____	_____
5. Do you blame the drinker's behavior on his or her companions?	_____	_____
6. Are plans frequently upset or meals delayed because of the drinker?	_____	_____
7. Do you make threats, such as: "If you don't stop drinking, I'll leave you"?	_____	_____
8. Do you secretly try to smell the drinker's breath?	_____	_____
9. Are you afraid to upset someone for fear it will set off a drinking bout?	_____	_____
10. Have you been hurt or embarrassed by a drinker's behavior?	_____	_____
11. Are holidays and gatherings spoiled because of someone's drinking?	_____	_____
12. Have you considered calling the police for help in fear of abuse?	_____	_____
13. Do you search for hidden alcohol?	_____	_____
14. Do you often ride in a car with a driver who has been drinking?	_____	_____
15. Have you refused social invitations out of fear or anxiety that the drinker will cause a scene?	_____	_____
16. Do you sometimes feel like a failure when you think of the lengths to which you have gone to control the drinker?	_____	_____
17. Do you think that if the drinker stopped drinking, your other problems would be solved?	_____	_____
18. Do you ever threaten to hurt yourself to scare the drinker?	_____	_____
19. Do you feel angry, confused, or depressed most of the time?	_____	_____
20. Do you feel there is no one who understands your problems?	_____	_____
TOTAL	_____	_____

Interpretation

If you answered yes to three or more of these questions, Al-Anon or Alateen may be able to help. You can contact Al-Anon or Alateen by looking in your local telephone directory or by writing to Al-Anon Family Group Headquarters, Inc., 1600 Corporate Landing Parkway, Virginia Beach, VA 23454–5617, or you may call (888) 4AL-ANON.

To Carry This Further . . .

Sometimes the decision to seek help from a support group is a difficult one. If you answered yes to any of the questions above, spend a few moments reflecting on your responses. How long have you been experiencing problems because of someone else's drinking? How would sharing your feelings with others—people who have dealt with very similar problems—help you cope with your own situation? Knowing you're not alone can often be a great relief; it's up to you to take the first step.

chapter nine

Rejecting Tobacco Use

Chapter Objectives

On completing this chapter, you will be able to:

▌ examine smoking rates among demographic groups, student groups on your campus, and groups in different states, and speculate on the underlying reasons for these trends.

▌ identify techniques used by the tobacco industry to encourage people to smoke.

▌ critically evaluate tobacco advertisements to determine what audience particular ads target, and what messages they send to consumers.

▌ administer the 10-item Hooked on Nicotine Checklist (HONC) to friends who smoke to determine the existence and depth of dependence.

▌ explain the bolus theory, the adrenocorticotropic hormone (ACTH) theory, and the self-medication theory of nicotine addiction.

▌ explain the particulate phase and the gaseous phase of tobacco smoke and identify the primary components of each.

▌ describe the relationship between smoking and cardiovascular disease.

▌ trace the role of smoking in the development of respiratory-tract cancer.

▌ identify smoking-cessation aids, including various nicotine delivery techniques and describe steps that smokers can take to reduce or eliminate their use of tobacco.

▌ describe how parents of young children can discourage tobacco use in the future.

▌ explain the dangers of secondhand smoke and develop steps to reduce your exposure to it.

Eye on the Media

Tobacco Industry Denies Ads Target Kids

On various occasions during the past 8 years the tobacco industry has run television commercials intended to "educate" the public about the fundamental changes that the industry has undertaken in terms of marketing, particularly in light of charges that the industry previously targeted children in an attempt to develop a new generation of smokers. In these commercials several changes were described, all of which were attributed to the 1998 settlement (formally signed in 1999) reached between the tobacco industry and the states' attorneys general stemming from a massive class action suit to recoup Medicaid money. There was no mention in the commercials that the original agreement reached between the states and the tobacco industry in June of 1997 was much more restrictive and closely reflective of the intent of the court in curbing the marketing activities of the tobacco industry. The more permissive 1998 settlement, known as the Master Settlement Agreement (MSA), arose when the tobacco industry promised to vigorously fight the 1997 agreement in court. Thus, compromises favoring the tobacco industry were made by the states to save time and resources that would otherwise be lost to additional litigation.

The accompanying chart shows selected examples of the differences between the 1997 agreement and the final 1999 settlement. Because of the tobacco industry's ability to afford media exposure, the American public will continue to be led to believe that the tobacco industry complied completely with the intent of the courts.

In yet a more current example of the tobacco industry's relationship to media exposure, RJR withdrew its corporate sponsorship of NASCAR's premier racing series, the Winston Cup Series. By finally complying with the 1999 Master Settlement Agreement RJR can redirect hundreds of millions of dollars once spent on NASCAR into other areas of media exposure, such as advertisements in magazines popular with teens (such as *Sports Illustrated* and *Hot Rod*) and point-of-purchase displays in convenience stores and drug stores.

Source:
Wakefield, MA, et al. "Tobacco Industry Marketing of Point of Purchase after the 1999 MSA Billboard Ban," *AJPH* 9, No. 6, June 2002.

Master Settlement Agreement (MSA)

Restriction	1997 Agreement	1999 (MSA)
Outdoor and Transit Ads	Bans all outdoor and transit ads	Allows signs of up to 14 sq feet on any building or property where tobacco products are sold, including those near schools and playgrounds. Bans other billboards and transit ads.
Cartoons and Human Images	Banned	Allows human images, such as the Marlboro man. Bans cartoons.
Brand Name Sponsorships	Banned	Each company allowed one brand name sponsorship of an event or series of events. Prohibits events in which contestants are under 18 years of age.
Free Samples	Banned	Free samples allowed in adult-only facilities.

Tobacco Use in American Society

If you were to visit certain businesses, entertainment spots, or sporting events in your community, you might leave convinced that virtually every adult is a tobacco user. Certainly, for some segments of society, tobacco use is the rule rather than the exception. You may be quite surprised, however, to find out that the great majority of adults do not use tobacco products.

Table 9.1 displays current cigarette smoking by males and females for each state.[2] Note that Kentucky, a major tobacco-producing state, has the highest percentage of smokers (32.6 percent), whereas Utah, a state in which nearly three-fourths of the residents are Mormons and thus refrain from tobacco and alcohol use, reports the smallest percentage of tobacco uses (12.7 percent). How does your home state compare?

Following the Surgeon General's 1964 report (the first official statement of concern by the federal government regarding the dangers of smoking),[3] the prevalence of smoking began a decline that lasted until 1991, when a leveling off was noted that lasted for the next

Table 9.1 Current Cigarette Smoking by Sex and State: 2002

[In percent. Current cigarette smoking is defined as persons who reported having smoked 100 or more cigarettes during their lifetime and who currently smoke every day or some days. Based on the Behavioral Risk Factor Surveillance System, a telephone survey of health behaviors of the civilian, noninstitutionalized U.S. population, 18 years old and over; for details, see source]

State	Total	Male	Female	State	Total	Male	Female	State	Total	Male	Female
U.S.	23.1	25.9	20.9	KS	22.1	23.2	20.9	ND	21.5	23.1	20.0
				KY	32.6	34.8	30.5	OH	26.6	28.4	25.0
AL	24.4	27.5	21.6	LA	23.9	26.6	21.5	OK	26.7	29.7	23.8
AK	29.4	31.9	26.7	ME	23.6	26.4	21.1	OR	22.4	24.6	20.2
AZ	23.5	27.0	20.1	MD	22.0	25.7	18.6	PA	24.6	26.1	23.2
AR	26.3	28.7	24.1	MA	19.0	20.2	18.0	RI	22.5	24.3	20.9
CA	16.4	19.7	13.3	MI	24.2	25.1	23.5	SC	26.6	29.1	24.4
CO	20.4	21.4	19.4	MN	21.7	24.3	19.4	SD	22.6	25.6	19.7
CT	19.5	20.6	18.4	MS	27.4	33.2	22.2	TN	27.8	31.0	24.9
DE	24.7	25.4	24.1	MO	26.6	29.6	23.9	TX	22.9	26.8	19.1
DC	20.4	23.8	17.5	MT	21.3	21.3	21.4	UT	12.7	14.2	11.3
FL	22.1	23.6	20.7	NE	22.8	26.3	19.4	VT	21.2	21.5	20.9
GA	23.3	26.8	20.0	NV	26.0	28.5	23.5	VA	24.6	28.5	20.9
HI	21.1	26.2	16.0	NH	23.2	23.9	22.6	WA	21.5	23.6	19.4
ID	20.6	21.6	19.7	NJ	19.1	20.4	17.9	WV	28.4	29.8	27.2
IL	22.9	26.1	19.8	NM	21.2	23.3	19.3	WI	23.4	25.4	21.4
IN	27.7	29.8	25.8	NY	22.4	25.9	19.3	WY	23.7	25.3	22.0
IA	23.1	26.3	20.2	NC	26.4	30.7	22.3				

Source: U.S. Centers for Disease Control and Prevention, Atlanta, GA, *Morbidity and Mortality Weekly Report,* Vol. 52, No. 53, January 9, 2004

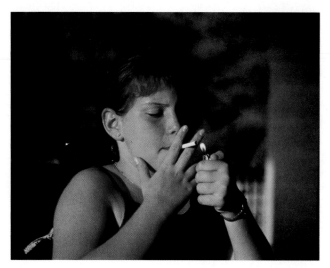

Smoking is a learned behavior and most smokers begin as kids.

Table 9.2 Patterns of Cigarette Smoking

Prevalence by Sex		
Total	Men	Women
22.5	25.2	20.0

Note: Subjects have smoked more than 100 cigarettes and reported smoking every day or some days.

Percentage by Ethnicity and Race

Total	White	Black	Hispanic	American Indian or Alaska Native	Asian or Pacific Islander
22.5	23.6	22.4	16.7	40.8	13.3

Note: Subjects have smoked more than 100 cigarettes and smoked at the time of the survey.
Cigarette smoking among adults—United States, 2002. *MMWR*, Vol. 53, No. 20, May 28, 2004.

three years. Since 1994 the percentage of the population who smoke has declined slowly but progressively. Current statistics reveal that 22.5 percent of American adults smoke cigarettes on a daily or near-daily basis. Men are more likely to smoke (25.9 percent) than are women (20.9 percent).[2] When subsegments of the population, based on race and ethnicity, were studied it was found that whites and blacks were essentially smoking with the same prevalence (23.6 percent and 22.4 percent). At the same time, Hispanics were considerably less likely to smoke (16.7 percent), while American Indians and Alaska Natives (40.8 percent) were more likely to smoke. Persons of Asian or Pacific Island descent were the Americans least likely to smoke (13.3 percent) (see Table 9.2).[4]

Cigarette Smoking among College Students

Until very recently, the rate of cigarette smoking among college graduates was lower than that reported for the population as a whole, and it was significantly lower than the rate for persons with very little formal education. In fact, the prevalence of smoking among college students decreased progressively from 21 percent in 1964 to 14 percent in 1995.[5] However, an upward trend in cigarette use by college students has been noted, with a recent study indicating that 31.4 percent had smoked within the preceding month.[6] In contrast, a downward trend in smoking by 12th-graders has been reported for five out of six consecutive years (1998–2004), with 25.0 percent smoking during the past month in 2004.[7] Because the majority of today's college students graduated from high school during these years, we could have expected a progressive decline in

college student smoking. Such has not been the case, however, suggesting that factors encountered after matriculation are fostering smoking among college students. This is, in fact, possible since among the 2004 12th-graders with college aspirations, only 21.6 percent were cigarette smokers.[7]

When a college community is viewed as a whole regarding which segments of the student body are most likely to smoke, there appears to be a direct relationship between the level of alcohol consumption and cigarette smoking. Additional direct relationships appear between smoking and other drug use and in housing where smoking is permitted. Similar, although perhaps less influential, relationships are seen among tobacco use and coping style, depression, and perceptions of life satisfaction.[8]

The historically predictable relationship between higher levels of completed education and the lessened likelihood of smoking remains clearly evident even today. For example, when comparing the percentage of heavy smokers (a pack or more per day) on the basis of education completed, the influence of education is evident—less than high school (37.5m/31.3f percent), high school graduate (32.0m/26.2f percent), some college (25.4m/21.9f percent), and college graduate (11.0m/10.7f percent).[9] Unfortunately, the more recently reported incidence of smoking among college students (2004) seems to indicate that today's college students are smoking at a level more characteristic of high school dropouts from two decades ago.

The most disturbing aspect of the increase in reported smoking among college students, beyond the

A Simple Dependency Test Regarding Your Relationships with Cigarettes

To nonsmokers it must seem that smokers would realize the existence of their dependency on cigarettes; however, such might not be the case. The Hooked On Nicotine Checklist (HONC) appearing below is a simple way to determine whether a cigarette-based dependency exists. If you are a smoker, answer each question asked by the HONC in an honest manner; then give careful consideration to your findings. If you are a nonsmoker, ask a smoker to complete the HONC and share responses to each item with you—a good discussion could ensue.

Nicotine Addiction's 10 Warning Signs

HONC - H ooked O n N icotine C hecklist

1.	Have you ever tried to quit but couldn't?
2.	Do you smoke now because it is really hard to quit?
3.	Have you ever felt like you were addicted to tobacco?
4.	Do you ever have strong cravings to smoke?
5.	Have you ever felt like you really needed a cigarette?
6.	Is it hard to keep from smoking in places where you are not supposed to, like school?

In answering the last four questions, when you tried to stop smoking, or when you have not used tobacco for a while . . . .

7.	Did you find it hard to concentrate?
8.	Did you feel more irritable?
9.	Did you feel a strong need or urge to smoke?
10.	Did you feel nervous, restless or anxious because you couldn't smoke?

Answering "yes" to any one of these 10 questions indicates that you may already be hooked on nicotine and are chemically dependent. Think about it! Your "yes" answer is your own honest self-assessment that you have already lost the freedom and ability to simply and effortlessly walk away. Two-thirds of all teens whom you see smoking regularly will spend their entire life as slaves to nicotine.

Source: HONC - (Hooked on Nicotine Checklist). Tobacco Control, Sept. 2002 Dr. JR Difranza, *Development of Symptoms of Tobacco Dependency in Youths. Reliability Study of HONC Factors*—July 2002. Created by www.WhyQuit.com. Join us for motivation, education, and support!

eventual influence it will have on health and life expectancy, is its negation of the traditional belief that the college and university experience "protected" this segment of the society from making some ill-informed choices. As recently as the mid-1990s it was still possible to believe that the college population was "too well informed" and "too future oriented" to engage widely in an addictive behavior that fosters dependence, compromises health, and eventually shortens life. Today that proposition seems to lack some of its former validity, but one hopes that the corner is being turned.

Other Demographic Factors Influencing Tobacco Use

In addition to gender, race, ethnicity, and education level, other demographic facts appear to influence the extent to which smoking occurs. Included among these factors are the age groups into which persons fall, the region of the country in which they live, the size of their communities, and their employment status.

If age grouping is begun with 18- to 25-year-olds and progresses to 65 years of age and older, the general trend is for the percentage of persons smoking (during the past month) within each group to go down. For example, among the younger age group, 18- to 24-year-olds, 32.4 percent of males and 24.6 percent of females reported having smoked during the preceding month, whereas among the 25- to 34-year-olds, 27.5 percent of males and 21.6 percent of females smoked during the preceding month, and in the 45- to 64-year-old group, 24.5 percent of males and 21.1 percent of females smoked during the preceding month. In comparison, in the oldest age group, the 65-year-olds and older, only 10.1 percent of males and 8.6 percent of females smoked cigarettes within the preceding 30 days. Most likely over the course of time, both quitting and premature death serve to reduce the percentage of smokers.

Comparing smoking during the preceding month among people in different regions of the country reveals that persons living in the north central portion of the country are the most likely to smoke (26 percent). In contrast, persons living in the West are least likely to have smoked during the preceding month (20.0 percent). People in the South (25.4 percent) and the Northeast (23.9 percent) fall in between.[9] In terms of population density, one might be surprised to learn that persons living outside metropolitan areas are more likely to have smoked during the preceding month (30.5 percent), whereas persons living in small metropolitan areas (27.2 percent) and large metropolitan areas (26.5 percent) are less likely to have smoked during the same period.[10]

Employment status also affects the likelihood of regular smoking. Persons who are employed part-time are more likely to have smoked during the previous month (31.2 percent) than are people who are employed full-time (25.5 percent)—most likely reflecting the greater opportunity of the former group to smoke, since today's work place is increasingly a smoke-free environment. In stark contrast to those who have some degree of employment, the unemployed are by far the most likely to have smoked during the preceding month (48.2 percent.)[11] This fact may reflect not only the lower level of education found among this group but also the immediate gratification that smoking brings to persons who may have little opportunity to seriously pursue long-range goals and the postponed gratification that striving for such goals can often require.

Marketing of Tobacco Products

Shredded plant material, wrapped in paper or leaf, ignited with a flame, and then placed on or near the delicate tissues of the mouth. . . what other human behavior does this resemble? If you answered *None!* to this question, then you appreciate that smoking is unique, and, therefore, that it must be learned. How it is learned is currently a less than fully understood process that most likely requires a variety of stimuli ranging from modeling to actual experimentation. The role of advertising as a source of models has long been suspected and intensely debated. Today, as in the past, controversy surrounds the intent of the tobacco industry's advertising. Are the familiar logos seen in a variety of media intended to challenge the brand loyalty of those who have already decided to smoke, as the industry claims? Or are the ads intended to entice new smokers, older children and young adolescents, in sufficient numbers to replace the 3,000 smokers who die each day from the consequences of tobacco use? This latter objective is now known, by admission of the tobacco industry, to have been pursued for decades. Its effectiveness has also been documented. The cartoon character Joe Camel was an especially successful tool for enticing children and teens to begin smoking.

Over the years the tobacco industry has used all aspects of mass media advertising, including radio, television, print, billboards, and sponsorship of televised athletic events and concerts, to sell its products. In addition, it has often distributed free samples and sold merchandise bearing the company or product logo.

Today the tobacco industry has been denied access to television and radio, and it can no longer distribute free samples to minors, but the industry continues to be active and innovative in other aspects of the media to which it has access. For example, Philip Morris contemplated the introduction of an upscale lifestyle magazine to be provided free to over 1 million smokers. Interestingly, the magazine would feature articles about healthful activities that many longtime smokers would be unable to engage in because of the effects of smoking.

In the 9 months following the 1998 settlement, the tobacco industry increased their magazine advertising budget by 30 percent over presettlement levels in magazines with 15 percent or more youth (under 18 years of age) readership, even though they had agreed to discontinue advertising in youth-oriented publications. Most recently, increased tobacco advertising has been noted in magazines that appeal specifically to younger women, working women, fans of hip-hop music, and women of color.

The development of nonmarket brands of cigarettes for free distribution to patrons of bars and restaurants who are attempting to "bum" cigarettes represents a second form of "advertising." This "premarketing" introduction of a prototype brand technically does not violate the law regarding the distribution of samples. To date, several hundred establishments in several major cities have participated.

A final current example of the tobacco industry's subtle but effective presence in the mind of the public is that of tobacco use in motion pictures. In spite of a 1990 tobacco industry policy and the 1999 Master Settlement Agreement, both of which prohibit "brand placement" of tobacco products in films, cigarette and cigar smoking continue to be disproportionately represented in current films. Unfortunately, children and adolescents can easily identify with these

Thanks, But No Cigar

If one were to judge on the basis of the number of newly opened cigar stores and clubs catering to cigar smokers, as well as the highly visible magazine *Cigar Aficionado,* one could conclude that cigar smoking was the hottest trend in tobacco use. To a degree this contention is true when one considers that in 1991 only 2.2 percent of the adult population smoked cigars on a regular basis, whereas by 1998 the size of the cigar-smoking population had risen to 5.2 percent. However, the most recent data available (2002) suggest only a slight increase, to 5.4 percent. We can hope that this very small increase suggests a possible leveling off of the cigar craze of the 1990s.

In any case, cigar smokers who continue to smoke and those of you who might be interested in this form of tobacco use should consider the following information from the American Lung Association:

- *Secondhand (sidestream) cigar smoke is more poisonous than secondhand cigarette smoke is.* The smoke from one cigar equals that of three cigarettes. Carbon monoxide emissions from one cigar are 30 times higher than those for one cigarette.

- *Cigar smoking can cause cancer of the larynx (voice box), mouth, esophagus, and lungs.* Cancer death rates for cigar smokers are 34 percent higher than those for nonsmokers.

- *Ninety-nine percent of cigar smokers have atypical cells found in the larynx.* These cells are the first step toward malignancy (cancer).

- *Cigar smokers are three to five times more likely to die of lung cancer than are nonsmokers.*

- *Cigar smokers have five times the risk of emphysema compared to nonsmokers.*

- *Nicotine does not have to be inhaled to damage the heart and blood vessels.* It is absorbed into the bloodstream through the mucous membranes of the mouth. Nicotine increases the heart rate and constricts the blood vessels, which reduces blood flow to the heart.

characters (and their smoking), since they are generally depicted in a positive light. As an example, in a 2001 survey, two-thirds of the 43 movie stars most frequently named by 10-to 19-year-olds were seen smoking in their most recent films.[12] Perhaps even younger children were exposed to tobacco placement when Philip Morris was able to place its products in *Who Framed Roger Rabbit* and *The Muppet Movie.*[13]

Pipe and Cigar Smoking

Many people believe that pipe or cigar smoking is a safe alternative to cigarette smoking. Unfortunately, this is not the case. All forms of tobacco present users with a series of health threats (see the Star box).

When compared with cigarette smokers, pipe and cigar smokers have cancer of the mouth, throat, larynx (voice box), and esophagus at the same frequency. Cigarette smokers are more likely than are pipe and cigar smokers to have lung cancer, cancer of the larynx, chronic obstructive lung disease (COLD), also called chronic obstructive pulmonary disease (COPD), and heart disease. The cancer risk of death to pipe and cigar smokers is four times greater from lung cancer and

10 times greater from laryngeal cancer than it is for nonsmokers.

In comparison to cigarette smokers, pipe and cigar smokers are considerably fewer in number. Interestingly, cigar smoking enjoyed a resurgence through much of the 1990s. However, during 1998–1999 a substantial decline in sales of premium cigars occurred. Whether this downturn represents an emerging dissatisfaction with cigars as an enjoyable use of tobacco or simply reflects adjustments in the import market remains uncertain. In 1995 cigars generated sales of $1 billion, mainly to younger adults, including a very small but growing percentage of women.

Perhaps because of the increase in cigar smoking noted above, the National Cancer Institute commissioned the first extensive study of regular cigar smoking. That report confirmed and expanded on the health risks identified in earlier smaller studies.[14] In a study conducted in England, 7,735 middle-aged male cigar and pipe smokers were followed for nearly 22 years. Evaluation of the morbidity and mortality data collected determined that cigar and pipe smokers showed an increased risk for major coronary heart disease events and stroke events and an increased mortality rate for cardiovascular disease and for overall mortality.[15]

In response to the recognition of these risks, the FTC now requires that cigar manufacturers disclose the tobacco content and additives in their products. Most recently the FTC announced its intention of requiring five rotating health warnings to appear on cigars, including two that have been currently agreed on by the FTC and major cigar manufacturers: *Cigars Are Not a Safe Alternative to Cigarettes* and *Cigar Smoking Can Cause Cancer of the Mouth and Throat, Even If You Don't Inhale.*

The use of smokeless tobacco, a third alternative to cigarette smoking, is discussed later in the chapter.

Tobacco Use and the Development of Dependence

Although not true for every tobacco user (see the discussion of "chippers" later in this section), the vast majority of users, particularly cigarette smokers, will develop a dependency relationship with the nicotine contained in tobacco. This state of **dependence** causes users to consume greater quantities of nicotine over extended periods of time, further endangering their health.

Dependence can imply both a physical and psychological relationship. Particularly with cigarettes, *physical dependence* or *addiction,* with its associated *tolerance, withdrawal,* and **titration,** is strongly developed by 40 percent of all smokers. The development of addiction reflects a strong genetic predisposition to physical dependence.[16] Most of the remaining population of smokers will experience lesser degrees of physical dependence. Psychological *dependence* or *habituation,* with its accompanying psychological components of *compulsion* and *indulgence,* is almost universally seen.

Compulsion is a strong emotional desire to continue tobacco use despite restrictions on smoking and the awareness of health risks. Very likely, users are "compelled" to engage in continual tobacco use in fear of the unpleasant physical, emotional, and social effects that result from discontinuing use. In comparison to compulsion, indulgence is seen as "rewarding" oneself for aligning with a particular behavior pattern—in this case, smoking. Indulgence is made possible by the existence of various reward systems built around the use of tobacco, including a perceived image, group affiliation, and even appetite suppression intended to foster weight control.

Much to the benefit of the tobacco industry, dependence on tobacco is easily established. Many experts believe that physical dependence on tobacco is far more easily established than is physical dependence on alcohol, cocaine (other than crack), or heroin. Of all people who experiment with cigarettes, 85 percent develop various aspects of a dependence relationship.

A small percentage of smokers, known as "chippers," can smoke on occasion without becoming dependent. Most likely, chippers respond differently to environmental

cues than do more dependent smokers,[17] thus smoking less frequently. They may be truly "social smokers" in that they smoke only with a few selected friends or in a very limited number of places. Unfortunately, many inexperienced smokers feel that they too are only social smokers; however, a few months or even a few days, of this type of occasional smoking could be a transitional period into a dependence pattern of tobacco use.

Sandwiched between regular smokers and chippers is a newly emerging group of smokers—part-time smokers. Today these smokers constitute about 20 percent of all smokers.[18] The practice most likely reflects the reality of the high cost of cigarettes and restrictions in the workplace. The health effects of this form of smoking appear to be the same as seen in regular smokers.

Theories of Nicotine Addiction

The establishment and maintenance of physical dependence or addiction is less than fully understood. Most experts, however, believe that for a specific individual, addiction has a multifaceted etiology, or cause, with increasing attention being directed toward a genetic basis for addiction. Accordingly, several theories have been proposed to explain the development of dependence. We present a brief account of some of these theories. Readers are reminded that many of these theories are technically sophisticated and only a most basic description can be provided in a personal health textbook. The more emotional aspects of dependence formation are discussed later in the chapter.

Genetic Influences

Although the specific genetic pathways that influence both the initiation and maintenance of smoking (or other forms of tobacco use) are less than fully understood, a role for genetic influence is evident. Applying new statistical techniques to earlier studies of smoking patterns in families and between identical twins, it is now believed that initiation and maintenance of initial smoking is 60 percent driven by genetic influences.[19] Of course, the smoking of the first few cigarettes is a choice made by beginning smokers. In a yet-to-be-determined percentage of beginning smokers, the *initiation* of smoking, or the desire to continue with this new

---

Key Terms

dependence a physical and/or psychological need to continue the use of a drug

titration (tie **tray** shun) the particular level of a drug within the body; adjusting the level of nicotine by adjusting the rate of smoking

A smoker inhales about 70,000 times during the first year of smoking, resulting in a nicotine addiction that often lasts a lifetime.

nicotine (a ball or bolus) that reaches the brain and results in a period of neurohormonal excitement. The smoker perceives this period of stimulation as pleasurable but, unfortunately, short-lived. Accordingly, the smoker attempts to reestablish this pleasurable feeling by again inhaling and sending another bolus of nicotine on its way to the brain. The 70,000 or more inhalations during the first year of smoking serve to condition the novice smoker, resulting in a lifelong pattern of cigarette dependence. The level needed for arousal is different for each individual smoker, depending on the length of addiction, the level of tolerance, genetic predisposition, and environmental and personal stimuli.

Recognition of two types of smokers emerges from an understanding of the bolus theory of smoking. *Peak smokers* are those smokers who become dependent on the arousal of pleasure centers in the brain (see page 286) that are stimulated by the rapid increase of nicotine levels following inhalation and distribution of nicotine within the CNS. In contrast, the *trough maintenance smokers* maintain an even consistently higher level of nicotine titration in order to avoid the negative consequences of withdrawal. In other words, some smokers enjoy the consequences (arousal) caused by arrival of the bolus, whereas others so dislike the feelings caused by dissapation of the bolus that they inhale to avoid these unpleasant feelings.

Adrenocorticotropic Hormone (ACTH) Theory

Yet another theory of dependence suggests that nicotine stimulates the release of adrenocorticotropic hormone (ACTH) from the anterior pituitary, or "master gland" of the endocrine system (see Chapter 3) causing the release of **beta endorphins** (naturally occurring opiatelike chemicals) that produce mild feelings of euphoria. Perhaps this stresslike response mechanism involving ACTH accounts for the increased energy expenditure seen in smokers and thus their tendency to maintain a lower body weight. Others, however, have questioned the ability of nicotine to stimulate endorphin release.[21]

When these physiological responses are viewed collectively, nicotine may be seen as biochemically influencing brain activity by enhancing the extent and strength of various forms of "communication" between different brain areas and even glands of the endocrine system. If this

behavior, is underlined by a genetic predisposition to neurohormonally "appreciate" the stimulating effects of nicotine. Once smoking has been so easily and successfully initiated, the continuation of smoking is then *maintained* by the same, or closely related, genetic predisposition for neurohormonal excitation of the central nervous system. The "hook" for a lifetime of smoking is, thus, set in large part by a genetic susceptibility.[20] The remaining influence needed for initiation and maintenance of initial smoking is 20 percent environmental and 20 percent the unique needs of individuals.[19]

Once the relatively brief period of initial exposure (initiation) and early maintenance is passed, the role of genetic influences may be even more powerful—providing 70 percent of the maintenance stimulus required over decades of smoking. Environmental and personality factors subside accordingly.[19]

Bolus Theory

In the **bolus theory** of nicotine addiction, one of the oldest and most general theories of addiction, each inhalation of smoke releases into the blood a concentrated quantity of

Key Terms

bolus theory a theory of nicotine addiction based on the body's response to the bolus (ball) of nicotine delivered to the brain with each inhalation of cigarette smoke

beta endorphins mood-enhancing, pain-reducing, opiatelike chemicals produced within the smoker's body in response to the presence of nicotine is the case, it is apparent why, once addicted, the functioning of the smoker's control systems is much altered in comparison with that of nonsmokers.

Self-Medication Theory

Another explanation of the addiction to smoking, called *self-medication,* suggests that nicotine, through the effects of mood-enhancing dopamine, may allow smokers to "treat" feelings of tiredness, lack of motivation, or even depression.[22] In other words, a smoke lifts the spirits, if only briefly. Eventually, however, smokers become dependent on tobacco as a "medication" to make themselves feel better. Thus, because tobacco is a legal drug that is readily available, it becomes preferred to prescription medications and illegal drugs, such as cocaine and the stimulants, that elevate mood.

Regardless of the mechanism involved, as tolerance to nicotine develops, smoking behavior is adjusted to either maintain arousal or prevent the occurrence of withdrawal symptoms. At some point, however, the desire for constant arousal is probably superseded by the smoker's desire not to experience withdrawal.

The importance of nicotine as the primary factor in establishing dependence on tobacco is supported by research that demonstrates that smokers will not select a nontobacco cigarette if a tobacco cigarette is available. Even tobacco cigarettes with a very low level of nicotine seem to be unacceptable to most smokers, as do cigarettes with very low nicotine but with high tar content. Interestingly, users of low-nicotine cigarettes tend to inhale more frequently and deeply to obtain as much nicotine as possible.

Even more impressive (and alarming) regarding nicotine's dependency-producing power, is seen in conjunction with the small amount of time needed to become dependent. Using the HONC instruments described in the Star box on page 281, it is now established that beginning smokers (recall that most smokers begin during adolescence) become dependent on cigarettes within 3 weeks to 3 months of smoking on as little as two cigarettes per day. Males are more likely to be a bit more resistant to dependency, taking a month or two, whereas females can become dependent in a matter of a very few days of initial experimentation.[23]

 TALKING POINTS A smoker says that she does not consider smoking to be a form of drug use. She becomes angry at the suggestion that cigarettes are part of a drug-delivery system. How would you respond to her position?

Acute Effects of Nicotine on Nervous System Function

In comparison with the more chronic effects of nicotine on the central nervous system (CNS) that may eventually result in physical dependence or addiction, nicotine also produces changes of short duration. In the CNS, nicotine activates receptors within the nucleus accumbens (a reward center) and the locus caeruleus (a cortical activating center) of the brain. Stimulation of the brain is seen by changes in electroencephalogram (EEG) patterns, reflecting an increase in the frequency of electrical activity. This is part of a general arousal pattern signaled by the release of the neurotransmitters **norepinephrine,** dopamine, acetylcholine, and serotonin. Heavy use of tobacco products, resulting in high levels of nicotine in the bloodstream, eventually produces a blocking effect as more and more receptor sites for these neurotransmitters are filled. The result is a generalized depression of the CNS.

The level of plasma nicotine associated with normal levels of heavy smoking (one to two packs per day) would not likely produce the depressive effect just described. However, in chain smokers (four to eight packs per day), plasma nicotine levels would be sufficient to have a depressive influence on nervous system function. In fact, it has been suggested that chain smoking is driven by the fruitless effort to counter the depressive influence of chronically excessively high levels of nicotine. In contrast to chain smokers, inexperienced smokers, lacking tolerance, can quickly reach a blood level of nicotine sufficient enough to activate the brain's vomiting centers. This response is a built-in protective mechanism against nicotine poisoning.

In carefully controlled studies involving both animals and humans, nicotine increased the ability of subjects to concentrate on a task. However, the duration of this improvement was limited. Most people would agree that this brief benefit is not enough to justify the health risks associated with chronic tobacco use.

Non–Nervous-System Acute Effects of Nicotine

Outside the CNS, nicotine affects the transmission of nerve signals at the point where nerves innervate muscle tissue (called the *neuromuscular junction*) by mimicking the action of the neurotransmitter acetylcholine. Nicotine occupies receptor sites at the junction and prevents the transmission of nerve impulses from nerve cell to muscle cell.

Nicotine also causes the release of epinephrine from the adrenal medulla (see Chapter 3), which results in an increase in respiration rate, heart rate, blood pressure, and coronary blood flow. These changes are accompanied by

> **Key Terms**
>
> **norepinephrine** (nor epp in **eff** rin) an adrenalinlike chemical produced within the nervous system

the constriction of the blood vessels beneath the skin, a reduction in the motility in the bowel, loss of appetite, and changes in sleep patterns.

Although a lethal dose of nicotine could be obtained through the ingestion of a nicotine-containing insecticide, to "smoke oneself to death" in a single intense period of cigarette use would be highly improbable. In humans, 40 to 60 mg (.06–.09 mg/kg) is a lethal dose. A typical cigarette supplies .05 to 2.5 mg of nicotine, and that nicotine is relatively quickly broken down for removal from the body.

Psychosocial Factors Related to Dependence

Recall that a psychological aspect of dependence (habituation) exists and is important in maintaining the smoker's need for nicotine. Both research and general observation support many of the powerful influences this aspect of dependence possesses, especially for beginning smokers, before the onset of physical addiction. Consequently, in the remainder of this section, we explore nonphysiological factors that may contribute to the development of this aspect of dependence.

Modeling

Because tobacco use is a learned behavior, it is reasonable to accept that modeling acts as a stimulus to experimental smoking. **Modeling** suggests that susceptible people smoke to emulate, or model their behavior after, smokers whom they admire or with whom they share other types of social or emotional bonds. Particularly for young adolescents (ages 14 to 17), smoking behavior correlates with the smoking behavior of slightly older peers and very young adults (ages 18 to 22), older siblings, and, most important, parents. Negative parental influences on cigarette smoking by their children include their own smoking status, and/or their failure to clearly state their disapproval of smoking.[24] Further, for parents who smoke, it is important that they cease smoking before their children turn 8 years of age if they wish to maximize an antismoking message.

Key Terms

modeling the process of adopting the admired behavioral patterns of another person

Smoker with arm patch

Modeling is particularly evident when smoking is a central factor in peer group formation and peer group association and can lead to a shared behavioral pattern that differentiates the group from others and from adults. Further, when risk-taking behavior and disregard for authority are common to the group, smoking becomes the behavioral pattern that most consistently identifies and bonds the group. Particularly for those young people who lack self-directedness or the ability to resist peer pressure, initial membership in a tobacco-using peer group may become inescapable. The ability to counter peer pressure is a salient component of successful anti-smoking programs for use with older children and younger adolescents.

In addition, when adolescents have lower levels of self-esteem and are searching for an avenue to improve self-image, a role model who smokes is often seen as tough, sociable, and sexually attractive. These three traits have been played up by the tobacco industry in their carefully crafted advertisements. In fact, teens from any background may see the very young and attractive models used in tobacco (and beer) advertisements as being more peerlike in age than they really are. FCC regulations require that models for both products be 21 years of age or older, regardless of how youthful they might (and the advertisers hope they do) appear to older children and young adolescents. (See the Learning from Our Diversity box on page 287 for a counterapproach to the acceptance of tobacco.)

Manipulation

In addition to modeling as a psychosocial link with tobacco use, cigarette use may meet the beginning smoker's need to manipulate something and at the same time provide the manipulative "tool" necessary to offset boredom, feelings of depression, or social immaturity. Clearly the availability of affordable smoking paraphernalia provides smokers with ways to reward themselves. A new cigarette lighter, a status brand of tobacco, or a beach towel with a cigarette's logo are all reinforcements to some smokers. Fortunately, the last item will become increasingly harder to find since logos can no longer be placed on items such as beach towels. For others, the ability to take out a cigarette or fill a pipe adds a measure of structure and control to situations in which they might otherwise feel somewhat ill at ease. The cigarette becomes a readily available and dependable "friend" to turn to during stressful moments.

Susceptibility to Advertising

The images of the smoker's world portrayed by the media can be particularly attractive. For adolescents, women, minorities, and other carefully targeted groups of adults, the tobacco industry has paired suggestions of a better life with the use of its products. To these users and potential users, the self-reward of power, liberation, affluence, sophistication, or adult status is achieved by using the products that they are told are associated with these desired states. Thus the self-rewarding use of tobacco products becomes a means of hoped-for achievement.

With this multiplicity of forces at work, we can understand why so many who experiment with tobacco use find that they quickly, in combination with genetic predisposition, become emotionally dependent on tobacco. Human needs, both physiological and psychosocial, are many and complex. Tobacco use meets the needs on a short-term basis, whereas dependence, once established, replaces these needs with a different, more immediate set of needs.

Despite the satisfaction of the dependency that continued smoking brings, approximately 80 percent of adult smokers have, on at least one occasion, expressed a desire to quit, and the majority of these have actually attempted to become nonsmokers. Today, with the over-the-counter availability of transdermal nicotine patches, nicotine-containing gum, prescription medications such as antidepressants, and nicotine inhalers, the number of smokers making concerted and repeated attempts to stop smoking is up considerably over that seen in the past. It therefore seems apparent that tobacco use is a source of **dissonance.** This dissonance stems from the need to deal emotionally with a behavior that

> ### Key Terms
>
> **dissonance** (**dis** son ince) a feeling of uncertainty that occurs when a person believes two equally attractive but opposite ideas

is both highly enjoyable and highly dangerous but known to be difficult to stop. The degree to which this dissonance exists probably varies from user to user.

Preventing Teen Smoking

Even before the 1997 release of tobacco industry documents confirming the targeting of young adolescents, the federal government stated its intention to curb these cigarette advertisements. In August 1995 the FDA described the specific actions that it hoped it would be given authority to implement. These policies were, in large part, incorporated into *Healthy People 2000* and retained in *Healthy People 2010*. If these policies, in combination with other initiatives, are effective, the adolescent smoking rate will be lowered to no more than 16 percent by 2010.

1. Limit tobacco advertising in publications that appeal to teens and restrict billboards with tobacco-related content to no closer than 1,000 feet of schools and playgrounds. (An August 1995 study in California found that stores near schools displayed significantly more tobacco-related advertisements than those farther from schools.)
2. Restrict the use of logo and other tobacco-related images on nontobacco-related products, such as towels, T-shirts, and caps.
3. Bar certain sources of access to tobacco products, such as mail order sales, the distribution of free samples, and vending machines.
4. Halt sponsorship of high-visibility events, such as auto racing and athletic contests in which brand names appear on highly televised surfaces, including hoods, fenders, uniforms, and arena sign boards. (It is estimated that the Marlboro logo is seen 5,933 times during the course of a 90-minute televised Nextel Cup auto race.)
5. Require merchants to obtain proof of age when selling tobacco products to adolescents. (This particular component of the initial plan became law in 1997. Merchants are required to validate the age of people whom they suspect to be younger than 27 years of age before selling cigarettes to those 18 years of age and older. If found in violation, both the salesperson and the store owner will be fined $500.)

By mid-1998 the federal government's desire to reduce youth smoking through implementation of the steps just described was mired in a larger package of tobacco-related policies being debated in Congress. This undertaking was related to the class action suit filed by all 50 (46 as a single large class and 4 as a smaller class) states against the tobacco industry in an attempt to recoup Medicaid expenditures for treating tobacco-related illnesses. As Congress attempted to construct a settlement that would be acceptable to all parties, the impasse fragmented attempts to reduce youth smoking. Unfortunately, this outcome diluted some restrictions on tobacco advertisements, as well as the FDA's ability to reduce smoking by defining cigarettes as drug delivery systems. In fact, in 2000 the United States Supreme Court ruled that the FDA lacked the regulatory authority to bring tobacco products under its control, unless Congress was willing to rescind laws that currently define tobacco as an agricultural product that can be freely marketed to persons 18 years of age or older. (If defined as a drug delivery system, cigarettes would be obtainable only with a physician's prescription, which would essentially prevent, or greatly limit, children's access to them.)

As noted earlier in the chapter, the Master Settlement Agreement (1999), which required the tobacco industry to pay the states 246 billion dollars, was able to restrict some forms of youth-oriented advertising and fund antismoking education, which may accomplish some of the changes initially proposed. Unfortunately, during the economic downturn, many states have used or borrowed against the funds to meet taxation shortfalls.

Early Childhood Intervention

Although significant concern centers on the onset of smoking behavior by adolescents in the 11- to 14-year-old age group and later teen years, the decision to smoke (or use other forms of tobacco) may be made at a much earlier age. Accordingly, parents (and other adults) who do not want their children to smoke or use tobacco in other forms should begin educating their children as preschoolers and certainly by school age. The following recommendations, and many additional ones as well, can be found in *A Parent's Guide to Prevention,* available from the National Clearinghouse for Alcohol and Drug Information.

When dealing with preschool children, it should be remembered that facts are unlikely to be comprehended. Accordingly, the following activities are suggested:

- Set aside regular time when you can give your child your full attention. Playing and reading together builds a strong parent-child bond.
- Point out poisonous and harmful substances that can be found in the home.
- Explain how medicines can be harmful if used incorrectly.
- Provide guidelines that teach the child what kind of behavior is expected.
- Encourage the child to follow instructions.
- Help the child learn decision-making skills; give positive feedback when appropriate decisions have been made.

For children in kindergarten through third grade, new skills and insights need to be developed to deal with drugs, including tobacco products. Adults should attempt to:

- Help the child recognize and understand family rules.
- Discuss how television advertisements try to persuade people to buy their products.
- Practice ways in which the child can say no to other people.
- Develop a "helper" file made up of the names and phone numbers of people the child can turn to when confronted by others who want them to try smoking or smokeless tobacco.

As children approach the preteen years, more focused presentations can be made regarding the dangers associated with smoking and the use of other substances. Adults working with children in grades four through six should focus on the following activities:

- Create special times when an adult is available to talk with the child about whatever he or she wants to talk about.
- Encourage participation in a variety of activities that are both fun and allow the child to meet new friends.
- Teach the child how drugs, including tobacco products, are promoted and how their messages can be "defused."
- Continue to assist the child in learning how to say no.
- Become acquainted with the parents of the child's friends so that you will be able to work with them in support of antismoking activities in the community.
- Participate in providing support for supervised activities for children of this age.

Although nothing is certain regarding the decision that older preadolescents or teens make about beginning to smoke, the activities just listed may be effective in countering the influences of the peer group and the mass media.

Tobacco: The Source of Physiologically Active Compounds

When burned, the tobacco in cigarettes, cigars, and pipe mixtures is the source of an array of physiologically active chemicals, many of which are closely linked to significant changes in normal body structure and function. At the burning tip of the cigarette, the 900° C (1,652° F) heat oxidizes tobacco (as well as paper, wrapper, filter, and additives). With each puff of smoke, the body is exposed to approximately 4,700 chemical compounds, hundreds of which are known to be physiologically active, toxic, and carcinogenic. These chemicals have their origins in the tobacco or have been introduced as additives, pesticides, and other agricultural chemicals. An annual 70,000 puffs

Table 9.3 Partial Listing of Toxic and Carcinogenic Components of Cigarette Smoke

Agent

Agent	
Carbon Monoxide	1
Nitrogen Oxides (NO$_x$)	2
Hydrogen Cyanide	3
Formaldehyde	4
Acrolein	5
Acetaldehyde	6
Ammonia	7
Hydrazine	8
Vinyl Chloride	9
Benzo[a]pyrene	10
Aromatic Amines	11
Aromatic Nitrohydrocarbons	12
Polonium-210	13
Nickel	14
Arsenic	15
Cadmium	16

Nontobacco Sources of Selected Chemical Compounds Found in Tobacco Smoke

1. released by internal combustion engines (cars, trucks, buses, etc.)
2. released by internal combustion engines
3. burning of polyurethane foam (insulating material)
4. released by internal combustions and the burning of many forms of building materials
5. burning of fat (e.g., barbecuing of meats)
6. released by internal combustion engines
7. found in fertilizers, many cleaning agents, and released during decomposition of organic material
8. rocket fuel exhaust
9. released by burning plastics
10. produced when grilling meats and found in wood smoke and soot
11. released during the decomposition of organic material
12. found in fumes produced by the incineration of municipal wastes
13. released into air during radioactive decay
14. leakage from/burning of nickel-cadmium batteries
15. found in localized ground-water areas
16. found in pesticides and batteries, and released by municipal waste incineration

Source: Mulcahy S. *The Toxicology of Cigarette Smoke and Environmental Tobacco Smoke*, A Review of Cigarette Smoke and Its Toxicological Effects, www.csn.ul.ie/-stephen/reports/bc4927.html.

taken in by the one-pack-a-day cigarette smoker results in an environment that makes the most polluted urban environment seem clean by comparison.

Table 9.3 presents a partial list of toxic and carcinogenic compounds of tobacco smoking. In addition to tobacco smoke, these materials, and hundreds of others not listed above, are routinely found within many materials used in industrial and residential settings.

Particulate Phase

Cigarette, cigar, and pipe smoke can be described on the basis of two phases. These phases include a particulate phase and a gaseous phase. The **particulate phase** includes **nicotine,** water, and a variety of powerful chemicals known collectively as tar. **Tar** includes phenol, cresol, pyrene, DDT, and a benzene-ring group of compounds that includes benzo[a]pyrene. Most of the carcinogenic compounds are found within the tar. A person who smokes one pack of cigarettes per day collects four ounces of tar in his or her lungs in a year. Only the gases and the smallest particles reach the small sacs of the lungs, called the *alveoli,* where oxygen exchange occurs. The carcinogen-rich particles from the particulate phase are deposited somewhere along the air passage leading to the lungs.

Gaseous Phase

The **gaseous phase** of tobacco smoke, like the particulate phase, is composed of a variety of physiologically active compounds, including carbon monoxide, carbon dioxide, ammonia, hydrogen cyanide, isopyrene, acetaldehyde, and acetone. At least 60 of these compounds have been determined to be **carcinogens,** or co-carcinogenic promoters, thus capable of stimulating the development of cancer. Carbon monoxide is, however, the most damaging compound found in this component of tobacco smoke. Its effect is discussed next.

Carbon Monoxide

Like every inefficient engine, a cigarette, cigar, or pipe burns (oxidizes) its fuel with less than complete conversion into carbon dioxide, water, and heat. As a result of this incomplete oxidation, burning tobacco forms **carbon monoxide (CO)** gas. Carbon monoxide is one of the most harmful components of tobacco smoke.

Carbon monoxide is a colorless, odorless, tasteless gas that possesses a very strong physiological attraction for hemoglobin, the oxygen-carrying pigment on each red blood cell. When CO is inhaled, it quickly bonds with hemoglobin and forms a new compound, carboxyhemoglobin. In this form, hemoglobin is unable to transport oxygen to the tissues and cells where it is needed.

Although it is true that normal body metabolism always keeps an irreducible minimum of CO in our blood (0.5–1 percent), the blood of smokers may have levels of 5–10 percent CO saturation.[25] We are exposed to additional CO from environmental sources such as automobiles and buses and other combustion of fossil fuels. When we consider the combination of a smoker's CO with environmental CO, we are not surprised that smokers more easily become out of breath than nonsmokers do. The half-life of CO combined with hemoglobin is approximately 4 to 6 hours. Most smokers replenish their level of CO saturation at far shorter intervals than this.

As mentioned, the presence of excessive levels of carboxyhemoglobin in the blood of smokers leads to shortness of breath and lowered endurance. Because an adequate oxygen supply to all body tissues is critical for normal functioning, any oxygen reduction can have a serious impact on health. Brain function may be eventually reduced, reactions and judgment are dulled, and of course, cardiovascular function is impaired. Fetuses are especially at risk for this oxygen deprivation (hypoxia) because fetal development is so critically dependent on a sufficient oxygen supply from the mother.

Illness, Premature Death, and Tobacco Use

For people who begin tobacco use as adolescents or young adults, smoke heavily, and continue to smoke, the likelihood of premature death is virtually ensured. Two-pack-a-day cigarette smokers can expect to die 7 to 8 years earlier than their nonsmoking counterparts will. (Only nonsmoking-related deaths that can afflict smokers and nonsmokers alike keep the difference at this level rather than much higher.) Not only will these people die sooner, but they will also probably be plagued with painful, debilitating illnesses for an extended time. Smoking is responsible for nearly 440,000 premature deaths each year.[26] Table 9.4 presents an overview of illnesses known to be caused or worsened by tobacco use.

Cardiovascular Disease

Although cancer is now the leading cause of death for Americans under 80 years of age, cardiovascular disease is the leading cause of death among all adults, accounting

---

Key Terms

particulate phase portion of the tobacco smoke composed of small suspended particles

nicotine physiologically active, dependence-producing drug found in tobacco

tar a chemically rich, syrupy, blackish-brown material obtained from the particulate matter within cigarette smoke when nicotine and water are removed

gaseous phase portion of the tobacco smoke containing carbon monoxide and many other physiologically active gaseous compounds

carcinogens environmental agents, including chemical compounds within cigarette smoke, that stimulate the development of cancerous changes within cells

carbon monoxide (CO) chemical compound that can "inactivate" red blood cells

Table 9.4 Selected Established and Suspected Health Effects of Cigarette Smoking

Category of Condition	Established and Suspected Effects
1 Lung Disease	lung cancer, chronic obstructive lung disease; increased severity of asthma; increased risk of developing various respiratory infections
2 Cancer Risk	esophageal, laryngeal, oral, bladder, kidney, stomach, pancreatic, vulvar, cervical, and colorectal cancers
3 Heart Disease	coronary heart disease; angina pectoris; heart attack; repeat heart attack; arrhythmia; aortic aneurysm; cardiomyopathy
4 Peripheral Vascular Disease	pain and discomfort in the legs and feet resulting from restricted blood flow into the extremities
5 Skin Changes	wrinkling; fingernail discoloration; psoriasis; palmoplantar pustulosis
6 Surgical Risk	need for more anesthesia; increased risk of postsurgical respiratory infection; increased need for supplemental oxygen following surgery; delayed wound healing
7 Orthopedic Problems	disc degeneration; less successful back surgery; musculoskeletal injury; delayed fracture healing
8 Rheumatologic Conditions	osteoporosis and osteoarthritis
9 Environmental Tobacco Smoke and Pediatric Illnesses	infections of the lower respiratory tract; more severe asthma; middle ear infections; Crohn's disease and ulcerative colitis; sudden infant death syndrome; impaired delivery of oxygen to body tissues
10 Complications in Obstetrics and Gynecology	infertility; miscarriage; fetal growth retardation; prematurity; stillbirth; transmission of HIV to the fetus from the infected biological mother; birth defects; intellectual impairment of offspring; sudden infant death syndrome; earlier menopause
11 Male Infertility and Sexuality Dysfunctions	decreased sperm motility; decreased sperm density; impotence
12 Neurological Disorders	transient ischemic attack; stroke; worsened multiple sclerosis
13 Brain and Behavior	depression
14 Abnormalities of the Ears, Nose, and Throat	snoring and hearing loss
15 Eyes	cataracts; complications from Graves' disease; macular degeneration; optic neuropathy
16 Oral Health	periodontal disease
17 Endocrine System	increased metabolic rate; blood-sugar abnormalities; increased waist-to-hip ratio; redistribution of body fat
18 Gastrointestinal Diseases	stomach and duodenal ulcers; Crohn's disease
19 Immune System	impaired humoral and cell-mediated immunity
20 Emergency Medicine	injuries from fires; occupational injuries

Source: Kapier KN, et al. *Cigarettes: What the Warning Label Doesn't Tell You.* American Council on Science and Health, 1997.

Note: Recently *The 2004 United States Surgeon General's Report: The Health Consequences of Smoking* added abdominal aneurysms, periodontal disease, and myeloid leukemia to the list of illnesses and diseases attributed to smoking and listed in Table 9.4.

for 927,448 deaths in the United States in 2004.[27] Tobacco use, and cigarette smoking in particular, is clearly one of the major factors contributing to this cause of death. Although overall progress is being made in reducing the incidence of cardiovascular-related deaths, tobacco use impedes these efforts. So important is tobacco use as a contributing factor in deaths from cardiovascular disease that the cigarette smoker more than doubles the risk of experiencing a **myocardial infarction,** the leading cause of death from cardiovascular disease. Smokers also increase their risk of **sudden cardiac death** by two to four times. Fully one-third of all cardiovascular disease can be traced to cigarette smoking.

The relationship between tobacco use and cardiovascular disease is centered on two major components of tobacco smoke: nicotine and carbon monoxide.

Nicotine and Cardiovascular Disease

The influence of nicotine on the cardiovascular system occurs when it stimulates the nervous system to release norepinephrine. This powerful stimulant increases the heart rate. In turn, an elevated heart rate increases cardiac output,

Key Terms

myocardial infarction heart attack; the death of heart muscle as a result of a blockage in one of the coronary arteries

sudden cardiac death immediate death resulting from a sudden change in the rhythm of the heart

A healthy lung (right) vs. the lung of a smoker (left).

thus increasing blood pressure. The extent to which this is dangerous depends in part on the coronary circulation's ability to supply blood to the rapidly contracting heart muscle. The development of **angina pectoris** and the possibility of sudden heart attack are heightened by this sustained elevation of heart rate, particularly in those individuals with existing coronary artery disease (see Chapter 10).

Nicotine is also a powerful vasoconstrictor of the peripheral blood vessels. As these vessels are constricted by the influence of nicotine, the pressure against their walls increases. Research shows that irreversible atherosclerotic damage to major arteries also occurs with smoking.

For over a decade it has been known that nicotine also increases blood **platelet adhesiveness.** As the platelets become more and more likely to "clump," a person is more likely to develop a blood clot. In people already prone to cardiovascular disease, more rapidly clotting blood is an unwelcome liability. Heart attacks occur when clots form within the coronary arteries or are transported to the heart from other areas of the body.

In addition to other influences on the cardiovascular system, nicotine possesses the ability to decrease the proportion of high-density lipoproteins (HDLs) and to increase the proportion of low-density lipoproteins (LDLs) and very-low-density lipoproteins that constitute the body's serum cholesterol. Low-density lipoproteins appear to support the development of atherosclerosis and are clearly increased in the bloodstreams of smokers. (See Chapter 10 for further information about cholesterol's role in cardiovascular disease.)

Carbon Monoxide and Cardiovascular Disease

A second substance contributed by tobacco influences the type and extent of cardiovascular disease found among tobacco users. Carbon monoxide interferes with oxygen transport within the circulatory system.

As described earlier in the chapter, carbon monoxide is a component of the gaseous phase of tobacco smoke and readily joins with the hemoglobin of the red blood cells. Carbon monoxide has an affinity for hemoglobin 206 times that of oxygen. Once the hemoglobin of a red cell has accepted carbon monoxide molecules, the hemoglobin is transformed into carboxyhemoglobin. Thereafter, the carboxyhemoglobin permanently weakens the red blood cell's ability to transport oxygen. So long as smoking continues, these red blood cells remain relatively useless during the remainder of their 120-day lives. Levels of carboxyhemoglobin in heavy smokers are associated with significant increases in the incidence of myocardial infarction.

When a person has impaired oxygen-transporting abilities, physical exertion becomes increasingly demanding on both the heart and the lungs. The cardiovascular system will attempt to respond to the body's demand for oxygen, but these responses are themselves impaired as a result of the influence of nicotine on the cardiovascular system. If tobacco does create the good life, as advertisers claim, it also unfortunately lessens the ability to participate actively in that life.

Key Terms

angina pectoris (an **jie** nuh **peck** tor is) chest pain that results from impaired blood supply to the heart muscle

platelet adhesiveness tendency of platelets to clump together, thus enhancing the speed at which the blood clots

Oral cancer may appear near the edge of the mouth as well as inside the oral cavity.

Cancer

Over the past 60 years, research from the most reputable institutions in this country and abroad has consistently concluded that tobacco use is a significant factor in the development of virtually all forms of cancer and the most significant factor in cancers involving the respiratory system.

In describing cancer development, the currently used reference is 20 pack-years, or an amount of smoking equal to smoking one pack of cigarettes a day for 20 years. Thus the two-pack-a-day smoker can anticipate cancer-related tissue changes in as few as 10 years, while the half-pack-a-day smoker may have 40 years to wait. Regardless, the opportunity is there for all smokers to confirm these data by developing cancer as predicted. It is hoped that most people will think twice before disregarding this evidence.

Data supplied by the American Cancer Society (ACS) indicate that during 2004 an estimated 1,372,910 Americans developed cancer.* These cases were nearly equally divided between the sexes and resulted in approximately 570,280 deaths. In the opinion of the ACS, 30 percent of all cancer cases are heavily influenced by tobacco use. Lung cancer alone accounted for about 172,570 of the new cancer cases and 163,510 deaths in 2004. Fully 87 percent of men with lung cancer were cigarette smokers.[26] A genetic "missing link" between smoking and lung cancer was established, when mutations to an important tumor suppressor gene were identified. If it was necessary to have a final "proof" that smoking causes lung cancer, that proof appears to be in hand.

Cancer of the entire respiratory system, including lung cancer and cancers of the mouth and throat accounted for about 184,800 new cases of cancer and 168,140 deaths.[26] Despite these high figures, not all smokers develop cancer.

---

*Excluding cases of nonmelanoma skin cancer.

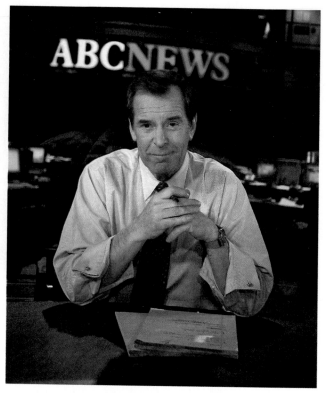

Peter Jennings, who died of lung cancer in 2005.

Respiratory Tract Cancer

Recall that tobacco smoke produces both a gaseous and a particulate phase. As noted, the particulate phase contains the tar fragment of tobacco smoke. This rich chemical environment contains more than four thousand known chemical compounds, hundreds of which are known to be carcinogens.

In the normally functioning respiratory system, particulate matter suspended in the inhaled air settles on the tissues lining the airways and is trapped in **mucus** produced by specialized *goblet cells*. This mucus, with its trapped impurities, is continuously swept upward by the beating action of hairlike **cilia** of the ciliated columnar epithelial cells lining the air passages (Figure 9-1). On reaching the throat, this mucus is swallowed and eventually removed through the digestive system.

> **Key Terms**
>
> **mucus** clear, sticky material produced by specialized cells within the mucous membranes of the body; mucus traps much of the suspended particulate matter within tobacco smoke
>
> **cilia** (**sill** ee uh) small, hairlike structures that extend from cells that line the air passages

Figure 9-1 Tissue changes associated with bronchogenic carcinoma (lung cancer).

When tobacco smoke is drawn into the respiratory system, however, its rapidly dropping temperature allows the particulate matter to accumulate. This brown, sticky tar contains compounds known to harm the ciliated cells, goblet cells, and the basal cells of the respiratory lining. As the damage from smoking increases, the cilia become less effective in sweeping mucus upward to the throat. When cilia can no longer clean the airway, tar accumulates on the surfaces and brings carcinogenic compounds into direct contact with the tissues of the airway.

At the same time that the sweeping action of the lining cells is being slowed, substances in the tar are stimulating the goblet cells to increase the amount of mucus they normally produce. The "smoker's cough" is the body's attempt to remove this excess mucus.

With prolonged exposure to the carcinogenic materials in tar, predictable changes will begin to occur within the respiratory system's basal cell layer (Figure 9-1). The basal cells begin to display changes characteristic of all cancer cells. In addition, an abnormal accumulation of cells occurs. When a person stops smoking, preinvasive lesions do not repair themselves as quickly as once thought.[28]

By the time lung cancer is usually diagnosed, its development is so advanced that the chance for recovery is very poor. Still today, only 15 percent of all lung cancer victims survive for 5 years or more after diagnosis.[26] Most die in a very uncomfortable, painful way.

Cancerous activity in other areas of the respiratory system, including the larynx, and within the oral cavity (mouth) follows a similar course. In the case of oral cavity cancer, carcinogens found within the smoke and within the saliva are involved in the cancerous changes. Tobacco users, such as pipe smokers, cigar smokers, and users of smokeless tobacco, have a higher (4 to 10 times) rate of cancer of the mouth, tongue, and voice box.

In addition to drawing smoke into the lungs, tobacco users swallow saliva that contains an array of chemical compounds from tobacco. As this saliva is swallowed, carcinogens are absorbed into the circulatory system and transported to all areas of the body. The filtering of the blood by the liver, kidneys, and bladder may account for the higher-than-normal levels of cancer in these organs among smokers. Smoking may also accelerate the rate of pancreatic cancer development.

As reported earlier in the chapter, documents released in 1997 from within the tobacco industry clearly show that the major tobacco companies were aware of tobacco's role in the development of cancer and had made a concerted effort to deprive the American public access to such knowledge.

Chronic Obstructive Lung Disease

Chronic obstructive lung disease (COLD), also known as chronic obstructive pulmonary disease (COPD), is a disorder in which the amount of air that flows in and out of the lungs becomes progressively limited. COLD is a disease state that is made up of two separate but related diseases: **chronic bronchitis** and **pulmonary emphysema.**

With chronic bronchitis, excess mucus is produced in response to the effects of smoking on airway tissue, and the walls of the bronchi become inflamed and infected. This produces a characteristic narrowing of the air passages. Breathing becomes difficult, and activity can be severely restricted. With cessation of smoking, chronic bronchitis is reversible.

Emphysema causes irreversible damage to the tiny air sacs of the lungs, the **alveoli.** Chest pressure builds when air becomes trapped by narrowed air passages (chronic bronchitis) and the thin-walled sacs rupture. Emphysema patients lose the ability to ventilate fully. They feel as though they are suffocating. You may have seen people with this condition in malls and other locations as they walk slowly by, carrying or pulling their portable oxygen tanks.

More than 10 million Americans suffer from COLD. It is responsible for a greater limitation of physical activity than any other disease, including heart disease. COLD patients tend to die a very unpleasant, prolonged death, often from a general collapse of normal cardiorespiratory function that results in congestive heart failure (see Chapter 10).

Additional Health Concerns

In addition to the serious health problems stemming from tobacco use already described, other health-related changes are routinely seen. These include a generally poor state of nutrition, a decline in insulin sensitivity, a decline in short-term memory, the gradual loss of the sense of smell, and premature wrinkling of the skin. Tobacco users are also more likely to experience strokes (a potentially fatal condition), lose bone mass leading to osteoporosis, experience more back pain and muscle injury, and find that fractures heal more slowly. Further, smokers who have surgery spend more time in the recovery room. Although not perceived as a health problem by people who continue smoking in order to control weight, smoking does appear to minimize weight gain. In studies using identical twins, twins who smoked were six to eight pounds lighter than their nonsmoking siblings. Current understanding about why smoking results in lower body weight is less than complete. One factor may be an increase in Basal Metabolic Rate (BMR) (see Chapter 6) brought about by the influence of nicotine on sympathetic nervous system function. Additionally, smokers have a fourfold greater risk of developing serious gum (periodontal) disease, now thought to be a risk factor for cardiovascular disease. Also, smokers may need supplementation for two important water-soluble vitamins, vitamin C and vitamin B.

Smoking and Reproduction

In all its dimensions, the reproductive process is impaired by the use of tobacco, particularly cigarette smoking and environmental tobacco smoke in close proximity to pregnant women.[29] Problems can be found in association with infertility, problem pregnancy, breast-feeding, and the health of the newborn. So broadly based are reproductive problems and smoking that the term *fetal tobacco syndrome* or *fetal smoking syndrome*[30] is regularly used in clinical medicine. Some physicians even define a fetus being carried by a smoker as a "smoker" and, upon birth, as a "former smoker."

Infertility

Recent research indicates that cigarette smoking by both men and women can reduce levels of fertility. Among men, smoking adversely affects blood flow to erectile tissue, reduces sperm motility, and alters sperm shape, and it causes an overall decrease in the number of viable sperm. Among women, the effects of smoking are seen in terms of abnormal ovum formation, including a lessened ability on the part of the egg to prevent polyspermia, or the fertilization by multiple sperm. Smoking also negatively influences estrogen levels, resulting in underdevelopment of the uterine wall and ineffective implantation of the fertilized ovum. Lower levels of estrogen may also influence the rate of transit of the fertilized egg through the fallopian tube, making it arrive in the uterus too early for successful implantation or, in some cases, restricting movement to the point that an **ectopic, or tubal, pregnancy** may develop. Also, the early onset of menopause is associated with smoking.

Although causative pathways remain somewhat unclear, the influences of smoking are noted in two aspects of male infertility, sperm degradation and erectile dysfunction. In the former cases, several chemicals in tobacco smoke are able to cross the blood-testis barrier and structurally

---

Key Terms
chronic bronchitis persistent inflammation and infection of the smaller airways within the lungs
pulmonary emphysema an irreversible disease process in which the alveoli are destroyed
alveoli (al **vee** oh lie) thin, saclike terminal ends of the airways; the site at which gases are exchanged between the blood and inhaled air
ectopic (tubal) pregnancy pregnancy resulting from the implantation of the fertilized ovum within the inner wall of the fallopian tube

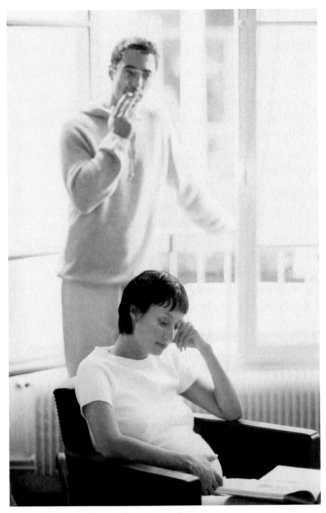

To protect the health of the developing fetus, pregnant women and those around them should refrain from smoking.

alter the DNA of the genetic material within the sperm. The presence of abnormal sperm in the male compromises the chances of fertilization. In erectile dysfunction, smoking, most likely through the effects of nicotine on blood-flow dynamics, decreases blood flow into the erectile tissues of the penile shaft, resulting in the inability to obtain or sustain an erection.[31, 32]

Problem Pregnancy

The harmful effects of tobacco smoke on the course of pregnancy are principally the result of the carbon monoxide and nicotine to which the mother and her fetus are exposed. Carbon monoxide from the incomplete oxidation of tobacco is carried in the maternal blood to the placenta, where it diffuses across the placental barrier and enters the fetal circulation. Once in the fetal blood, the carbon monoxide bonds with the fetal hemoglobin to form fetal carboxyhemoglobin. As a result of this exposure to carbon monoxide, the fetus is progressively deprived of normal oxygen transport and eventually becomes compromised by chronic **hypoxia.**

Nicotine also exerts its influence on the developing fetus. Thermographs of the placenta and fetus show signs of marked vasoconstriction within a few seconds after inhalation by the mother. This constriction further reduces the oxygen supply, resulting in hypoxia. In addition, nicotine stimulates the mother's stress response, placing the mother and fetus under the potentially harmful influence of elevated epinephrine and corticoid levels (see Chapter 3). Any fetus exposed to all of these agents is more likely to be miscarried, stillborn, or born prematurely. Even when carried to term, children born to mothers who smoked during pregnancy have lower birth weights and may show other signs of a stressful intrauterine life.

Breastfeeding

Women who breast-feed their infants and continue to smoke continue to expose their children to the harmful effects of tobacco smoke. It is well recognized that nicotine appears in breast milk and thus is capable of exerting its vasoconstricting and stress-response influences on nursing infants. Mothers who stop smoking during pregnancy should be encouraged to continue to refrain from smoking while they are breastfeeding.

Neonatal Health Problems

Babies born to women who smoked during pregnancy are, on average, shorter and have a lower birth weight than do children born to nonsmoking mothers. During the earliest months of life, babies born to mothers who smoke experience an elevated rate of death caused by sudden infant death syndrome. Statistics also show that infants are more likely to develop chronic respiratory problems, more frequent colic, be hospitalized, and have poorer overall health during their early years of life. Problems such as those just mentioned may also be seen in children of nonsmoking mothers, when they were exposed prenatally to environmental tobacco smoke. In addition, environmental tobacco smoke exposure extending beyond the home and into the workplace may increase the probability of problem pregnancies and neonatal health problems. Most recently, the interest in the effects of tobacco smoke on pregnancy has been extended to include behavioral differences in infants born to women who smoked during pregnancy.[33]

Parenting, in the sense of assuming responsibility for the well-being of children, does not begin at birth, but

---

Key Terms

hypoxia oxygenation deprivation at the cellular level

during the prenatal period. In the case of smoking, this is especially true. Pregnant women who continue smoking are disregarding the well-being of the children they are carrying. Other family members, friends, and coworkers who subject pregnant women to cigarette, pipe, or cigar smoke are, in a sense, exhibiting their own disregard for the health of the next generation.

Oral Contraceptives and Tobacco Use

Women who smoke and use oral contraceptives, particularly after age 35, are placing themselves at a much greater risk of experiencing a fatal cardiovascular accident (heart attack, stroke, or **embolism**) than are oral contraceptive users who do not smoke. This risk of cardiovascular complications increases further for oral contraceptive users 40 years of age or older. Women who both smoke and use oral contraceptives are four times more likely to die from myocardial infarction (heart attack) than are women who only smoke. Because of this adverse relationship, *it is strongly recommended that women who smoke not use oral contraceptives.*

Combining Tobacco and Alcohol Use

Although there are exceptions to every generalization, it is very common to see tobacco and alcohol being used by the same people, often at the same time. Younger people who use both tobacco and alcohol are also more likely to use additional drugs. Accordingly, both tobacco and alcohol are considered *gateway drugs* because they are often introductory drugs that "open the door" for a more broadly based polydrug use pattern (see Chapter 7).

Beyond the potential for polydrug use initiated by the use of tobacco and alcohol is the simple reality that the use of both tobacco products and alcoholic beverages is associated with a wide array of illnesses and with premature death. As you have seen in this chapter and in Chapter 8 regarding alcohol use, the negative health impact of using both is significant. When use is combined, of course, the risks of living less healthfully and dying prematurely are accentuated.

Smokeless Tobacco Use

As the term implies, smokeless tobacco, such as Skoal and Copenhagen, is not burned; rather, it is placed into the mouth. Once in place, the physiologically active nicotine and other soluble compounds are absorbed through the mucous membranes and into the blood. Within a few minutes, chewing tobacco and snuff generate blood levels of nicotine in amounts equivalent to those seen in cigarette smokers.

Chewing tobacco is taken from its foil pouch, formed into a small ball (called a "wad," "chaw," or "chew"), and placed into the mouth. Once in place, the bolus of tobacco is sucked and occasionally chewed, but not swallowed.

Snuff, a more finely shredded smokeless tobacco product, is marketed in small round cans. Snuff is formed into a small mass (or "quid") for dipping or used in prepackaged pouches. The quid or pouch is placed between the jaw and the cheek; the user sucks the quid or pouch, then spits out the brown liquid. Snuff, as once used, was actually a powdered form of tobacco that was inhaled through the nose.

Although smokeless tobacco would seem to free the tobacco user from many of the risks associated with smoking, chewing and dipping are not without their own substantial risks. The presence of *leukoplakia* (white spots) and *erythroplakia* (red spots) on the tissues of the mouth indicate precancerous changes. In addition, an increase in **periodontal disease** (with the pulling away of the gums from the teeth, resulting in later tooth loss), the abrasive damage to the enamel of the teeth, and the high concentration of sugar in processed tobacco all contribute to dental problems among users of smokeless tobacco. In

Key Terms

embolism a potentially fatal condition in which a circulating blood clot lodges in a smaller vessel

periodontal disease destruction of soft tissue and bone that surround the teeth those who develop oral cancer, the risk is dramatically heightened if the cancer metastasizes from the site of origin in the mouth to the brain. Clearly, users should be aware of any signs of damage being done by their use of smokeless tobacco. (See the Changing for the Better box.) The validity of this warning was made clear in 1998 when about half of smokeless-tobacco-using major league baseball players were found to have tobacco-related lesions when oral examinations were performed by team dentists on the first day of spring training.

In addition to the damage done to the tissues of the mouth, the need to process the inadvertently swallowed saliva that contains dissolved carcinogens places both the digestive and urinary systems at risk of cancer.

In the opinion of health experts, the use of smokeless tobacco and its potential for life-threatening disease is very real and should not be disregarded. Consequently, television advertisements have been banned, and the following warnings have been placed in rotation on all smokeless tobacco products:

> WARNING: THIS PRODUCT MAY CAUSE MOUTH
> CANCER
> WARNING: THIS PRODUCT MAY CAUSE GUM
> DISEASE AND TOOTH LOSS
> WARNING: THIS PRODUCT IS NOT A SAFE ALTER-
> NATIVE TO CIGARETTE SMOKING

Clearly, smokeless tobacco is a dangerous product, and little doubt exists that continued use of tobacco in this form is a serious problem to health in all its dimensions.

The Risks of Involuntary (Passive) Smoking

The smoke generated by the burning of tobacco can be classified as either **mainstream smoke** (the smoke inhaled and then exhaled by the smoker) or **sidestream smoke** (the smoke that comes from the burning end of the cigarette, pipe, or cigar that simply disperses into the air without being inhaled by the smoker). When either form of tobacco smoke is diluted and stays within a common source of air, it can eventually be referred to as **environmental tobacco smoke.** All three forms of tobacco smoke lead to involuntary or passive smoking and can present health problems for both nonsmokers and smokers. (See the Discovering Your Spirituality box on page 300.)

Surprisingly, mainstream smoke makes up only 15 percent of our exposure to the harmful substances associated with involuntary smoking. Sidestream smoke is responsible for 85 percent of the harmful substances associated with secondhand smoke exposure. Because it is not filtered by the tobacco, the filter, or the smoker's body, sidestream smoke contains more free nicotine and produces higher yields of

carbon dioxide and carbon monoxide. Much to the detriment of nonsmokers, sidestream smoke has a much higher quantity of highly carcinogenic compounds, called *N-nitrosamines,* than mainstream smoke has.

Current scientific opinion suggests that smokers and nonsmokers are exposed to very much the same smoke when tobacco is used within a common airspace. The important difference is the quantity of smoke inhaled by smokers and nonsmokers. It is likely that for each pack of cigarettes smoked by a smoker, nonsmokers who must share a common air supply with the smokers involuntarily smoke the equivalent of three to five cigarettes per day. Even today, because of the small size of the particles produced by burning tobacco, environmental tobacco smoke cannot be completely removed from a workplace, restaurant, or shopping mall by the most effective ventilation system.

Recently reported research indicates that involuntary smoke exposure may be responsible for 35,000 to 40,000 premature deaths per year from heart disease among nonsmokers in the United States.[26] Other estimates range upward to 53,000 premature deaths when lung cancer and COPD are included. In addition, large numbers of people exposed to involuntary smoke develop eye irritation, nasal symptoms, headaches, and a cough. Furthermore, most nonsmokers dislike the odor of tobacco smoke.

For these reasons, state, local, and private-sector initiatives to restrict smoking have been introduced. Most buildings in which people work, study, play, reside, eat, or shop now have some smoking restrictions. Some have complete smoking bans. Nowhere is smoking more noticeably prohibited than in the U.S. airline industry. Currently, smoking is banned on all domestic plane flights of less than 6 hours, and major American airlines have extended the ban on smoking to international flights as well.

Involuntary smoking poses major threats to nonsmokers within residential settings. Spouses and children of smokers are at greatest risk for involuntary smoking. Scientific studies suggest that nonsmokers married to smokers are three times more likely to experience heart attacks than nonsmoking spouses of nonsmokers, and the former have a 30 percent greater risk of lung cancer than do the latter. However, a recent study of 35,561 nonsmoking spouses of

---

Key Terms

mainstream smoke smoke inhaled and then exhaled by a smoker

sidestream smoke smoke that comes from the burning end of a cigarette, pipe, or cigar

environmental tobacco smoke tobacco smoke, regardless of its source, that stays within a common source of air

The Hidden Price Tag of Smoking

"I started to hug him but felt myself drawing back. It was almost like a reflex action." Those are the words of a young woman after greeting her brother when he returned home from his first semester at college. The young man had recently become a smoker, and his sister was reacting to the strong smell of smoke on his clothes and hair.

Dramatic as it may sound, smoking does set up barriers between people. First, there's the health issue. Some nonsmokers are adamant about not wanting people they care about to smoke. They also want to protect their children from this danger. And they certainly don't want to breathe in smoke themselves. So, at a family gathering, a smoker may want to have a cigarette after dinner, in the living room with everyone else. But the nonsmokers say no—go outside if you want to smoke. In the process, a birthday dinner or a special holiday is marred by this disagreement.

Whether the person is a family member or a friend, it's difficult to feel close to someone who's doing something you disapprove of—such as smoking. But, from the smoker's point of view, it's hard to feel good about someone who acts superior and doesn't accept you as you are. What do children think about all this? Does a "good" aunt or uncle smoke? If smoking is bad, as a little girl constantly hears at school and at home, why does her favorite uncle smoke?

On the job, smoking has gone the way of the three-martini lunch. It's just not politically correct. In fact, many companies have a no-smoking policy, or smoking is allowed in designated areas only. Ever drive by a big factory or office building and see a group of people standing outside, perhaps huddled under umbrellas? They're not organizing a strike—they're having a smoke. Once again, the smoker feels isolated.

Just as in the family group, the smoker feels the judgment of others—only now it's her boss or secretary who's frowning.

In addition to the more modest work-site restrictions just described, today the hammer has fallen even harder on the heads of smokers—companies are beginning to reject job applications from smokers. (It's hard to hide the telltale signs of smoking and relatively easy to learn from references whether an applicant is a smoker.) Additionally, companies have begun terminating employees who smoke, even when they don't smoke at work. Some companies will pay for smoking-cessation assistance, so long as the employees remain active participants in the program and eventually quit smoking. Countersuits brought by rejected applicants and terminated employees will certainly begin filtering through the court system, but until final rulings are made, smokers should be prepared for increasing discrimination.

The price of smoking is hard to measure. The damage to the smoker's health is beyond dispute. But the spiritual and psychological costs are also real. How does it feel to always be the outsider? The unaccepted? Why does the smoker have to take the chance of missing an exciting play in the stadium to go smoke a cigarette? Or feel the resentment of others at work because he leaves to take a smoking break every hour? Many who have stopped smoking—often after several attempts—say that they thought about more than their health in deciding to quit. They thought about many situations—involving family, outdoor activities, and work—before they threw away the pack and said: "That was my last cigarette."

smoking partners failed to show significantly higher death rates from heart disease, lung cancer, and COPD than did nonsmoking spouses in nonsmoking relationships.[34] It should be noted, however, that between the time of publication of the study and October of 2004, dozens of letters to the editor were sent to the *British Medical Journal*, publisher of the original study. A substantial number of these letters called attention to flaws in the design of the study, faulty statistical interpretation, and a potential conflict of interest between the authors and the tobacco industry.

In spite of what may or may not be the effects of passive smoking on the nonsmoking partners of smokers, the effects of environmental tobacco smoke on the health of children seems well established. The children of parents who smoke are twice as likely as children of nonsmoking parents to experience bronchitis or pneumonia during the first year of life. In addition, throughout childhood these children will experience more wheezing, coughing, and sputum production than will children whose parents do not smoke. Otitis media (middle ear infection), one of the most frequently seen conditions in pediatric medicine, is also significantly more common in children under age 3 who reside with one or more adults who smoke.

In July 1998, the tobacco industry challenged in court the salient 1993 EPA report that was the basis for restricting smoking in a wide array of public places and work sites. The federal judge who heard the case concluded that the principal study used in the report was flawed in its methodology and that its conclusions therefore were of questionable validity. Since this decision, the scientific community has documented to a very substantial degree the inherent dangers of passive or environmental tobacco smoke to the health of nonsmokers and smokers alike. Accordingly, restrictions on public smoking have been large scale and continue to be imposed. These restrictions include statewide bans on smoking in public places in California, Connecticut, Delaware, Florida, Idaho, Maine, Massachusetts, New York, Rhode Island, South Dakota, and Utah. Additionally, many cities and towns have enacted their own bans, particularly in states that have no statewide bans. Examples are Anchorage, Tempe, Boulder, Honolulu, Fort Wayne (IN), Albuquerque, Columbus (OH), Eugene, and Austin.[35]

Although the United States does not have a single encompassing ban on smoking in public places, several countries have enacted such bans. Among them are Australia, Italy, Scotland, England, Cuba, Ireland, Uganda, Greece, Sweden, and Romania.

Many colleges and universities are instituting bans on smoking near the entrances to classroom buildings and residence halls. At Ball State University, cigarettes must be extinguished within 30 feet of an entrance. This restriction on smoking reflects the fact that environmental tobacco smoke accumulates under overhangs and in alcoves.

New Product Development

The development of new products by the tobacco industry also attests, in an interesting way, to the inherent dangers of tobacco use long known by the tobacco industry (and forcibly admitted to the public in the 1999 tobacco settlement). The products include the development of Eclipse (by R.J. Reynolds), a cigarette that heats rather than burns most of its tobacco. According to its manufacturer, Eclipse is the first cigarette that produces smoke so low in carcinogens that it is the "next best choice" to quitting. This latter contention certainly states in a null manner something about cigarettes marketed before the development of Eclipse. Unfortunately for customers who switched to Eclipse in search of a safe cigarette, the claims made by the company about the cigarette's low carcinogenic composition proved inaccurate (or purposefully false). Most likely the end of the "safe cigarette" is in sight.

Another recently introduced cigarette, Accord, features a "smoking system" intended to reduce the production of sidestream smoke. This system uses a battery-powered device into which a special small cigarette is inserted. The smoker inhales through the device, and the cigarette is electrically ignited only when actively inhaled.

Three additional new products appeared in 2003, including Advance, cigarettes with "Trionic" filters supposedly capable of extracting more toxins than any filter to date; Omni, a brand advertised to significantly reduce selected carcinogens, nitrosamines, and catechols, the "major causes of lung cancer" according to their advertisements; and Quest, a brand intended to lead smokers to "nicotine free smoking." It should be noted that none of these new brands can deliver anything approaching a safe cigarette, nor are they intended to assist smokers in becoming nonsmokers.

Another addition to the new products recently introduced by the tobacco industry are self-extinguishing (reduced-ignition-propensity, or RIP) cigarettes that are necessary for continuing sales in the state of New York. The technology for this form of fire-risk-reducing cigarette, that largely extinguishes a burning cigarette if not inhaled upon within 60 seconds, has been available for several years, although not introduced by the tobacco industry until required to do so by New York.

A more alarming new product introduced by the tobacco industry is that of flavored cigarettes, such as Camel Exotic Blend. The manufacturer of this brand, R.J. Reynolds, contends that they are on the market to offer established smokers a greater choice of products, but their appeal appears instead to be aiming at young, beginning smokers.

Nontobacco Sources of Nicotine

Regardless of whether they are intended as aids to smoking cessation or only supplemental forms of nicotine for use when smoking is not permitted, numerous new forms of nicotine delivery systems have appeared in the marketplace in recent years. An area of growing concern is, of course, that these nontobacco delivery sources of nicotine could provide introductory exposure to nicotine, at a tragically early age, for the next generation of nicotine-dependent youth. Included among these nontobacco sources of nicotine are multiple flavors of nicotine suckers, nicotine-flavored gum, nicotine straws, nicotine-enhanced water (Nico Water), inhalers, sprays, drops, lozenges, and transdermal patches. To date, only Nico Water has been formally addressed by the Food and Drug Administration (and their request for control was rejected by the courts), other than those that came into the marketplace as prescription-only or approved OTC products.

Stopping What You Started

Experts in health behavior contend that before people will discontinue harmful health behaviors, such as tobacco use, they must appreciate fully what they are expecting of themselves. This understanding grows in relationship to the following:

1. *Knowledge* about the health risks associated with tobacco use
2. *Recognition* that these health risks are applicable to all tobacco users
3. *Familiarity* with steps that can be taken to eliminate or reduce these risks
4. *Belief* that the benefits to be gained by no longer using tobacco will outweigh the pleasures gained through the use of tobacco
5. *Certainty* that one can start and maintain the behaviors required to stop or reduce the use of tobacco

These steps combine both knowledge and desire (or motivation). Being knowledgeable about risks, however, will not always stop behaviors that involve varying degrees of psychological and physical dependence. The 75 percent failure rate thought to be common among tobacco-cessation programs suggests that the motivation is not easy to achieve

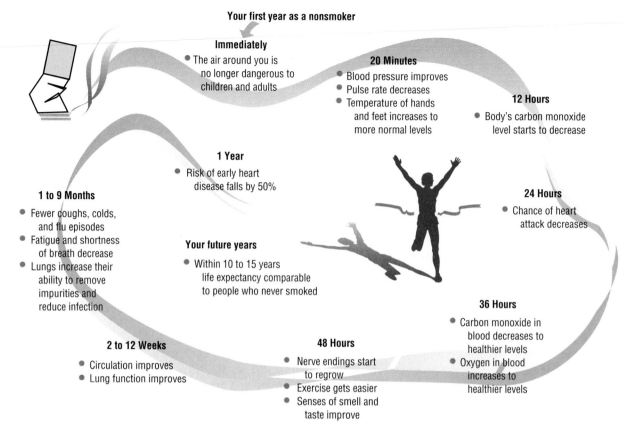

Your first year as a nonsmoker

Immediately
- The air around you is no longer dangerous to children and adults

20 Minutes
- Blood pressure improves
- Pulse rate decreases
- Temperature of hands and feet increases to more normal levels

12 Hours
- Body's carbon monoxide level starts to decrease

1 Year
- Risk of early heart disease falls by 50%

1 to 9 Months
- Fewer coughs, colds, and flu episodes
- Fatigue and shortness of breath decrease
- Lungs increase their ability to remove impurities and reduce infection

Your future years
- Within 10 to 15 years life expectancy comparable to people who never smoked

24 Hours
- Chance of heart attack decreases

2 to 12 Weeks
- Circulation improves
- Lung function improves

48 Hours
- Nerve endings start to regrow
- Exercise gets easier
- Senses of smell and taste improve

36 Hours
- Carbon monoxide in blood decreases to healthier levels
- Oxygen in blood increases to healthier levels

Figure 9-2 The health benefits of quitting smoking begin immediately and become more significant the longer you stay smoke-free

or maintain. In fact, on the basis of information reported by the Hazelden Foundation, for persons who are successful in quitting, approximately 18.6 years elapse between the first attempt to stop and the actual time of quitting. The many health benefits of quitting smoking are shown in Figure 9-2.

A variety of smoking-cessation programs exist, including those using highly organized formats, with or without the use of prescription or OTC nicotine replacement systems. In past years, most of the 1.3 million people who managed to quit smoking each year did so by throwing away their cigarettes (going cold turkey) and paying the physical and emotional price of waiting for their bodies to adjust to life without nicotine. Today, however, the use of nicotine replacement products in combination with external smoking cessation approaches, such as those described later in this chapter, or the use of prescription medication, such as antidepressants, is more common. The Changing for the Better box on page 303 provides a plan for smoking cessation that incorporates nicotine replacement products.

Programs to help people stop their tobacco use are available in a variety of formats, including educational programs, behavior modification, aversive conditioning, hypnosis, acupuncture, and various combinations of these approaches. (See Considering Complementary Care on page 304.) Programs are offered in both individual and group settings and are operated by hospitals, universities, health departments, voluntary health agencies, churches, and private practitioners. The better programs will have limited success rates—20–50 percent as measured over one year (with self-reporting), whereas the remainder will have even poorer results. If results are monitored using the assessment of nicotine breakdown products in the blood, the effectiveness rate of these programs falls even lower, as some "successful" self-reporters are not completely honest in their reporting of cessation.

Two methods for weaning smokers from cigarettes to a nontobacco source of nicotine are nicotine-containing chewing gum (Nicorette) and transdermal patches, in either prescription or OTC versions (Nicoderm, Nicotrol, Habitrol, Prostep, and others), using either single-strength or step-down formulas. A brief description of both gum and the transdermal patch is provided next, although subtle variations exist between prescription and OTC formulations and between brands.

Nicotine-Containing Chewing Gum Correct use of nicotine-containing chewing gum requires an immediate cessation of smoking, an initial determination of dosage (4 mg or 2 mg of nicotine per piece), knowledge of the appropriate manner of chewing each piece of gum, the appropriate time to chew each piece, the maximum number of pieces to be chewed each day, and time to begin withdrawal from the therapy. When used in combination with physician guidance or program support provided by the manufacturer, cessation using nicotine-containing gum may have a success rate of 40 percent or more, based on blood evaluation. Nicotine-containing chewing gum therapy ranges in cost from an initial $60 kit to weekly refills of approximately $30.

Transdermal Nicotine Patches   The more recently developed transdermal (through the skin) nicotine patches appear to be less effective (25 percent) than does the gum just described, but in many ways the patches are more easily used. If a step-down version (21 mg, 14 mg, 7 mg) is employed, determinations must be made as to the appropriate initial dosage (based on number of cigarettes smoked per day and body weight), the length of time at the initial dosage before stepping down, and the manner of withdrawal after a usual 8- to 12-week treatment period. The single-dose (15 mg) version, of course, eliminates the step-down component. Costs associated with transdermal nicotine replacement therapy are similar to those for the gum-based program.

In addition to the nicotine-replacement therapies already described, a nicotine inhaler and spray have been

---

Changing for the Better

Countdown to Quit Day: A Plan for Smoking Cessation

I started smoking at parties to feel more relaxed. Now I smoke at least a pack a day, and I'm afraid I'm hooked for life. How do I get myself off tobacco?

Make a decision to quit smoking on a particular day during the next week. Then use the following steps to begin preparing yourself for that day.

Five Days before Quit Day

- Keep a daylong record of each cigarette you smoke. List the time you smoked, whom you were with, and why you decided to light up (for example, for stimulation, tension reduction, or social pleasure, or because you had a craving or wanted something to do with your hands). Once you know why you smoke, you can plan intervention strategies for use during the two-minute periods of craving you will feel during the first weeks of your smoke-free life.
- Contact your physician to help you decide whether to use prescription or OTC nicotine-replacement therapy. Make sure you understand all directions for its safe and effective use.
- Draw up a contract in which you formally state your intention to quit smoking. Sign and date the contract and clearly display it in your home or workplace.

Four Days before Quit Day

- Solicit support from family, friends, and coworkers by sharing your intention with them and asking for their help and encouragement.
- Organize your intervention strategies and assemble needed supplies, such as gum, bottled water, diet soda, handwork (for example, needlepoint or wood carving), and walking shoes.

Three Days before Quit Day

- Review your quitting contract and touch bases with several people in your support group to bolster your resolve.
- Study all nicotine-replacement therapy product information and any material supplied by your physician.
- Continue preparing your intervention supplies.

- Reschedule your personal calendar and work schedule to minimize situations that could tempt you to smoke during the first several days of your smoke-free life.

Two Days before Quit Day

- Continue or revisit any earlier tasks that you have not yet finished.
- Practice your intervention strategies as appropriate. For example, map out a safe walking route and practice your deep-breathing exercises.
- Obtain a large glass or other container, such as an empty milk jug, that will serve as a bank into which you will deposit daily the money that you would have otherwise spent on cigarettes.
- If you feel comfortable doing so, construct a yard sign to inform outsiders that your home is a smoke-free environment and to report your daily success toward a smoke-free life.
- Smoke-proof your home and workplace by removing and destroying all materials and supplies associated with tobacco use, saving only enough tobacco products needed for today and tomorrow.

One Day before Quit Day

- Complete all preparations described above, including the almost total removal and destruction of smoking-related materials.
- As the end of the day approaches, review your contract and call a few people in your support network for last-minute words of encouragement.
- Smoke your last cigarette and flush any remaining cigarettes down the toilet.
- Begin your nicotine-replacement therapy as directed by your physician or by product insert information.
- Publicly display your yard sign, if you decided to make one.
- Retire for the night and await your rebirth in the morning as a former smoker.

InfoLinks

www.philipmorrisusa.com/en/health_issues/quitting_smoking.asp

Hypnotism: A Solution for Smokers?

On at least one occasion each year a "professional" hypnotist visits the community in which we (the authors) live. A large advertisement appears in the local paper a day or two before his visit to identify his location (usually a motel conference room) and the problems (obesity and smoking) that his brand of hypnosis proves effective against. The cost of a one-time session generally ranges between $30 (for one condition) and $50 (for both conditions), with a discount for groups of two or more preregistered persons. Effective rates are generally stated to be 97.5% for weight reduction and 98% for smoking abatement. The term "effective" is, of course, never defined.

In terms of smoking abatement, what about the services of a clinically trained and hospital-based psychologist who specializes in the use of hypnosis? Does hypnosis of this type have efficacy in smoking abatement—either as a sole treatment modality or in combination with other therapies?

In an attempt to answer this question, a Med-Line search using the key word "hypnosis" was conducted with the following results. In the time period between January and August 2000, 68 studies addressing the clinical application of hypnosis were published in the medical literature. Of these, three studies were related to the use of hypnosis in smoking abatement. Two of the three studies reported involved the meta-analysis of 59 and 9 earlier studies, respectively. On the basis of 59 earlier studies, the authors of the largest of the current studies concluded that "hypnosis cannot be considered a specific and efficacious treatment for smoking cessation." They did acknowledge that hypnosis is "possibly efficacious," but only when cognitive/behavioral and educational intervention that often accompanies hypnosis is included in the study.[1] The authors of the second and smallest (9 earlier studies) of the current studies concluded that they were unable to show "that hypnotherapy has a greater effect on 6-month quit rates than did other interventions or no treatment."[2] A more recent Med-line review of hypnosis-based smoking-cessation studies shows that very few were undertaken since 2000. Again, results that were reported were, at best, cautiously optimistic, but in most studies the number of persons treated was small, sessions were few in number, and self-reporting was the principal means of assessing results.

Authors of the various, Med-line studies all concluded that more and better-designed studies on hypnosis-based smoking cessation were needed.

Searches involving the Web sites of The National Center for Complementary and Alternative Medicine and American Psychological Association failed to identify studies related to hypnosis and smoking cessation.

[1] Green JP, Lynn SJ. Hypnosis and suggestion-based approaches to smoking cessation: An examination of the evidence. *Int J Clin Hypn* 48(2): 195–224. 2000.
[2] Abbot NC, et al. Hypnotherapy for smoking cessation. *Cochrane Data Base Syst Rev* 2000.

approved (in prescription form) by the FDA. Because of the large surface area of the lungs and rapid absorption into the blood, inhalation-based delivery of nicotine has become a very attractive alternative to transdermal and oral routes of replacement.

In all delivery forms and formulations, nicotine replacement therapy can be associated with contraindications and adverse reactions, including skin irritation, redness, and irregular heart rates. People who are concerned that nicotine-replacement therapies are simply a "trade-off" of addictions (from cigarettes to gum, patches, or a nasal spray) should remember that while using the therapy the former smoker is no longer being exposed to carbon monoxide and carcinogens, and the step-down feature allows for a gradual return to a totally nicotine-free lifestyle. Therefore, a short period of cross-addiction should be viewed simply as the cost of recovery.

Recently developed prescription medications used in combination with other cessation methods improve the latter's effectiveness rate to somewhat above the 40 percent (perhaps approaching 50 percent) level reported for nicotine-containing chewing gum, according to a blood-based assessment. These drugs affect receptors in the CNS, reducing the pleasurable effects of nicotine and thus decreasing dependency. Among the more recently "discovered" prescription medications for smoking cessation is methoxsalen. Although intended for the treatment of psoriasis, a skin condition, this medication has been found to constructively alter the breakdown of nicotine in persons who have a particular genetic mutation that lessens their need for frequent cigarettes. Another recently approved drug for use in smoking cessation is varenicline. On the basis of clinical trials, it is reported that nearly one-half of all persons receiving the drug were able to cease smoking. Should this efficacy carry over into long-term trials, this medication would equal or most likely exceed the most effective approaches now available.

Several additional nicotine-free prescription medications to aid smoking cessation have now been approved or are nearing approval. These agents can be used alone or with nicotine replacement therapy. Zyban and Wellbutrin are antidepressant drugs that increase the production of dopamine, a neurotransmitter. Production of dopamine

Table 9.5 How Methods of Smoking Cessation Stack Up

Of the nation's estimated 48 million smokers, 70% want to quit, and 46% try each year. Only 1 in 40 succeeds. Federal guidelines, based on published studies, estimate varied success rates for a number of medications designed to help smokers quit.

Medications	Nicotine gum	Nicotine inhaler	Buproprion SR (Zyban)	Nicotine spray	Nicotine patch	Combination
Number of studies	13	4	2	3	27	3
Five-month quit rate	23.7%	22.8%	30.5%	30.5%	17.7%	28.6%
Advantage	Can be used to offset cravings	Mimics smoking	Nonnicotine, an antidepressant	Higher nicotine levels	Private, one/day	Combines benefits
Disadvantage	Poor taste	Low nicotine levels	Must screen for seizures	Irritation, sneezing	Skin irritation	Not FDA-approved
Over the Counter (OTC) or prescription (Rx)	OTC	Rx	Rx	Rx	Both	Both

Source: *Treating Tobacco Use and Dependence.* U.S. Public Health Service: John Hughes, University of Vermont, November 2000.

declines when a smoker quits, creating the craving to smoke. Prozac, the serotonin-reuptake inhibitor antidepressant approved for the treatment of depression, bulimia nervosa, PMS, and obsessive-compulsive disorder, has also shown promise as an adjunct to smoking cessation. See Table 9.5 for a comparison of various cessation approaches.

In a recent meta-analysis of smoking cessation program success involving African Americans, it was found that there is no statistically significant difference between the success of this racial group and others. Of interest, however, was a finding that church-based programs might be more successful for smoking cessation than previously recognized.

Tobacco Use: A Question of Rights

For those readers who have found themselves involved (or nearly so) in confrontation situations involving smokers' versus nonsmokers' rights, we hope the following section allows you to see more clearly the positions that you have taken. For those who have somehow remained removed from this discussion, consideration of these issues now may be good preparation for the future. Regardless, consider these two important questions:

1. To what extent should smokers be allowed to pollute the air and endanger the health of nonsmokers?
2. To what extent should nonsmokers be allowed to restrict the personal freedom of smokers, particularly since tobacco products are sold legally?

At this time, answers to these questions are only partially available, but one trend is developing: the tobacco user is being forced to give ground to the nonsmoker. Today, in fact, it is becoming more a matter of where the smoker will be allowed to smoke, rather than a matter of where smoking will be restricted. Smoking is currently becoming less and less tolerated. The health concerns of the majority are prevailing over the dependence needs of the minority.

 TALKING POINTS You're having a discussion with a friend about life insurance and mention that you get a 10-percent reduction in your annual premium because you're a nonsmoker. Your friend, who is a smoker, becomes annoyed and says that this is just one example of how smokers are penalized. How would you respond?

Taking Charge of Your Health

- Commit yourself to establishing a smoke-free environment in the places where you live, work, study, and recreate.

- Support friends and acquaintances who are trying to become smoke-free.

- Support legislative efforts, at all levels of government, to reduce your exposure to environmental tobacco smoke.

- Be civil toward tobacco users in public spaces, but respond assertively if they infringe on smoke-free spaces.

- Support agencies and organizations committed to reducing tobacco use among young people through education and intervention.

SUMMARY

- The percentage of American adults who smoke is continuing to decline.
- In spite of a reversal on the part of more recent college graduates, cigarette smoking has traditionally been inversely related to the level of formal education.
- A number of demographical variables influence the incidence of tobacco use.
- The tobacco industry continues to aggressively market its products to potential smokers.
- Multiple theories regarding nicotine's role in dependence have been advanced, including a better understanding of the proportional influences of genetics, environment, and personality.
- Nicotine exerts acute effects both within the central nervous system and on a variety of other tissues and organs.
- Tobacco smoke can be divided into gaseous and particulate phases. Each phase has its unique chemical composition.
- Thousands of chemical components and hundreds of carcinogenic agents are found in tobacco smoke.
- Nicotine and carbon monoxide have predictable effects on the function of the cardiovascular system.
- The development of nearly one-third of all cancers can be attributed to tobacco use, and virtually every form of cancer is found more frequently in smokers than in nonsmokers.

- Chronic obstructive lung disease (COLD), also called chronic obstructive pulmonary disease (COPD), is a likely consequence of long-term cigarette smoking, with early symptoms appearing shortly after beginning regular smoking.
- Smoking alters normal structure and function of the body, as seen in a wide variety of noncardiovascular and noncancerous conditions, such as infertility, problem pregnancy, and neonatal health concerns. Additional health concerns include the diminished ability to smell, periodontal disease, vitamin inadequacies, and bone loss leading to osteoporosis.
- The use of smokeless tobacco carries its own health risks, including oral cancer.
- The presence of secondhand smoke results in involuntary (or passive) smoking by those who must share a common air source with smokers. This secondhand smoke threatens the health of the spouse, children, and coworkers of the smoker.
- Stopping smoking can be undertaken in any one of several ways, including the use of nicotine-replacement products, such as nicotine-containing gum, transdermal nicotine patches, and nicotine inhalers, as well as medications that influence the recognition of neurotransmitters that bring pleasure to smokers.

REVIEW QUESTIONS

1. What percentage of the American adult population smoke? In what direction has change been occurring?
2. What is the current direction that adolescent smoking is taking?
3. What was the outcome of the class action suit brought by the 46 states, and what was the effect of the Master Settlement Agreement (1999) on the ability of the tobacco industry to market its products?
4. In comparison to cigarettes, what health risks are associated with pipe and cigar smoking?
5. What are the two principal dimensions of nicotine dependence? What are specific aspects seen within physical dependence?
6. Identify each of the theories of nicotine dependence discussed in the chapter.
7. How do modeling and manipulation explain the development of emotional dependence on tobacco?
8. In the amount consumed by the typical smoker, what is the effect of nicotine on central nervous system function? How does this differ in chain smokers?

9. What effects does nicotine have on the body outside of the central nervous system? How does the influence of nicotine resemble that associated with the stress response?
10. What is the principal effect of carbon monoxide on cardiac function?
11. What influences does passive smoking have on nonsmoking adult partners of smokers? On their children?
12. How is the federal government attempting to limit the exposure that children and adolescents currently have to tobacco products and tobacco advertisements?
13. How might concerned parents begin to "tobacco proof" their children to keep them from becoming smokers in the future?
14. What prescription and OTC products are now available to assist smokers in quitting?
15. What percentage of smokers are able to quit, and what is the best way to confirm that quitting has occurred?

ENDNOTES

1. Wakefield MA, et al. Tobacco industry marketing of point of purchase after the 1999 MSA billboard ban. *AJPH* 9, No. 6 June 2002.
2. U.S. Centers for Disease Control and Prevention. *MMWR*, Vol 52, No. 53. January 9, 2004.
3. U.S. Department of Health and Human Services. *Smoking and Health: Report of the Advisory Committee to the Surgeon General of the Public Health Service.* Public Health Service. 1964.
4. Cigarette smoking among adults—United States, 2002. *MMWR*, Vol. 53, No. 20. May 28, 2004.
5. National Center for Health Statistics, United States, *Health, 1998, with Socioeconomic Status and Health Chartbook.* NCHS, 1998.

6. Substance Abuse and Mental Health Service Administration. *Results from the 2003 National Survey on Drug Use and Health: National Findings.* NSDUH Series H-25, DHHS Publication No. SMA 04-3964, 2004.

7. Johnston LD, et al. *Monitoring the Future national results on adolescent drug use: Overview and key findings, 2004.* NIH Publication No. 05-5726. National Institute on Drug Abuse, 2005.

8. Patterson F, et al. Cigarette smoking practices among American college students: Review and future directions. *J Am Coll Health,* 2004 Mar-Apr; 52(5): 203–210.

9. Schoenborn CA, Jackline VL, Barnes PM. *Cigarette Smoking Behavior of Adults: United States, 1998.* Advanced Data from Vital and Health Statistics, No. 331. Division of Interview Statistics, National Center for Vital Statistics, February 2003.

10. *National Household Survey on Drug Abuse—Main Findings 1998* (H-11). Substance Abuse and Mental Health Services. Department of Health and Human Services, 2000.

11. *National Survey on Drug Use and Health 2002–2003* (formerly called the *National Survey On Drug Abuse*) (G-30), Substance Abuse and Mental Health Services, Department of Health and Human Services, 2004.

12. Tickle JJ, et al. Favorite movie stars, their tobacco use in contemporary movies and its association with adolescent smoking. *Tob Control.* 2001 Mar 10(1):16–22.

13. *More Antismoking Issues in Movies and TV.* TobaccoFree.org. The Foundation for a Smokefree America, www.tobaccofree.org/films.htm, 2005.

14. Burns DM, et al. *Cigars: Health Effects and Trends.* Cancer Monograph Series (No. 9) National Cancer Institute, 1998.

15. Shaper AG, Wannamethee SG, Walker M. Pipe and cigar smoking and major cardiovascular events, cancer incidence, and all-cause mortality in middle-aged British men. *In J Epidemiol.* 2003 Oct; 32(5): 802–808.

16. Zickler P. Evidence builds that genes influence cigarette smoking. *NIDA Notes* 2000; 15(3):1–15.

17. Sasyette MA, et al. A multi-dimensional analysis of cue-elicited craving in heavy smokers and tobacco chippers. *Addiction* 2001; 96(10):1419–1432.

18. Hassmiller KM, et al. Nondaily smokers: Who are they? *Am J Public Health* 2003 Aug; 93(8):1321–1327.

19. Sullivan PF, Kendler KS. The genetic epidemiology of smoking. *Nicotine Tob Res, Suppl.* 2:51–57, 1999.

20. Sullivan PF, et al. Candidate genes for nicotine dependence via linkage, epistasis, bioinformatics. *Am J Med Genet B Neuropsychiatr Genet.* 2004 Apr 1; 126(1):23–36.

21. Pomerleau OF. Endogenous opioids and smoking: A review of progress and problems. *Psychoneuroendocrinology.* 1998 Feb; 23(2):115–130.

22. Balfour DJ, Ridkey DL. The effects of nicotine on neural pathways implicated in depression. *Pharmacol Biochem Behav.* 2000; 66(1):79–85.

23. DiFranza JR, et al. Development of symptoms of tobacco dependency in youth: 30-month follow-up from the DANDY study. *Tob Control* 2002; 11(3):228–235.

24. Bricker JB, et al. Nine-year prospective relationship between parental smoking cessation and children's daily smoking. *Addiction* 2003; 98(5):585–593.

25. Saladin KS. *Anatomy and Physiology: The Unity of Form and Function* (4th ed.). New York: McGraw-Hill, 2007.

26. American Cancer Society. *Cancer Facts and Figures—2005.* Atlanta: Cancer Society, 2005.

27. American Heart Association: *Heart Disease and Stroke Statistics—2005 Update,* 2004.

28. Lam S, et al. Sex-related differences in bronchial epithelial changes associated with tobacco smoking. *L Natl Cancer Inst.* 91(8):691–696, April 1999.

29. Habek D, et al. Fetal tobacco syndrome and perinatal outcome. *Fetal Diagn Ther* 2002 November-December; 17(6):367–371.

30. DiFranza JR, Aligne CA, Weitzman M. Prenatal and postnatal environmental tobacco smoke exposure: children's health. *Pediatrics* 2004 Apr; 113(4 Suppl): 1007–1015.

31. Sepaniak S, et al. Negative impact of cigarette smoking on male fertility: From spermatozoa to the offspring. *J Obstet Biol Reprod.* 2004 Sept; 33(5):384–390.

32. Gades NM, et al. Association between smoking and erectile dysfunction: A population-based study. *Am J Epidemiol.* 2005 Feb 15; 16(4):341–351.

33. Maughan B, et al. Prenatal smoking and early childhood conduct problems: Testing genetic and environmental explanations of the association. *Arch Gen Psychiatry* 2004 Aug; 61(8):836–843.

34. Enstrom JE, Kabat GC. Environmental tobacco smoke and tobacco related mortality in a prospective study of Californians, 1990–1998. *BMJ* 2003 May; 326(7398): 1048–1057.

35. Smoke Free USA. www.smokefreeworld.com/usa.sjtml, 2005.

Sold only online by its developer, a new smokeless cigarette contains tobacco but is neither lighted nor heated in any manner. In the absence of any burning or heating, there is no smoke, tar, and carbon monoxide. This product is the Aeros Smokeless Cigarette, and it was developed by Woodleaf Corporation of Newport Beach, California. Online promotional material suggests that Aeros was developed over 8 years in conjunction with FDA criteria for a smokeless cigarette.

The Aeros cigarette is described as being a sealed plastic tube containing a tightly packed carefully formulated tobacco mixture. "Smoking" the Aeros involves cutting both ends of the plastic tube and inhaling through the appropriate opened end. Over the course of about 8 inhalations the user enjoys the aroma, taste, and nicotine of the tobacco, without the health-detracting particulate and gaseous components of normal cigarettes. The developer assures the "smoker" that no tobacco touches the lips. Data provided by an independent laboratory reports that 0 milligrams of tar and .05 milligrams of nicotine are delivered by each cigarette. The FDA appears to concur with the developer's contention that the Aeros Smokeless Cigarette could be legally used in all traditional nonsmoking environments.

personal assessment

How much do you know about cigarette smoking?

Are the following assumptions about smoking true or false? Take your best guess, and then read the answer to the right of each statement.

Assumption

1. There are now safe cigarettes on the market.

2. A small number of cigarettes can be smoked without risk.

3. Most early changes in the body resulting from cigarette smoking are temporary.

4. Filters provide a measure of safety to cigarette smokers.

5. Low-tar, low-nicotine cigarettes are safer than high-tar, high-nicotine brands.

6. Mentholated cigarettes are better for the smoker than are nonmentholated brands.

7. It has been scientifically proven that cigarette smoking causes cancer.

8. No specific agent capable of causing cancer has ever been identified in the tobacco used in smokeless tobacco.

9. The cure rate for lung cancer is so good that no one should fear developing this form of cancer.

10. Smoking is not harmful as long as the smoke is not inhaled.

11. The "smoker's cough" reflects underlying damage to the tissue of the airways.

12. Cigarette smoking does not appear to be associated with damage to the heart and blood vessels.

13. Because of the design of the placenta, smoking does not present a major risk to the developing fetus.

14. Women who smoke cigarettes and use an oral contraceptive should decide which they wish to continue, because there is a risk in using both.

15. Air pollution is a greater risk to our respiratory health than is cigarette smoking.

16. Addiction, in the sense of physical addiction, is found in conjunction with cigarette smoking.

Discussion

F Depending on the brand, some cigarettes contain less tar and nicotine; none are safe, however.

F Even a low level of smoking exposes the body to harmful substances in tobacco smoke.

T Some changes, however, cannot be reversed—particularly changes associated with emphysema.

T However, the protection is far from adequate.

T Many people, however, smoke low-tar, low-nicotine cigarettes in a manner that makes them just as dangerous as stronger cigarettes.

F Menthol simply makes cigarette smoke feel cooler. The smoke contains all the harmful agents found in the smoke from regular cigarettes.

T Particularly lung cancer and cancers of the larynx, esophagus, oral cavity, and urinary bladder.

F Unfortunately, smokeless tobacco is no safer than the tobacco that is burned. The user of smokeless tobacco swallows much of what the smoker inhales.

F Approximately 15% of people who have lung cancer will live the 5 years required to meet the medical definition of "cured."

F Because of the toxic material in smoke, even its contact with the tissue of the oral cavity introduces a measure of risk in this form of cigarette use.

T The cough occurs in response to an inability to clear the airway of mucus as a result of changes in the cells that normally keep the air passages clear.

F Cigarette smoking is in fact the single most important risk factor in the development of cardiovascular disease.

F Children born to women who smoked during pregnancy show a variety of health impairments, including smaller birth size, premature birth, and more illnesses during the first year of life. Smoking women also have more stillbirths than do nonsmokers.

T Women over 35 years of age, in particular, are at risk of experiencing serious heart disease should they continue using both cigarettes and an oral contraceptive.

F Although air pollution does expose the body to potentially serious problems, the risk is considerably less than that associated with smoking.

T Dependence, including true physical addiction, is widely recognized in cigarette smokers.

Preventing Diseases

Part Four consists of four chapters that focus on disease prevention. Each illness you contract or develop can harm your health in each of its dimensions; therefore, prevention should be a high priority.

1. **Physical Dimension**

   We usually associate illness with pain, fear, discomfort, and limitations. But paradoxically, health problems can also improve the physical dimension of health. For example, exposure to certain infectious diseases may allow your body to develop immunity. Illness can also force you to rest, reduce your workload, and reconsider your health behavior. Weight loss, smoking cessation, improved dietary practices, genetic counseling, or a renewed commitment to fitness may follow your recovery from an illness.

2. **Emotional Dimension**

   Emotionally healthy people feel good about themselves and others and are able to cope with most of life's demands. Being diagnosed with an illness or disease can jeopardize your emotional resources. You may feel anxious, isolated, and vulnerable. Fortunately, many diseases can be prevented or at least managed or treated successfully.

3. **Social Dimension**

   People rarely face an illness or manage a chronic health condition alone. People who have heart disease, cancer, diabetes, or HIV infection often join support groups or establish friendships with others who have the same condition. In addition, you probably interact with people during activities aimed at preventing diseases. For example, you might exercise with a partner or meet people at a weight-loss group.

4. **Intellectual Dimension**

   We can best use our intellect when we are free from health problems. In some cases, diseases or medications can impair our intellectual functioning. However, managing a condition or recovering from an illness can allow you to learn about your body, your personality, and the health care system. Learning how to reduce your risk of certain diseases will also require you to draw on your intellectual resources.

5. **Spiritual Dimension**

   Your ability to serve others can be hindered by an illness or chronic condition. In addition, your faith can be shaken when a family member falls ill or when you are diagnosed with a serious disease. For most people, however, this initial questioning leads to an even stronger faith or spirituality than they had before the experience.

6. **Occupational Dimension**

   Diseases and your efforts to prevent them can have a significant effect on your job performance. If you have an acute illness, you probably will not be able to work temporarily. If you have a chronic condition or disease, you must try to manage it well enough that you are still able to work. Some conditions are so severe that employment becomes impossible. However, your efforts to prevent illness, such as fitness activities, will enhance your job performance.

chapter ten

Enhancing Your Cardiovascular Health

Chapter Objectives

On completing this chapter, you will be able to:

▎ describe the prevalence of cardiovascular disease compared to other diseases.

▎ list the cardiovascular disease risk factors and distinguish between those that can and cannot be modified.

▎ explain how each of the modifiable cardiovascular disease risk factors can be changed.

▎ explain atherosclerosis and the factors that are involved in causing it.

▎ list and describe the different forms of cardiovascular disease.

▎ explain the different forms of treatment for coronary heart disease.

▎ distinguish between the different types of stroke.

▎ explain the recommendations for prevention and treatment of hypertension.

Eye on the Media

The Pressure Is Building

A recent *Time* magazine cover story, "The Stealth Killer," discussed the growing problem of hypertension in the United States. Current estimates suggest that 65,000,000 Americans have this condition, and the rates are projected to keep increasing. One of the issues discussed in the article was the concept that hypertension is a "silent" process. In other words, people cannot feel high blood pressure; rather, it has to be measured to be detected. One of the principal reasons for the projected increased prevalence of hypertension is that obesity is strongly related to hypertension. Obesity rates have reached epidemic proportions in our country, including increased levels in children.

One of the most alarming aspects of this is that children are now being diagnosed with type 2 diabetes and hypertension, which typically was first observed in adults aged 40 years and older. The long-term consequences of hypertension—both financial and health-related—will be tremendously magnified if hypertension occurs 20 years earlier than usual.

Source: "Blowing a Gasket," *Time,* December 6, 2004. Volume 164, Number 23.

This section of the book contains four chapters that deal with diseases. Although uninformed people claim that "there is nothing you can do to avoid disease," ample evidence indicates that positive personal health choices can help reduce your risk of developing many diseases, from cardiovascular disease to cancer to sexually transmitted diseases, including HIV and AIDS.

In this chapter we explain what you can do to reduce your risk of developing cardiovascular disease. Prevention efforts are most effective when started in childhood, but it is never too late to adopt a wellness lifestyle. Quitting smoking, becoming physically active, following a nutritious, low-fat diet, and controlling your blood pressure are important ways of reducing your risk of heart disease and improving your overall health.

Great progress has been made with respect to **cardiovascular** disease (CVD), the focus of this chapter. Although heart disease continues to be the number-two killer of Americans under the age of 80 (behind cancer), between 1990 and 2000 the death rates from CVD declined 17 percent.[1] Still, CVD claimed about 1.4 million lives in 2002.[1] By comparison, cancer caused 557,271 deaths, accidents caused 106,742, Alzheimer's disease caused 58,866, and HIV/AIDS caused 14,095. This means CVD caused 38 percent of all deaths, or one out of every 2.6 deaths in 2002. Today, more than 2,600 Americans die each day of CVD, an average of one death every 34 seconds. Cardiovascular diseases claim more lives each year than the next five leading causes of death combined.

This chapter provides material to help you understand how the heart works. Beyond this, it will help you identify your CVD risk factors and suggest ways you can alter certain lifestyle behaviors to reduce your risk of developing heart disease.

Prevalence of Cardiovascular Disease

Cardiovascular diseases were directly related to 38 percent of deaths in the United States in 2002 and indirectly related to a large percentage of additional deaths.[1] Fortunately, the rate of deaths from coronary heart disease has been falling. If all major forms of CVD were eliminated, life expectancy in the United States would increase by almost 7 years (see Figure 10-1 and Table 10.1).[1]

Key Terms

cardiovascular pertaining to the heart (cardio) and blood vessels (vascular)

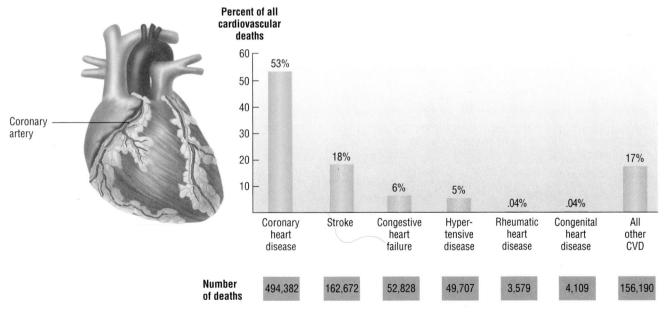

Figure 10-1 Of the 923,467 deaths in the United States in 2002* resulting from cardiovascular diseases, nearly half were attributable to heart attack.[1]

(*The most recent year for which statistics are available.)

Table 10.1 Estimated Prevalence of Major Cardiovascular Diseases*

Hypertension	65,000,000
Coronary heart disease	13,000,000
Stroke	5,400,000
Rheumatic heart disease	1,800,000
Congenital heart disease	1,000,000
Congestive heart failure	4,900,000
TOTAL	91,100,000

*70,100,000 people total. The sum of the individual estimates exceeds 70,100,000 because so many people have more than one cardiovascular disorder.

Normal Cardiovascular Function

The cardiovascular system, also called the *circulatory system,* uses a muscular pump to send a complex fluid on a continuous trip through a closed system of tubes. The pump is the heart, the fluid is blood, and the closed system of tubes is the network of blood vessels.

The Vascular System

The term *vascular system* refers to the body's blood vessels. Although we might be familiar with the arteries (vessels that carry blood away from the heart) and the veins (vessels that carry blood to the heart), arterioles, capillaries, and venules are also part of the vascular system. Arterioles are the smaller-diameter extensions of arteries. These arterioles lead eventually to capillaries, the smallest extensions of the vascular system. At the capillary level, oxygen, food, and waste are exchanged between cells and the blood.

After the blood leaves the capillaries and begins its return to the heart, it drains into small veins, or venules. The blood in the venules flows into increasingly larger vessels called *veins.* Blood pressure is highest in arteries and lowest in veins, especially the largest veins, which empty into the right atrium of the heart.

The Heart

The heart is a four-chambered pump designed to create the pressure required to circulate blood throughout the body. Usually considered to be about the size of a person's clenched fist, this organ lies slightly tilted between the lungs in the central portion of the **thorax.** The heart does not lie completely in the center of the chest. Rather, approximately two-thirds of the heart is to the left of the body midline and one third is to the right.[2]

Two upper chambers, called *atria,* and two lower chambers, called *ventricles,* form the heart. The thin-walled atrial chambers are considered collecting chambers, whereas the thick-walled muscular ventricles are considered the pumping chambers. The right and left sides of the heart are divided by a partition called the *septum.* Study Figure 10-2 and follow the flow of blood through the heart's four chambers.

> **Key Terms**
>
> **thorax** the chest; portion of the torso above the diaphragm and within the rib cage

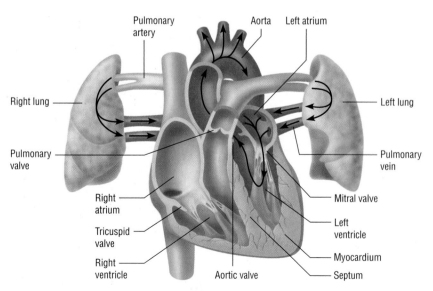

Figure 10-2 The heart functions like a complex double pump. The right side of the heart pumps deoxygenated blood to the lungs. The left side of the heart pumps oxygenated blood through the aorta to all parts of the body. Note the thickness of the walls of the ventricles. These are the primary pumping chambers.

To function well, the heart muscle must receive adequate amounts of oxygen. The two main **coronary arteries** (and their many branches) accomplish this. These arteries are located outside of the heart. If the coronary arteries are diseased, a heart attack (myocardial infarction) is possible.

Heart Stimulation

The heart contracts and relaxes through the delicate interplay of **cardiac muscle** tissue and cardiac electrical centers, called *nodes*. Nodal tissue generates the electrical impulses necessary to contract heart muscle.[3] The heart's electrical activity is measured by an instrument called an *electrocardiograph (ECG or EKG),* which provides a printout called an *electrocardiogram* that can be evaluated to determine cardiac electrical functioning.

Blood

The average-sized adult has approximately 5 quarts of blood in his or her circulatory system. Blood's functions, which are performed continuously, are quite similar to the overall functions of the circulatory system and include the following:

- Transportation of nutrients, oxygen, wastes, hormones, and enzymes
- Regulation of water content of body cells and fluids
- Buffering to help maintain appropriate pH balance of body fluids

- Regulation of body temperature; the water component in the blood absorbs heat and transfers it
- Prevention of blood loss; by coagulating or clotting, the blood can alter its form to prevent blood loss through injured vessels
- Protection against toxins and microorganisms, accomplished by chemical substances called *antibodies* and specialized cellular elements circulating in the bloodstream.

Cardiovascular Disease Risk Factors

As you have just read, the heart and blood vessels are among the most important structures in the human body. By protecting your cardiovascular system, you lay the groundwork for a more exciting, productive, and energetic life. The best time to start protecting and improving your cardiovascular system is early in life, when

---

Key Terms

coronary arteries vessels that supply oxygenated blood to heart muscle tissues

cardiac muscle specialized muscle tissue that forms the middle (muscular) layer of the heart wall

---

Risk Factors for Cardiovascular Disease

Factors You Cannot Change

- Increasing age
- Male gender
- Heredity (including race)

Factors You Can Change ("Big Six" Risk Factors)

- Tobacco smoke
- Physical inactivity
- High blood cholesterol level
- High blood pressure
- Diabetes mellitus
- Obesity and overweight

Contributing Factor

- Individual response to stress

lifestyle patterns are developed and reinforced. (See Learning from Our Diversity on page 315.) Of course, it is difficult to move backward through time, so the second-best time to start protecting your heart is today. Improvements in certain lifestyle activities can pay significant dividends as your life unfolds. (Complete the Personal Assessment on pages 335–336 to estimate your risk for heart disease.)

The American Heart Association encourages people to protect and enhance their heart health by examining the ten cardiovascular risk factors that are related to various forms of heart disease. A *cardiovascular risk factor* is an attribute that a person has or is exposed to that increases the likelihood that he or she will develop some form of heart disease. Three risk factors are those you will be unable to change. An additional six risk factors are those you can clearly change. One final risk factor is thought to be a contributing factor to heart disease. These risk factors are summarized in the Star box above. Let's look at these three groups of risk factors separately.

Risk Factors That Cannot Be Changed

The four risk factors that you cannot change are increasing age, male gender, heredity, and race. Despite the fact that these risk factors cannot be changed, your knowledge that they might be an influence in your life should encourage you to make a more serious commitment to the risk factors you *can* change.

Increasing Age

Heart disease tends to develop gradually over the course of one's life. Although we may know of a person or two who experienced a heart attack in their 20s or 30s, most of the serious consequences of heart disease become evident as we age. For example, nearly 84 percent of people who die from heart disease are aged 65 and older.

Male Gender

Before age 55, men have a greater risk of heart disease than women do. Yet when women move through menopause (typically in their 50s), their rates of heart disease become similar to men's rates (see the Star box on page 317). It is thought that women have a degree of protection from heart disease because of their natural production of the hormone estrogen during their fertile years.

Heredity

Obviously, you have no input in determining who your biological parents are. Like increasing age and male gender, this risk factor cannot be changed. By the luck of the draw, some people are born into families where heart disease has never been a serious problem, whereas others are born into families where heart disease is quite prevalent. In this latter case, children are said to have a genetic predisposition (tendency) to develop heart disease as they grow and develop throughout their lives. These people have every reason to be highly motivated to reduce the risk factors they can control.

Race is also a consideration related to heart disease. The prevalence of hypertension among African Americans is among the highest in the United States.[1] More than one in every three African Americans has hypertension (two out of every three over age 65).[4] Hypertension significantly increases the risk of heart disease, stroke, and kidney disease. Fortunately, as you will soon read, hypertension can be controlled through a variety of methods. It is especially important for African Americans to take advantage of every opportunity to have their blood pressure measured so that preventive actions can be started immediately if necessary.

Risk Factors That Can Be Changed

Six cardiovascular risk factors are influenced, in large part, by our lifestyle choices. These risk factors are tobacco smoke, physical inactivity, high blood cholesterol level, high blood pressure, diabetes mellitus, and obesity and overweight.[3] Healthful behavior changes you make concerning these "big six" risk factors can help you protect and strengthen your cardiovascular system.

Women and Heart Disease

Is heart disease mainly a problem for men? According to the American Heart Association, the answer is no. In fact, data indicate that 53 percent of all cardiovascular disease deaths occur in women. Sixty-three percent of women who died suddenly of coronary heart disease had no previous symptoms. Also, 38 percent of women who have a heart attack will die within 1 year, compared with 25 percent of men. A total of 60 percent of the deaths from stroke and high blood pressure are in women, compared with 40 percent in men. Coronary heart disease is the leading cause of death of American women (254,630 deaths in 2000).[1]

For many years, it was thought that men were at much greater risk than women were for the development of cardiovascular problems. Today it is known that young men are more prone to heart disease than young women are, but once women reach menopause (usually in their early to middle 50s), their rates of heart-related problems quickly equal those of men.

The protective mechanism for young women seems to be the female hormone estrogen. Estrogen appears to help women maintain a beneficial profile of blood fats. When the production of estrogen is severely reduced at menopause, this protective factor no longer exists. Prescribing postmenopausal hormone replacement therapy (PHT) was a common practice by many physicians in treating a number of factors in postmenopausal women. One of the benefits of PHT was considered to be prevention of cardiovascular diseases. However, in 2002 a major clinical research trial was stopped owing to the finding that more women on PHT were experiencing heart attacks and strokes. Thus, the American Heart Association now recommends that PHT should not be used for the purpose of preventing cardiovascular diseases. Certainly, PHT may still be utilized for other purposes (i.e., relief of menopausal symptoms or osteoporosis prevention). Women prescribed PHT need to be aware of the increased risk for cardiovascular disease in evaluating its value. Certainly, much more research is underway that may influence the use of PHT in the future.[2]

Young women should not rely solely on naturally produced estrogen to prevent heart disease. The general recommendations for maintaining heart health—good diet, adequate physical activity, monitoring blood pressure and cholesterol levels, controlling weight, avoiding smoking, and managing stress—will benefit women at every stage of life.

[1]American Heart Association, *Statistical Fact Sheet: Women and Cardiovascular Diseases,* 2003.
[2]www.americanheart.org/presenter.jhtml? identifer=4536, July 21, 2003.

Tobacco Smoke

Approximately, 48.5 million adults (22.5 percent) in the United States smoke cigarettes and 30.3 percent of male and 24.6 percent of female high school students are smokers.[5] Smokers have a heart attack risk that is more than twice that of nonsmokers. Smoking cigarettes is the major risk factor associated with sudden cardiac death. In fact, smokers have two to four times the risk of dying from sudden cardiac arrest than do nonsmokers. Smokers who experience a heart attack are more likely to die suddenly (within an hour) than are those who don't smoke.

Smoking also adversely affects nonsmokers who are exposed to environmental tobacco smoke. Studies suggest that the risk of death caused by heart disease is increased about 30 percent in people exposed to secondhand smoke in the home. The risk of death caused by heart disease may even be higher in people exposed to environmental tobacco smoke in work settings (for example, bars, casinos, enclosed offices, some bowling alleys and restaurants), since higher levels of smoke may be present at work than at home. Because of the health threat to nonsmokers, restrictions on indoor smoking in public areas and business settings are increasing tremendously in every part of the country.

For years it was commonly believed that if you had smoked for many years, it was pointless to try to quit; the damage to one's health could never be reversed. However, the American Heart Association now indicates that by quitting smoking, regardless of how long or how much you have smoked, your risk of heart disease declines rapidly.

This news is exciting and should encourage people to quit smoking, regardless of how long they have smoked. Of course, if you have started to smoke, the healthy approach would be to quit now . . . before the nicotine controls your life and leads to heart disease or damages your lungs or leads to lung cancer. (For additional information about the health effects of tobacco, see Chapter 9.)

 TALKING POINTS A friend complains of not being able to quit smoking after several serious attempts. How could you direct this person toward a new approach?

Physical Inactivity

Lack of regular physical activity is a significant risk factor for heart disease. Regular aerobic exercise (discussed in Chapter 4) helps strengthen the heart muscle, maintain healthy blood vessels, and improve the ability of the vascular system to transfer blood and oxygen to all parts of the body. In addition, physical activity helps lower overall blood cholesterol levels for most people, encourages weight loss and retention of lean muscle mass, and allows people to moderate the stress in their lives.

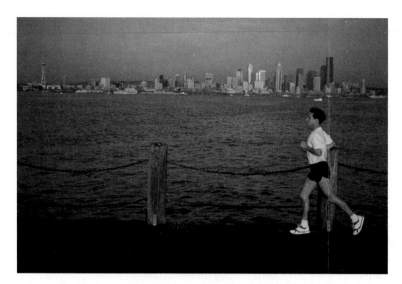

Regular physical activity helps prevent heart disease and also has many other health and functional benefits.

With all the benefits that come with physical activity, it amazes health professionals that so many Americans refuse to become regularly active. The Centers for Disease Control and Prevention[6] reports that 60 percent or more of American adults do not achieve the recommended amount of physical activity each week and that 25 percent of Americans age 18 or older report no leisure-time physical activity. In terms of relative risk for developing CVD, physical inactivity is comparable to high blood pressure, high blood cholesterol, and cigarette smoking.

Critical findings reported in the year 2000 from the highly respected Harvard Alumni Health Study[7,8] support the contention that physical activity is closely associated with decreased risk of coronary heart disease. After monitoring Harvard alumni for nearly 20 years in a variety of epidemiological studies, researchers confirmed that sustained, vigorous physical activity produces the strongest reductions in CVD. Light and moderate physical activities such as golf, gardening, and walking are helpful in reducing CVD, but more vigorous activities (such as jogging, swimming, tennis, stair climbing, or aerobics) produce greater reductions in CVD.[7] Additionally, Harvard researchers found that physical activity produced reductions in CVD whether the daily activity comes in one long session or in two shorter sessions of activity.[8] The "bottom line" is this: to reduce your chances of experiencing CVD, you must engage in some form of regular, sustained, physical activity (see the Discovering Your Spirituality box on page 319).

If you are middle-aged or older and have been inactive, you should consult with a physician before starting an exercise program. Also, if you have any known health condition that could be aggravated by physical activity, check with a physician first (see Chapter 4 for more information).

 TALKING POINTS You've started exercising many times by yourself, but you can't seem to stick to it. How would you convince a new friend that you can help each other get started on regular physical activity and keep it up?

High Blood Cholesterol Level

The third controllable risk factor for heart disease is high blood cholesterol level. Approximately 107 million American adults have a total cholesterol level of greater than 200 mg/dl (about 38 million have levels greater than 240 mg/dl). Generally speaking, the higher the blood cholesterol level, the greater the risk for heart disease. Table 10.2 shows ranges for cholesterol levels. When high blood cholesterol levels are combined with other important risk factors, the risks become much greater.

Fortunately, blood cholesterol levels are relatively easy to measure. Many campus health and wellness centers provide cholesterol screenings for employees and students. These screenings help identify people whose

Table 10.2 Classification of Total Cholesterol, Triglycerides, and HDL Cholesterol. All values expressed in mg/dL.

	Normal or Desirable	Borderline-High	High
Total cholesterol	< 200	200–239	≥ 240
Triglycerides	< 150	150–199	≥ 200

	Low	Normal	High
HDL cholesterol	< 40	40–59	≥ 60

Getting a Spiritual Lift through Physical Activity

Pick up almost any book on exercise, and you'll read about the "feel good" effect. It's what happens when you start doing any type of aerobic activity, such as walking, running, or swimming. First you'll notice physical changes. You've got more energy. You're sleeping better. Maybe you're even a little less grouchy.

But something else is happening, too. Gradually, your outlook seems more positive. Things you couldn't even think about doing a few weeks ago seem possible. You find yourself thinking about starting to write poetry, figuring out what you want to do with your life, improving your grades, or making new friends. That's the feel-good effect spilling over into all areas of your life.

After a few weeks of starting your exercise program, you've dropped a few pounds and your clothes feel more comfortable. But how you think about yourself is changing, too. Maybe you're paying more attention to your appearance. Or you're eating in a healthier way—almost without thinking about it. What's happening is that your self-image is improving. The idea of taking care of yourself is starting to grow, so how you look, what you eat, and how you spend your time are becoming important.

Joining in physical activities with family or friends offers more than the obvious physical and social benefits. Canoeing, playing volleyball in the back yard, or backpacking builds connections. You see others in a new way, relate to them differently, gain new insights, and find ways to help others. People and experiences you may have taken for granted take on a new dimension, and you appreciate them more.

Some people get a spiritual lift from the great outdoors. Wilderness hiking, for example, transports you to a different setting. The quietness, beauty, and solitude can be soothing to the soul. You're looking at the sky, trees, and water. You're enjoying a very peaceful time. This feeling may seem to disappear as soon as you get back to your dorm, but it may make the things you need to deal with there a little easier.

To experience this type of spiritual lift, you don't have to become a marathon runner or climb a mountain. Start going for long walks—alone or with a friend. Start a group that plays games, such as basketball, tennis, or volleyball. Try going for an early morning swim. Get into bicycling. The spiritual effects may be hard to measure, but they'll surprise and reward you.

---

cholesterol levels (or profiles) may be dangerous. Medical professionals have linked people's diets with their cholesterol levels. People with high blood cholesterol levels are encouraged to consume a heart-healthy diet (see Chapter 5) and to become physically active. In recent years, researchers have developed a variety of drugs that are very effective at lowering cholesterol levels. In a later section in this chapter, you will read more about cholesterol, particularly the cholesterol carrying compounds—lipoproteins.

High Blood Pressure

The fourth of the six cardiovascular risk factors that can be changed is high blood pressure, or hypertension. Approximately 65 million Americans have hypertension, one-third of whom have not been diagnosed. High blood pressure can seriously damage a person's heart and blood vessels. High blood pressure causes the heart to work much harder, eventually causing the heart to enlarge and weaken. High blood pressure increases the risk of stroke, heart attack, congestive heart failure, and kidney disease.

When high blood pressure is seen with other risk factors, the risk for stroke or heart attack is increased tremendously. As you will soon see, this "silent killer" is easy to monitor and can be effectively controlled through a variety of approaches.

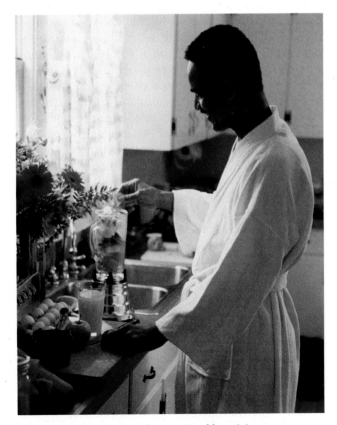

Preparing healthy food can be an enjoyable activity.

Diabetes Mellitus

Diabetes mellitus (discussed in detail in Chapter 12) is a debilitating chronic disease that has a significant effect on the human body. Approximately 17 million Americans have diabetes, one-third of whom have not been diagnosed. In addition to increasing the risk of developing kidney disease, blindness, and nerve damage, diabetes increases the likelihood of developing heart and blood vessel diseases. More than 65 percent of people with diabetes die of some type of heart or blood vessel disease. The cardiovascular damage is thought to occur because of the abnormal levels of cholesterol and blood fat found in individuals with diabetes. With weight management, exercise, dietary changes, and drug therapy, diabetes can be relatively well controlled in most people. Despite careful management of this disease, diabetic patients remain quite susceptible to eventual heart and blood vessel damage.[9]

 TALKING POINTS How would you show support for a friend who is struggling with the dietary requirements of diabetes?

Obesity and Overweight

According to the 2002 National Health and Nutrition Survey, approximately 65 percent of American adults are overweight, and 30 percent are obese. Even if they have no other risk factors, obese people are more likely than are nonobese people to develop heart disease and stroke. Obesity, particularly if of the abdominal form, places considerable strain on the heart, and it tends to worsen both blood pressure and blood cholesterol levels. Obese men and women can expect a greater risk of heart disease, diabetes, gallbladder disease, osteoarthritis, respiratory problems, and certain cancers.[10] Maintaining body weight within a desirable range minimizes the chances of obesity ever happening. To accomplish this, you can elect to make a commitment to a reasonably sound diet and an active lifestyle.

 TALKING POINTS How could you tactfully bring up a friend's weight problem to show concern for his or her health?

Another Risk Factor That Contributes to Heart Disease: Individual Response to Stress

The American Heart Association identifies one other risk factor that is associated with an increased risk of heart disease. This risk factor is one's *individual response to stress*.

Unresolved stress over a long period may be a contributing factor to the development of heart disease. Certainly, people who are unable to cope with stressful life experiences are more likely to develop negative dependence behaviors (for example, smoking, underactivity, poor dietary practices), which can then lead to cardiovascular problems through changes in blood fat profiles, blood pressure, and heart workload. (Chapter 3 covers ways of coping with stress.)

Forms of Cardiovascular Disease

The American Heart Association describes six major forms of CVD as coronary heart disease, hypertension, stroke, congenital heart disease, rheumatic heart disease, and congestive heart failure. These six diseases account for over 75 percent of the deaths caused by CVD. Additionally many other diseases influence the heart and blood vessels, such as peripheral vascular disease and arrhythmias. (These CVDs are discussed later in the chapter.)

A person may have just one of these diseases or a combination of forms at the same time. Each form exists in varying degrees of severity. All forms are capable of causing secondary damage to other body organs and systems.

Coronary Heart Disease

This form of CVD, also known as *coronary artery disease,* involves damage to the vessels that supply blood to the heart muscle. The bulk of this blood is supplied by the coronary arteries. Any damage to these important vessels can cause a reduction of blood flow (with its vital oxygen and nutrients) to specific areas of heart muscle. The ultimate result of an inadequate blood supply is a heart attack.

Atherosclerosis

The principal cause of coronary heart disease is **atherosclerosis** (Figure 10-3). Atherosclerosis produces a narrowing of the coronary arteries. This narrowing stems from the long-term buildup of fatty deposits, called *plaque,* on the inner walls of the arteries. This buildup reduces the blood supply to specific portions of the heart. Often arteries of the heart can become totally blocked (occluded) owing to a clot so that all blood supply is stopped. Heart muscle tissue begins to die when it is

---

Key Terms

atherosclerosis the buildup of plaque on the inner walls of arteries

---

Figure 10-3 Progression of atherosclerosis. This diagram shows how plaque deposits gradually accumulate to narrow the lumen (interior space) of an artery. Shown enlarged here, coronary arteries are only as wide as a pencil lead.

Labels: Connective tissue / Smooth muscle / Lumen / Endothelial cell / Plaque accumulation

deprived of oxygen and nutrients. This damage is known as **myocardial infarction.** In lay terms, this event is called a heart attack. (Changing for the Better explains how to recognize the signs of a heart attack and what to do next.)

Within the past five years, researchers have found that a high blood level of the amino acid **homocysteine** may be related to an increased risk of CHD. It is thought that high concentrations of homosysteine may accelerate the atherosclerotic plaque formation process that clogs the artery passageways.[11] For persons who did not exhibit any

> **Key Terms**
>
> **myocardial infarction** heart attack; the death of part of the heart muscle as a result of a blockage in one or more of the coronary arteries
>
> **homocysteine** an amino acid found in the bloodstream; high levels of homocysteine are thought to be related to an increased risk of coronary heart disease

of the traditional CHD risk factors (perhaps as many as 50 percent of the people who get heart attacks), the possibility that a blood test might identify this marker for heart disease was seen as good news.[11] If a person has a high homocysteine level, the theory is that he or she could probably lower the level by taking a multivitamin or by increasing the intake of certain B vitamins, especially B6, B12, and folic acid (folate). At the time of this writing, however, physicians and scientists are not fully convinced that this is a sound strategy.

While the jury remains undecided regarding the benefits of lowering homocysteine levels, a second possible marker for heart disease has emerged. This marker is a compound called **C-reactive protein.**[12] This protein is a byproduct of the inflammation process. Persons who have elevated levels of C-reactive protein appear to be at greater risk of CHD than those with low levels. Research is presently underway to determine what causes C-reactive protein to reach high levels and for potential treatments. Some promising reports have emerged suggesting that statin medications (used to treat blood cholesterol abnormalities) may help reduce C-reactive protein levels.

Cholesterol and Lipoproteins   For many years, scientists have known that atherosclerosis is a complicated disease that has many causes. Some of these causes are not well understood, but others are clearly understood. Cholesterol, a soft, fatlike material, is manufactured in the liver and small intestine and is necessary in the formation of sex hormones, cell membranes, bile salts, and nerve fibers. Elevated levels of serum cholesterol (200 mg/dl or more for adults aged 20 and older, and 170 mg/dl or more for young people under age 20) are associated with an increased risk of developing atherosclerosis.

Initially, most people can help lower their serum cholesterol level by adopting three dietary changes: lowering their intake of saturated fats, lowering their intake of dietary cholesterol, and lowering caloric intake to a level that does not exceed body requirements. The aim is to reduce excess fat, cholesterol, and calories in our diet while promoting sound nutrition. By carefully following such a diet, people with high serum cholesterol levels may be able to reduce their cholesterol levels by 30 to 55 mg/dl. However, dietary changes do not affect people equally; some will experience greater reductions than others. Some will not respond at all to dietary changes and may need to take cholesterol-lowering medications and increase physical activity.

Cholesterol is attached to structures called *lipoproteins.* Lipoproteins are particles that circulate in the blood and transport lipids (including cholesterol).[3] The two major classes of lipoproteins are **low-density lipoproteins (LDLs)** and **high-density lipoproteins (HDLs).** A person's total cholesterol level is essentially determined by the amount of the LDLs and HDLs in a measured sample of blood. For example, a person's total cholesterol level of 200 mg/dl could be represented by an LDL level of 130 and an HDL level of 40, or an LDL level of 120 and an HDL level of 60. (Note that additional forms of lipoproteins do exist and carry some of the cholesterol in the blood; thus, the total cholesterol value is greater than the sum of LDL and HDL.)

After much study, researchers have determined that high levels of LDL are a significant cause of atherosclerosis. This makes sense, because LDLs carry the greatest percentage of cholesterol in the bloodstream. LDLs are more likely to deposit excess cholesterol into the artery walls. This contributes to plaque formation. For this reason, LDLs are often called the "bad cholesterol."[1] Borderline-high LDL levels (above 130 mg/dl) and high LDL levels (above 160 mg/dl) are determined partly by inheritance, but they are also clearly associated with smoking, poor dietary patterns, obesity, and lack of exercise.

In contrast, high levels of HDLs (60 mg/dl or higher) are related to a decrease in the development of atherosclerosis. HDLs are thought to transport cholesterol out of the bloodstream. Thus HDLs have been called the "good cholesterol." Certain lifestyle alterations, such as quitting smoking, reducing obesity, regular aerobic-type exercise, and consumption of monounsaturated dietary fats, help many people increase their level of HDLs.

Improving cholesterol levels is a significant step in reducing the risk of death from coronary heart disease. Since 1980 the percentage of American adults with high cholesterol has dropped from 27.8 percent to 18 percent. The main reason for this decrease was the introduction of the National Cholesterol Education Program in the mid-1980s. Before this program was instituted, measurement of blood cholesterol was not a routine part of health screenings. The recommendations from this program were updated in 1993 and then most recently in 2001. It is now recommended that all

---

Key Terms

C-reactive protein a chemical compound found in the blood that is associated with inflammation; high levels are related to increased risk of coronary heart disease

low-density lipoprotein (LDL) the type of lipoprotein that transports the largest amount of cholesterol in the bloodstream; high levels of LDL are related to heart disease

high-density lipoprotein (HDL) the type of lipoprotein that transports cholesterol from the bloodstream to the liver, where it is eventually removed from the body; high levels of HDL are related to a reduction in heart disease

Americans over the age 19 be tested for LDL, HDL, and triglycerides. Although identification and treatment of those with high total and LDL cholesterol levels remain important, the most recent report recommends more intensive therapy for individuals with multiple-risk factors for coronary artery disease. For people with elevated cholesterol levels, a 1 percent reduction in serum cholesterol level yields about a 2 percent reduction in the risk of death from heart disease. Thus a 10–15 percent cholesterol reduction can reduce risk by 20–30 percent.[13] The National Cholesterol Education Program has specific recommendations for improving your blood cholesterol concentration. The recommendations begin with what we call "therapeutic lifestyle changes," which include dietary modification, weight reduction for those overweight or obese, and regular physical activity. If the therapeutic lifestyle changes are not completely effective or if the individual is at increased risk for coronary artery disease, then lipid-lowering medications are recommended. Among the most potent of these is a group of drugs called "statins." These medications have been shown to lower the risk of death from heart disease.

Angina Pectoris   When coronary arteries become narrowed, chest pain, or angina pectoris, is often felt. This pain is caused by a reduced supply of oxygen to heart muscle tissue. Usually, a coronary artery disease patient feels angina when he or she becomes stressed or exercises too strenuously. Angina reportedly can range from a feeling of mild indigestion to a severe viselike pressure in the chest. The pain may extend from the center of the chest to the arms and even up to the jaw. Generally, the more severe the blockage, the more pain is felt.

Some cardiac patients relieve angina with the drug nitroglycerin, a powerful blood vessel dilator. This prescription drug, available in slow-release transdermal (through the skin) patches or small pills that are placed under the patient's tongue, causes a major reduction in the workload of the heart muscle. Other cardiac patients may be prescribed drugs such as **calcium channel blockers** or **beta blockers.**

Emergency Response to Heart Crises

Heart attacks need not be fatal. The consequences of any heart attack depend on the location of the damage to the heart, the extent to which heart muscle is damaged, and the speed with which adequate circulation is restored. Injury to the ventricles may very well prove fatal unless medical countermeasures are immediately undertaken. Recognizing a heart attack is critically important. (See Changing for the Better on page 321)

Cardiopulmonary resuscitation (CPR) is one of the most important immediate countermeasures that trained people can use when confronted with a person having a heart attack. Public education programs sponsored by the

Heart Disease: A Family Affair

When it comes to cardiovascular health, arming yourself with information is the first step. As with most health conditions, learning your family's medical history is a great way to start. Talk to parents, grandparents, aunts, and uncles to find out if there's a history of heart attack, stroke, or other cardiovascular disease in your family.

American Red Cross and the American Heart Association teach people how to recognize, evaluate, and manage heart attack emergencies. CPR trainees are taught how to restore breathing (through mouth-to-mouth resuscitation) and circulation (through external chest compression) in people who require such emergency countermeasures. Frequently, colleges offer CPR classes through health science or physical education departments. We encourage each student to enroll in a CPR course. Additionally, automated external defibrillators are now located in many public buildings. Studies have reported that survival rates of those in cardiac arrest is greater than 90 percent when defibrillation is provided within the first minute.[14]

Diagnosis

A blood test, measuring cardiac muscle enzymes (markers of damage to the heart muscle), is usually performed initially. After a person's vital signs have stabilized, further diagnostic examinations can reveal the type and extent of damage to heart muscle. Initially an ECG might be taken, which may be able to identify if areas of ischemia (insufficient blood flow) or damage has occurred to the heart muscle. Another test which may be used is echocardiography. This procedure can also detect ischemia. The diagnostic ability of both of these tests is improved if used in conjunction with exercise (that is, stress ECG or stress echocardiography). This test analyzes the electrical activity of the heart. Heart catheterization, also called *coronary arteriography,* is a minor surgical procedure that starts by placing a thin plastic tube into an arm or leg artery. This tube, called a *catheter,* is guided through the artery until it

---

Key Terms

calcium channel blockers   drugs that reduce the workload of the heart; used in the treatment of blood pressure and the long-term management of angina pectoris

beta blockers   drugs that reduce the workload of the heart, which reduces blood pressure and decreases the occurrence of angina pectoris reaches the coronary circulation, where a radiopaque dye is then released. X-ray pictures called *angiograms* then record the progress of the dye through the coronary arteries. Areas of blockage are relatively easily identified.

Some newer techniques for noninvasive diagnosis of coronary artery disease are positron emission tomography (PET), electron beam computed tomography (EBCT), and magnetic resonance imaging (MRI). Now PET, EBCT, and MRI can be used to illustrate the anatomy of coronary arteries and the function of the heart, enabling physicians to evaluate such problems as valvular disease and cardiac shunts.

Nuclear medicine is another important tool in the diagnosis of cardiac disease. Nuclear medicine uses radiopharmaceuticals such as thallium-201 and technetium-99m sestamibi to evaluate perfusion of the heart muscle. Physicians use such tools to study the function of the heart and diagnose cardiac problems.

Treatment

After the extent of damage has been determined, a physician or team of physicians can decide on a medical course of action. Treatments can be divided into two broad categories: surgical and nonsurgical.

Surgical Treatments   Currently popular is an extensive form of surgery called **coronary artery bypass surgery.** An estimated 515,000 bypass surgeries were performed in 2002. The purpose of such surgery is to detour (bypass) areas of coronary artery obstruction by usually using a section of an artery from the patient's chest (the internal mammary artery) and grafting it from the aorta to a location just beyond the area of obstruction. Multiple areas of obstruction result in double, triple, or quadruple bypasses.

Surgeons have recently begun performing heart bypass surgery through a 3-inch incision in the rib cage, along with two to four small incisions in the patient's chest, rather than the traditional large, 12- to 15-inch incision. Physicians manipulate the coronary arteries through the small ports, and they view their work through a fiber-optic camera called a *thoracoscope.* This new technique results in much less pain and blood loss, a shorter hospital stay, and a quicker recovery for the patient. This method has been nicknamed "keyhole" surgery and is still considered to be somewhat experimental.

Angioplasty

In 2002, about 657,000 people with heart disease underwent angioplasty. Angioplasty is an alternative to bypass surgery, involving the use of a coronary catheter (described earlier) to place a doughnut-shaped "balloon" directly into the narrowed coronary artery (Figure 10-4). When this balloon is inflated, plaque and fatty deposits are compressed against the artery walls, widening the space through which blood flows. These balloons usually remain within the artery for less than a minute. Renarrowing of the artery will occur in about one-quarter of angioplasty patients. Many patients are now having a stent (small mesh tube) inserted in the region where the coronary artery was enlarged by the balloon. Recently, these stents were being coated with drugs to prevent blood clotting at this site.

Balloon angioplasty can be used for blockages in the heart, kidneys, arms, and legs. The decision whether to have

---

Key Terms

coronary artery bypass surgery a surgical procedure designed to improve blood flow to the heart by providing alternative routes for blood to take around points of blockage

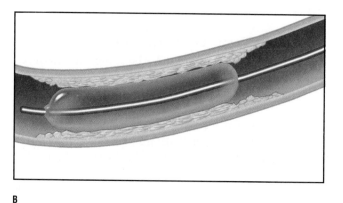

A   **B**

Figure 10-4   Angioplasty. A: A "balloon" is surgically inserted into the narrowed coronary artery. **B:** The balloon is inflated, compressing plaque and fatty deposits against the artery walls.

angioplasty or bypass surgery can be a difficult one to make.

In the past 10 years, a number of devices have been developed to remove the diseased material inside a coronary artery. These are called atherectomy devices. Inserted through a leg artery and held in place by a tiny inflated balloon, these motor-driven cutters shave off plaque deposits from inside the artery. A nose cone in the scraper unit stores the plaque until the device is removed.

The use of laser beams to dissolve plaque that blocks arteries has been slowly evolving. The FDA has approved three laser devices for use in clogged leg arteries. In 1992 the FDA approved the use of an excimer laser for use in coronary arteries. Other devices used to open coronary arteries are being researched. These techniques include thermal, photochemical, or acoustical energy to reduce the plaque.

Heart Transplants and Artificial Hearts

For approximately 30 years, surgeons have been able to surgically replace a person's damaged heart with that of another human being. Although very risky, these transplant operations have added years to the lives of a number of patients who otherwise would have lived only a short time. In 2002, doctors performed 2,057 heart transplants in the United States.[1]

Artificial hearts have also been developed and implanted in humans. These mechanical devices have extended the lives of patients and have also served as temporary hearts while patients wait for a suitable donor heart. One of the important difficulties with artificial heart implantation has been the control of blood clots that may form, especially around the artificial valves. Blood clots can cause heart attacks or strokes that can be fatal.

Nonsurgical Treatments

Platelet Inhibitors Platelets are part of the physiological pathway that produces blood clots. This new class of drugs has been shown to prevent the formation of blood clots, a major cause of heart attacks, chest pain, and artery tightening after angioplasty. It is well established that platelet inhibitors reduce heart attacks in patients with unstable angina, or severe chest pain, by about half.[3] Observers say this new class of drugs will have a tremendous effect on the treatment of heart problems.

Aspirin Studies released in the late 1980s highlighted the role of aspirin in reducing the risk of heart attack in men who had no history of previous attacks. Specifically, the studies concluded that for men with hypertension, elevated cholesterol levels, or both, taking one aspirin per day was a significant factor in reducing their risk of heart attack. Aspirin works by making the blood less able to clot, which reduces the likelihood of blood vessel blockages. Experts currently disagree about the age at which this preventive action should begin. The safest advice is to check with your physician before starting aspirin therapy.

Likewise, it now appears that women who take aspirin on a regular basis are less likely to have a heart attack than are women who do not take aspirin. However, women should first consult with their physicians about the correct dosage and the best way to use aspirin to protect their cardiovascular health.[15]

Alcohol For years, scientists have been uncertain about the extent to which alcohol consumption is related to a reduced risk of heart disease. The current thinking is that moderate drinking (defined as no more than two drinks per day for men and one drink per day for women) is related to a lower heart disease risk (see the Star box on page 326). However, the benefit is much smaller than proven risk-reduction behavior such as stopping smoking, reducing cholesterol level, lowering blood pressure, and increasing physical activity. Experts caution that heavy drinking increases cardiovascular risks and that nondrinkers should not start to drink just to reduce heart disease risk.

Hypertension

Just as your car's water pump recirculates water and maintains water pressure, your heart recirculates blood and maintains blood pressure. When the heart contracts, blood is forced through your arteries and veins. Your blood pressure is a measure of the force that your circulating blood exerts against the interior walls of your arteries and veins.

Blood pressure is measured with a *sphygmomanometer*. A sphygmomanometer is attached to an arm-cuff device that can be inflated to stop the flow of blood temporarily in the brachial artery. This artery is a major supplier of blood to the lower arm. It is located on the inside of the upper arm, just above the elbow.

A health professional using a stethoscope listens for blood flow while the pressure in the cuff is released. Two pressure measurements are recorded: The **systolic pressure** is the highest blood pressure against the vessel walls during the heart contraction, and the **diastolic pressure** is the lowest blood pressure against the vessel walls when the heart relaxes (between heartbeats). Expressed in units of millimeters of mercury, blood pressure is recorded as the systolic pressure over the diastolic pressure, for example, 115/82.

Key Terms

systolic pressure (sis **tol** ick) blood pressure against blood vessel walls when the heart contracts

diastolic pressure (**dye** uh stol ick) blood pressure against blood vessel walls when the heart relaxes

Can Alcohol Be Good for Your Heart?

You have probably seen the controversial headlines over the past couple of years, stating that moderate consumption of alcohol may reduce your risk of coronary heart disease. Such research is controversial because experts fear this may encourage problem drinkers or turn abstainers into problem drinkers.

Nevertheless, the evidence is strong that drinking alcohol in moderate amounts indeed reduces the risk of heart attack and death from coronary heart disease. The best evidence comes from population studies that show a reduction in coronary risk among moderate drinkers when compared with abstainers. The results are similar in both men and women, and among various ethnic groups. Moderate drinking is typically defined as one or two daily drinks for men and one for women.

Three possible explanations for the cardiovascular benefits are (1) that alcohol raises the level of protective high-density lipoprotein (HDL) cholesterol in the blood, making atherosclerosis less likely, (2) that alcohol inhibits blood clotting by helping to dissolve clots in blood vessels, and (3) other substances in the alcoholic beverage may have antioxidant properties.

Researchers are looking at specific types of alcohol, such as red wine, but the results are not yet strong enough to justify recommending that people switch to wine from beer or liquor. It appears that the benefits come from any type of alcohol product.

The American Heart Association* makes the following recommendations:

- The beneficial effects of alcohol are limited to one or two drinks a day.

- Heavier consumption is related to many health problems, including alcoholism, high blood pressure, obesity, stroke, breast cancer, suicide, and accidents.

- Pregnant women should not use alcohol.

- Do not drink alcohol if you take aspirin on a regular basis. Check with your physician.

InfoLinks

www.americanheart.org/presenter.jhtml?/identifier=4422

*American Heart Association, Alcohol and Heart Disease. *Circulation* 94:3023–3025, 1996.

Although a blood pressure of less than 120/80 is considered "normal" for adults, lower values do not necessarily indicate a medical problem. In fact, many young college women of average weight display blood pressures that seem to be relatively low (100/60, for example), yet these lowered blood pressures are quite "normal" for them.

Hypertension refers to a consistently elevated blood pressure. Generally, concern for high blood pressure begins when a person has a systolic reading of 140 or above or a diastolic reading of 90 or above, although now one is considered to have prehypertension if their systolic pressure is between 120–139 or their diastolic pressure is between 80–89. Table 10.3 shows the classifications for blood pressure.

Based on data from 1999–2000, approximately one in every three adults has hypertension.[16] In the United States, more men have hypertension than women until age 55, when women surpass men. In terms of prevalence for United States adults age 20 and older, non-Hispanic black females have the highest rate (45 percent) of hypertension. Thirty-one percent of non-Hispanic white males and 33 percent of non-Hispanic white females have high blood pressure. Among Hispanic males in the United States, 28 percent have hypertension; 29 percent of Hispanic females have high blood pressure.[1]

The causes of 90–95 percent of the cases of hypertension are unknown, called essential hypertension. However, the health risks are real. Throughout the body, long-term hypertension makes arteries and arterioles become less elastic and thus incapable of dilating under a heavy workload. Brittle, calcified blood vessels can burst unexpectedly and produce serious strokes (brain accidents), kidney failure (renal accidents), or eye damage **(retinal hemorrhage).** Furthermore, it appears that blood clots are more easily formed and dislodged in a vascular system affected by

Table 10.3 Blood Pressure Classification

Blood Pressure (mm Hg)	Normal	Prehypertension	Hypertension
Systolic (top number)	less than 120	120–139	140 or higher
Diastolic (bottom number)	less than 80	80–89	90 or higher

High blood pressure, or hypertension, is defined in an adult as a systolic pressure of 140 mm Hg or higher and/or a diastolic pressure of 90 mm Hg or higher. Blood pressure is measured in millimeters of mercury (mm Hg).

InfoLinks

www.nhlbi.nih.gov/guidelines/hypertension/index.htm

Key Terms

retinal hemorrhage uncontrolled bleeding from arteries within the eye's retina

Using Meditation to Lower Hypertension

In the practice of Western medicine, the most frequently used methods for reducing hypertension are medical approaches (taking various drugs that lower blood pressure) and lifestyle changes (losing excess weight, reducing sodium intake, increasing exercise, and drinking less alcohol). Practitioners of Eastern medicine might employ some of the lifestyle changes used in the West, but they would also be likely to recommend some form of meditation to help reduce blood pressure.

Meditation refers to an activity that produces a mental state of alert relaxation. While the body rests, the mind remains active. As it is practiced in the West, meditation is usually employed twice a day for 15–20 minutes at a time. The person sits still with eyes closed and repeats a soothing sound (mantra). This permits the body to relax and release stressful sensations, allowing the body and mind to exist in a state of balance.[1]

Meditation is taught in its various forms through noncredit courses at universities, local mental health centers, health clubs, or commercial stress management or relaxation centers. Students can take classes in the movement forms of meditation, such as the Chinese martial art tai chi, the Japanese martial art aikido, yoga, and the walking meditation of Zen Buddhism. There are many books, audiotapes, and videotapes available that promise to teach meditation. One of the most well-known books (*The Relaxation Response*, Avon Books) is by Harvard cardiologist Herbert Benson.

The important question remains: How successful is meditation in reducing hypertension? The answer is that meditation can be helpful and should be used in combination with other therapeutic approaches. A particular benefit of meditation is that it does not come with any of the side effects of drugs. One study, conducted at California's West Oakland Health Center,[1] found that people age 55 and over who learned transcendental meditation and practiced it every day for 3 months lowered their systolic blood pressure by 11 points and their diastolic pressure by 6 points. This drop in blood pressure was thought to reduce the likelihood of stroke by 35–40% and the risk of congestive heart failure by 20–45%. Similar drops in blood pressure have been found in other controlled studies.

How meditation works to control hypertension is not fully understood. It may be that meditation alters the stress response (see Chapter 3) and that this lowers blood pressure. It may be that meditation causes people to curb many of their unhealthy behaviors, and the reduction in lifestyle excesses (overeating, overdrinking, underactivity) may cause the blood pressure to drop.

The National Institutes of Health is currently supporting research to further study the impact of meditation on hypertension. Increasingly, researchers are finding major connections between the mind and the heart.[2] Certainly, meditation won't effectively control every case of hypertension, but it may be a very useful approach for many people with hypertension.

[1]Meditation lowers blood pressure as well as drugs. *Tufts University Diet and Nutrition Letter*, January 1997; Vol. 14: No. 11, p. 3
[2]The mind and the heart: They really are connected. *Tufts University Health and Nutrition Letter*, August 2000; Vol. 18: No. 6, pp. 1–5.

---

hypertension. Thus hypertension can be a cause of heart attacks. Clearly, hypertension is a potential killer.

Hypertension is referred to as "the silent killer" because people with hypertension often are not aware that they have the condition. People with this disorder cannot feel the sensation of high blood pressure. The condition does not produce dizziness, headaches, or memory loss unless one is experiencing a medical crisis. Because it is a silent killer, it is estimated that 30 percent of the people who have hypertension do not realize they have it. Eleven percent know they have hypertension but are not taking any measures to reduce it. Twenty-six percent are on medication but do not keep their hypertension under control. Just 34 percent of people with hypertension are aware that they have high blood pressure *and* have it under control with medication.[17]

Hypertension is not thought of as a curable disease; rather, it is a controllable disease. When therapy is stopped, the condition returns. As a responsible adult, you should use every opportunity you can to measure your blood pressure regularly.

Prevention and Treatment

Weight reduction, physical activity, moderation in alcohol use, and the dietary approaches to stop hypertension (DASH eating plan) are all recommended to reduce hypertension. These lifestyle modifications are now recommended therapy for individuals classified as prehypertensive. For overweight or obese people, a reduction in body weight may produce a significant drop in blood pressure. Physical activity helps lower blood pressure by expending calories (which may lead to weight loss in those who are overweight or obese) and through other physiological changes that affect the circulation. Moderation in alcohol consumption helps reduce blood pressure in some people.

The restriction of sodium (salt) in the diet also helps some people reduce hypertension. Interestingly, this

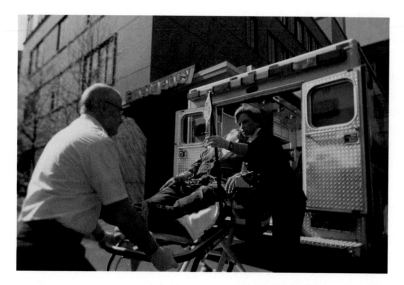

Emergency response teams help keep cardiac patients alive during transit to a medical facility.

strategy is effective only for those who are **salt sensitive** —estimated to be about 25 percent of the population. Reducing salt intake would have little effect on the blood pressure of the rest of the population. Nevertheless, because our daily intake of salt vastly exceeds our need for salt, the general recommendation to curb salt intake still makes good sense. The DASH eating plan also recommends foods that are rich in potassium and calcium.

Many of the stress reduction activities we discuss in Chapter 3 are receiving increased attention in the struggle to reduce hypertension. In recent years, behavioral scientists have reported the success of meditation, biofeedback, controlled breathing, and muscle relaxation exercises in reducing hypertension (see Considering Complementary Care on page 327). Look for further research findings in these areas in the years to come.

Drugs used to lower high blood pressure are called *antihypertensives. Diuretic drugs* work by stimulating the kidneys to eliminate more fluid, thereby reducing blood volume. *Vasodilators* relax the smooth muscle in the walls of blood vessels (especially the arterioles), allowing the vessels to dilate (widen). Also used are calcium channel blockers, beta blockers, angiotension converting enzyme (ACE) inhibitors, and other drugs that work in various ways to relax blood vessels. The most disturbing aspect of drug therapy for hypertension is that many patients refuse to take their medication on a consistent basis, probably because of the mistaken notion that "you must feel sick to be sick."

Some people taking these medications report uncomfortable side effects, including depression, reduced libido (sex drive), muscle weakness, impotence, dizziness, and fainting. Thus the medication's side effects may seem worse than the disease. This is all the more reason to emphasize the lifestyle modifications described earlier. Because of the poor record of patient compliance with hypertension drug therapy, many television and radio public service announcements are geared to the hypertensive patient. Nutritional supplements, such as calcium, magnesium, potassium, and fish oil, have not proven to be effective and reliable in lowering blood pressure.

Stroke

A third major CVD is stroke. *Stroke* is a general term for a wide variety of crises (sometimes called *cerebrovascular accidents* [*CVAs*] or brain attacks) that result from blood vessel damage in the brain. African Americans have a 60 percent greater risk of stroke than white Americans do, probably because African Americans have a greater likelihood of having hypertension than do white Americans. About 700,000 (200,000 of which are recurrent events) people suffer a stroke in the United States each year, and of these, about a quarter die. A total of 162,672 Americans died of stroke in 2002.[1] Just as the heart muscle needs an adequate blood supply, so does the brain. Any disturbance in the proper supply of oxygen and nutrients to the brain can pose a threat.

Key Terms

salt sensitive term used to describe people whose bodies overreact to the presence of sodium by retaining fluid, thus increasing blood pressure

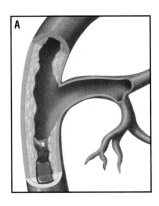

Thrombus
A clot that forms within a narrowed section of a blood vessel and remains at its place of origin.

Embolus
A clot that moves through the circulatory system and becomes lodged at a narrowed point within a vessel.

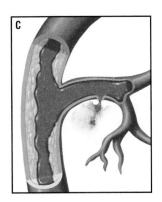

Hemorrhage
The sudden bursting of a blood vessel.

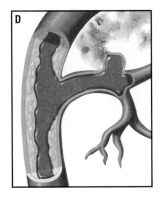

Aneurysm
A sac formed when a section of a blood vessel thins and balloons; the weakened wall of the sac can burst, or rupture, as shown here.

Figure 10-5   Causes of stroke

Cerebrovascular Occlusions

Perhaps the most common form of stroke results from the blockage of a cerebral (brain) artery. Similar to coronary occlusions, **cerebrovascular occlusions** can be started by a clot that forms within an artery, called a *thrombus,* or by a clot that travels from another part of the body to the brain, called an *embolus* (Figure 10-5 A and B). The resultant accidents (cerebral thrombosis or cerebral embolism) cause more than 85 percent of all strokes. The portion of the brain deprived of oxygen and nutrients can literally die.

Cerebral Hemorrhage

A third type of stroke can result from an artery that bursts to produce a crisis called *cerebral hemorrhage* (Figure 10-5 C). Damaged, brittle arteries can be especially susceptible to bursting when a person has hypertension.

Cerebral Aneurysm

A fourth form of stroke is a *cerebral aneurysm.* An aneurysm is a ballooning or outpouching on a weakened area of an artery (Figure 10-5 D). Aneurysms may occur in various locations of the body and are not always life threatening. The development of aneurysms is not fully understood, although there seems to be a relationship between aneurysms and hypertension. It is quite possible that many aneurysms are congenital defects. In any case, when a cerebral aneurysm bursts, a stroke results. See Changing for the Better on page 330 to learn the warning signs of stroke.

Diagnosis

A person who reports any warning signs of stroke or periods of temporary lack of bloodflow to a region of the brain, called a **transient ischemic attack (TIA),** is given a battery of diagnostic tests, which could include a physical examination, a search for possible brain tumors, tests to identify areas of the brain affected, electroencephalogram, cerebral arteriography, and a **CAT** (computerized axial tomography) **scan** or MRI (magnetic resonance imaging) **scan.** Many other tests can also be used.

Treatment

Researchers recently made a breakthrough in the treatment of stroke, with the discovery that the clot-dissolving drug tissue plasminogen activators (TPA) and the cell-rebuilding drug citicoline could reduce the severity of strokes.

> **Key Terms**
>
> **cerebrovascular occlusions** (ser ee bro **vas** kyou lar) blockages to arteries supplying blood to the cerebral cortex of the brain; cause of the most common type of stroke
>
> **transient ischemic attack (TIA)** (**tran** see ent iss **key** mick) strokelike symptoms caused by temporary spasm of cerebral blood vessels
>
> **CAT scan** computerized axial tomography scan; an x-ray procedure designed to illustrate structures within the body that would not normally be seen through conventional x-ray procedures
>
> **MRI scan** magnetic resonance imaging scan; an imaging procedure that uses a giant magnet to generate an image of body tissue

In the past, physicians essentially waited for a stroke to end before assessing damage and beginning rehabilitation. Now, experts find that TPA can actually reduce the severity of a stroke as it is occurring. TPA was previously used to dissolve clots in the treatment of heart attacks. This same effect, applied during a stroke, can help prevent brain cells from "starving" to death because of a lack of blood supply. TPA is useful only for strokes caused by clots (embolism or thrombosis).

As a result, experts are reclassifying stroke as a medical emergency that must be treated as quickly as possible. To be effective, TPA must be administered in the first 3 hours of the stroke. After that time, brain cells have been damaged and TPA can worsen the damage. Because 700,000 people suffer strokes and about one-quarter of these die each year, TPA has the potential to save thousands of lives a year.

Other treatment after a stroke depends on the nature and extent of the damage the patient has suffered. Some patients require surgery (to repair vessels and relieve pressure) and acute care in the hospital.

The advances made in the rehabilitation of stroke patients are amazing. Although some severely affected patients have little hope of improvement, our continuing advances in the application of computer technology to such disciplines as speech and physical therapy offer encouraging signs for stroke patients and their families.

Congenital Heart Disease

A congenital defect is one that is present at birth. About 36,000 babies are born each year with one of at least 35 recognized congenital heart defects. In 2001, a total of 4,109 infants died from congenital heart disease.[1]

A variety of abnormalities may be produced by congenital heart disease, including valve damage, holes in the walls of the septum, blood vessel transposition, and an underdevelopment of the left side of the heart. All of these problems ultimately prevent a newborn baby from receiving adequate oxygenation of tissues throughout the body. A bluish skin color (cyanosis) is seen in some infants with such congenital heart defects.

The cause of congenital heart defects is not clearly understood, although one cause, rubella, has been identified. The fetuses of mothers who contract the rubella virus during the first three months of pregnancy are at great risk of developing congenital rubella syndrome (CRS), a catch-all term for a wide variety of congenital defects, including heart defects, deafness, cataracts, and mental retardation. Other hypotheses about the development of congenital heart disease implicate environmental pollutants, maternal use of drugs, including alcohol, during pregnancy, and unknown genetic factors (see the Star box on page 331).

Treatment of congenital defects usually requires surgery, although some conditions may respond well to drug therapy. Defective blood vessels and certain malformations of the heart can be surgically repaired. This surgery is so successful that many children respond quickly to the increased circulation and oxygenation. Many are able to lead normal, active lives.

Rheumatic Heart Disease

Rheumatic heart disease is the final stage in a series of complications started by a streptococcal infection of the

---

Key Terms

rheumatic heart disease chronic damage to the heart (especially the heart valves) resulting from a streptococcal infection within the heart; a complication of rheumatic fever

Risk Factors for Congenital and Rheumatic Heart Disease

Risk Factors for Congenital Heart Disease
Fetal exposure to rubella, other viral infections, pollutants, alcohol, or tobacco smoke during pregnancy

Risk Factors for Rheumatic Heart Disease
Streptococcal infection

Common Symptoms of Strep Throat
Sudden onset of sore throat, particularly with pain when swallowing
Fever
Swollen, tender glands under the angle of the jaw
Headache
Nausea and vomiting
Tonsils covered with a yellow or white pus or discharge

throat (strep throat). The Star box lists common symptoms of strep throat. This bacterial infection, if untreated, can result in an inflammatory disease called *rheumatic fever* (and a related condition, *scarlet fever*). Rheumatic fever is a whole-body (systemic) reaction that can produce fever, joint pain, skin rashes, and possible brain and heart damage. A person who has had rheumatic fever is more susceptible to subsequent attacks. Rheumatic fever tends to run in families. About 1.8 million Americans suffer from various stages of rheumatic heart disease. In 2002, this disease killed 3,579 people.

Damage from rheumatic fever centers on the heart's valves. For some reason the bacteria tend to proliferate in the heart valves. Defective heart valves may fail either to open fully (stenosis) or to close fully (insufficiency). A physician initially might diagnose valve damage when she hears a backwashing or backflow of blood (a **murmur**). Further tests, including chest X rays, cardiac catheterization, and echocardiography, can reveal the extent of valve damage. After it is identified, a faulty valve can be replaced surgically with a metal or plastic artificial valve or a valve taken from an animal's heart.

Congestive Heart Failure

Congestive heart failure is a condition in which the heart lacks the strength to continue to circulate blood normally throughout the body. During congestive heart failure, the heart continues to work, but it cannot function well enough to maintain appropriate circulation. Venous blood flow starts to "back up." Swelling occurs, especially in the legs and ankles. Fluid can collect in the lungs and cause breathing difficulties and shortness of breath, and kidney function may be damaged. In 2001, congestive heart failure led to 52,828 deaths in the United States.[1]

Congestive heart failure can result from heart damage caused by congenital heart defects, lung disease, rheumatic fever, heart attack, atherosclerosis, or high blood pressure. Generally, congestive heart failure is treatable through a combined program of rest, proper diet, modified daily activities, and the use of appropriate drugs. Without medical care, congestive heart failure can be fatal.

Other Heart Diseases

Peripheral Artery Disease

Peripheral artery disease (PAD), also called *peripheral vascular disease* (*PVD*), is a blood vessel disease characterized by pathological changes to the arteries and arterioles in the extremities (primarily the legs and feet but sometimes the hands). PAD affects approximately 10 million Americans. These changes result from years of damage to the peripheral blood vessels. Important causes of PAD are cigarette smoking, a high-fat diet, obesity, and sedentary occupations. In some cases, PAD is aggravated by blood vessel changes resulting from diabetes.

PAD severely restricts blood flow to the extremities. The reduction in blood flow is responsible for leg pain or cramping during exercise, numbness, tingling, coldness, and loss of hair on the affected limb. The most serious consequence of PAD is the increased likelihood of developing ulcerations and tissue death. These conditions can lead to gangrene and may eventually necessitate amputation.

Key Terms

murmur an atypical heart sound that suggests a backflow of blood into a chamber of the heart from which it has just left

congestive heart failure inability of the heart to pump out all the blood that returns to it; can lead to dangerous fluid accumulations in veins, lungs, and kidneys

peripheral artery disease (PAD) atherosclerotic blockages that occur in arteries that supply blood to the legs and arms

PAD is treated in multiple ways, including efforts to improve blood lipid levels (through diet, exercise, or drug therapy), to reduce hypertension, to reduce body weight, and to eliminate smoking. Blood vessel surgery may be a possibility.

Arrhythmias

Arrhythmias are disorders of the heart's normal sequence of electrical activity that are experienced by more than 2 million Americans. They result in an irregular beating pattern of the heart. Arrhythmias can be so brief that they do not affect the overall heart rate. Some arrhythmias, however, can last for long periods of time and cause the heart to beat either too slowly or too fast. A slow beating pattern is called **bradycardia** (fewer than 60 beats per minute), and a fast beating pattern is called **tachycardia** (more than 100 beats per minute).

Hearts that beat too slowly may be unable to pump a sufficient amount of blood throughout the body. The body becomes starved of oxygen, and loss of consciousness and even death can occur. Hearts that beat too rapidly do not allow the ventricles to fill sufficiently. When this happens, the heart cannot pump enough blood throughout the body. The heart becomes, in effect, a very inefficient machine. It beats rapidly but cannot pump much blood from its ventricles. This pattern may lead to fibrillation, which is the life-threatening, rapid uncoordinated contractions of the heart. Interestingly, whether the heart pumps too slowly or too rapidly, the result is the same: inadequate blood flow throughout the body.

The person most prone to arrhythmia is a person with some form of heart disease, including atherosclerosis, hypertension, or inflammatory or degenerative conditions. The prevalence of arrhythmia tends to increase with age. Certain congenital defects may make a person more likely to have an arrhythmia. Some chemical agents, including high or low levels of minerals (potassium, magnesium, and calcium) in the blood, addictive substances (caffeine, tobacco, other drugs), and various cardiac medications, can all provoke arrhythmias.

Arrhythmias are most frequently diagnosed through an ECG (electrocardiogram), which records electrical activity of the heart. After diagnosis, a range of therapeutic approaches can be used, including simple monitoring (if the problem is relatively minor), drug therapy, use of a pacemaker, or the use of implantable defibrillators.

Related Cardiovascular Conditions

Besides the cardiovascular diseases already discussed, the heart and blood vessels are also subject to other pathological conditions. Tumors of the heart, although rare, occur. Infectious conditions involving the pericardial sac that surrounds the heart (*pericarditis*) and the innermost layer of the heart (*endocarditis*) are more commonly seen. Some people develop serious diseases of the heart valves. In addition, inflammation of the veins (*phlebitis*) is troublesome to some people.

Key Terms

bradycardia slowness of the heartbeat, as evidenced by a resting pulse rate of less than 60

tachycardia excessively rapid heartbeat, as evidenced by a resting pulse rate of greater than 100

Taking Charge of Your Health

- Complete the Personal Assessment on pages 335–336 to determine your risk for heart attack and stroke.

- Review the Food Guide Pyramid in Chapter 5 (page 109), and make changes to your diet so that it is more "heart healthy."

- Begin or continue an aerobic exercise program that is appropriate for your current fitness level.

- If you are a smoker, resolve to quit smoking. Visit your physician to talk about safe and effective approaches. Begin putting your plan into action.

- Develop a plan to lower your dietary intake of fat to keep your blood cholesterol level low.

- Have your blood pressure checked, and review your weight, physical activity, alcohol intake, and salt intake to determine whether you can make changes in any of these areas.

- If you are overweight or obese, develop a plan to combine dietary changes and increased physical activity to lose weight gradually but steadily.

SUMMARY

- Cardiovascular diseases are responsible for more disabilities and deaths than any other disease.
- The vascular system refers to the body's blood vessels, including arteries, veins, arterioles, capillaries, and venules.
- A cardiovascular risk factor is an attribute that a person has or is exposed to that increases the likelihood of heart disease.
- The "big six" risk factors are tobacco smoke, physical inactivity, high blood cholesterol level, high blood pressure, diabetes mellitus, and obesity and overweight. These are risk factors that can be changed.
- Smokers have a heart attack risk that is more than twice that of nonsmokers. However, the risk of heart disease declines rapidly if the smoker quits.
- Regular aerobic exercise helps strengthen the heart muscle, maintain healthy blood vessels, and improve the vascular system's ability to transport blood and oxygen to the body.

- People with high blood cholesterol should eat a heart-healthy diet and become physically active.
- The six major forms of cardiovascular disease are coronary artery disease, hypertension, stroke, congenital heart disease, rheumatic heart disease, and congestive heart failure.
- Each form of heart disease develops in a unique way and requires specialized treatment.
- Moderate alcohol consumption may be related to a lower risk of heart disease. However, heavy drinking increases cardiovascular disease risk.
- Weight reduction, physical activity, lowering alcohol use, sodium restriction, meditation, and antihypertensive drugs are often used to control hypertension.
- Other heart diseases include peripheral artery disease and heart arrhythmias.

REVIEW QUESTIONS

1. Identify the principal components of the cardiovascular system. Trace the path of blood through the heart and cardiovascular system.
2. How much blood does the average adult have? What are some of the important functions of blood?
3. Define *cardiovascular risk factor*. What relationship do risk factors have to cardiovascular disease?
4. Identify the risk factors for cardiovascular disease that cannot be changed. Identify the risk factors that can be changed. Identify the risk factor that is a contributing factor.
5. Describe the relationship between smoking and heart disease, including the role of environmental tobacco smoke. Explain the cardiovascular benefits of quitting smoking.

6. What is C-reactive protein? What role might it play regarding cardiovascular disease?
7. What are the six major forms of cardiovascular disease? For each of these diseases, describe the disease, its cause (if known), and its treatment. Describe some additional CVDs.
8. Describe how high-density lipoproteins differ from low-density lipoproteins.
9. What problems does atherosclerosis produce?
10. Why is hypertension called the "silent killer"? What serious health problems can hypertension cause?
11. What are the warning signals of stroke? Identify and describe each of the four types of stroke.
12. What is a heart arrhythmia and what are its consequences? Identify the two main heart arrhythmia patterns.

ENDNOTES

1. American Heart Association. *Heart Disease and Stroke: Statistical Update.* AHA, 2005.
2. Thibodeau GA, Patton KT. *Structure and Function of the Human Body* (11th ed.). St. Louis, MO: Mosby-Year Book, 2000.
3. Brubaker PH, Kaminsky LA, Whaley MH. *Coronary Artery Disease.* Champaign, IL: Human Kinetics, 2002.
4. American Heart Association: www.americanheart.org/hbp/risk_afam.html, July 21, 2003.
5. Centers for Disease Control and Prevention. www.cdc.gov/tobacco/oshsummary02.htm, July 16, 2003.
6. Centers for Disease Control and Prevention. *CDC's National Physical Activity Initiative Fact Sheet.* November 17, 1999.
7. Sesso HD, Paffenbarger RS, Lee I. Physical activity and coronary heart disease in men: The Harvard alumni health study. *Circulation,* 2000; Vol. 102, pp. 975–980.
8. Lee I, Sesso HD, Paffenbarger RS. Physical activity and coronary heart disease in men: Does the duration of exercise episodes predict risk? *Circulation,* 2000; Vol. 102, pp. 981–986.
9. Diabetes and heart disease: New strategies emerge. *Harvard Heart Letter,* July 2000; Vol. 10: No. 11. pp. 1–4.
10. National Institutes of Health. *Clinical Guidelines on the Identification, Evaluation, and Treatment of Overweight and Obesity in Adults.* 1998.
11. American Heart Association. Homocyst(e)ine, diet, and cardiovascular diseases. *Circulation,* 1999; Vol. 99, pp. 178–182.
12. American Heart Association. Markers of Inflammation and Cardiovascular Disease. *Circulation,* 2003; Vol. 107, pp. 499–511.
13. Cholesterol: Up with the good. *Harvard Health Letter,* July 1995; Vol. 5; No. 11. pp. 3–4.
14. American Heart Association/American College of Sports Medicine. Automated external defibrillators in health/fitness facilities. *Circulation,* 2002; Vol. 105, pp. 1147–1150.

15. Women and heart disease. *Harvard Heart Letter,* February 2000; Vol 10: No. 5, pp. 1–4.
16. National Center for Health Statistics. *Health, United States,* 2002.
17. National Heart, Lung, and Blood Institute. *The Seventh Report of the Joint National Committee on* Prevention, Detection, Evaluation, and Treatment of High Blood Pressure (JNC 7). www.nhlbi.nih.gov/guidelines/hypertension/index.htm, July 21, 2003.

As We Go to Press

The American Heart Association Journal *Hypertension*[1] recently published a study that reported that women who use acetaminophen, ibuprofen, or naproxen (all frequently used analgesic medications) had a greater risk for developing hypertension. Use of aspirin was not associated with developing hypertension. Certainly, as with all early studies on a topic, more research is necessary to fully understand the issues. At this time, women who regularly use any of these medications should consult with their physicians.

[1]Forman, JP, Stampfer MJ, Curhan GC, in *Hypertension* (Journal of the American Heart Association) 46: 1–8, 2005.

personal assessment

What is your risk for heart disease?

Cholesterol

Your serum cholesterol level is

0	190 or below
+ 2	191 to 230
+ 6	231 to 289
+12	290 to 319
+16	Over 320

Your HDL cholesterol is

− 2	Over 60
0	45 to 60
+ 2	35 to 44
+ 6	29 to 34
+ 12	23 to 28
+ 16	Below 23

Smoking

In the past, you

0	Never smoked, or quit more than 5 years ago
+ 1	Quit 2 to 4 years ago
+ 3	Quit about 1 year ago
+ 6	Quit during the past year

You now smoke

+ 9	1/2 to 1 pack a day
+ 12	1 to 2 packs a day
+ 15	More than 2 packs a day

The quality of the air you breathe is

0	Unpolluted by smoke, exhaust, or industry at home and at work
+ 2	Live or work with smokers in unpolluted area
+ 4	Live and work with smokers in unpolluted area
+ 6	Live or work with smokers **and** live or work in air-polluted area
+ 8	Live **and** work with smokers **and** live and work in air-polluted area

Blood Pressure

Your blood pressure is

0	120/75 or below
+ 2	120/75 to 140/85
+ 6	140/85 to 150/90
+ 8	150/90 to 175/100
+ 10	175/100 to 190/110
+ 12	190/110 or above

Exercise

Your exercise habits are

0	Exercise vigorously 4 or 5 times a week
+ 2	Exercise moderately 4 or 5 times a week
+ 4	Exercise only on weekends
+ 6	Exercise occasionally
+ 8	Little or no exercise

Weight

Your weight is

0	Always at or near ideal weight
+ 1	Now 10% overweight
+ 2	Now 20% overweight
+ 3	Now 30% or more overweight
+ 4	Now 20% or more overweight and have been since before age 30

Stress

You feel overstressed

0	Rarely at work or at home
+ 3	Somewhat at home but not at work
+ 5	Somewhat at work but not at home
+ 7	Somewhat at work **and** at home
+ 9	Usually at work **or** at home
+ 12	Usually at work **and** at home

Diabetes

Your diabetic history is

0	Blood sugar always normal
+ 2	Blood glucose slightly high (prediabetic) or slightly low (hypoglycemic)
+ 4	Diabetic beginning after age 40 requiring strict dietary or insulin control
+ 5	Diabetic beginning before age 30 requiring strict dietary or insulin control

Alcohol

You drink alcoholic beverages

0	Never or only socially, about once or twice a month, or only one 5-ounce glass of wine or 12-ounce glass of beer or 1½ ounces of hard liquor about 5 times a week
+ 2	Two to three 5-ounce glasses of wine or 12-ounce glasses of beer or 1½-ounce cocktails about 5 times a week
+ 4	More than three 1½-ounce cocktails or more than three 5-ounce glasses of wine or 12-ounce glasses of beer almost every day

Interpretation

Add all sources and check below.

0 to 20: **Low risk.** Excellent family history and lifestyle habits.

21 to 50: **Moderate risk.** Family history or lifestyle habits put you at some risk. You might lower your risks and minimize your genetic predisposition if you change any poor habits.

51 to 74:   **High risk.** Habits and family history indicate high risk of heart disease. Change your habits now.

Above 75:   **Very high risk.** Family history and a lifetime of poor habits put you at very high risk of heart disease. Eliminate as many of the risk factors as you can.

To Carry This Further . . .

Were you surprised with your score on this assessment? What were your most significant risk factors? Do you plan to make any changes in your lifestyle to reduce your cardiovascular risks? Why or why not?

chapter eleven

Living with Cancer

Chapter Objectives

On completing this chapter, you will be able to:

▌ describe cancer statistics and identify groups who are at high risk for developing particular forms of cancer.

▌ explain the role of cell regulation in the development of cancer, and discuss the relationship of genetic mutations, viral infections, and carcinogens to the loss of cell regulation.

▌ name specific steps that individuals can take to aid in early detection of specific cancers, including breast cancer, melanoma, and testicular cancer.

▌ discuss the importance of medical screening for specific cancers, and identify several procedures used to screen for particular forms of cancer.

▌ offer several lifestyle changes that effectively reduce your cancer risk.

▌ summarize the status of our current "War on Cancer."

Eye on the Media

Support Is Just a Click Away

Support groups are composed of people who come together to help one another through the demands of a chronic health condition. These groups have traditionally been organized by institutions in the local health care community, such as hospitals, by the local affiliates of national organizations, such as the American Cancer Society, or by citizens who have the same chronic condition. Today, however, more and more support group members are connected not by physical proximity but by the Internet.

Health self-help groups on the Internet develop in one of two ways. The first occurs when a brick-and-mortar organization, such as a national agency or health care institution, develops a support group for its homepage. The second way is for a person with the condition (or a family member of that person) to organize an online group.

You can find a health support group simply by surfing the net. Or you can be referred to a site by a health care professional, friend, family member, colleague, or someone with a similar condition. You can also go to the homepage of a medical institution or a national agency to find out if it provides a support group link.

For someone with a newly diagnosed chronic condition, the initial contact with a support group may be made to get information about the condition and its treatment. For others, it is a way of connecting with other people who have the condition. Web support groups provide windows to the outside world, particularly for those whose conditions limit their mobility and social contacts. The Internet support group transcends the restrictions of various diseases to make new connections possible.

Note that online support groups' members are rarely physicians or other highly trained health professionals, so you shouldn't rely on this source for specific technical information. Instead, your main sources of information about medical management of a chronic condition should be your health care providers. Seasoned members of support groups need to remind themselves that newly diagnosed members are inexperienced and vulnerable. It will take them time to adjust to the frankness and clinical sophistication demonstrated by some group members in addressing their health problems.

Some hospitals provide laptop computers to patients so they can maintain contact with their support groups. In this way, health care institutions are encouraging patients to support their efforts and, perhaps, helping them recover more quickly.

Most people can attest to the disruptive influence an illness can have on their ability to participate in day-to-day activities. When we are ill, school, employment, and leisure activities are replaced by periods of lessened activity and even periods of bed rest or hospitalization. When an illness is chronic, the effect of being ill may extend over long periods, perhaps even an entire lifetime. People with chronic illness must eventually find a balance between day-to-day function and the continuous presence of their condition. Cancer is usually a chronic illness.

In spite of our understanding of its relationship to human health and our ceaseless attempts to prevent and cure it, progress in the "war on cancer" has been relatively limited. In this regard, cancer is clearly an "expensive" condition, both in terms of its human consequences and its monetary costs. It is estimated that 1,372,910 people developed cancer in 2005. Once diagnosed, approximately 64 percent (adjusted for other causes of death) of this group will be alive 5 years later.[1] This 5-year period, called *relative survivability,* includes "persons who are living 5 years after diagnosis, whether disease free, in remission, or under treatment with evidence of cancer."[1] If one limits 2005's new cases to those forms of cancer for which early detection through screening is applicable (breast, colon, rectum, cervix, prostate, oral cavity, and skin), 85 percent will be alive after 5 years. Understandably, the term *cured* is used guardedly, since an initially diagnosed case of cancer can affect survivability beyond the end of the 5-year time period. Regardless of survivability, for those who develop cancer, the physical, emotional, and social costs will be substantial.

The financial cost of cancer to society is also troublesome. The National Institutes of Health (NIH) estimates that in 2004 alone cancer cost the American economy 189.8 billion dollars, including 95.2 billion for loss of productivity due to death, 69.4 billion for direct medical costs, and 15.5 billion for indirect costs due to loss of productivity during treatment and recovery.[1] Not reflected in this total is the sizable amount of money spent on primary cancer prevention, such as school-based programs, public education efforts, and lobbying efforts intended to remove harmful products and pollutants from the environment.

No single explanation can be given for why progress in eliminating cancer has been so limited. It is a combination of factors, including the aging of the population, continued use of tobacco, the high-fat American diet, the continuing urbanization and pollution of our environment, the lack of health insurance for an estimated 45 million Americans to pay for early diagnosis and proper treatment,[2] or simply our delayed recognition of cancer's true role in deaths once ascribed to other causes. Regardless, we continue to be challenged to control this array of abnormal conditions that we collectively call cancer. There is, however, increasing optimism that with new pharmacological agents and the development of vaccines to prevent and treat cancers real progress will finally be made.

 TALKING POINTS A close friend justifies her high cancer-risk lifestyle by saying that "Everyone will die of something." How would you counter this point?

Chemotherapy is a treatment for many types of cancer.

Cancer: A Problem of Cell Regulation

Just as a corporation depends on individuals to staff its various departments, the body depends on its basic units of function, the cells. Cells band together as tissues, such as muscle tissue, to perform a prescribed function. Tissues in turn join to form organs, such as the heart, and organs are assembled into the body's several organ systems, such as the cardiovascular system. Such is the "corporate structure" of the body.

If individuals and cells are the basic units of function for their respective organizations, the failure of either to perform in a prescribed, dependable manner can erode the overall organization to the extent that it might not be able to continue. Cancer, the leading cause of death among adults under 80 years of age,[3] is a condition reflecting cell dysfunction in its most extreme form. In cancer, the normal behavior of cells ceases.

Cell Regulation

Most of the body's tissues lose cells over time. This continual loss requires that replacement cells come from areas of young and less specialized cells. The process of specialization required to turn the less specialized cells into mature cells is controlled by genes within the cells. On becoming specialized, these newest cells copy, or replicate, themselves. These two processes are carefully monitored by the cells' **regulatory genes.** Failure to regulate replication and specialization results in abnormal, or potentially cancerous, cells.

In addition to genes that regulate replication and specialization, cells also have genes designed to repair mistakes in the copying of genetic material (the basis of replication) and genes to suppress the growth of abnormal cells should it occur. Thus, repair genes and tumor suppressor genes, such as the *p53* gene (altered or missing in half of all cancers), can also be considered regulatory genes in place to prevent the development of abnormal cells. Should these genes fail to function properly, resulting in the development of malignant (cancerous) cells, the immune system (see Chapter 13) will ideally recognize their presence and remove them before a clinical (diagnosable) case of cancer can develop.

Because, when they are not working properly, replication, specialization, repair, and suppressor genes can become cancer-causing genes, or **oncogenes,** these four types of genes can also be referred to as **proto-oncogenes,** or potential oncogenes.[4] How proto-oncogenes become oncogenes is a question that cannot be completely answered at this time. Regardless, abnormal cells produce abnormal proteins, and the absence of normal proteins alters the body's ability to function appropriately, from the molecular to the organ system level.

Oncogene Formation

All cells have proto-oncogenes, so what events alter otherwise normal regulatory genes, causing them to become cancer-causing genes? Three mechanisms, genetic mutations, viral infections, and carcinogens, have received much attention.

Genetic mutations develop when dividing cells miscopy genetic information. If the gene that is miscopied is a gene that controls specialization, replication, repair, or tumor suppression (a proto-oncogene), the oncogene that results will allow the formation of cancerous cells. A variety of factors, including aging, free radical formation, and radiation, are associated with the miscopying of the complex genetic information that constitutes the genes found within the cell, including those intended to prevent cancer.

In both animals and humans, cancer-producing viruses, such as the feline leukemia virus in cats and the human immunodeficiency virus (HIV) and multiple forms of the human papilloma virus (HPV) in humans (see Chapter 13), have been identified. These viruses seek out cells of a particular type, such as cells of the immune system or the lining of the cervix, and substitute some of their genetic material for some of the cells' thus converting them into virus-producing cells. In so doing, they convert proto-oncogenes into oncogenes. Once converted into oncogenes, the altered genes are passed on through cell division.

A third possible explanation for the conversion of proto-oncogenes into oncogenes involves the presence of environmental agents known as *carcinogens.* Over an extended period, carcinogens, such as chemicals found in tobacco smoke, polluted air and water, toxic wastes, and even high-fat foods, may convert proto-oncogenes into oncogenes. These carcinogens may work alone or in combination with co-carcinogenic promoters (see Chapter 9, Table 9.3) to alter the genetic material, including regulatory

---

Key Terms

regulatory genes genes that control cell specialization, replication, DNA repair, and tumor suppression

oncogenes faulty regulatory genes that are believed to activate the development of cancer

proto-oncogenes (pro toe **on** co genes) normal regulatory genes that may become oncogenes

genes, within cells. Thus people might develop lung cancer only if they are exposed to the right combination of carcinogens over an extended period.

You may already see that some of the specific risk factors in each area—such as radiation in the development of mutations, sexually transmitted viruses in cancers of the reproductive tract, and smoking-introduced carcinogens in the development of lung cancer—can be moderated by adopting health-promoting behaviors.

Our understanding of the role of genes in the development of cancer is expanding rapidly. Through ongoing research, including the Human Genome Project, the scientific community has now identified dozens of genes that function as oncogenes in a variety of cancers. On occasion the public learns the identity of selected oncogenes. Very likely many readers have heard of the *BRCA1* and *BRCA2* genes associated with breast and ovarian cancer, the RAS oncogene thought to influence 30 percent of all cancers, and the *p53* suppressor oncogene that may be involved in more cancers than is any other single oncogene. As geneticists continue to build on the base established by the Human Genome Project and in doing so discover additional genetic links to cancer, the possibility of some form of oncogene suppressor technology becomes a more realistic possibility in the war against cancer.

In light of the complexity of cancer, some people in the scientific community believe that cancer can never be truly prevented. Rather, they feel that the ability to stop and then reverse cancerous changes at an early stage of development is more likely than is the prevention of this complex disease process. However, this text addresses the concepts of prevention in the belief that prevention-based practices reflect our personal contribution to the "war on cancer."

Attachment
Attachment to the basement membrane (a physical barrier that separates tissue components) is the first step.

Local breakdown
Once cancer cells are attached, they break through with the help of an enzyme.

Blood vessel
Cancer cells move into a blood vessel and spread to other parts of the body.

Secondary tumor
Cancer cells then move through the blood and lymph system to form a secondary tumor at another site in body.

Figure 11-1 How cancer spreads. Locomotion (movement) is essential to the process of metastasis (spread of cancer). Scientists have identified a protein that causes cancer cells to grow arms, or pseudopodia, enabling them to move to other parts of the body.

The Cancerous Cell

Compared with noncancerous cells, cancer cells function in similar and dissimilar ways. It is the dissimilar aspects that often make them unpredictable and difficult to manage.

Perhaps the most unusual aspect of cancerous cells is their infinite life expectancy. Specifically, it appears that cancerous cells can produce an enzyme, *telomerase,* that blocks the cellular biological clock that informs normal cells that it is time to die.[5] In spite of this ability to live forever, cancer cells do not necessarily divide more quickly than normal cells do. In fact, they can divide at the same rate or even on occasion at a slower rate.

In addition, cancerous cells do not possess the *contact inhibition*[6] (a mechanism that influences the number of cells that can occupy a particular space at a particular time) of normal cells. In the absence of this property, cancer cells accumulate, altering the functional capacity of the tissue or organ they occupy. Further, the absence of

cellular cohesiveness[6] (a property seen in normal cells that "keeps them at home") allows cancer cells to spread through the circulatory or lymphatic system to distant points via **metastasis** (Figure 11-1). Interestingly, once migrating cancer cells arrive at a new area of the body, they "rediscover" their cellular cohesive capabilities. A final unique characteristic of cancerous cells is their ability to command the circulatory system to send them additional blood supply to meet their metabolic needs and to provide additional routes for metastasis. This *angiogenesis*[6]

Key Terms

metastasis (muh **tas** ta sis) the spread of cancerous cells from their site of origin to other areas of the body capability of cancer cells makes them extremely hardy compared with noncancerous cells.

Staging Cancer

In light of the interesting capabilities of malignant cells just described, it is critically important in the diagnosis and treatment of cancer that *oncologists* (physicians who have specialized in the care of cancer patients) know not only the type of cancer but also its extent. The latter determination is reflected in the concept of "staging" cancer.

For purposes of effective communication regarding the staging of cancer, the international medical community has adopted the *TNM* staging system.[1] This system first identifies the extent of a malignancy as to whether it is primary (T), whether it has or has not progressed to regional lymph node involvement (N), and the presence or absence of metastasis (M). On establishing a TNM profile of the tumor, a numerical stage (I, II, III, or IV) is determined. This categorization reflects: (I) *in situ* or "at the point of origin", (II) *Local*—an invasive cancer confined to the organ of origin, (III) *Regional*—cancer extended into the immediately neighboring tissue or into regional lymph nodes, and (IV) *Distant*—cancer extended to distant parts of the body, either by discontinuous metastasis or through the lymphatic drainage to distant nodes.

On the basis of the system described above, important decisions regarding treatment, management, and prognosis (survivability) of the cancer are made—information important to all persons involved in the medical care to be received.

Benign Tumors

Noncancerous, or **benign,** tumors can also form in the body. These **tumors** are usually enclosed by a membrane and do not spread from their point of origin. Benign tumors can be dangerous when they crowd out normal tissue within a confined space.

Types of Cancer

Again, for the purposes of effective diagnosis and appropriate treatment, cancers can be named or labeled on the basis of their cell type of origin (such as hepatoma) and/or the organ in which they are located (such as the liver). To the medical community, the name of cancers, based on the cell type of origin, is most often used in making determination regarding diagnosis and treatment, whereas for the general public, the labeling of cancer on the basis of the organ of origin is more familiar and understandable. In this section the labeling based on the cell type of origin is given brief consideration, while the body of the chapter describes cancer based on its organ of

origin. In some cases labeling may also be extended back to embryonic germ layer of origin, but this is beyond the scope of this textbook.

For the majority of physicians and the patients with whom they must communicate, descriptions of cancer based on the organ of origin are technically adequate and, with explanation to patients, understandable. In the list that follows, several cell- or tissue-based cancers are discussed.

carcinoma—Found most frequently in the skin, nose, mouth, throat, stomach, intestinal tract, glands, nerves, breasts, urinary and genital structures, lungs, kidneys, and liver; approximately 85 percent of all malignant tumors are classified as carcinomas

sarcoma—Formed in the connective tissues of the body; bone, cartilage, and tendons are the sites of sarcoma development; only 2 percent of all malignancies are of this type

melanoma—Arises from the melanin-containing cells of skin; found most often in people who have had extensive sun exposure, particularly a deep, penetrating sunburn; although once rare, the amount of this cancer has increased markedly in recent years; remains among the most deadly forms of cancer

neuroblastoma—Originates in the immature cells found within the central nervous system; neuroblastomas are rare; usually found in children

adenocarcinoma—Derived from cells of the endocrine glands

hepatoma—Originates in cells of the liver; although not thought to be directly caused by alcohol use, seen more frequently in people who have experienced **sclerotic changes** in the liver

leukemia—Found in cells of the blood and blood-forming tissues; characterized by abnormal, immature white blood cell formation; several forms are found in children and adults

lymphoma—Arises in cells of the lymphatic tissues or other immune system tissues; includes lymphosarcomas and Hodgkin's disease; characterized by abnormal white cell production and decreased resistance

---

Key Terms

benign noncancerous; tumors that do not spread

tumor mass of cells; may be cancerous (malignant) or noncancerous (benign)

sclerotic changes (skluh **rot** ick) thickening or hardening of tissues

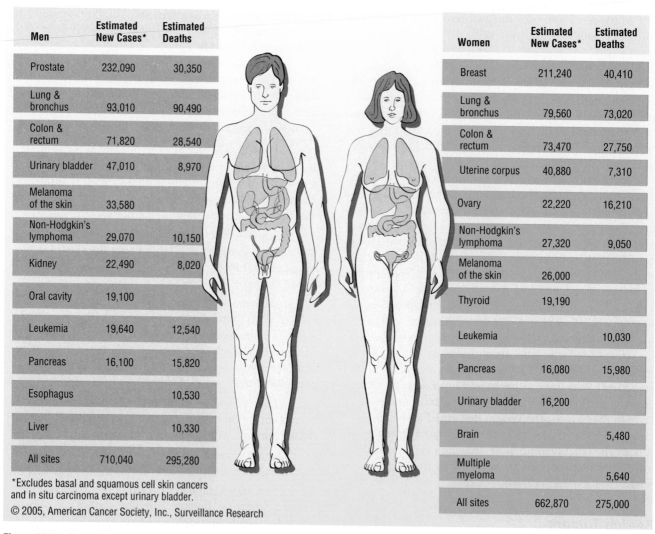

Men	Estimated New Cases*	Estimated Deaths
Prostate	232,090	30,350
Lung & bronchus	93,010	90,490
Colon & rectum	71,820	28,540
Urinary bladder	47,010	8,970
Melanoma of the skin	33,580	
Non-Hodgkin's lymphoma	29,070	10,150
Kidney	22,490	8,020
Oral cavity	19,100	
Leukemia	19,640	12,540
Pancreas	16,100	15,820
Esophagus		10,530
Liver		10,330
All sites	710,040	295,280

*Excludes basal and squamous cell skin cancers and in situ carcinoma except urinary bladder.

© 2005, American Cancer Society, Inc., Surveillance Research

Women	Estimated New Cases*	Estimated Deaths
Breast	211,240	40,410
Lung & bronchus	79,560	73,020
Colon & rectum	73,470	27,750
Uterine corpus	40,880	7,310
Ovary	22,220	16,210
Non-Hodgkin's lymphoma	27,320	9,050
Melanoma of the skin	26,000	
Thyroid	19,190	
Leukemia		10,030
Pancreas	16,080	15,980
Urinary bladder	16,200	
Brain		5,480
Multiple myeloma		5,640
All sites	662,870	275,000

Figure 11-2 These 2005 estimates of new cases of cancer and deaths from cancer reveal some significant similarities between men and women. Note that lung cancer is the leading cause of cancer deaths for both genders.

Figure 11-2 presents information about the estimated new cases of cancer and deaths from cancer at various sites in both men and women.[1] Table 11.1 shows that cancer incidence and mortality rates vary among different racial and ethnic groups.

Cancer at Selected Sites in the Body

A second and more familiar way to describe cancer is on the basis of the organ site at which it occurs. The following discussion relates to some of these more familiar sites. A lack of space, in combination with the wide arrays of human cancers, limits the number of specific malignancies that can be described. Remember also that regular screening procedures can lead to early identification of

cancer at these sites. (See Changing for the Better box on page 345.)

Lung Cancer

Lung cancer is one of the most lethal and frequently diagnosed forms of cancer. Primarily because of the advanced stage of the disease at the time symptoms first appear, only 15 percent of all people with lung cancer (all stages) survive 5 years beyond diagnosis.[1] By the time a person is sufficiently concerned about having a persistent cough, blood-streaked sputum, and chest pain, it is often too late for treatment to be effective. This failure to be able to diagnose lung cancer in its earlier stages could, however, begin to change. Currently the National Cancer Institute is studying the efficacy of *spiral CT scans* in detecting lung

Table 11.1 Incidence and Mortality Rates* by Site, Race, and Ethnicity, US, 1997–2001

Incidence	White	African American	Asian American and Pacific Islander	American Indian and Alaska Native	Hispanic/Latino[†]
All sites					
Males	556.5	689.2	385.9	263.2	419.8
Females	429.8	400.1	302.8	222.5	309.9
Breast (female)	141.7	119.9	96.8	54.2	89.6
Colon & rectum					
Males	63.1	72.9	56.3	38.3	49.6
Females	45.9	56.5	38.6	32.7	32.5
Lung & bronchus					
Males	77.9	117.2	60.5	46.0	45.2
Females	51.3	54.5	28.5	23.4	23.9
Prostate	167.4	271.3	100.7	51.2	140.0
Stomach					
Males	10.8	18.8	21.9	15.7	17.8
Females	5.0	9.9	12.4	8.9	10.0
Liver & intrahepatic bile duct					
Males	7.2	11.8	21.1	8.3	13.5
Females	2.9	3.9	7.7	4.8	5.8
Uterine cervix	8.9	11.8	9.5	6.0	16.2

Mortality	White	African American	Asian American and Pacific Islander	American Indian and Alaska Native	Hispanic/Latino[†]
All sites					
Males	245.5	347.3	151.2	167.0	174.0
Females	165.5	196.5	100.5	113.4	111.6
Breast (female)	26.4	35.4	12.6	13.6	17.3
Colon & rectum					
Males	24.8	34.3	15.8	17.1	18.0
Females	17.1	24.5	10.8	11.7	11.6
Lung & bronchus					
Males	76.6	104.1	40.2	49.8	39.6
Females	41.6	39.9	19.2	26.6	14.9
Prostate	28.8	70.4	13.0	20.2	23.5
Stomach					
Males	5.8	13.3	11.9	7.3	9.7
Females	2.8	6.3	7.0	4.1	5.3
Liver & intrahepatic bile duct					
Males	6.1	9.3	15.6	8.3	10.6
Females	2.7	3.8	6.6	4.3	5.1
Uterine cervix	2.6	5.6	2.8	2.8	3.6

*Per 100,000, age-adjusted to the 2000 US standard population.

[†]Hispanic/Latinos are not mutually exclusive from whites, African Americans, Asian Americans, and Pacific Islanders, and American Indians and Alaska Natives.

Source: Ries LAG, Eisner MP, Kosary CL, Hankey BF, Miller BA, Clegg L, Mariotto A, Fay MP, Feuer EJ, Edwards BK (eds). *SEER Cancer Statistics Review, 1975–2001,* National Cancer Institute, Bethesda, MD: 2004. http://seer.cancer.gov/csr/1975_2001. American Cancer Society, Surveillance Research, 2005.

tumors earlier than can be done by conventional chest x-rays. However, an initial assessment of the technology questions its cost-effectiveness and potential for excessive false-positive findings.

Risk Factors

Today it is known that genetic predisposition is important in the development of lung cancer. Perhaps, in fact, the majority of people who develop this form of cancer have an inherited "head start." When people who are genetically at risk also smoke, their level of risk for developing lung cancer is significantly greater than it is for nonsmokers. Of particular interest at this time are multiple genes on chromosome 3. Damage to three tumor suppressors on this chromosome is found in virtually every case of small-cell lung cancer and 90 percent of nonsmall-cell lung cancer. Most of the remaining lung cancer cases appear in people who smoke but are not genetically predisposed.

Cigarette smoking is the single most important behavioral factor in the development of lung cancer. For men who smoke, the rate of lung cancer is 22 times higher than it is for men who do not smoke. For women who smoke, the rate is 12 times higher than for women who do not smoke. Smokers account for nearly 87 percent of all cases of lung cancer, and lung cancer itself produces at least 30 percent of all cancer-caused deaths.[1]

Since 1987, lung cancer has exceeded breast cancer as the leading cause of cancer death in women, although more new cases of breast cancer than lung cancer are diagnosed each year. The incidence of lung cancer in men has shown a gradual decline over the last several years that parallels their declining use of tobacco products. In comparing 2003 estimated new cases of lung cancer in women with 2005 data, it appears for the first time that the incidence of lung cancer has also begun declining in women.[4] One hopes that this decline in new cases of lung cancer in women reflects a continuing decline in tobacco use.

Environmental agents, such as radon, asbestos, and air pollutants, make a smaller contribution to the development of lung cancer. Radon alone may be the principal causative agent in most lung cancer found in nonsmokers.

Prevention

The preceding information clearly suggests that not smoking or quitting smoking (see page 301) and avoidance of second-hand smoke (see page 299) are the most important factors in the prevention of lung cancer. In addition, place of residence, particularly as it relates to air pollution, is a long-suspected risk factor for lung cancer.[7] Nonsmokers who are considering living with a smoker or working in a confined area where second-hand smoke is prevalent should carefully consider the risk of developing lung cancer. A recent study does, however, lessen concern over moderate alcohol use and the risk of developing lung cancer.[8]

Treatment

The prognosis for surviving lung cancer remains extremely guarded. Depending on the type of lung cancer, its extent, and factors related to the patient's overall health, various combinations of surgery, radiation, and chemotherapy remain the physicians' primary approach to treatment. Today, for persons with early-stage lung cancer, chemotherapy, following surgery, has increased survivability slightly. Additionally, an experimental vaccine (GVAX) now in the early stages of testing has shown extremely encouraging results in patients with non-small-cell lung cancer, the most common form of the disease.[9] Also, a once-promising drug, Iressa, used as a last-resort drug by terminally ill lung cancer patients, now seems far less promising after subsequent study, thus is basically ineffective against the lethality of advanced lung cancer.

Breast Cancer

Surpassed only by lung cancer, breast cancer is the second leading cause of death from cancer in women. It is the third leading cause of cancer deaths overall. Nearly one in eight women will develop breast cancer in her lifetime, resulting in an estimated 211,240 new invasive cases and 40,410 deaths in 2005.[1] In men, an estimated 1,690 new cases and 460 deaths occurred in 2005.[1] (See Learning from Our Diversity on page 346.) As women age, their risk of developing breast cancer increases. Regardless of age, however, waiting to learn whether a suspicious lump is benign or is a relatively harmless fluid-filled cyst is stressful. Early detection is the key to complete recovery. Ninety-seven percent of women who discover their breast cancer before it has spread (metastasized) survive more than 5 years.[1]

Risk Factors

Although all women and men are at some risk of developing breast cancer, the following groups of women have a higher risk.

- Women whose menstrual periods began at an early age, or whose menopause occurred late (although the former may be more important than the latter is)
- Women who had no children, had their first child later in life, or did not nurse[10]
- Women who have used hormone replace therapy (HRT)—particularly combined estrogen and progestin[11]
- Women who have a high degree of breast density (high level of glandular tissues relative to fat) or biopsy-established hyperplasia[1]
- Women whose diets are high in saturated fats, who are sedentary, or who are obese after menopause[12] (particularly central body cavity obesity; see Chapter 6)
- Women who carry the BRCA1 and/or BRCA2 mutated tumor suppressor genes, or those with a strong family history of breast cancer

As mentioned above, significant concern exists regarding the long-term use of hormone replacement therapy and the development of breast cancer in postmenopausal women. In fact, in a government-sponsored study (Women's Health Initiative Study) the link appeared so strongly and early that the study was terminated much earlier than had been planned. Researchers found that tumor development in women taking HRT versus those on a placebo was more common, that tumors were larger at diagnosis, and that tumors were more often invasive.[11] Many physicians are now advising that HRT be used only on a very short-term basis to relieve the symptoms of menopause, rather than the much longer period of time previously deemed appropriate.

Screening Guidelines for the Early Detection of Cancer in Asymptomatic People

Site	Recommendation
Breast	• Yearly mammograms are recommended starting at age 40. The age at which screening should be stopped should be individualized by considering the potential risks and benefits of screening in the context of overall health status and longevity. • Clinical breast exams should be part of a periodic health exam, about every 3 years for women in their 20s and 30s, and every year for women 40 and older. • Women should know how their breasts normally feel and report any breast change promptly to their health care providers. Breast self-exam is an option for women starting in their 20s. • Women at increased risk (e.g., family history, genetic tendency, past breast cancer) should talk with their doctors about the benefits and limitations of starting mammography screening earlier, having additional tests (i.e., breast ultrasound and MRI), or having more frequent exams.
Colon and rectum	Beginning at age 50, men and women should begin screening with 1 of the examination schedules below: • A fecal occult blood test (FOBT) or fecal immunochemical test (FIT) every year • A flexible sigmoidoscopy (FSIG) every 5 years • Annual FOBT or FIT and flexible sigmoidoscopy every 5 years* • A double-contrast barium enema every 5 years • A colonoscopy every 10 years *Combined testing is preferred over either annual FOBT or FIT, or FSIG every 5 years, alone. People who are at moderate or high risk for colorectal cancer should talk with a doctor about a different testing schedule.*
Prostate	The PSA test and the digital rectal examination should be offered annually, beginning at age 50, to men who have a life expectancy of at least 10 years. Men at high risk (African American men and men with a strong family history of 1 or more first-degree relatives diagnosed with prostate cancer at an early age) should begin testing at age 45. For both men at average risk and high risk, information should be provided about what is known and what is uncertain about the benefits and limitations of early detection and treatment of prostate cancer so that they can make an informed decision about testing.
Uterus	**Cervix:** Screening should begin approximately 3 years after a woman begins having vaginal intercourse, but no later than 21 years of age. Screening should be done every year with regular Pap tests or every 2 years using liquid-based tests. At or after age 30, women who have had 3 normal test results in a row may get screened every 2 to 3 years. Alternatively, cervical cancer screening with HPV DNA testing and conventional or liquid-based cytology could be performed every 3 years. However, doctors may suggest a woman get screened more often if she has certain risk factors, such as HIV infection or a weak immune system. Women 70 years and older who have had 3 or more consecutive normal Pap tests in the last 10 years may choose to stop cervical cancer screening. Screening after total hysterectomy (with removal of the cervix) is not necessary unless the surgery was done as a treatment for cervical cancer. **Endometrium:** The American Cancer Society recommends that at the time of menopause all women should be informed about the risks and symptoms of endometrial cancer, and strongly encouraged to report any unexpected bleeding or spotting to their physicians. Annual screening for endometrial cancer with endometrial biopsy beginning at age 35 should be offered to women with or at risk for hereditary nonpolyposis colon cancer (HNPCC).
Cancer-related checkup	For individuals undergoing periodic health examinations, a cancer-related checkup should include health counseling, and depending on a person's age, and gender, might include examinations for cancers of the thyroid, oral cavity, skin, lymph nodes, testes, and ovaries, as well as for some nonmalignant diseases.

American Cancer Society guidelines for early cancer detection are assessed annually in order to identify whether there is new scientific evidence sufficient to warrant a reevaluation of current recommendations. If evidence is sufficiently compelling to consider a change or clarification in a current guideline or the development of a new guideline, a formal procedure is initiated. Guidelines are formally evaluated every 5 years regardless of whether new evidence suggests a change in the existing recommendations. There are 9 steps in this procedure, and these "guidelines for guideline development" were formally established to provide a specific methodology for science and expert judgment to form the underpinnings of specific statements and recommendations from the Society. These procedures constitute a deliberate process to ensure that all Society recommendations have the same methodological and evidence-based process at their core. This process also employs a system for rating strength and consistency of evidence that is similar to that employed by the Agency for Health Care Research and Quality (AHCRQ) and the US Preventive Services Task Force (USPSTF).

Learning from our Diversity

Breast Cancer: A Rare Diagnosis in Men

With all the attention given to breast cancer in women—in the news, by physicians, and by research foundations—you may be surprised to learn that men are also diagnosed with this condition. For every 100 women who develop breast cancer, however, only one case is reported among men. Estimates for the year 2005 suggest that no more than 1,690 American men will develop breast cancer. When compared to the 211,240 cases anticipated in women during the same year, the rarity of breast cancer in men becomes apparent.

The typical male breast cancer victim is usually older than 60 and often has a family history of the disease. The *BRCA2* tumor suppressor gene mutation is also found within the victim's genetic linage. In some cases, the male breast cancer victim has the inherited condition of Klinefelter's syndrome, in which a second X (or female) sex chromosome is present. The presence of the extra sex chromosome produces enhanced estrogen within the male body, resulting in adolescent development of prominent breasts and a higher risk of breast cancer later in life. Other conditions, such as various forms of liver disease, also result in higher levels of estrogen and, eventually, a greater risk of male breast cancer.

In most ways male breast cancer is very similar in type to that seen in women. Infiltrating ductal cancer, ductal carcinoma in situ, and a form of cancer arising from the ducts immediately beneath the nipple (Paget's disease) have been reported. Because of this close similarity to female breast cancer, medical management of male breast cancer closely parallels that seen in women. Surgery (a modified radical mastectomy), chemotherapy, external radiation, and hormonal therapy are used alone or in combination. The latter therapy may include not only drugs to block the influence of estrogen on estrogen-sensitive cancer cells, but removal of testicles as well. As with virtually all forms of cancer, early diagnosis and treatment are of critical importance.

InfoLinks

www.cancernet.nci.nih.gov

The effects of environmental pollutants and regional influences have also been investigated as causative factors in the development of breast cancer. Environmental pollutants vary from region to region and are influenced by a number of factors, including the type of industrial and agricultural activity in a particular area. A wide array of regional factors may be involved, including genetic background of people in a given area and lifestyle differences involving diet, alcohol consumption, and exercise patterns.

The role of genetic predisposition in the development of breast cancer has also received considerable attention. For example, a small percentage (perhaps 5 percent) of women with breast cancer have inherited or developed mutations in one or both of two tumor suppressor genes (proto-oncogenes), *BRCA1* and *BRCA2*. Discovered in 1994 and 1995, respectively, and currently the focus of extensive research, more than 200 mutations in these genes have been identified. In a study involving 5,000 Ashkenazi Jews (Jews of Central and Eastern European descent) living in the Washington, D.C., area, mutation in the *BRCA1* gene resulted in a 56 percent greater chance of developing breast cancer by age 70 (versus a 13 percent greater risk for people without a mutated version of the gene).[13] In the years since these genes' identification, studies have been ongoing in an attempt to more accurately define the level of risk for developing breast cancer among women who carry one or both *BRCA 1* or *2* mutations. The desirability of fine-tuning the level of risk holds important implications in establishing recommendations for screening and in the development of public education programs.[14] Both of these genes are also associated with increased risk of developing ovarian cancer (see page 352) and, perhaps, prostate cancer in men.

Uncertainty exists regarding the use of screening tests to determine the status of the *BRCA1* and *BRCA2* oncogenes. Central to this concern is that a complex set of circumstances must accompany the genetic mutation for breast or ovarian cancer to actually develop. Therefore, it cannot be definitively determined whether a given carrier of a mutated gene will actually develop cancer.

In addition to the much-studied *BRCA1* and *2* genes discussed above, other genetic mutations have been implicated in the development of breast cancer, thus complicating further all aspects of screening, treatment, prevention, and public education. Among these additional mutations is one that influences a protein (MAP kinase) that functions as a "chemical switch" in controlling cell replication. In cancer patients with extra copies of the *HER-2* gene, cancerous cells are less likely to respond to chemotherapy. Yet another involves a portion of a gene (*CYP17*) that plays a role in the synthesis of estrogen, and a fourth mutation results in the malfunction of the important APC tumor suppressor gene.

The Personal Assessment on pages 367–368 may be helpful in determining your relative level of risk of developing breast cancer.

Prevention

As already discussed, a variety of risk factors are thought to be important in the development of most cases of breast cancer. Accordingly, some degree of prevention is possible when factors such as diet; alcohol use; physical activity level; decisions about contraception, pregnancy, and breastfeeding; occupational exposure to toxins; and even place of residence are considered.

For women who have a primary family history of breast cancer (sisters, mother, or grandmothers with the disease) and who have been found to carry one or both of the BRCA genes, an extreme form of prevention is also possible— **prophylactic mastectomy.** In this surgical procedure, both noncancerous breasts are removed, in an attempt to eliminate the possibility of future cancer development. When carefully planned, breast reconstruction surgery can be undertaken immediately, with satisfactory results. A high level of satisfaction (70 percent) was found among women who had undergone this procedure.[15] Accordingly some physicians, however, recommend against the surgery, preferring to monitor susceptible women very carefully and frequently.

One important consideration related to this procedure is that not every person who carries a mutated tumor suppressor gene will develop cancer, making the surgery unnecessary.

At the present time pharmacological prevention represents the newest approach to reducing the incidence of breast cancer. Two medications, Evista, or raloxifene (a drug developed for use in osteoporosis prevention), and tamoxifen (an estrogen-receptor blocker developed for use in the treatment of cancer) have been found to be effective in lowering the risk of cancer in high-risk women. However, a warning (August 2000) from the FDA reminds physicians that tamoxifen can have serious side effects, including the development of uterine cancer and potentially fatal blood clots. That said, however, it is now believed that 2.47 million women could benefit by using tamoxifen for breast cancer protection.[16]

Early Detection: Breast Self-Examination

For several decades a fundamental component of early detection of breast cancer has been breast self-examination (BSE). Generally recommended for women 20 years of age and older, the procedure was to be performed during the menstrual period or during the day immediately following the end of the menstrual period, when estrogen levels are at their lowest and cystic activity in breast tissue is minimal (or on the same day of each month by postmenopausal women). The proper technique is illustrated in the Changing for the Better box on page 348. Although breast self-examination is an easily learned technique, today its value is being strongly challenged by researchers in both this country and in China. It has, in fact, become the contention of some that teaching BSE to another generation of women is a misuse of time and money that could be better spent on other screening techniques. Others, however, feel that women who know the technique should not be discouraged from using BSE, but they also should be regularly reminded of its significant limitations in finding tumors. In 2003, the American Cancer Society (ACS) revised its recommendation for breast cancer screening to better address the doubts regarding BSE's limitations. Specific to BSE the following statement summarizes the ACS's position.

> Previously, the guidelines (for BSE) recommended women perform breast self-exam every month. Now, (we) recommend that, beginning in their 20s, women should be told about the benefits and limitations of BSE, and that it is acceptable for women to choose not to do BSE, or to do it occasionally. The importance of promptly reporting changes to a physician is emphasized
>
> The reason for this change is that research has shown that BSE plays a very small role in detecting breast cancer compared with self-awareness.

However, since 2003, the ACS appears to have retained a more supportive stance on BSE than its 2003 statement suggests. The following statements from 2001 appear to reflect what one might call "the working perception" of BSE on the part of individuals at the American Cancer Society.[17]

> Breast self-exam is useful before age 40 to help a woman learn what her breast feels like when it's normal," notes Robert Smith of the ACS. "That way, she can have an idea of whether a lump she encounters is something that she should see her doctor about." . . . "And it can help with early detection of the small number of breast cancers found in that under 40 age group," adds Smith. "After 40, we should not expect much added benefit from BSE, but we do expect a little, and that little is to provide a safety net for some women whose breast cancers aren't picked up by mammography," explains Smith. . . . "The bottom line is that in breast cancer early detection is better than later detection, and BSE helps with early detection," notes Smith. "BSE is a prudent thing to do; it's worth the time and effort to teach and to use.

In any case, monthly BSE can be viewed as an adjunct to regularly scheduled breast examinations conducted by a physician (CBE) and to the routine use of mammography. Breast self-examination also reinforces the importance of

---

Key Terms

prophylactic mastectomy surgical removal of the breasts to prevent breast cancer in women who are at high risk of developing the disease

Breast Self-Examination

I've never felt confident about doing a breast self-exam. What is the proper technique?

The following explains how to do a breast self-examination:

1. In the shower: Examine your breasts during a bath or shower; hands glide more easily over wet skin. With your fingers flat, move gently over every part of each breast. Use right hand to examine left breast, left hand for right breast. Check for any lump, hard knot, or thickening. This self-examination should be done monthly, preferably a day or two after the end of the menstrual period.

2. Before a mirror: Inspect your breasts with arms at your sides. Next, raise your arms high overhead. Look for any changes in contour of each breast, a swelling, dimpling of skin, changes in the nipple. Then rest palms on hips, and press down firmly to flex your chest muscles. Left and right breast will not exactly match—few women's breasts do.

3. Lying down: To examine your right breast, put a pillow or folded towel under your right shoulder. Place right hand behind your head—this distributes breast tissue more evenly on the chest. With left hand, fingers flat, press gently in small circular motions around an imaginary clock face. Begin at outermost top of your right breast for 12 o'clock, then move to 1 o'clock, and so on around the circle back to 12 o'clock. A ridge of firm tissue in the lower curve of each breast is normal. Then move in an inch toward the nipple; keep circling to examine every part of your breast, including the nipple. This requires at least three more circles. Now slowly repeat the procedure on your left breast with a pillow under your left shoulder and left hand behind head. Notice how your breast structure feels. Finally, squeeze the nipple of each breast gently between thumb and index finger. Any discharge, clear or bloody, should be reported to your doctor immediately.

Breast cancer can occur in men, too, and they should perform this examination monthly. Regular examination will teach you what is normal for you and will give you confidence in your examination.

InfoLinks

www.mskcc.org

breast health and thus the importance of regularly scheduled comprehensive breast cancer screening.

In light of the concern regarding the role of BSE in early cancer detection, the second rung of early detection, Clinical Breast Examination (CBE), is also being critically reviewed because of the lack of standard procedures for conducting the examination. Steps are being taken to develop standardized protocols.[18] Currently, the ACS appears to remain totally committed to the importance of CBE.

Early Detection: Mammography

Although researchers once disagreed about the age at which women should begin routine mammography and the extent to which mammography is effective in finding masses in dense breast tissue, today mammograms are physicians' best tool for the early detection of breast cancer. Accordingly, the American Cancer society recommends that mammography begin at age 40.

Whether women begin routine mammography at 40, as advised by the ACS, or as early as 35 years of age, particularly women with previous symptoms or a family history of breast disease, women should continue these examinations on an annual basis. Recommendations regarding mammography for older women (65+) are, however, a bit more individually determined and should be discussed annually with physicians. For older women, overall health status and expectations for reaching a normal life expectancy are weighed relative to the lessening cost-effectiveness of mammography.

Because of the important role routine mammography plays in the early identification of breast lesions, the Mammography Quality Standards Act (MQSA), formulated by the FDA (April 1998), is a valuable step toward ensuring that mammography is performed by experienced technicians, using correctly calibrated equipment, and interpreted by skilled radiologists. Every woman should be certain that her mammography is being performed in a MQSA-certified facility. However, even when interpreted by experienced radiologists, mammograms are at times difficult to read, and tumors will therefore be missed. In fact, misinterpreted mammograms represent the most common basis for medical malpractice suits in radiology and perhaps in all aspects of medicine as practiced in the United States.

To secure the highest quality images for interpretation, the soft-tissue X-ray-based mammography of the past is increasingly supplemented by newer technologies, including MRI, contrast media-based MRI, ultrasound, and the Image-Checker, in which MRI images are quickly checked against a computerized library of normal breast images, and any suspicious areas are "tagged" for further evaluation, including biopsy. Magnetic Resonance Imaging (MRI) technology is, however, very expensive and is generally used with women who have already had breast cancer or have strong family history (occurring in a mother or sister) of the disease. Ideally these newer approaches will identify tumors in their earliest stages of development and reduce the percentage of false-positive results associated with traditional mammography procedures.

Treatment

Regardless of the method of detection, if a lump is found, a breast biopsy can determine whether the lump is cancerous. If the lump is cancerous but localized, treatment is highly effective, with cure rates at nearly 100 percent. The most frequently used treatments are **lumpectomy** combined with radiation, lumpectomy without radiation, and mastectomy. The use of chemotherapy following surgery is strongly advocated as well. Today the injection of a radioactive "tag" before surgery allows identification of the nearest lymph node (the *sentinel node*) to which breast cancer cells may have spread, thus allowing the surgeon to spare noncancerous nodes. When the cancer is invasive or has metastasized, more radical surgery (mastectomy with lymph node removal) combined with chemotherapy and/or various forms of radiation may be the most effective course of treatment.

When drug therapy is deemed desirable in treating breast cancer, oncologists may consider two drugs that have recently become available or whose earlier protocols have been redefined. The first, tamoxifen, discussed earlier in terms of breast cancer prevention, is a hormonelike drug that prevents estrogen from stimulating cancer cell growth. The use of tamoxifen has proven highly effective in women who have the type of breast cancer stimulated by the presence of estrogen. Used for many years for more localized tumors, today the use of tamoxifen has been extended to the treatment of highly metastasized breast cancers. Tamoxifen's ability to stimulate uterine cancer development, blood clots, strokes, and cataracts, however, is a potentially serious side effect of the drug's use and must be closely monitored.

The second drug, herceptin, is an antibody-like agent used in combination with other chemotherapeutic drugs in highly advanced breast cancer. This newly approved drug interferes with the activity of a protein produced by the *HER-2* oncogene that normally fosters tumor cell division.

As we would expect, additional cancer treatment and prevention drugs are becoming available. Two such drugs, Fermara and Arimidex, which belong to a class of drugs called *aromatase inhibitors,* reduce or stop the production of estrogen. Currently researchers are determining the manner in which these drugs will join (or replace) tamoxifen in the treatment of breast cancer.[19]

Cervical Cancer

In 2005 an estimated 10,370 new cases of cancer of the cervix (the anatomical neck of the uterus) occurred in the United States.[1] Fortunately, the death rate from cervical cancer has dropped greatly since 1950, largely because of

---

Key Terms

lumpectomy a surgical treatment for breast cancer in which a minimal amount of breast tissue is removed; when appropriate, this procedure is an alternative to mastectomy, in which the entire breast and underlying tissue are removed the **Pap test.** This test screens for precancerous cellular changes (called *cervical intraepithelial neoplasia,* or *CIN*) and malignant cells. If malignant cells are found, it is hoped that they represent only cancer in situ (at the site of origin), rather than a more advanced invasive stage of the disease. Unfortunately, this simple and relatively inexpensive screening test is still underused, particularly in women over age 60, the group in which cervical cancer is most frequently found.

Risk Factors

Because of the clear association between sexually transmitted infections and cervical cancer, risk factors for this form of cancer include early age of first intercourse, large number of sexual partners, history of infertility (which may indicate chronic pelvic inflammatory disease), and clinical evidence of *human papillomavirus* (*HPV*) infections (see page 428 in Chapter 13). For patients with previous HPV infections or whose sexual history suggests a higher risk for HPV, a ThinPrep Pap test has been shown effective in detecting the DNA from four HPVs that are known to be cancer causing, while being as easy to use as the more widely used Pap smear. Today the test is approved only for identifying HPV infection, but it is also capable of detecting both chlamydia and gonorrhea. At the time of writing, clinical trials are underway on vaccines designed to protect against some HPV infections. Initial human studies have been highly effective in preventing infections from the most virulent of the HPVs.[18] On the basis of these trials it has been shown that the vaccines are approximately 93 percent effective against HPVs 16 and 18 (the most virulent of the 15 human cancer-causing HPVs), are well tolerated, and remain effective for at least 5 years.[20]

In addition to sexual history, cigarette smoking and socioeconomic factors are also risk factors for cervical cancer. The latter most likely relates to less frequent medical assessment, including infrequent Pap tests. (The Personal Assessment on page 367 will help women evaluate their risk of developing cervical cancer.)

 TALKING POINTS Three risk factors are associated with HPV-induced cervical cancer: early age of first sexual intercourse, higher-than-average number of partners, and lack of protection against sexually transmitted diseases (for example, condoms). How would you introduce this topic to a teenage daughter, sister, or niece?

Prevention

Sexual abstinence is the most effective way of reducing the risk of developing cervical cancer (for example, Catholic nuns have extremely low rates of cervical cancer). However, abstinence is unlikely to be the choice for most women; other alternatives include fewer sexual partners,

What Pap Smear Results Mean

Pap smear results and their meanings can include:

- **Normal.** The cervical cells are healthy.

- **Unsatisfactory for evaluation.** The slide can't be read. Causes include douching, bleeding, infection, or not enough cells on the slide. The test should probably be repeated in 2–3 months.

- **Benign.** The Pap smear showed infection, irritation, or normal cell repair. If you have an infection, you might need medication.

- **Ascus.** The Pap smear showed some abnormal changes in the cells, but the cause is not clear. Infection is a common cause.

- **Low-grade changes.** You might have been infected with the human papilloma virus (HPV). Some types of the virus are associated with an increased risk for cancer of the cervix. Your health care provider will recommend specific follow-up. This might include another Pap smear or a colposcopy—a look at the cervix with a high-power microscope.

- **High-grade changes.** The cells of the cervix can progress toward cancer, but they aren't cancer yet. Fewer than half of the women with this test will develop cancer. Colposcopy is needed. Biopsy and treatment might be necessary.

more careful selection of partners to minimize contact with those at high risk, the use of condoms, and the use of spermicides. In addition, of course, regular medical assessment, including annual Pap tests (and the ThinPrep Pap test), represents prevention through early detection. Of course, when widely available, the HPV vaccine will further increase prevention.

Early Detection

At this time, the importance of women having Pap tests for cervical cancer performed on a regular basis cannot be overemphasized. However, the specific scheduling of cervical screening is undergoing adjustment. For young sexually active women, initial screening using the Pap smear (preferably in combination with the ThinPrep) should be undertaken within 3 years of first exposure. For young women not sexually at risk, or for women who have had a hysterectomy, the initial screening with the Pap smear can be determined in consultation with

Key Terms

Pap test a cancer-screening procedure in which cells are removed from the cervix and examined for precancerous changes health care providers. Once initiated, however, following three consecutive annual negative tests, the interval between tests may be increased upon discussion with health care providers. The American Cancer Society estimates that cervical cancer claimed the lives of 3,710 women in 2005.

The Pap test is not perfect, however. When tests are read in laboratories highly experienced in interpreting Pap slides, about 7 percent will be false negatives, resulting in a 93 percent accuracy rate. In less-experienced laboratories, false negatives may be as high as 20 percent. (The Star box on page 350 explains what the possible Pap smear results mean.) In addition, not all women whose test results are accurately assessed as abnormal receive adequate follow-up care, nor do they have subsequent Pap tests regularly enough. On a more positive note, potentially more effective tests have been developed and are gaining acceptance. AutoPap and PAPNET provide automated tests analyses, and ThinPrep represents a new technology that identifies DNA from important cancer-causing HPV. Some, however, fear that ThinPrep and the automated Pap tests are too expensive and lack data from large-scale studies of effectiveness.

In addition to changes discovered by a Pap test, symptoms that suggest potential cervical cancer include abnormal vaginal bleeding between periods and frequent spotting.

Treatment

Should precancerous cellular changes (CIN) be identified, treatment can include one of several alternatives. Physicians can destroy areas of abnormal cellular change using cryotherapy (freezing), electrocoagulation, laser destruction, or surgical removal of abnormal tissue. More advanced (invasive) cancer of the cervix can be treated with a hysterectomy combined with other established cancer therapies. A combination of radiation and chemotherapy is the most effective treatment for cervical cancer.

Uterine (Endometrial) Cancer

The American Cancer Society estimates that in 2005, 40,880 cases of uterine cancer (cancer within the inner wall of the body of the uterus, rather than within the cervix or neck of the uterus) were diagnosed in American women. In addition, 7,310 women died of the disease.[1] Although African Americans have a lower incidence of uterine cancer than white women do, their death rate is nearly twice as high.[21]

Risk Factors

Unlike cervical cancer, in which a strong viral link has been identified, the principal risk factor related to the development of endometrial cancer is a high estrogen level.

Accordingly, the following factors are related to higher levels of estrogen and, thus, to the development of endometrial cancer:

- Early menarche (early onset of menstruation)
- Late menopause
- Lack of ovulation (infertility)
- Never having given birth
- Estrogen replacement therapy (ERT not moderated with progesterone)
- Use of tamoxifen (a drug used in breast cancer therapy)
- History of polycystic ovary syndrome
- Hereditary nonpolyposis colon cancer

To some degree, endometrial cancer is seen more frequently in people who are diabetic, obese, hypertensive, or who have gallbladder disease.

Prevention

The risk factors associated with high levels of estrogen are areas in which prevention might be targeted. In addition, the need for regular gynecological care that includes pelvic examination is a principal factor in minimizing the risk of uterine cancer. Pregnancy and the use of oral contraceptives both provide some protection from endometrial cancer.[1] Some degree of prevention may also be accomplished through a diet high in phytoestrogens that may provide an antiestrogenic effect. Soy-based foods, soy-enriched foods, coffee, and orange juice have low to moderate amounts and types of phytoestrogens.[22]

Early Detection

Compared with cervical cancer, which is routinely identified through Pap tests, endometrial cancer is much more likely to be suspected on the basis of symptoms (irregular or postmenopausal bleeding) and confirmed by biopsy. Although more invasive, biopsy is a more effective method than ultrasound to diagnose uterine cancer.

Treatment

The treatment for early or localized endometrial cancer is generally surgical removal of the uterus (hysterectomy). Other therapies, such as radiation, chemotherapy, and hormonal therapy, may then be added to the treatment regimen. However, in terms of hormone replacement therapy (HRT), in which estrogen is combined with a synthetic progesterone, the FDA, The National Institute on Aging, and various medical associations now advise that no women 65 or older with an intact uterus should take HRT owing to several concerns, including an increased risk for endometrial cancer. For women who are undergoing menopause and experiencing troublesome symptoms such as night sweats and hot flashes, HRT should be used in the smallest doses that provide relief and for the shortest duration of time possible.

Vaginal Cancer

Although rare, cancer of the vagina (the passage leading to the uterus) is of concern to a particular group of women: the daughters of more than 3 million mothers who were given the drug DES (diethylstilbestrol) to prevent miscarriages. Because of the effects of DES on the development of the fetal reproductive system, these daughters face the risk of developing a form of vaginal (and cervical) cancer called *clear cell cancer*. The medical community has been following large groups of daughters to better assess their level of risk. In a longitudinal study that followed such women and a control group of 1,374 unexposed agemates, the risk of developing vaginal cancer was two to four times higher in the affected group than it was in women whose mothers were not given DES.[23]

Outside this unique group of women, vaginal cancer is relatively rare. The American Cancer Society estimates that in 2005, there were 2,140 new cases diagnosed, and 810 women died as the result of vaginal cancer.[1] Early detection can be accomplished using a Pap test when vaginal wall cell samples are taken. Treatment centers on surgical removal of the vagina and associated lymph nodes. Other supportive therapies may also be included in the treatment regimen.

Ovarian Cancer

Since the death in 1989 of actress Gilda Radner, a star in the early years of *Saturday Night Live,* public awareness of ovarian cancer has increased in the United States. The American Cancer Society estimates that in 2005, there were 22,200 new cases diagnosed, and 16,210 women died of the disease.[1] Most cases develop in women over age 40 who have not had children or began menstruation at an early age. The highest rate is in women over age 60. Today ovarian cancer causes more deaths than does any other form of female reproductive system cancer.

For a relatively small percentage of all women (10 percent), the inheritance of either the *BRCA1* or *BRCA2* suppressor gene mutation (see page 346) significantly increases the risk of developing both breast and ovarian cancer. Today it is estimated that about 20 percent of all cases of ovarian cancer stem from these genetic mutations.

Beyond the 20 percent of cases attributed to genetic mutations, what might account for the majority of ovarian cancers? A number of studies, with varying degrees of assurance, suggested that decades of estrogen replacement therapy (ERT) used to counter symptoms of menopause, maintain bone mass, and provide hormonal protection from heart disease could be responsible for the majority of ovarian cancers.[24] As mentioned in conjunction with endometrial cancer, hormone replacement therapy is now used for only the briefest period of time.

Prevention

Methods of preventing or lowering the risk of developing ovarian cancer are very similar to those recommended for breast cancer. These include using oral contraceptives, giving birth and breast-feeding (for at least 3 months), reducing dietary fat intake, abstaining from alcohol use, and performing regular physical activity.

For the small group of women with a strong family history of ovarian cancer, a **prophylactic oophorectomy** should be seriously considered. In this surgical procedure, both ovaries are removed. Carefully monitored hormone replacement therapy is then used to provide the protective advantages of estrogen in maintaining cardiovascular health and bone density.

Early Detection

Because of its vague symptoms, ovarian cancer has been referred to as a *silent cancer*. Women in whom ovarian cancer has been diagnosed often report that the only symptoms of their cancer's presence were digestive disturbances, gas, urinary incontinence, stomach distention and crampy abdominal pain over a few short weeks. The last symptom should be medically evaluated immediately.[25]

Two recently approved and now available screening tests for ovarian cancer and other cancers, the CA125 and CA125 II, detect specific proteins (antigens) produced by malignant cells. More routine use of these tests is anticipated.

For women with a strong family history of ovarian cancer (four primary family members who have had breast or ovarian cancer, with two or more cases occurring before age 50) or women of Ashkenazi Jewish descent (see page 346), genetic screening, newly available screening tests, and transvaginal ultrasound screening are likely to be recommended. These women may also be referred for participation in one of several prevention trials now under way.

Treatment

At this time, treatment of ovarian cancer requires surgical removal of the ovary, followed by aggressive use of chemotherapy. Use of the chemotherapeutic drug Taxol,

---

Key Terms

prophylactic oophorectomy surgical removal of the ovaries to prevent ovarian cancer in women at high risk of developing the disease

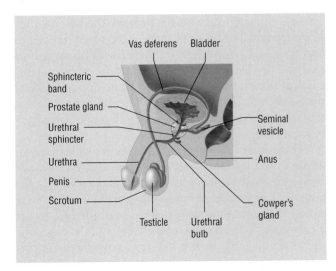

Figure 11-3 Location of the prostate gland within the male reproductive system

Symptoms of Prostate Disease

- Difficulty urinating
- Frequent urination, particularly at night
- Continued wetness for a short time after urination
- Blood in the urine
- Low-back pain
- Ache in the upper thighs

obtained from the bark and needles of the Pacific yew tree, results in a 50 percent survival rate 19 months after the completion of therapy. Most recently, use of an experimental three-drug combination—cyclophosphamide, paclitaxel, and cisplatin—has resulted in a 70 percent survival rate 22 months after chemotherapy.

Prostate Cancer

If the names Bob Dole, General Norman Schwarzkopf, Jerry Lewis, and Colin Powell are familiar, then you know four older men who have been diagnosed with and treated for prostate cancer. In fact, prostate cancer is so common that in 2005 an estimated 232,090 new cases were diagnosed, and 30,500 men died of the disease.[1] Prostate cancer is the second leading cause of cancer deaths in American men, exceeded only by lung cancer deaths. Cancer of the prostate is the most common form of cancer in men and a leading cause of death from cancer in older men.

The prostate gland is a walnut-size gland located near the base of the penis. (See Figure 11-3.) It surrounds the neck of the bladder and the urethra. The prostate secretes a number of components of semen, such as nutrients used to fuel sperm motility.

Risk Factors

Compared with other cancers, the risk factors for prostate cancer are less clearly defined. The most predictable risk factor is age. Nearly 80 percent of all prostate cancer cases are diagnosed in men over 65 years of age; however, cases in men under age 50 are not infrequent. African American men and men with a family history of prostate cancer are at greater risk of developing this form of cancer [167.4/100,000 (W) versus 271.3/100,000 (AA)].[1] A link between prostate cancer and dietary fat intake, including excessive red meat and dairy product consumption, has also been suggested. With the discovery of the *BRCA1* and *BRCA2* genes related to breast and ovarian cancer, a genetic link with prostate cancer was also established. Men with one of these genetic mutations have an increased risk of developing prostate cancer.

Prevention

Although the American Cancer Society does not specifically address prevention of prostate cancer, prevention is not an unrealistic goal. Clearly, moderation of dietary fat intake is a preventive step. Increased dietary intake levels of vitamin E and the micronutrient selenium have been shown to play a preventive role in prostate cancer. In addition, effective treatment of benign prostatic hyperplasia (BPH) (prostate enlargement) with the drug Proscar (finasteride) has proven effective in preventing low-grade tumors in clinical trials.[26]

Early Detection

The symptoms of prostate disease, including prostate cancer, are listed in the Star box. A physician should be consulted if any of these symptoms appear, particularly in men aged 50 or older. Screening for prostate cancer should begin by age 40. This screening consists of an annual rectal examination performed by a physician and a blood test, the **prostate-specific antigen (PSA) test,** administered every 2 years. Although the initial version of

Key Terms
prostate-specific antigen (PSA) test a blood test used to identify prostate-specific antigen, an early indicator that the immune system has recognized and mounted a defense against prostate cancer

the PSA test was very successful in diagnosing prostate cancer, new, age-specific test values are now employed. These new interpretive standards allow increased specificity in determining risk. This said, however, the PSA test continues to deliver both false negative and false positive results. Currently debate is occurring within the medical community regarding the need to increase rigor (lower the upper limits of "normal") of PSA levels and, even more important, the need to look more closely at the suddenness at which levels increase.

Another version of the PSA test has also been developed. This test can identify the "free" antigen most closely associated with the more aggressive forms of prostate cancer, thus cutting down on the false positives and extensive use of biopsies. In addition, an ultrasound rectal examination is used in men whose PSA scores are abnormally high. In spite of the important contribution made by the PSA test, concern is being expressed about the possibility of overtreating 30 percent of men in the 60–84 age group, particularly in light of the side effects of treatment described below.[27]

Treatment

Today prostate cancer is treated surgically, or through the use of external radiation or the implantation of radioactive seeds (brachytherapy) into the gland, in combination with relatively short-term use of hormonal therapy. Of course, each form of treatment carries the potential for side effects, including an 80 percent chance of impotence over a 10-year period;[27] incontinence with surgery; diarrhea and tiredness with external radiation; some anal discomfort in association with the implantation of radioactive seeds into the prostate with internal radiation; and thinning of bones in conjunction with longer term hormone therapy.

One form of prostate cancer grows so slowly that men whose cancer is of this type, whose tumors are very localized, and whose life expectancy is less than 10 years at the time of diagnosis, do not receive treatment but rather are closely monitored for any progression of the cancer. For men who have the more aggressive form of the cancer, or whose tumor is no longer localized, physicians can employ a range of therapies, including surgery, radiation, chemotherapy, and hormonal therapy. In addition, an experimental vaccine has recently been tested on humans with promising results.[28] The 5-year survival rate for men with localized prostate cancer is very high. In terms of treatment type, the choice of treatment to be employed can be influenced by the physician being consulted. A recent survey of urologists and radiation oncologists found the urologists (who are surgeons) strongly favor a surgical approach, while radiologists favor radiation. Accordingly, second opinions and/or enrollment in clinical trials are highly recommended.

Changing for the Better

Testicular Self-Examination

I feel unsure about how to perform a testicular self-exam. What is the correct method?

Your best hope for early detection of testicular cancer is a simple 3-minute monthly self-examination. The following explains how to do a testicular self-examination. The best time is after a warm bath or shower, when the scrotal skin is most relaxed.

1. Roll each testicle gently between the thumb and fingers of both hands.
2. If you find any hard lumps or nodules, you should see your doctor promptly. They may not be malignant, but only your doctor can make the diagnosis.

After a thorough physical examination, your doctor may perform certain x-ray studies to make the most accurate diagnosis possible.

Monthly testicular self-examinations are as important for men as breast self-examinations are for women.

InfoLinks

www.mskcc.org/document/WICTEST.htm

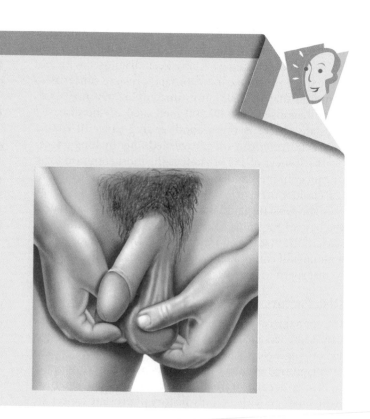

Testicular Cancer

Cancer of the testicle is among the least common forms of cancer; however, it is the most common solid tumor in men ages 15 to 34. Awareness of this type of cancer was raised in 1996 and 1997, when seven-time winner of the Tour de France Lance Armstrong and champion figure skater Scott Hamilton were diagnosed with testicular cancer. In both men, chronic fatigue and abdominal discomfort were the first symptoms of the disease. The American Cancer Society estimates that in 2005 testicular cancer was diagnosed in 8,010 men and caused the deaths of 390.[1]

Four forms of testicular cancer have been described: seminoma, teratoma, carcinoma, and choriocarcinoma. The most prevalent, seminoma, forms in the seminiferous tubules (where sperm originate) and is generally first observed during testicular self-examination as a small, hard mass on the side (or near the front) of the testicle. Fortunately, this form of testicular cancer is now highly curable.

Risk Factors

Risk factors for testicular cancer are variable, ranging from family history to environmental factors. The disease is more frequently seen in white Americans and in men whose testicles were undescended during childhood. Additional risk factors, such as difficulty during the mother's pregnancy, elevated temperature in the groin, and mumps during childhood, have been reported. The incidence of this cancer has been increasing in recent decades, while a corresponding drop in sperm levels has also been observed. Although no single explanation can be given for these changes, environmental factors such as agricultural pesticide toxicity may be involved. Once pesticides are concentrated in the tissues of the human body, during pregnancy they mimic estrogen. This, in turn, may lead to testicular dysgenesis syndrome, or the failure of the testicles to develop normally.[29]

Testicular cancer is more frequently seen among white-collar workers than among people in blue-collar occupations. The suspicion that testicular cancer is linked to vasectomies appears to be unfounded.

Prevention

Because risk factors for testicular cancer are so variable, prevention is limited to regular self-examination of the testicles. Symptoms such as fatigue, abdominal discomfort, and enlargement of the testicle should be reported to a physician, since these can be associated with other disease processes. A male infant with one or both testicles in the undescended position (resulting in an empty scrotum) should be seen promptly by a physician so that corrective procedures can be undertaken.

Early Detection

In addition to the fatigue and abdominal distress reported by both Armstrong and Hamilton, other symptoms of testicular cancer include a small, painless lump on the side or near the front of the testicle, a swollen or enlarged testicle, and a heaviness or dragging sensation in the groin or scrotum. The importance of testicular self-examination, as well as early diagnosis and prompt treatment, cannot be overemphasized for men in the at-risk age group of 15 to 34 years. The Changing for the Better box on page 354 explains how to perform a testicular self-examination.

Treatment

Depending on the type, stage, and degree of localization of the tumor, surgical intervention generally includes removal of the testicle, spermatic cord, and regional lymph nodes. Chemotherapy and radiation might also be used. Today, treatment is very effective, with 96 percent of all testicular cancer patients surviving 5 years and 99.4 percent surviving 5 years when the cancer was localized at the time of diagnosis.[1] It should be noted, however, that concern exists regarding the development of other forms of cancer, such as leukemia, later in life.

Colorectal Cancer

Cancer of the colon and rectum (colorectal cancer) cause the second greatest number of cancer deaths (56,290 in 2005), second only to lung cancer. In the most general sense, two types of tumors, carcinoma and lymphoma, can be found in both the colon and rectum. However, even within the most common form of colorectal cancer, there may subtle difference in type of tumors (or their origins) which influence the degree of potential spread and, thus, the nature of treatment itself. Fortunately, when diagnosed in a localized state, colorectal cancer has a relatively high survival rate (90 percent when localized, and 63 percent for all stages).[1]

Risk Factors

Underlying the development of colorectal cancer are at least two potentially important areas of risk: genetic susceptibility and dietary patterns. Genes have recently been discovered that lead to familial colon cancer and familial polyposis (abnormal tissue growth that occurs before the formation of cancer) and are believed to be responsible for the tendency of colorectal cancer to run in families. Dietary risk factors include diets that are high in saturated fat from red meat and low in fruits and vegetables, which contain antioxidant vitamins and fiber. In regard to fiber's ability to prevent colorectal cancer, however, the ability of dietary fiber, when taken in supplement form, is in question.

Prevention

Small outpouchings in the lower intestinal tract wall, called *polyps,* are frequently important in the eventual development of colorectal cancer. Prompt removal of polyps has been shown to lower the risk of colorectal cancer. Further, some evidence indicates that the development of colorectal cancer may be prevented or slowed through regular exercise, the regular use of low-dose (81 mg) aspirin (consistently for at least two decades), an increase in dietary calcium intake, and long-term folic acid supplementation. Additionally, oral contraceptive use may be protective for women.

Again, routine screening for colorectal cancer should be considered a form of prevention, much as PSA testing is for prostate cancer and mammography is for breast cancer.

Early Detection

Symptoms of colorectal cancer include bleeding from the rectum, blood in the stool, and a change in bowel habits. In addition, a family history of inflammatory bowel disease, polyp formation, or colorectal cancer should make one more alert to symptoms.[1] In people over age 50, any sudden change in bowel habits that lasts 10 days or longer should be evaluated by a physician. The American Cancer Society recommends preventive health care that includes digital (manual) rectal examination after age 40, a stool blood test after age 50, and sigmoidoscopy every 3 to 5 years and **colonoscopy** every 10 years after age 50. However, in March of 2005, the American College of Gastroenterology proposed that, because of the higher incidence of colorectal cancer in African Americans, routine colonoscopy should begin at age 45 for this group rather than at age 50.

Some experts question the advisability of using **sigmoidoscopy** as the routine screening procedure for colorectal cancer in comparison to using colonoscopy, which can more effectively find distal (higher up in the colon) cancerous changes.

Although colonoscopy is currently the "gold standard" in the screening for colorectal cancer, new technologies are on the horizon. Four alternatives include the Pre-Gen-Plus test that identifies cancer-indicating DNA mutations appearing in stool samples; a yet-named blood test capable of identifying "loss of imprinting" (LOI) factor associated with a high risk for colorectal cancer; virtual colonoscopy using a miniaturized camera that can, after being swallowed, be followed as it moves through the lower intestinal tract, generating digitized pictures of the entire colon; and CT colonography (CTC), which uses serial tomography (a form of CAT scan) to visualize the colon, thus eliminating the need to scope the colon.

It should be noted, that the digital stool-sample test, used as the only stool-sample test by most doctors and

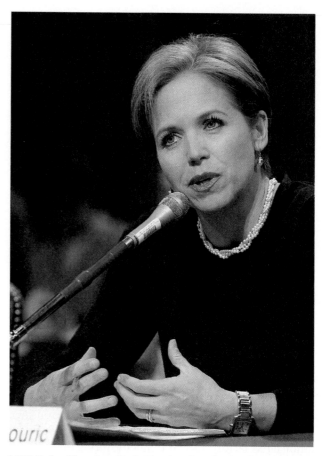

NBC Today Show host Katie Couric, whose husband died of colon cancer, testified on Capitol Hill March 6, 2000, before a Senate Special Committee on Aging hearing that focused on the importance of colorectal cancer screening tests. (AP Photo/Dennis Cook)

taken during physical examinations,[30] as well as the newer test to find traces of cancer cell DNA in the stool,[31] have both been found to be less effective than previously believed.

Treatment

When one or more of these screening procedures suggests the possibility of disease within the lower intestinal tract,

---

Key Terms

colonoscopy (co lun **os** ko py) examination of the entire length of the colon, using a flexible fiberoptic scope to inspect the structure's inner lining

sigmoidoscopy examination of the sigmoid colon (lowest section of the large intestine), using a short, flexible fiberoptic scope a careful visual evaluation of the entire length of the colon will be undertaken. During colonoscopy, areas of concern can be biopsied and the presence of a malignancy confirmed. Upon diagnosis, a localized and noninvasive malignancy will be removed surgically. When an invasive tumor is identified, supportive treatment with radiation or chemotherapy is necessary. Metastatic cancer requires chemotherapy. New guidelines regarding screening for metastatic tumors arising from a primary colorectal cancer are being formulated. These guidelines are meant to remind physicians that metastatic tumors are unlikely to be found through use of colonoscopy.

Pancreatic Cancer

Pancreatic cancer is one of the most lethal forms of cancer, with a survival rate of only 4 percent 5 years after diagnosis.[1] Because of this gland's important functions in both digestion and metabolic processes related to glucose utilization, its destruction by a malignancy leaves the body in a state incompatible with living.

In 2005 an estimated 32,180 new cases of pancreatic cancer were diagnosed, and 31,800 deaths occurred.[1]

Risk Factors

Pancreatic cancer is more common in men than women, occurs more frequently with age, and develops most often in African American men. Smoking is clearly a risk factor for this form of cancer, with smokers more than twice as likely to develop the disease. Other risk factors have been tentatively suggested, such as chronic inflammation of the pancreas (pancreatitis), diabetes mellitus, alcohol-induced liver deterioration (cirrhosis), obesity, and high-fat diets.[1] Relatively little else is known about risk factors and, thus, prevention.

Prevention

Not smoking and abstaining from alcohol use are the most effective steps toward preventing this form of cancer. Further, reducing the risk of type 2 diabetes mellitus, through weight loss and exercise, would also make an important contribution to prevention. Annual medical examinations are, of course, associated with overall cancer prevention.

Early Detection

Early detection of this cancer is difficult because of the absence of symptoms until late in its course. Perhaps for people with a history of chronic pancreatitis, physicians might consider routine ultrasound assessment or computerized axial tomography scans (CAT scans). Once symptoms appear, a biopsy is performed.

Treatment

At this time there is no effective treatment for pancreatic cancer. Surgical removal of malignant sites within the gland, in addition to radiation and chemotherapy, is usually tried. Certainly, if a particular patient with pancreatic cancer qualifies, enrollment in a clinical trial would be worth consideration.

Lymphatic Cancer

In 1996 sports fans were saddened by the news that National Hockey League great Mario Lemieux had been diagnosed with cancer of the lymphatic system, the basis of the body's immune capabilities. Lemieux's cancer was Hodgkin's disease, a form of lymphoma. Following treatment in 1996, he appears to be in complete remission. In fact, in 2001 he resumed his playing career, but has since retired.

An estimated 63,740 new cases of lymphoma (7,350 cases of Hodgkin's disease and 56,390 cases of non-Hodgkin's lymphoma) were diagnosed in 2005. The number of deaths from both forms of lymphoma was near 20,610.[1] The incidence of Hodgkin's disease has declined over the last 30 years, while the incidence of non-Hodgkin's disease has nearly doubled, but is now holding steady.[1]

Risk Factors

Risk factors for lymphoma are difficult to determine. Some possible factors are a general reduction in immune protection, exposure to toxic environmental chemicals such as pesticides and herbicides, and viral infections. As you will learn in Chapter 13, the virus that causes AIDS (HIV) is a leukemia/lymphoma virus that was initially called HTLV-III (human T-cell leukemia/lymphoma virus-type III). A related leukemia/lymphoma virus, HTLV-I, is also suspected in the development of lymphatic cancer. The Epstein-Barr (EBV) virus may also play a role in lymphatic cancer development.

Prevention

Beyond limiting exposure to toxic chemicals and sexually transmitted viruses, few recommendations can be made about prevention. Again, early detection and diagnosis can serve as a form of prevention, since early-stage cancer is more survivable than advanced disease.

Early Detection

Unlike other cancers, the early symptoms of lymphoma are diverse and similar to symptoms of other illnesses, most of which are not serious. These symptoms include enlarged lymph nodes (frequently a sign of any infection that the immune system is fighting), fever, itching, weight loss, and anemia.

Treatment

Although surgery (beyond a biopsy) is usually not associated with the treatment of lymphoma, a variety of other therapies are employed. Depending on the stage and type of lymphoma, therapy may involve only radiation treatment of localized lymph nodes, as is seen in non-Hodgkin's lymphoma. Radiation combined with chemotherapy is generally used in the treatment of late-stage non-Hodgkin's lymphoma. More recently, other therapies, including more aggressive chemotherapy, monoclonal antibody therapy, and bone marrow and stem cell transplantation, have been employed.

After completion of therapy, 1-year survival rates for Hodgkin's disease are near 95 percent and near 77 percent for non-Hodgkin's lymphoma. By the end of 5 years, these rates have dropped to 84 percent and 55 percent, respectively.[1] Lower rates of survival are seen at 10 years and beyond.

Skin Cancer

Thanks largely to our desire for a fashionable tan, many teens and adults have spent more time in the sun (and in tanning booths) than their skin can tolerate. As a result, skin cancer, once common only among people who had to work in the sun, is occurring with alarming frequency. In 2005, more than 1 million Americans developed basal or squamous cell skin cancer, and 59,580 cases of highly dangerous malignant melanoma were diagnosed.[1]

Deaths from skin cancer do occur, with 10,590 estimated in 2005. More than 80 percent of these deaths were the result of malignant melanoma.

Risk Factors

Severe sunburning during childhood and chronic sun exposure during adolescence and younger adulthood are largely responsible for the "epidemic" of skin cancer being reported. The current emphasis on screening for skin cancer may also be increasing the incidence of early-stage cancer being reported. Progress is being made in deterring people from pursuing the perfect tan. The American Academy of Dermatology reports that the incidence of deliberate tanning is down, and the use of sunscreens has increased. Occupational exposure to some hydrocarbon compounds can also cause skin cancer.

In spite of the progress reported by the American Academy of Dermatology, Americans continue to seek natural sources of sun or tanning salons for cosmetically related tanning, or they find that their exposure cannot be avoided owing to the nature of their jobs. In regard to "purposeful tanning" either outdoors or indoors, recent research has given some creditability to the contention that tanning is emotionally "addictive."[32] Researchers are now beginning to see this factor as a detrimental player in ongoing efforts to persuade the public to increase their avoidance of ultraviolet radiation exposure.

For those who must or choose to seek extended periods of time in the sun, the most recently established UV (ultraviolet) Index, The New Global Solar UV Index, can

The New Global Solar UV Index	
Exposure category	**Index number**
Low	1–2
Moderate	3–5
High	6–7
Very high	8–10
Extreme	11+
Source: EPA	

be found above. This daily index for your ZIP code (in the United States) can be accessed online at www.epa.gov/sunwise/uvindex.html. It is also often given on local television stations or in some local newspapers.

Prevention

Prevention of skin cancer should be a high priority for people who enjoy the sun or must work outdoors. The use of sunscreen with a sun protection factor (SPF) of 15 or greater is very important. In addition, parents can help their children prevent skin cancer later in life by restricting their outdoor play from 11:00 A.M. to 2:00 P.M., requiring them to wear hats that shade their faces, and applying a sunscreen with an SPF of 15 regardless of skin tone. An evaluation of sunscreen effectiveness studies by Sloan-Kettering Cancer Center, however, suggests that sunscreens provide little protection against the deeply penetrating UV-A rays associated with the development of melanoma in susceptible people, and less protection than once thought against the UV-B rays associated with burning and wrinkling of the skin. Practicing dermatologists nonetheless continue to recommend their use. Regardless of the extent to which sunscreens provide protection, users are reminded that the level of protection provided is not doubled by simply doubling the SPF—for example, a sunscreen carrying an SPF of 30 does not provide twice the protection provided by a product with an SPF of 15. Therefore, the compliant use of a SPF-15 product is deemed not only appropriate but can also save money over the more expensive products with a higher SPF rating.

A further rationale for preventing the development of skin cancer is the recently described relationship between skin cancer and the heightened probability of developing other forms of cancer later in life. Research suggests that people who have had skin cancer carry a 20–30 percent greater risk of developing other types of cancer than do people who have never developed skin cancer.[33] (The Personal Assessment on page 367 will help you determine your risk of developing this kind of cancer.)

Self-Examination for Melanoma

Through a routine physical exam, my brother found out he has melanoma. How should I check myself for this condition?

How to look for melanoma

1. Examine your body front and back in the mirror, then right and left sides with arms raised.

2. Bend your elbows and carefully look at your palms, forearms, and under your upper arms.

3. Look at the backs of your legs and feet, the spaces between your toes, and the soles of your feet.

4. Examine the back of your neck and scalp with a hand mirror. Part your hair for a closer look.

5. Finally, check your back and buttocks with a mirror.

What to look for
Potential signs of malignancy in moles or pigmented spots:

Asymmetry
One half unlike the other half

Irregularity
Border irregular or poorly defined

Color
Color varies from one area to another; shades of tan, brown, or black

Size
Diameter larger than 6 mm, as a rule (diameter of a pencil eraser)

Early Detection

Although many doctors do not emphasize this point enough, the key to the successful treatment of skin cancer is early detection. For basal cell or squamous cell cancer, a pale, waxlike, pearly nodule or red, scaly patch may be the first symptom. Other types of skin cancer may be indicated by a gradual change in the appearance of an existing mole. A physician should be consulted if such a change is noted. Melanoma usually begins as a small, molelike growth that increases progressively in size, changes color, ulcerates, and bleeds easily. To help detect melanoma, the American Cancer Society recommends using the guidelines below:

A is for asymmetry.

B is for border irregularity.

C is for color (change).

D is for a diameter greater than 6 mm.

E is for elevation (raised margins).

Figure 11-4 shows a mole that would be considered harmless and one that clearly demonstrates the ABCDE characteristics just described. (Changing for the Better shows how to make a regular inspection of the skin.)

Most recently, a relationship between the presence of abnormal moles, called *dysplastic nevi* (flat, irregularly shaped, mottled in color, with irregular edges), and the risk of developing malignant melanoma has been established. By counting these "indicator moles," physicians can judge the relative risk of developing this serious form of skin cancer before it first appears.

A   B

Figure 11-4 **A:** Normal mole. This type of lesion is often seen in large numbers on the skin of young adults and can affect any body site. Note its symmetrical shape, regular borders, uniform color, and relatively small size (about 6 millimeters). **B:** Malignant melanoma. Note its asymmetrical shape, irregular borders, uneven color, and relatively large size (about 2 centimeters).

Treatment

When nonmelanoma skin cancer is found, an almost 100 percent cure rate can be expected. Treatment of these skin cancers can involve surgical removal by traditional excising or laser vaporization, destruction by burning or freezing, or destruction using x-ray therapy. When the more serious melanomas are found at an early stage, a high cure rate (95 percent) is accomplished using the same techniques. However, when malignant melanomas are more advanced, extensive surgery and chemotherapy are necessary. The 5-year survival rate for regionalized forms of the disease drops to 60 percent, and, unfortunately, long-term disease recovery is uncommon (16 percent).[1]

However, a new treatment for malignant melanoma offers a ray of hope to people with the disease. Among the more promising of these is a combination therapy using interleukin-2, an immune system chemical that stimulates various "killer cells" within the immune system and a drug that activates phagocyctic cells within the immune system. Additionally, a vaccine has been developed that stimulates the immune system to attack the melanoma cells more aggressively. This treatment-centered (rather than prevention-centered) vaccine uses components of the patient's own cancer cells to mobilize more white blood cells and produce more antibodies to fight the cancer.

The Future of Cancer Prevention, Diagnosis, and Treatment

It has been over 35 years since President Nixon (1971) declared a national "War On Cancer," and today the results are both encouraging and discouraging. On the positive side

Cancer's Seven Warning Signals

Listed below are the seven warning signs of cancer, which the acronym CAUTION will help you remember:

1. **C**hange in bowel or bladder habits
2. **A** sore that does not heal
3. **U**nusual bleeding or discharge
4. **T**hickening or lump in the breast or elsewhere
5. **I**ndigestion or difficulty in swallowing
6. **O**bvious change in a wart or mole
7. **N**agging cough or hoarseness

If you have a warning signal for more than 5 days, see your doctor!

impressive technological advances have been and continue to be made in the diagnosis and treatment of cancer. As mentioned throughout the chapter, new screening procedures as well as treatment protocols seem to appear at a consistent rate. Additionally, the death rates from a variety of cancers have fallen, including a 70 percent decrease in the rate for Hodgkin's disease and a 14 percent decline in the death rate for breast cancer. Death rates for cervical, stomach, uterine, colon, bladder, and thyroid cancers have also fallen. Particularly important is a general increase in the public's awareness of cancer prevention and early detection.

On the negative side is the reality that cancer is not only a biological disease but also a disease (or more than 100 diseases) with strong sociopolitical implications. Central to this area are factors such as the inability of the majority of Americans to make needed changes in lifestyle in regard to smoking, alcohol use, exercise, weight management, and dietary practices. Also impeding progress is the absence of health care insurance for 45 million Americans, which prevents early diagnosis and treatment of cancer. In fact, virtually every cancer in adults is negatively affected by one or more of these largely modifiable complicating factors.

In addition to factors such as the lack of health insurance for millions of Americans and the inability (or unwillingness) of large segments of the American population to modify current lifestyles, a third force, the federal government, is also potentially negatively affecting the war against cancer. In letter dated January 25, 2005, a coalition of 40 organizations working to win the cancer war (including the American Cancer Society, the American College of Surgeons, and the Cancer Research and Prevention Foundation) called on the President to reconsider his planned overall cut in the Fiscal Year 2006 budget of the National Cancer Institute (NCI). The coalition, *One Voice Against Cancer,* reminded the administration that the NCI's goal of eliminating death and suffering from cancer by 2015 will incur egregious damage from a yearly parade of budget reductions.[34]

Facing a cancer diagnosis can be overwhelming. Your stress levels may skyrocket. You may be asking yourself questions such as how you'll be able to deal with uncertainty about your future, the unpredictability of the disease, disability, and the emotions you're feeling. Spiritual resources can help you cope with your health changes and ease the difficult journey that is just beginning.

In addition to traditional religious aids such as prayer, trusting and supportive relationships with people can help you find the emotional resilience to bounce back from the daily challenges of living with a life-threatening illness. Perhaps most significant is an individual or group—from a church or synagogue or from the secular community—that provides spiritual and emotional support. When you and your family affiliate with a local or online cancer support group, for example, the mutual sharing based on a common experience can be uplifting in constructing a secular "community of faith." You and your loved ones can obtain strength and direction in reaching out to others who possess an empathetic understanding of the disease. You won't feel as though you're facing hardships alone. Becoming open to assistance and gaining acceptance of your illness can lead to a sense of inner peace and a willingness to explore new interests and abilities.

In addition, you may reduce stress and find spiritual fulfillment in looking outward to focused involvement with other persons who need assistance, children, or pets. Care-giving activities offer you a renewed sense of value of your own ability to stay healthy and functional while providing a constructive emotional escape from the demands placed on you by your illness. Even as you must accept new physical limitations, you can maintain a sense of self-reliance and a positive spiritual and emotional outlook on life.

In the final analysis, the "war" remains very challenging: progress is being made, setbacks occur, and the victory remains far from being in hand. The "Big C" remains.

Prevention through Risk Reduction

Because cancer will probably continue to be the second most common cause of death among all adults, you should explore ways to reduce your risk of developing cancer. The following factors, which could make you vulnerable to cancer, can be controlled or at least recognized.

- *Know your family history.* You are the recipient of the genetic strengths and weaknesses of your biological parents and your more distant relatives. If you are able to determine that cancer is prevalent in your family medical history, you cannot afford to disregard this fact. It may be appropriate for you to be screened for certain types of cancer more often or at a young age. The importance of family history was clearly seen in our discussion of the *BRCA1/BRCA2* inheritance pattern and related decisions about prophylactic mastectomy and prophylactic oophorectomy.

- *Select and monitor your occupation carefully.* Because of recently discovered relationships between cancer and occupations that bring employees into contact with carcinogenic agents, you must be aware of the risks posed by certain job selections and assignments. Worksites where you will come into frequent contact with pesticides, strong solvents, volatile hydrocarbons, and airborne fibers could pay well but also shorten your life. The importance of this point is evident in reviewing the current list of environmental carcinogens studies funded by the National Cancer Institute. Included are studies that focus on indoor air pollution (tobacco smoke and cooking oils), dust (cotton, grain, plastic, and wood), organic solvents (benzene, carbon tetrachloride, toluene, xylene, and chlordane), organophosphates (diazinon, dichlorvos, malathion, triazines, and cyaniazine), polybrominated biphenyls, polychlorinated biphenyls, fumigants (ethylene), water pollution (chloride, phosphene, and fluoride), petroleum products (diesel fuel, gasoline, jet fuel), radiation (radon, neutron therapy, and reactor accidents), biological agents (chlamydia, HIV/HPV, helicobacter, hepatitis B and C) and radioisotopes (iodine and radium).

- *Do not use tobacco products.* You may want to review Chapter 9 on the overwhelming evidence linking all forms of tobacco use (including smokeless tobacco) to the development of cancer. Smoking, along with obesity, is so detrimental to health that it is considered a co-number-one preventable cause of death.

- *Monitor environmental exposure to carcinogens.* When one considers carcinogenic concerns related to types of employment, residential radon levels, ozone depletion leading to increased exposure to solar radiation, and environmental tobacco smoke (Chapter 9), one realizes that the environment holds great potential as a source of carcinogenic exposure. To the extent to which it is possible to select the environment in which you will reside, work, and recreate, you should add selecting a low-risk environment to your list of cancer-prevention activities.

- *Follow a sound diet.* As mentioned in conjunction with folic acid and colorectal cancer and high-fat diets and prostate cancer, dietary patterns are known to play both a causative and a preventive role in cancer. (Review Chapter 5 for information about dietary practices and the incidence of various diseases,

The Macrobiotic Diet

As common and potentially serious as cancer is, it is not a condition likely to be treated exclusively with alternative therapies. However, the use of a *macrobiotic diet* has been used by some cancer patients with anecdotal reports of success.

When the macrobiotic diet was introduced into the United States from Asia in the 1960s, it was first viewed as nutritionally deficient in comparison to all recognized forms of dietary intake, including the more restrictive forms of vegan vegetarianism. Central to the diet was the extensive (if not total) reliance on brown rice, seaweed, and a fish-based gruel. It also involved restrictions regarding food preparation, such as the type of cookware to be used.

Today the typical macrobiotic diet has been nutritionally enhanced to derive 50% of its calories from whole grains, 25–30% from vegetables, 5–10% from soups of various types, and 5–10% from beans and sea vegetables. It also features highly specific "macrobiotic" lifestyle guidelines, such as when eating is to occur, the rate at which food is to be chewed, hours of sleep required, and restrictions on the types of clothing materials and cosmetics to be used. This complex program must be learned through careful study at an organization such as the Kushi Institute, established by Michio Kushi, who introduced macrobiotics into this country from Japan.

In an attempt to evaluate the merits of the macrobiotic diet, studies of macrobiotic-based cancer treatment plans were funded by the National Center for Complementary and Alternative Medicine (NCCAM) in 1993—one at the University of Minnesota (directed by Michio Kushi's son) and a second at the University of Colorado (Denver). On February 25, 2002, the NCCAM Advisory Committee and researchers met for an initial assessment of the macrobiotic diet study. During the meeting, nine Best Case Series (BCS) participant reports from an initial group of 18 participants were reviewed, and 6 participants gave personal accounts to the review panel. From these sources of information, serious methodological flaws were noted, including a virtual absence of medical records and X-rays on any of the 9 participants, the variety of ways in which diets were composed and prepared, and the absence of any oncology-based assessment before or during the study period. Of 6 participants that addressed the committee, all 6 reported (and demonstrated on assessments) an improved quality of life, while 2 had apparently lived longer than generally expected for persons with their forms of cancer. For the remaining 4 participants, survivability expectations could not be determined.

In light of the use of the Best Case Series format and the absence of various controls, the conclusion reached by the advisory committee was for continuation of the study using a prospective model involving approximately 30 subjects, including a methodology that minimized the concerns regarding medical assessment, standardization of the diet, assessment of compliance, medical assessment of the patients' malignancy status at selected time intervals, and each participant's final outcome.

InfoLinks

www.macrobiotics.org/whatmacro.html

---

including cancer. In that chapter, the role of fruits and vegetables known to be sources of cancer-preventing phytochemicals is introduced. Good sources include a wide variety of fruits and vegetables, particularly the cruciferous vegetables, including cauliflower, broccoli, and brussels sprouts, and fruits high in beta-carotene, vitamin C, and fiber.)

Should research demonstrate an even clearer role for nutrients, **chemoprevention** may become an even more widely practiced component of cancer prevention (see Considering Complementary Care above). Chemoprevention is not limited to food items and dietary supplements but can also involve pharmaceutical agents, such as aspirin, estrogen replacement therapy, and hormone replacement therapy.

- *Control your body weight.* For women, obesity is related to a higher incidence of cancer of the uterus, ovary, and breast because obesity correlates with high estrogen levels. Maintaining a desirable body weight could improve overall health and lead to more successful management of cancer should it develop. Additionally, consider carefully whether you want to follow the currently popular high-protein, high-fat diets (Chapter 6), given their recognized carcinogenic potential.

- *Exercise regularly.* Chapter 4 discusses in detail the importance of regular moderate exercise to all aspects of health, including reducing the risk of chronic illnesses. Moderate exercise increases the body's ability to deliver oxygen to its tissues and thus to reduce the formation of cancer-enhancing free radicals formed

Key Terms

chemoprevention cancer prevention using food, food supplements, and medications thought to bolster the immune system or reduce the damage caused by carcinogens during incomplete oxidation of nutrients. Moderate exercise also stimulates the production of enzymes that remove free radicals.

- *Limit your exposure to the sun.* It is important to heed this message even if you enjoy many outdoor activities. Particularly for people with light complexions, the radiation received through chronic exposure to the sun may foster the development of skin cancer.
- *Consume alcohol in moderation, if at all.* People who consume a lot of alcohol have an increased prevalence of several types of cancer, including cancer of the oral cavity, larynx, and esophagus. Whether this results directly from the presence of carcinogens in alcohol or is more closely related to the alcohol user's tendency to smoke has not yet been established.

Cancer and Wellness

When you carefully consider the preceding suggestions, you will clearly see that you can do a great deal to prevent or at least minimize the development of cancer. A wellness-oriented lifestyle is the best weapon in your "personal war against cancer." However, all risk factor reduction is relative. Observation and experience tell us that life cannot be totally structured around the desire to achieve maximum longevity or reduce morbidity at all costs. Most people need to strike a balance between life that is emotionally, socially, and spiritually satisfying and life that is structured solely for the purpose of living a long time and minimizing exposure to illness. Regardless of our personal lifestyles, however, we can educate others, provide comfort and support to those who are living with cancer, and support the funding of continuing and innovative new cancer research.

 Taking Charge of Your Health

- Stay attuned to media reports about cancer so that you can make informed choices.
- Support agencies devoted to the prevention of cancer.

- Monitor your work, home, and recreational environments to determine whether they are placing you at risk for cancer.
- Perform regular self-examinations for forms of cancer that can be detected through these techniques.

- Undergo the recommended cancer screening procedures for your age and sex.
- If you have cancer, participate actively in your own treatment.

SUMMARY

- More than 1.25 million people in the United States develop cancer each year.
- Cancer is a condition in which the body is unable to control the specialization, replication, and repair of cells or the suppression of abnormal cell formation.
- Genes that control the replication, specialization, and repair of cells and the suppression of abnormal cellular activity have the potential to become oncogenes and thus can be considered proto-oncogenes.
- A variety of agents, including genetic mutations, viruses, and carcinogens, stimulate the conversion of regulatory genes (proto-oncogenes) into oncogenes.
- Cancer can be described on the basis of the type of tissue from which it originates and on the basis of its location within the body.
- Cigarette smoking and genetic predisposition are both related to the development of lung cancer.
- Most cases of breast cancer do not demonstrate a clear familial pattern that suggests a genetic predisposition, although some do.

- Long-term exposure to high levels of estrogen is an important risk factor for breast cancer.
- Mammograms are an important component of breast cancer identification. Drugs capable of preventing breast cancer are available; however, their use is being carefully studied.
- Regular use of Pap tests is related to the early detection of cervical cancer. Sexually transmitted viral infections are strongly suspected of causing cervical cancer.
- For women at high risk of HPV infections, screening for infections may be as effective in cervical cancer detection as the Pap test.
- Uterine (endometrial) cancer is more common than cervical cancer. High levels of estrogen are strongly associated with this form of cancer.
- A group of women who are the daughters of mothers given the drug DES during pregnancy have a high incidence of vaginal cancer.
- Ovarian cancer is often "silent" in its presentation of symptoms.
- The excessively long use of HRT is a strongly suspected cause of uterine cancer.

- Prostate cancer is the second leading cause of cancer deaths in men.
- The PSA test improves the ability to diagnose prostate cancer. Age, high-fat diets, and inheritance of a mutated suppressor gene are known risk factors.
- Regular self-examination of the testicles leads to early detection of testicular cancer. Environmental factors may be associated with an increasing rate of testicular cancer.
- Colorectal cancer has a strong familial link and is seen in populations that consume diets high in fat and low in fruits and vegetables. Polyp formation is associated with an increased risk of this form of cancer.
- Colonoscopy is the most effective method of detecting polyps and colorectal cancers.
- Pancreatic cancer is very difficult to survive, in part because of the absence of symptoms early in the disease's course.

- Lymphatic cancers display a wide array of initial symptoms that reflect failure of the immune system to function fully. Viral infections and environmental toxins are suspected causative agents.
- Basal cell and squamous cell carcinomas are highly curable forms of skin cancer when detected early. Malignant melanoma is life threatening if not detected early.
- Skin cancer prevention requires protection from excessive ultraviolet ray exposure.
- Early detection based on self-examination and screening is the basis for the identification and successful treatment of many cancers.
- Risk reduction, through living a wellness lifestyle, remains at the heart of cancer prevention.

REVIEW QUESTIONS

1. What is the relationship between regulatory genes and tumor suppressor genes in the development of cancer? Why are regulatory genes called both proto-oncogenes and oncogenes?
2. What properties do cancer cells possess that are lacking in normal cells?
3. What are some of the major types of cancer, based on the tissue from which they originate? What are some of the more familiar cancers based on organ of origin?
4. What are the principal factors that contribute to the development of lung cancer? Of breast cancer? What is prophylactic mastectomy and who might consider its use?
5. When should regular use of mammography begin, and which women should begin using it earliest?
6. What important information can be obtained with the use of Pap tests? What innovations are associated with the ThinPrep Pap Test?

7. Why is ovarian cancer described as a "silent" cancer?
8. How does the PSA test contribute to the early detection of prostate cancer?
9. What are the steps for effective self-examination of the breasts and testicles? What is the current status of breast self-examination?
10. What signs indicate the possibility that a skin lesion has become cancerous?
11. Why is pancreatic cancer among the most lethal of all cancers?
12. What is now known about the effectiveness of the macrobiotic diet as a cancer treatment?
13. What are the risk reduction activities identified in this chapter?

ENDNOTES

1. American Cancer Society. *Cancer Facts & Figures 2005.* American Cancer Society, 2005.
2. *Number of Americans Without Insurance Reaches Highest Level on Record.* Center on Budget and Policy Priorities. August 27, 2004. www.cbpp.org/8-26-04health.htm.
3. *Estimated Cancer Cases and Deaths by Sex, for All Sites, US, 2005.* American Cancer Society, 2005. www.cancer.org/ docroot/MED/content/downloads/MED_1_1xOFF2005_ Estimated_New_Cases_Death_by_Sex_USasp.
4. Rieger PT. The biology of cancer genetics. 2004. *Semin Oncol Nursing.* Aug; 20(3):145–154.
5. Gilley D, Tanaka H, Herbert BS. Tolmere dysfunction in aging and cancer. 2005. *Int J Biochem Cell Biol.* May; 37(5): 1000–1013.
6. Bertino JR (Ed.). *Encyclopedia of Cancer* (2nd ed.) (Vols 1–4.). Philadelphia: Academic Press, 2002.

7. Pope CA, et al. Lung cancer, cardiopulmonary mortality and long-term exposure to fine particulate air pollution. *JAMA,* 2002; 287(9):1132–1141.
8. Djousse L, et al. Alcohol consumption and risk of lung cancer: The Framingham Study. *J Natl Cancer Inst;* 2002, 94(24):1877–1882.
9. Nemunaitis J, et al. Granulocyte-marcophage colony-stimulating factor gene-modified autologous tumor vaccines in non-small-cell lung cancer. *J Natl Cancer Inst.* 2004; 96(4):326–331.
10. Collaborative Group on Hormonal Factors in Breast Cancer. Breast cancer and breast-feeding reanalysis of individual data from 47 epidemiological studies in 30 countries, including 50,302 women with the disease. *Lancet.* 2002. 360(9328):203–210.

11. Chlebowski RT. Influence of estrogen plus progestin on breast cancer and mammography in healthy post-menopausal women: The Women's Health Initiative Randomized Trial. *JAMA*. 2003. 289(24):3243–3253.

12. Folsom AR, et al. Association of general and abdominal obesity with multiple health outcomes in older women: The Iowa Women's Health Study. *Arch Intern Med*. 2000. 160(14): 2117–2128.

13. Krainer M, et al. Differential contributions of *BRCA1* and *BRCA2* to early-onset breast cancer. *N Engl J Med*. 1997. 336(20):1416–1421.

14. McClain MR, et al. Adjusting the estimated proportion of breast cancer cases associated with *BRAC1* and *BRCA2* mutations: Public health implications. *Genet Med* 2005. Jan; 7(1):28–33.

15. Spear SL, Carter ME, Schwarz K. Prophylactic mastectomy: Indications, options, and reconstruction alternatives. *Plast Reconstr Surg*. 2005. 115(3):891–909.

16. Freedman AN, et al. Estimates of the number of U.S. women who could benefit from tamoxifen for breast cancer prevention. *J Natl Cancer Inst*. 2003. 95(7):526–532.

17. Smith R. Breast self-exam is too valuable to discard, experts say. *ACS News Center*. 2001. June 28. www.cancer.org/NWS/content/update/NWS_1_1xU_Breast_Self_Exam_Is_T...

18. McDonald S, Saslow D, Alciati MH. Performance and reporting of clinical breast examination: A review of the literature. 2004. *CA Cancer J Clin*. 54(6):345–361.

19. Henderson IC. Aromatase inhibitors in the management of early breast cancer: Optimizing the clinical benefit. *Semin Oncol*. 2004. 31(6 Suppl 12):31–34.

20. Harper DM, et al. Efficacy of a bivalent L1 viruslike particle vaccine in prevention of infection with human papillomavirus 16 and 18 in young women: A randomized controlled trial. *Lancet*. 2004. 364(9447):1757–1765.

21. American Cancer society. Cancer *Facts & Figures 2003*. American Cancer Society, 2003.

22. Horn-Ross PL, et al. Phytoestrogen intake and endometrial cancer risk. *J Natl Cancer Inst*. 2003. 95(15):1158–1164.

23. Hatch EE, et al. Incidence of squamous neoplasia of the cervix and vagina in women exposed prenatally to dietrhylstilbestrol (United States). *Cancer Causes Control*. 2001. 12(9):837–845.

24. Folson AR, Anderson JP, Ross JA. Estrogen replacement therapy and ovarian cancer. *Epidemiology*. 2004. 15(1):100–104.

25. Yawn BP, Barrette BA, Wollan PC. Ovarian cancer: The neglected diagnosis. *Mayo Clin Proc*. 2004. 79(10):1277–1282.

26. Thompson IM, et al. The influence of finasteride on the development of prostate cancer. *N Engl J Med*. 2003. 349(3):215–224.

27. Etzioni R, et al. Overdiagnosis due to prostate-specific antigen screening: Lessons from U.S. prostate cancer incidence trends. *J Natl Cancer Inst*. 2002. 94(3):981–990.

28. Fong L, Small EJ. Immunotherapy for prostate cancer. *Semin Oncol*. 2003. 30(5):649–658.

29. Brucker-Davis F, Pointis G, Fenichel P. Update on cryptorchidism: Endocrine, environmental, and therapeutic aspects. *Endocrinol Invest*. 2003. 26(6):575–587.

30. Collins JF, et al. Accuracy of screening for fecal occult blood on a single stool sample obtained by digital rectal examination: a comparison with recommended sampling practice. *Ann Intern Med*. 2005. 142(2):81–85.

31. Imperiale TF, et al. Fecal DNA versus fecal occult blood for coleroctal-cancer screening in an average-risk population. *N Engl J Med*. 2004. 351(26):2704–2714.

32. Feldman SR, et al. Ultraviolet exposure is a reinforcing stimulus in frequent indoor tanners. *Am Acad Dermatol*. 2004. 51(1):45–51.

33. Rosenberg CA, et al. Association of nonmelanoma skin cancer with second maligance. *Cancer*. 2004. 100(1):130–138.

34. *January 25, 2005, Letter to The Honorable George W. Bush*. One Voice Against Cancer. www.dragonflydc.com/ovac/link.html

As We Go to Press

Over the past three decades the 5-year survival rate for breast cancer has clearly improved, with 97 percent of women diagnosed with localized tumors alive at 5 years following the end of treatment in comparison to 91 percent in the 1970s. For women with regional involvement at diagnosis, today 80 percent are alive after 5 years in comparison to 68 percent during the earlier period. This improvement in survival rate raises the question whether it is the result of better treatment or earlier diagnosis, when tumors are smaller and more likely localized.

To test this question, researchers examined 260,000 excised breast tumors. When survival data were adjusted for tumor size and localization versus regionalization, the roles of tumor size and treatment advances could be more clearly determined. For example, for women with small localized tumors (1 centimeter or less) 61 percent of the increase in survivability was accounted for by the improved ability to identify more tumors earlier than was previously possible. For localized tumors that were larger (2.5 centimeters or larger) at diagnosis, 50 percent of the improvement in survivability was due to earlier diagnosis. When regionalized tumors were examined, a similar pattern was seen with 76 percent of the improved survivability accounted for by earlier diagnosis—a result most pronounced in women 65 years of age and older.

In the final analysis, there is no question that treatment modalities have improved over the last 30 years. However, the role of earlier diagnosis has been more important, and the availability and utilization of mammography is the single salient factor.

personal assessment

Are you at risk for skin, breast, or cervical cancer?

Some people may have a higher than average risk of developing particular types of cancer. These people can be identified by certain risk factors.

This simple self-testing method is designed by the American Cancer Society to help you assess your risk factors for three common types of cancer. These are the major risk factors but by no means represent the only ones that might be involved.

Check your response to each risk factor. Add the numbers in the parentheses to arrive at a total score for each cancer type. Find out what your score means by reading the information in the "Interpretation" section. You are advised to discuss the information with your physician if you are at a higher risk.

Skin Cancer

1. Frequent work or play in the sun
   - A. Yes (10)
   - B. No (1)

2. Work in mines, around coal tars, or around radioactivity
   - A. Yes (10)
   - B. No (1)

3. Complexion—fair skin or light skin
   - A. Yes (10)
   - B. No (1)

YOUR TOTAL POINTS _____

Explanation

1. Excessive ultraviolet light causes skin cancer. Protect yourself with a sunscreen.
2. These materials can cause skin cancer.
3. Light complexions need more protection than others.

Interpretation

Numerical risks for skin cancer are difficult to state. For instance, a person with a dark complexion can work longer in the sun and be less likely to develop cancer than can a light-complected person. Furthermore, a person wearing a long-sleeved shirt and a wide-brimmed hat may work in the sun and be less at risk than is a person who wears a bathing suit and stays in the sun for only a short period. The risk increases greatly with age.

The key here is if you answered "yes" to any question, you need to realize that you have above-average risk.

Breast Cancer

1. Age group
   - A. 20–34 (10)
   - B. 35–49 (40)
   - C. 50 and over (90)

2. Race/nationality
   - A. Asian American (5)
   - B. African American (20)
   - C. White (25)
   - D. Mexican American (10)

3. Family history of breast cancer
   - A. Mother, sister, or grandmother (30)
   - B. None or unknown (10)

4. Your history
   - A. No breast disease (10)
   - B. Previous noncancerous lumps or cysts (25)
   - C. Previous breast cancer (100)

5. Maternity
   - A. First pregnancy before age 25 (10)
   - B. First pregnancy after age 25 (15)
   - C. No pregnancies (20)

YOUR TOTAL POINTS _____

Interpretation

Under 100	Low-risk women should follow the 2005 ACS cancer screening guidelines. Note that the role of BSE has been redefined. Consult your physician's possible modifications to this protocol.
100–199	Moderate-risk women should consult their physicians to determine whether the ACS guideline should be followed as stated or, possibly, be modified in terms of scheduling or procedures employed. Note that the role of BSE has been redefined.
200 or more	High-risk women should consult their physicians to determine whether the ACS guidelines should be followed as stated or, very likely, be modified in terms of scheduling or procedures employed. Note that the role of BSE has been redefined.

Cervical Cancer*

1. Age group
    A. Less than 25 (10)
    B. 25–39 (20)
    C. 40–54 (30)
    D. 55 and over (30)

2. Race/nationality
    A. Asian American (10)
    B. Puerto Rican (20)
    C. African American (20)
    D. White (10)
    E. Mexican American (20)

3. Number of pregnancies
    A. 0 (10)
    B. 1 to 3 (20)
    C. 4 and over (30)

4. Viral infections
    A. Herpes and other viral infections or ulcer formations on the vagina (10)
    B. Never (1)

5. Age at first intercourse
    A. Before 15 (40)
    B. 15–19 (30)
    C. 20–24 (20)
    D. 25 and over (10)

6. Bleeding between periods or after intercourse
    A. Yes (40)
    B. No (1)

YOUR TOTAL POINTS _____

Explanations

1. The highest occurrence is in the 40-and-over age group. The numbers represent the relative rates of cancer for different age groups. A 45-year-old woman has a risk three times higher than that of a 20-year-old.
2. Puerto Ricans, African Americans, and Mexican Americans have higher rates of cervical cancer.
3. Women who have delivered more children have a higher occurrence.
4. Viral infections of the cervix and vagina are associated with cervical cancer.
5. Women with earlier intercourse and with more sexual partners are at a higher risk.
6. Irregular bleeding may be a sign of uterine cancer.

Interpretation/To Carry This Further . . .

40–69	This is a low-risk group. Ask your doctor for a Pap test. You will be advised how often you should be tested after your first test.
70–99	In this moderate-risk group, more frequent Pap tests may be required.
100 or higher	You are in a high-risk group and should have a Pap test (and pelvic examination) as advised by your doctor.

Regardless of score, you should discuss with your physician the desirability of the ThinPrep Pap test (or one similar to it); it is designed to identify the presence of DNA from one or more of the HPV strains associated with cervical cancer.

*Lower portion of uterus. These questions would not apply to a woman who has had a complete hysterectomy.

chapter twelve

Managing Chronic Conditions

Chapter Objectives

On completing this chapter, you will be able to:

▌ explain the difference between acute and chronic medical conditions.

▌ describe the genetic causes and the symptoms of several inherited conditions.

▌ discuss treatment options for a number of congenital abnormalities.

▌ explain the difference between Type 1 and Type 2 diabetes, and discuss the importance of physical activity and diet in remaining glucose tolerant as we get older.

▌ evaluate your home or residence hall for sources of allergens that might trigger asthma.

▌ explain what an autoimmune/hypersensitivity disorder is, and describe several such disorders, with their symptoms and possible treatment protocols.

▌ recognize signs of degenerative diseases, including Parkinson's Disease and Alzheimer's Disease, and offer support to persons suffering from these disorders as well as to their caregivers.

Eye on the Media

Fibromyalgia: More Questions Than Answers

"Is it a real illness?" is a frequently asked question in media reports on fibromyalgia, a chronic disorder characterized by widespread musculoskeletal pain. Because there is not yet convincing physiological evidence for the symptoms suffered by people with fibromyalgia, even some physicians question its existence. But experts who have spent years studying this controversial illness say that 3 to 6 million Americans suffer from fibromyalgia syndrome, or FMS. Media coverage on Internet sites, in journals, and in newspapers currently reflects our better understanding of underlying problems that trigger fibromyalgia symptoms and the medication and nondrug approaches, such as exercise, that can help many patients feel better.

FMS, which has no known cause or cure, is a frustrating and perplexing illness. It includes pain involving the tender points at the junctures between muscles and tendons. The spectrum of symptoms may also include chronic fatigue, headaches, flulike symptoms, nonrestorative sleep, morning stiffness, impaired memory and concentration, and depression. It is called a syndrome rather than a disease, because the symptoms vary from person to person.

One frustrating aspect of the disorder stems from the perception among the general public (and some health care providers) that fibromyalgia is a psycho-somatic problem, an emotional problem that manifests as a physical one. This perception can add to patients' emotional suffering. Although people with FMS often are anxious and depressed, most authorities believe that those feelings are the result rather than the cause of the problem.

According to coverage in *The New York Times* and cnn.com, environmental influences such as stress may play a part in FMS. Patients often report that their chronic pain is preceded by a mental or physical trauma, such as an auto accident, or a serious infection, such as Lyme disease. Despite considerable investigation, researchers have been unable to identity any infectious organism as a cause of fibromyalgia.

Increasingly, serious media coverage has helped develop a more comprehensive understanding of this disorder as well as competence to manage the illness over the long term. Information and support for those who suffer from FMS are available through websites such as www.niams.nih.gov, www.arthritis.org, www.drlowe.com, and www.mdadvise.com.

In clinical medicine, thousands of diseases, illnesses, and conditions can be diagnosed and treated. For ease of communication, these diseases and illnesses have been individually named and categorized. We have chosen a set of categories—*genetic/inherited, congenital, metabolic, autoimmune, degenerative, and infectious*—and a sample of conditions that we believe you will be interested in learning about. Knowledge of these conditions will increase your understanding of chronic disease processes and how they differ from infectious diseases. Where appropriate, you will also find useful information about risk factors and lifestyle changes you can make to reduce your risk of developing a chronic condition.*†

The first five categories of conditions—genetic/inherited, congenital, metabolic, autoimmune, and **degenerative**—are discussed in the sections that follow. They have in common a slow, gradual course of development and remain a part of people's lives for long periods of time; thus they are said to be **chronic** conditions. Conversely, the infectious diseases are often quickly contracted and, once treatment has begun, stay active for a limited amount of time. These are referred to as the **acute** conditions (although HIV/AIDS is now defined as a chronic condition because of its extended duration). This sixth category, the infectious conditions, comprises illnesses caused by pathogenic organisms often transmitted from person to person. These conditions are discussed separately, in Chapter 13. The worldwide HIV/AIDS epidemic, the increasing threat of infectious diseases contracted from animals from distant areas of the world, and the comeback of familiar infections that are now resistant to antibiotics make this separate coverage necessary.

Three types of chronic conditions—obesity, cardiovascular disease, and cancer—are also addressed separately (in Chapters 6, 10, and 11, respectively) because of their importance to so many families and to the health of the nation. Many other chronic conditions are addressed in appropriate chapters throughout the book. For example, low-back pain is discussed in Chapter 4, osteoporosis in Chapter 4, and chronic obstructive lung disease in Chapter 9. Even though these conditions are not discussed in this chapter, they too fit into one or more of the categories described and are either chronic or acute in nature.

Chronic Disease Prevention

With the well-deserved emphasis placed on the prevention of heart disease and cancer, you might expect that virtually all diseases are preventable if you follow a wellness lifestyle. While it is true that many conditions are strongly linked to the lifestyle choices you make, we know little about how to prevent most of the chronic diseases described in this chapter. Learning about these conditions reminds us that even the most carefully tended human body is vulnerable to the effects of aging and the array of diseases that, in many cases, we do not yet understand. Accordingly, we are challenged to move beyond our perception of health as the absence of disease and illness. As we first discussed in Chapter 1, only then can we see that the value of health is not what it prevents, but rather what it makes possible—a life characterized by growth and development through each stage of the life cycle (see Discovering Your Spirituality on page 371).

Genetic/Inherited Conditions

Genetic or inherited conditions can occur in any of three ways: (1) abnormal genetic material (genes) are transmitted from one or both biological parents at conception; (2) abnormal genetic material is formed by mutation of normal genetic material at a very early stage of cellular replication and, subsequently, passed on with each cell doubling; or (3) an abnormal number of chromosomes—more or fewer than the normal number of 46—is inherited or formed. We will present several conditions from this broad category, including Klinefelter's syndrome, Turner's syndrome, cystic fibrosis, and Duchenne muscular dystrophy.

In discussing chronic diseases, other than the more prominent ones such as cardiovascular disease, cancer, and diabetes mellitus, we must note that few requirements for reporting the incidence of such diseases exist (unlike infectious diseases). For example, only 4 states keep records of autoimmune diseases such as lupus; fewer than 10 monitor developmental disabilities; and fewer than one-half of the states report on asthma. Because of these

---

*Only a clinician can diagnose and treat these conditions. The information contained in this chapter is intended only to inform.

†We have placed each condition into its most appropriate category. However, the characteristics of a given condition may overlap with those in a second group. We will point this out when it occurs.

Key Terms

degenerative a slow but progressive deterioration of the body's structure or function

chronic develops slowly and persists for an extended period of time

acute having a sudden onset and a prompt resolution

Chronic Illness—The End or a Turning Point?

Most people diagnosed with a chronic illness go through a period of serious adjustment. For college students, the necessary adaptations feel particularly burdensome because so few of their peers are faced with equal demands. Not only must self-care routines be changed, but the help of others may be necessary to carry out that care. The limitations imposed by a chronic illness can restrict the activities and behavior of the affected individual and his or her family and friends. Financial matters (including the ability to afford medications), the need to see physicians frequently, and insurance issues add to the person's stress. When young people's lives change so profoundly, they can feel isolated and singled out in a negative way.

People respond to the diagnosis of a chronic illness in various ways. Frequently, their first reaction is denial. When this occurs, care may be delayed. At the same time, school and work performance and relationships begin to suffer from the internalized stress. Eventually, though, denial gives way to anger, which is often directed at others. Common targets of this anger are people close to the ill person, such as family and friends. Then anger broadens to include the world or God (for "letting these things happen"). Eventually, the demands of the illness, combined with a sense of futility, give way to acceptance. At this stage, the individual's resourcefulness surfaces as he or she looks within for untapped sources of strength. Gradually, the person becomes open to the assistance offered by others, begins to discover new interests and abilities, and realizes that life is not over—just different.

The decision to accept the chronic condition often brings a sense of inner peace and allows for a new approach to living. People who believe that they will not be given a burden too great for them to bear may rise to the challenge and find a level of strength that they—and others—didn't know they had. With acceptance come new learning experiences. The person begins to understand the limitations of the body, to appreciate what true friendships are, and to recognize the importance of emotional resources once taken for granted. Even more significant is the realization that the spiritual dimension of health is bountiful. As the daily challenges of the illness continue, the person realizes that his or her personal beliefs and values have not only survived but are even stronger.

---

inadequacies it is likely that many chronic diseases are underestimated, so emerging trends are difficult to determine, and environmental factors associated with their development remain unrecognized.

Abnormal Number of Sex Chromosomes

At the time of conception (fertilization) an ovum (egg) from the biological mother containing 23 chromosomes is penetrated by a sperm from the biological father that also contains 23 chromosomes. This fusion of genetic material results in an initial human cell that contains 46 chromosomes, the number found in virtually every human cell. Of these 46 chromosomes, two are **sex chromosomes** (an X from the biological mother and an X or Y from the biological father). A normal male would thus possess a 44XY (44 nonsex chromosomes plus an X chromosome and a Y chromosome) chromosomal profile, and a normal female would be depicted as 44XX.[1] Occasionally people are born who possess more or fewer than the normal 46 chromosomes because they have more than or fewer than the normal 2 sex chromosomes.

Klinefelter's Syndrome

Klinefelter's syndrome is one condition in which an abnormal number of sex chromosomes is present. It occurs in males and is a relatively rare (1 in 1,000 male births)[2] condition in which a Y sex chromosome from the biological father is combined with two X sex chromosomes. Klinefelter's syndrome would be graphically depicted as 44XXY, for a total of 47 chromosomes. Advanced maternal age is thought to be related to the development of this syndrome.

Although they look normal at birth, male children with Klinefelter's syndrome gradually show signs of the condition by the time they reach puberty. Men with Klinefelter's syndrome are often tall, very thin, and have gynecomastia (breast enlargement). In addition, a small penis, small testicles, and underdeveloped secondary sexual characteristics are typical. Men with Klinefelter's syndrome are generally infertile and have some impairment in learning ability and personality adjustment. The unique components of Klinefelter's syndrome are thought to reflect the feminizing influence of the additional X chromosome.

Prevention, Diagnosis, and Management Klinefelter's syndrome cannot be cured. Testosterone therapy is often used to minimize feminization. Since some males with

---

Key Terms

sex chromosomes the X and Y chromosomes that determine sex; chromosomes other than the autosomes

Klinefelter's syndrome have minimal symptoms and are capable of spermatogenesis (sperm production), genetic counseling regarding reproduction is strongly advised.

Turner's Syndrome

Another genetic condition caused by an altered sex chromosome number is Turner's syndrome. It occurs in females (1 in 5,000 female births)[2] when one of the 2 X chromosomes is missing, resulting in a chromosomal number of 45. This pattern is graphically depicted as 44X0, with 0 reflecting the absence of the second X chromosome. Women with Turner's syndrome have equivalent versions of many of the problems seen in men with Klinefelter's syndrome: infertility, a characteristic body type, and diminished secondary sex characteristics. Treatment of Turner's syndrome involves the carefully coordinated use of growth hormone (GH), to stimulate growth in height and well-being in adulthood, and estrogen therapy to feminize the body.[3] The most effective management of Turner's syndrome involves a multidisciplinary team approach, including specialists from endocrinology, cardiology, audiology, plastic surgery, genecology, dentistry, and psychology.[4]

Inherited Genetic Mutations

Cystic Fibrosis

No inherited condition claims more children's and young adults' lives than does cystic fibrosis (CF). In the United States, in about 1 of every 2,000 live births an infant is born with this inherited condition. In past decades, life expectancy for children with cystic fibrosis was only about 8 years. Today, however, with a fuller understanding of the disease and with more effective forms of treatment, life expectancy has increased significantly, to about 30 years. Unfortunately, the disease is very demanding, and effective management requires daily intervention.

Cystic fibrosis causes a profound disruption in the function of the **exocrine glands** in several areas of the body. This impaired function is due to the body's inability to produce a protein that helps regulate chloride content within the secretory cells of various exocrine glands. In the absence of this protein, the glands cannot produce certain enzymes needed to carry out important bodily functions.

For example, CF impairs the ability of the pancreas, an exocrine gland, to produce digestive enzymes. CF is known to affect other exocrine glands as well. It reduces the ability of sweat glands to conserve electrolytes, the ability of mucous glands lining the airway to control mucus production, and the ability of secretory glands within the digestive tract to produce digestive enzymes. These impairments of normal function underlie significant problems in respiration and digestion.[5]

Prevention, Diagnosis, and Management   Although CF is sometimes not identified until later in life, the diagnosis is usually made during childhood. Infants and young children with CF present a combination of the following symptoms:

- Poor growth
- Frequent, foul-smelling stools
- Chronic coughing and wheezing
- Recurrent pneumonia
- Nasal polyps
- Enlarged fingertips
- Skin that has a salty taste

When CF is suspected on the basis of these symptoms, a diagnosis is made using a blood or saliva test. Today over 1,000 mutations to the CFTR gene on chromosome 7 have been identified as being potentially capable of causing cystic fibrosis. Of these 1,000 or more mutations, approximately 35 are clearly related to the classic expression of the disease. The remaining mutations, in various pairings, are more likely related to "nonclassic cystic fibrosis" and other cystic fibrosislike conditions, but not the absence of the protein that is missing in classic CF.[6]

The management of CF has improved dramatically in recent years. Diets designed to maintain weight and support growth, respiratory therapy to maintain the health of the airways, a newly approved inhaled antibiotic, a vaccine effective against CF's principal pneumonia-causing bacterium, and new drugs have improved the quality of life and increased the life expectancy of people with CF. On a few occasions, **gene replacement therapy** through inhalation of virus-containing microscopic beads of genetic material has been attempted, but the existence of lung disease is a major obstacle to the effective delivery of the beads. Accordingly, CF remains an incurable, life-shortening disease.

Like sickle-cell disease, which is described on the following page, CF shows a **recessive inheritance pattern.**

Key Terms

exocrine glands glands whose secretions are released through tubes or ducts, such as sweat glands

gene replacement therapy an experimental therapy in which a healthy human gene is incorporated into a harmless virus to be delivered to cells that have an abnormal version of the gene

recessive inheritance pattern the inheritance of traits whose expression requires that they be carried by both biological parents

Genetic testing can determine whether a person who is apparently free from CF might, in fact, carry a copy of the recessive gene. In addition, if an at-risk pregnancy has occurred, chorionic villus sampling or amniocentesis can be performed, although this carries a risk of miscarriage. When the embryo is positive for CF, parents can seek counseling regarding their options, including whether to continue the pregnancy.

Sickle-Cell Trait and Sickle-Cell Disease

Of all the chemical compounds found within the body, few occur in as many forms as hemoglobin, which helps bind oxygen to red blood cells. Two forms of hemoglobin are associated with *sickle-cell trait* and *sickle-cell disease.* With an occasional exception, it is African Americans who can possess either form of this abnormal hemoglobin. Those who inherit the trait form do not develop the disease but are capable of transmitting the gene for abnormal hemoglobin to their offspring. Those who inherit the disease form face a shortened life characterized by periods of pain and impairment called *crises.*

Approximately 8 percent of African Americans carry the recessive gene for sickle-cell trait; they experience little impairment, and they can transmit the gene to their children. For approximately 1.5 percent of African Americans, however, sickle-cell disease is a painful, incapacitating, and life-shortening condition. Red blood cells are elongated, crescent-shaped (or sickled), and unable to pass through the body's minute capillaries (Figure 12-1). The body responds to the presence of these abnormal red blood cells by removing them very quickly. This sets the stage for anemia—thus the condition is often called *sickle-cell anemia.* In addition to anemia, this form of the condition is associated with many serious medical problems, including impaired lung function, congestive heart failure, gallbladder infections, bone changes, abnormalities of the eyes and skin, and, occasionally, extremely serious pulmonary hypertension, for which all patients should be screened and treated.[7] Until recently, living beyond early adulthood was not possible. Today, however, with effective screening and new medications, people with sickle-cell disease may live to reach 50 years of age.[5]

Prevention, Diagnosis, and Management In about 1 percent of people with sickle-cell disease, a bone-marrow or stem-cell transplant may be able to give the body the ability to produce a normal form of hemoglobin. Early results are promising and raise hope of a "cure" of sorts, although the number of patients who might be helped by this therapy is small. In addition, a newly introduced drug, hydroxyurea, has provided some relief from the pain caused by the clogging of vessels and the discomfort of acute chest congestion. The drug also reduces the number of blood transfusions normally needed to relieve pain.

Recently it was found that long-term transfusions can increase the risk of heart and liver damage, but its benefits outweigh this risk.

Screening to determine whether a woman or her partner carries the recessive gene may be the only key for preventing sickle-cell trait and disease. Genetic counseling can then help couples weigh the risk of passing on the gene to their children. Today, for couples at risk for passing on the gene, an ovum can be fertilized **in vitro,** the resulting embryo can then be tested, and if the ovum is found to be free of the condition it can be implanted in the uterus. This eliminates the need for any decision regarding a therapeutic abortion. (The Star box on page 374 provides useful information about genetic counseling.)

Sex Chromosome–Linked Inherited Genetic Mutations

Duchenne Muscular Dystrophy

Genetic mutations located on a maternal sex chromosome (which is always an X chromosome) present a unique problem for male offspring. The crux of the problem lies in the male's inability to "offset" or "override" the mutated gene's influence because he lacks a second X chromosome containing a normal version of the mutated gene. Females can carry the mutated gene but may not be affected by the abnormal trait because they have a normal second X chromosome.

Figure 12-1 A sickled (crescent-shaped) red blood cell in a person with sickle-cell disease. The red blood cells are elongated and thus cannot pass through the body's minute capillaries, causing periods of pain and impairment called *crises.*

> **Key Terms**
>
> **in vitro** outside the living body, in an artificial environment

Duchenne muscular dystrophy (DMD) is an inherited condition in which muscle fibers lack the ability to produce a protein called *dystrophin,* which is necessary for normal muscular function. In the absence of this protein, skeletal muscles deteriorate, impairing the ability to stand, walk, and, eventually, even breathe. Death occurs prematurely, generally because of respiratory collapse. Some people with DMD die during their teen years and some live to reach their 30s, but most die in their 20s.

Prevention, Diagnosis, and Management Muscular dystrophy can be relatively easily diagnosed by an experienced physician, but the symptoms are usually not apparent until after the age of 2. Before this age the signs of the disease are unlikely to be recognized, unless parents' concern about delayed walking prompts them to have the child seen by a physician. After age 2, however, falls, changes in gait, the development of distinct scoliosis (spinal curvature), and the appearance of muscle wasting become obvious, and the disease is identified. The diagnosis is generally made using a blood test that assesses the level of creatine kinase, an enzyme that leaks out of the muscle in response to the inadequate presence of dystrophin. Abnormally high levels of creatine kinase confirm the diagnosis.

The medical management of DMD centers on the prompt and effective use of physical therapy and occupational therapy to maintain the highest level of function possible. By the teen years, people with DMD usually can no longer walk and have begun to use a wheelchair. Scoliosis can be surgically corrected to provide relief from chest compression caused by the increasing rotation of the spine. Some people choose to use mechanical ventilation when breathing is no longer possible. Even with the best care, however, the course of the disease is irreversible. That said, however, gene therapy to correct the genetic error responsible for muscular dystrophy was attempted in 1999. Three years later some evidence of the stem cells' nuclei could be found within the muscle; however, the number of nuclei was deemed insufficient enough to be responsible for the limited improvement found in the patient's MD status.[8] Since then stem-cell transplantation research for the treatment of MD has been largely confined to animal-based models.

Several other forms of MD exist, including Becker, limb girdle, and a rare adult-onset form (Miyoshi myopathy). In very rare cases, muscular dystrophy is seen in females. The occurrence of the disease in females is almost certainly caused by a mutation in the person's genetic makeup that takes place during an early stage of development, rather than by inheritance.

Congenital Abnormalities

The second group of conditions, congenital abnormalities, refers to abnormalities that are present at birth. These conditions are caused by inappropriate changes in tissues (and thus in organs and organ systems) during embryonic development. Although both inherited (genetic) and congenital conditions are present at birth, congenital abnormalities differ in that they do not involve an atypical number of chromosomes, or an inherited chromosomal abnormality.

During the first 3 months of pregnancy (the first trimester), the embryo is "constructed" within the protective confines of the uterus. Tissues, organs, and organ systems are formed and take their proper positions according to the complex genetic blueprint established at conception. The embryo will be fully formed by the end of this 3-month period. Subsequent enlargement (growth) and refinement (maturation) will occur during the fetal period, which comprises the second and third trimesters.

A congenital abnormality is a condition caused by the inappropriate or incomplete development of a particular embryonic structure or the failure of a structure to function properly at birth. In the section that follows, we will describe selected types of congenital abnormalities. Some congenital abnormalities are so severe that they are incompatible with life, even within the uterus. Thus the embryo is spontaneously aborted by the body (this event is commonly known as a *miscarriage*). Some other congenital abnormalities are life threatening, but the pregnancy can be carried to full term. And in many other cases the abnormality is recognized early in the child's life and can be corrected, or may even be so minor that it is not problematic.

No single factor is responsible for causing congenital abnormalities. They generally form early in pregnancy, during the critical weeks when the embryo's organs are being formed. They may be the result of genetic mutation or environmental factors, such as infections and drugs. Most congenital abnormalities, however, are caused by a complex interplay of factors, some genetic and some environmental. Thus their cause is considered to be **multifactorial.**

Talipes (Clubfoot)

Talipes (clubfoot) is among the most common congenital abnormalities, affecting 1 of every 1,000 infants (Figure 12-2). A clubfoot is turned so that the heel points inward while the rest of the foot points inward and downward. The arch of the foot is prominent, and the muscles of the lower leg appear atrophied. This form of talipes is the most common form of the abnormality. Although there appears to be a genetic predisposition for talipes, the specific cause or causes are unknown. Late first-trimester amniocentesis (at 13 weeks) also may foster the formation of talipes.[9]

Figure 12-2 An infant with talipes (clubfoot). Treatment for this common congenital abnormality usually begins soon after birth, using plaster casts and manipulation of the foot. Surgery can be performed to give the foot a more normal appearance.

Prevention, Diagnosis, and Management

Treatment of talipes begins soon after birth, with a combination of manipulation of the foot followed by a series of plaster casts. You may have seen infants in lower-leg casts that contain a spacer board between one leg and the other. When the foot is profoundly deformed, tendon reassignment surgery can be performed to give the foot a more normal appearance. Some forms of talipes have responded well to stretching exercises performed regularly, combined with splinting or casting if necessary.

Cleft Palate and Cleft Lip

In the early weeks of embryonic life, the structures of the face, including the lips and roof of the mouth, form as separate halves on each side of the midline. Failure of the upper lip to fuse results in a split or cleft lip. Failure of the roof of the mouth to fuse causes cleft palate. One of these conditions (or both) occurs in about 1 of every 800 live births.

Although a genetic predisposition may be a factor in some cases of cleft lip and palate, the cause of these conditions is unknown. Environmental factors, such as the use of certain medications during pregnancy, alcohol use, and smoking, may contribute to varying degrees.[10]

If a child's cleft lip or cleft palate is not corrected, he or she may have trouble eating or speaking clearly. In addition,

---

Key Terms

multifactorial requiring the interplay of many factors; refers to the cause of a disease or condition

Figure 12-3 An infant with cleft lip and cleft palate. This common congenital abnormality is repaired before the child is 2 years old. Surgical correction is usually quite successful, both cosmetically and functionally.

cosmetic concerns may be at issue, an adequate bone foundation for tooth stability may not be established, and significant hearing loss may occur.[10] For these reasons, surgery is recommended to correct both conditions and prevent these difficulties. Figure 12-3 shows a child with cleft lip and cleft palate before surgery.

Prevention, Diagnosis, and Management

Cleft lip and cleft palate are diagnosed at delivery, when the newborn is screened for the presence of these and other abnormalities. A diverse team of health care specialists then assists parents in understanding the condition(s) and in planning the infant's presurgical and postsurgical care. This medical team would include a plastic surgeon, pediatrician, otolaryngologist (nose/throat specialist), speech pathologist, audiologist (hearing specialist), dentist, dietitian, and nurse. These health care professionals will collectively determine the child's treatment plan.

Surgery to repair a cleft lip is usually performed when the infant is 3 to 4 months old, whereas surgery to repair a cleft palate is usually completed before the child reaches his or her second birthday. If the nasal passages and throat structures are involved, additional surgeries may be required to achieve the high level of success that characterizes today's medical care of these facial abnormalities.

Patent Foramen Ovale (PFO)

During intrauterine life, blood flow in the fetal heart bypasses the right ventricle, the chamber that normally pumps unoxygenated blood to the lungs for oxygenation (see Chapter 10). The lungs are bypassed because the fetus is in effect "under water" and, thus, cannot use its lungs. A hole (the foramen ovale) in the interatrial septum, the wall that divides the upper right chamber of the heart from the upper

left chamber, provides the necessary passageway around the lungs. At the time of birth, however, when the fetus begins to breathe air, this hole is normally closed by a small flap of tissue. The blood is then redirected from the right atrium into the right ventricle to be sent to the lungs.[11]

In about 1 in 5 live births, the foramen ovale fails to close completely, without any apparent leakage of blood. In the absence of other cardiac abnormalities, this patent foramen ovale does not cause any problems, is rarely identified, and, thus, prompts no medical attention. In some infants or children, however, a patent foramen ovale may leak, allowing unoxygenated blood to flow into the left atrium and then into the left ventricle of the heart and out into the general circulation. This leakage may result in some **cyanosis** and cause a heart murmur to develop.[11]

Prevention, Diagnosis, and Management

Patent foramen ovale is usually diagnosed by the child's primary care physician. No treatment is needed unless other heart abnormalities exist or the volume of unoxygenated blood reaching the left side of the heart is too great. Interestingly, a relationship between patent foramen ovale-type opening between the atria (the two upper chambers) of the heart and persons with chronic migraine headaches has been noted. In approximately 12 percent of persons with this form of headache congenital openings of this type are found to exist, and their surgical closure significantly reduces the occurrence of migraines.[12]

The possible worsening of the leakage of PFO (both diagnosed and undiagnosed) in adults who regularly scuba dive has recently caused concern. Researchers speculate that pressure changes on the chest wall may increase the risk of blood moving from the right (venous side) of the heart into the left (arterial) side of the heart, thus increasing the risk of decompression illness as small nitrogen bubbles are distributed throughout the body by the arterial blood flow.[13] Experts disagree somewhat about whether scuba divers should undergo an echocardiogram to test for the presence of a patent foramen ovale. If you are concerned, discuss the issue with your physician.

Scoliosis

Most cases of scoliosis (abnormal lateral spinal curvatures) have no known cause and are thus classified as *idiopathic*. For a small percentage, particularly when present

---

Key Terms

cyanosis blue coloration of the lips, skin, and nail beds caused by inadequate oxygenation of the blood

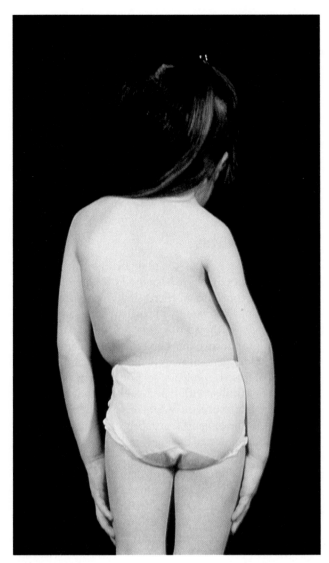

Figure 12-4 Evidence of scoliosis is commonly noted in late childhood or early adolescence.

postural problems, including uneven positioning of the shoulder blades and a "rib hump" deformity. In addition, the changing shape of the chest compresses the heart, lungs, and related structures that pass through the middle of the chest. Increasing disfiguration and discomfort accompany each degree of additional curvature and rotation.

Prevention, Diagnosis, and Management

For most people with scoliosis, the curvature that initially develops during the preteen years progressively worsens until the spine stops growing after puberty. Since treatment is the key to preventing these problems, most American elementary schools screen students between the 4th and 6th grades to identify children who need additional evaluation. Children should be screened every 6 to 9 months until growth of the spine slows and then stops. Curvatures of 20 degrees but less than 30 degrees when initially diagnosed may require treatment but will generally not progress after skeletal growth stops. Curvatures greater than 30 degrees will, however, usually continue to increase well after skeletal growth has stopped and into adulthood unless effective treatment is undertaken. (Changing for the Better above lists several signs of scoliosis.)

at birth, a genetic basis is thought to exist. In general, curvatures that are less than 10 degrees (or 20 degrees and nonprogressive) are considered postural malalignments and do not require treatment.

Most spinal curvatures begin as a lateral deviation of the spine (curvature to the side) in either the thoracic (upper back) or lumbar (lower back) region (Figure 12-4). The normally aligned spine above or below the initial curvature then begins to curve in the opposite direction to offset the original curvature. This eventually gives the spine an "S" shape. If it is not corrected, the increasing curvature of the spine causes the vertebrae that form the spinal column to rotate. As the vertebrae rotate forward, the ribs follow accordingly, eventually altering the entire architecture of the chest cavity. This causes noticeable

In this country, scoliosis is treated by orthopedic surgeons. Once the spine has been radiographically evaluated and the precise nature of the condition determined, one of the following three treatment options is chosen:

- *Do nothing.* Depending on the patient's age and the degree of curvature, it may be appropriate to do nothing and simply monitor the condition to see whether further change occurs.
- *Use a brace.* In children and adolescents, a curve in the mild range (between 25 and 35 degrees) is most effectively treated by bracing the back with a specially fitted metal brace for 23 hours per day. This treatment continues until the spine has moved into acceptable alignment.
- *Undergo surgery.* When a curvature in a preteen or adolescent is near or beyond 45 degrees, the treatment of choice may well be surgical realignment of several vertebrae within and beyond the curvature.

A recently completed longitudinal study could significantly alter both the role of the school in screening for scoliosis and aspects of the treatment. This study involved three groups of school students: one composed of children with untreated scoliosis; a second group with treated scoliosis; and a third group without scoliosis. At the end of a half-century of periodic assessments, no significant differences were found between the treated and untreated scoliosis groups in terms of functionality, both physically and emotionally. Nor did either scoliosis group differ significantly from their nonscoliosis classmates, using the same criteria. The nonscoliosis group members did, however, show somewhat less impairment than their scoliosis counterparts.[14] The authors concluded that the routine screening by schools might well be curtailed. Others, however, have questioned whether today's children would accept the deformities that were apparently acceptable to the children of 50 years ago.

Only about 2 percent of females and 1 percent of males have scoliosis. For those who do, however, new options regarding treatment could be forthcoming.

Metabolic Disorders

The third category of chronic conditions is metabolic. Metabolic disorders are caused by the body's inability to control chemical processes that regulate the building up (anabolism) and tearing down (catabolism) of tissue. Diabetes mellitus type 2 and diabetes mellitus type 1 are, perhaps, the most familiar of the metabolic disorders.

Congenital abnormalities, which you learned about in the last section, are caused by abnormal structure that leads to abnormal function. The metabolic disorders, on the other hand, are caused directly by abnormal function. The body is unable to normally utilize various nutrients in the growth and repair of tissues and in the regulation of body processes. The conditions described in this section have clear metabolic components. They may also have some characteristics that overlap with other categories of conditions. For example, a genetic predisposition is associated with non-insulin-dependent diabetes mellitus (type 2), and an autoimmune response with type 1.[15]

Diabetes Mellitus

Before beginning a discussion of diabetes mellitus, we will review the names that have been used over the years to describe this serious and an increasingly widespread medical condition. There are two principal forms of diabetes mellitus: *type 2* (the most common form) and *type 1* (a less common form); this book uses these names. However, some older persons refer to diabetes mellitus in both its principal forms simply as "sugar diabetes." Other people might be familiar with type 2, the type that usually begins during adulthood, as "adult-onset diabetes mellitus" and type 1 as "juvenile-onset diabetes mellitus," since this form most often begins during childhood. Persons with a fuller understanding of diabetes' physiology might call type 2 "non-insulin-dependent diabetes mellitus," since extrinsic (outside) sources of insulin are not required; they might call type 1 "insulin-dependent diabetes mellitus," since it requires extrinsic sources of insulin in its management.

Type 2 Diabetes Mellitus

In people who do not have diabetes mellitus, the body's need for energy is met through the "burning" of glucose (blood sugar) within the cells. Glucose is absorbed from the digestive tract and carried to the cells by the blood or stored in the liver as glycogen for later conversion back to glucose.[11] Glucose passes into the cell through a transport system that moves the glucose molecule across the cell's membrane. Activation of this glucose transport mechanism requires the hormone **insulin** (Figure 12-5).

> **Key Terms**
>
> **insulin** a hormone produced by the islet cells of the pancreas that is necessary for the normal utilization of glucose

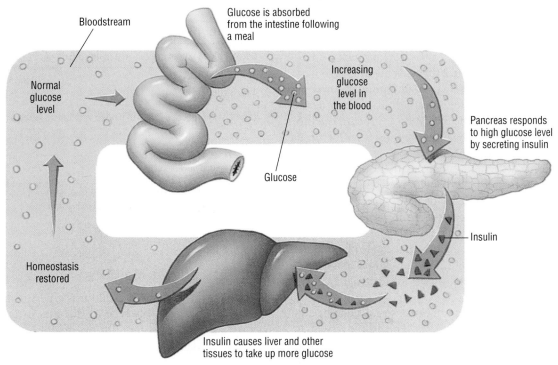

Figure 12-5 Normal blood glucose regulation. The secretion of insulin is regulated by a mechanism that tends to reverse any deviation from normal. Thus an increase in blood glucose level triggers secretion of insulin. Since insulin promotes glucose uptake by cells, blood glucose level is restored to its lower, normal level.

Specific receptor sites for insulin can be found on the cell membrane. Insulin is also required for the conversion of glucose into glycogen in the liver and for the formation of fatty acids in adipose cells. Insulin is produced in the islet cells of the pancreas. The release of insulin from the pancreas corresponds to the changing levels of glucose within the blood.[11]

In adults, and tragically in an increasing percentage of children and adolescents, with a genetic predisposition for developing non-insulin-dependent type 2 diabetes, trigger mechanisms (most likely obesity and inactivity) begin a process through which the body cells become increasingly less sensitive to the presence of insulin. The growing ineffectiveness of insulin in moving glucose into cells causes the buildup of glucose in the blood. Elevated levels of glucose in the blood give rise to **hyperglycemia,** a hallmark symptom of type 2 diabetes mellitus.

In response to this buildup, the kidneys begin the process of filtering glucose from the blood. Excess glucose then spills over into the urine. This removal of glucose in the urine is a second important symptom of adult-onset diabetes. Increased thirst, a third symptom of developing diabetes, occurs in response to the movement of fluid from extracellular spaces into the circulatory system to maintain homeostasis.[16]

Prevention, Diagnosis, and Management

For many adults with type 2 diabetes or with a prediabetic status often referred to as "glucose intolerance" or "lowered insulin insensitivity,"[11] dietary modification (with an emphasis on monitoring total carbohydrate intake, not just sugar), weight loss, and regular exercise, is the only treatment required to maintain an acceptable level of glucose. Weight loss improves the condition by "releasing" more insulin receptors, and exercise increases the actual number of receptor sites. With better insulin recognition, the person can return to a more normal state of functioning.

For people whose condition is more advanced, dietary modification, increased activity, and weight loss alone will not be effective in managing the condition, and oral drugs that stimulate insulin output, called hypoglycemic agents, will be required. Increasingly, very aggressive management, including drugs and insulin, is

Key Terms

hyperglycemia the condition of having an abnormally high blood glucose level successfully reducing risks associated with the disease. Many persons, however, have difficulty controlling blood sugar levels even with the use of insulin.

Today, the role of obesity in the development of prediabetes and eventually type 2 diabetes mellitus is so well established, and the percentage of the population with these conditions is increasing so rapidly, that a new term, *diabesity*[17] (a.k.a. Metabolic Syndrome), is being used to call the public's attention even more closely to the need for better weight management.

In addition to genetic predisposition and obesity as important factors in type 2 diabetes mellitus, unresolved stress appears to play a role in the development of hyperglycemic states. Although stress alone probably cannot produce a diabetic condition, it is likely that stress can induce a series of endocrine changes that can lead to a state of hyperglycemia. Depression too can elevate blood glucose levels and thus increase the risk of expressing type 2 diabetes.

Diabetes in both forms can cause serious damage to several important body structures. The extent to which people with diabetes develop these pathological changes can be markedly influenced by the nature of their particular condition and the type of management with which they comply. Today, in addition to the 18 million persons known to have type 2 diabetes, there are perhaps 41 million people in a prediabetic state and 5.2 million undiagnosed for either type 2 diabetes or the prediabetic state.[17] Particularly distressing is the rate of increase noted among Hispanic Americans, especially those of Mexican decent. Their rate of increase (double that of the population as a whole) may be explained on the basis of a unique genetic marker recently discovered. Once fully understood, this genetic uniqueness may add further insight into the pathology of diabetes mellitus type 2.

Because of the increased incidence in diabetes mellitus type 2, the medical community is now recommending routine blood glucose screening for persons age 25 and older and is urging the establishment of a more rigorous standard for defining normal blood glucose levels. Of course, prevention is always the best solution. Currently the American Diabetes Association (ADA) recommends a blood glucose of 90–130 mg/dl between meals and a level less than 180 mg/dl at 2 hours after beginning a meal. (See Table 12.1 for a variation on these recommendations.)

A second important biomedical index to maintain, in addition to blood glucose, in the prevention type 2 is that of blood pressure. Today, for persons of susceptibility, it is now advised that pressure readings be 135 or less over 80 or less. (Changing for the Better on page 381 presents a wellness plan for preventing this type of diabetes.)

Table 12.1 Normal and Target Blood Glucose Ranges (mg/dL)

Normal blood glucose levels in people who do not have diabetes	
Upon waking (fasting)	70 to 110
After meals	70 to 140

Target blood glucose levels in people who have diabetes	
Before meals	90 to 130
1 to 2 hours after the start of a meal	less than 180
Hypoglycemia (low blood glucose)	70 or below

Source: National Diabetes Information Clearinghouse (NIDC). Hypoglycemia. 2003. www.diabetes.niddk.nih.gov/dm/pubs/hypoglycemia/index.htm.

Type 1 Diabetes Mellitus

A second type of diabetes mellitus is type 1 diabetes mellitus. The onset of this type of diabetes usually occurs before age 35, most often during childhood. In contrast to type 2 diabetes, in which insulin is produced but is ineffective because of insensitivity, in type 1 diabetes the body produces no insulin at all. Destruction of the insulin-producing cells of the pancreas by the immune system (possibly in search of a viral infection within the islet cells of the pancreas) accounts for this sudden and irreversible loss of insulin production.[18]

Prevention, Diagnosis, and Management

In most ways the two forms of diabetes are similar, with the important exception that type 1 always requires the use of insulin from an outside source (see the Star box on page 382). Today this insulin is obtained from either animals or genetically engineered bacteria. It is taken by injection (one to four times per day) or through the use of an insulin pump, which provides a constant supply of insulin. Delivery of insulin by inhalation has recently been introduced. Transdermal delivery of insulin (by a patch) is also an option. Development of the glucometer, a highly accurate device for measuring the amount of glucose in the blood, allows better management of this condition. Progress toward development of an immunization for type 1 diabetes mellitus and in vitro pancreas cell transplantation also has occurred.

An even more recently introduced variation of a transplant-based treatment (or cure) of diabetes mellitus type 1 is the use of cadaver islet cells. These cells are harvested from the pancreas of a nondiabetic deceased donor and implanted into the pancreas of a person with diabetes mellitus type 1. This experimental procedure is under refinement.[19]

With both forms of diabetes mellitus, sound dietary practices, planned activity, and control of stress are important for keeping blood glucose levels within a normal range. When diabetes mellitus is not properly managed,

A Wellness Plan for Preventing Type 2 Diabetes Mellitus

I've recently been diagnosed with Type 2 diabetes. How can I live well with this condition?

The rate at which Americans develop non-insulin-dependent diabetes mellitus (type 2) is on the rise, partly because the population is aging. The disease typically affects older people and thus is sometimes called *adult-onset diabetes.* African Americans, Hispanic Americans, and Native Americans are at greater risk than are members of other ethnic groups, but anyone can develop the disease. There is no fool-proof way to prevent diabetes, but you can take steps to lower your risk.

- Obesity and Overweight
  Not all obese people become diabetic, but 90 percent of people with diabetes are overweight. In addition, body fat distribution is important—those who are heavy around the middle ("apple shaped") are more susceptible to the disease than those whose fat is stored in the buttocks and thighs ("pear shaped"). Evidence indicates that both men and women who gain weight in adulthood increase their risk of diabetes. A recent study conducted at Harvard University showed that women who had gained 11 to 17 pounds since age 18 doubled their risk of diabetes; those who had gained between 18 and 24 pounds tripled their risk.

  If diabetes runs in your family and you are overweight, you are four times as likely to become diabetic as a person with neither risk factor and twice as likely as a person with only one of these risk factors. Whatever your family history, staying within a healthy weight range and losing weight if you are overweight (see Chapter 6) will lower your risk of diabetes. If you tend to weight-cycle (repeatedly lose weight and then gain it back), keep trying. It is not true, as was once believed, that weight-cycling (yo-yo dieting) is in itself harmful to health.

- Genetics
  Some progress has been made in identifying the genes that pre-dispose a person to become obese or develop diabetes, but many more years of research will undoubtedly be required before this knowledge is of any practical use. As already mentioned, a family history of diabetes puts you at increased risk. This does not mean that people with a family history are certain to develop diabetes. But if the disease runs in your family, you should try to reduce other risk factors.

- Diet
  Following a sound diet is a worthwhile step toward preventing dia-betes. A semivegetarian diet (see Chapter 5) is known to lower the risk of heart disease and cancer and may also lower the risk of di-abetes. It is low in fat, especially animal fat, and rich in fruits, grains, vegetables, and low-fat or nonfat dairy products. Such a diet is unlikely to promote weight gain and often promotes weight loss. It also provides the vitamins, minerals, and other nutrients you need to help prevent chronic diseases.

- Exercise
  Direct evidence shows that regular physical activity helps prevent diabetes. In one study, researchers from the University of California at Berkeley and Stanford University found that men who were very active—expending 3,500 calories in exercise per week—were only half as likely to develop diabetes as men who were sedentary, expending less than 500 calories per week in leisure-time activity. In fact, those who benefited most from exer-cise were those at highest risk for diabetes.

  Other strong evidence indicates that vigorous exercise has a protective effect against diabetes in both women and men. This is not just because exercise can promote weight loss—physical activity lowers blood sugar whether or not you lose weight.

- Vitamin and Mineral Supplements
  There is no evidence that any supplement can prevent diabetes, despite manufacturers' claims for chromium and other supple-ments. People with diabetes are often deficient in some vitamins and minerals, such as vitamin E, zinc, magnesium, and occasion-ally chromium. But these deficiencies may be caused in part by a reduced ability to absorb and utilize these nutrients. Thus they may be a result of the disease, not the cause.

- Smoking
  Smoking boosts your risk of diabetes and exacerbates the disease if you already have it. If you are a smoker, do whatever it takes to quit (see Chapter 9). Diabetes is just one of the many serious threats to your health that will be greatly reduced if you stop smoking now.

- Stress
  Stress negatively influences type 2 diabetes mellitus in two ways. First, with regard to physiological function, the body's natural re-sponse to stress (see Chapter 3) increases the level of glucose and free fatty acids in the blood, thus placing greater than normal de-mands on the diabetic's already compromised insulin response. Second, during periods of stress people with diabetes may not maintain the level of control over their condition that is normally in place. This can occur in different ways. For example, while stressed, they may be too occupied to monitor blood glucose lev-els on a regular basis, they may alter their dietary patterns in a less than healthful manner, or they may decrease their level of physical activity and thus lower their level of insulin sensitivity.

  When taken in combination, the detrimental influence of stress and the control of type 2 diabetes mellitus demand advanced cop-ing capabilities on the part of the person with this form of dia-betes. Chapter 3 of your textbook discusses at length ways in which persons can increase their ability to prevent stress, moder-ate its intensity, or expend the high blood glucose levels found in association with the stress response.

Differences between Types of Diabetes Mellitus

Insulin-Dependent (Type 1)

(These symptoms usually develop rapidly.)

- Extreme hunger
- Extreme thirst
- Frequent urination
- Extreme weight loss
- Irritability
- Weakness and fatigue
- Nausea and vomiting

Non-Insulin-Dependent (Type 2)

(These symptoms usually develop gradually.)

- Any of the symptoms for insulin-dependent diabetes
- Blurred vision or a change in sight
- Itchy skin
- Tingling or numbness in the limbs

If you notice these symptoms occurring, bring them to the attention of your physician.

Common Complications of Diabetes

- Cataract formation
- Glaucoma
- Blindness
- Dental caries
- Stillbirths/miscarriages
- Neonatal deaths
- Congenital defects
- Cardiovascular disease
- Kidney disease
- Gangrene
- Impotence

---

several serious problems can result, including blindness, gangrene, kidney disease, and heart attack. These and other common complications of diabetes are listed in the Star box. People who cannot establish good control of the disease are likely to die prematurely.

Hypoglycemia (Classic, Reactive, and Functional)

When people with type 1 diabetes do not eat enough, exercise too much, or take too much insulin, they may develop excessively low levels of blood sugar (blood glucose), resulting in a state of **classic hypoglycemia.** In nondiabetic people, difficulty maintaining high enough blood glucose levels may also be associated with drug use, liver damage, partial removal of the stomach, fasting, pancreatic tumors, and rare forms of adrenal and breast tumors, or as a prediabetic symptom.[20] People who have classic hypoglycemia experience headaches, mild confusion, low energy levels, anxiety, sweating, and tremors. They may look pale and behave somewhat abnormally. The blood glucose ranges shown in Table 12.1 on page 380 are applicable to both the diagnosis of hypoglycemia and the management of diabetes. The form of hypoglycemia just described is the form seen routinely by

medical personnel and on occasion by classroom teachers, coaches, and the parents of children with type 1 diabetes.

A rare form of hypoglycemia called *reactive hypoglycemia* is seen in people who are hypersensitive to the presence of sugar in the blood. In these people, a meal that is high in simple carbohydrates (sugars) stimulates excessive insulin production. This insulin removes blood sugar too quickly, leading to a state of hypoglycemia. People with reactive hypoglycemia have the same symptoms seen in hypoglycemia caused by other factors.

Prevention, Diagnosis, and Management

Before reactive hypoglycemia can be definitively diagnosed, the many other causes of low blood sugar (including diabetes mellitus) must first be ruled out. Treatment of reactive hypoglycemia involves dietary modification centered on the consumption of frequent, small meals that contain high levels of complex carbohydrates and few simple carbohydrates. These dietary modifications make the movement of glucose into the bloodstream more gradual, thus eliminating high glucose loads. This "spacing out" of glucose delivery to the blood reduces the body's tendency to over-produce insulin.

In the 1970s the diagnosis of hypoglycemia was made by some physicians to placate patients who complained of vague symptoms of anxiety, moodiness, fatigue, and a loss

---

Key Terms

hypoglycemia the condition of having an abnormally low blood glucose level of interest in normal activities. Once clinical conditions such as depression were ruled out, patients were told that they "must be experiencing hypoglycemia." Patients were then put on a special diet and assured that they would begin to feel better "now that the problem was known." In many cases, patients reported dramatic improvement. Thus hypoglycemia was, for the better part of a decade, much more "common" than it is now believed to be. Today, this less frequently seen, yet still controversial, hypoglycemia is referred to as *functional hypoglycemia* by some. Central to its clear substantiation is a normal blood glucose reading at the time of symptoms (which can be difficult to obtain) and suggestions of a psychiatric illness on a valid mental health inventory.[21]

Autoimmune/Hypersensitivity Disorders

In Chapter 13 you'll learn more about the immune system. Until that time, the immune system can be described as an integrated collection of tissues, organs, and specific areas of endocrine (ductless) cells working to protect the body from foreign protein. On occasion, however, the immune system fails to recognize the body's own protein as being familiar (self) and mistakenly identifies its own protein as foreign (other) and begins attacking it in an attempt to "protect" the body. When this begins, an **autoimmune disorder** has begun. In this section of the chapter, examples of the autoimmune response will be described.

Fibromyalgia

Fibromyalgia syndrome (FMS) is a chronic condition with symptoms that are so complex an affected person might never be diagnosed and treated despite years of discomfort. For the 2 percent of the adult population believed to have FMS, intermittent periods of morning stiffness, muscle pain, fatigue, numbness and tingling, poor sleep, chronic headaches, jaw discomfort, and many other problems are often seen simply as signs of aging or stress. To trained physicians (often rheumatologists), however, these symptoms may indicate FMS. Accordingly, this syndrome can be diagnosed and effectively treated. Of course, other chronic conditions can coexist with FMS.

The cause of fibromyalgia is unclear at this time. Theories focus on immune system dysfunction (autoimmunity), altered neurotransmitter regulation, hormonal abnormalities (cortisol and HGH), and subtle brain dysfunction. Additionally, certain trigger events—infections, emotional stress, physical trauma such as a fall—thyroid dysfunction, and connective tissue disorders, such as lupus (see page 386), may cause or exacerbate FMS.[22]

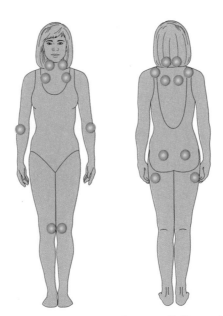

Figure 12-6 Tenderpoint locations Persons with fibromyalgia experience tenderness in at least 11 of the 18 tenderpoint locations.

Prevention, Diagnosis, and Management

Preventive measures for fibromyalgia syndrome might be to reduce stress, avoid infections, and maintain a high level of overall health. Another preventive strategy is the appropriate diagnosis and treatment of associated conditions, such as lupus, rheumatoid arthritis, and thyroid disease.

The diagnosis of FMS is based on medical history and the assessment of discomfort in 18 so-called *tenderpoint locations* (see Figure 12-6). For research purposes, people who experience pain in at least 11 of the 18 tender points are diagnosed with FMS. A lower number of "hits" is considered to be diagnostic in a nonresearch setting. Most people with chronic discomfort will be found to have several tender points during the examination. People who lack tender points and morning stiffness, but have other symptoms of FMS, may have chronic fatigue syndrome (CFS).[23]

The treatment of fibromyalgia centers on improving sleep and reducing pain. Physicians can prescribe medications to enhance the effectiveness of sleep-inducing neurotransmitters (such as serotonin and norepinephrine). Nonsteroidal anti-inflammatory drugs (NSAIDs), such as ibuprofen, are used for pain relief. Mild sedatives and

> **Key Terms**
>
> **autoimmune disorders** disorders caused by the immune system's failure to recognize the body as "self"; thus the body mounts an attack against its own cells and tissues

Figure 12-7 Common asthma triggers. If you have asthma, do you know which triggers are troublesome for you?

muscle relaxants are also employed. Other therapies include synthetic narcotics or transdermal patches for pain relief, acupuncture, and therapeutic massage.

The prognosis for people with FMS is unclear, since few long-term studies have been carried out. For most patients, the condition will remain chronic, with periods of remission and active discomfort occurring intermittently. Whether daily functioning will be significantly impaired later in life remains to be seen.

Asthma

Bronchial asthma is a chronic respiratory disease characterized by acute attacks of breathlessness and wheezing caused by chronic airway inflammation with episodes of narrowing of the bronchioles. Although the mechanisms associated with asthmatic attacks are understood, the reason that some people develop a high level of immune system hypersensitivity is not fully known. The identification of a gene (which may be one of several) related to asthma suggests a genetic predisposition that is expressed during exposure to one or more triggering agents, or allergens.

Two main types of asthma have been identified: extrinsic and intrinsic. In extrinsic asthma, allergens such as pollen, dust mites, mold spores, animal fur or dander, and feathers produce sudden and severe bronchoconstriction that narrows the airways. Increased sputum production further narrows the bronchioles and restricts the passage of air. This narrowing fosters the development of chronic inflammation of the airways, which is the most damaging aspect of asthma. Wheezing is most pronounced when the person attempts to exhale air through the narrowed air passages. For many people with asthma, exercise, cigarette smoke, and certain foods or drugs can cause an asthma attack (Figure 12-7). Physicians once suspected that immunizations (for measles, mumps, and rubella) predisposed people to extrinsic asthmatic attacks by hypersensitizing the immune system, but this view currently finds lessened support.[24]

The incidence of extrinsic asthma increased within the general population and particularly among children during the 1980s and 1990s. Today that increase has leveled. That said, however, asthmatic attacks account for nearly one-fifth of the pediatric emergency room visits in this country. Minority children, in particular, are most at risk of developing asthma and dying from its complications. Underlying this increased risk for asthma among minority children is a combination of factors.

Among the environmental factors potentially causing this increase are the diminished quality of both outdoor and indoor urban air quality (acidic particles), high levels of urban violence (stress), and overexposure to ozone in high-density traffic areas. However, genetic predisposition may also play an important role in this increase; studies comparing asthma levels among children of different races who share the same environment consistently find higher rates among minority children than their non-minority classmates. A final environmental factor that may account for some of the reported increase is the more complete reporting of acute asthmatic attacks and deaths (by hospital ERs) without, unfortunately, the much-needed increase in initial diagnosis and medical management that would have prevented the acute attacks and death.

Intrinsic asthma, the less common form, has similar symptoms but is caused by stress, frequent respiratory tract infections, hormone replacement therapy (for postmenopausal women),[25] or possibly by the aftereffects of maternal antibiotic during pregnancy. Allergens play a lesser role in this form of asthma, which may be more strongly influenced by genetic predisposition for a hypersensitive immune response to foreign protein (allergens).

Prevention, Diagnosis, and Management

Prevention or effective management of asthma is often possible using a combination of approaches. Most important, of course, is the maintenance of high-level wellness through a healthful lifestyle that includes a sound diet, regular exercise, and effective stress management. Each person who has asthma should work with his or her physician to develop a sound, individually tailored management plan. If you have asthma, complete the Personal Assessment on page 387 to determine whether you are doing all you can to manage your condition effectively.

A number of components can be included in an asthma management plan. Exercises that are well tolerated, such as swimming, can help maintain a more normal level of respiratory function. Immunotherapy, in which the patient with extrinsic asthma is desensitized through injections of weakened allergens, is often attempted. In addition, the careful use of corticosteroid drugs several times per day by inhalation reduces inflammation. Additional drugs have recently been introduced. Among these are *antileukotrienes* that reduce the immune system's ability to foster inflammation, a new class of engineered antibodies that bind to natural antibodies, thus preventing the activation of mast cells that trigger the asthmatic response,[26] and others that reduce the effects of exercise and cold air that frequently trigger asthma attacks.

Changing for the Better

Tips for Controlling Exercise-Induced Asthma

I've been jogging every day for the past 3 years and recently found out that I have asthma. How can I keep jogging without triggering asthma attacks?

- Obtain a treatment and prevention plan from your physician.
- Alert instructors and coaches about the existence of any treatment plan.
- Medicate before exercising according to your physician's instruction.
- Warm up slowly to increase heart rate gradually and cool down slowly after exercise.
- Carry your bronchodilator with you at all times if one was prescribed.
- Wear a scarf or mask over your mouth and nose during cold weather to warm and moisten the air you breathe.
- Wear an allergy mask over the mouth and nose when exercising during pollen season.

Despite the use of older drugs, such as the bronchodilators that open constricted airways, and the newer drugs that counter specific allergens or immune system-based inflammation, asthma remains a serious and potentially fatal condition. Each year in this country, several thousand people die as the result of asthma attacks. Some experts believe that this number could be reduced if physicians were more aggressive in their treatment of the bronchial inflammation component of the condition.

People with exercise-induced asthma (EIA), a common type of extrinsic asthma, should take several important steps when attempting to exercise (see Changing for the Better).

Many children who have asthma manage well with the proper use of exercise and medication. They may experience less asthma, or none at all, when they reach adulthood.

Crohn's Disease

A wide array of chronic conditions that involve the gastrointestinal system are collectively referred to as *inflammatory bowel disease (IBD)*. One type of IBD is Crohn's disease, an erosive deterioration of the inner surface and muscular layer of the intestinal wall that affects nearly 500,000 Americans, many of whom are of traditional college age. The disease most often affects the terminal end of the small intestine and the beginning of the large intestine, or colon. When the disease is active (it frequently has long periods of remission), symptoms include abdominal pain in the lower right quadrant, fever, diarrhea, weight loss, and rectal bleeding that leads to anemia.

Although the cause of Crohn's disease is not fully understood, an autoimmune response, a genetic predisposition, and a history of emotional stress may be the principal factors. Multiple forms of Crohn's disease are thought to exist, with each reflecting different genetic components. Genes located on a variety of chromosomes are under investigation.[27] Because of the array of conditions that constitute IBD and the complex etiology of each condition, it is difficult to account for the disproportionate incidence of Crohn's (and IBD) among women, and particularly among minority women. Within the latter, younger Jewish women are disproportionately represented.

Prevention, Diagnosis, and Management

When a patient reports the symptoms just described, the physician quickly suspects some form of IBD, such as Crohn's disease. Accordingly, blood tests are ordered and a complete series of gastrointestinal (GI) X-rays is taken. Additional diagnostic procedures could include a CT scan of the GI tract, endoscopic examination of the colon, and a biopsy of the intestinal wall. Positive results of these tests confirm the diagnosis of Crohn's disease.[5]

Currently the most effective treatment for Crohn's and rheumatoid arthritis is the use of Remicade, an antibody to tumor necrosis factor (TNF). TNF is an immune system component that, in Crohn's disease, attacks the lining of the intestinal tract. Although still approved for use, Remicade now carries two new cautionary labels—one warning against an increased risk of fatal blood and central nervous system conditions and the second against an increased risk of lymphoma. A not-yet released medication, ABT-874, which influences other aspects of immune system function, has also shown promise in clinical trials.[28]

Although Crohn's disease can often be well managed, intestinal obstructions can occur owing to the progressive thickening of the intestinal wall in the area of inflammation. Surgery may be necessary to remove the obstruction. However, obstructions may form in neighboring areas of the intestinal tract, requiring additional surgery. **Fistulas** can develop between the intestinal tract wall and adjacent structures, such as the vagina or the urinary bladder. These, too, can be corrected surgically. People with Crohn's disease may encounter further complications, including gallstones, arthritis, and chronic irritation of the skin. (Changing for the Better offers suggestions for managing Crohn's disease and other inflammatory bowel diseases.)

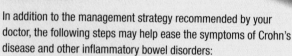

Changing for the Better

Managing Inflammatory Bowel Disease

What are the most important steps I should take to control my inflammatory bowel disease?

In addition to the management strategy recommended by your doctor, the following steps may help ease the symptoms of Crohn's disease and other inflammatory bowel disorders:

- Eat a low-fat diet. Avoid cream, butter, whole milk, and high-fat salad dressings, cheeses, and meats.
- Eat more high-fiber foods, such as fruits, grains, and vegetables. This should help if you are constipated. But take a gradual approach. Sudden increases in fiber may cause gas and diarrhea.
- Avoid sorbitol, a sugar substitute used in many products; it can cause diarrhea. Fructose, found in fruits and often in processed foods, may also be a problem.
- Try switching to lactose-free milk in case you have trouble digesting milk sugar.
- Cut down on or eliminate alcohol and caffeine.
- If you are taking medications, particularly antibiotics, ask your doctor if they could exacerbate the disease.
- Try eating several small meals a day rather than two or three large ones.
- If emotional stress is involved, try dealing with it directly by talking with a counselor.
- Regular exercise and other lifestyle alterations may help.

Systemic Lupus Erythematosus (SLE)

Systemic lupus erythematosus, or simply *lupus*, is one of the most familiar autoimmune disorders or connective tissue disorders. These conditions are caused by an extensive and inappropriate attack by the body's immune system on its own tissues, which then serve as **self-antigens.** (See Chapter 13 for a discussion of the immune response.)

The word **systemic** refers to the widespread destruction of fibrous connective tissue and other tissues.

Key Terms

fistula a fissure, break, or hole in the wall of an organ

self-antigens the cells and tissues that stimulate the immune system's autoimmune response

systemic (sis **tem** ic) distributed or occurring throughout the entire body system

Erythematosus (*erythema*- means "red") refers to the reddish rash that imparts a characteristic "mask" to the face of a person with SLE. The disease is seen in women 25 times more often than in men, and it first appears during young adulthood, although it is now known that autoantibodies may first appear in the blood as much as a decade before the first observable symptoms of SLE appear.[29] (See Learning from Our Diversity on page 388.) Particularly interesting within this gender inequity is the higher incidence of lupus reported among African American women and women of Hispanic and Asian origin than among other women.

The course of systemic lupus erythematosus is gradual, with intermittent periods of inflammation, stiffness, fatigue, pleurisy (chest pain), and discomfort over wide areas of the body, including muscles, joints, and skin. Similar changes may take place in the tissues of the nervous system, kidneys, and heart.[5]

Researchers do not know why the immune system attacks the body in such an extensive and aggressive way. It is likely, however, that a combination of genetic predisposition, hormones (estrogen), chronic emotional stress (see Chapter 3), ultraviolet radiation (including sunlight), and an earlier viral infection may be involved in its development.

 TALKING POINTS You learn that two young women who are your coworkers have recently been diagnosed with lupus and Crohn's disease, respectively. How can you be supportive of them? What would you say to them about their conditions, particularly on days when it is obvious that they are not feeling well?

Prevention, Diagnosis, and Management

A physician may suspect lupus based on the patient's description of her symptoms and make a diagnosis using a number of laboratory tests, including the identification of an SLE factor in the blood. A skin biopsy may be taken to confirm structural changes in the connective tissue layer below the skin.

Management of lupus generally involves the occasional or long-term use of nonsteroidal anti-inflammatory drugs (NSAIDs), malarial drugs for the skin rash, and a low dose of prednisone (a corticosteroid) to reduce fever, treat episodes of pleurisy, and minimize certain neurological symptoms. The immune system itself may be medically suppressed as well. These treatments must be carefully monitored because they have serious side effects. *Plasmapheresis*, a plasma exchange procedure, in which various immune system components are filtered from the blood, has also been employed in the treatment of SLE.

Management of lupus centers on the prevention of episodes of the disease called *flares*. These periods of active lupus are often triggered by exposure to the sun, periods of fatigue, or an infectious disease, all of which should be avoided as much as possible.

Multiple Sclerosis (MS)

For proper nerve conduction to occur within portions of the brain and the spinal cord, an insulating sheath of myelin must surround the neurons (nerve cells). In the progressive disease multiple sclerosis (MS), the cells that produce myelin are destroyed, myelin production ceases, and the underlying nerves are badly damaged.

Neurological functioning eventually becomes so disrupted that vital functions are significantly impaired. The cause of MS is not known. Research continues to focus on virus-induced autoimmune mechanisms in which T cells attack viral-infected myelin-producing cells. The virus most strongly suspected at this time is the Epstein-Barr virus, because antibodies for the Epstein-Barr Nuclear Antigen (EBNA) are found in higher than normal levels in people with diagnosed MS.[30] Some immune system evidence of this virus can be found in about 90 percent of all Americans, but not at the levels associated with MS.

Prevention, Diagnosis, and Management

Multiple sclerosis usually appears for the first time during the young adult years. It may take one of four forms, depending on the interplay of periods of stabilization (remitting), renewed deterioration (relapsing), and continuous deterioration (progressive) combinations of the above. The initial symptoms of the condition are often visual impairment, prickling and burning in the extremities, and an altered gait. In its most advanced stages, movement is greatly impaired, and mental deterioration may be present. It should be noted, however, that MS may be a "silent epidemic" among children, including those younger than 10 years of age.[31] To facilitate a more timely diagnosis of MS, children showing mild tremors or reporting intermittent dimming of vision should be seen by a pediatric neurologist. It is currently estimated that over 20,000 American children may have early-onset MS.

The definitive diagnosis of MS is made through MRI scans for lesions (areas of myelin erosion) in the spinal nerves or the brain. Additionally, a newly developed blood test can assist physicians in determining at what point in time assertive medical management of patients should begin following the initial presentation of symptoms.[32]

Treatment of MS is aimed at reducing the severity of symptoms and extending the periods of remission. Today a variety of therapies are used, including immune system-targeted drugs, steroid drugs, drugs to relieve muscle spasms, a medication to fight fatigue, injections of nerve blockers, and physical therapy.

The development of immune system-related medications is at the center of the fight against MS. Until very recently, four immune system-related medications, Avonex, Betaserone, Coplaxone, and Tysabri (a.k.a. Antegren), were at the forefront of treating MS. Tydabri, however, was voluntarily withdrawn from the marketplace because of a small number of fatal reactions. The remaining three medications (sometimes called the A, B, C of MS treatment) remain highly effective, depending on the specific form of MS being addressed, in delaying the onset of the most debilitating symptoms.

Additional medications are available to address complications of MS, such as spasticity. Also, initial studies involving the implantation of stem cells into mice has proven promising in reducing the number of brain lesions, as has the use of statins (cholesterol-lowering drugs) in MS-developing laboratory mice. To date, this represents the closest approximation of "prevention" that has been obtained in the field of MS treatment.

Psychotherapy is an important adjunct to the treatment of MS. Profound periods of depression often accompany the initial diagnosis of this condition. Emotional support is helpful in dealing with the progressive impairment associated with the condition.

Degenerative Diseases

A fifth category of chronic conditions is that of degenerative diseases. Conditions within this category are among the most debilitating of all chronic conditions in that they generally appear late in life, in conjunction with the overall frailty of advanced age, and thus put great demand on caregivers. Eventually, expensive institutional care is required when the level of debilitation prevents the afflicted persons from meeting the activities of daily living (ADL) or even maintaining a sense of self and of the world in which they live. Paramount among these degenerative conditions are Parkinson's disease and Alzheimer's disease.

Parkinson's Disease

Once called "shaking palsy," Parkinson's disease is now recognized as a specific neurological disorder belonging to a family of conditions called *motor system disorders*. Parkinson's disease involves the chronic progressive loss of dopamine production within specific areas of the brain. These areas, called the substantia nigra and striatum, transmit signals required to produce purposeful muscle activity that leads to more highly coordinated movement. The four primary signs of the disease reflect this loss of muscular coordination: (1) tremor or trembling in the hands, arms, legs, jaw, and face; (2) rigidity or stiffness of the limbs or trunk; (3) slowness of movement; and (4) postural instability and impaired balance. As these symptoms worsen, people with Parkinson's disease become progressively less able to talk, walk, and perform simple tasks associated with daily living.[11]

Parkinson's-like symptoms are associated with other conditions, such as head injury, tumors, prolonged use of tranquilizers, and manganese and carbon monoxide poisoning. The labels *Parkinson's syndrome* and *atypical Parkinson's* are used to describe these conditions. It is believed that as many as one in five elderly Americans shows some Parkinsonian signs.

Actor Michael J. Fox has Parkinson's disease, and actively supports research for a cure.

About 500,000 Americans have been diagnosed with primary Parkinson's disease, and about 50,000 new cases are diagnosed annually. The exact number of people with this condition has always been difficult to establish with certainty, since some people assume that these changes are the result of aging and thus do not seek medical evaluation. The incidence of Parkinson's disease is the same in men and women. The condition is usually first seen in people over age 50, with 60 being the average age at first diagnosis. Compared with African Americans and Asian Americans, whites are more likely to be diagnosed with Parkinson's disease. A relatively small percentage of people develop the disease as early as age 40. Slightly fewer cases of Parkinson's disease are seen among smokers than among nonsmokers (the risks of smoking, however, greatly outweigh the slightly lower risk of Parkinson's disease among smokers). Additionally, for women, fewer cases of Parkinson's disease are seen in those who consume little or no caffeine but at the same time use hormone replacement therapy (HRT). However, a higher incidence of the disease is seen in women who both consume caffeine and use HRT, thus suggesting a caffeine-estrogen interplay. Caffeine consumption seems unrelated to the occurence of Parkinson's disease in males.[33]

Three explanations of the cause of Parkinson's disease have been proposed. The first involves the formation of highly excited unstable chemical compounds known as *free radicals*. With aging, the formation of these highly unstable free radicals increases, and they accumulate within a large variety of body tissues. These free radicals seek stability by physically altering the chemical structure of tissues with which they have contact, including the cells of the substantia nigra. Once damaged, the cells of the substantia nigra and striatum die; thus their dopamine production is lost and the symptoms of Parkinson's appear.

The second possible explanation relates to environmental toxins that are known to produce Parkinson's-like symptoms in humans. However, no widely occurring environmental toxins of this nature have been discovered that could account for the large number of cases of Parkinson's disease in this country and around the world. This theory was, however, given support by a recent twin study that found that, in comparison to other conditions known to have strong inherited underpinnings, a notably lower-than-anticipated incidence of Parkinson's disease was found in twinned siblings.[34]

The third theory about the cause of Parkinson's disease suggests an inherited predisposition associated with genetic material found within the mitochondria of cells. Mitochondria are cell structures in which energy is produced to fuel specific cellular tasks, such as the production of dopamine. In 1997 a mutated gene was identified within the mitochondrial DNA of members of a family with a long history of Parkinson's disease. Currently, however, a genetic basis for Parkinson's is thought most likely only in those cases of the disease that occur in persons considerably younger than typical victims and often with a substantial family history of the condition—perhaps 10 percent of all cases of Parkinson's disease.

Prevention, Diagnosis, and Management

Parkinson's disease is usually diagnosed by a neurologist after the patient is referred by a primary care physician. Although there is no single test for diagnosing Parkinson's disease, medical imaging, such as CT scans and MRI scans, may be helpful in ruling out conditions that mimic the disease.

Several medications are used to delay the progression of the disease. Most of these drugs affect dopamine production. Two drugs, carbidopa/levodopa, an older medication, and tolcapone (Tasmar), a newer drug, enhance the conversion of levodopa into dopamine. A third drug, Requip, a dopamine agonist, is available for use in combination with older levodopa-enhancing medications. This combination appears to delay the onset of the more severe symptoms of Parkinson's disease. As helpful as these medications are, however, their influence is temporary and at best only slows the progress of the disease.

Although only in the earliest stage of human trials, a compound derived from glial cells, called GDNF, has shown a clear ability to increase dopamine production while at the same time reducing the limitations in the loss of motor control initially present.[35] Considerable research and development remains to be done on this new treatment approach.

 TALKING POINTS Your grandmother seems increasingly frustrated by your grandfather's "clumsiness" and has complained that he is becoming increasingly unsteady and nervous. What might you say to her about his condition? What would you suggest she say to him?

At this time a radically different form of treatment for Parkinson's disease is under refinement. A **xenotransplant**-based technique has been developed through which fetal pig cells are transplanted into the brains of Parkinson's patients for the purpose of reestablishing functional dopamine-producing cells in the areas of the brain deprived of this ability by the disease. In the limited number of persons having had this procedure, levels of success are sufficiently high enough to encourage continued study, in spite of some ethical and safety (animal-to-human virus transmission) concerns regarding the use of animal tissues.[36]

Additionally, in some cases electrodes have been surgically implanted into the brain. This procedure appears to reduce tremors to the extent that affected people can achieve and maintain a more functional level of activity for as long as 2 years.

Alzheimer's Disease (AD)

Although it affects only 1–2 percent of elderly people, organic brain syndrome, in either its acute or chronic form, is a collection of incapacitating, heart-rending, and costly afflictions. **Alzheimer's disease** is the best known of these conditions, affecting approximately 4 to 5 million adults in this country and perhaps as many as 10 million worldwide. Today, more than ever before, it is *the* disease associated with aging.

Key Terms

xenotransplant a transplant of tissue from an animal, such as a pig, to a human recipient

Alzheimer's disease adult-onset form of dementia resulting from loss of acetylcholine production within specific areas of the brain

---

The initial signs of Alzheimer's disease are often subtle and may be confused with mild depression or frontotemporal dementia (FTD), a collection of degenerative brain disorders. At this stage of the disease process, however, the person might have some difficulty answering questions like these:

- Where are we now?
- What month is it?
- What is today's date?
- When is your birthday?
- Who is the president?

During the ensuing months, people with this condition experience greater memory loss, confusion, and **dementia.** In the most advanced stage, people with Alzheimer's disease are incontinent (unable to control bladder and bowel function), display infantile behavior, and finally become totally incapacitated as a result of the destruction of brain tissue. Patients with advanced Alzheimer's disease usually must be institutionalized.

Several theories have been advanced about the cause of Alzheimer's disease. Increasing evidence indicates that genetic mutations on chromosomes 1, 14, 19, or 21 may encourage the development of the disease. Other theories suggest links between Alzheimer's disease and abnormal protein development, deficiencies in acetylcholine (a neurotransmitter) production, loss of nicotine receptors in specific areas of the brain, abnormal blood flow, or exposure to infectious agents or toxins.

In the current classification system for AD, two principal categories are used, *early-onset AD* (before age 65) and *late-onset AD* (after age 65). Early-onset AD, encompassing types 1, 3, and 4, accounts for approximately 25 percent of all AD patients and is clearly an inherited form of the disease. Chromosomes 1 (*PSEN2* gene), 14 (*PSEN1* gene), and 21 (*APP* gene) have been identified as factors in this form of the disease. Late-onset AD, designated as type 2, the most prevalent form of the disease, is less clearly understood from a genetic point of view, although chromosome 19 (*APOE*) is believed to be involved.[37]

Prevention, Diagnosis, and Management

The precise diagnosis of Alzheimer's disease and similar disorders is difficult to make before the patient dies. Only during an autopsy can the characteristic signs of the disease—*neurofibrillary tangles* (twisted strands of neuronal material) and *senile plaque* (compressed masses of cellular material, badly damaged nerve fibers, and a core composed of *beta amyloid protein*)—be identified to confirm the diagnosis. Before death, all other conditions capable of causing dementia must be individually ruled out. Thus, tentative or probable diagnosis of Alzheimer's disease is made by a process of elimination. Newer medical imaging technologies, such as MRIs and PET scans, have become so refined that it is now *nearly* possible to confirm the diagnosis of Alzheimer's disease before death. Today these technologies have been combined with the application of selected memory tests allowing clinicians to clearly view subtle signs of diminished functional activity in specific areas of the brain. Using this approach, the ability to predict the development of Alzheimer's disease, particularly in persons with a known genetic marker for the condition, may be at hand.

Effective drugs to treat Alzheimer's disease have not yet been developed. That said, four drugs (tacrine, donepezil, rivastigmine, and galantamine) provide temporary improvement in intellectual function in mild to moderate AD by inhibiting the enzyme that breaks down the neurotransmitter *acetylcholine,* whose diminished availability is the basis of Alzheimer's disease. A fifth medication, menantine, used in moderate to severe AD, functions by blocking glutamate, a substance capable of damaging neurons. Many additional drugs are in various stages of development.

At this time, a wide array of studies attempting to link behavioral patterns to the prevention of cognitive diseases that occur with aging and decline, including the development of AD, are underway. Among these are studies assessing the role of fatty acids (particularly n-3 omega fatty acid) in preventing cognitive decline,[38] the role of exercise (particularly walking) in improving cognitive capabilities in aging adults,[39] and the contributions of regular light alcohol consumption in protecting against Alzheimer's-like conditions.[40] Additional studies in the same vein include those related to the effectiveness of NSAID (nonsteroidal anti-inflammatory drugs) in preventing cognitive decline, as well as their interactions with other AD-approved medications,[41] the ability of antioxidant vitamins (carotenes, vitamin C, and vitamin E) to prevent dementia,[42] and the role of high-dose HRT in the cause or exacerbation of cognitive decline, including AD.[43]

In addition to the speculative preventive approaches just described, vaccines for the prevention of Alzheimer's disease are now in clinical trials. These vaccines utilize a

---

> **Key Terms**
>
> **dementia** the loss of cognitive abilities, including memory and reason

synthetic version of the beta-amyloid protein to stimulate an immune response against the beta-amyloid that occurs in conjunction with the disease. On the basis of the initial human trials, immunizations appear safe, but their effectiveness requires continuing study.

A Final Thought about Health and Chronic Conditions

In this chapter we have addressed different types of chronic conditions, many of which have their onset in younger adulthood. Recall the definitions of health, both traditionally and developmentally oriented, that were introduced in Chapter 1. For persons diagnosed with any of the illnesses presented here, the traditional definitions of health could easily label them as being "sick," "ill," or "unhealthy." From a developmental perspective, however, these persons almost certainly hold aspirations of living the fullest life possible, in light of the limitations imposed by their medical conditions. To do this, they must reassess the aspirations held for them by society and the life experiences they envisioned for themselves. Once having made these reassessments, and not always easily, they begin applying resources less dependent on the structure and function of the body, but more in tune with the resources of the mind, intellect, spirit, and the supportive presence of other people. As these alternative centers of resourcefulness become more easily recognizable and skillfully and comfortably called on, the ability to engage more and more fully in life increases. Thus, these people experience an increasing number of "good days" and a greater sense of being healthy—even though the body (and perhaps society) may disagree.

Taking Charge of Your Health

- Stay attuned to media reports about chronic conditions so that you can make informed choices.

- Support agencies devoted to the prevention of chronic health conditions.

- Monitor your work, home, and recreational environments to determine whether they are enhancing your risk for developing a chronic health condition.

- Undergo the recommended screening procedures and other preventive procedures related to chronic conditions for your age and sex.

- If you have a chronic condition, participate actively in your own treatment.

SUMMARY

- Chronic conditions can be classified into several categories: genetic/inherited, congenital, metabolic, autoimmune, and degenerative.
- Chronic conditions are those that develop slowly and last a long time, whereas acute conditions are those that develop quickly and are generally resolved in a short period of time.
- Klinefelter's syndrome is a genetic condition caused by the presence of one or more additional X chromosomes; it results in feminization of the male body.
- Turner's syndrome occurs in females who lack 1 of the normal 2 X chromosomes, resulting in a total of 45 chromosomes, rather than 46.
- Cystic fibrosis is caused by the inheritance of a recessive gene that prevents the body from producing a protein required for the normal function of exocrine glands.
- Sickle-cell disease results from inheriting a gene for an abnormal form of hemoglobin associated with crescent-shaped red blood cells that have limited oxygen transport capabilities. People with sickle-cell trait are carriers of the abnormal hemoglobin gene.
- Duchenne muscular dystrophy is an X-linked recessive trait, thus seen almost exclusively in males, in which the body lacks the ability to produce dystrophin. The disease causes a progressive loss of muscular control and premature death.
- Talipes (clubfoot) is a common congenital abnormality in which, during embryonic formation of the lower extremity, the foot is turned inward and tipped into a clearly abnormal position.
- Cleft palate and cleft lip are caused by lack of fusion in the bones of the face during embryonic formation of the mouth and nasal cavity.
- Patent foramen ovale is a congenital heart abnormality in which a hole linking the right atrium to the left atrium fails

to close completely at birth, allowing unoxygenated blood to enter the systemic circulation.

- Scoliosis, an abnormal lateral curvature of the spine, can begin to develop before birth; thus it is classified as a congenital abnormality, although most cases develop during later childhood and adolescence.
- Diabetes mellitus type 2, or non-insulin-dependent diabetes mellitus, occurs when the body's cells lose the ability to recognize insulin and thus are unable to utilize blood glucose normally. Hispanic Americans appear particularly susceptible to the development of type 2 diabetes.
- Type 1 diabetes, or insulin-dependent diabetes mellitus, occurs when the cells of the pancreas are destroyed, thus depriving the body of insulin, the hormone needed for the normal utilization of blood glucose.
- Reactive hypoglycemia is a relatively rare condition in which a high level of glucose in the blood after a meal stimulates the overproduction of insulin; thus glucose is removed from the blood too quickly, and the amount of glucose in the blood falls to an abnormally low level.
- Fibromyalgia is characterized by stiffness, poor sleep, chronic headaches, and other symptoms. Diagnosis is based on soreness in specific tender-point locations. Treatment is primarily aimed at reducing discomfort and enhancing sleep.
- Asthma is a chronic respiratory disease characterized by acute attacks of respiratory hypersensitivity causing abnormal narrowing of the airways. Minority children experience asthma more frequently than do other children, even those living under similar environmental conditions.
- Crohn's disease, a type of inflammatory bowel disease, results from the erosion of the inner and middle layers of the intestinal tract wall, leading to pain, fever, weight loss, and rectal bleeding that causes anemia.
- Systemic lupus erythematosus is an autoimmune disorder in which the body's own immune system attacks connective tissue in the skin, muscles, nervous system, kidneys, and other areas. Minority women are particularly susceptible to the development of SLE.
- Multiple sclerosis is thought to be an autoimmune disorder in which the body loses the ability to produce myelin, an insulation material needed for proper conduction of nerve impulses.
- Parkinson's disease is characterized by loss of fine muscular control caused by the gradual cessation of dopamine production within the brain.
- Alzheimer's disease is a form of dementia (or loss of cognitive ability) caused by the gradual loss of the brain's ability to produce acetylcholine, a neurotransmitter essential for normal mental functioning.

REVIEW QUESTIONS

1. Identify and describe the five categories of chronic conditions presented in this chapter.
2. What is the genetic basis of Turner's syndrome? Klinefelter's syndrome? What physical features characterize persons with Turner's syndrome and Klinefelter's syndrome?
3. Cystic fibrosis is a *recessive genetic disorder;* explain this term. What functional difficulties are experienced by people with cystic fibrosis? What is the condition's long-term prognosis?
4. What complex protein structure is present in an abnormal form in people with sickle-cell disease? What shape are the red blood cells in people with this condition? Why are genetic screening and counseling considered important for sickle-cell disease and trait?
5. Duchenne muscular dystrophy is an *X-linked recessive disorder;* explain this term. Which gender carries this trait, and which is affected by it?
6. What is the function of the foramen ovale in the fetal heart? What recreational pursuit may be compromised by the presence of a patent foramen ovale?
7. What are the differences between type 2 diabetes and type 1 diabetes? How do the treatments for these conditions differ?
8. How does a person with reactive hypoglycemia respond physiologically to a large blood glucose load?
9. Identify three symptoms that characterize fibromyalgia. What role do tender points play in the diagnosis and treatment of fibromyalgia?
10. How are intrinsic asthma and extrinsic asthma similar? In what important way are they different? In what population group is this increase most noticeable and distressful? What factors might account for this increase?
11. How is Crohn's disease different from other forms of inflammatory bowel disease? What is currently believed to be the cause of Crohn's disease?
12. Systemic lupus erythematosus is an *autoimmune disorder;* explain this term. What environmental factors seem to trigger outbreaks or "flares" of SLE? In what gender is SLE most prevalent, and to what extent is it seen among members of minorities?
13. In multiple sclerosis, what important material associated with nervous system function cannot be produced? Why does the body lose its ability to produce this important material? To what important immune system chemical are several of the more effective MS drugs related?
14. What neurotransmitter is inadequately produced in people with Parkinson's disease? In which specific area of the brain is the production of this neurotransmitter lost? How do drugs used to manage the condition work?
15. Alzheimer's disease is classified as a form of *dementia;* explain this term. Which neurotransmitter is involved in Alzheimer's disease? How effective is drug treatment? What are the long-term consequences of Alzheimer's disease?

ENDNOTES

1. Nader S. *Human Biology* (8th ed.). New York: McGraw-Hill, 2004.
2. Griffiths AJF, et al. *An Introduction to Genetic Analysis* (7th ed.). New York: W. H. Freeman & Co., 2000.
3. Bertelloni S, et al. Growth and puberty in Turner's syndrome. *J Pediatr Endocrinol Metab*. March 2003. Suppl 2:307–313.
4. Karnis MF, Reindollar RH. Turner syndrome in adolescence. *Obstet Gynecol Clin North Am*. 2003. 30(2):303–320.
5. Kasper DL, et al. *Harrison's Principles of Internal Medicine* (16th ed.). New York: McGraw-Hill, 2004.
6. Groman JD, et al. Variant cystic fibrosis phenotypes in the absence of CFTR mutations. *N Engl J Med*. 2002. 347(6):401–407.
7. Gladwin MT, et al. Pulmonary hypertension as a risk for death in patients with sickle cell disease. *N Engl J Med*. 2004. 350(9):886–895.
8. Sohn RL, Gussoni E. Stem cell therapy for muscular dystrophy. *Expert Opin Biol Ther*. 2004. 4(1):1–9.
9. Philip J, et al. Late first-trimester invasive prenatal diagnosis: Results of an international randomized trial. *Obstet Gynecol*. 2004. 103(6):1164–1173.
10. Kummer AW, Lourinia K. *Cleft Palate and Craniofacial Abnormalities*. Clifton Park, NY: Delmar Publishers, 2000.
11. Saladin KS. *Anatomy and Physiology: The Unity of Form and Function* (4th ed.). New York: McGraw-Hill, 2007.
12. Azarbal B, et al. Association of interatrial shunts and migraine headaches: Impact of transcather closure. *J Am Coll Cardiol*. 2005. 45(4):496–492.
13. Torti SR, et al. Risk of decompression illness among 230 divers in relation to the presence and size of patent foramen ovale. *Eur Heart J*. 2005. 25(12):1014–1020.
14. Weinstein SL, et al. Health and function of patients with untreated idiopathic scoliosis: A 50-year natural history. *JAMA*. 2003. 289(5):559–567.
15. Hamann B. *Disease Identification, Prevention, and Control* (2nd ed.). New York: McGraw-Hill, 2001.
16. Sherwood L. *Human Physiology: From Cell to Systems* (5th ed.). Belmont, CA: Thomson-Brooks/Cole, 2004.
17. Kaufman F. *Diabesity*. New York: Bantam, 2005.
18. Rasilainen S, et al. Mechanisms of beta cell death during restricted and unrestricted enterovirus infection. *J Med Virol*. 2004. 72(3):451–461.
19. Hering BJ, et al. Single-donor, marginal-dose islet transplantation in patients with type 1 diabetes. *JAMA*. 2005. 293(&):830–835.
20. National Diabetes Information Clearinghouse (NIDC). Hypoglycemia. 2005. www.diabetes/niddk.nih.gov/dm/pubs/hypoglycemia/index.htm.
21. Snorgaard O. Functional hypoglycemia. Fancy or fact? *Ugeskr Laeger*. 1992. 154(36):1423–1429.
22. Nampiaparampil DE, Shmerling RH. A review of fibromyalgia. *Am J Manag Care*. 2004. 10(11 Pt 1):794–800.
23. Richardson RD, Engel CC, Jr. Evaluation and management of medically unexplained physical symptoms. *Neurologist*. 2004. 10(1):18–30.
24. McKeever TM, et al. Vaccination and allergic disease: A birth cohort study. *Am J Public Health*. 2004. 94(6):985–989.
25. Barr RG, et al. Prospective study of postmenopausal hormone use and newly diagnosed asthma and chronic obstructive pulmonary disease. *Arch Inter Med*. 2004. 164(4):379–386.
26. Riccioni G, et al. Advances in therapy with antileukotriene drugs. *Ann Clin Lab Sci*. 2004. 34(4):379–387.
27. Pierik M, et al. The IBD international genetics consortium provides further evidence for linkage of IBD4 and shows gene-environment interaction. *Inflamm Bowel Dis*. 2004. 11(1):1–7.
28. Mannon PJ, et al. Anti-interleukin-12 antibody for active Crohn's disease. *N Engl J Med*. 2004. 351(20):2069–2079.
29. Arbuckle MR, et al. Development of autoantibodies before clinical onset of systemic lupus erythematosus. *N Engl J Med*. 2003. 349(16):1526–1533.
30. Haahr S, et al. The role of late Epstein-Barr infection in multiple sclerosis. *Acta Neurol Scand*. 2004. 109(4):270–275.
31. Ruggieri M. Multiple sclerosis in children under 10 years of age. *Neurol Sci*. 2004. 25 Suppl 4:S326–335.
32. Berger T, et al. Antimyelin antibodies as a predictor of clinically definite multiple sclerosis after a first demyelinating event. *N Engl J Med*. 2003. 349(2):139–145.
33. Ascherio A, et al. Coffee consumption, gender, and Parkinson's disease mortality in the cancer prevention study II cohort: The modifying effects of estrogen. *Am J Epidemiol*. 2004. 160(10):977–984.
34. Wirdefeldt K, et al. No evidence for heritability of Parkinson disease in Swedish twin study. *Neurology*. 2004. 63(2):305–311.
35. Slevin JT, et al. Improvement of bilateral motor function in patients with Parkinson disease through the unilateral intraputaminal infusion of glial cell line-derived neurotropic factor. *J Neurosurg*. 2005. 102(2):216–222.
36. Sayles M, Jain M, Barker RA. The cellular repair of the brain in Parkinson's disease—past, present and future. *Transpl Immunol*. 2005. 12(3-4):321–342.
37. Alzheimer's disease—genetic home reference. U.S. National Library of Medicine. 2005. March 18. www.ghr.nlm.nih.gov/condition=alzheimerdisease.
38. Bourre JM. Roles of unsaturated fatty acids (especially omega-3 fatty acids) on the brain at various ages and during ageing. *J Nutr Health Aging*. 2004. 8(3):163–174.
39. Knoops KT, et al. Mediterranean diet, lifestyle factors, and 10-year mortality in elderly European men and women. *JAMA*. 2004. 292(12):1433–1439.
40. Letenneur L, Larrieu S, Barberger-Gateau P. Alcohol and tobacco consumption as risk factors of dementia: A review of epidemiological studies. *Biomed Pharmacother*. 2004. 58(2):95–105.
41. Imbimbo BP. The potential role of nonsteroidal anti-inflammatory drugs in treating Alzheimer's disease. *Expert Opin Investig Drugs*. 2004. 13(11):1469–1481.

42. Moreira PI, et al. Oxidative damage and Alzheimer's disease: Are antioxidant therapies useful? *Drug News Perspect.* 2005. 18(1):13–19.

43. Henderson VW, at al. Postmenopausal hormone therapy and Alzheimer's disease risk: Interaction with age. *J Neurol Neurosurg Psychiatry*. 2005. 76(1):103–105.

As We Go to Press . . .

Three respected health organizations (American Diabetes Association, European Association for the Study of Diabetes, and American Heart Association) are involved in a controversy regarding the role of "metabolic syndrome" in the prevention of heart disease. Metabolic syndrome (aka Syndrome X or diabesity) is a collection of conditions, including abdominal obesity, hypertension, elevated cholesterol, and glucose intolerance (insulin insensitivity), that is considered by cardiologists to be a "disease" that predisposes a person to cardiovascular disease. Cardiologists, and the American Heart Association, await the availability of a new medication, rimonabant (Acomplia), which will allow them to "treat" metabolic syndrome in a more comprehensive manner. Rimonabant has shown effectiveness in smoking abatement and weight management.

Aligned on the other side of the metabolic syndrome controversy are two diabetes groups that believe that the newly emerging emphasis on metabolic syndrome, as if it were a valid disease entity, is distracting the medical community's focus on more widely recognized cardiovascular disease, such as coronary artery disease, and perhaps is taking attention away from the focused attempt to deal with glucose insensitivity, a long-recognized indicator for diabetes mellitus.

personal assessment

Are you managing your asthma effectively?

Place a check mark next to each statement that applies to you.

Reducing or Avoiding Asthma Triggers

_____ I have identified my asthma triggers.

_____ I do not smoke, and I avoid environmental tobacco smoke as much as possible.

_____ I use and properly maintain an air filter and an air conditioner to keep my home cleaner and more comfortable.

_____ I avoid vacuuming, or I use a dust mask.

_____ I avoid mowing the lawn, or I use a dust mask.

_____ I avoid wood stoves and fireplaces.

_____ I use dustproof encasings on my pillows, mattress, and box spring.

_____ I use a dehumidifier as necessary in my home to reduce indoor mold.

_____ I use window shades or curtains made of plastic or other washable material for easy cleaning.

_____ My closets contain only needed clothing; clothing I do not currently wear is stored in plastic garment bags.

_____ I do not sleep or lie down on upholstered furniture.

_____ If I have a pet, it does not sleep in or go into the bedroom.

_____ I avoid perfume and cologne, cleaning chemicals, paint, and talcum powder as much as possible.

Preventing and Managing Asthma Attacks

_____ I have learned everything I can about asthma.

_____ I take medications as prescribed by my physician whether or not I am having an attack.

_____ I carry my inhaler with me at all times.

_____ I have asked my physician to help me develop a crisis plan for managing a severe asthma attack.

_____ I keep emergency numbers by the phone.

_____ I have learned about my asthma medications and know how quickly they should work.

_____ I use a peak flow meter to anticipate and respond quickly to asthma attacks.

Interpretation

17 or more items checked: You are doing a great job avoiding asthma triggers and preventing and managing asthma attacks.

14 to 16 items checked: In many ways you are doing a good job of managing your asthma. However, you may be unnecessarily exposing yourself to common asthma triggers, or your plan for preventing and managing asthma attacks may need some work.

13 or fewer items checked: You could be managing your asthma much more effectively. Modify your home and activities as necessary to avoid common asthma triggers. Talk to your physician right away about establishing an asthma management plan and an emergency plan. Remember, asthma can be fatal, and poor preventive asthma management is an important contributing factor. Don't let it happen to you!

To Carry This Further . . .

Discuss this assessment with other members of your family or your roommates. Secure their cooperation in helping you maintain a clean home free of dust, pet hair, smoke, and other asthma triggers. Make sure they know what to do to help you in case of a severe asthma attack.

chapter thirteen

Preventing Infectious Diseases

Chapter Objectives

On completing this chapter, you will be able to:

▌ describe the movement of a cold virus through each link in the chain of infectious disease.

▌ explain why persons with HIV/AIDS do not generally progress beyond the clinical stage of their disease.

▌ develop and then implement a plan to protect (or enhance) your immune system.

▌ assess your own immunizations status, and make arrangements for any additional immunizations such as flu shots.

▌ understand and describe the importance of frequent hand washing, particularly during the cold and flu season.

▌ recognize the importance of testing dead birds found on campus or in your neighborhood for the presence of the West Nile virus.

▌ identify those forms of hepatitis that are potentially sexually transmitted, in comparison to those that are not.

▌ take proper precautions to protect yourself from HIV/AIDS and other sexually transmitted diseases.

Eye on the Media

From Fear to Hope—AIDS in the News

In the early days of news coverage about AIDS, magazines like *Time* and *Newsweek* ran articles called: "The AIDS Epidemic," "Epidemic of Fear," "Plague Mentality," "Fear of Sex," "The Growing Threat," "A Spreading Scourge," "The New Untouchables," "AIDS Spreading Panic Worldwide," "A Grim Race Against the Clock," and "The Lost Generation." The titles reflected fear of the unknown, a new killer disease.

When the case of Kimberley Bergalis broke into the news in 1991, a routine visit to the dentist was suddenly fraught with risk. Bergalis was the first American to die of AIDS after being infected by her dentist, Dr. David Acer. Four of Acer's other patients became infected with AIDS—all traced back to Acer. The public's reaction was near-hysteria. *Time* ran an article called "Should You Worry About Getting AIDS from Your Dentist?" People started asking their dentists (and other doctors) about their use of sterile precautions and even whether they had been tested for HIV.

By 1996, when the "cocktail" approach to AIDS treatment started showing remarkably good results, Magic Johnson was on the cover of both *Time* and *Newsweek* the same week. After more than 4 years of retirement from pro basketball—and the announcement that he had tested positive for HIV—he was back in the game. The secret to his survival? New drug treatments, a healthy diet, regular exercise, support from family and friends, and a positive attitude.

By the late 1990s, many news articles reflected a more hopeful tone: "Living Longer with AIDS," "Hope with an Asterisk," "Are Some People Immune?" and "What—I'm Gonna Live?" Doctors, too, are feeling more positive about the disease. As one AIDS specialist said: "I go to work feeling like there's something I can do for my patients."

For people with HIV/AIDS in the most highly developed countries, the future holds different things. For some, who can't afford or tolerate the new drugs, it's still a matter of waiting to die. Others feel that they've been given a second chance. They can think about having relationships again—something many put on hold when they learned they were HIV positive. They can make plans for what they want to do with the rest of their lives—however long that may be.

Most people with HIV/AIDS are buying time—hoping for the big breakthrough, the cure for AIDS. They're trying new drug treatments, hoping that one treatment won't disqualify them from the next one. They're watching TV news, reading the newspapers, and using the Internet with greater attention. Will protease-inhibiting drugs be the answer? Are the even newer antiviral medications the breakthrough hoped for? Is a vaccine on the horizon?

Today, the media are calling our attention to yet other aspects of the AIDS pandemic. For the more developed countries, the failure of younger gays and bisexuals to protect themselves from exposure to HIV has led to a reversal in the progress made over the last 20 years. In ways all too familiar to public health professionals, a younger generation can too easily forget the progress against disease and premature death made by those who came before, and in doing so, unravel the threads of progress.

Increasingly, media attention has also been focused on the plight of the millions of HIV/AIDS victims in third world countries, particularly in Africa and areas of Asia. Television increasingly exposes the suffering in countries where diagnosis is inadequately undertaken and, once done, virtually no effective treatment exists for those infected.

Beyond the suffering and limited hope for those infected, the media has also publicized the plights of the tens of thousands of orphaned children in these areas whose parents have died from AIDS. Our federal government and pharmaceutical industry has been exposed to this suffering as well, and initial responses are being mustered.

At the midpoint of the first decade of the new century, most major media outlets carry relatively little news regarding HIV/AIDS in the United States. Whether this situation reflects the transition of the disease from "infectious" to its present status of a "chronic condition," to date no vaccine has proven to be safe and effective against HIV in humans. Other than reporting on the global spread of HIV/AIDS and the recent discovery of a few cases of a drug-resistant form of the virus in persons either entering or reentering the country, the media has reduced its focus on HIV/AIDS.

Sources: Gayle HD. Curbing the global AIDS epidemic. *N Engl J Med* 348(18):1802–1805. 2003. Klausner RD, et al. Medicine. The need for a global HIV vaccine enterprise. *Science* 300(5628): 2036–2039. 2003.

In the 19ᵗʰ century, infectious diseases were the leading cause of death. These deaths came after exposure to the organisms that produced such diseases as smallpox, tuberculosis (TB), influenza, whooping cough (pertussis), typhoid, diphtheria, and tetanus. However, since the early 1900s, improvements in public sanitation, the widespread use of antibiotic drugs, and vaccinations have considerably reduced the number of people who die from infectious diseases. People now die more often from chronic disease processes.

Today, however, we have a new respect for infectious diseases. By the end of 2004, 39.4 million people worldwide were living with HIV/AIDS, with long-range projections pointing to 70 million in the absence of effective prevention programs. We are witnessing the resurgence of TB. We recognize the role of pelvic infections in infertility. We also know that failure to fully immunize children has laid the groundwork for a return of whooping cough, polio, and other serious childhood diseases. In fact, some experts suggest that because of HIV/AIDS and the emergence and reemergence of infectious diseases, today's young adults may have a lower life expectancy than did the generation immediately ahead of them.

Several new types of infectious disease have appeared, and new concerns have been raised about the spread of familiar infectious diseases:

- The extremely virulent viruses, such as the Ebola virus in Zaire, which is fatal to 75 percent of those who contract it, for which we do not have an immunization and whose transmission is not fully understood
- The increasing resistance of bacteria such as *Staphylococcus aureus, Enterococcus,* and *Mycobacterium* (which causes tuberculosis) to antibiotics as the result of overuse and improper use, as well as the biological "redesign" of the organisms themselves

- The now-completed cross-country march of the mosquitoborne West Nile virus, and the importation of SARS (sudden acute respiratory syndrome) into Canada and the United States from Asia
- The transmission of infectious organisms through contaminated food, improper preparation of food, and contamination of water

Infectious Disease Transmission

Infectious diseases can generally be transmitted from person to person, although the transfer is not always direct. Infectious diseases can be especially dangerous because they can spread to large numbers of people, producing epidemics or **pandemics.** The following sections explain the process of disease transmission and the stages of infection.

Pathogens

For a disease to be transferred, a person must come into contact with the disease-producing agent, or **pathogen,** such as a virus, bacterium, or fungus. When pathogens enter our bodies, the pathogens can sometimes resist

---

Key Terms

pandemic an epidemic that has crossed national boundaries, thus achieving regional or international status (HIV/AIDS is a pandemic)

pathogen a disease-causing agent

Table 13.1 Pathogens and Common Infectious Diseases

Pathogen	Description	Representative Disease Processes
Viruses	Smallest common pathogens; nonliving particles of genetic material (DNA) surrounded by a protein coat	Rubeola, mumps, chicken pox, rubella, influenza, warts, colds, oral and genital herpes, shingles, AIDS, genital warts
Prion	Potentially self-replicating protein, lacking both DNA and RNA, viruslike in size, clinically called TSE (transmissible spongiform encephalopathies)	Creutzfeldt-Jakob disease, Gerstmann-Straussler-Scheinker syndrome, "mad cow" disease (bovine spongiform encephalopathy)
Bacteria	One-celled microorganisms with sturdy, well-defined cell walls; three distinctive forms: spherical (cocci), rod shaped (bacilli), and spiral shaped (spirilla)	Tetanus, strep throat, scarlet fever, gonorrhea, syphilis, chlamydia, toxic shock syndrome, Legionnaires' disease, bacterial pneumonia, meningitis, diphtheria, food poisoning, Lyme disease
Fungi	Plantlike microorganisms; molds and yeasts	Athlete's foot, ringworm, histoplasmosis, San Joaquin Valley fever, candidiasis
Protozoa	Simplest animal form, generally one-celled organisms	Malaria, amebic dysentery, trichomoniasis, vaginitis
Rickettsia	Viruslike organisms that require a host's living cells for growth and replication	Typhus, Rocky Mountain spotted fever, rickettsialpox
Parasitic worms	Many-celled organisms; represented by tapeworms, leeches, and roundworms	Dirofilariasis (dog heartworm), elephantiasis, onchocerciasis

body defense systems, flourish, and produce an illness. We commonly call this an *infection.* Because of their small size, pathogens are sometimes called *microorganisms,* or *microbes.* Table 13.1 describes infectious disease agents and some of the illnesses they produce.[1]

Chain of Infection

The movement of a pathogenic agent through the various links in the chain of infection (Figure 13-1) explains how diseases spread.[1] Not every pathogenic agent moves all the way through the *chain of infection,* because various links in the chain can be broken. Therefore, the presence of a pathogen creates only the potential for causing disease.

Agent

The first link in the chain of infection is the disease-causing **agent.** Whereas some agents are very **virulent** and lead to serious infectious illnesses such as HIV, which causes AIDS, others produce far less serious infections, such as the common cold. Through mutation, some pathogenic agents, particularly viruses, can become more virulent.

Reservoir

Infectious agents require the support and protection of a favorable environment to survive. This environment forms the second link in the chain of infection and is called the *reservoir.* For many of the most common infectious diseases, the reservoirs are the bodies of people who are already infected. Here the agents thrive before being spread to others. These infected people are, accordingly,

the hosts for particular disease agents. In some infectious illnesses a person's reservoir status may be restored after treatment and apparent recovery from the original infection. This is because some pathogens, particularly viruses, can remain sequestered (hidden), emerging later to give rise to another infection. The herpes viruses are often sequestered.

For other infectious diseases, however, the reservoirs are the bodies of animals. Bird flu is a well-known animal-reservoir disease. The infected birds are not always sick and do not always show symptoms similar to those seen in infected people.

The third type of reservoir in which disease-causing agents can live is in a nonliving environment, such as the soil. The spores of the tetanus bacterium, for example, can survive in soil for up to 50 years, entering the human body in a puncture wound.

Portal of Exit

For pathogenic agents to cause diseases and illnesses in others, they must leave their reservoirs. Thus the third link in the chain of infection is the *portal of exit,* or the point at which agents leave their reservoirs.

Key Terms

agent the causal pathogen of a particular disease

virulent (**veer** yuh lent) capable of causing disease

Figure 13-1   The six links in the chain of infection. The example above shows a rhinovirus, which causes the common cold, being passed from one person to another. I. the *agent* (pathogen) is a rhinovirus; 2. the *reservoir* is the infected person; 3. the *portal of exit* is the respiratory system (coughing); 4. the *mode of transmission* is indirect hand contact; 5. the *portal of entry* is the mucous membranes of the uninfected person's eye; 6. the virus now has a *new host*.

The principal portals of exit are familiar—the digestive system, urinary system, respiratory system, reproductive system, and the blood, especially with infectious diseases that infect humans.

Mode of Transmission

The fourth link in the chain of infection is the *mode of transmission,* or the way in which pathogens move from reservoirs to susceptible hosts. Two principal methods are direct transmission and indirect transmission.

We see three types of direct transmission in human-to-human transmission. These include contact between body surfaces (such as kissing, touching, and sexual intercourse), droplet spread (inhalation of contaminated air droplets), and fecal-oral spread (feces on the host's hands are brought into contact with the new host's mouth), as could occur when changing the diaper of an infected infant.

Indirect transmission between infected and uninfected people occurs when infectious agents travel by means of nonhuman materials. Vehicles of transmission include inanimate objects (known as *fomites*), such as water, food, soil, towels, clothing, and eating utensils.

Infectious agents can also be indirectly transmitted through vectors. The term *vector* describes living things, such as insects, birds, and other animals, that carry diseases from human to human. An example of a vector is the deer tick, which transmits Lyme disease.

Airborne indirect transmission includes the inhalation of infected particles that have been suspended in an air source for an extended time. Unlike droplet transmission, in which both infected and uninfected people must be in close physical proximity, noninfected people can become infected through airborne transmission by sharing air with infected people who were in the same room hours earlier. Viral infections such as German measles can be spread this way.

Portal of Entry

The fifth link in the chain of infection is the *portal of entry.* As with the portals of exit, portals of entry have three primary methods that allow pathogenic agents to enter the bodies of uninfected people. These are through the digestive system, respiratory system, and reproductive system. In addition, a break in the skin provides another portal of entry. In most infectious conditions, the portals of entry are the same systems that served as the portals of exit from the infected people. In HIV, however, we see cross-system transmission. Oral and anal sex allow infectious agents to pass between the warm, moist tissues of the reproductive and digestive systems.

The New Host

All people are, in theory, at risk for contracting infectious diseases and thus could be called susceptible hosts. In practice, however, factors such as overall health, acquired immunity, health care services, and health-related behavior can affect susceptibility to infectious diseases.

Stages of Infection

When a pathogenic agent assaults a new host, a reasonably predictable sequence of events begins. That is, the disease moves through five distinctive stages.[1] You may be able to recognize these stages of infection each time you catch a cold.

1. *The incubation stage.* This stage lasts from the time a pathogen enters the body until it multiplies enough to produce signs and symptoms of the disease. The duration of this stage can vary from a few hours to many months, depending on the virulence of the organisms, the concentration of organisms, the host's level of immune responsiveness, and other health problems. This stage has been called a *silent stage.* The pathogen can be transmitted to a new host during this stage, but this is not likely. A host may be infected during this stage but not be infectious. HIV infection is an exception to this rule.

2. *The prodromal stage.* After the incubation stage, the host may experience a variety of general signs and symptoms, including watery eyes, runny nose, slight fever, and overall tiredness for a brief time. These symptoms are nonspecific and may not be severe enough to force the host to rest. During this stage the pathogenic agent continues to multiply. Now the host is capable of transferring pathogens to a new host, but this is not yet the most infectious stage of an infectious disease. One should practice self-imposed isolation during this stage to protect others. Again, HIV infection is different in this stage.

3. *The clinical stage.* This stage, also called the *acme* or *acute stage,* is often the most unpleasant stage for the host. At this time the disease reaches its highest point of development. Laboratory tests can identify or analyze all of the clinical (observable) signs and symptoms of the particular disease. The likelihood of transmitting the disease to others is highest during this peak stage; all of our available defense mechanisms are in the process of resisting further damage from the pathogen.

4. *The decline stage.* The first signs of recovery appear during this stage. The infection is ending or, in some cases, falling to a subclinical level. People may suffer a relapse if they overextend themselves.

5. *The recovery stage.* Also called the *convalescence stage,* this stage is characterized by apparent recovery from the invading agent. The disease can be transmitted during this stage, but this is not probable. Until the host's overall health has been strengthened, he or she may be especially susceptible to another (perhaps different) disease pathogen. Fortunately, after the recovery stage, further susceptibility to the pathogenic agent is typically lower because the body has built up immunity. This buildup of immunity is not always permanent; for example, many sexually transmitted diseases can be contracted repeatedly.

We will discuss HIV/AIDS later in the chapter; for now, however, we need to note that this critically important pandemic infectious disease does not easily fit into the five-step model of infectious diseases just presented. In individuals infected with HIV there is an initial asymptomatic *incubation stage,* followed by a *prodromal stage* characterized by generalized signs of immune system inadequacy. However, once the level of specific protective cells of the immune system declines to the point that the body cannot be protected from opportunistic diseases, and the label AIDS is assigned, the five-stage model becomes less easily applied.

Body Defenses: Mechanical and Cellular-Chemical Immune Systems

Much as a series of defensive alignments protect a military installation, so too is the body protected by sets of defenses. These defenses can be classified as either mechanical or cellular-chemical (Figure 13-2). Mechanical defenses are first-line defenses, because they physically separate the internal body from the external environment. Examples include the skin, the mucous membranes of the respiratory and gastrointestinal tracts, earwax, the hairs and cilia that filter incoming air, and even tears. These defenses serve primarily as a shield against foreign materials that may contain pathogenic agents. These defenses can, however, be disarmed, such as when tobacco smoke kills the cilia that protect the airway, resulting in chronic bronchitis, or when contact lenses reduce tearing, leading to irritation and eye infection.

The second component of the body's protective defenses is the cellular-chemical system or, more commonly, the **immune system.** The cellular-chemical component

Key Terms

immune system the system of cellular and chemical elements that protects the body from pathogens, abnormal cells, and foreign protein

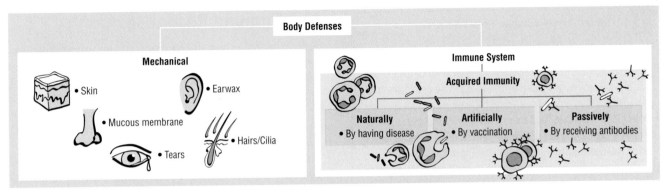

Figure 13-2 The body has a variety of defenses against invading organisms. Mechanical defenses are the first line of protection, since they separate the internal body from the external environment. The immune system defenses include chemicals and specialized cells that provide protection from a vast array of antigens.

is far more specific than the mechanical defenses. Its primary mission is to eliminate microorganisms, foreign protein, and abnormal cells from the body. A wellness-oriented lifestyle, including sound nutrition, effective stress management, and regular exercise, supports this important division of the immune system. The microorganisms, foreign proteins, or abnormal cells that activate this cellular component are collectively called *antigens.*[2]

Divisions of the Immune System

Closer examination of the immune system, or cellular-chemical defenses, reveals two separate but highly cooperative groups of cells. One group of cells originates in the fetal thymus gland and has become known as *T cell-mediated immunity,* or simply **cell-mediated immunity.** The second group of cells that makes up cellular immunity are the B cells (bursa of Fabricius), which are the working units of **humoral immunity.**[3] Cellular elements of both cell-mediated and humoral immunity are found within the bloodstream, the lymphatic tissues of the body, and the fluid that surrounds body cells.

Although we are born with the structural elements of both cell-mediated and humoral immunity, developing an immune response requires that components of these cellular systems encounter and successfully defend against specific antigens. When the immune system has done this once, it is, in most cases, primed to respond quickly and effectively if the same antigens appear again. This confrontation produces a state of **acquired immunity (AI).**[1] Acquired immunity develops in different ways, as shown in Figure 13-2.

- **Naturally acquired immunity (NAI)** develops when the body is exposed to infectious agents. Thus when we catch an infectious disease, we fight the infection and in the process become immune (protected) from developing that illness if we encounter these agents

again. For example, when a child catches chicken pox and recovers, it is unlikely that the child will develop a subsequent case of chicken pox. Before the advent of immunizations, this was the only way of developing immunity.

- **Artificially acquired immunity (AAI)** occurs when the body is exposed to weakened or killed infectious agents introduced through vaccination or immunization. As in NAI, the body fights the infectious agents and records the method of fighting the agents. Young children, older adults, and adults in high-risk occupations should consult their physicians about immunizations.

Key Terms

cell-mediated immunity also called *T cell-mediated immunity;* is principally provided by the immune system's T cells, both working alone and in combination with highly specialized B cells

humoral immunity also called *B cell-mediated immunity;* is responsible for the production of critically important immune system elements known as *antibodies*

acquired immunity (AI) the major component of the immune system; forms antibodies and specialized blood cells capable of destroying pathogens

naturally acquired immunity (NAI) a type of acquired immunity resulting from the body's response to naturally occurring pathogens

artificially acquired immunity (AAI) a type of acquired immunity resulting from the body's response to pathogens introduced into the body through immunizations

---

- **Passively acquired immunity (PAI),** a third form of immunity, results when antibodies are introduced into the body. These extrinsic antibodies are for a variety of specific infections, and they are produced outside the body (either in animals or by the genetic manipulation of microorganisms). When introduced into the human body, they provide immediate protection until the body can develop a more natural form of immunity. This form of short-term but immediate protection is provided when the emergency room staff administers a tetanus-toxoid "booster." Note that in PAI no actual pathogenic agents are introduced into the body—only the antibodies against various forms of disease-causing agents.

Regardless of how infectious agents are acquired, either through naturally acquired immunity (NAI) or through artificially acquired immunity (AAI), the result is an "arming" of the body's own immune system. This process is frequently labeled as *active immunity*. This contrasts to passively acquired immunity (PAI) in which the body "borrows" another's immune elements without actual involvement of the body's own immune system. The latter case is called *passive immunity.*[4]

In addition to the forms of immunity just described, unborn infants are also provided with a period of short-term immunity via the biological mothers' immune system elements crossing the placental barrier (see Chapter 17) and then following birth via breast milk. This *maternal immunity,* however, gradually deteriorates but is concurrently being replaced by the child's own increasingly functional immune system.

Collectively, these forms of immunity can provide important protection against infectious disease.

The Immune Response

Fully understanding the function of the immune system requires a substantial understanding of human biology and is beyond the scope of this text. Figure 13-3 presents a simplified view of the immune response.

When antigens (whether microorganisms, foreign protein, or abnormal cells) are discovered within the body, various types of white blood cells confront and destroy some of these antigens. Principal among these blood cells are the *macrophages* (very large white blood cells) that begin ingesting antigens as they are encountered. In conjunction with this "eating" of antigens, macrophages display segments of the antigen's unique protein coat on their outer surface. Now in the form of macrophage/antigen complexes, macrophages transport their captured antigen identifiers to awaiting T cells, whose recognition of the antigen will initiate the full cell-mediated immune response. This involves the specialization of "basic" T cells into four forms: helper T cells, killer T cells, suppressor T cells, and memory T cells.

Once helper T cells have been derived from "parent" T cells by the presence of the macrophage/antigen complex, they notify a second component of cellular immunity, the killer T cells. Killer T cells produce powerful chemical messengers that activate specific white blood cells that destroy antigens through the production of caustic chemicals called cytotoxins, or "cell poisons." In addition to the helper T cells' activation of killer T cells, helper T cells also play a critical role in the activation of B cells, principal players in the expression of humoral immunity.

Activation of the humoral immunity component of the overall immune response involves the helper T cells' ability to construct a working relationship among themselves, the macrophage/antigen complexes (mentioned earlier), and the small B cells. Once these three elements have been constituted into working units, the B cells are transformed into *plasma cells*. Plasma cells then utilize the information about the antigen's identity to produce massive numbers of **antibodies.** On release from the plasma cells, these antibodies then circulate throughout the body and capture free antigens in the form of *antigen/antibody complexes.*[4] The "captured" antigens are now highly

> **Key Terms**
>
> **passively acquired immunity (PAI)** temporary immunity achieved by providing extrinsic antibodies to a person exposed to a particular pathogen
>
> **antibodies** chemical compounds produced by the body's immune system to destroy antigens and their toxins

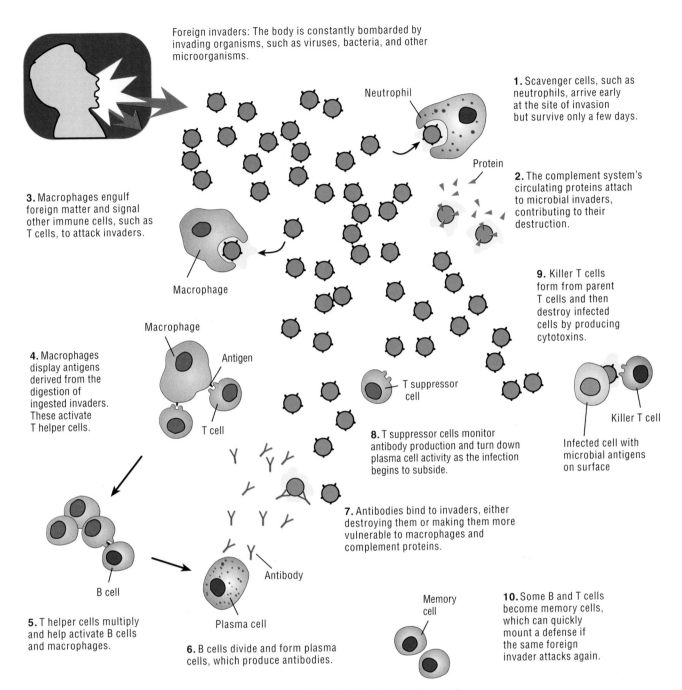

Foreign invaders: The body is constantly bombarded by invading organisms, such as viruses, bacteria, and other microorganisms.

Neutrophil

1. Scavenger cells, such as neutrophils, arrive early at the site of invasion but survive only a few days.

Protein

2. The complement system's circulating proteins attach to microbial invaders, contributing to their destruction.

3. Macrophages engulf foreign matter and signal other immune cells, such as T cells, to attack invaders.

Macrophage

9. Killer T cells form from parent T cells and then destroy infected cells by producing cytotoxins.

Macrophage

Antigen

T suppressor cell

Killer T cell

4. Macrophages display antigens derived from the digestion of ingested invaders. These activate T helper cells.

T cell

8. T suppressor cells monitor antibody production and turn down plasma cell activity as the infection begins to subside.

Infected cell with microbial antigens on surface

7. Antibodies bind to invaders, either destroying them or making them more vulnerable to macrophages and complement proteins.

Antibody

B cell

Plasma cell

Memory cell

10. Some B and T cells become memory cells, which can quickly mount a defense if the same foreign invader attacks again.

5. T helper cells multiply and help activate B cells and macrophages.

6. B cells divide and form plasma cells, which produce antibodies.

Figure 13-3 Biological warfare. The body commands an army of defenders to reduce the danger of infection and guard against repeat infections. Antigens are the ultimate targets of all immune responses.

susceptible to a variety of white blood cells that ingest or chemically destroy these infectious agents.

To assure that the response to the presence of the antigen can be appropriately controlled, a third group of T cells, the suppressor T cells, have been formed by the activation of parent T cells. These suppressor T cells monitor the outcome of the humoral response (antibody formation) and, when comfortable with the number of

antibodies produced, turn off further plasma cell activity. The fourth group of specialized T cells, the memory T cells, record this game plan for fighting the antigen invasion so that any subsequent similar invasion will be quickly fought.

An additional group of cells that operates independently from the T cell/B cell interplay just described are the *natural killer* (NK) cells. These immune cells continuously

Learning from Our Diversity

Infectious Disease: A Challenge for Older Adults

It's not always easy for young adults in excellent health to recover quickly and completely from some infectious diseases. Later in life the recovery often becomes much more difficult and in some cases impossible. For a variety of reasons older adults do not respond to infectious conditions with the same resiliency as they once did.

Central to this issue is the gradual degradation of the immune system over time. For reasons not fully understood, the immune system loses both its ability to recognize the presence of pathogens that have entered the body and its ability to mount an effective response against them. Particularly important in this regard are the decreased prevalence of active immune system cells and the inability of existing immune cells to respond effectively. Whether this reduced level of immune protection is a "programmed" aspect of aging (all human life does end at some point in time) or whether it reflects a process that is preventable (perhaps through lifestyle modifications) remains hotly debated. Perhaps no group of older adults is at greater risk because of a compromised immune system than are those with AIDS. The nearly 80,000 persons over age 50 with this immune system–destroying disease have a decreased ability to resist all infectious conditions, even when their HIV levels are suppressed through drug therapy.

In addition to the normal aging of their immune systems, older adults are generally afflicted with a variety of chronic conditions. The presence of multiple chronic illnesses (known as comorbidity) places the body under great stress, which also undermines the immune system. The combined effects of these conditions result in damage to different organ systems of the body—most importantly, the cardiovascular system, the respiratory system, and the renal system. Any time these systems are compromised by the effects of illness, either chronic or acute, the body becomes particularly vulnerable to infectious agents that routinely exist in our environment.

Compounding this situation is the inability of many older adults to understand the potential seriousness of infections at this stage of their lives. They may even have a false sense of confidence that their bodies are just as "good" at warding off infections as they once were. In addition, a lack of social support, isolation from health care facilities, and the inability to afford expensive prescription medication together make important medical care less available at a time when it could be effective.

When these factors are combined, as they are for many older adults, serious and even fatal infectious conditions become a reality. Therefore, anyone who is responsible for the health and well-being of older persons needs to understand their susceptibility to infectious conditions and recognize the fact that timely and competent care is of critical importance.

---

patrol the blood and intracellular fluids looking for abnormal cells, including cancer cells and viral-infected cells. When these are found, the NK cells attack them with destructive cytotoxins in a process called *lysing*.[4] (Can you think of a popular household sanitizing product that uses a version of *lysing* in its brand name?)

Clearly, without a normal immune system employing both cellular and humoral elements, we would quickly fall victim to serious and life-shortening infections and malignancies. As you will see later, this is exactly what occurs in many people infected with HIV (see Learning from Our Diversity).

Emerging medical technology holds promise for repairing damaged immune systems. In a current form of treatment, *adult stem cells* are harvested from nondiseased tissues of a person's body or from a biologically related family member and used to replace damaged or diseased cells within the immune system.[5] A second form of immune system repair involves harvesting *cord blood (stem) cells* taken from the umbilical cord blood collected and "banked" at birth. After careful matching, these cells can be transplanted into a recipient in anticipation that they will specialize into the cell type needed by the damaged or diseased immune system.[6] The virtual absence of any specialization in stem cells at the time of harvesting provides an opportunity for the highly generic stem cells to develop into immune system cells once transplanted into the recipient's body. Perhaps the most interesting use of this technology first occurred in October 2000, when a young cancer victim's immune system was restarted via a stem cell transplant obtained from her newborn brother, who was conceived for the purpose of being a stem cell donor. It should be noted, however, that this was a highly unusual procedure. Considerable controversy now surrounds the use of stem cells obtained from embryonic or fetal tissue sources. Even though these are considered to be the "best" stem cells, restrictions by the federal government (and several states) on their collection and use have forced clinicians to use stem cells from the sources mentioned earlier, as well as from cadavers. In spite of federal government restrictions on funding of embryonic stem cell research, however, some states have undertaken its funding to advance the application of this form of immune system–based therapy.

Immunizations

Although the incidence of several childhood communicable diseases is at or near the lowest level ever, we are risking a resurgence of diseases such as measles, polio, diphtheria, and rubella. The possible increase in childhood infectious illnesses is based on the disturbing finding that only 79 percent (range 67.5–93 percent, depending on state of residence) of American preschoolers are adequately immunized, which is principally due to the failure of many parents to complete their children's immunization programs. Today health professionals are attempting to raise the level of immunization to 90 percent of all children under the age of 2 years.

Vaccinations against several potentially serious infectious conditions are available and should be given. These include the following:

- *Diphtheria:* A potentially fatal illness that leads to inflammation of the membranes that line the throat, to swollen lymph nodes, and to heart and kidney failure
- *Whooping cough:* A bacterial infection of the airways and lungs that results in deep, noisy breathing and coughing
- *Hepatitis B:* A viral infection that can be transmitted sexually or through the exchange of blood or bodily fluids; seriously damages the liver
- *Haemophilus influenzae type B:* A bacterial infection that can damage the heart and brain, resulting in meningitis, and can produce profound hearing loss
- *Tetanus:* A fatal infection that damages the central nervous system; caused by bacteria found in the soil
- *Rubella (German measles):* A viral infection of the upper respiratory tract that can cause damage to a developing fetus when the mother contracts the infection during the first trimester of pregnancy
- *Measles (red measles):* A highly contagious viral infection leading to a rash, high fever, and upper respiratory tract symptoms
- *Polio:* A viral infection capable of causing paralysis of the large muscles of the extremities
- *Mumps:* A viral infection of the salivary glands
- *Chicken pox:* A varicella zoster virus spread by airborne droplets, leading to a sore throat, rash, and fluid-filled blisters
- *Pneumococcal infection:* A bacterium capable of causing infections, including pneumonia, heart, kidney, and middle ear infections

Parents of newborns should take their infants to their family-care physicians, pediatricians, or well-baby clinics operated by county health departments to begin the immunization process. The Children's Immunization Schedule shown on the Online Learning Center is recommended by the American Academy of Pediatrics, the American Academy of Family Physicians, and the Centers for Disease Control and Prevention. As children quickly discover, and parents already know, most of today's immunizations are administered by injection. To improve compliance with the immunization schedule (some parents have a fear of "shots" resulting from early childhood experiences and thus avoid completing the schedule), researchers are attempting to develop a single immunization that would combine many individual vaccines. In addition, research is being conducted on new delivery systems, including a skin patch, nasal spray, and vaccine-enriched foods, such as potatoes.

 TALKING POINTS Through community service work, you meet a couple that say that they have not had their children immunized and don't see the reason for doing so. How would you explain the importance of having this done?

In recent years concern has arisen regarding the role of childhood immunizations in the development of other serious childhood physical and emotional health problems, such as type 1 diabetes mellitus, asthma, autism, and sudden infant death syndrome (SIDS). At this time studies investigating the possible relationship between recommended immunizations and conditions mentioned above have found no demonstrable cause-and-effect relationships. Persons interested in more in-depth information regarding adverse affects and contraindications associated with immunizations, the Vaccine Adverse Events Reporting System (VAERS), administered by the Food and Drug Administration (FDA) and the CDC, is in the public domain. Like other reporting systems, the VAERS has limitations; however, information from a wide array of research studies can be readily obtained through the system.[7]

Although immunization is universally viewed as important for infants and children, adults have immunization needs that can be unmet. Accordingly, the CDC's National Immunization Program has just released its first immunization schedule for adults. Table 13.2 lists the eight immunizations that should be updated or initially received by adults. Adults are particularly underprotected in regard to diphtheria and tetanus.[8,9]

Table 13.2 Recommended Adult Immunization Schedule by Vaccine and Age Group. United States: October 2004—September 2005

Vaccine ▼ / Age group (yrs) ▶	19–49	50–64	≥ 65
Tetanus, Diphtheria (Td)*	1 dose booster every 10 years		
Influenza	1 dose annually	1 dose annually	
Pneumococcal (polysaccharide)	1 dose		1 dose
Hepatitis B*	3 doses (0, 1–2, 4–6 months)		
Hepatitis A*	2 doses (0, 6–12 months)		
Measles, Mumps, Rubella (MMR)*	1 or 2 doses	1 dose	
Varicella*	2 doses (0, 4–8 weeks)		
Meningococcal (polysaccharide)	1 dose		

Legend:

For all persons in this group

For persons lacking documentation of vaccination or evidence of disease

For persons at risk (i.e., with medical/exposure indications)

*Covered by the Vaccine Injury Compensation Program.
www.cdc.gov/nip/recs/adult-schedule.pdf

The Recommended Adult Immunization Schedule is Approved by the Advisory Committee on Immunization Practices (ACIP), the American College of Obstetricians and Gynecologists (ACOG), and the American Academy of Family Physicians (AAFP)

This schedule indicates the recommended age groups for routine administration of currently licensed vaccines for persons aged ≥19 years. Licensed combination vaccines may be used whenever any components of the combination are indicated and when the vaccine's other components are not contraindicated. Providers should consult manufacturers' package inserts for detailed recommendations. Physicians should report all clinically significant postvaccination reactions to the Vaccine Adverse Event Reporting System (VAERS). Reporting forms and instructions on filing a VAERS report are available by telephone, 800-822-7967, or from the VAERS Web site at www.vaers.org.

Information on how to file a Vaccine Injury Compensation Program claim is available at www.hrsa.gov/osp/vicp or by telephone, 800-338-2382. To file a claim for vaccine injury, contact the U.S. Court of Federal Claims, 717 Madison Place, N.W., Washington, DC 20005, telephone 202-219-9657.

Additional information about the vaccines listed above and contraindications for immunization is available at www.cdc.gov/nip or from the National Immunization Hotline, 800-232-2522 (English) or 800-232-0233 (Spanish).

Causes and Management of Selected Infectious Diseases

This section focuses on some of the common infectious diseases and some diseases that are less common but serious. You can use this information as a basis for judging your own disease susceptibility.

The Common Cold

The *common cold,* an acute upper-respiratory-tract infection, must reign as humankind's supreme infectious disease. Also known as **acute rhinitis,** this highly contagious viral infection can be caused by any of the nearly 200 known rhinoviruses. Colds are particularly common when people spend time in crowded indoor environments, such as classrooms.

The signs and symptoms of a cold are fairly predictable. Runny nose, watery eyes, general aches and pains, a listless feeling, and a slight fever all may accompany a cold in its early stages. Eventually the nasal passages swell, and the inflammation may spread to the throat. Stuffy nose, sore throat, and coughing may follow (Table 13.3). The

Washing your hands often is the best way to prevent the common cold.

senses of taste and smell are blocked, and appetite declines.

> ### Key Terms
>
> **acute rhinitis** the common cold; the sudden onset of nasal inflammation

Table 13.3 Is It a Cold or the Flu?

	Cold	Flu
Symptoms		
Fever	Rare	Characteristic, high (102°–104° + F); lasts 3–4 days
Headache	Rare	Prominent
General aches, pains	Slight	Usual; often severe
Fatigue, weakness	Quite mild	Can last up to 2–3 weeks
Extreme exhaustion	Never	Early and prominent
Stuffy nose	Common	Sometimes
Sneezing	Usual	Sometimes
Sore throat	Common	Sometimes
Chest discomfort, cough	Mild to moderate; hacking cough	Common; can become severe
Complications	Sinus congestion, earache	Pneumonia, bronchitis; can be life threatening
Prevention	Avoidance of infected people	Annual vaccination; amantadine or rimantadine (antiviral drugs)
Treatment	OTC products for symptom relief	Amantadine or rimantadine within 24–48 hours after onset of symptoms

Note: The need to consult a physician as the result of complications that might arise during the course of a cold or flu is not unknown. During the course of a cold any of the following should be called to the attention of a physician: (1) when a cold fails to resolve within 5 to 7 days, (2) when an elevated temperature develops (above 103°F), or (3) when a "deep chest" cough develops that produces either a brownish-tinged sputum or does not respond to OTC cough medication. Similar complications can occur in conjunction with the flu and require consultation with a physician. In addition, prolonged vomiting and diarrhea also should be called to the attention of a physician. Upon contracting the flu, children, older adults, pregnant women, and all persons with chronic conditions such as diabetes mellitus, cardiovascular diseases, and malignancies should be carefully monitored and complications should be promptly reported to a physician.

Everyone, at one time or another, thinks about how to prevent a cold or how to recover from one. For many people the use of herbal or homeopathic products seems worthy of consideration. Four such products are routinely suggested as being effective in the prevention and/or recovery from colds (and in some cases the flu).

Echinacea, a dietary supplement derived from the roots of the purple coneflower *(Echinacea purpursa),* is purported to be effective in strengthening the immune system and in so doing reducing the number of colds typically contracted during the course of a year. However, in an article appearing in the *New England Journal of Medicine* (July, 2005), researchers at the University of Virginia reported that echinacea was ineffective in the prevention of colds.

Elderberry, in extract form, represents a second herbal product whose ability to prevent the development of colds and influenza has been reported. Additionally, elderberry extract has been reported to be effective in reducing the duration of flu-related symptoms from the usual 6 days to as few as 2 days. Mild gastrointestinal complications have also been reported in conjunction with elderberry extract use if taken without food in the stomach.

Goldenseal, an herbal product, is generally taken in combination with echinacea. It is believed that goldenseal has some antibacter-

ial efficacy, as well as the ability to stimulate the production of mucus within the respiratory track. To date no antiviral capabilities have been demonstrated with goldenseal, so a direct influence on cold and flu agents seems unlikely. Herbalists suggest that goldenseal detoxifies the body in some fashion.

Oscillococcinum, a nonherbal homeopathic flu medication popular in Europe, contains small quantities of duck liver (see the discussion of homeopathic medication in Chapter 18). Underlying the purported effectiveness of oscillococcinum is its vaccinelike protection resulting from a heightened immune system response to the minuscule amount of flu virus contained in the infected duck liver.

Remember that neither dietary supplements nor homeopathic medications must undergo the rigorous clinical trials required by the FDA for prescriptions medications. Nor do they need to meet the standards for safety and effectiveness required by the FDA for OTC products. Anecdotal information and studies conducted in other countries are the primary basis for the claims made for these products.

When you notice the onset of symptoms, you should begin managing the cold promptly. After a few days, most of the cold's symptoms subside. In the meantime, you should isolate yourself from others, drink plenty of fluids, eat moderately, and rest.

In addition to the unpleasantness of the symptoms associated with colds, these nearly universal respiratory infections are also expensive. Collectively, colds cost the American economy 40 billion dollars annually, owing to lost work and out of pocket expenditures on cold medications, including 2.19 billion for cold remedies and 1.88 billion for cough drops.[10]

At this time there is no effective way to prevent colds. In 1999 a medication, pleconaril, appeared to be effective in reducing the extent and duration of colds once initial symptoms had developed. However, in 2002 the FDA denied approval of pleconaril (brand name Picovir) owing, in part, to adverse reactions in some women using the drug and oral contraceptives; and the possibility of developing resistance to the drug within the family of viruses for which it is intended.

Some of the many OTC cold remedies can help you manage a cold. These remedies will not cure your cold but may lessen the discomfort associated with it. Nasal decongestants, expectorants, cough syrups, and aspirin or acetaminophen can give some temporary relief.

Follow label directions carefully. (For herbal and homeopathic remedies, see Considering Complementary Care.)

If a cold persists, as evidenced by prolonged chills, fever above 103 degrees Fahrenheit, chest heaviness or aches, shortness of breath, coughing up rust-colored mucus, or persistent sore throat or hoarseness, you should contact a physician. Because we now consider colds to be transmitted most readily by hand contact, you should wash your hands frequently.

Two factors seem predictable in terms of "preventing" colds. The first involves the less than average number of colds seen in children between 6 and 11 years of age, who had attended larger preschool programs (more than six other children).[11] The second factor involved a lower than average number of colds in adults (average age of 48) who exercised at the higher levels of intensity (based on current exercise guidelines from the U.S. Surgeon General).[12] A third factor, the use of large doses of vitamin C supplements to prevent colds or shorten their duration, is far less predictable than long thought. In a 2004 meta-analysis of 29 studies involving 11,077 persons using vitamin C supplementation of 200 mg or more (up to 4 grams) daily, upon onset of symptoms, showed no significant benefit over placebo users in regard to criteria for duration and severity.[13]

How to Wash Your Hands

The manner in which the hands are washed is as important as frequency is. Because of the preventive role of effective hand washing in the prevention of cold and influenza transmission, the CDC has formulated guidelines for handwashing.

1. Hands transmit infectious agents when they touch the eyes, nose, or mouth.

2. Hands should be washed:

   • before, during, and after you prepare food.

   • before you eat and after you use the bathroom.

   • after handling animals or animal waste.

   • when your hands are dirty.

   • more frequently when someone in your home is sick.

   • immediately following a period of frequent handshaking.

3. Effective handwashing involves the following steps:

   • First wet your hands and apply liquid soap or clean bar soap (place bar soap back on rack, thus allowing bar to dry).

   • Next, rub your hands vigorously together and scrub all hand surfaces.

   • Continue for 10–15 seconds.

   • Rinse well and dry with clean towel.

Source: "HandWashing: An Ounce of Prevention Keeps the Germs Away." National Center for Infectious Disease. CDC. 2000. www.cdc.gov/ncidod/op/handwashing.htm.

Influenza

Influenza is also an acute contagious disease caused by viruses. Some influenza outbreaks have killed many people, such as the influenza pandemics of 1889 to 1890, 1918 to 1919, 1957 and 2003/2004. The viral strains that produce this infectious disease have the potential for more severe complications than the viral strains that produce the common cold. The viral strain for a particular form of influenza enters the body through the respiratory tract. After brief incubation and prodromal stages, the host develops signs and symptoms not just in the upper respiratory tract but throughout the entire body. These symptoms include fever, chills, cough, sore throat, headache, gastrointestinal disturbances, and muscular pain. (See Table 13.3 on page 409.)

Antibiotics are generally not prescribed for people with influenza, except when the patient has a possible secondary bacterial infection. Physicians may recommend only aspirin, fluids, and rest. Parents are reminded not to give aspirin to children because of the danger of Reye's syndrome. Reye's syndrome is an aspirin-enhanced complication of influenza in which central nervous system changes can occur, including brain swelling. For a person seeking a quicker resolution to the debilitating symptoms of flu, four antiviral medications are currently available; two are intended for influenza virus type A and two for both virus types A and B. Specific recommendations regarding use of these prescription medications, including age limitations, also exist.[14]

Most young adults can cope with the milder strains of influenza that appear each winter or spring. However, pregnant women and older people—especially older people with additional health complications, such as heart disease, kidney disease, emphysema, and chronic bronchitis—are not as capable of handling this viral attack. People who regularly come into contact with the general public, such as teachers, should also consider annual flu shots.

Today approximately 70 million Americans receive annual "flu shots." In past years, these annual immunizations, tailored to work against the flu viruses anticipated for the coming flu season, were principally received by adults over 50 years of age and others with special needs. During the flu epidemic of 2003/2004 younger adults moved into the recipient population. The nation's supply of 89 million doses of vaccine proved inadequate.

The 2004/2005 flu season will go down as one of the most difficult in recent memory, particularly since flu strains that arrived that season were less virulent than had been predicted. Rather, the anticipated supply of 100 million doses of vaccine that should have been in place for the beginning of the season did not materialize because the FDA curtailed production at a major facility in the United Kingdom. As a result, available vaccine was rationed, some vaccine was purchased from other countries, and, finally, the amount of vaccine in each dose was reduced by one half and administered, with acceptable levels of protection, by under-the-skin injection rather than deep-muscle injection.[15]

Concern about coming flu seasons is beginning to shift focus from the more familiar A and B viral strains to a pandemic involving mutating forms of the avian (bird) flu.[16] This highly virulent form of flu is now primarily spread from birds (chicken and ducks) to humans (and other animals such as cats, pigs, and dogs) having contact with viral-infested droppings. Additional mutation of the virus is anticipated, very likely in a manner giving rise to human-to-human transmission. Should human transmission become well established, a global pandemic would surely follow. Currently, the supply of antiviral medication is grossly inadequate to even treat the American population.

In the near future, the term *flu shot* may be less frequently heard. In June of 2003, the FDA approved the sale of Flumist, a nasal spray inhalation delivery system for influenza vaccine. Its use is approved for people ages 5 to 49. Its use is not, at this time, recommended for persons most in need of the highest level of protection.

The flu season generally runs from November through February, with nearly 115,000 persons developing clear symptoms of influenza, and 36,000 dying from its complications.

Tuberculosis

Experts considered *tuberculosis* (*TB*), a bacterial infection of the lungs resulting in chronic coughing, weight loss, and sometimes death, to be under control in the United States until the mid-1980s. The number of cases surged then, however, with a peak of 26,283 cases in 1992. The number has declined since then, with 14,874 cases reported in 2003, a 9 percent decline from 2000.[17] However, public health officials must continually monitor this infectious disease, because people immigrate to the United States from areas of the world in which TB is considerably more common and because drug-resistant strains of the bacterium continue to develop. Drug-resistant TB takes two forms, monodrug resistant and multidrug resistant. The former involves a resistance to isoniazid (but not Rifampin), whereas the latter is resistant to both drugs. The international medical community is calling for the development of additional drugs to treat TB in an attempt to manage the growing drug-resistant populations. Worldwide TB infects 8.7 million people annually and kills 2 million.

Tuberculosis thrives in crowded places where infected people are in constant contact with others, since TB is spread by coughing. This includes prisons, hospitals, public housing units, and even college residence halls. In such settings, a single infected person can spread the TB agents to many others.

When healthy people are exposed to TB agents, their immune systems can usually suppress the bacteria well enough to prevent symptoms from developing and to reduce the likelihood of infecting others. When the immune system is damaged, however, such as in some older adults, malnourished people, and those who are infected with HIV, the disease can become established and eventually be transmitted to other people at risk.

As previously mentioned, multidrug-resistant (MDR) TB has become a problem. Increasingly prevalent in this country, MDR tuberculosis is the result of patients' inability to follow their physicians' instructions when initially treated (for whatever reason), inadequate treatment by physicians, and increased exposure of HIV-infected people to TB. Only 50 percent of people with this form of TB can be cured. Some believe that MDR tuberculosis will be the next epidemic in this country.

Health officials are again requesting that TB testing programs be implemented and that infected people be identified, isolated, and brought into treatment. A new serum-based TB screening test, ELISPOT, has been developed. Similar to the screening test used to detect HIV infection, this test identifies T cells that have been sensitized to an antigen component of the principal tuberculosis bacterium, mycobacterium. This test is more accurate in identifying infected persons than the older and more familiar skin tests.

Pneumonia

Pneumonia is a general term that describes a variety of infectious respiratory conditions. There are bacterial, viral, fungal, rickettsial, mycoplasmal, and parasitic forms of pneumonia. However, bacterial pneumonia is the most common form and is often seen with other illnesses that weaken the body's immune system. In fact, pneumonia is so common in the frail older adult that it is often the specific condition causing death. *Pneumocystis carinii* pneumonia, a parasitic form, is important today because it is a principal opportunistic infection associated with AIDS in HIV-infected people.

Older adults with a history of chronic obstructive lung disease, cardiovascular disease, diabetes, or alcoholism often encounter a potentially serious midwinter form of pneumonia known as *acute (severe) community-acquired pneumonia*. Characteristics of this condition are the sudden onset of chills, chest pain, and a cough producing sputum. In addition, a symptom-free form of pneumonia known as *walking pneumonia* is also commonly seen in adults and can become serious without warning.

As the number of older Americans grows, recommendations regarding immunization against pneumococcal pneumonia have been established and vaccination programs undertaken. Today, these recommendations encourage vaccination beginning at 50 years of age. The cost effectiveness of pneumonia immunizations for older adults, and particularly for minority older adults, is well established. The first known drug-resistant strains of pneumonia have been identified in this country. As a result, some experts are calling for an even more comprehensive vaccination plan for older adults.

Mononucleosis

College students who contract **mononucleosis ("mono")** can be forced into a long period of bed rest during a

---

Key Terms

mononucleosis ("mono") a viral infection characterized by weakness, fatigue, swollen glands, sore throat, and low-grade fever semester when they can least afford it. Other common diseases can be managed with minimal disruption, but the overall weakness and fatigue seen in many people with mono sometimes require a month or two of rest and recuperation.

Mono is a viral infection in which the body produces an excess of mononuclear leukocytes (a type of white blood cell). After uncertain, perhaps long, incubation and prodromal stages, the acute symptoms of mono can appear, including weakness, headache, low-grade fever, swollen lymph glands (especially in the neck), and sore throat. Mental fatigue and depression are sometimes reported as side effects of mononucleosis. After the acute symptoms disappear, the weakness and fatigue usually persist— perhaps for a few months.

Mono is diagnosed by its characteristic symptoms. The Monospot blood smear can also be used to identify the prevalence of abnormal white blood cells. In addition, an antibody test can detect activity of the immune system that is characteristic of the illness.

This disease is most often caused by an Epstein-Barr virus (EBV), so antibiotic therapy is not recommended. Treatment usually includes bed rest and the use of OTC remedies for fever (aspirin or acetaminophen) and lozenges for sore throat. Corticosteroid drugs can be used in extreme cases. Rupture of the spleen is an occasional, but serious, consequence of the condition, particularly in persons who are too physically active during their recovery. Adequate fluid intake and a well-balanced diet are also important in the recovery stages of mono. Fortunately, the body tends to develop NAI (naturally acquired immunity) to the mono virus, so repeat infections of mono are unusual. However, persons on immunosuppressant drugs, such as Remicade for Crohn's disease, are somewhat likely to experience a recurrence of mononucleosis or other EBV-related infections.

For years, mono has been labeled the "kissing disease"; however, mono is not highly contagious and is known to be spread by direct transmission in ways other than kissing. No vaccine has been developed for mononucleosis. The best preventive measures are the steps that you can take to increase your resistance to most infectious diseases: (1) eat a well-balanced diet, (2) exercise regularly, (3) sleep sufficiently, (4) use health care services appropriately, (5) live in a reasonably healthful environment, and (6) avoid direct contact with infected people.

Chronic Fatigue Syndrome

Chronic fatigue syndrome (CFS) may be the most perplexing "infectious" condition physicians see. First identified in 1985, this mononucleosislike condition is most often seen in women in their 30s and 40s. People with CFS, often busy professional people, report flulike symptoms, including severe exhaustion, fatigue, headaches, muscle aches, fever, inability to concentrate, allergies, intolerance to exercise, and depression. Examinations of the first people with CFS revealed antibodies to the Epstein-Barr virus. Thus observers assumed CFS to be an infectious viral disease (and initially called it *chronic Epstein-Barr syndrome*).

In the years since its first appearance, the condition has received great attention that has produced considerable confusion over its exact nature. In fact, several theories have been advanced to identify the cause (or causes) of CFS.[18] As suggested above, some experts believe an infectious agent may be partially responsible, possibly a virus such as EBV, cytomegalovirus, herpes simplex 1 and 2, or human herpes virus 6. To date no specific virus has been consistently isolated. A second explanation involves an extended challenge to the immune system, possibly activated by an initial viral infection and resulting in the overproduction of immune system chemicals that produce flulike symptoms. A final CFS model suggests the involvement of one or more factors, including emotional, environmental, genetic, and infectious factors. In this model, a stresslike response is believed to disrupt the appropriate interplay among the pituitary, hypothalamus, and adrenal glands (see Chapter 3), thus reducing cortisol production. On the basis of this explanation, other conditions, such as fibromyalgia (see Chapter 12), are related to CFS.

Regardless of its cause or causes, CFS is extremely unpleasant for people who have it. Those experiencing the symptoms over an extended time need to see a physician experienced in dealing with CFS (see Discovering Your Spirituality on page 414).

Bacterial Meningitis

Since approximately 1995, a formerly infrequently seen but potentially fatal infectious disease, *meningococcal meningitis*, has appeared on college campuses, suggesting that college students are currently at greater risk of contracting the disease than are their noncollege peers. Particularly interesting is the fact that among college students, the risk of contracting this infection on campus is highest for those students living in residence halls, suggesting that close living quarters, as well as sharing cigarettes and beverages, kissing (exchanging infectious oral fluids), and contact with students from other areas of the world favor transmission of the bacteria. Since many colleges and universities require that first-year students reside in residence halls, it is in this group that the

> **Key Terms**
>
> **chronic fatigue syndrome (CFS)** an illness that causes severe exhaustion, fatigue, aches, and depression; mostly affects women in their 30s and 40s

Living with an Infectious Disease—Life Is Not Over, Just Different

A chronic infectious disease can wear down your body and your spirit. First, you've got to deal with the pain, fatigue, and medicinal side effects associated with the condition. But you also need to learn to adapt everything—your routine, your relationships, and your work—to the illness. As the quality of your life changes dramatically, you may feel depressed, frustrated, and alone. What is the best way to handle the different aspects of your life as you learn to cope with a long-term illness such as chronic fatigue syndrome, hepatitis, or HIV? Will it ever be possible to enjoy a full life again?

Your workplace may present the first big challenge. Since your energy level will be decreased by your illness, you may have trouble completing tasks on time and handling your normal workload. Your allotted sick time and vacation days may be used up quickly for doctor's appointments, hospitalizations, and those days when you are simply too exhausted to go to work. Your coworkers and your supervisor may discriminate against you in subtle ways, making you feel that you're not doing your fair share. The best way to handle these challenges is to maintain a positive and friendly attitude, carefully manage your time off, promote open communication with your employer, and do your best to produce quality work even when you're not feeling well.

Your intimate relationships may also be strained. Your partner may not understand the new limits your illness places on your activities, especially if you were very active before. The best approach is open and honest communication. Try to dispel (or come to terms with) any fears your partner may have about your illness. Take all necessary precautions to avoid infecting your partner if the disease is transmissible. Also, reassure your partner that you're taking these precautions so that he or she won't become ill. Make a point of including your partner in your daily routines. Keep him or her informed of all doctor's appointments, procedures you must undergo, and any news of progress or setbacks. Share your feelings as a way of reducing anxiety for both of you. Create adaptations so that you can still enjoy a romantic relationship. Make the most of your time together, and find new ways to enjoy each other's company.

If you have children, they will also be affected by your illness. Young children may not understand why you can't take them for a sled ride when you feel sick or why you can't go to a school play because of a doctor's appointment. It's best to let children know that their fears and anxieties are valid and that you want them to share them with you. Tell them about your prognosis, taking care not to make any false promises of recovery if that is not expected. Spend time with each child—helping with homework, reading a story, or doing light chores around the house. Always allow the child to ask questions.

From your home to your workplace, your life will change along with your condition. As you adapt to your new situation, it is important to:

- *Be your own best friend.* Eat well, exercise as much as you can, rest when you need to, and follow the treatments prescribed by your physician.
- *Know and understand your limits.* Don't feel guilty about not doing things you used to do before you got sick. Instead, set goals and handle responsibilities as your condition allows.
- *Find new things to do for fun.* This is a good time to start a new hobby that's relaxing. You can also make adaptations so that you can continue activities you've always enjoyed. Maybe you can't run 3 miles a day, but an after-dinner walk might be a pleasant substitute.
- *Communicate openly with others.* Share your feelings respectfully, and allow others around you to share theirs. Together, you can calm your fears, instill hope in each other, and foster a sense of belonging.
- *Remain positive.* Remember, life is not over—just different. Look forward to the good days, when you feel well, and take advantage of them. Create new ways to fulfill your needs and desires. Remain positive about the future and your treatment. New discoveries do occur, and treatments are always evolving. However, be realistic about your situation. Joining a support group may be one of the best things you can do for yourself.

What you learn about yourself throughout your illness may surprise you. You may discover a strength of spirit you never knew you had. Some days may be very hard, but somehow you get through them. You may see life in a new way—slowing down and taking pleasure in a job well done, enjoying friendships more, listening to your inner voice, spending time with your children, taking a second look at nature, and being thankful for today and tomorrow.

---

incidence of meningococcal meningitis is highest. Additionally, this group of students is most likely to be in large section lecture classes and take meals in large dining facilities. Annually, about 150 cases of meningococcal meningitis occur on American college campuses, resulting in 15 deaths per year. Understandably, more and more colleges and universities are requiring, as a condition of admission, documentation of immunization against bacterial meningitis. Additionally, a growing number of states are requiring that health care providers provide clearly stated information regarding the value of meningococcal meningitis immunization. Some people, however have questioned the cost-effectiveness of immunizing all entering college students.

Meningococcal meningitis is a bacterial infection of the thin membranous coverings of the brain. In its earliest stages, this disease can easily be confused with the flu. Symptoms usually include a high fever, severe headache, stiff neck, nausea with vomiting, extreme tiredness, and the formation of a progressive rash. For about 10 percent of people who develop this condition, the infection is fatal, often within

24 hours. Therefore the mere presence of the symptoms described above signals the need for immediate medical evaluation. If done promptly, treatment is highly effective.

Lyme Disease

Lyme disease is an infectious disease that has become a significant health problem in eastern, southeastern, upper Midwestern, and West Coast states, with 21,273 cases in 2003. The significant increase in the number of cases of Lyme disease since 1992 (when 9,909 cases were reported) most likely reflects widening geographical distribution of the disease, a greater awareness of its symptoms by the general public, and more consistent reporting by physicians. This bacterial disease results when infected blacklegged ticks (also called deer ticks), usually in the nymph (immature) stage, attach to the skin and inject the infectious agent as they feed on a host's blood. The deer ticks become infected by feeding, as larvae, on infected white-footed mice.

The symptoms of Lyme disease vary but typically appear within 30 days as small red bumps surrounded by a circular red rash at the site of bites. The red rash has been described as being like a "bulls eye" in appearance—a pale center surrounded by a reddish margin. Flulike symptoms, including chills, headaches, muscle and joint aches, and low-grade fever, may accompany this acute phase. A chronic phase develops in about 20 percent of untreated infected persons. This phase may produce disorders of the nervous system, heart, or joints. Fortunately, Lyme disease can be treated with antibiotics. Unfortunately, however, no immunity develops, so infection can recur. Some physicians order tests and begin antibiotic therapy too quickly. The basis of treatment should be the appearance of clinical symptoms, not simply the reporting of a tick bite. Lyme disease may be more difficult to diagnose in children than in adults.

People who live in tick-prone areas, including near small urban/suburban wood lots, and participate in outdoor activities can encounter the nearly invisible tick nymphs. These people should check themselves frequently to be sure that they are tick-free. They should tuck shirts into pants, tuck pants into socks, and wear gloves and hat when possible. They should shower after coming inside from outdoors and check clothing for evidence of ticks. Pets can carry infected ticks into the house. If you find ticks, carefully remove them from the skin with tweezers and wash the affected area. There is no vaccine available for humans, so prevention is very important. Repellants containing DEET or permethrin are effective in repelling ticks; they should be used according to directions on the label. A form of "natural" prevention seems to occur in conjunction with frequent noninfected tick exposure in the past, but this should not discourage persons from using preventive measures.[20]

The tick that carries Lyme disease has also been found to be responsible for a potentially fatal bacterial infection called *human granulocytic ehrlichiosis* (*HGE*). This disease is associated with high fever, headache, muscle aches, and chills. HGE is successfully treated with doxycycline, an antibiotic that can also be used in the treatment of Lyme disease. People with these symptoms who live in areas of the country where Lyme disease is reported should make certain that their physician considers HGE in the diagnosis and treatment of their symptoms.

Hantavirus Pulmonary Syndrome

Since 1993 a small but rapidly growing number of people have been dying of extreme pulmonary distress caused by the leakage of plasma into the lungs. In the initial cases, the people lived in the Southwest, had been well until they began developing flulike symptoms over one or two days, then quickly experienced difficulty breathing, and died only hours later. Epidemiologists quickly suspected a viral agent such as the *hantavirus,* known to exist in Asia and, to a lesser degree, in Europe. Exhaustive laboratory work led to the culturing of the virus and confirmed that all of these patients had been infected with an American version of the hantavirus. Researchers identified this latest infectious condition as *hantavirus pulmonary syndrome.*

Today hantavirus pulmonary syndrome has been reported in areas beyond the Southwest, including most of the western states and some of the eastern states. The common denominator in all these areas is the presence of deer mice. We now know that this common rodent serves as the reservoir for the virus. In fact, so common is the mouse that in 2000 the National Park Service began warning hikers, campers, and off-road bikers that hantavirus probably existed in every national park and that caution should be taken to avoid high-risk sites.

The virus moves from deer mice to humans when people inhale dust contaminated with dried virus-rich rodent urine or saliva-contaminated materials, such as nests. Health experts now warn people who live in areas with deer mouse populations (most of the United States) to be extremely careful when cleaning houses and barns in which deer mouse droppings are likely to be found. If you must remove rodent nests, wear rubber gloves, pour a disinfectant or bleach on the nests and soak them thoroughly, and finally, pick up the nests with a shovel and

> **Key Terms**
>
> **Lyme disease** a bacterial infection transmitted by deer ticks

burn them or bury them in holes that are several feet deep. These procedures should greatly reduce the airborne spread of the viral particles.

As humans and their domesticated animals encroach on the habitat of wild animals, which serve as reservoirs for infectious agents, transmission from wild animals to domesticated animals is also possible, if not probable.[21] In terms of hantavirus, curtailing the entry of domesticated animals into the nesting areas of deer mice, although difficult, may be prudent.

Because there is no vaccine for hantavirus pulmonary syndrome, people who likely have been exposed to the infected excrement of deer mice should seek early evaluation of flulike symptoms.

West Nile Virus

First detected in New York City in 1999, the *West Nile virus* was, by the summer of 2000, identified in six eastern states—New York, Connecticut, New Jersey, Maryland, Rhode Island, and Massachusetts. By the end of 2002 the West Nile virus had spread westward and to include 34 states. By the end of 2003, the West Nile virus had been found in all but 2 of the 48 contiguous U.S. states. During the summer and early fall months of 2002 and 2003, the number of newly reported cases and deaths doubled weekly. During the infectious season of 2004, the number of cases of West Nile decreased in comparison to the previous year (2003: 9,858 cases and 262 deaths / 2004: 2,282 cases reported and 77 deaths). A combination of temperature, rainfall, and aggressive community control of mosquitoes was a factor in the decline.

This vector-borne infectious virus is transmitted from a reservoir, most often birds, by mosquitoes that in turn infect humans.[1] Human-to-human transmission (via mosquitoes) apparently does not occur. West Nile virus infection involves flulike symptoms, including fever, headache, muscle ache, fatigue, and joint pain. In young children, persons with immune systems weakened by HIV, and older adults, West Nile virus infection may involve encephalitis, a potentially fatal inflammation of the brain. Physicians recommend that any unusual neurological symptoms be considered as a possible West Nile infection. The West Nile virus deaths that have occurred since the infection's initial appearance in 1999 have been the result of encephalitis.

In an attempt to determine the extent of the West Nile virus range, public health officials throughout the United States have tested mosquitoes, sentinel chickens, crows, other birds, cows, and other animals, including humans. Additionally, mosquito habitats are being treated in an attempt to reduce the vector population. Public service announcements focusing on protection against mosquito bites are routinely made in high-risk areas. Additionally, a newly developed immunization that protects birds is being field tested.

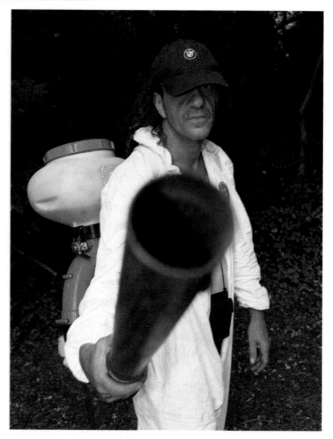

West Nile virus control efforts in Staten Island.

In the period 1999–2003, additional aspects of the disease were reported to the CDC, including the presence of the virus in blood transfusions. (Today, clinically recovered patients cannot give blood for 60 days following release from the hospital.) The West Nile virus has also been isolated from breast milk, and cases of prenatal transmission have been confirmed. Additionally, a new test to accurately screen for infected blood has been developed, as has a new diagnostic test that significantly reduces the time needed to obtain confirmation of the West Nile virus.

Tampon-Related Toxic Shock Syndrome

Toxic shock syndrome (TSS) made front-page headlines in 1980, when the CDC reported a connection between TSS and the presence of a specific bacterial agent (*Staphylococcus*

Key Terms

toxic shock syndrome (TSS) a potentially fatal condition caused by the proliferation of certain bacteria in the vagina that enter the general blood circulation

Signs and Symptoms of Toxic Shock Syndrome

- Fever (102°F or above)
- Headache
- Vomiting
- Sore throat
- Diarrhea
- Muscle aches
- Sunburnlike rash
- Low blood pressure
- Bloodshot eyes
- Disorientation
- Reduced urination
- Peeling of skin on the palms of the hands and soles of the feet

aureus) in the vagina associated with the use of tampons. (In addition to tampon misuse–induced TSS, the condition can be caused in conjunction with nasal packing following surgery, infected burns, and subcutaneous abscesses.)

TSS causes the signs and symptoms listed in the Star box. Superabsorbent tampons can irritate the vaginal lining three times more quickly than regular tampons do. This vaginal irritation is aggravated when the tampon remains in the vagina for a long time (more than five hours). When this irritation begins, the staphylococcal bacteria (which are usually present in the vagina) have relatively easy access to the bloodstream. When these bacteria proliferate in the circulatory system, their resultant toxins produce a massive T cell response (see pages 404–406), in which powerful cytotoxins and other immune system chemicals, including tumor necrosis factor and interleukins, are produced. These immune system products exacerbate the effects of the bacterial toxin on body tissues. A woman with TSS can die, usually as a result of cardiovascular failure, if left untreated. Fortunately, less than 10 percent of women diagnosed as having TSS die.

In comparison to other infectious diseases, the incidence of TSS is limited. During the 1980s and through most of the 1990s, the rate of infection was 1/100,000 women. However, in recent years the rate of infections has increased to 5/100,000. This increase is believed to reflect the relaxed vigilance of women, in combination with earlier age of menstruation. Accordingly, premenopausal women should review (or learn anew) the recommendations for appropriate use of tampons.

These recommendations include: (1) tampons should not be the sole form of sanitary protection used, and (2) tampons should not remain in place for too long. Women should change tampons every few hours and intermittently use sanitary napkins. Tampons should not be used during sleep. Some physicians recommend that tampons not be used at all if a woman wants to be extraordinarily safe from TSS.

 TALKING POINTS As a parent you are preparing yourself to discuss menstruation with your rapidly maturing daughter. What would you say regarding the safe use of tampons?

Hepatitis

Hepatitis is an inflammatory process in the liver that can be caused by several viruses. Types A, B, C (once called non-A and non-B), D, and E have been recognized. Hepatitis can also be caused indirectly from abuse of alcohol and other drugs. General symptoms of hepatitis include fever, nausea, loss of appetite, abdominal pain, fatigue, and jaundice (yellowing of the skin and eyes).[1]

Type A hepatitis is often associated with consuming fecal-contaminated food, such as raw shellfish raised in fecal-contaminated water, raw vegetables field-washed in contaminated water, or contaminated drinking water. As an example, in November of 2003, 520 patrons of a Chi-Chi's Mexican restaurant near Pittsburgh became ill and 3 died as a result of eating contaminated green onions. Poor sanitation, particularly in the handling of food and diaper-changing activities, has produced outbreaks in child care centers. Experts estimate that up to 200,000 people per year experience this infection. This number far exceeds the reported 26,000 to 27,000 cases per year, suggesting that a very large reservoir exists among children, who are routinely asymptomatic before 6 years of age. Therefore, it is currently recommended that children living in states with high levels of reported hepatitis A be vaccinated, as well as children with weakened immune systems, and those who will travel outside the United States.

Type B hepatitis (HBV) is spread in various ways, including sexual contact, intravenous drug use, tattooing, body piercing, and even sharing electric razors. On the basis of these modes of transmission, college students should be aware of the potential risk that they too carry for HBV infection. Beyond the risk factors just identified, medical and dental procedures are also a potential means of transmitting the virus, including patient to practitioner, and practitioner to patient transmission. Chronic HBV infection has been associated with liver cirrhosis and is the principal cause of liver cancer. An effective immunization for hepatitis B is now

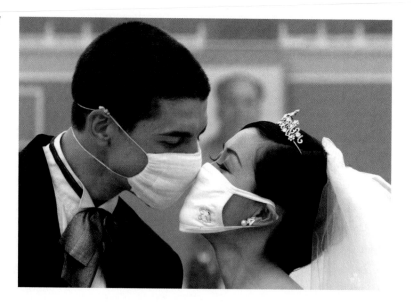

Attempts to prevent contracting SARS were widespread in China during 2003, as seen in this wedding photograph from Beijing.

available; thus, the incidence of HBV in children and adolescents has dropped by one-fifth since 1999. However, an increase has been noted in people over 19 years of age. Although it is given during childhood, it should be seriously considered for older unvaccinated people and college students. In 2002 the American Academy of Pediatrics recommended that all newborns be immunized before leaving the hospital. A new vaccine against both hepatitis A and B is now available. Earlier concerns regarding hepatitis B vaccine and multiple sclerosis have been largely dismissed.

Hepatitis C is contracted in ways similar to hepatitis B (sexual contact, tainted blood, and shared needles). In the absence of immunization, the pool of infected people is in excess of 4 million, and the death rate is expected to climb. Currently a dual-drug therapy for HCV involving multiple forms of interferon in combination with the drug ribavirin is the treatment of choice. Many infected persons remain asymptomatic for decades, and many persons infected with HCV recover from this liver-threatening infection. People in the latter group appear to have a genetically based ability to stimulate a high level of natural killer cells (NK cells) within the immune system.[22] In a recent study, a two-drug combination treatment resulted in a virus-free state for nearly 60 percent of a large group of infected persons treated for 1 year. In spite of encouraging news such as this, recovery from HCV infection seems less likely the case for infected African Americans, a phenomenon that cannot currently be explained.

The newly identified type D (delta) hepatitis is very difficult to treat and is found almost exclusively in people already suffering from type B hepatitis, since the hepatitis D virus requires the presence of the hepatitis B virus in order to gain full pathogenicity. This virus, like type B hepatitis and HIV, makes unprotected sexual contact, including anal and oral sex, very risky. Hepatitis E, associated with water contamination, is rarely seen in this country other than in people returning from hepatitis E virus-endemic areas of the world.

Sudden Acute Respiratory Syndrome (SARS)

In February 2003, the world became aware of a previously unknown respiratory disease, initially thought to be a form of pneumonia. This disease, characterized by high fever (100.4+°F), chills, headaches, and, a few days later, a dry cough, was, in fact, a new viral disease, *Sudden Acute Respiratory Syndrome (SARS)*. First reported in Hanoi, then in Singapore, mainland China, and other Asian countries, the disease quickly presented in Europe and North America. In actuality, the disease had first appeared in a rural area of China, during the fall of 2002, but the Chinese government had apparently chosen not to disseminate this information.

With the rapid spread of SARS, the World Health Organization and CDC issued travel advisories against unnecessary travel to several areas and cities of Asia, as well as to Toronto, Canada. At the same time, scientists isolated the virus responsible for the respiratory disease and identified it as a member of the coronavirus family—a viral family with links to upper respiratory infection (colds). This particular virus, however, apparently entered the human germ pool in conjunction with the eating of civet cats—a delicacy in China—again demonstrating that many infectious conditions in humans have their origins in other animals— **zoonosis.** There still, however, remains some doubt as to whether the civet cat is the principal reservoir of the SARS virus or if rats or other rodents living in close proximity infect both the civet cat and humans.

With news of the SARS outbreak, the international scientific community began a cooperative effort to understand the disease's human-to-human transmission. It was quickly determined that the virus was transmitted by respiratory droplets. It was further determined that the frail, the elderly, and the young were at greatest risk, as well as persons in direct contact with symptomatic persons (family members and hospital staff). Soon thereafter, a diagnostic test was developed and treatment protocols became more focused and effective. These developments, in combination with concerted public health measures regarding the recognition of symptoms and curtailment of transmission opportunities, led to a rapid decline of reported new cases. On June 5, 2003, the World Health Organization declared that SARS had peaked and was subsiding in all infected areas. By the WHO-defined end of the pandemic, August 15, 2003, 33 people in the United States had been infected and no one died, while worldwide 8,422 had been infected and 916 had died.[23] Clearly, in terms of a potentially pandemic disease, the global village had been condensed in size by international travel and commerce.

However, between late summer of 2003 and early fall of 2004, evidence of a greater understanding of SARS virology, as well as its transmission, treatment, and confinement became apparent. On October 6, 2004, the CDC announced that the outbreak of laboratory-acquired SARS cases in China had been controlled and that there were no known cases of SARS anywhere in the world.[24]

Monkeypox

During the summer of 2003, yet another example of a zoonosis, monkeypox, occurred in this country. Specifically, in three Midwest states a viral infection similar to smallpox and characterized by fever, rash, chills, and aches was diagnosed in 49 persons, with probable cases in 91 additional persons in other states. The common thread in all cases proved to be the purchase of pet prairie dogs from a variety of retailers. These retailers had, however, received their "dogs" from a single supplier in Illinois—"Phil's Pocket Pets."

Since the monkeypox virus is endogenous to Africa, and these prairie dogs came from the United States, what had served as the reservoir for the virus? The answer was eventually determined to be the large Gambian rat (apparently another "pocket pet") imported from Ghana in Africa. Apparently physical contact, in some fashion, had occurred between the two different types of animals, thus

providing a mode of transmission. Fortunately, no deaths were reported among the persons contracting the disease.

As mentioned in conjunction with hantavirus transmission, the interplay among wild animals, domesticated animals, and humans is also applicable to monkeypox. Initially seen in terms of prairie-dog-to-human transmission, experts view the popularity of hedgehogs as pockets pets to be the basis of a future version of monkeypox.[25]

Bird (Avian) Influenza

As noted earlier in the chapter, countries are interconnected to such an extent that emerging infections can be spread globally in a matter of days, if not hours. Because of this, the probability of future pandemics—including one of *bird (avian) flu*—is nearing certainty. Based on extrapolations from the 1918 influenza pandemic and taking into account improvements in health care, the most conservative estimates of deaths if (some experts confidently say "when") avian flu reaches pandemic levels are a billion people ill, with 2 to 7 million deaths. Two highly respected experts in infectious disease epidemiology have separately predicted that one-quarter to one-third of the world's population would become ill and 180 million deaths would result. The financial costs would be in the tens of billions of dollars.[26]

Bird flu first reached the public in 2003 when health officials in Laos, Cambodia, Vietnam, and eventually nearly a dozen more Asian countries reported the wholesale death of millions of chickens and, by the end of 2004, the death of 45 humans—all infected with new orthomyxovirus, H5N1, a highly virulent mutated version of the avian virus associated with the Hong Kong bird flu epidemic of 1997. In this latest case, the 45 deaths represented about three-fourths of the infected people seen during that year.

Because the highly virulent H5N1 has now acquired genetic material from widening array of animal hosts (chickens, ducks, turkeys, and other birds, and possibly cats) and could comingle with the less virulent but human-to-human transmissible avian virus (H7), the probability of a "super version" is high. To date killing or immunizing fowl has been the principal method of minimizing bird-to-human transmission,[27] but human-to-human transmission would be extremely difficult to curtail. Thus, as the world awaits coming flu seasons, vaccine experimentation is underway,[28] and several

---

Key Terms

zoonosis the transmission of diseases from animals to humans

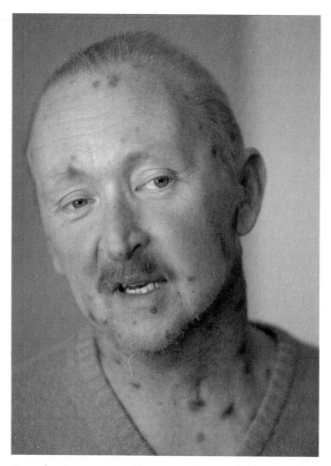

Kaposi's sarcoma, a rare skin cancer, is frequently seen in persons with AIDS.

countries, including the United States and Canada, have begun stockpiling antiviral medications.

AIDS

AIDS (*acquired immunodeficiency syndrome*) has become the most devastating infectious disease in recent history and it is virtually certain to be among the most devastating diseases in history unless a cure is forthcoming. Setting aside for the present the international scope of the HIV/AIDS epidemic, statistics for the United States alone paint a distressing picture. On the basis of data reported through December 2003, a total of 929,985 Americans have been diagnosed with AIDS, and 524,060 have died from its effects (or 56.3 percent of all cases).[29] Table 13.4 shows the estimated numbers of persons living with HIV/AIDS at the end of 2003, by race/ethnicity, sex, and transmission category in 33 confidential name-based reporting areas. Note that for adolescents and adults, male-to-male homosexual contact, female heterosexual contact, and male injected drug use are the leading means

of transmission. It was recently reported that the rate of infection has, over the past decade, doubled for black Americans (from 1 to 2 percent), while holding steady at 0.2 percent for whites.

In addition to the human tragedy suggested by these statistics, the financial cost of treating the HIV/AIDS epidemic is sizable. Today it is estimated that annual medical care costs (including medications) for an infected individual is approximately $20,000, and that over $13 billion is expended annually by the public and third-party funding sources. Although these costs appear to be falling gradually owing to the effectiveness of newer medications, the buying power of AIDS advocacy groups, the movement of older medications into generic status, and efforts on the part of the pharmaceutical industry to lower costs, the financial burden that AIDS places on the health care system makes the disease demanding for all Americans.

Cause of AIDS

AIDS is the disease caused by HIV, a virus that attacks the helper T cells of the immune system (see pages 404–406). When HIV attacks helper T cells, people lose the ability to fight off a variety of infections that would normally be easily controlled. Because these infections develop while people are vulnerable, they are collectively called *opportunistic infections*. HIV-infected (HIV+) patients become increasingly vulnerable to infection by bacteria, protozoa, fungi, and several viruses. A variety of malignancies also develop during this period of immune-system vulnerability.

HIV+ with AIDS was originally diagnosed based on the presence of specific conditions. Among these were *Pneumocystis carinii* pneumonia and Kaposi's sarcoma, a rare but deadly form of skin cancer. Gradually, experts recognized that additional conditions were associated with advancing deterioration of the immune system and thus added them to the list of AIDS conditions. This list now includes almost 30 definitive conditions, with more conditions being added as they become apparent. Among the conditions found on the current version of the list are toxoplasmosis within the brain, cytomegalovirus retinitis with loss of vision, lymphoma involving the brain, recurrent salmonella blood infections, and a wasting syndrome that includes invasive cervical cancer in women, recurrent pneumonia, and recurrent tuberculosis. Today, however, experts tend to assign the label of HIV+ with AIDS to HIV-infected people when their level of helper T cells drops below 250 cells per cubic milliliter of blood, regardless of whether specific conditions are present.

Spread of HIV

HIV cannot be contracted easily in comparison to other infectious conditions such as colds, flu, and some childhood infections that can spread quickly within a classroom or office complex. The chances of contracting HIV through

Table 13.4 Estimated Numbers of Persons Living with HIV/AIDS at the End of 2003 (by race/ethnicity, sex, and transmission category—33 areas with confidential name-based HIV infection reporting)

Transmission category	White, not Hispanic No.	%	Black, not Hispanic No.	%	Hispanic No.	%	Asian/Pacific Islander No.	%	American Indian/Alaska Native No.	%	Total[a] No.	%
Male adult or adolescent												
Male-to-male sexual contact	86,674	76	50,675	47	20,498	60	809	67	840	61	160,433	62
Injection drug use	10,550	9	23,658	22	6,365	19	141	12	210	15	41,207	16
Male-to-male sexual contact and injection drug use	10,431	9	7,817	7	2,165	6	48	4	187	14	20,773	8
Heterosexual contact	5,178	5	23,513	22	4,814	14	190	16	122	9	34,124	13
Other[b]	1,524	1	1,198	1	276	1	28	2	19	1	3,071	1
Subtotal	114,358	100	106,861	100	34,118	100	1,216	100	1,379	100	259,609	100
Female adult or adolescent												
Injection drug use	6,625	34	13,244	23	1,957	23	51	14	164	34	22,173	25
Heterosexual contact	12,494	64	43,957	75	6,498	75	290	81	306	64	63,981	73
Other[b]	447	2	1,118	2	183	2	18	5	7	2	1,787	2
Subtotal	19,566	100	58,319	100	8,638	100	359	100	477	100	87,940	100
Child (<13 yrs at diagnosis)												
Perinatal	636	84	2,591	94	443	91	15	76	15	88	3,720	92
Other[c]	118	16	165	6	42	9	5	24	2	12	342	8
Subtotal	754	100	2,756	100	485	100	20	100	17	100	4,062	100
Total[d]	**134,678**		**167,938**		**43,241**		**1,595**		**1,873**		**351,614**	

[a]Includes 2,289 persons of unknown race or multiple races
[b]Includes hemophilia, blood transfusion, perinatal, and risk factors not reported or not identified
[c]Includes hemophilia, blood transfusion, and risk factors not reported or not identified
[d]Includes 4 persons of unknown sex. Because column totals were calculated independently of the values for the subpopulations, the values in each column may not sum to the column total.

casual contact with HIV-infected people at work, school, or home are extremely low or nonexistent. HIV is known to be spread only by direct sexual contact involving the exchange of bodily fluids (including blood, semen, and vaginal secretions), the sharing of hypodermic needles, transfusion of infected blood or blood products, and perinatal transmission (from an infected mother to a fetus or newborn baby). For HIV to be transmitted, it must enter the bloodstream of the noninfected person, such as through needles or tears in body tissues lining the rectum, mouth, or reproductive system. Current research also indicates that HIV is not transmitted by sweat, saliva, tears, or urine, although the virus may be found in very low concentrations in these fluids. The virus cannot enter the body through the gastrointestinal system because digestive enzymes destroy the virus. An exception to this generalization, however, might exist, as studies conducted in Africa indicate that transmission can occur in conjunction with breast-feeding infants.[30] A second exception involves the transmission of HIV between infected persons and their uninfected sexual partners during episodes of unprotected oral sex when the uninfected persons have evident gingivitis and bleeding gums.[31]

Women are at much greater risk than men are of contracting HIV through heterosexual activity because of the higher concentration of lymphocytes in semen ($\pm$ 10 million lymphocytes/tsp) than in vaginal secretions ($\pm$ 1,200 thousand lymphocytes/tsp). This susceptibility is evidenced in part by the increasing percentage of women with AIDS who were infected through heterosexual contact—from 8 percent in 1981, to 19 percent in 1993, and 73 percent in 2003.[29] Women under age 25 contract the virus principally through heterosexual contact. Figure 13-4 shows the estimated number of new cases of HIV worldwide.

Signs and Symptoms of HIV Infection

Most people infected with HIV initially feel well and have no symptoms (that is, they are asymptomatic). Experts generally consider the *incubation stage* for HIV infection to be 6 months to 10 or more years, with the average

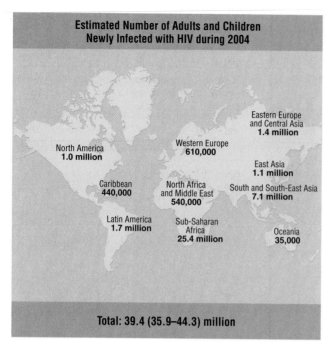

Estimated Number of Adults and Children Newly Infected with HIV during 2004

North America 1.0 million

Western Europe 610,000

Eastern Europe and Central Asia 1.4 million

East Asia 1.1 million

Caribbean 440,000

North Africa and Middle East 540,000

South and South-East Asia 7.1 million

Latin America 1.7 million

Sub-Saharan Africa 25.4 million

Oceania 35,000

Total: 39.4 (35.9–44.3) million

Figure 13-4 For every person counted in these statistics, there is a face and a story. What are you doing to protect yourself from HIV (AIDS)?

approximately 6 years. Despite the long period between infection and the first clinical observation of damage to the immune system, antibodies to HIV may appear within several weeks to three months of contracting the virus. Of course, relatively few people are tested for HIV infection at any time during the incubation period. Thus infected people could remain asymptomatic (currently described as HIV+ without symptoms) and be carriers of HIV for years before they experience signs of illness sufficient to warrant a physical examination. In light of the long

incubation of HIV infection and the relatively small percentage of the general public yet tested, the cost-effectiveness of very widescale HIV screening has received renewed interest.[32] On the basis of new research, the CDC is reevaluating its current, and more restrictive, guidelines regarding screening populations.

Without symptoms of immune-system deterioration or AIDS-testing results, sexually active people need to redefine the meaning of monogamy. Couples must now account for the sexual partners they have both had over the past 10 years. Unfortunately, people do this so infrequently that some observers are labeling today's young adults "a generation in jeopardy."

Most people infected with HIV, in the absence of early screening and prophylactic drug treatment, eventually develop signs and symptoms of a more advanced stage of the disease. These *prodromal stage* signs and symptoms include tiredness, fever, loss of appetite and weight, diarrhea, night sweats, and swollen glands (usually in the neck, armpits, and groin). At this point, they are said to be HIV+ with symptoms. (See Table 13.5.)

Given sufficient time, perhaps as long as 15 years, most infected people without prophylactic drug treatment move beyond HIV with symptoms into the *acute stage*. At this point, the label HIV+ with AIDS is applied, either on the basis of clinically defined conditions or more likely on the basis of a helper T cell count below 250 per cubic milliliter of blood. A normal helper T cell range is 800 to 1,000. The efficacy of treatment is based in part on improvements in the T cell count over time.

A small percentage of infected people can suppress the infection and have survived for over two decades without developing AIDS, but experts do not fully understand this ability (possibly attributing it to a suppressor compound formed by specific immune system cells).

Table 13.5 The Spectrum of HIV Infection

	HIV+ without symptoms (asymptomatic)	HIV+ with symptoms	HIV+ with AIDS
External signs	No symptoms Looks well	Fever Night sweats Swollen lymph glands Weight loss Diarrhea Minor infections Fatigue	Kaposi's sarcoma *Pneumocystis carinii* pneumonia and/or other predetermined illnesses Neurological disorders One or more of an additional 30+ diagnosable conditions or a helper T cell count falls below 250 per cubic milliliter
Incubation	Invasion of virus to 10 years	Several months to 10 or more years	Several months to 10–12 or more years
Internal level of infection	Antibodies are produced Immune system remains intact Positive antibody test	Antibodies are produced Immune system weakened Positive antibody test	Immune system deficient Positive antibody test
Infectious?	Yes	Yes	Yes

Diagnosis of HIV Infection

HIV infection is diagnosed through a clinical examination, laboratory tests for accompanying infections, and an initial screening test. Should the initial screening test produce a negative result, persons at risk for infection should be rescreened in 3 to 6 months. For persons reluctant to present themselves for screening in a clinical setting, home screening tests are also available. Regardless, once initial screening has been undertaken, to eliminate the small chance of a false positive having occurred, more sensitive tests can be administered, including the enzyme-linked immunosorbent assay (ELISA) and Western blot test. Although expensive and not completely reliable, even more recently developed tests are now available. One of these tests identifies the existence of viral mutations known to be drug resistant, while another helps determine whether a particular drug will function in suppressing the contracted viral strain. This information helps physicians structure treatment protocols.

Treatment of HIV and AIDS

There is no cure for HIV infection and the resultant AIDS. It is critically important, however, that treatment begin upon diagnosis, or at least no later than the time at which the T cell count reaches 250/cubic milliliters of blood. Current treatment uses a combination of drugs drawn principally from two distinct groups: the *reverse-transcriptase inhibitors* (divided into two classes, nucleoside analogs and nonnucleoside analogs reverse-transcriptase inhibitors) and the *protease inhibitors.*

The reverse-transcriptase inhibitors block the action of reverse transcriptase, an enzyme the virus requires to replicate itself within the host's infected T helper cells. Currently a combination of two of the many available reverse-transcriptase inhibitors is used to formulate a portion of the drug "cocktail" employed in treating HIV infection.

Introduction of the protease inhibitors, in combination with the reverse-transcriptase inhibitors, has revolutionized the treatment of HIV infection. These drugs inhibit the ability of the virus to undertake the replication process. In most treatment protocols, one protease inhibitor is combined with two reverse-transcriptase inhibitors to complete the drug cocktail.

More recently, new combination protease inhibitor-based products have reached the market. These products that combine two or more protease inhibitors are intended to reduce the number of pills taken daily by HIV+ persons. Prior to the development of these products, a regimen of taking twenty or more pills needed to be followed each day. This demanding regimen leads to a high degree of *noncompliance,* or failure to follow directions, sometimes resulting in the cessation of medication use.

In addition to reverse-transcriptase inhibitors and protease inhibitors, three recently introduced types of medications have been developed to further enhance the battle against HIV/AIDS. Now, newer and even more potent "cocktails" are developed by combining both older and new medication. The treatment is deemed highly active antiretroviral therapy, or *HAART.* HAART has proven highly effective in extending the life of many persons with HIV/AIDS by significantly reducing the level of HIV (viral load) in the body. Decision as to what a given patient's HAART will consist of is determined by factors such as the viral load data and the presence of preexisting conditions.

In the final analysis, however, as effective as HAART is in improving the length and quality of life for persons with HIV/AIDS, mortality concerns remain, and life expectancy is compromised. The inability of persons with AIDS to move into and through the *decline stage* and on to the *recovery stage* reflects the relationship between the disease and the immune system itself.

In addition to the antiviral drugs, physicians also have a variety of medications to treat the symptoms associated with various infections and malignancies that make up AIDS. These drugs, of course, cannot reverse HIV status or cure AIDS. Researchers continue to search for vaccines to prevent HIV infection. Currently, several HIV vaccines are in the initial stage (Phase I) of human trial. One vaccine, under development by Merck Pharmaceuticals, has recently entered Phase II trials after showing considerable promise in initial trials. Of the two vaccines to reach Phase III trials (the most extensive trials before FDA approval for marketing), one was deemed unsuccessful, and trials using the second are ongoing.

The reality of HIV/AIDS in Africa and Asia is only now being recognized worldwide. With an estimated 25.4 million infected persons in sub-Saharan Africa and an additional 7.1 million infected persons in Southeast Asia, the need for a vaccine specific to the viral strains of these areas is growing rapidly.[33] Conversely, in the absence of a vaccine (and the inability to effectively treat those currently infected), it is projected that African life expectancy will drop to 29 years and that more than 29 million orphans will need care. Similar consequences are expected in areas of Asia.

Developing a safe, effective, and affordable vaccine (as has been done for other infectious diseases) remains difficult because of the unique ability of HIV to alter its outer coat and quickly incorporate its genetic material into the host's helper T cells' genetic material, thus preventing the immune system from developing immune recognition.

Prevention of HIV Infection

Can HIV infection be prevented? The answer is a definite yes. HIV infection rates on college campuses are considered low (approximately 0.2 percent), but students can be at risk. Every person can take several steps to reduce the risk of contracting and transmitting HIV. All these steps require understanding one's behavior and the methods by which HIV can be transmitted. Some appropriate steps for college-aged people are abstinence, safer sex, sobriety, and communication with potential sexual partners. To ensure the greatest protection from HIV, one should abstain from sexual activity.

Changing for the Better on page 425 lists recommendations for safer sex, sobriety, and the exchange of honest, accurate information about sexual histories.

However, it is increasingly apparent that it is difficult (or nearly impossible) for people to remember and then apply these guidelines. Accordingly, the CDC is beginning a gradual "reversal of course" away from an emphasis on prevention toward a medical model based on testing, contact identification, and individual counsel. Initial testing, the beginning point of this model, will initially occur in homeless shelters, drug treatment centers, jails, and in conjunction with prenatal care. A 2005 recommendation by the CDC added a new dimension to possible adoption of a medical model for HIV/AIDS prevention. This recommendation suggests that all persons potentially exposed to possible HIV infection through rape, accident (needle pricks or blood splatter to the eyes), occasional drug use, or unprotected intercourse be immediately started on a drug cocktail within 72 hours and continued for 28 days in hopes of preventing infection.[34] At this point, the effectiveness of this prophylactic approach is based on positive results using primates and the monkey form of HIV.

The role of prevention may become even more critical than it is now if an initial case of a drug-resistant form of HIV is proven to be more than an anomaly. This situation relates to an HIV infection in a New York City patient who failed to respond to three of the established drug protocols and progressed to AIDS within a few months.[35] The person involved was described as a male in his 40s, sexually promiscuous (anal intercourse), and a user of methamphetamine, but who apparently had a normal immune system before becoming infected. Clinicians in San Diego reported that they too may be dealing with a similar situation. Other HIV/AIDS experts believe that this situation does not represent the beginning of a drug-resistant form of the HIV-1 virus but is a true anomaly.

 TALKING POINTS In a job interview with a representative from a large pharmaceutical company, you are asked about your feelings regarding the affordability of HIV/AIDS medications in third world countries. What would your response be?

Sexually Transmitted Diseases

Sexually transmitted diseases (STDs) were once called venereal diseases (for Venus, the Roman goddess of love). Today the term *venereal disease* has been superseded by the broader terms *sexually transmitted disease* or *sexually transmitted infections*. Experts currently emphasize the successful prevention and treatment of STDs rather than the ethics of sexuality. Thus one should consider the following points: (1) By age 25 years approximately one-third of all adults will have contracted a sexually transmitted disease—most often chlamydia, herpes simplex, or human papillomavirus infection; (2) a person can have more than one STD at a time; (3) the symptoms of STDs can vary over time and from person to person; (4) the body develops little immunity for STDs; and (5) STDs can predispose people to additional health problems, including infertility, birth defects in their children, cancer, and long-term disability. In addition, the risk of HIV infection is higher when sexual partners are also infected with STDs. Several of the most common STDs are summarized in Table 13.6.

This section focuses on the STDs most frequently diagnosed among college students (chlamydia, gonorrhea, human papillomavirus infection, herpes simplex, syphilis, and pubic lice). (Complete the Personal Assessment on page 437 to determine your risk of contracting an STD. See Changing for the Better on page 425 for safer sex practices.)

Chlamydia (Nonspecific Urethritis)

Chlamydia is thought to be the most prevalent STD in the United States today. Chlamydia infections occur an estimated 5 times more frequently than does gonorrhea and up to 10 times more frequently than syphilis. Because of its high prevalence in sexually active adolescents (310,505 cases in 2003),[36] they should be screened for chlamydia twice a year, even in the absence of symptoms. Because chlamydia frequently accompanies gonorrheal infections, a dual therapy is often appropriate when gonorrhea is found. Sexually active people in the 20- to 24-year age range (with 324,411 cases of chlamydia in 2003)[36] should also be

> **Key Terms**
>
> **sexually transmitted diseases (STDs)** infectious diseases that are spread primarily through intimate sexual contact
>
> **chlamydia** the most prevalent sexually transmitted disease; caused by a nongonococcal bacterium

Average Number of Sexual Partners

- Women
- Men

3% 3% | 31% 20% | 36% 21% | 20% 23% | 6% 16% | 3% 17%

| 0 | 1 | 2–4 | 5–9 | 10–20 | 21 or more |

Figure 13-5 Average number of sexual partners men and women have had since age 18. The fewer the number of partners you've had, the lower your risk of contracting HIV or an STD.

Source: RT Michael, JH Gagnon, EO Laumann, G Kolata: *Sex in America: A definitive study.*

considered for routine screening, particularly if they have a history of multiple sex partners and have not practiced a form of barrier contraception (see Figure 13-5).

Chlamydia trachomatis is the bacterial agent that causes the chlamydia infection. Chlamydia is the most common cause of nonspecific urethritis (NSU). NSU describes infections of the **urethra** and surrounding tissues that are not caused by the bacterium responsible for gonorrhea. About 80 percent of men with chlamydia display gonorrhealike signs and symptoms, including painful urination and a whitish pus discharge from the penis. As in gonorrheal infections and many other STDs, most women report no overt signs or symptoms. A few women might exhibit a mild urethral discharge, painful urination, and swelling of vulval tissues. The recommended treatment for chlamydia is either a single dose of azithromycin (1 g) or doxycycline (100 mg) given orally twice a day for 7 days. The infected person should carefully comply with instructions to abstain from sexual intercourse.[47]

Both sexual partners should receive treatment to avoid the ping-pong effect—the back-and-forth reinfection that occurs among couples when only one partner receives treatment. Furthermore, as with other STDs, having chlamydia once does not effectively confer immunity.

Unresolved chlamydia can lead to the same negative health consequences that result from untreated gonorrheal infections. In men the pathogens can invade and damage the deeper reproductive structures (the prostate

gland, seminal vesicles, and Cowper's glands). Sterility can result. The pathogens can spread further and produce joint problems (arthritis) and heart complications (damaged heart valves, blood vessels, and heart muscle tissue).

In women the pathogens enter the body through the urethra or the cervical area. If the invasion is not properly

Key Terms

urethra (yoo **ree** thra) the passageway through which urine leaves the urinary bladder

Table 13.6 Summary of Common Sexually Transmitted Diseases

STD	Pathogen Name/Type	Symptoms
Chlamydia	*Chlamydia trachomatis* bacterium	Most women report no overt signs or symptoms. In men, gonorrhealike signs and symptoms include painful urination and a whitish pus discharge from the penis
Human papillomavirus (HPV, genital warts)	Human papillomavirus	Genital warts (condylomata acuminata), pinkish-white lesions in raised clusters on the penis, scrotum, labia, cervix, or around the anus.
Gonorrhea	*Neisseria gonorrhoea* bacterium	In men, a milky-white discharge from the penis, painful urination; women tend to be asymptomatic but can report frequent, painful urination, with a slimy yellow-green discharge from the vagina or urethra.
Herpes	Herpes simplex 1 virus (HSV-1) produces labial herpes; herpes simplex 2 virus (HSV-2) produces genital herpes	HSV-1 produces common fever blisters or cold sores around the lips and oral cavity; HSV-2 produces similar blisterlike lesions in the genital area, swollen lymph glands, muscular aches and pains, and fever.
Syphilis	*Treponema pallidum* bacterium	Primary stage marked by appearance of small, painless red pustule on skin or mucous membrane anywhere on body 10 to 90 days after exposure; forms a painless but highly infectious ulcer called a *chancre;* heals spontaneously in 4 to 8 weeks. If not treated, progresses to secondary, latent, and late stages.
Pubic lice	Pubic louse (insect)	Intense itching in the genital region.

Source: Centers for Disease Control and Prevention. "Sexually Transmitted Disease Treatment Guidelines 2002." *MMWR* 51: (No. RR-6) [1–80], 2002.

treated, it can reach the deeper pelvic structures, producing a syndrome called **pelvic inflammatory disease (PID).** The infection may attack the inner uterine wall (endometrium), the fallopian tubes, and any surrounding structures to produce this painful syndrome. A variety of further complications can result, including sterility, ectopic

Key Terms

pelvic inflammatory disease (PID) an acute or chronic infection of the peritoneum or lining of the abdominopelvic cavity and fallopian tubes; associated with a variety of symptoms or none at all and a potential cause of sterility

Table 13.6 *Continued*

Modes of Transmission	Treatment	Consequences if Not Treated
Sexual intercourse; can be transmitted to newborn during vaginal birth	Azithromycin: 1 g orally in a single dose Doxycycline: 100 mg orally twice a day for 7 days Erythromycin and ofloxacin are alternative medications.	In men, damage to prostate gland, seminal vesicles, and Cowper's glands; sterility; joint problems; heart complications. In women, PID; infection of uterine wall (endometrium), fallopian tubes, and surrounding structures; sterility and peritonitis.
Sexual activity	*Patient-Applied:* Podofilox solution or gel: applied by swab or finger twice a day for 3 days Imiquimod 5% cream: applied by finger 3 times a week for 16 weeks *Provider-Administered:* Cryotherapy: with liquid nitrogen or cryoprobe Podophyllin resin: small amount applied directly to each wart within a relatively small area TCA or BCA: applied in liquid form, repeated weekly if necessary Surgical removal: scissors, shave excision, curettage, or electrosurgery	In women, precancerous changes in the cervix; can become large enough to block the birth canal. In both sexes can become large enough to block the anus.
Sexual activity; oral sex can produce a gonorrheal infection of the throat; can be transmitted to the rectal areas of both sexes; can be transmitted to a newborn during birth	Cefixine: 400 mg orally (single dose) or Ceftriaxone: 125 mg IM (single dose) or Ciprofloxacin: 500 mg orally (single dose) or Ofloxacin: 400 mg orally (single dose) + azithromycin or doxycycline	Nausea, vomiting, fever, tachycardia (rapid heart beat), infection of upper or lower genital tract; can spread to tissues surrounding liver, peritoneum, heart, joints, or other structures.
Direct contact with a person who has an active infection; shared drinking glasses or utensils; intimate sexual contact; condoms may provide insufficient protection	*Initial Infection* (episodic and suppressive therapy protocols required later): Acyclovir: 400 mg orally 3/day (7–10 days) Acyclovir: 200 mg orally 5/day (7–10 days) Famciclovir: 250 mg orally 3/day (7–10 days) Valacyclovir: 1 g orally 2/day (7–10 days)	Recurrent infections are shorter and less severe than the initial episode.
Sexual intercourse	*Primary and Secondary:* Benzathine penicillin G: 2.4 million units IM (single dose) *Latent (early):* Benzathine penicillin G: 2.4 million units IM (single dose) *Latent (late):* Benzathine penicillin G: 7.2 million units (3 doses of 2.4 million once/week)	Secondary stage: general malaise, loss of appetite, fever, headache, hair loss, bone and joint pain, rash, sores in mouth and throat. Late (tertiary) stage: soft, rubbery tumors anywhere on the body that ulcerate and heal with scarring; damage to CNS and heart; disability; premature death.
Sexual contact; contact with contaminated bedsheets and clothes	Permethrin: 1% cream (applied for 10 minutes/washed off) Lindane: 1% shampoo (applied for 4 minutes/washed off) or Pyrethrins with piperonyl butoxide: (applied for 10 minutes/washed off) Bedding/clothing: wash (machine)/dry (hot cycle); no body contact for 72 hours	Lice rarely carry disease, but the itching they cause can be embarrassing and uncomfortable.

(tubal) pregnancies, and **peritonitis.** Infected women can transmit a chlamydia infection to the eyes and lungs of newborns during a vaginal birth. Detecting chlamydia and other NSUs early is of paramount concern for both men and women.

> **Key Terms**
>
> **peritonitis** (pare it ton **eye** tis) inflammation of the peritoneum, or lining of the abdominopelvic cavity

Human Papillomavirus

The appearance of another STD, **human papillomavirus (HPV),** is unwanted news. Because HPV infections are generally asymptomatic, the exact extent of the disease is unknown. A study of a group of sexually active college women found HPV infection in approximately 20 percent of the women. HPV-related changes to the cells of the cervix are found in nearly 5 percent of the Pap smears taken from women under age 30. Researchers currently believe that risk factors for HPV infection in women include: (1) sexual activity before age 20, (2) intercourse with three or more partners before age 35, and (3) intercourse with a partner who has three or more partners. The extent of HPV infection in men is even less clearly known, but it is probably widespread.

HPV infection is alarming because some of the more than 50 forms of the virus are strongly associated with precancerous changes to cells lining the cervix, illustrating the importance of new viral pap smears (see Chapter 11). Additionally, visible genital warts (cauliflowerlike, raised, pinkish-white lesions) are associated with viral forms 6 or 11, while viral forms 16, 18, 31, 33, and 35 foster changes in other areas (Figure 13-6). Found most commonly on the penis, scrotum, labia, cervix, and around the anus, these lesions represent the most common symptomatic viral STD in this country. Although most genital wart colonies are small, they may become very large and block the anus or birth canal during pregnancy.

Treatment for HPV, including genital warts, may include patient-applied gels or creams or physician-administered cryotherapy, topical medication, or surgery (see Table 13.6). Regardless of treatment, however, the viral colonies will probably return. One should use condoms to attempt to prevent transmission of HPV.

As noted in Chapter 11, in conjunction with cervical cancer, a vaccine effective for HPV 16 and 18 has been approved for use. Additional vaccines are under development, some intended for use in newly infected patients, some for long-established infections but before clear changes in the cervical lining cells occur, and others for more advanced cervical cancer.[38] Most of the last two classes of vaccines are for treatment rather than prevention of HPV infections.

Gonorrhea

Another extremely common (600,000 cases/year estimated and 335,104 cases reported in 2003[39]) STD, *gonorrhea* is caused by a bacterium *(N. gonorrhoea).* The incidence of gonorrhea rose 18 percent between 1997 and 2001, perhaps, in part, because of decreasing fear of HIV/AIDS brought about by the effectiveness of the protease inhibitors being widely reported at that time. However, since 2001 the reported cases of gonorrhea have declined.[39] In men this bacterial agent can produce a milky-white discharge from the penis, accompanied by painful urination. About 80 percent of men who contract gonorrhea report varying degrees of these symptoms. This figure is approximately reversed for women: Only about 20 percent of women are symptomatic and thus report varying degrees of frequent, painful urination, with a slimy yellow-green discharge from the vagina or urethra. Oral sex with an infected partner can produce a gonorrheal infection of the throat (pharyngeal gonorrhea). Gonorrhea can also be transmitted to the rectal areas of both men and women.

An interesting finding relative to gonorrhea in adolescents suggests that the incidence of gonorrhea within the adolescent population correlated closely with the consumption of beer, suggesting that alcohol consumption fosters a higher level of high-risk sexual behavior, including earlier onset of sexual activity, an increased number of partners, and less selectivity in choosing those partners.

Figure 13-6 A human papillomavirus infection (genital warts)

Key Terms

human papillomavirus (HPV) sexually transmitted viruses, some of which are capable of causing precancerous changes in the cervix; causative agent for genital warts

With heavy consumption of beer on many college campuses, this finding does not bode well for the highly asymptomatic female population.

Physicians diagnose gonorrhea by culturing the bacteria. Because of the paired occurrence of chlamydia and gonorrhea, dual therapy with doxycycline or azithromycin in combination with ofloxacin (see Table 13.6) is used in susceptible populations, particularly adolescent women. Outside of these groups, recommended treatment for uncomplicated cases involves the use of one of several antimicrobial drugs. Although prevalent in other areas of the world, drug-resistant strains are not extensive in the United States. This said, however, it should be noted that a clear increase in drug-resistant strains has been reported along the West Coast, in various Pacific areas, such as Hawaii, other Pacific Islands, and Asia. Infected persons who might have contracted the disease while in these areas should report this information to their physicians.

Testing for gonorrhea is included as a part of prenatal care so that infections in mothers can be treated before they give birth. If the birth canal is infected, newborns can easily contract the infection in the mucous membranes of the eye.

Herpes Simplex

Public health officials think that the sexually transmitted genital herpes virus infection rivals chlamydia as the most prevalent STD. To date about 45 million Americans have been diagnosed, although the asymptomatic (thus undiagnosed) population could increase this figure substantially. *Herpes* is really a family of more than 50 viruses, some of which produce recognized diseases in humans (chicken pox, **shingles** mononucleosis, and others). One subgroup, called herpes simplex 1 virus (HSV-1), produces an infection called *labial herpes* (oral or lip herpes). Labial herpes produces common fever blisters or cold sores around the lips and oral cavity. Herpes simplex 2 virus (HSV-2) is a different strain that produces similar clumps of blisterlike lesions in the genital region (Figure 13-7). Laypeople call this second type of herpes the STD type, but both types produce identical clinical pictures. About 5 to 30 percent of cases are caused by HSV-1. Oral-genital sexual practices most likely account for this crossover infection.

Herpes appears as a single sore or as a small cluster of blisterlike sores. These sores burn, itch, and (for some) become very painful. The infected person might also report swollen lymph glands, muscular aches and pains, and fever. Some patients feel weak and sleepy when they have blisters. The lesions may last from a few days to a few weeks. Viral shedding lasts a week on average; then the blisters begin scabbing, and new skin is formed. Even when the patient has become asymptomatic, viral transmission is still possible.

Herpes is an interesting virus for several reasons. It can lie dormant for long periods. For reasons not well understood but perhaps related to stress, diet, or overall

Figure 13-7 A severe herpes infection

health, the viral particles can be stimulated to travel along the nerve pathways to the skin and then create an active infection. Thus herpes can be considered a recurrent infection. Fortunately for most people, recurrent infections are less severe than the initial episode and do not last as long. Recommended treatment for an initial outbreak of herpes calls for the use of one of three medications: acyclovir, famcyclovir, or valacyclovir. These medications are taken orally, multiple times each day, for 7 to 10 days (see Table 13.6). Because herpes may occur at intervals following initial treatment, two choices exist. One is to treat each recurrence as it arises (episodic recurrent treatment), and the second is to attempt to suppress recurrence through continuous use of medication (daily suppressive therapy) (see Table 13.6). The treatment choices described above appear to be equally effective for HSV-1 and HSV-2. Additionally, physicians may recommend other medications

> ### Key Terms
>
> **shingles** painful fluid-filled skin eruptions along underlying sensory nerve pathways—caused by reactivation of once-sequestered herpes zoster (chicken pox) virus

for relief of various symptoms. Genital herpes is almost always diagnosed through a clinical examination.

At this time a much anticipated Phase III trial is under way in which a large number of women, known to be free of both HSV-1 and HSV-2, are testing a new vaccine manufactured by GlaxoSmith Kline Biologicals. Earlier, but in much smaller trials, it was found that the vaccine was effective in providing protection for about 70 percent of the female subjects but was almost completely ineffective for males. The current trial, still ongoing, is being conducted to confirm these initial findings.

Currently, the best method of preventing herpes infection is to avoid all direct contact with a person who has an active infection. Do not kiss someone with a fever blister—or let them kiss you (or your children) if they have an active lesion. Do not share drinking glasses or eating utensils. Check your partner's genitals. Do not have intimate sexual contact with someone who displays the blisterlike clusters or rash. Condoms are only marginally helpful and cannot protect against lesions on the female vulva or the lower abdominal area of men. Be careful not to infect yourself by touching a blister and then touching any other part of your body. Changing for the Better gives helpful advice about talking with your partner if you have genital herpes. Note that valacyclovir is more effective than other medications. Intended as a prophylactic medication (to be taken daily), valacyclovir does reduce the incidence of viral shedding, but it does not completely suppress episodes of recurrent herpes.[40]

Newborn babies are especially susceptible to the virus if they come into contact with an active lesion during birth. Newborns have not developed the defense capabilities to resist the invasion. They can quickly develop a systemic (general) infection (neonatal herpes) that is often fatal or local infections that produce permanent brain damage or blindness. Fortunately, most of these problems can be prevented through proper prenatal care. A cesarean delivery can be performed if viral particles might be present at birth, although this is done less often today than in the past.

Syphilis

Like gonorrhea, *syphilis* is caused by a bacterium *(Treponema pallidum)* and is transmitted almost exclusively by sexual intercourse. The incidence of syphilis, a CDC-reportable disease, is far lower than that of gonorrhea. In 1950 a record 217,558 cases of syphilis were reported in this country. The number of cases then fell steadily to fewer than 80,000 cases in 1980. From 1980 through 1990 the incidence climbed, reaching nearly 140,000 cases in 1990. Another decline then began, and in 1993 the number of cases dropped to 101,259. In 2000 the CDC re-

Changing for the Better

Talking with Your Partner about Herpes

My girlfriend told me she has herpes and said she's "taking care of everything." What can I do to get things out in the open?

Although herpes rarely has serious consequences, the lesions are infectious and tend to reappear. It is important to talk openly with your partner about this sexually transmitted disease. Here are some tips to make things easier:

- *Educate yourself.*
  Be aware that herpes is rarely dangerous. Learn when the disease is most contagious (during the eruption and blister stage), and realize that herpes can be spread even during the noneruption, nonblister periods—traditionally defined as safe periods.
- *Choose the right time to talk.*
  Discuss herpes with your partner only after you have gotten to know each other.
- *Listen to your partner.*
  Be prepared to answer any questions that he or she may have.
- *Together, put things in perspective.*
  Keep a positive outlook.
  Remember that you are not alone.
  Be aware that using a condom and abstaining from coitus during the most infectious period can prevent transmission of the disease.
  Although there is no known cure, research continues on an antiviral drug.
  Join a local support group together.

InfoLinks

www.herpeszone.com/MainMenu.htm

ported that syphilis had fallen to the lowest level (5,972) in 42 years. By 2003, however, reported syphilis cases had risen to 7,177, with increases across all racial and ethnic groups, with the exception of African Americans.[41]

Whether the upward trend in the number of reported syphilis cases continues remains to be seen. As has been true for most of the last decades a high percentage of cases have been associated with HIV infections, largely among gay men in several larger cities. (See the Star box on page 431 for more information on this disease.) Observers have noted an alarming increase in infant syphilis in children born to mothers who use drugs and support their habit through sexual activity. For additional information on symptoms, mode of transmission, treatment, and the consequences of not treating syphilis, see Table 13.6, on pages 426 and 427.

Syphilis

Syphilis is a serious disease that, left untreated, can cause death. The chance of contracting syphilis during a single sexual encounter with an infected partner is now about 30%. Syphilis takes a well-established course after it is contracted.

Infection

The syphilis bacterium, *Treponema pallidum,* is a spirochete. It is transmitted from an infected person to a new host through intimate contact. Moist, warm tissue, such as that lining the reproductive, urinary, and digestive tracts, offers an ideal environment for the agent.

Incubation

Syphilis incubates without symptoms for 10 to 90 days, followed by the characteristic primary stage of the disease.

Primary Stage

The primary stage of syphilis lasts 1 to 5 weeks. A small, raised, painless sore called a *chancre* forms at this time. This highly infectious lesion is not easily identified in 90% of women and 50% of men; thus these people generally do not seek treatment. The chancre heals in 4 to 8 weeks.

Secondary Stage

The extremely contagious secondary stage of the disease occurs 6 to 12 weeks after initial infection. The infectious agents are now systemic, so symptoms may include a generalized body rash, a sore throat, or a patchy loss of hair. A blood test (VDRL) will be positive, and treatment can be effectively administered. If untreated, the second stage subsides within 2 to 6 weeks. A pregnant woman can easily transmit syphilis to her fetus during this stage. Congenital syphilis often results in stillbirth or an infant born with a variety of life-threatening complications. Early treatment of infected pregnant women can prevent congenital syphilis.

Latent Stage

After the secondary stage subsides, an extended period of noninfectiousness occurs. The infectious agents remain dormant within the body cells, and the infected person displays few clinical signs during this state.

Late Stage

Syphilis can recur for a third time 15 to 25 years after initial contact. In late-stage syphilis, tissue damage is profound and irreversible. The person suffers damage to the cardiovascular system, central nervous system, eyes, and skin, and death from the effects of the disease is likely.

Treatment

Depending on the stage, syphilis is treated with varying doses of Benzathine penicillin G. See Table 13.6 for protocol specifics.

Pubic Lice

Three types of lice infect humans: the head louse, the body louse, and the pubic louse all feed on the blood of the host. Except for the relatively uncommon body louse, these tiny insects do not carry diseases. They are, however, very annoying.

Pubic lice, also called *crabs,* attach themselves to the base of the pubic hairs, where they live and lay their eggs (nits). These eggs move into a larval stage after one week; after two more weeks, they develop into mature adult crab lice.

People usually notice they have a pubic lice infestation when they suffer intense itching in the genital region. Prescription and OTC creams, lotions, and shampoos are usually effective in killing both the lice and their eggs, although some reports suggest that lice are becoming resistant to OTC treatments.

Lice are not transmitted exclusively through sexual contact but also by contact with contaminated bedsheets and clothes. If you develop a pubic lice infestation, you must thoroughly treat yourself, your clothes, your sheets, and your furniture.

Vaginal Infections

Two common pathogens produce uncomfortable *vaginal infections.* The first is the yeast or fungus pathogen *Candida (Monilia) albicans,* which produces the yeast infection often called *thrush.* These organisms, commonly found in the vagina, seem to multiply rapidly when some unusual stressor (pregnancy, use of birth control pills or antibiotics, diabetes) affects a woman's body. This infection, now called *vulvovaginal candidiasis* (*VVC*), is signaled by a white or cream-colored vaginal discharge that resembles cottage cheese. Vaginal itching and vulvar swelling are also commonly reported. Current treatment is based on the use of one of several prescription and OTC azole drugs. For women who have recurrent VVC, some degree of prophylactic suppression of candidiasis seems possible. Weekly use of a prescription antifungal medication (fluconazole) for periods of 6, 9, and 12 months managed to keep slightly over 40 percent of a group of women with recurrent VVC free of infection for 12 months; higher percentages of infection-free patients were found at 6 and 9 months.[42] Success after 12 months was not determined.

Nonprescription azole-based products offer effective home treatment. One should first consult with a physician before using these new products for the first time. (Men rarely report this monilial infection, although some may report mildly painful urination or a barely noticeable discharge at the urethral opening or beneath the foreskin of the penis.)

The protozoan *Trichomonas vaginalis* also produces a vaginal infection. This parasite can be transmitted through sexual intercourse or by contact with contaminated (often damp) objects, such as towels, clothing, or toilet seats, that may contain some vaginal discharge. In women, this infection, called *trichomoniasis,* or "trich," produces a foamy, yellow-green, foul-smelling discharge that may be accompanied by itching, swelling, and painful urination. Although topically applied treatments with limited effectiveness for trichomoniasis are available, only one highly effective oral medication is currently on the market. Men infrequently contract trichomoniasis but may harbor the organisms without realizing it. They also should be treated to minimize reinfection of partners.

The vagina is warm, dark, and moist, an ideal breeding environment for a variety of organisms. Unfortunately, some highly promoted commercial products seem to increase the incidence of vaginal infections. Among these are tight panty hose (without cotton panels), which tend to increase the vaginal temperature, and commercial vaginal douches, which can alter the acidic level of the vagina. Both of these products might promote infections. Women are advised to wipe from front to back after every bowel movement to reduce the opportunity for direct transmission of pathogenic agents from the rectum to the vagina. Avoiding public bathrooms when possible is also a good practice. Of course, if you notice any unusual discharge from the vagina, you should report this to your physician.

Cystitis and Urethritis

Cystitis, an infection of the urinary bladder, and urethritis, an infection of the urethra, occasionally can be caused by a sexually transmitted organism. Such infections can also be caused by the organisms that cause vaginitis and organisms found in the intestinal tract. A culture is required to identify the specific pathogen associated with a particular case of cystitis or urethritis. The symptoms are pain when urinating, the need to urinate frequently, a dull aching pain above the pubic bone, and the passing of blood-streaked urine.

Physicians can easily treat cystitis and urethritis with antibiotics when the specific organism has been identified. The drug Monurol, which requires only a single dose, has proved effective. Few complications result from infections that are treated promptly. If cystitis or urethritis is left untreated, the infectious agent could move upward in the urinary system and infect the ureters and kidneys. These upper-urinary-tract infections are more serious and require more extensive evaluation and aggressive treatment. Therefore one should obtain medical care immediately upon noticing symptoms.

A study involving urinary tract infections in mice, whose urinary tract infections are virtually identical to those in humans, demonstrated that the bacteria involved often avoid complete antibiotic elimination. This occurs when the bacteria clump into pods that are then covered by a "bio-film" produced by the organisms. The film retards further antibody effectiveness, allowing the infection to be re-established when antibiotics have been cleared from the body.

Preventing cystitis and urethritis depends to some degree on the source of the infectious agent. One can generally reduce the incidence of infection by urinating completely (to fully empty the urinary bladder), particularly following intercourse, and by drinking ample fluids to flush the urinary tract. Drinking cranberry juice has been found to reduce urinary tract infections. Prevention of urinary tract infections cannot be disregarded, from both medical and cost perspectives. As noted, untreated cystitis and urethritis can be the basis of serious damage to the kidneys. These two infections combined are the second greatest cause of antibiotic use—which is both costly and increasingly losing effectiveness.

 TALKING POINTS Honesty regarding past sexual experiences is a critical issue in the decision to introduce sexual intimacy into a new relationship. What questions would you feel comfortable being asked by another person, and what questions would you be prepared to ask that person?

Nosocomial Infections

Where would you have to have been to have contracted a *nosocomial infection?* The answer is a hospital, a clinic, or a nursing home, or the office of a health care provider. Nosocomial infections are infections spread in conjunction with the delivery of health care services—most often from providers to patients or from patients to other patients. Persons who are hospitalized are particularly vulnerable to the development of a potentially fatal nosocomial infection.

Each year approximately 2.2 million persons develop an infection directly linked to the health care system, including 780,000 in association with operations. Contact with infectious agents occurs in a variety of ways, including the failure of personnel to wash or glove their hands properly prior to conducting examinations, the use of contaminated medical equipment such as endoscopes and catheters, failure to maintain sterile operating areas during surgery, receiving intravenous medications contaminated during their manufacture, contact with visitors who are infectious, sharing a semiprivate room with an infectious roommate, and even from the clothing of physicians and other staff members.

Two factors make today's nosocomial infections particularly serious. The first, of course, is that these infections strike people who by virtue of being institutionalized are less than healthy. Second is the fact that the organisms most frequently associated with these infections are among the most pathogenic with which we have contact, staphylococcus aureus and enterococcus faecium, both of which are (or nearly are) resistant to vancomycin, our most potent antibiotic.

Today, disease control officials debate the generally stated mortality (32,000 deaths/year) attributed to nosocomial infections. Some experts suggest that a relatively large percentage of the hospital and nursing home infections are in patients who are already terminal or so frail that infection was only an exacerbating factor in their demise. Accordingly, they believe that these deaths should not be included in the mortality statistics associated with nosocomial infections.

Because of the potential seriousness of nosocomial infections, persons entering the health care arena should discuss infection control with their physician, including the proper procedures for self-care, the possible need for greater isolation while an in-patient, and the desirability of restricting visitation.

Taking Charge of Your Health

- Since microorganisms develop resistance to antibiotics, continue taking all such medications until gone, even when the symptoms of the infection have subsided.
- Check your current immunization status to make sure you are protected against preventable infectious diseases.

- If you are a parent, take your children to receive their recommended immunizations as necessary.
- Because of the possibility of contracting HIV/AIDS and sexually transmitted diseases, incorporate disease prevention into all your sexual activities.

- Use the Personal Assessment on page 437 to determine your risk of contracting a sexually transmitted disease.
- If you have ever engaged in high-risk sexual behavior, get tested for HIV.

SUMMARY

- We have made progress in reducing the incidence of some forms of infectious disease, but other infectious conditions are becoming more common.
- A variety of pathogenic agents are responsible for infectious conditions.
- A chain of infection with six potential links characterizes every infectious condition.
- One can acquire immunity for some diseases through both natural and artificial means. Children should be immunized according to a schedule.
- The immune system's response to infection relies on cellular, chemical, and humoral elements.
- The common cold and influenza produce many similar symptoms but differ in their infectious agents, incubation period, prevention, and treatment.
- Tuberculosis and pneumonia are potentially fatal infections of the respiratory system.
- Mononucleosis and chronic fatigue syndrome are infections that produce chronic tiredness.
- Bacterial meningitis, a potentially fatal infection of the linings that cover the brain, is of increasing concern on college campuses.

- Lyme disease is a bacterial infection contracted through outdoor activities.
- Hantavirus pulmonary syndrome is caused by a virus carried by ticks; human-to-human transmission has also been reported.
- West Nile virus is a vectorborne infection that is distributed throughout the United States.
- Toxic shock syndrome is a bacterial infection generally arising from the improper use of tampons.
- Hepatitis B (serum hepatitis) is a bloodborne infectious condition that produces serious liver damage. Other varieties are hepatitis A, C, D, and E.
- SARS, a potentially fatal respiratory infection, has reached North America from Asia.
- Monkeypox and bird (avian) flu reflect the ability of infectious agents to move from animals to humans.
- HIV/AIDS is a widespread, incurable viral disease transmitted through sexual activity, through intravenous drug use, in infected blood products, or across the placenta during pregnancy.
- HIV and AIDS are currently best treated with a drug cocktail, using protease inhibitors and reverse-transcriptase

inhibitors; an effective vaccine for prevention has not been developed. Concerns are rising regarding the unchecked spread of HIV/AIDS in areas of Africa and Asia.

- There are a variety of sexually transmitted conditions, many of which do not produce symptoms in most infected women and many infected men.

- Nosocomial infections are infections that develop in conjunction with the delivery of health care services, most often in hospitals and nursing homes.

REVIEW QUESTIONS

1. What are the agents responsible for the most familiar infectious conditions?
2. Describe the six links in the chain of infection.
3. What are the two principal cellular/chemical components of the immune system, and how do they cooperate to protect the body from infectious agents, foreign protein, and abnormal cells?
4. How are the common cold and influenza similar? How do they differ in their causative agents, incubation period, prevention, and treatment?
5. What symptoms make mononucleosis and chronic fatigue syndrome similar? What aspects of each are different?
6. Why is bacterial meningitis of greater concern on the college campus than elsewhere?
7. Why is outdoor activity a risk factor for contracting Lyme disease?
8. What role do birds play in the transmission of the West Nile virus? What insect is the vector?

9. In what way is toxic shock syndrome most directly linked to the menstrual cycle?
10. How is hepatitis B transmitted, and which occupational group is at greatest risk of contracting this infection? How do forms A, C, D, and E compare with hepatitis B?
11. What is SARS? Where was its site of origin, and how did it most likely reach North America?
12. How is HIV transmitted? How are HIV/AIDS currently treated, and how effective is the treatment? In what areas of the world does the HIV/AIDS epidemic seem virtually unchecked?
13. What specific infectious diseases could be classified as STDs?
14. Why are women more often asymptomatic for STDs than men?
15. What is a nosocomial infection, and in what settings are nosocomial infections most likely to develop?

ENDNOTES

1. Hamann B. *Disease Identification, Prevention, and Control* (2nd ed.). New York: McGraw-Hill, 2001.
2. Salidin KS. *Anatomy and Physiology: Unity of Form and Function,* 4th ed. New York: McGraw-Hill, 2007.
3. Parkham P. *The Immune System* (2nd ed.). New York: Garland Publishing, 2004.
4. Vander A, Sherman J, Luciano D. *Human Physiology: The Mechanisms of Body Function* (9th ed.). New York: McGraw-Hill, 2003.
5. Schonberger S, et al. Transplantation of haematopoietic stem cells derived from cord blood, bone marrow or peripheral blood: A single centre matched-pair analysis in a heterogeneous risk population. *Klin Padiatr.* 2004. 216(6):356–363.
6. Warwick R, Armitage S. Cord blood banking. *Best Pract Res Clin Obstet Gynaecol.* 2004. 18(6):995–1011.
7. Varricchio F, et al. Understanding vaccine safety information from the Vaccine Adverse Event Reporting System. *Pediatr Infect Dis* J. 2004. 23(4):287–294.
8. McQuillan GM, et al. Serologic immunity to diphtheria and tetanus in the United States. *Ann Intern Med.* 2002. 136(9);660–666.
9. Kruszon-Moran DM, McQuyillan GM, Chu SY. Tetanus and diphtheria immunity among females in the United States: Are recommendations being followed? *Am J Obstet Gynecol.* 2004. 190(4):1070–1076.

10. Fendrick AM, et al. The economic burden of non-influenza-related viral respiratory tract infections in the United States. *Arch Intern Med.* 2003. 163(4): 487–494.
11. Douglas RM, et al. Vitamin C for preventing and treating the common cold. *Cochrane Database Syst Rev.* 2004. (4): CD000980.
12. Ball TM, et al. Influence of attendance at day care on the common cold from birth through 13 years of age. *Arch Pediatr Adolesc Med.* 2002. 156(2):121–126.
13. Matthews CE, et al. Moderate to vigorous physical activity and risk of upper-respiratory tract infection. *Med Sci Sports Exer.* 2002. 34(8):1242–1248.
14. Guidelines & Recommendations. *Influenza antiviral medications:* 2004–2005 *interim chemoprophylaxis and treatment guidelines.* November 2004. www.cdc.gov/flu/professionals/treatment/0405_antiviralguide.htm.
15. Belshe RB, et al. Serum antibody responses after intradermal vaccination against influenza. *N Engl J Med.* 2004. 351(22):2286–2294.
16. Stohr K. Avian influenza and pandemics—research needs and opportunities. *N Engl J Med.* 2005. 352(4):405–407.
17. *Reported Tuberculosis in the United States, 2003.* U.S. Department of Health and Human Services, CDC. September 2004.

18. *Chronic Fatigue Syndrome, NIAID Fact Sheet*. 2004. National Institute of Allergy and Infectious Diseases. U.S. Department of Health and Human Services. www.niaid.nih.gov/factsheets/cfs.htm.

19. Scott RD, et al. Vaccinating first-year college students living in dormitories for Meningococcal disease: An economic analysis. *Am J Prev Med.* 2002. 23(2):98–105.

20. Burke G, et al. Hypersensitivity to ticks and Lyme disease risk. *Emerg Infect Dis.* 2005. 11(1):36–41.

21. Zeier M, et al. New ecological aspects of hantavirus infection: A change of a paradigm and a challenge—a review. *Virus Genes.* 2005. 30(2):157–180.

22. Khakoo SI, et al. HLA and NK cell inhibitory receptor genes in resolving hepatitis C virus infection. *Science.* 2004. 305(5685):872–874.

23. World Health Organization. *Summary Table of SARS Cases by Country, 1 November 2002–7 August 2003.* August 15, 2003. www.who.int/entity/crs/sars/country/en/country200308_15.pdf.

24. Centers for Disease Control and Prevention, Department of Health and Human Services. *Current SARS Situation.* October 6, 2004. www/cdc.gov/ncidod/sars/situation.htm.

25. Riley PY. Hedgehog zoonoses. *Emerg Infect Dis.* 2005. 11(2):1–5.

26. Specter M. Nature's bioterrorist: Is there any way to prevent a deadly avian-flu pandemic? *The NewYorker.* Feb. 28, 2005. pp 50–61.

27. Larkin M. Avian flu: Sites seek to respond and reassure. *Lancet Infect Dis.* 2005. 5(3):141–142.

28. Quirk M. USA to manufacture two million doses of pandemic flu vaccine. *Lancet Infect Dis.* 2005. 4(11):654.

29. Centers for Disease Control and Prevention, Department of Health and Human Services. *HIV/AIDS Surveillance Report.* 2003 (Vol 15).

30. Coutsoudis A. Infant feeding dilemmas created by HIV: South African experiences. *J Nutr.* 2005. 135(4):956–959.

31. Edwards S, Crane C. Oral sex and the transmission of viral STIs. *JAMA.* 1998. 74(1):6–10.

32. Sanders GD, et al. Cost-effectiveness of screening for HIV in the era of highly active antiretroviral therapy. *N Engl J Med.* 2005. 352(6):570–585.

33. *Adults and Children Estimated to Be Living with HIV/AIDS, End 2004.* AIDS epidemic update: December 2004. www.unaids.org/wad2004/EPIupdate2004_html_enEPI04_13_en.htm.

34. Valdiserri RO. A future free of HIV: What will it take? *J Public Health Manag Pract.* 2005. 11(1):1–3.

35. Berkhout B, de Rhonde A, van der Hoek L. Aggressive HIV-1? *Retrovirology.* 2005. 2(1):13.

36. Centers for Disease Control and Prevention. "Sexually Transmitted Disease Treatment Guidelines 2002." *MMWRSI:* No. RR-6, 1–80, 2002.

37. Centers for Disease Control and Prevention. *Chlamydia—Reported Cases and Rates per 100,000 Population by Age and Sex. United States 1999–2003.* www.cdc.gov/std/stats/tables/table10.htm.

38. American Cancer Society. What's new in cervical cancer research and treatment? *Cancer Reference Information.* www.cancer.org/docroot/CRI/content/CRI_2_4_6X_Whats_new_in_cervical_cancer.

39. Centers for Disease Control and Prevention. *Gonorrhea—Reported Cases and Rates per 100,000 Population by Age and Sex: United States 1999–2003.* www.cdc.gov/std/stats/tables/table20.htm.

40. Chakrabarty A, et al. Valacycolovir for the management of herpes viral infections. *Skin Therapy Lett.* 2005. 10(1):1–4.

41. Centers for Disease Control and Prevention. *Primary and Secondary Syphilis—Reported Cases by Race/Ethnicity, Age Group and Sex: United States 1999–2003.* www.cdc.gov/std/stats/tables/table34a.htm.

42. Sobel JD, et al. Maintenance fluconazole therapy for recurrent vulvovaginal candidiasis. *N Engl J Med.* 2004. 351(9): 876–883.

As We Go to Press

Infectious diseases once common but now rare can, under certain circumstances, return with a vengeance. Cholera, a gastrointestinal bacterial infection that produces rapid and fatal diarrhea-induced dehydration is such a disease. When an outbreak of cholera develops it signals that human drinking water or food has been contaminated with human or animal waste. Cholera is currently occurring in several West African nations in conjunction with heavy rains that wash untreated sewage into wells and other drinking water sources. Compounding the problem are the mass migrations of displaced people fleeing politically induced hostilities and their settlement in over-burdened refugee camps. Young children and the frail elderly are particularly vulnerable to the effects of cholera.

At the time of this writing, the United Nations describes the growing incidence of cholera as being an "upsurge" and is responding with antidiarrhea medications and, most important, uncontaminated drinking water supplies. Unfortunately, these supplies are not always effective, because of inadequately functioning health care delivery systems.

personal assessment

What is your risk of contracting a sexually transmitted disease?

A variety of factors interact to determine your risk of contracting a sexually transmitted disease (STD). This inventory is intended to provide you with an estimate of your level of risk.

Circle the number in each row that best characterizes you. Enter that number on the line at the end of the row (points). After assigning yourself a number in each row, total the number appearing in the points column. Your total points will allow you to interpret your risk for contracting an STD.

Age
						Points
1	3	4	5	3	2	_____
0–9	10–14	15–19	20–29	30–34	35+	

Sexual Practices
0	1	2	4	6	8	_____
Never engage in sex	One sex partner	More than one sex partner but never more than one at a time	Two to five sex partners	Five to ten sex partners	Ten or more sex partners	

Sexual Attitudes
0	1	8	1	7	8	_____
Will not engage in nonmarital sex	Premarital sex is okay if it is with future spouse	Any kind of premarital sex is okay	Extramarital sex is not for me	Extramarital sex is okay	Believe in complete sexual freedom	

Attitudes toward Contraception
1	1	6	5	4	8	_____
Would use condom to prevent pregnancy	Would use condom to prevent STDs	Would never use a condom	Would use the birth control pill	Would use other contraceptive measure	Would not use anything	

Attitudes toward STD
3	3	4	6	6	6	_____
Am not sexually active so I do not worry	Would be able to talk about STD with my partner	Would check out an infection to be sure	Would be afraid to check out an infection	Can't even talk about an infection	STDs are no problem— easily cured	

YOUR TOTAL POINTS _____

Interpretation
5–8	Your risk is well below average
9–13	Your risk is below average
14–17	Your risk is at or near average
18–21	Your risk is moderately high
22+	Your risk is high

To Carry This Further . . .
Having taken this Personal Assessment, were you surprised at your level of risk? What is the primary reason for this level? How concerned are you and your classmates and friends about contracting an STD?

part five

Sexuality and Reproduction

Sexuality is an important part of our being. It colors the way we interact with the world around us and affects our goals, relationships, and roles in society.

1. **Physical Dimension**

   Sexuality is closely related to the physical dimension of health. For example, our bodies mature at puberty, we respond to sexual arousal, we make choices about contraception and pregnancy, and we adjust our sexual behavior as we age. Sexual experiences and relationships can be very complex and demanding because they are fueled by energy and time. They are enhanced when the body is well maintained, rested, and relatively free from illness.

2. **Emotional Dimension**

   One of the most stressful aspects of life is sexual intimacy. Feelings about your own sexual behavior can range from exhilaration to ambivalence to depression. Being comfortable with your sexuality comes from being guided by your core values, knowing how to express your sexual feelings openly, being able to set limits when appropriate, and understanding how to communicate effectively with your partner.

3. **Social Dimension**

   Because sexuality often involves interaction with others, the development of social skills in this area is imperative. For many, dating is an excellent arena in which to establish specific social skills. As a relationship becomes more serious, communication skills will grow. These skills are important factors in the process of mate selection and marriage for those who choose this path.

4. **Intellectual Dimension**

   As a relationship matures, opportunities abound for contemplation, analysis, and reflection. You may have to sort through your feelings, examine your values, and use lessons from past experiences as you take part in this process of introspection. You will also draw on your intellectual resources as you learn about reproductive anatomy, fertility, sexual response, contraception, and birth.

5. **Spiritual Dimension**

   As an intimate relationship progresses, you may have to explore your feelings about your sense of morality, the appropriateness of premarital sex, or the value of fidelity in a marriage or other long-term committed relationship. Dating, courtship, and particularly marriage offer opportunities to enhance your spirituality by extending sympathy, support, and love to another person. Some people even find the sexual act itself to be a way of expressing their spirituality.

6. **Occupational Dimension**

   Decisions about reproduction can have a significant effect on your occupational dimension of health. Women who are pregnant may have to work even when they are not feeling well. Then they must decide how much time to take off work after the child is born. They and their partners must also make difficult choices about long-term child care arrangements. The decisions they make will affect their occupational satisfaction and sense of fulfillment.

chapter fourteen

Exploring the Origins of Sexuality

Chapter Objectives

On completing this chapter, you will be able to:

▌ describe the genetic basis and the gonadal basis of sexuality.

▌ describe the psychosexual bases of sexuality, including gender identity, gender preference, gender adoption, and initial adult gender identification.

▌ define androgyny and discuss its role in our society.

▌ examine your attitudes toward masculine and feminine roles in our society.

▌ explain the structure and function of the male reproductive and female reproductive systems.

▌ discuss the issues related to male and female circumcision.

▌ trace the stages of the menstrual cycle.

▌ identify techniques for reducing menstrual pain.

▌ analyze the risks and benefits of hormone replacement therapy for reducing the symptoms of menopause.

▌ differentiate among the terms *reproductive sexuality*, *genital sexuality*, and *expressionistic sexuality*.

Eye on the Media

Responsible Sexual Behavior by 2010

Be on the lookout for media reports that feature progress on the nation's health objectives for the year 2010. The government's *Healthy People 2010* report, a comprehensive, public health planning document for the United States, lists 467 health objectives in 28 focus areas. Especially significant for young adults (and their parents) are reports that indicate progress made toward national goals in the area of "responsible sexual behavior." Responsible sexual behavior is one of the 10 leading health indicators that are thought to be able to provide a snapshot of the health of the Nation.[1]

Success in the area of responsible sexual behavior is largely determined by progress made in two key objectives:

Objective 25-11: *Increase the proportion of adolescents who abstain from sexual intercourse or use condoms if currently sexually active.* Objective 13-6a: *Increase the proportion of sexually active persons who use condoms.* These two key objectives were thought to be particularly important because of their overall ability to influence trends in sexual behavior, unintended pregnancies, sexually transmitted diseases, and HIV/AIDS.

[1]U.S. Department of Health and Human Services. *Healthy People 2010: understanding and improving health,* 2nd ed. Washington DC: U.S. Government Printing Office, November 2000.

Early in this new millennium, we have reached a better understanding of both the biological and psychosocial factors that contribute to the complex expression of our sexuality. As a society, we are now inclined to view human behavior in terms of a complex script written on the basis of both biology and conditioning.

Reflecting this understanding is the way in which we use the words *male* and *female* to refer to the biological roots of our sexuality and the words *man* and *woman* to refer to the psychosocial roots of our sexuality. In this chapter, we explore human sexuality as it relates to the dynamic interplay of the biological and psychosocial bases that form our masculinity or femininity.

Biological Bases of Human Sexuality

Within a few seconds after the birth of a baby, someone (a doctor, nurse, or parent) emphatically labels the child: "It's a boy," or "It's a girl." For the parents and society as a whole, the child's biological sexuality is being displayed and identified. Another female or male enters the world.

Genetic Basis

At the moment of conception, a Y-bearing or an X-bearing sperm cell joins with the X-bearing ovum to establish the true basis of biological sexuality.[1] A fertilized ovum with sex chromosomes XX is biologically female, whereas a fertilized ovum bearing the XY sex chromosome is biologically male. Genetics forms the most basic level of an individual's biological sexuality.

Gonadal Basis

The gonadal basis for biological sexuality refers to the growing embryo's development of *gonads*.[2] Male embryos develop testes about the 7th week after conception, and female embryos develop ovaries about the 12th week after conception.

Structural Development

The development of male or female reproductive structures is initially determined by the presence or absence of hormones produced by the developing testes—androgens and müllerian inhibiting substance (MIS). With these hormones present, the male embryo starts to develop male reproductive structures (penis, scrotum, vas deferens, seminal vesicles, prostate gland, and Cowper's glands).

Because the female embryo is not exposed to these male hormones, it develops the characteristic female repro-ductive structures: uterus, fallopian tubes, vagina, labia, and clitoris.

Biological Sexuality and the Childhood Years

The growth and the development of the child in terms of reproductive organs and physiological processes have traditionally been thought to be "latent" during the childhood years. However, a gradual degree of growth occurs in both girls and boys. The reproductive organs, however, undergo faster growth at the onset of puberty and achieve their adult size and capabilities shortly thereafter.

Puberty

The entry into puberty is a gradual maturing process for young girls and boys. For young girls, the onset of menstruation, called *menarche,* occurs at about age 12 or 13 but may come somewhat earlier or later.[3] Early menstrual cycles tend to be anovulatory (ovulation does not occur). Menarche is usually preceded by a growth spurt that includes the budding of breasts and the growth of pubic and underarm hair.[4]

Young males follow a similar pattern of maturation, including a growth spurt followed by a gradual sexual maturity. However, this process takes place about 2 years later than it does in young females. Genital enlargement, underarm and pubic hair growth, and a lowering of the voice commonly occur. The male's first ejaculation is generally experienced by the age of 14, most commonly through **nocturnal emission** or masturbation. For many young boys, fully mature sperm do not develop until about age 15.

Reproductive capability declines only gradually over the course of the adult years. In the woman, however, the onset of **menopause** signals a more direct turning off of the reproductive system than is the case for the male adult. By the early to mid-50s, virtually all women have entered a postmenopausal period, but for men, relatively high-level **spermatogenesis** may continue for a decade or two.[4]

Key Terms

nocturnal emission ejaculation that occurs during sleep; "wet dream"

menopause decline and eventual cessation of hormone production by the female reproductive system

spermatogenesis (sper mat oh **jen** uh sis) process of sperm production

---

The story of sexual maturation and reproductive maturity cannot, however, be solely focused on the changes that take place in the body. Now we will discuss the psychosocial processes that accompany the biological changes.

 TALKING POINTS Your 12-year-old son comes to you and says that all of his male friends are starting to grow facial hair. He is worried that his own beard will never begin. What could you say to him that could ease his fears?

Psychosocial Bases of Human Sexuality

If you visualized growth and development of sexuality as a ladder (Figure 14-1), one vertical rail of the ladder would represent our biological sexuality. Arising at various points along this rail would be rungs representing the sequential unfolding of the genetic, gonadal, and structural components. These biological bases of our sexuality can be considered the "hard-wired" parts of our sexuality. They are rooted in the linkages of our parents' genetic backgrounds. These are the parts of our sexuality over which we have little control.

Because humans, more so than any other life form, can rise above a life centered on reproduction, we have a second dimension or rail to our sexuality—our **psychosocial sexuality.** The reason we possess the ability to be more than reproductive beings is a question for the theologian or the philosopher. We are considerably more complex than the hard-wired functions determined by biology. The process that transforms a male into a man and a female into a woman begins at birth and continues to influence us throughout the course of our lives.

It is during this transformation into a man or woman that we humans have some ability to influence our gender development. Here is where we occasionally are able to make decisions that influence both the way we view ourselves as men or women and the way we are viewed as men or women by others. This is the part of our sexuality that is not completely hard-wired by our genetic background.

Gender Identity

Although expectant parents may prefer to have a child of a particular **gender,** they frequently must wait until the birth of the baby to have their question answered. External genitals "cast the die," and femininity or masculinity begins to receive its traditional reinforcement by the parents and society in general. By the 18th month, typical children have both the language and the insight to correctly identify their gender. They have established a **gender identity.**[5] The first rung rising from the psychosocial rail of the ladder has been climbed.

Gender Preference

During the preschool years, children receive the second component of the scripting required for the full development of psychosocial sexuality—**gender preference.** Gender preference refers to the emotional and intellectual acceptance of one's birth gender. Reaching this rung on the psychosocial rail of the ladder takes place during the preschool years, when nearly every boy prefers being a boy and nearly every girl prefers being a girl.

Late adolescence — Initial Adult Gender Identification

Gender adoption

Pubescence — Structural maturation

Preadolescence — Gender adoption

Childhood — Gender preference

Early childhood — Gender identity

Structural development

Intrauterine — Gonadal sexuality

Genetic sexuality

Biological sexuality / Psychosocial sexuality

Figure 14-1 Our sexuality develops through biological and psychosocial stages.

Key Terms

psychosocial sexuality masculine and feminine aspects of sexuality

gender general term reflecting a biological basis of sexuality; the male gender or the female gender

gender identity recognition of one's gender

gender preference emotional and intellectual acceptance of one's own gender

---

During the preschool years, parents typically begin to control the child's exposure to experiences traditionally reserved for children of the opposite gender. This is particularly true for boys; parents often stop a boy's play activities if they perceive them as being too feminine. (Note: The concept of gender preference is not to be confused with sexual preference. Sexual preference refers to a sexual and/or emotional attraction to sexual partners. Sexual preference is discussed in Chapter 15 in a section entitled "Sexual Orientation.")

Attitudes toward gender roles have become more flexible in recent years. Many parents now allow their children to pursue the activities they enjoy, regardless of whether the activities were once considered strictly masculine, such as playing baseball or building a model airplane, or feminine, such as growing flowers or cooking.

Parents should not become alarmed if their children or teenagers experiment with their gender identity through their appearance or activities. Such experimentation is natural and a part of finding the gender identity that best fits them. Such children often become very secure in their gender identity as adults.

With the recent acceleration in the importance of competitive sports for women, many of the skills and experiences once reserved for boys are now being fostered in young girls. What effect, if any, this movement will have on the speed at which gender preference is reached will be a topic for further research.

Gender Adoption

The process of reaching an initial adult gender identification requires a considerable period of time. The specific knowledge, attitudes, and behavior characteristic of adults must be observed, analyzed, and practiced. The process of acquiring and personalizing these "insights" about how men and women think, feel, and act is reflected by the term **gender adoption,** the first and third rungs below the initial adult gender identification rail of the ladder in Figure 14-1.

In addition to constructing a personalized version of an adult sexual identity, the child and particularly the adolescent must construct a gender schema for a member of the opposite gender. Clearly, the world of adulthood, with its involvement with intimacy, parenting, and employment, requires that men know women and women know men. Gender adoption provides an opportunity to begin constructing the equally valuable "pictures" of what the genders are like.

Initial Adult Gender Identification

By the time young people have climbed all of the rungs of the sexuality ladder, they have arrived at the chronological point in the life cycle when they need to construct an initial

adult **gender identification.** You might notice that this label seems remarkably similar to the terminology used to describe one of the developmental tasks being used in this textbook. In fact, the task of forming an initial adult identity is closely related to developing an initial adult image of oneself as a man or a woman. Although most of us currently support the concept of "person" in many gender-neutral contexts (for some very valid reasons), we still must identify ourselves as either a man or a woman.

Androgyny: Sharing the Pluses

Our society has increasingly accepted an image of a person who possesses both masculine and feminine qualities. This accepted image has taken years to develop because our society traditionally has reinforced rigid masculine roles for men and rigid feminine roles for women.

In the past, from the time a child was born, we assigned and reinforced only those roles and traits that were thought to be directly related to his or her biological gender. Boys were not allowed to cry, play with dolls, or help in the kitchen. Girls were not encouraged to become involved in sports; they were told to learn to sew, cook, and baby-sit. Men were encouraged to be strong, expressive, dominant, aggressive, and career oriented, whereas women were encouraged to be weak, shy, submissive, passive, and home oriented.

These traditional biases have resulted in some interesting phenomena related to career opportunities. Women were denied jobs requiring above-average physical strength, admittance into professional schools requiring high intellectual capacities, such as law, medicine, and business, and entry into most levels of military participation. Likewise, men were not encouraged to enter traditionally feminine careers, such as nursing, clerical work, and elementary school teaching.

For a variety of reasons, the traditional picture has changed. **Androgyny,** or the blending of both feminine and masculine qualities, is more clearly evident in our

---

Key Terms

gender adoption the long process of learning the behavior that is traditional for one's gender

gender identification achievement of a personally satisfying interpretation of one's masculinity or femininity

androgyny (an **droj** en ee) the blending of both masculine and feminine qualities

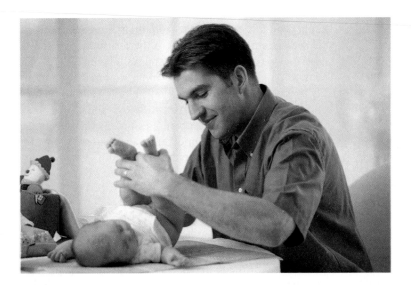

Just as women have broken into traditionally male careers, many men have taken on jobs and tasks that were once considered women's exclusive domain.

society now than ever before. Today it is quite common to see men involved in raising children (including changing diapers) and doing routine housework. It is also quite common to see women entering the workplace in jobs traditionally managed by men and participating in sports traditionally played by men. Men are not scoffed at when they are seen crying after a touching movie. Women are not laughed at when they choose to assert themselves. The disposal of many sexual stereotypes has probably benefited our society immensely by relieving people of the pressure to be 100 percent "womanly" or 100 percent "macho."

Research data suggest that androgynous people are more flexible and independent, have greater self-esteem, have more positive attitudes toward sexuality, and show more social skills and motivation to achieve.[5] (Complete the Personal Assessment on page 459 to explore your own attitudes about sexuality and sex roles.)

 TALKING POINTS How could you demonstrate to your grandmother that the blending of gender roles is a positive development?

Reproductive Systems

The most familiar aspects of biological sexuality are the structures that compose the reproductive systems. Each structure contributes in unique ways to the reproductive process. Thus with these structures, males have the ability to impregnate. Females have the ability to become pregnant, give birth, and nourish infants through breast-feeding. In addition, many of these structures are associated with non-reproductive sexual behavior.

Male Reproductive System

The male reproductive system consists of external structures of genitals (the penis and scrotum) and internal structures (the testes, various passageways or ducts, seminal vesicles, the prostate gland, and the Cowper's glands) (Figure 14-2A).

Male newborn babies are routinely circumcised by all Muslims and Jews. Millions of infants are circumcised in the United States and Canada annually. However, this routine practice has become a controversial subject.[6] Many researchers argue that male circumcision should no longer be an automatic choice, but rather that parents should consider the pros and cons. (See the Star box on page 446 for a look at this debate.)

The Testes

The *testes* (also called *gonads* or *testicles*) are two egg-shaped bodies that lie within a saclike structure called the *scrotum*. During most of fetal development, the testes lie within the abdominal cavity. They descend into the scrotum during the last two months of fetal life.

The testes are housed in the scrotum because a temperature lower than the body core temperature is required for adequate sperm development. The walls of the scrotum are composed of contractile tissue and can draw the testes closer to the body during cold temperatures (and sexual arousal) and relax during warm temperatures. Scrotal contraction and relaxation allow a constant, productive temperature to be maintained in the testes (Figure 14-2B).

A cross-sectional view of a single testis reveals an intricate network of structures called *seminiferous tubules*. Within these 300 or so seminiferous tubules, the process of sperm production (spermatogenesis) takes place. Sperm cell development starts at about age 11 in boys and is

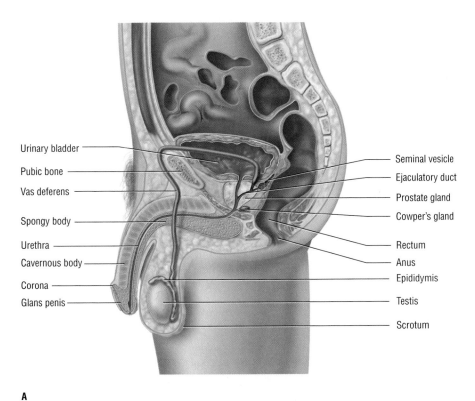

Figure 14-2 The male reproductive system. **A:** Side view, **B:** Front view.

Urinary bladder

Pubic bone

Vas deferens

Spongy body

Urethra

Cavernous body

Corona

Glans penis

Seminal vesicle

Ejaculatory duct

Prostate gland

Cowper's gland

Rectum

Anus

Epididymis

Testis

Scrotum

A

Shaft of penis

Glans penis

Scrotum

Anus

B

influenced by the release of the hormone **ICSH (interstitial cell-stimulating hormone)** from the pituitary gland. ICSH does primarily what its name suggests: it stimulates specific cells (called *interstitial cells*) within the testes to begin producing the male sex hormone *testosterone*. Testosterone in turn is primarily responsible for the gradual

Key Terms

ICSH (interstitial cell-stimulating hormone)
(in ter **stish** ul) a gonadotropic hormone of the male required for the production of testosterone

Male Circumcision: No Longer an Automatic Choice

Should newborn boys still be routinely circumcised? Researchers no longer think so. For example, a committee of the Canadian Paediatric Society recently studied the issue and concluded that newborns should not be routinely circumcised. The study compared the costs and complications of the procedure itself, the incidence of urinary tract infections, sexually transmitted diseases, and cancer of the penis in both circumcised and uncircumcised males, and of cervical cancer in their partners. The committee concluded that routine circumcision cannot be justified.[1] This recommendation echoes that of the American Academy of Pediatrics and the Canadian Paediatric Society.

Another study reported that the rate of penile cancer in fact is lower in circumcised men, but that this difference alone is not sufficient to justify routine circumcision. Other researchers are more vehement, calling circumcision the mutilation of healthy organs. If parents do decide on circumcision, it should be performed only by a trained surgeon in a medical institution, since 85 percent of complications and nearly all disastrous circumcisions are performed by traditional, but medically untrained, circumcisers.[2] In addition, the surgeon should have adequate training in pain relief for this treatment, in view of the overwhelming evidence that newborn circumcision is painful.[3] The parents, in consultation with their physician, should make the final decision.

[1]Anonymous. Neonatal circumcision revisited. Fetus and Newborn Committee, Canadian Paediatric Society (review) *Can Med Assoc J* 1996 March 15; 154(6): 769–780.

[2]Azdemir E. Significantly increased complication risks with mass circumcisions. *Br J Urol* 1997; 80(1): 136–139.

[3]Howard CR, el al. Neonatal circumcision and pain relief: Current training practices. Pediatrics 1998; 101 (3, part 1 of 2): 423–428.

development of the male secondary sex characteristics at the onset of puberty. By the time a boy is approximately fifteen years old, sufficient levels of testosterone exist so that the testes become capable of full spermatogenesis.

Before the age of about 15 most of the sperm cells produced in the testes are incapable of fertilization. The production of fully mature sperm *(spermatozoa)* is triggered by another hormone secreted by the brain's pituitary gland—**FSH (follicle-stimulating hormone).** FSH influences the seminiferous tubules to begin producing spermatozoa capable of fertilization.

Ducts

Spermatogenesis takes place around the clock, with hundreds of millions of sperm cells produced daily. The sperm cells do not stay in the seminiferous tubules but rather are transferred through a system of *ducts* that lead into the epididymis. The epididymis is a tubular coil that attaches to the back side of each testicle. These collecting structures house the maturing sperm cells for 2 to 3 weeks. During this period the sperm finally become capable of motion, but they remain inactive until they mix with the secretions from the accessory glands (the seminal vesicles, prostate gland, and Cowper's glands).

Each epididymis leads into an 18-inch passageway known as the *vas deferens.* Sperm, moved along by the action of hairlike projections called *cilia,* can also remain in the vas deferens for an extended time without losing their ability to fertilize an egg.

Seminal Vesicles

The two vasa deferens extend into the abdominal cavity, where each meets with a *seminal vesicle*—the first of the three accessory structures or glands. Each seminal vesicle contributes a clear, alkaline fluid that nourishes the sperm cells with fructose and permits the sperm cells to be suspended in a movable medium. The fusion of a vas deferens with the seminal vesicle results in the formation of a passageway called the *ejaculatory duct.* Each ejaculatory duct is only about one inch long and empties into the final passageway for the sperm—the urethra.

Prostate Gland

The ejaculatory duct is located within the second accessory gland—the *prostate gland* (see Figure 14-2). The

---

Key Terms

FSH (follicle-stimulating hormone) a gonadotropic hormone required for the initial development of ova (in the female) and sperm (in the male)

prostate gland secretes a milky fluid containing a variety of substances, including proteins, cholesterol, citric acid, calcium, buffering salts, and various enzymes. The prostate secretions further nourish the sperm cells and also raise the pH level, making the mixture quite alkaline. The alkalinity permits the sperm to have greater longevity as they are transported during ejaculation through the urethra, out of the penis, and into the highly acidic vagina.

Cowper's Glands

The third accessory gland, the *Cowper's glands,* serves primarily to lubricate the urethra with a clear, viscous mucus. These paired glands empty their small amounts of preejaculatory fluid during the arousal stage of the sexual response cycle. Alkaline in nature, this fluid also neutralizes the acidic level of the urethra. Viable sperm cells can be suspended in this fluid and can enter the female reproductive tract before full ejaculation by the male.[7] This may account for many of the failures of the "withdrawal" method of contraception.

The sperm cells, when combined with secretions from the seminal vesicles and the prostate gland, form a sticky substance called **semen.**[8] Interestingly, the microscopic sperm actually makes up less than 5 percent of the seminal fluid discharged at ejaculation. Contrary to popular belief, the paired seminal vesicles contribute about 60 percent of the semen volume, and the prostate gland adds about 30 percent.[1] Thus the fear of some men that a **vasectomy** will destroy their ability to ejaculate is completely unfounded (see Chapter 16).

During *emission* (the gathering of semen in the upper part of the urethra), a sphincter muscle at the base of the bladder contracts and inhibits semen from being pushed into the bladder and urine from being deposited into the urethra.[9] Thus semen and urine rarely intermingle, even though they leave the body through the same passageway.

Penis

Ejaculation takes place when the semen is forced out of the *penis* through the urethral opening. The involuntary, rhythmic muscle contractions that control ejaculation result in a series of pleasurable sensations known as *orgasm.*

Key Terms

semen a secretion containing sperm and nutrients discharged from the urethra at ejaculation

vasectomy a surgical procedure in which the vasa deferens are cut to prevent the passage of sperm from the testicles; the most common form of male sterilization

The urethra lies on the underside of the penis and extends through the three cylindrical chambers of erectile tissue (two *cavernous bodies* and one *spongy body*). Each of these three chambers provides the vascular space required for sufficient erection of the penis. When a male becomes sexually aroused, the areas become congested with blood (*vasocongestion*). After ejaculation or when a male is no longer sexually stimulated, these chambers release the blood into the general circulation and the penis returns to a **flaccid** state.

The *shaft* of the penis is covered by a thin layer of skin that is an extension of the skin that covers the scrotum. This loose layer of skin is sensitive to sexual stimulation and extends over the head of the penis, except in males who have been circumcised. The *glans* (or head) of the penis is the most sexually sensitive (to tactile stimulation) part of the male body. Nerve receptor sites are especially prominent along the *corona* (the ridge of the glans) and the *frenulum* (the thin tissue at the base of the glans).

Later in life, men begin to experience some changes in their reproductive system. The level of androgens, or male hormones, decreases with age, and the size of the prostate gland often increases. A deficiency of androgens has been found to cause health concerns in older men, including a lack of strength and energy, changes in mood, lower interest in sex, decreased bone density, and a decrease in muscle mass.[10]

As a result, researchers are studying the benefits and risks of androgen replacement therapy in older men, similar to the hormone replacement therapy given to women. The benefits are an increase in bone and muscle mass, improved muscular and cardiovascular function, improved sexual function, and an overall better sense of well-being. The possible risks include an increased incidence of prostate disease, cardiovascular disease, and liver disease.[10,6] Androgen replacement therapy is available through prescription injections, transdermal patches, oral pills, and most recently through a gel applied daily to the upper arm, shoulders, or abdomen.[11]

Another steroid hormone, DHEA, is believed by some to reverse the aging process and revitalize sexual function (see Considering Complementary Care on page 447).

Female Reproductive System

The external structures (genitals) of the female reproductive system consist of the mons pubis, labia majora, labia minora, clitoris, and vestibule (Figure 14-3). Collectively these structures form the *vulva* or vulval area.

Mons Pubis

The *mons pubis* is the fatty covering over the pubic bone. The mons pubis (or mons veneris, "mound of Venus") is covered by pubic hair and is quite sensitive to sexual stimulation.

Labia Majora and Labia Minora

The *labia majora* are large longitudinal skin folds that cover the entrance to the vagina, whereas the *labia minora* are the smaller longitudinal skin folds that lie within the labia majora. These hairless skin folds of the labia minora join at the top to form the *prepuce.* The prepuce covers the glans of the *clitoris,* which is the most sexually sensitive part of the female body.

Clitoris

In terms of its tactile sensitivity, the *clitoris* is the most sensitive part of the female genitals. It contains a glans and a shaft, although the shaft is below the skin surface. It is composed of erectile tissue that can become engorged with blood. It is covered by skin folds (the clitoral prepuce) and can collect **smegma** beneath these tissue folds.[5]

Vestibule

The *vestibule* is the region enclosed by the labia minora. Evident here are the urethral opening and the entrance to the vagina (vaginal orifice). Also located at the vaginal opening are the *Bartholin's glands,* which secrete a minute amount of lubricating fluid during sexual excitement.

The *hymen* is a thin layer of tissue that stretches across the opening of the vagina. Once thought to be the only indication of virginity, the intact hymen rarely covers the vaginal opening entirely. Openings in the hymen are necessary for the discharge of menstrual fluid and vaginal secretions. Many hymens are stretched or torn to full opening by adolescent physical activity or by the insertion of tampons. In women whose hymens are not fully ruptured, the first act of sexual intercourse will generally accomplish this. Pain may accompany first intercourse in females with relatively intact hymens.

The internal reproductive structures of the female include the vagina, uterus, fallopian tubes, and ovaries.

Vagina

The *vagina* is the structure that forms a canal from the orifice, through the vestibule, to the uterine cervix.

Key Terms

flaccid (**fla** sid) nonerect; the state of erectile tissue when vasocongestion is not occurring

smegma cellular discharge that can accumulate beneath the clitoral hood or the foreskin of an uncircumcised penis

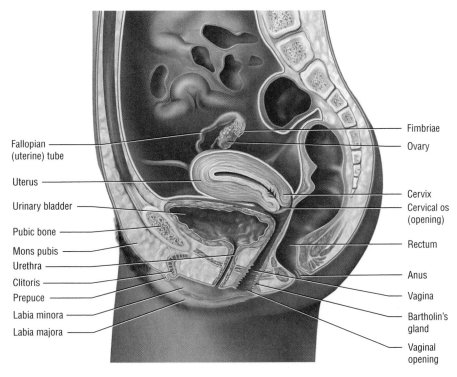

Figure 14-3 The female reproductive system. **A:** Side view, **B:** Front view.

Fallopian (uterine) tube

Uterus

Urinary bladder

Pubic bone

Mons pubis

Urethra

Clitoris

Prepuce

Labia minora

Labia majora

Fimbriae

Ovary

Cervix

Cervical os (opening)

Rectum

Anus

Vagina

Bartholin's gland

Vaginal opening

A

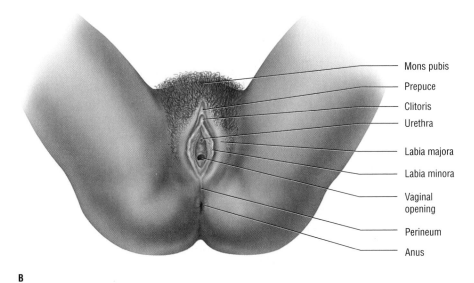

Mons pubis

Prepuce

Clitoris

Urethra

Labia majora

Labia minora

Vaginal opening

Perineum

Anus

B

Normally the walls of the vagina are collapsed, except during sexual stimulation, when the vaginal walls widen and elongate to accommodate the erect penis. Only the outer third of the vagina is especially sensitive to sexual stimulation. In this location, vaginal tissues swell considerably to form the **orgasmic platform.** [12] This platform constricts

Key Terms

orgasmic platform expanded outer third of the vagina, which grips the penis during sexual intercourse

Female Circumcision

Although commonly referred to as female circumcision, the practice of surgically altering a young girl's vulva is more appropriately called female genital cutting (FGC) or female genital mutilation (FGM). This procedure is practiced in twenty-eight African countries, several countries in the Middle East, and among some Muslims in Indonesia and Malaysia.[1] Some cases have been documented in the United States.[2] Typically, the procedure takes one of three forms: the removal of the clitoral hood (circumcision), the removal of the clitoris and perhaps the labia minora (clitoridectomy), and the drastic removal of the clitoris, inner lips, and part of the outer lips (infibulation).

For people from Western cultures, these practices may seem barbaric. Often performed by native women with crude instruments in unsanitary conditions, FGC takes place without the use of anesthetics. Female infants or young girls are subjected to this ritualistic cutting. Obvious dangers include severe bleeding, infection, and the formation of scar tissue.[3]

Infibulation is sometimes extended to incorporate the sewing together the remaining parts of the labia majora. This is thought to ensure virginity in a woman, but poses major risks when a newlywed husband tries to force his penis through the sewn area. Sometimes a midwife must first cut through the scar tissue to open the entrance to the vagina. Years after FGC, women face the possibility of serious complications with childbirth.

It is estimated that FGC and FGM have taken place on 100 million women worldwide.[1] At face value, these procedures may seem gruesome to us in the West, yet we must pause to consider imposing our values on other cultures . . . cultures that readily accept these acts as important to the foundations of their belief systems.[3] To many of us, these procedures represent a sexist devaluation of women. Yet this is normative behavior for groups of people who believe in carrying traditional values for their society. FGC and FGM pose real ethical dilemmas for those of us in Western cultures. What are your thoughts on this?

[1]Hyde JS, DeLamater JD. *Understanding Human Sexuality*, 8th ed. New York: McGraw-Hill, 2003.
[2]Crooks R, Baur K. *Our Sexuality*, 9th ed. Belmont, CA: Wadsworth, 2004.
[3]Masters WH, Johnson VE, Kolodny RC. *Human Sexuality*, 5th ed. Boston: Addison Wesley, 1997.

the vaginal opening and in effect "grips" the penis (or other inserted object)—regardless of its size. Thus the belief that a woman receives considerably more sexual pleasure from men with large penises is not supported from an anatomical standpoint.

Uterus

The *uterus* (or *womb*) is approximately the size and shape of a small pear. This highly muscular organ is capable of undergoing a wide range of physical changes, as evidenced by its enlargement during pregnancy, its contraction during menstruation and labor, and its movement during the orgasmic phase of the female sexual response cycle. The primary function of the uterus is to provide a suitable environment for the possible implantation of a fertilized ovum, or egg. This implantation, should it occur, takes place in the innermost lining of the uterus—the *endometrium*. In the mature female, the endometrium undergoes cyclic changes as it prepares a new lining on a near-monthly basis.

The lower third of the uterus is called the *cervix*. The cervix extends slightly into the vagina. Sperm can enter the uterus through the cervical opening, or *cervical os*. Mucous glands in the cervix secrete a fluid that is thin and watery near the time of ovulation. Mucus of this consistency apparently facilitates sperm passage into the uterus and deeper structures. However, cervical mucus is much thicker during portions of the menstrual cycle when pregnancy is improbable, and during pregnancy, to protect against bacterial agents and other substances that are especially dangerous to the developing fetus.

The upper two-thirds of the uterus is called the *corpus* or *body*. This is where the fertilized ovum generally implants into the uterus.

Fallopian Tubes

The upper portion of the uterus opens into *two fallopian tubes*, sometimes called *oviducts* or *uterine tubes*, each about four inches long. The fallopian tubes are each directed toward an ovary. They serve as a passageway for the ovum in its weeklong voyage toward the uterus. In most cases, conception takes place in the upper third of the fallopian tubes.

Ovaries

The *ovaries* are analogous to the testes in the male. Their function is to produce the ovum, or egg. Usually, one ovary produces and releases just one egg each month. Approximately the size and shape of an unshelled almond, an ovary produces viable ova in the process known as *oogenesis*.

The ovaries also produce the female sex hormones through the efforts of specific structures within the ovaries. These hormones play multiple roles in the development of female secondary sex characteristics, but their primary function is to prepare the endometrium of the uterus for possible implantation of a fertilized ovum. In the average healthy female, this preparation takes place

Menstrual cycle

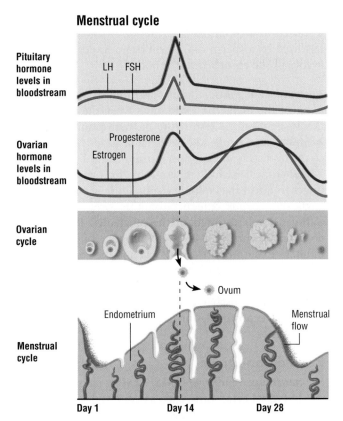

Pituitary hormone levels in bloodstream

LH   FSH

Ovarian hormone levels in bloodstream

Progesterone

Estrogen

Ovarian cycle

Ovum

Endometrium

Menstrual flow

Menstrual cycle

Day 1   Day 14   Day 28

Figure 14-4   The menstrual cycle involves the development and release of an ovum, supported by hormones from the pituitary, and the buildup of the endometrium, supported by hormones from the ovary, for the purpose of establishing a pregnancy.

about 13 times a year for a period of about 35 years. At menopause, the ovaries shrink considerably and stop nearly all hormonal production.

Menstrual Cycle

Each month or so, the inner wall of the uterus prepares for a possible pregnancy. When a pregnancy does not occur (as is the case throughout most months of a woman's fertile years), this lining must be released and a new one prepared. The breakdown of this endometrial wall and the resultant discharge of blood and endometrial tissue is known as *menstruation* (or *menses*) (Figure 14-4). The cyclic timing of this is controlled by a woman's hormones.

Girls generally have their first menstrual cycle, the onset of which is called *menarche,* around age 12 or 13. However, menarche ranges widely, from about age 9 to 17 years.[4] Over the past few decades, the age of menarche has been dropping gradually. This drop appears to be related to heredity, improved overall health, better childhood nutrition, and increased caloric intake. These factors in combination produce the increased body weight evident today in

Endometriosis

Endometriosis is a condition in which endometrial tissue that normally lines the uterus is found growing within the pelvic cavity. Because the tissue remains sensitive to circulating hormones, it is the source of pain and discomfort during the latter half of the menstrual cycle. Endometriosis is most commonly found in younger women and is sometimes related to infertility in women with severe cases.

In addition to painful cramping before and during menstruation, the symptoms of endometriosis include low-back pain, pain during intercourse, painful bowel movements, heavy menstrual flow, and difficulty becoming pregnant. Many women with endometriosis, however, experience no symptoms.*

Treatment of endometriosis largely depends on its extent. Drugs to suppress ovulation, including birth control pills, may be helpful in mild cases. For more severe cases, surgical removal of the tissue or a hysterectomy may be necessary. For some women, endometriosis is suppressed during pregnancy and does not return after pregnancy.

*Health guide A–Z: Endometriosis. WebMDHealth. www.my.webmd.com/hw/endometriosis/hw103000.asp, September 5, 2005.

many young adolescent girls that seems to trigger an earlier menarche.

After a girl first menstruates, her cycles may be anovulatory for a year or longer before a viable ovum is released during her cycle. She will then continue this cyclic activity until age 45 to 55.

This text refers to a menstrual cycle that lasts 28 days. Be assured that few women display absolutely perfect 28-day cycles. Most women fluctuate by a few days to a week or more around this 28-day pattern.

It is not uncommon for some women to experience irregular cycles (cycles that differ in length) and even occasional mid-cycle spotting (small amounts of reddish discharge). These events are most likely to occur in young women who are just establishing their cycles, women who are approaching or moving through menopause, and women who are just starting to use hormone-based contraceptive methods. Major life changes, certain illnesses and medications, and unresolved stress can also affect the length of a woman's cycle. Any woman who experiences a significant, dramatic change from her usual pattern should contact her physician or health care practitioner.[5]

Your knowledge about the menstrual cycle is critical for your understanding of pregnancy, contraception, menopause, and issues related to the overall health and comfort of women (see the Star box on this page for a discussion of endometriosis). Although seemingly complicated, each segment of the cycle can be studied separately for better understanding.

The menstrual cycle can be thought of as occurring in three segments or phases: the menstrual phase (lasting about one week), the preovulation (also lasting about one week), and the postovulation phase (lasting about two weeks). Day 1 of this cycle starts with the first day of bleeding, or menstrual flow.

Menstrual Phase   The *menstrual phase* signals the woman that a pregnancy has not taken place and that her uterine lining is being sloughed off. During a 5- to 7-day period, a woman will discharge about one-fourth to one-half cup of blood and tissue. (Only about one ounce of the menstrual flow is blood.) The menstrual flow is heaviest during the first days of this phase. Because the muscular uterus must contract to accomplish this tissue removal, some women have uncomfortable cramping during menstruation. Most women, however, report more pain and discomfort during the few days before the first day of menstrual flow. (See the discussion of menstrual pain on page 453.)

Today's methods of absorbing menstrual flow include the use of internal tampons and external pads. Caution must be exercised by the user of tampons to prevent the possibility of toxic shock syndrome (TSS) (see Chapter 13). Because menstrual flow is a positive sign of good health, women are encouraged to be normally active during menstruation.

Preovulation Phase   The *preovulation phase* of the menstrual cycle starts about the time menstruation stops. Lasting about one week, this phase is first influenced by the release of follicle-stimulating hormone (FSH) from the pituitary gland. FSH circulates in the bloodstream and directs the ovaries to start the process of maturing approximately 20 primary ovarian *follicles*. Thousands of primary egg follicles are present in each ovary at birth. These follicles resemble shells that house immature ova. As these follicles ripen under FSH influence, they release the hormone *estrogen*. Estrogen's primary function is to direct the endometrium to start the development of a thick, highly vascular wall. As FSH secretions are reduced, the pituitary gland prepares for the surge of the **luteinizing hormone (LH)** required to accomplish ovulation.[13]

In the days immediately before ovulation, one of the primary follicles (called the *graafian follicle*) matures fully. The other primary follicles degenerate and are absorbed by the body. The graafian follicle moves toward the surface of the ovary. When LH is released in massive quantities on about day 14, the graafian follicle bursts to release the fully mature ovum. The release of the ovum is called **ovulation.** Regardless of the overall length of a woman's cycle, ovulation occurs 14 days before her first day of menstrual flow.

The ovum is quickly captured by the fingerlike projections (*fimbriae*) of the fallopian tubes. In the upper third of the fallopian tubes, the ovum is capable of being fertilized in a 24- to 36-hour period. If the ovum is not fertilized by a sperm cell, it will begin to degenerate and eventually be absorbed by the body.

Postovulation Phase   After ovulation, the *postovulation phase* of the menstrual cycle starts when the remnants of the graafian follicle restructure themselves into a **corpus luteum.** The corpus luteum remains inside the ovary, secreting estrogen and a fourth hormone called *progesterone.* Progesterone, which literally means "for pregnancy," continues to direct the endometrial buildup. If pregnancy occurs, the corpus luteum monitors progesterone and estrogen levels throughout the pregnancy. If pregnancy does not occur, high levels of progesterone signal the pituitary to stop the release of LH and the corpus luteum starts to disintegrate on about day 24. When estrogen and progesterone levels diminish significantly by day 28, the endometrium is discharged from the uterus and out the vagina. The postovulation phase ends, and the cycle is complete.

Related Conditions

Premenstrual Syndrome (PMS)   PMS is characterized by psychological symptoms, such as depression, lethargy, irritability, and aggressiveness, or somatic symptoms, such as headache, backache, asthma, acne, and epilepsy, that recur in the same phase of each menstrual cycle, followed by a symptom-free phase in each cycle. Some of the more frequently reported symptoms of PMS include tension, tender breasts, fainting, fatigue, abdominal cramps, and weight gain.

The cause of PMS appears to be hormonal. Perhaps a woman's body is insensitive to a normal level of progesterone, or her ovaries fail to produce a normal amount of progesterone. These reasons seem plausible because PMS-type symptoms do not occur during pregnancy, during which natural progesterone levels are very high, and because women with PMS seem to feel much better after receiving high doses of natural progesterone in suppository

---

Key Terms

luteinizing hormone (LH) (**loo** ten eye zing) a gonadotropic hormone of the female required for fullest development and release of ova; ovulating hormone

ovulation the release of a mature egg from the ovary

corpus luteum (kore pus **loo** tee um) cellular remnant of the graafian follicle after the release of an ovum

I am a 24-year-old woman who has a great amount of menstrual pain. What can I do to lessen this pain?

The medical term is *dysmenorrhea,* but most women know it as menstrual cramps, and most women suffer from it at one time or another. Fortunately, the medical profession seems to be paying more attention to this problem, and various treatments are being studied. Currently, the most popular treatments still seem to be exercise and prostaglandin inhibitors.

The periodic cramps can occur before and during the menstrual phase, when the uterus must contract to remove the uterine lining. These contractions are produced by prostaglandin hormones normally found in the body. The problem occurs when the body produces an excess of one of the prostaglandin hormones, and the result is excessive cramping and pain. Thus prostaglandin-inhibiting medications can be used to reduce the body's production of prostaglandins and thereby reduce the intensity of cramping. Antiprostaglandin medications include ibuprofen, aspirin, and some prescription medications.

Before beginning treatment, however, the first step is to see a physician to rule out other causes of the dysmenorrhea. If other underlying causes are eliminated, consider the following treatment suggestions:

- Consume a well-balanced diet, with limited salt and sugar intake. Reduce spicy foods, and drink six to eight glasses of water per day.
- Consider taking aspirin, ibuprofen, other over-the-counter medications, or prescription medications, with your physician's guidance. Do not take aspirin if you are allergic to aspirin or have anemia, ulcers, or intestinal bleeding.
- Try taking a warm bath or placing a hot water bottle on your abdomen.

Try the following exercise routine that targets menstrual cramping.

- Lie face up with the legs and knees bent; perform abdominal breathing about 10 times. Feel the abdomen slowly inflate and then slowly fall.
- Stand and hold the back of a chair; lift one heel off the floor, then the other. Repeat 20 times.
- Lie on your back; lift and bring your knees to your chin; repeat 10 times.

Other treatments currently being explored include herbal remedies, acupuncture, transcutaneous electrical nerve stimulation, and microwave diathermy.

---

form. When using oral contraceptives that supply synthetic progesterone at normal levels, many women report relief from some symptoms of PMS. However, the effectiveness of a common form of treatment, progesterone suppositories, is now being questioned (see Changing for the Better).

Until the effectiveness of progesterone has been fully researched, the medical community is unlikely to treat PMS through any approach other than a relatively conservative treatment of symptoms with the use of analgesic drugs (including prostaglandin inhibitors), diuretic drugs, dietary modifications (including restriction of caffeine and salt), vitamin B_6 therapy, exercise, and stress-reduction exercises. The exact nature of PMS has been further complicated by the classification of severe PMS as a mental disturbance by some segments of the American Psychiatric Association.

Fibrocystic Breast Condition In some women, particularly those who have never been pregnant, stimulation of the breast tissues by estrogen and progesterone during the menstrual cycle results in an unusually high degree of secretory activity by the cells lining the ducts. The fluid released by the secretory lining finds its way into the fibrous connective tissue areas in the lower half of the breast, where in pocketlike cysts the fluid presses against neighboring tissues. Excessive secretory activity produces in many women a benign fibrocystic breast condition characterized by swollen, firm, or hardened tender breast tissue before menstruation.

Researchers have begun to describe the importance of a healthy diet in preventing fibrocystic breast condition, in particular a low-fat, low-salt, low-red-meat diet that is rich in whole grains, fish, and chicken. The reduction or elimination of caffeine found in coffee, tea, soft drinks, and chocolate might also help reduce these benign breast changes. In some cases, vitamin E and vitamin B-complex supplementation have helped.[5] Women with more extensive fibrocystic conditions can be treated with drugs that have a "calming" effect on progesterone production. Occasional draining of cysts can bring relief.

Amenorrhea

Amenorrhea is a condition characterized by the absence of menstruation. The lack of menstruation, if not caused by aging or pregnancy, is categorized as either primary or secondary amenorrhea.[9] *Primary amenorrhea*

Key Terms

amenorrhea the absence of menstruation

Alternatives to Hormone Replacement Therapy

Recall from Chapter 10 that recent studies now question the benefits of hormone replacement therapy (HRT) for postmenopausal women. For the past few decades, it was thought that HRT not only helped women find relief from the uncomfortable symptoms of menopause (hot flashes, night sweats, vaginal dryness, mood swings, and insomnia) but that HRT also helped protect women from osteoporosis, and most importantly, cardiovascular disease.

However, in the largest study of its kind to examine the impact of HRT (specifically the most popular estrogen-progestin combination) on women's health, the National Heart, Lung, and Blood Institute found that HRT actually *increased* the incidence of breast cancer, heart attacks, blood clots, and strokes. Although the increase was not large (for example, women taking hormones were less than a tenth of 1 percent more likely to have a heart attack), it was enough to have this aspect of the Women's Health Initiative stopped in 2002, 3 years before completion of the study.[1] More recently, additional analysis of the data found that the estrogen-progestin pills can cause an aggressive form of breast cancer to develop.[2] Furthermore, the combination pills can encourage the breast tissue to become more dense, thus making it more difficult for physicians to detect tumors when they develop.[2]

It appears that taking an estrogen-only pill does not have the effect on the development of breast cancer as much as the combined estrogen-progestin regimen does. A 2003 study of 975 postmenopausal women taking various combinations of hormone replacement therapy indicated that women taking estrogen alone had no appreciable increase in breast cancer, even if they had been using estrogen for many years.[3] However, the estrogen-only approach is recommended for women who have had hysterectomies, since estrogen taken by itself seems to play a role in causing uterine cancer.

Since the 2002 report[1], many women have stopped taking the combined estrogen-progesterone pills for menopausal symptoms. For women who still want this form of HRT, physicians generally recommend they take the lowest dosage for the least amount of time. Thus, women might think in terms of taking HRT for 2 to 5 years, not for a lifetime.

Another consequence of the recent concern is the increased interest in alternative approaches to HRT. For concerns about osteoporosis, there are alternative prescription drugs that can be helpful including alendronate (Fosamax) or raloxifens (Evista). A diet that adds calcium-rich foods (dairy products, leafy green vegetables, and sardines) in combination with Vitamin D promotes bone density. Weight-bearing exercise, such as walking and weight lifting, encourages bone growth as well.

Hot flashes and night sweats result from changing estrogen levels and are, perhaps, the most challenging acute symptoms to control. However, reducing the intake of spicy foods, caffeine, and alcohol may help. Vitamin E and soy products help some women, and the use of certain herbs (especially black cohosh) is being studied. For some women, the use of a prescription antidepressant (such as Prozac or Paxil) may reduce hot flashes.

Vaginal dryness can be helped by the use of over-the-counter lubricants and moisturizers, vaginal estrogen creams, and regular sexual activity. Insomnia can be countered with the use of good sleeping patterns (consistent bedtime hour, a small glass of warm milk, reduced caffeine, alcohol, and food intake before bed). Cardiovascular concerns at menopause can be reduced by a healthy lifestyle that includes not smoking, consuming healthy foods, monitoring blood cholesterol levels, and getting regular exercise.

Interestingly, physical activity cuts across most of the issues related to menopause. Physical activity has been demonstrated to help sleep patterns, provide emotional balance, encourage mental acuity, and bolster cardiovascular functioning. Physical activity also makes many people feel better about their bodies and, thus, become potentially more interested in sexual activity that can help maintain vaginal lubrication.

[1]Writing Group for the Women's Health Initiative Investigators. Risks and benefits of estrogen plus progestin in healthy postmenopausal women: principal results from the Women's Health Initiative Randomized Controlled Trial. *Journal of the American Medical Association,* Vol 288: No 3 (July 17, 2002), 321–333.
[2]Chlebowski RT, et al. Influence of estrogen plus progestin on breast cancer and mammography in healthy postmenopausal women: The Women's Health Randomized Trial. *Journal of the American Medical Association,* Vol 289: No 24 (June 25, 2003), 3243–3253.
[3]Li Cl, et al. Relationship between long durations and different regimens of hormone therapy and risk of breast cancer. *Journal of the American Medical Association,* Vol 289: No 24 (June 25, 2003), 3254–3263.

occurs when girls have passed the age of 16 and have never menstruated. Perhaps these girls have not yet reached a critical body weight (with the increased ratio of body fat) to trigger the menstrual cycle to begin. Additionally, some girls may have inherited a familial tendency to mature later than most of their peers. At an appropriate time for their bodies, these girls will start to menstruate. However, in cases where the primary amenorrhea is determined to be caused by hormonal deficiencies or abnormal body structure, hormone therapy can be quite useful.

Secondary amenorrhea occurs when a previously menstruating woman ceases to menstruate. Likely reasons for secondary amenorrhea include pregnancy, breastfeeding, or the use of hormonal contraceptives. Less common reasons could be linked to unresolved stress, a reduction in body fat, hormonal irregularities, or serious athletic training. Other causes could be anorexia (see Chapter 6) or the female athlete syndrome (see Chapter 4). If a woman has not menstruated in 6 months and is not pregnant, not breastfeeding, and not using hormonal contraceptives, she should consult with her physician or medical care professional.[9]

Learning from Our Diversity

No Fear of 50: The New Model for Menopause

Just a generation ago, menopause was regarded almost as a dreaded disease by many women—not to mention the men who were married to them. It was seen not just as the end of fertility but as the loss of youth, attractiveness, femininity, sex appeal, and sexual enjoyment. Both women and their husbands dreaded the onset of hot flashes, mood swings, depression, and loss of sex drive that were commonly believed to be every woman's fate during premenopause. In the minds not just of middle-aged women but also of men and young people, the definition of menopause was "old."

That was then; this is now. With the first women of the baby boom generation dealing with menopause, it's a whole new story. The generation that said it would never get old is not taking menopause on the chin—instead, today's women are fighting back, with every weapon at their command. Regular exercise and stress reducers like meditation and yoga go a long way toward easing the emotional swings associated with menopause—and a balanced diet, rich in healthful sources of calcium, helps stabilize mood and prevent osteoporosis. For some women, hormone replacement therapy (HRT) is helpful in alleviating unpleasant symptoms of menopause and in reducing bone loss. However, recent concerns over HRT have caused other women to opt not to use HRT and instead pursue treatments offered by alternative medicine, or simply let nature take its course.

Many of the "new" 50-plus women are treating menopause as a natural process instead of a disease. Rather than using menopause as an excuse to stop exercising and eating healthfully, these women and thousands of others see it as a compelling reason to stay fit.

With their children grown and gone, midlife women who have spent decades raising a family now find that they have time to themselves—and for themselves. Career women, whether they're mothers or not, have usually achieved their major goals or are in sight of them, and they no longer need to make an all-out push to scale the corporate or professional ladder. There's more time for friendships, for hobbies and interests, for travel, and for contemplating instead of competing. There's more time for the healthful, self-nuturing pursuits that help ease the transition into menopause. And there's more life to be lived than at any time in the past. No longer considered the figurative end of a woman's life, menopause now is increasingly regarded as a passage into the next stage, with all the challenges and rewards it offers.

Increasingly, physicians are rejecting the "menopause as disease" model in favor of a more positive approach that empowers women to manage this stage of their lives proactively instead of being overwhelmed or overmedicated by it. Women of the baby boom generation may be aging—but they're not doing it passively.

Menopause

For the vast majority of women in their late 40s through their mid-50s, a gradual decline in reproductive system function, called *menopause*, occurs. Menopause is a normal physiological process, not a disease process. It can, however, become a health concern for some middle-aged women who have unpleasant side effects resulting from this natural ending of ovum production and menstruation.

As ovarian function and hormone production diminish, the hypothalamus, ovaries, uterus, and other estrogen-sensitive tissues must adjust. The extent of menopause as a health problem is determined by the degree to which **hot flashes,** night sweats, insomnia, vaginal wall dryness, depression and melancholy, breast changes, and the uncertainty of fertility are seen as problems.

Many of today's midlife women are likely to find menopause to be a relatively positive experience. The end of fertility, combined with children leaving home, makes the middle years a period of personal rediscovery for many women (see Learning from Our Diversity).

For women who are troubled by the changes brought about by menopause, physicians may prescribe **hormone replacement therapy (HRT).** This can relieve many symptoms and offer benefits to help reduce the incidence of osteoporosis (see Chapters 4 and 5). However, HRT has recently been found to increase the risk of breast cancer and cardiovascular problems.[14,15] These concerns have caused many women to reconsider their use of HRT. (The Star box on page 454 takes a closer look at HRT.)

> ### Key Terms
>
> **hot flashes** unpleasant, temporary feelings of warmth experienced by women during and after menopause, caused by blood vessel dilation
>
> **hormone replacement therapy (HRT)** medically administered hormones to replace hormones lost as the result of menopause

Additional Aspects of Human Sexuality

Earlier in this chapter, we identified the biological and psychosocial bases of our sexuality. In this section we explore three additional aspects of our sexuality—reproductive, genital, and expressionistic—around which many of our important decisions in life are made.* With these new perspectives in mind, you will be better able to see the complexity associated with our development as productive and satisfied beings.

Reproductive Sexuality

Of these three aspects of sexuality, *reproductive sexuality* reflects the most basic level of sexuality over which the adult must exercise discretion and display insight. Simply stated, reproductive sexuality is related to your knowledge of, desire for, and ability to participate in the act of *procreation*. Pregnancy, delivery, natural childbirth, breast-feeding, fertility control, and pregnancy termination are terms related to this dimension of sexuality. Demographic data indicate that most (but not all) of you will choose to be active in this dimension of your sexuality by becoming parents.

Genital Sexuality

Genital sexuality refers to the nonreproductive use of the reproductive organs. In comparison with the concept of reproductive sexuality, genital sexuality implies recreation and communication rather than procreation. The behaviors and meanings associated with the terms *orgasm, having sex, making love, oral-genital sex,* and *sexual responsiveness* are genital in their orientation.

In the most positive sense, sexual experiences that are genitally oriented should be sensual, erotic, and stimulating and should give the individual a sense of release. Genital sexuality reflects our gift to ourselves and to our partners as well. However, many forms of genital sexuality may not be condoned by certain groups of people or religions.

For some, genital sexuality can be a volatile experience. Far too frequently a genitally centered sexual experience results in an unanticipated and unwanted pregnancy. In such circumstances the couple, or more often the female acting alone, is forced to make decisions that could significantly affect the future. An unexpected pregnancy, even for a relatively mature college person, may result in a series of compromises. In addition, the close association between genital sexuality and sexually transmitted diseases (including HIV infection) makes some sexual activities potentially dangerous.

For some people, genital sexuality becomes the mode of communication with which they feel most comfortable. In such cases, partners may know each other only in a very limited way. Growth in sexual technique may readily

---

*We cite no specific source for the terms *reproductive sexuality, genital sexuality,* and *expressionistic sexuality.* They are labels we and our colleagues use in instructional units associated with human sexuality.

occur within the context of a genitally centered relationship, but a fully developed relationship will not be formed. Genitally based relationships are rarely elevated to a much higher level.

Expressionistic Sexuality

Expressionistic sexuality represents the most broadly based dimension of yourself as a man or woman. (See Discovering Your Spirituality on page 456.) As the name implies, this is your expression of your current gender schema. Cognitively, *affectively*, and behaviorally, you are playing out your initial adult gender identification. The way you dress, the occupation you pursue, and the leisure activities you develop are all aspects of this dimension of your sexuality.

Expressionistic sexuality encompasses the reproductive and genital dimensions of your sexuality, but it is more. It is the sexuality that will serve you most fully for the rest of your life. Most adults probably are conventional in their patterns of expressionistic sexuality, yet many people also express a variety of additional patterns (see Chapter 15).

Taking Charge of Your Health

- Take the Personal Assessment on page 459 to determine how traditional or nontraditional your attitudes are toward sexuality.

- If you wish to become more flexible and expand your social skills, identify ways in which you can increase your androgynous behavior. For example, learn to cook, expand your assertiveness skills, do volunteer work with children, join a club sports team, or learn how to invest in the stock market.

- Most college sexuality textbooks encourage readers to become familiar with their external reproductive "body parts." If you believe that this is important, study the illustrations in this chapter, find a handheld mirror, undress, and identify these structures as best you can.

- If you are a woman who has a significant amount of menstrual pain, try some of the treatment suggestions in this chapter.

- If you are a man who is essentially "clueless" about the menstrual cycle and would like to understand it much better, study the information in this chapter. If you have a very close female friend and you wish to validate some of this information, ask her (diplomatically, of course) if you could get her "impressions" of this natural phenomenon.

SUMMARY

- The biological basis of human sexuality includes genetic, gonadal, and structural components.
- The structural basis of sexuality begins as the male and female reproductive structures develop in the growing embryo and fetus. Structural sexuality changes as one moves through adolescence and later life.
- The psychosocial basis of human sexuality includes gender identity, gender preference, gender adoption, and initial adult gender identification.
- Androgyny is the blending of feminine and masculine qualities.
- The male and female reproductive structures are external and internal. The complex functioning of these structures is controlled by hormones.
- The menstrual cycle's primary functions are to produce ova and to develop a supportive environment for the fetus in the uterus.

- Endometriosis is a condition in which endometrial tissue that normally lines the uterus grows within the pelvic cavity, causing pain before and during menstruation and can lead to infertility.
- Fibrocystic breast condition is characterized by swollen, firm, or hardened tender breast tissue before menstruation.
- Hormone replacement therapy has benefits in treating the symptoms of menopause and of PMS but may carry risks for some women.
- Reproductive sexuality refers to aspects of sexuality related to procreation.
- Genital sexuality refers to the nonreproductive use of the reproductive organs.
- Expressionistic sexuality is the cognitive, affective, and behavioral expression of your gender.

REVIEW QUESTIONS

1. Describe the following foundations of our biological sexuality: the genetic basis, the gonadal basis, and structural development.
2. Define and explain the following terms: gender identity, gender preference, gender adoption, and initial adult gender identification.
3. Define androgyny and explain its advantages.
4. Identify the major components of the male reproductive system. Trace the passageway for sperm.
5. Identify the major components of the female reproductive system. Trace the passageway for ova.
6. Identify and describe the four main hormones that control the menstrual cycle.
7. What are some of the nonpharmacologic techniques for reducing the symptoms of PMS?
8. What are the symptoms of fibrocystic breast condition and endometriosis?
9. Describe the difference between primary and secondary amenorrhea.
10. Name two circumstances in which hormone replacement therapy might be prescribed for women.
11. What is expressionistic sexuality?
12. What is genital sexuality?
13. What is reproductive sexuality?

ENDNOTES

1. Thibodeau GA, Patton KT. *Anatomy and Physiology* (5th ed.). St. Louis, MO: Mosby, 2003.
2. Sherwood L. *Human Physiology: From Cells to Systems* (5th ed.). Belmont, CA: Brooks/Cole, 2004.
3. Hyde JS, DeLamater JD. *Understanding Human Sexuality* (9th ed.). McGraw-Hill, 2006.
4. Allgeier ER, Allgeier AR. *Sexual Interactions* (5th ed.). New York: Houghton Mifflin, 2000.
5. Crooks R, Baur K. *Our Sexuality* (9th ed.). Belmont, CA: Wadsworth, 2004.
6. LeVay S, Valente, SM. *Human Sexuality*. Sunderland, MA: Sinauer Associates, Inc., 2003.
7. Kelly GF. *Sexuality Today: The Human Perspective* (8th ed.). New York: McGraw-Hill, 2006.
8. Masters WH, Johnson VE, Kolodny RC. *Human Sexuality* (5th ed.). Boston: Addison Wesley, 1997.
9. Strong B, DeVault C, Sayad BW, Yarber WL. *Human Sexuality: Diversity in Contemporary America* (5th ed.). New York: McGraw-Hill, 2005.
10. Barclay L. *Unisex Hormones?* WebMd Medical News Archive, May 4, 2001, www.webmd.com/content/article/32/1728_79051.htm, accessed July 10, 2003.
11. Manos A. *FDA Approves Gel to Treat Low Testosterone Levels,* WebMd Medical News Archive, March 2, 2000, www.my.webmd.com/content/article/22/1728_55404.htm, accessed July 10, 2003.
12. Greenberg JS, Bruess CE, Haffner DW. *Exploring the Dimensions of Human Sexuality* (2nd ed.). Boston: Jones and Bartlett, 2004.
13. Hatcher RA, et al. *Contraceptive Technology* (18th ed.). New York: Ardent Media, 2004.
14. Writing Group for the Women's Health Initiative Investigators. Risks and benefits of estrogen plus progestin in healthy postmenopausal women: Principal results from the Women's Health Initiative Randomized Controlled Trial. *JAMA (Journal of the American Medical Association),* Vol 288: No 3 (July 17, 2002), 321–333.
15. Hormone therapy is no heart helper. *Harvard Heart Letter,* Vol 13: No 2 (October 2002), 2–4.

personal assessment

Sexual attitudes: a matter of feelings

Respond to each of the following statements by selecting a numbered response (1–5) that most accurately reflects your feelings. Circle the number of your selection. At the end of the questionnaire, total these numbers for use in interpreting your responses.

1 Agree strongly
2 Agree moderately
3 Uncertain
4 Disagree moderately
5 Disagree strongly

Men and women have greater differences than they have similarities.	1	2	3	4	5
Homosexuality and bisexuality are immoral and unnatural.	1	2	3	4	5
Our society is too sexually oriented.	1	2	3	4	5
Pornography encourages sexual promiscuity.	1	2	3	4	5
Children know far too much about sex.	1	2	3	4	5
Education about sexuality is solely the responsibility of the family.	1	2	3	4	5
Dating begins far too early in our society.	1	2	3	4	5
Sexual intimacy before marriage leads to emotional stress and damage to one's reputation.	1	2	3	4	5
Sexual availability is far too frequently the reason that people marry.	1	2	3	4	5
Reproduction is the most important reason for sexual intimacy during marriage.	1	2	3	4	5
Modern families are too small.	1	2	3	4	5
Family planning clinics should not receive public funds.	1	2	3	4	5
Contraception is the woman's responsibility.	1	2	3	4	5
Abortion is the murder of an innocent child.	1	2	3	4	5
Marriage has been weakened by the changing role of women in society.	1	2	3	4	5
Divorce is an unacceptable means of resolving marital difficulties.	1	2	3	4	5
Extramarital sexual intimacy will destroy a marriage.	1	2	3	4	5
Sexual abuse of a child does not generally occur unless the child encourages the adult.	1	2	3	4	5
Provocative behavior by the woman is a factor in almost every case of rape.	1	2	3	4	5
Reproduction is not a right but a privilege.	1	2	3	4	5

YOUR TOTAL POINTS _____

Interpretation

20–34 points	A very traditional attitude toward sexuality
35–54 points	A moderately traditional attitude toward sexuality
55–65 points	A rather ambivalent attitude toward sexuality
66–85 points	A moderately nontraditional attitude toward sexuality
86–100 points	A very nontraditional attitude toward sexuality

To Carry This Further . . .

Were you surprised at your results? Compare your results with those of a roommate or close friend. How do you think your parents would score on this assessment?

chapter fifteen

Understanding Sexual Behavior and Relationships

Chapter Objectives

On completing this chapter, you will be able to:

▌ identify the four stages of the human sexual response pattern.

▌ indicate how the stages of the sexual response pattern differ between men and women.

▌ identify several of the common sexual performance difficulties, their possible causes, and their therapies.

▌ define the three most common sexual orientations.

▌ differentiate between transsexualism, transgenderism, and transvestism.

▌ identify how aging affects sexual performance in both women and men.

▌ define *passionate love* and *companionate love.*

▌ point out how *mutual monogamy* and *serial monogamy* differ.

▌ discuss the general makeup of each of the five forms of marriage presented.

▌ describe the importance of communication in a relationship, and identify any five positive strategies couples can use to communicate better.

Eye on the Media

Advertising to Gays and Lesbians

An evolving form of advertising is currently being seen in the United States and abroad. This approach depicts gays and lesbians in positive ways (that is, successful, attractive, happy); a far cry from historic, stereotypical views. What do these ads look like? You might be surprised, since the sexual orientation implications are frequently subtle and hidden.

To learn more about the blending of gay advertising into mainsteam media advertising, search the Web using "gay advertising" as key words. One site you will likely find is the Web site for The Commercial Closet Association, a nonprofit educational and journalism organization that "works to improve public opinion of the lesbian, gay, bisexual, and transgender community through more informed GLBT portrayals in the powerful medium of advertising."[1] This Web site provides up-to-date reports, critiques, visitor reviews, live video lectures, and guidelines and resources for advertisers and the ad agencies they use. At this site, you can see the Commercial Closet's top 10 ads that feature advertising to gays and lesbians, and see its list of "leaders and laggards" in gay advertising. You can also see video clips of many of these commercials. You might be surprised at how mainstream these commercials appear.

[1]The Commercial Closet. *Mission Statement,* www.commercialcloset.com, May 1, 2005.

As we begin a new century and a new millennium, we have reached a greater understanding of the psychosocial factors that contribute to the complex expression of our sexuality. In this chapter, we explore human sexuality as it relates to the dynamic interplay of the psychosocial bases of sexual behavior and relationships. We begin by examining the human sexual response pattern.

The Human Sexual Response Pattern

Although history has many written and visual accounts of the human's ability to be sexually aroused, it was not until the pioneering work of Masters and Johnson[1] that the events associated with arousal were clinically documented. These researchers posed the following five questions, which gave direction to a series of studies involving the scientific evaluation of human sexual response.

Do the Sexual Responses of Men and Women Have a Predictable Pattern?

The answer to the first question posed by the researchers was an emphatic *yes*. A predictable sexual response pattern was identified;[1] it consists of an initial **excitement stage**, a **plateau stage**, an **orgasmic stage**, and a **resolution stage.** Each stage involves predictable changes in the structural characteristics and physiological function of reproductive and nonreproductive organs in both the male and female. These changes are shown in Figure 15-1.

Is the Sexual Response Pattern Stimuli-Specific?

The research of Masters and Johnson[1] clearly established a *no* answer to the second question concerning stimuli specificity. Their findings demonstrated that several senses can supply the stimuli necessary for initiating the sexual response pattern. Although touching activities might initiate arousal in most people and maximize it for the vast majority of people, in both men and women, sight, smell, sound, and *vicariously formed stimuli* can also stimulate the same sexual arousal patterns.

What Differences Occur in the Sexual Response Pattern?

Differences Between Men and Women

In response to the third question, several differences are observable when comparing the sexual response patterns of men and women:

- With the exception of some late adolescent males, the vast majority of men are not multiorgasmic. The **refractory phase** of the resolution stage prevents most men from experiencing more than one orgasm in a short time, even though sufficient stimulation is available.

- Women possess a **multiorgasmic capacity.** Masters and Johnson found that as many as 10–30 percent of all female adults routinely experience multiple orgasms.

- Although they possess multiorgasmic potential, some 10 percent of all women are *anorgasmic*—that is, they never experience an orgasm.[1] For many of these women, orgasms can be experienced when masturbation, rather than **coitus,** provides the stimulation.

- When measured during coitus, men reach orgasm far more quickly than do women. However, when masturbation is the source of stimulation, women reach orgasm as quickly as men.

More important than any of the differences pointed out is the finding that the sexual response patterns of men and women are far more alike than they are different. Not only do men and women experience the four basic stages of the response pattern, but they also have similar responses in specific areas, including the **erection** and

---

Key Terms

excitement stage initial arousal stage of the sexual response pattern

plateau stage second stage of the sexual response pattern; a leveling off of arousal immediately before orgasm

orgasmic stage third stage of the sexual response pattern; the stage during which neuromuscular tension is released

resolution stage fourth stage of the sexual response pattern; the return of the body to a preexcitement state

refractory phase that portion of the male's resolution stage during which sexual arousal cannot occur

multiorgasmic capacity potential to have several orgasms within a single period of sexual arousal

coitus (**co** ih tus) penile-vaginal intercourse

erection the engorgement of erectile tissue with blood; characteristic of the penis, clitoris, nipples, labia minora, and scrotum

---

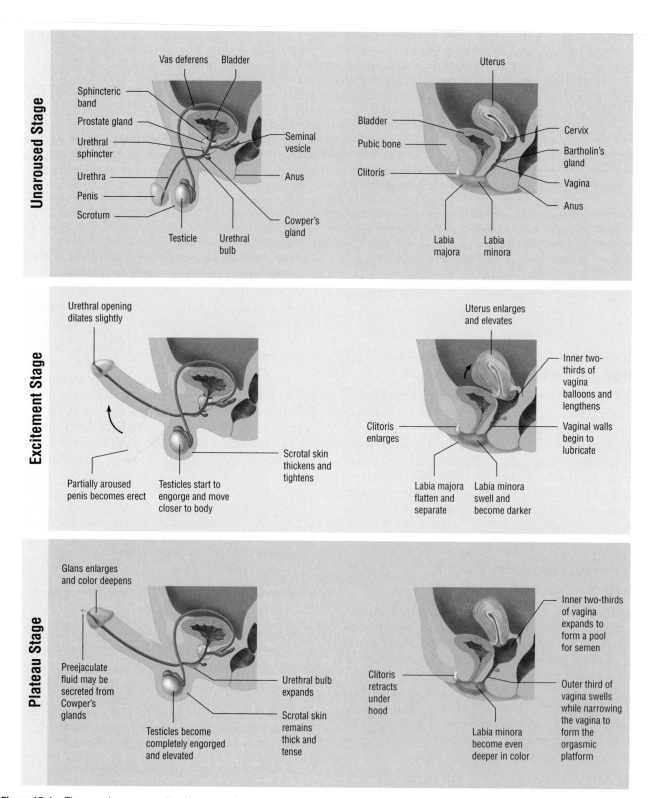

Figure 15-1 The sexual response pattern in men and women

Orgasmic Stage

SENSATION OF ORGASM

Prostatic portion of urethra fills with semen

Contractions occur in upper part of vas deferens

Sphincteric band contracts

Urethral sphincter contracts

Seminal vesicle contracts

Urethral bulb expands further

Prostate gland contracts

Uterine contractions occur

Clitoris remains under hood

Contractions occur in anal sphincter

Contractions in outer third of the vagina occur rhythmically 3 to 15 times; the first of these contractions are spaced at 0.8-second intervals; later contractions are weaker and occur more slowly

EJACULATION

Semen is expelled; the first 2 or 3 contractions are strong and spaced 0.8 seconds apart

Sphincteric band remains contracted

Semen is released as urethral sphincter relaxes

Urethral bulb contracts

Pelvic floor muscles contract

BREAST CHANGES

① **Unaroused stage**

② **Excitement stage**
Breast size increases; nipples become erect; veins become more visible

③ **Plateau and orgasmic stages**
Breast size increases more; areola increases in size (making nipples appear less erect); skin color may become flushed from vasocongestion

Resolution Stage

Rapid partial decrease in size of penis; then slow return to unaroused state and size

Scrotal skin relaxes

Testicles return to normal size and position

Uterus returns to normal position

Cervical canal enlarges

Inner two-thirds of vagina returns to normal in 5 to 8 minutes

Clitoris quickly returns to normal position and slowly returns to unaroused state

Outer third of vagina quickly returns to normal

Labia majora and minora slowly return to unaroused position and color

Figure 15-1 *Continued*

Drugs for Erectile Dysfunction

Within the last decade, three prescription drugs for erectile dysfunction (ED) have been developed and marketed for men. The oldest drug, Viagra (Pfizer Pharmaceuticals), came on the market in 1998. A second drug, Levitra (GlaxoSmithKline), was approved by the Food and Drug Administration in 2003, and the newest drug, Cialis (Eli Lilly & Company), came on the market in 2004.

All three drugs act on an enzyme that helps relax small muscles in the penis and increase the flow of blood into the erectile chambers. Sexual stimulation is required for each of the drugs to work. The difference in the drugs is how long each drug can work and how

quickly it produces an erection. Reportedly, Viagra can produce the desired effect within a 4-hour period, Levitra can work for about 5 hours, and Cialis can work for up to 36 hours. Viagra can work in as quickly as 30 minutes, Levitra in about 15 minutes, and Cialis around 30 minutes or more. Men are encouraged to discuss possible side effects and health risks with their physicians before using these drugs.

In the near future, be on the lookout for the development of prescription drugs that enhance sexual desire and performance in women. Pharmaceutical companies stand to reap tremendous sales with effective drugs in this area.

---

tumescence of sexual structures; the appearance of a **sex flush;** the increase in cardiac output, blood pressure, and respiratory rate; and the occurrence of *rhythmic pelvic thrusting.*[1]

Differences among Subjects within a Same-Gender Group

When a group of subjects of the same gender was studied in an attempt to answer questions about similarities and differences in the sexual response pattern, Masters and Johnson noted considerable variation. Even when variables such as age, race, education, and general health were held constant, the extent and duration of virtually every stage of the response pattern varied.

Differences within the Same Individual

For a given person the nature of the sexual response pattern does not remain constant, even when observed over a relatively short period. A variety of internal and external factors can alter this pattern. The aging process, changes in general health status, levels of stress, altered environmental settings, use of alcohol and other drugs, and behavioral changes in a sexual partner can cause one's own sexual response pattern to change from one sexual experience to another. (Sexual performance difficulties and therapies are discussed in the Star box on page 465. For a discussion of aphrodisiacs, see Considering Complementary Care on page 466.)

What Are the Basic Physiological Mechanisms Underlying the Sexual Response Pattern?

The basic mechanisms in the fourth question posed by Masters and Johnson are now well recognized. One factor, *vasocongestion,* or the retention of blood or fluid within a

particular tissue, is critically important in the development of physiological changes that promote the sexual response pattern.[1] The presence of erectile tissue underlies the changes that can be noted in the penis, breasts, and scrotum of the male and the clitoris, breasts, and labia minora of the female.

A second mechanism now recognized as necessary for the development of the sexual response pattern is that of *myotonia,* or the buildup of neuromuscular tension within a variety of body structures.[2] At the end of the plateau stage of the response pattern, a sudden release of the accumulated neuromuscular tension gives rise to the rhythmic muscular contractions and pleasurable muscular spasms that constitute orgasm, as well as ejaculation in the male.[3]

What Role Is Played by Specific Organs and Organ Systems within the Sexual Response Pattern?

The fifth question posed by Masters and Johnson, which concerns the role played by specific organs and organ systems during each stage of the response pattern, can be readily answered by referring to the material presented in Figure 15-1. As you study this figure, remember that direct stimulation of the penis and either direct or indirect stimulation of the clitoris are the principal avenues toward orgasm. Also, intercourse represents only one activity that can lead to orgasmic pleasure.[4]

> **Key Terms**
>
> **sex flush** the reddish skin response that results from increasing sexual arousal

Sexual Performance Difficulties and Therapies

For all of the predictability of the human sexual response pattern, many people find that at some point in their lives, they are no longer capable of responding sexually. The inability of a person to perform adequately is identified as a sexual difficulty or dysfunction. Sexual difficulties can have a negative influence on a person's sense of sexual satisfaction and on a partner's satisfaction. Fortunately, most sexual difficulties can be resolved through strategies that use individual, couple, or group counseling. Most sexual performance difficulties stem from psychogenic factors.

Difficulty	Possible Causes	Therapeutic Approaches
Women		
Orgasmic Difficulties Inability to have orgasm	Lack of knowledge about female responsiveness; inadequate sexual arousal; interpersonal problems with partner; anxiety, fear, guilt, anger, poor self-concept	Counseling to improve a couple's communication; educating a woman and her partner about female responsiveness; teaching a woman how to experience orgasm through masturbation
Vaginismus Painful, involuntary contractions of the vaginal muscles	Previous traumatic experiences with intercourse (rape, incest, uncaring partners); fear of pregnancy; religious prohibitions; anxiety about vaginal penetration of any kind (including tampons)	Counseling to alleviate psychogenic causes; gradual dilation of the vagina with woman's fingers or dilators; systematic desensitization exercises; relaxation training
Dyspareunia Painful intercourse	Insufficient sexual arousal; communication problems with partner; infections, inflammation; structural abnormalities; insufficient lubrication	Individual and couple counseling with a focus on relaxation and communication; medical strategies to reduce infections and structural abnormalities; additional lubrication
Men		
Erectile Dysfunction Inability to achieve an erection (impotence)	Chronic diseases (including diabetes, vascular problems, and chemical dependencies); trauma; numerous psychogenic factors (including anxiety, guilt, fear, poor self-concept)	Medical intervention (including possible vascular surgery, drugs (see the Star Box on page 464), or the use of penile implants); couple counseling using sensate focusing, pleasuring, and relaxation strategies
Rapid Ejaculation Ejaculating too quickly after penile penetration; premature ejaculation	Predominantly psychogenic in origin; a man's need to prove his sexual prowess; anxiety associated with previous sexual experiences	Counseling to free the man from the anxiety associated with rapid ejaculation; altering coital position, masturbation before intimacy, use of the squeeze technique as orgasm approaches
Dyspareunia Painful intercourse	Primarily physical in origin; inability of the penile foreskin to retract fully; urogenital tract infections; scar tissue in seminal passageways; insufficient lubrication	Medical care to reduce infection or repair damaged or abnormal tissue; additional lubrication

Sexual Orientation

Sexual orientation refers to the direction in which people focus their sexual interests. People can be attracted to opposite-gender partners, same-gender partners, or partners of both genders.

Heterosexuality

Heterosexuality (or heterosexual orientation) refers to an attraction to opposite-gender partners. (*Heteros* is a Greek word that means "the other.") A heterosexual person is sometimes called *straight.* Throughout the world, this is the most common sexual orientation. For reasons related to species survival, heterosexuality has its most basic roots in the biological dimension of human sexuality. Beyond its biological roots, heterosexuality has significant cultural and religious support in virtually every country in the world. Worldwide, laws related to marriage, living arrangements, health benefits, child rearing, financial matters, sexual behavior, and inheritance generally support relationships that are heterosexual in nature. However, this may soon be changing. (See page 475 for information regarding same-sex marriage.)

Homosexuality

Homosexuality (or homosexual orientation) refers to an attraction to same-gender partners. The term *homosexuality* comes from the Greek word *homos,* meaning "same." The term *gay* can refer to males or females, whereas the word *lesbian* is used only in reference to females.[5]

The distinctions among the categories of sexual orientation are much less clear than their definitions might suggest. Most people probably fall somewhere along a continuum between exclusive heterosexuality and exclusive homosexuality. Kinsey in 1948 presented just such a continuum.[6]

Students often wonder "what makes a person gay?" This question has no simple answer. (College sexuality textbooks devote entire chapters to this topic.) Some research has pointed to differences in the sizes of certain brain structures as a possible biological or anatomical basis for homosexuality.[7] Other research proposes possible genetic, environmental, hormonal, or other foundations.

However, for sexual orientation in general, no single theory has emerged that fully explains this complex developmental process. The consensus of scientific opinion is that people do not choose their sexual orientation. Thus, being straight or being gay is something that "just happens." Most gays and lesbians report that no specific event "triggered" them into being gay. Many also indicate that they knew that their orientations were different from those of other children as far back as their prepuberty years.

Given the many challenges of being gay in a straight world, it would seem logical that gays and lesbians do not make conscious efforts to become gay. It is also highly unlikely that heterosexual persons actually choose to be straight. Sexual orientation is something that just unfolds. (See Discovering Your Spirituality for insight into some of the issues that gays and lesbians need to face.)

Although operational definitions of sexual orientation may vary from researcher to researcher, Kinsey estimated that about 2 percent of American females and 4 percent of American males were exclusively homosexual.[6,8] More recent estimates place the overall combined figure at about 10 percent of the population. Clearly the expression of same-gender attraction is not uncommon.

 TALKING POINTS How would you react if a close family member told you that he or she was gay? Could you be supportive or at least communicate your feelings without anger or criticism?

Bisexuality

People who have the ability to be attracted to either gender are referred to as *bisexuals*. Bisexuals may fall into one of three groups: those who are (1) genuinely attracted to both genders, (2) gay but also feel the need to behave heterosexually, or (3) aroused physically by the same gender but attracted emotionally to the opposite gender. Some people participate in a bisexual lifestyle for extended periods, whereas others move quickly to a more exclusive orientation. The size of the bisexual population is not accurately known.[9] (See Learning from Our Diversity on page 477, which describes some of the challenges for bisexual men and women.)

Gender Identity Issues

Gender identity refers to the recognition of oneself as a male or female. As noted in Chapter 14, this recognition initially takes place within about 18 months after birth. Most people then move through their lives, adopting many or all of the traditional gender roles for their biological sex. Most feel reasonably comfortable with who they are as a man or a woman.

However, this typical pattern does not occur for everyone: (a) Some individuals are not comfortable with their biological sex. They struggle with the issue of transsexualism. (b) Transgendered people prefer not conforming to society's traditional expectations for their sex. (c) Other individuals are comfortable with their gender identity but find sexual pleasure from dressing in clothes that are more culturally "appropriate" for the opposite gender. These persons engage in transvestism.

Transsexualism

Transsexualism is an uncommon sexual variation in which a person rejects his or her biological sexuality. The male transsexual believes that he truly is a "woman trapped in a man's body." He desires to be the woman who he knows he is. Likewise, the female transsexual believes that she is a male existing in a woman's body. She desires to be the man who she knows she is. (Note that sex therapists and psychiatrists do not view transsexuals as homosexual in their sexual orientation.)

For transsexuals, the periods of gender preference and gender adoption (see Chapter 14) are perplexing as they attempt, often with little success, to resolve the conflict between what their mind tells them is true and what their body displays. Adolescent and young adult transsexuals may cross-dress, undertake gay or lesbian relationships (which they view as heterosexual relationships), and experiment with hormone replacement therapy. Sometimes, transsexuals actively pursue a sex reassignment operation. Thousands of these surgeries have been performed at some of the leading medical centers in the United States. For more detailed information about transsexualism, including theories about the origins of transsexualism, you could consult a textbook used in college human sexuality courses or search the Internet for pertinent Web sites.

Transgenderism

People who are **transgendered** present appearances and personas that do not conform to the gender role expectations that society has established for their sex. Thus, transgendered persons tend to be nonconformists to traditional sex roles.[10] Transgendered women take on characteristics and mannerisms of men, and transgendered men take on characteristics and mannerisms of women. They might cross-dress on a full- or part-time basis, although they usually do not do this for sexual arousal purposes (as transvestites typically do).

Do transgendered persons differ from transsexuals? Yes, they are two different categories, according to sexuality experts.[10] The main distinction is that transgendered persons do not feel the need to surgically change their bodies to achieve the physical structures of the other sex. Transsexuals feel trapped in an opposite-sex body, and many would like to have their genitals and body appearance be consistent with the "sex they know themselves to be." However, transgendered individuals know and accept the sex to which they were born; yet they prefer to take on and display mannerisms of the other sex.

Transvestism

Public figures such as Dennis Rodman, Eddie Izzard, Harvey Fierstein, and RuPaul have turned a spotlight on cross-dressing, or transvestism. The term **transvestism** is typically used to describe a heterosexual male who, from time to time, dresses as a woman. (Some gay men and women enjoy cross-dressing on occasion.) The practice of transvestism can range from simple sexual gratification from the wearing of feminine clothing, to the expression of the feminine side of the individual's personality. Although many transvestites wish to express the feminine aspects of their personality, most are satisfied with their gender role and their biological gender. Many are married and may or may not have shared this aspect of their personality with their partner.

One large study found that typical cross-dressers are virtually indistinguishable from non-cross-dressing men in their personality traits, sexuality, and measures of psychological wellness.[11]

Years ago, psychologists attempted to cure cross-dressers, but today most have recognized that cross-dressing is lifelong and that they can obtain better results by teaching the cross-dresser to accept his feminine side.

It is rare for a female to be a transvestite, perhaps because the norms for women's clothing are far less restrictive than those for men.[12] For example, while it might be quite normal to see your grandmother wearing a flannel shirt and bluejeans around the house, it would be surprising for you to see your grandfather watching NFL football wearing a frilly negligee.

Patterns of Sexual Behavior

Although sex researchers may see sexual behavior in terms of the human sexual response pattern described earlier, most people are more interested in the observable dimensions of sexual behavior.

Celibacy

Celibacy can be defined as the self-imposed avoidance of sexual intimacy. Celibacy is synonymous with sexual abstinence. People could choose not to have a sexually intimate relationship for many reasons. For some,

---

Key Terms

transsexualism a sexual variation in which a person rejects his or her biological sexuality

transgendered refers to persons whose appearance and behaviors do not conform to society's traditional gender role expectations

transvestism atypical behavior in which a person derives sexual pleasure from dressing in the clothes of the opposite gender

---

celibacy is part of a religious doctrine. Others might be afraid of contracting a sexually transmitted disease. For most, however, celibacy is preferred simply because it seems appropriate for them. Celibate people can certainly have deep, intimate relationships with other people—just not sexual relationships. Celibacy may be short term or last a lifetime, and no identified physical or psychological complications appear to result from a celibate lifestyle.

 TALKING POINTS You have decided to remain celibate until you are ready to make a lifetime commitment to someone. How would you explain this to the person you are now dating?

Masturbation

Throughout recorded history, **masturbation** has been a primary method of achieving sexual pleasure. Through masturbation, people can explore their sexual response patterns. Traditionally, some societies and religious groups have condemned this behavior based on the belief that intercourse is the only "right" sexual behavior. With sufficient lubrication, masturbation cannot do physical harm. Today masturbation is considered by most sex therapists and researchers to be a normal source of self-pleasure.

Fantasy and Erotic Dreams

The brain is the most sensual organ in the body. In fact, many sexuality experts classify **sexual fantasies** and **erotic dreams** as forms of sexual behavior. Particularly for people whose verbal ability is highly developed, the ability to create imaginary scenes enriches other forms of sexual behavior.

Sexual fantasies are generally found in association with some second type of sexual behavior. When occurring before intercourse or masturbation, fantasies prepare a person for the behavior that will follow. As an example, fantasies experienced while reading a book may focus your attention on sexual activity that will occur later in the day.

When fantasies occur with another form of sexual behavior, the second behavior may be greatly enhanced by the supportive fantasy. Both women and men fantasize during foreplay and intercourse. Masturbation and fantasizing are inseparable activities.

Erotic dreams occur during sleep in both men and women. The association between these dreams and ejaculation resulting in a nocturnal emission (wet dream) is readily recognized in men. In women, erotic dreams can lead not only to vaginal lubrication but to orgasm as well.

Shared Touching

Virtually the entire body can be an erogenous zone when sensual contact between partners is involved. A soft, light touch, a slight application of pressure, the brushing back of a partner's hair, and gentle massage are all forms of communication that heighten sexual arousal.

Genital Contact

Two important purposes can be identified for the practice of stimulating a partner's genitals. The first is the tactile component of **foreplay.** Genital contact, in the form of holding, rubbing, stroking, or caressing, heightens arousal to a level that allows for progression into intercourse.

The second role of genital contact is that of *mutual masturbation to orgasm.* Stimulation of the genitals so that both partners have orgasm is a form of sexual behavior practiced by many people, as well as by couples during the late stage of a pregnancy. For couples not desiring pregnancy, the risk of conception is virtually eliminated when this becomes the form of sexual intimacy practiced.

As is the case in other aspects of intimacy, genital stimulation is best enhanced when partners can talk about their needs, expectations, and reservations. Practice and communication can shape this form of contact into a pleasure-giving approach to sexual intimacy.

Oral-Genital Stimulation

Oral-genital stimulation brings together two of the body's most erogenous areas: the genitalia and the mouth. Couples who engage in oral sex consistently report that this form of intimacy is highly satisfactory. Some people have experimented with oral sex and found it unacceptable, and some have never experienced this form of sexual intimacy. Some couples prefer not to participate in oral sex because they consider it immoral (according to religious doctrine), illegal (which it is in some states), or unhygienic (because of a partner's unclean genitals). Some

Key Terms
masturbation self-stimulation of the genitals
sexual fantasies fantasies with sexual themes; sexual daydreams or imaginary events
erotic dreams dreams whose contents elicit a sexual response
foreplay activities, often involving touching and caressing, that prepare individuals for sexual intercourse

couples may refrain because of the mistaken belief that oral sex is only for gays and lesbians. Regardless of the reason, a person who does not consider oral sex to be pleasurable should not be coerced into this behavior.

Because oral-genital stimulation can involve an exchange of body fluids, the risk of disease transmission is real. Small tears of mouth or genital tissue may allow transmission of disease-causing pathogens. Only couples who are absolutely certain that they are free from all sexually transmitted diseases (including HIV infection) can practice unprotected oral sex. Couples in doubt should refrain from oral-genital sex or carefully use a condom (on the male) or a latex square to cover the female's vulval area. Increasingly, latex squares (dental dams) can be obtained from drug stores or pharmacies. (Dentists may also provide you with dental dams, or you can make your own latex square by cutting a condom into an appropriate shape.)

Three basic forms of oral-genital stimulation are practiced by both heterosexual and homosexual couples.[10] **Fellatio,** in which the penis is kissed, licked, or sucked by the partner, is the most common of the three. **Cunnilingus,** in which the vulva of the female is kissed, licked, or penetrated by the partner's tongue, is only slightly less frequently practiced.

Mutual oral-genital stimulation, the third form of oral-genital stimulation, combines both fellatio and cunnilingus. When practiced by a heterosexual couple, the female partner performs fellatio on her partner while her male partner performs cunnilingus on her. Gay couples can practice mutual fellatio or cunnilingus.

Intercourse

Sexual intercourse (coitus) refers to the act of inserting the penis into the vagina. Intercourse is the sexual behavior that is most directly associated with **procreation.** For some, intercourse is the only natural and appropriate form of sexual intimacy.

The incidence and frequency of sexual intercourse is a much-studied topic. Information concerning the percentages of people who have engaged in intercourse is readily available in textbooks used in sexuality courses. Data concerning sexual intercourse among college students may be changing somewhat because of concerns about HIV infection and other STDs, but a reasonable estimate of the percentage of college students who have engaged in sexual intercourse is 60–75 percent.

These percentages reflect two important concepts about the sexual activity of college students. The first is that most college students are having intercourse. The second concept is that a large percentage (25–40 percent) of students are choosing to refrain from intercourse. Indeed, the belief that "everyone is doing it" may be a bit

shortsighted. From a public health standpoint, we believe it is important to provide accurate health information to protect those who choose to have intercourse and to actively support a person's right to choose not to have intercourse.

Sexually active couples need to share their expectations concerning techniques and the desired frequency of intercourse.[13] Even the "performance" factors, such as depth of penetration, nature of body movements, tempo of activity, and timing of orgasm are increasingly important to many couples. Issues concerning sexually transmitted diseases (including HIV infection) are also critically important for couples who are contemplating intercourse. These factors also need to be explored through open communication.

A variety of books (including textbooks) provide written and visually explicit information on intercourse positions. Four basic positions for intercourse—*man above, woman above, side by side,* and *rear entry*—each offer relative advantages and disadvantages.

Anal Sexual Activity

Some couples practice **anal intercourse,** in which the penis is inserted into the rectum of a partner. Anal intercourse can be performed by both heterosexual couples and gay men. According to a year 2000 report in the journal *Archives of Sexual Behavior,* about 20–25 percent of college students have experienced anal intercourse.[14] The anal sphincter muscles contract tightly and tend to resist entry. Thus, couples who engage in anal intercourse must do so slowly, gently, and with adequate amounts of water-based lubricants. Because of the danger of tearing tissues in the rectal area, HIV transmission risk is increased if the inserting male is infected.[3] Unless it is absolutely certain that both partners are uninfected, the inserting male should always wear a condom. Even with a condom, disease transmission is possible, since during anal intercourse, condoms are more likely to tear than during penis-vaginal intercourse. Couples practicing anal sex must not follow anal insertion with insertion into the

---

> **Key Terms**
>
> **fellatio** (feh **lay** she oh) oral stimulation of the penis
>
> **cunnilingus** (cun uh **ling** gus) oral stimulation of the vulva or clitoris
>
> **procreation** reproduction
>
> **anal intercourse** a sexual act in which the erect penis is inserted into the rectum of a partner

mouth or vagina because of the likelihood of transmitting infectious agents.

For many people, anal intercourse is not only unpleasant, but simply unnatural for humans. For others, the anal area is just another part of the human body that is especially sensitive to stimulation, and they enjoy the pleasurable sensations that come from intercourse or the insertion of a well-lubricated finger or sex toy. Some people enjoy kissing ("rimming") or touching in the anal area, but this should occur only when the anal area has been fully cleansed or covered with a sheet of protective plastic wrap. As with all sexual behavior, couples need to communicate clearly their feelings about any activity. If one partner is uncomfortable about an activity and wants to stop, his or her feelings must be supported by the other person. A desire for a particular sexual activity must not turn into sexual coercion or a sexual assault.

Until recently, thirteen states had laws on the books that banned **sodomy** (another term for anal sex as well as certain other sexual practices). However, a U.S. Supreme Court ruling *(Lawrence and Garner v Texas)* in June 2003 invalidated a Texas law that banned private consensual sex (in this case, sodomy) between adults of the same sex. Legal experts expect this Texas ruling to eventually invalidate the laws of the 12 other states that banned sodomy in one form or another.[15]

Secondary Virginity

Some individuals who have previously engaged in sexual intercourse have chosen to refrain from further sexual intercourse. They are said to be practicing **secondary virginity.** The practice of secondary virginity reflects a conscious choice for persons to wait until a time when they feel it's all right to resume intercourse.

The decision to be a secondary virgin can be made for a number of reasons. Some prefer to return to abstinence for moral or religious reasons, while others wish to wait until there is more commitment in the relationship. Some come to the realization that they are not yet physically or emotionally ready for intercourse. Others do not want to risk pregnancy or the possibility of contracting a sexually transmitted disease. Some do not have the time or energy needed to become involved in a sexual relationship.

Those who choose secondary virginity are quick to point out its advantages. They no longer worry about certain risks, such as pregnancy or developing an STD. They no longer have to worry about the expense of contraception or the side effects from certain forms of birth control. Some feel great relief knowing that they are successfully following their own moral compass or religious beliefs. By pursuing secondary virginity, they can focus a great deal more time and energy on other important aspects of their relationship.

Sexuality and Aging

Students are often curious about how aging affects sexuality. This is understandable because we live in a society that idolizes youth and demands performance. Many younger people become anxious about growing older because of what they think will happen to their ability to express their sexuality. Interestingly, young adults are willing to accept other physical changes of aging (such as the slowing down of basal metabolism, reduced lung capacity, and even wrinkles) but not those changes related to sexuality.

Research shows that, although sexual activity does decline with age, the capacity to enjoy sex is not altered, and a significant proportion of older adults remain sexually active.[16]

As with other aspects of aging, certain anatomical and physiological changes will be evident, but these changes do not necessarily reduce the ability to enjoy sexual activity.[17] Most experts in sexuality report that many older people remain interested in sexual activity. Furthermore, those who are exposed to regular sexual activity throughout a lifetime report being most satisfied with their sex lives as older adults.[10]

As people age, the likelihood of alterations in the male and female sexual response cycles increases. In the postmenopausal woman, vaginal lubrication commonly begins more slowly, and the amount of lubrication usually diminishes. However, clitoral sensitivity and nipple erection remain the same as in earlier years. The female capacity for multiple orgasms remains the same, although the number of contractions that occur at orgasm typically is reduced.

In the older man, physical changes are also evident. This is thought to be caused by the decrease in the production of testosterone between the ages of 20 and 60 years. After age 60 or so, testosterone levels remain relatively steady. Thus many men, despite a decrease in sperm production, remain fertile into their 80s.[10] Older men typically take longer to achieve an erection (however, they are able to maintain their erection longer before ejaculation), have fewer muscular contractions at orgasm, and ejaculate less forcefully than they once did. The volume of seminal fluid ejaculated is typically less than in earlier years, and its consistency is somewhat thinner. The resolution phase is usually longer in older men. In spite of these gradual

---

Key Terms

sodomy generally refers to anal or oral sex; a legal term whose definition varies from state to state

secondary virginity the discontinuation of sexual intercourse after initial exploration changes, some elderly men engage in sexual intercourse with the same frequency as do much younger men.

A significant proportion of older adults in nursing homes continue to be sexually active. Unfortunately, they face barriers such as a lack of privacy, chronic illness, lack of a willing partner, unsupportive attitudes of physicians and staff, feelings of unattractiveness, and a lack of knowledge about their own sexuality.[16]

Health care workers can help to remove these barriers by improving privacy, educating staff, arranging conjugal or home visits, encouraging several forms of sexual expression, and counseling interested patients.

Bonds between People

As people develop their relationships, they often form bonds that start with friendship and dating activities and then move toward intimacy and love. Let's explore these stepping stones.

Friendship

One of the exciting aspects of college life is that you will probably meet many new people, some of whom will become your best friends. Because of your common experiences, it is likely that you will keep in contact with a few of these friends for a lifetime. Close attachments to other people can have an important influence on all of the dimensions of your health.

What is it that draws friends together? With the exception of physical intimacy, many of the same growth experiences seen in dating and mate selection are also seen in the development of friendships. Think about how you and your best friend developed the relationship you now have. You probably became friends when you shared similar interests and experiences. Your friendship progressed (and even faltered at times) through personal gains or losses. In all likelihood, you cared about each other and learned to share your deepest beliefs and feelings. You cemented your bond by turning your beliefs into behaviors. You resolved conflicts (see the Star box).

Throughout the development of a deep friendship, the qualities of trust, tolerance, empathy, and support must be demonstrated. Otherwise the friendship can fall apart. You will soon note that the qualities seen in a friendship are very similar to the qualities noted in the upcoming description of companionate love (page 473). In both cases, people develop deep attachments through extensive familiarity and understanding.

Dating

A half-century ago, the events involved in a dating relationship were somewhat predictable. People met each

Resolving Conflict through Better Communication

Every relationship presents challenges to the individuals involved. Therapists would argue that couples who can learn to resolve conflict effectively have the best chance of maintaining long-term relationships. The hallmark of effective conflict resolution is that each person ends up feeling respected by his or her partner. Not surprisingly, this process is built on effective communication.

Here are some successful ways to communicate better to manage conflict:

- Show mutual respect. Remain calm.
- Identify and resolve the real issue.
- Be a good listener.
- Seek areas of agreement.
- Do not interrupt.
- Mutually participate in decision making.
- Be cooperative and specific.
- Focus on the present and future—not the past.
- Don't try to assign blame.
- Say what you are thinking and feeling.
- When talking, use sentences that begin with "I."
- Avoid using sentences that start with "You" or "Why."
- Set a time limit for discussing problems.
- Accept responsibility.
- Do something fun together.

other through their daily activities or groups of friends, and a formal request for a date was made. Ninety-nine times out of a hundred, the requestor was male and the invitee was female. After a period of formal and informal dates, the two made a commitment to steady dating or decided to "date around." If the relationship progressed, further commitments were made (for example, letter jackets, class rings, or other jewelry items were exchanged). After months or years of a committed relationship, the couple decided to get married. The man invariably asked for the woman's "hand" (after first receiving permission from her parents), and plans for a wedding ceremony were made.

Does this form of dating and mate selection exist as we move through the new millennium? For some couples, yes. The traditional way of dating and selecting a life partner works well for them. However, many young and midlife adults prefer a more flexible, less predictable format for dating and finding a person they might choose to marry. For example, more than ever, women are playing a more assertive role when it comes to initiating and establishing the ground rules for a relationship.

Interestingly, a large number of our students do not even like to use the word *dating* because it connotes a formalized pattern of behavior followed by their parents and grandparents. Many college students today seem to prefer "hanging out" with a group of 5 to 10 friends, instead of pairing off with a partner and doing only "couple activities."

When students do start to pair off and become exclusive in their dating, they tend to pursue a pattern called **serial monogamy.** In serial monogamy, a person dates one person exclusively until the relationship ends. Then another partner is found, and that couple dates exclusively for a period of time until that relationship eventually ends. In this pattern of dating, individuals do not date multiple people simultaneously. They go through mutually exclusive relationships, one after the other.

Students can fool themselves into believing that their dating patterns reflect **mutual monogamy.** Some couples believe that going out with another person as long as six months or a year reflects mutual monogamy. (Technically, for the six months or the year of going out, it can be called mutual monogamy.) When that relationship ends and a new one begins, however, the persons involved must understand that their dating pattern is developing into a serial pattern.

One critical health issue involved with serial monogamy is the increased possibility of exposure to infectious diseases, including all of the sexually transmitted diseases and HIV. While less risky than having indiscriminate sexual activities with multiple partners at the same time, serial monogamy still exposes a person to a new partner who may or may not be harboring a disease pathogen. Individuals who have a series of intimate relationships with multiple persons need to be especially vigilant in their safer sex practices. They need to understand clearly that their new partner could be exposing them to a rich pool of infectious diseases.

Intimacy

When most people hear the word **intimacy,** they immediately think about physical, sexual intimacy. However, sexuality experts and family therapists prefer to view intimacy more broadly, as any close, mutual, verbal or nonverbal behavior within a relationship. In this sense, intimate behavior can range from sharing deep feelings and experiences with a partner to sharing profound physical pleasures with a partner.

Intimacy is present in both love and friendship. You have likely shared intimate feelings with your closest friends, as well as with those you love. Intimacy helps us feel connected to others and allows us to feel the full measure of our own self-worth.

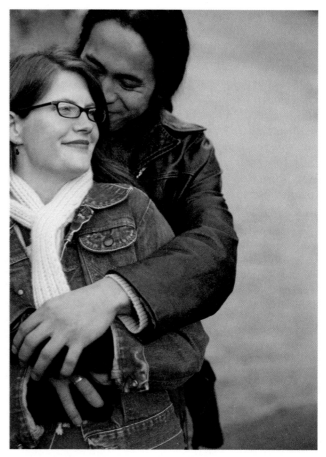

Companionate love is capable of sustaining mutual long-term growth.

TALKING POINTS Your teenage son equates intimacy with sex. How would you explain the emotional intimacy involved in marriage?

Love

Love may be one of the most elusive yet widely recognized concepts that describe some level of emotional attachment

Key Terms

serial monogamy a pattern of dating in which a person is involved in a series of exclusive relationships, one after the other

mutual monogamy a pattern of dating in which a person is involved exclusively with one partner

intimacy any close, mutual, verbal or nonverbal behavior within a relationship to another. Various forms of love include friendship and erotic, devotional, parental, and altruistic love. Other behavioral scientists[10] have focused primarily on two types of love most closely associated with dating and mate selection: *passionate love* and *companionate love.*

Passionate love, also described as romantic love or **infatuation,** is a state of extreme absorption in another. It is characterized by intense feelings of tenderness, elation, anxiety, sexual desire, and ecstasy. Often appearing early in a relationship, passionate love typically does not last very long. Passionate love is driven by the excitement of being closely involved with a person whose character is not fully known.

If a relationship progresses, passionate love is gradually replaced by companionate love. This type of love is a less intense emotion than passionate love. It is characterized by friendly affection and a deep attachment that is based on extensive familiarity with the loved one.[10] This love is enduring and capable of sustaining long-term mutual growth. Central to companionate love are feelings of empathy for, support of, and tolerance of the partner. (Complete the Personal Assessment on page 483 to determine whether you and your partner are truly compatible.)

Relationships and Lifestyles

A variety of formal and informal relationships and lifestyles exist in our society. Here are a few of the most common ones.

Marriage

Just as there is no single best way for two people to move through dating and mate selection, marriage is an equally variable undertaking. In marriage, two people join their lives in a way that affirms each as an individual and both as a legal pair. They are able to resolve issues constructively (see Changing for the Better). However, for a large percentage of couples, the demands of marriage are too rigorous, confining, and demanding. They will find resolution for their dissatisfaction through divorce or extramarital affairs. For most, though, marriage will be an experience that alternates periods of happiness, productivity, and admiration with periods of frustration, unhappiness, and disillusionment with the partner. Each marriage is unique. Each marriage provides an opportunity for the partners to share a lifetime of experiences.[17]

As we move through the early years of this new century, we see certain trends in marriage. The most obvious of these is the age at first marriage. Today men are waiting longer than ever to marry. Now the median

age at first marriage for men is 27 years.[18] In addition, these new husbands are better educated than in the past and are more likely to be established in their careers. Women are also waiting longer to get married and tend to be more educated and career oriented. Recent statistics indicate that the median age at first marriage for women is 25 years.[18]

Key Terms

infatuation an often shallow but intense attraction to another person

Recent statistics show that both men and women are waiting longer to get married.

Legalization of same-sex marriage would grant gay couples a wide range of legal and economic rights.

Marriage still appeals to most adults. Currently, 76 percent of adults aged 18 and older are married, widowed, or divorced.[19] Thus about one-quarter of today's adults have not married. Within the last decade, the percentage of adults who have decided not to marry has nearly doubled.

Gay and Lesbian Partnerships

To believe that adult partnerships are reserved only for heterosexual couples is to avoid reality. In the United States and in many parts of the world, gays and lesbians are forming partnerships that, in many ways, mimic those of heterosexuals. It no longer is unusual to see same-sex men and women openly living together in one household. Gay and lesbian couples buy houses together and share property rights. As businesses restructure their employee benefits packages, gays and lesbians are covering their partners on health care plans and making them beneficiaries on their insurance policies and retirement plans.

A search of the literature will indicate that gay and lesbian partnerships have many of the same characteristics and problems of heterosexual couples.[3] Like straight couples, they struggle with interpersonal issues related to their relationship and their lifestyle. They work to decide how best to juggle their financial resources, their leisure time, and their friends and extended families. If they live together in an apartment or house, they must decide how to divide the household tasks.

If children are present in the household, they must be cared for and nurtured. These children could have come from an adoption, a previous heterosexual relationship, or, in the case of a lesbian couple, from artificial insemination. Research indicates that children raised in lesbian or gay families overwhelmingly grow up with a heterosexual orientation, and are like other children from heterosexual families in terms of their adjustment, mental health, social skills, and peer acceptance.[3]

Same-Sex Marriage

One area in which gay and lesbian couples differ from heterosexual couples is in their ability to obtain a legal marriage. In the last few years, this inequity has been the focus of an intense national debate over same-sex marriage. The issues are complex, primarily because of the differences in state laws and the various courts' interpretations of those laws. At this point in the debate, here is where same-sex marriage stands.

If enacted, same-sex marriages would grant gay couples a legal marriage document that allows for an array of legal and economic benefits, including joint parental custody, insurance and health benefits, joint tax returns, alimony and child support, inheritance of property, hospital visitation rights, family leave, and a spouse's retirement benefits. (Social Security benefits come from a federal program and are not influenced by state laws.)

At the present time, only the state of Massachusetts has legalized gay marriage. The Massachusetts law came into effect in 2003, after a lengthy series of complex court battles. Ultimately, the Massachusetts Supreme Court determined that it was illegal (according to the state constitution) to deny gay couples the right to wed. In the year 2000, the Vermont legislature passed the nation's first "civil union" law, which granted legal status to gay and lesbian couples. Vermont's law confers on same-sex couples all the benefits that the state presently allows for heterosexual married couples. However, civil unions that take place in Vermont are not generally recognized in other states.

In early 2005, a San Francisco County Superior Court judge ruled that withholding marriage licenses from gay and lesbian couples constituted a violation of their civil rights under state law.[20] This ruling was expected to be appealed by those who felt it could undermine California's existing laws, which define marriage as between one man and one woman. Like Vermont, California already had a law that grants "domestic partner" benefits (but not marriage) to committed gay and lesbian couples who register with the state government. In April 2005, this law was upheld by the Court of Appeals for the Third Circuit thus keeping legal status for the 29,000 couples in California registered as domestic partners.[21]

In an attempt to counter the general push toward same-sex marriage, a number of states have passed so-called Defense of Marriage Acts (DOMAs). Voters in numerous states have passed laws that define marriage as the union between one man and one woman. It will be interesting to see how this debate evolves, since legal challenges to DOMAs are likely to occur in every state where these laws have been passed. The debate could encourage states to pass laws that support civil union or domestic partnerships, with the hopes of preserving bans on actual gay and lesbian marriages. Most observers believe that ultimately the U.S. Supreme Court will have to rule on the constitutionality of same-sex marriage.

Until that happens, some conservative members of the U.S. Congress are trying to rally support for a constitutional amendment that would ban gay marriage. This has been a challenging task indeed. While President George W. Bush has been somewhat reluctant to vigorously support such an amendment, he did "support the notion that marriage is between a man and a woman."[22]

Traditional Forms of Marriage

To describe the nature of marital relationships, we use the classic categories of marital relationships proposed by Cuber and Harroff.[23] These marriage types should not be viewed as either good or bad. Rather, you should recognize one simple reality: these marriages are routinely found and apparently meet the needs of the individuals involved.

Some of the types of marriages began in their current form. Others, however, evolved into their present form, having once been a very different type of marital relationship.

Interestingly, although Cuber and Harroff's classic descriptions that follow pertain to heterosexual marriages, it is quite likely that these forms of marriage would also apply to partnerships or marriages involving gay and lesbian couples. As you read this section, decide if you agree or disagree with this suggestion.

Conflict-Habituated Marriage

"We fought on our first date, our honeymoon was a disaster, and we've disagreed on everything of importance ever since." This frank description of a marital relationship characterized by confrontation, disagreement, and perhaps physical abuse reflects a *conflict-habituated marriage.* The central theme of this type of marital relationship is conflict, and its continuous presence suggests that the partners are making no attempt at resolution. Couples in long-term conflict-habituated marriages simply agree to disagree.

Devitalized Marriage

In the same way a dying person is said to possess failing signs, a *devitalized marriage* has lost its signs of life. Unlike the conflict-habituated marriage, which since its beginning was chronically impaired, the devitalized marriage was once a more active and satisfying marital relationship. However, the couple has lost its desire to keep the marriage dynamic.

The future of a devitalized marriage is difficult to predict. Some marriages of this type can be revitalized. Effective marriage counseling, a new job, or moving to a new community can rekindle a relationship. Other devitalized marriages are able to remain intact because one or both partners find vitality through an extramarital relationship. Some devitalized marriages persist at low levels of involvement and commitment with little hope for improvement. We would not be surprised if, for those of you who have witnessed the dissolution of your own or your parents' marriage, devitalization was an important factor in its ending.

Passive-Congenial Marriage

Passive means a low level of commitment or involvement, and the word *congenial* suggests warmth and friendliness. When these two words are combined as they are in *passive-congenial marriage,* they describe perfectly the type of marital relationship sought by some couples.

For some of today's young professionals, the passive-congenial marriage offers a safe harbor from the rigors encountered in the competitive world of corporate business. Children may not be valued "commodities" in the passive-congenial marriage. The added financial and personal stressors related to child rearing could compromise an established lifestyle. You may be able to construct

People whose sexual orientation is toward both men and women are termed bisexuals. This can be a confusing label, however. For example, if a man has had one sexual experience with a man, but all of his other sexual experiences are with women, does this mean he is a bisexual? And what about the woman who has sequential relationships with men, followed by an occasional relationship with a woman? Is she bisexual? What about people who are sexually attracted to one gender, but are emotionally more attracted to the other gender? The labels can get confusing and can make one wonder about the value of any label describing sexual orientation. This is just one of the many challenges facing bisexual people.

Some experts suggest that bisexuals (those who have had at least one sexual experience with a man and one with a woman) probably outnumber exclusive homosexuals (those who have had sexual experience *only* with persons of their own gender).[1] One might think that this larger group would be better understood by society, but that seems not to be the case. Bisexuals may have a larger field of potential partners, but this benefit may be offset by the difficulty of "fitting" into society.

Heterosexual people, gay males, and lesbians may not view bisexuality as acceptable, believing that the bisexual person is just incapable of making the decision to go one way or the other.[2] They may accuse the bisexual person of wanting the best of both worlds, as if "having it all" (in terms of sexual possibilities and experiences) is an inappropri-

ate, bad thing. Then there is the issue of telling a new dating partner that you are attracted to both men and women. Some new partners may find this reality a distinct "turnoff."

For these reasons, numerous college and university counseling centers are expanding their outreach programs to include programs for bisexual students. If you are interested, you might check into the offerings of your campus counseling center to see if they provide educational information, support groups, or specialized counseling for bisexual students. Many campuses also have student groups that focus on gay, lesbian, bisexual, and transgendered students.

Interestingly, it appears that more and more bisexual students are "coming out" despite the challenges they may face. Perhaps this has been encouraged by the public pronouncements of bisexuality by well-known movie stars, such as Drew Barrymore.[3] In the near future, we may find more public acceptance for people who are bisexual. Would you consider increased public acceptance of bisexuality to be a good or bad thing?

[1]Hyde JS, DeLamater JD. *Understanding Human Sexuality,* 9th ed. New York: McGraw-Hill, 2006.

[2]Kelly GF. *Sexuality Today: the Human Perspective,* 8th ed. New York: McGraw-Hill, 2006.

[3]Celebrity news. *Drew Barrymore: "I am bisexual,"* http://us. imdb.com/wn?20030717#6, July 23, 2003.

an image of a passive-congenial couple if you can picture two people meeting after work for a quiet dinner at a small restaurant, talking in muffled tones about their corporate battles, and planning their winter cruise.

Maintaining a passive-congenial marriage requires less time and energy than do other forms of marriage. For two people who feel certain that their major contributions to society will be made through their efforts in the workplace, this marriage may be ideal. Certainly you may know many couples who are choosing this increasingly popular form of marriage.

Total Marriage

In the *total marriage,* little remains of the unique identities the two people had before their marriage took place. For reasons that are probably lost to the subconscious mind, two people possessing individual personalities use marriage to fuse their identities into one identity—the total pair.

The total marriage requires that the individual partners set aside all aspirations for individual growth and development. Decisions are not made with "me" or even "you" as the center of attention. Rather, energies are

directed toward what is best for "us." Life outside the marital relationship and partner's presence does not exist, at least figuratively speaking. Eventually outsiders, when speaking about these individuals, can no longer truly speak about the man or the woman but are limited to speaking about the couple.

Vital Marriage

The *vital marriage* is intended to serve as an arena for the growth of both the individuals and the pair. The partners focus on "my growth," "your growth," and "our growth." In a vital marriage, personal goals may at times be subordinated for the good of the partner or the paired relationship. Yet both the partners (and the children) know that those once-subordinated goals will assume top priority when this becomes possible and desirable. The relationship has equality of opportunity.

In describing the vital marriage, we must point out that this type of marital relationship is not perfect, nor is it appropriate for all couples. In today's complex society, the vital marriage may be especially difficult to maintain (see Changing for the Better on page 478).

Divorce

Marriages, like many other kinds of interpersonal relationships, can end. Today, marriages—relationships begun with the intent of permanence "until death do us part"—end through divorce nearly as frequently as not.

Why should approximately half of marital relationships end? Unfortunately, marriage experts cannot provide one clear answer to this question. Rather, they suggest that divorce is a reflection of unfulfilled expectations for marriage on the part of one or both partners, including the following:

- The belief that marriage will ease your need to deal with your own faults and that your failures can be shared by your partner
- The belief that marriage will change faults that you know exist in your partner
- The belief that the high level of romance of your dating and courtship period will be continued through marriage
- The belief that marriage can provide you with an arena for the development of your personal power, and that once married, you will not need to compromise with your partner
- The belief that your marital partner will be successful in meeting all of your needs

If these expectations seem to be ones you anticipate through marriage, then you may find that disappointments will abound. To varying degrees, marriage is a partnership that requires much cooperation and compromise. Marriage can be complicated. Because of the high expectations that many people hold for marriage, the termination of marriage can be an emotionally difficult process to undertake (see Changing for the Better on page 479).

The American attitude toward divorce swung like a pendulum during the last century. Divorce has gone from being an embarrassing, painful ordeal, to a common, relatively simple legal procedure. More recently, some observers have begun to question the wisdom of no-fault divorce.

Our society is concerned about the well-being of children whose parents divorce. Different factors, however, influence the extent to which divorce affects children. Included among these factors are the gender and age of the children, custody arrangements, financial support, and the remarriage of one or both parents. Many children must adjust to accept their new status as a member of a blended family.

Singlehood

For many people, being single is a lifestyle that affords the potential for pursuing intimacy, if desired, and provides an uncluttered path for independence and self-directedness. Other people, however, are single because of divorce, separation, death, or the absence of an opportunity to establish a partnership. The U.S. Bureau of the Census indicates that 43 percent of women and 39 percent of men over the age of 18 are currently single.[19]

Single people can have many different living arrangements. Some single people live alone and choose not to share a household. Other arrangements for singles include cohabitation, periodic cohabitation, singlehood during the week and cohabitation on the weekends or during vacations, or the platonic sharing of a household with others. For young adults, large percentages of single men and women live with their parents.

Like living arrangements, the sexual intimacy patterns of singles are individually tailored. Some singles practice celibacy, others pursue intimate relationships in a **monogamous** pattern, and others have multiple partners. As in all interpersonal relationships, including marriage, the levels of commitment are as variable as the people involved.

Cohabitation

Cohabitation, or the sharing of living quarters by unmarried people, represents yet another alternative to marriage. According to the U.S. Census Bureau, the number of unmarried, opposite-gender couples living together totals over 4.8 million couples.[19] The number of reported same gender couples totaled nearly 600,000 in the year 2000.

Although cohabitation may seem to imply a vision of sexual intimacy between male and female roommates, several forms of shared living arrangements can be viewed as cohabitation. For some couples, cohabitation is only a part-time arrangement for weekends, during summer vacation, or on a variable schedule. In addition, **platonic**

Key Terms

monogamous (mo **nog** a mus) paired relationship with one partner

cohabitation sharing of a residence by unrelated, unmarried people; living together

platonic close association between two people that does not include a sexual relationship cohabitation can exist when a couple shares living quarters but does so without establishing an intimate relationship. Close friends, people of retirement age, and gay couples might all be included in a group called cohabitants.

How well do cohabitation arrangements fare against marriage partnerships in terms of long-term stability? A recent 2002 report prepared by the CDC's National Center for Health Statistics[24] indicated that unmarried cohabitations are generally less stable than marriages. The probability of a first marriage ending in separation or divorce within 5 years was found to be 20 percent, but the probability of a premarital cohabitation breaking up within 5 years was 49 percent. After 10 years, the probability of a first marriage ending was 33 percent, compared to 62 percent for cohabitations.

Single Parenthood

Unmarried young women continue to become pregnant and then become single parents in this country. There is also a significantly different form of single parenthood: the planned entry into single parenthood by older, better educated people, the vast majority of whom are women.

In contrast to the teenaged girl who becomes a single parent through an unwed pregnancy, the more mature woman who desires single parenting has usually planned carefully for the experience. She has explored several important concerns, including questions regarding how she will become pregnant (with or without the knowledge of a male partner or through artificial insemination), the need for a father figure for the child, the effect of single parenting on her social life, and, of course, its effect on her career development. When these questions have been resolved, no legal barriers stand in the way of her becoming a single parent.

A very large number of women and a growing number of men are actively participating in single parenthood as a result of a divorce settlement or separation agreement involving sole or joint custody of children. Increasing numbers of single persons are now adopting children. In the year 2000, single women headed up 7.6 million households with children under the age of 18. In contrast, single men headed up 1.8 million households in the year 2000 with children under age 18.[19]

Communication in Relationships

You may have noticed that one of the recurring messages in this chapter is the importance of effective communication between partners in a relationship. You saw the Star box (page 472) on resolving conflict through better communication. You also probably noticed the Changing for the Better boxes that discussed how to improve marriage (page 474), communication as the key to relationships (page 478), and how to cope with a breakup (page 479). Each of these behavior change boxes emphasized the value of effective communication. Furthermore, the chapter sections on friendship, dating, intimacy, love, and marriage become meaningless unless you realize that true satisfaction in these areas is grounded in effective communication.

When you think about it, effective communication is the basis for *all healthy relationships*. For this reason, we encourage all readers to take advantage of available opportunities to learn effective communication skills. You might find these opportunities in college courses that you select. Most speech and communication departments have courses in personal communication skills. Look for pertinent courses in psychology and counseling psychology departments. Most colleges and universities also offer one or more human sexuality courses in their psychology, sociology, or health science departments. The counseling center on your campus may offer programs that can improve your communication skills. Finally, your campus library or bookstore will have popular books that may be very useful.

Taking Charge of Your Health

- Take the Personal Assessment on page 483 to learn how compatible you and your partner are.

- If being around someone whose sexual orientation is different from yours makes you feel uncomfortable, focus on getting to know that person better as an individual.

- If you are in an unhealthy relationship, take the first step toward getting out of it through professional counseling or group support.

- If you are in a sexual relationship, communicate your sexual needs to your partner clearly. Encourage him or her to do the same so that you can have a satisfying sex life.

- Consider whether your lifetime plan will include singlehood, marriage, cohabitation, single parenthood, or a gay partnership. Evaluate your current plan in relation to that plan.

SUMMARY

- Men and women share the four stages of sexual response: excitement, plateau, orgasm, and resolution.
- Some differences have been shown in the sexual response patterns of men and women.
- Direct stimulation of the penis and direct or indirect stimulation of the clitoris are the principle avenues toward orgasm.
- The three sexual orientations are heterosexuality, homosexuality, and bisexuality.
- Celibacy is the self-imposed avoidance of sexual intimacy.
- Most sex therapists and researchers consider masturbation to be a normal source of self-pleasure.
- Shared touching, genital contact, oral-genital stimulation, and intercourse are common forms of sexual intimacy.
- Physiological changes may alter the way in which some older people perform sexually.
- The dating process has become more flexible and less formal and predictable during recent decades. Many young adults practice serial monogamy.

- Passionate love is gradually replaced by companionate love, which is characterized by deep affection and attachment.
- Intimacy is any close, mutual, verbal or nonverbal behavior within a relationship.
- Forms of marriage include conflict-habituated marriage, devitalized marriage, passive-congenial marriage, total marriage, and vital marriage.
- Although the legality of gay and lesbian marriages continues to be debated, committed relationships between members of the same sex often mimic the dynamics of heterosexual marriages.
- Although most people marry at some time in their lives, other relationships and lifestyles exist, including singlehood, cohabitation, and single parenthood.
- Most relationships can be improved through better communication.

REVIEW QUESTIONS

1. What similarities and differences exist between the sexual response patterns of males and females? Do both women and men experience vasocongestion and myotonia?
2. Explain the differences between heterosexuality, homosexuality, and bisexuality. How common is each of these sexual orientations in our society?
3. What is the general distinction between a transsexual person and a transgendered person?
4. Define celibacy, masturbation, sexual fantasies, erotic dreams, shared touching, genital contact, oral-genital stimulation, and sexual intercourse.
5. What precautions must be considered if a couple decides to engage in anal sexual activity?
6. Approximately what percentage of today's college students report having had sexual intercourse?

7. Identify the physiological changes that occur in men and women as they get older.
8. Identify and describe the five forms of marriage presented in this chapter.
9. What is meant by serial monogamy? What is meant by secondary virginity?
10. What are some differences between passionate love and companionate love?
11. In what ways do gay and lesbian partnerships differ from heterosexual partnerships?
12. Discuss current trends in the areas of singlehood, cohabitation, and single parenthood.
13. Describe the current status of the controversy over same-sex marriages.

ENDNOTES

1. Masters WH, Johnson VE. *Human Sexual Response.* Philadelphia: Lippincott, Williams and Wilkins, 1966.
2. Strong B, DeVault C, Sayad BW, Yarber, WL. *Human Sexuality: Diversity in a Contemporary America* (5th ed.). New York: McGraw-Hill, 2005.
3. Hyde JS, DeLameter JD. *Understanding Human Sexuality* (9th ed.). New York: McGraw-Hill, 2006.
4. Greenburg JS, Bruess CE, Haffner DW. *Exploring the Dimensions of Human Sexuality* (2nd ed.). Boston: Jones and Bartlett, 2004.
5. Kelly GF. *Sexuality Today: The Human Perspective* (8th ed.). New York: McGraw-Hill, 2006.
6. Kinsey AC, Pomeroy WB, Martin CE. *Sexual Behavior in the Human Male,* reprint edition. Bloomington, IN: Indiana University Press, 1998.

7. Allen LS, Gorski RA. Sexual orientation and the size of the anterior commisure in the human brain. *Pract Nat Acad Sci USA* 89(15):7199–7202, 1992.
8. Kinsey AC, et al. *Sexual Behavior in the Human Female,* reprint edition. Bloomington, IN: Indiana University Press, 1998.
9. Masters WH, Johnson VE, Kolodny RC. *Human Sexuality* (5th ed.). Upper Saddle River, NJ: Addison-Wesley, 1997.
10. Crooks RL, Baur K. *Our Sexuality* (9th ed.). Belmont, CA: Wadsworth, 2005.
11. Brown GR, et al. Personality characteristics and sexual functioning of 188 crossdressing men. *J Nervous Mental Dis* 185(5):265–273, 1996.
12. Allgeier ER, Allgeier AR. *Sexual Interactions* (5th ed.). New York: Houghton Mifflin, 2000.

13. LeVay S, Valente SM. *Human Sexuality.* Sunderland, MA: Sinauer Associates, 2002.

14. Baldwin JI, Baldwin JD. Heterosexual anal intercourse: An understudied, high-risk sexual behavior. *Archives of Sexual Behavior* 29(4): 357–373, 2000.

15. *Supreme Court Strikes Down Texas Sodomy Law,* www.cnn.com, July 22, 2003.

16. Richardson JP, Lazur A. Sexuality in the nursing home patient (review). *Am Family Phys* 51(1): 121–124, 1995.

17. McAnulty RD, Burnette MM. *Exploring Human Sexuality: Making Healthy Decisions* (2nd ed.). Boston: Allyn and Bacon, 2004.

18. U.S. Census Bureau. *Current Population Survey, March and Annual Social and Economic Supplements: 1970–2003,* cited in Fields, J. America's families and living arrangements: 2003. *Current Population Reports* (U.S. Census Bureau), P20-553, p.13, Washington, DC, 2003.

19. U.S. Census Bureau. *Statistical Abstract of the United States: 2004–2005,* ed. 124, Washington DC: 2004.

20. *Same-Sex Marriage Ruling Foreshadows Legal War,* www.cnn.com, April 8, 2005.

21. *California Court Upholds Domestic Partner Law,* www.cnn.com, April 8, 2005.

22. *Bush Uncertain about Gay Marriage Ban,* www.cnn.com, July 22, 2003.

23. Cuber J, Harroff P. *Sex and the Significant Americans.* New York: Penguin Books, 1965.

24. Bramlett MD, Mosher WD. *Cohabitation, Marriage, Divorce, and Remarriage in the United States.* U.S. Centers for Disease Control and Prevention, National Center for Health Statistics, Vital Health Statistics, 23(22), 2002.

personal assessment

How compatible are you?

This quiz will help test how compatible you and your partner's personalities are. You should each rate the truth of these twenty statements based on the following scale. Circle the number that reflects your feelings. Total your scores and check the interpretation following the quiz.

1 Never true
2 Sometimes true
3 Frequently true
4 Always true

	1	2	3	4
We can communicate our innermost thoughts effectively.	1	2	3	4
We trust each other.	1	2	3	4
We agree on whose needs come first.	1	2	3	4
We have realistic expectations of each other and of ourselves.	1	2	3	4
Individual growth is important within our relationship.	1	2	3	4
We will go on as a couple even if our partner doesn't change.	1	2	3	4
Our personal problems are discussed with each other first.	1	2	3	4
We both do our best to compromise.	1	2	3	4
We usually fight fairly.	1	2	3	4
We try not to be rigid or unyielding.	1	2	3	4
We keep any needs to be "perfect" in proper perspective.	1	2	3	4
We can balance the desires to be sociable and the need to be alone.	1	2	3	4
We both make friends and keep them.	1	2	3	4
Neither of us stays down or up for long periods.	1	2	3	4
We can tolerate the other's mood without being affected by it.	1	2	3	4
We can deal with disappointment and disillusionment.	1	2	3	4
Both of us can tolerate failure.	1	2	3	4
We can both express anger appropriately.	1	2	3	4
We are both assertive when necessary.	1	2	3	4
We agree on how our personal surroundings are kept.	1	2	3	4

YOUR TOTAL POINTS _____

Interpretation

20–35 points   You and your partner seem quite incompatible. Professional help may open your lines of communication.

36–55 points   You probably need more awareness and compromise.

56–70 points   You are highly compatible. However, be aware of the areas where you can improve.

71–80 points   Your relationship is very fulfilling.

To Carry This Further . . .

Ask your partner to take this test too. You may have a one-sided view of a "perfect" relationship. Even if you scored high on this assessment, be aware of areas where you can still improve.

chapter sixteen

Managing Your Fertility

Chapter Objectives

On completing this chapter, you will be able to:

- explain the difference between the terms *birth control and contraception.*
- define the *theoretical effectiveness* and the *use effectiveness* of contraceptive methods and why they differ.
- discuss the advantages and disadvantages of each form of birth control.
- describe the five methods of periodic abstinence.
- explain how a woman can determine the days in which she is most fertile.
- identify the many ways in which contraceptive hormones can be delivered to females.
- differentiate between the combined oral contraceptive pill and the minipill.
- identify the circumstances under which emergency contraception might be used.
- identify and explain the procedures for male and female sterilization.
- understand which abortion procedures are used in each trimester of pregnancy.

Eye on the Media

Information Online—Birth Control and Sexuality

The Internet offers a number of resources for locating information about contraception, birth control and related topics. Planned Parenthood Federation of America provides one of the most comprehensive sites at www.plannedparenthood.org. If you are looking for birth control information, click on this site's "Frequently Asked Questions," "Fact Sheets," "Sexual Health Glossary," and "Links." You will be able to learn about pregnancy determination, options concerning pregnancy, sexually transmitted diseases, laws in your state concerning teens' access to birth control and abortion services, and how to get access to contraception. Planned Parenthood believes that when people are empowered with knowledge, they are better able to make sound decisions about their health and sexuality.

Four other sites offer information about sexuality and reproductive choices. The Alan Guttmacher Institute site (www.agi-usa.org) is dedicated to protecting the reproductive choices of women and men throughout the world by disseminating the results of scientific research. The Guttmacher Institute's menu of options includes law and public policy, abortion, pregnancy and birth, prevention and contraception, sexual behavior, and STDs and youth.

The American Social Health Association (www.ashastd.org) is dedicated to stopping the spread of sexually transmitted diseases. ASHA's Web site provides comprehensive information about all aspects of STDs. Additionally, ASHA operates a network of national hotlines that answer over 2 million calls each year.

The Sex Information and Education Council of the United States (SIECUS) is a nonprofit organization dedicated to developing, collecting, and disseminating information about sexuality. This organization (www.siecus.org) promotes comprehensive sexuality education and distributes thousands of pamphlets, booklets, and bibliographies each year to professionals and the general public.

If you want to search for information about certain sexuality topics from a prolife perspective, you might wish to examine the Web site for The Ultimate Pro-life Resource List at www.prolifeinfo.org. This site is supported by the nonprofit Women and Children First organization and provides links to information related to abortion alternatives, *Roe v. Wade*, euthanasia and assisted suicide, pregnancy help, prolife news and prolife organizations.

There's More to Sex Than You Thought . . .

Are you ready for sex? If you're not sure, take time to think it over. If you start having sex before you're ready, you might feel guilty. You might feel bad because you realize this step isn't right for you now. Or your religious upbringing may make you feel as though you're doing something wrong. You also may not be ready for the emotional aspects of a sexual relationship. Most important, you will probably have difficulty handling the complexities of an unplanned pregnancy or a sexually transmitted disease.

If you do feel ready for sex, you still have a choice. Sex may be OK for you now. It may be personally fulfilling, something that enhances your self-esteem. Alternatively, you can choose to abstain from sex until later—another way of enhancing your self-esteem. You'll feel empowered by making the decision for yourself, rather than doing what is expected. Being strong enough to say "no" can also make you feel good about yourself. For some, making this decison may reflect a renewed commitment to spiritual or religious concerns.

If you're married, sex is a good way of connecting as a couple. It's something that the two of you alone share. It's a time to give special attention to each other—taking a break from the kids, your jobs, and your other responsibilities. It's a way of saying: "This relationship is important—it's something I value."

Going through a pregnancy together is another opportunity for closeness. From the moment you know that you're going to be parents, you're connected in a new way. Your focus becomes the expected child. You'll watch the fetus grow on ultrasound, go to parenting and Lamaze classes together, visit the doctor together, mark the various milestones, and share new emotions. When your child is born, you'll be connected as never before.

Whether you're thinking about starting to have sex, making the decision to wait, or examining the sexual life you have now, you can't ignore the possibilities and the consequences. Is the time right for you? Are you doing this for yourself or for someone else? What do you think you will gain from waiting? Do you expect your future partner to also have made the decision to wait? What do you expect to get from a sexual relationship—pleasure, intimacy, love? What do you expect to give? Do you want an emotional commitment? Do you view sex and love as inseparable? Do you understand how sex can enhance your spirituality? Taking time to consider these questions can make you feel good about yourself—no matter what you decide.

How you decide to control your fertility will have an important effect on your future. Your understanding of information and issues related to fertility control will help you make responsible decisions in this complex area.

In the beginning of this chapter, we discuss the difference between birth control and contraception and introduce the concept of contraceptive effectiveness rates. We also take a look at why people use birth control. Then we discuss in detail the many birth control methods available today.

Birth Control versus Contraception

Any discussion about the control of your **fertility** should start with an explanation of the subtle differences between the terms **birth control** and **contraception.** These terms reflect different perspectives about fertility control. *Birth control* is an umbrella term that refers to all the procedures you might use to prevent the birth of a child. Birth control includes all available contraceptive measures, as well as sterilization and abortion procedures.

Contraception is a much more specific term for any procedure used to prevent the fertilization of an ovum. Contraceptive measures vary widely in the mechanisms they use to accomplish this task. They also vary considerably in their method of use and their rate of success in preventing conception. A few examples of contraceptives are condoms, hormonal contraceptives, spermicides, and diaphragms.

Beyond the methods mentioned, certain forms of sexual behavior not involving intercourse could be considered forms of contraception. For example, mutual masturbation by couples virtually eliminates the possibility of pregnancy. This practice, as well as additional forms of sexual expression other than intercourse (such as kissing, touching, and massage), has been given the generic term **outercourse.** Outercourse protects against unplanned pregnancy and may also significantly reduce the transmission of sexually transmitted diseases, including HIV infection (see Discovering Your Spirituality above).

Key Terms

fertility the ability to reproduce

birth control all the methods and procedures that can prevent the birth of a child

contraception any method or procedure that prevents fertilization

outercourse sexual activity that does not involve intercourse

I have a new girlfriend and I think we are moving closer and closer to having sex. I know we should talk about birth control and disease prevention, but I don't know how to start. What should I do?

If you believe there is even a chance you will engage in any kind of sex, or if you think your partner may pursue sex with you, you should be prepared and discuss the possibility before being swept along by the heat of an encounter. In addition, you and your partner will feel more comfortable about your relationship and your sexual activity if you first discuss your feelings about contraception, disease prevention, and pregnancy. Consider the following topics:

- First, the fact that you are discussing contraception together does not necessarily mean that you will engage in sex. In addition, you can discuss abstinence as a very effective form of contraception.
- Discussing contraception and disease prevention with your partner is not rude. It is simply common sense.
- Talking about contraception is a way of sharing responsibility and intimacy. It can bring you closer.
- Which type(s) of contraception will you use? See the section below, Selecting Your Contraceptive Method, for help in making your choices.
- If you feel unsure about how to broach the subject or are undecided about any of the issues, consider discussing the subject with

a counselor or physician before you talk with your partner.

- Sort out your own feelings and understand all the alternatives, including their advantages and disadvantages, before you open the discussion.
- Pick the right occasion. Don't wait until you have begun sexual activity.
- Both partners have dignity and worth, and should be treated with dignity. If you and your boyfriend or girlfriend are discussing contraception and you have different views, you each have the right to your opinions. If necessary, you can agree to disagree.
- Listen carefully and ask questions. Speak honestly about your own feelings and beliefs.
- Who will pay for the contraceptive method? Will both partners share the cost?
- What will both of you do if the female partner becomes pregnant?

Have you discussed these issues in the past before initiating sex with a partner? Do you plan to discuss these issues in the future?

InfoLinks

www.arhp.org/success

Reasons for Choosing to Use Birth Control

People use birth control for many reasons. Many career-minded individuals carefully plan the timing and spacing of children to best provide for their children's financial support without sacrificing their job status. Others choose methods of birth control to ensure that they will never have children. Some use birth control methods to permit safe participation in a wide variety of sexual behaviors. Fear of contracting a sexually transmitted disease prompts some people to use particular forms of birth control (see Changing for the Better above).

Financial and legal considerations can be significant factors in the choice of certain birth control methods. Many people must of necessity take the cost of a method into account when selecting appropriate birth control. The cost of sterilization and abortion can prohibit some low-income people from choosing these alternatives, especially because federal funds do not support such procedures. A number of states have established statutes and policies that make contraceptive information and medical services relatively difficult to obtain.

Another important consideration in the use of birth control methods is the availability of professional services. An example of the effect of this factor may be the selection of birth control methods by college students. Some colleges and universities provide contraceptive services through their student health centers. Students enrolled in these schools have easy access to low-cost, comprehensive contraceptive services. Students enrolled in colleges that do not provide such complete services may find that access to accurate information and clinical services is difficult to obtain and that private professional services are expensive.

For many people, religious doctrine will be a factor in their selection of a birth control method. One example is the opposition of the Roman Catholic Church and other religious groups to the use of contraception other than natural family planning.

Theoretical Effectiveness versus Use Effectiveness

People considering the use of a contraceptive method need to understand the difference between the two effectiveness rates given for each form of contraception. *Theoretical*

Table 16.1 Effectiveness Rates of Birth Control for 100 Women during 1 Year of Use

Method	Estimated Effectiveness		Advantages	Disadvantages
	Theoretical	Use		
No method (chance)	15%	15%	Inexpensive	Totally ineffective
Withdrawal	96%	73%	No supplies or advance preparation needed; no side effects; men share responsibility for family planning	Interferes with coitus; very difficult to use effectively; women must trust men to withdraw as orgasm approaches
Periodic abstinence Calendar Standard days method Basal body temperature Cervical mucus method Symptothermal	91%–99%	75%	No supplies needed; no side effects; men share responsibility for family planning; women learn about their bodies	Difficult to use, especially if menstrual cycles are irregular, as is common in young women; abstinence may be necessary for long periods; lengthy instruction and ongoing counseling may be needed
Cervical cap (no previous births)	91%	85%	No health risks; helps protect against some STDs and cervical cancer	Limited availability in some areas
Spermicide (gel, foam, suppository, film)	92%	71%	No health risks; helps protect against some STDs; can be used with condoms to increase effectiveness considerably	Must be inserted 5 to 30 minutes before coitus; effective for only 30 to 60 minutes; some concern about nonoxynol-9
Diaphragm with spermicide	94%	84%	No health risks; helps protect against some STDs and cervical cancer	Must be inserted with jelly or foam before every act of coitus and left in place for at least 6 hours after coitus; must be fitted by health care personnel; some women may find it awkward or embarrassing to use; some concern about nonoxynol-9
Sponge (no previous births) (previous births)	91% 80%	84% 77%	Easy to use; not messy; protection is good for 24 hours and multiple acts of intercourse; no prescription required	Not reusable; contraceptive protection is reduced for women with previous births; some concern about nonoxynol-9
Male condom Male condom with spermicide	98% 99%	85% 95%	Easy to use; inexpensive and easy to obtain; no health risks; very effective protection against some STDs; men share responsibility for family planning	Must be put on just before coitus; some men and women complain of decreased sensation; some concern about nonoxynol-9
Female condom	95%	79%	Relatively easy to use; no prescription required; polyurethane is stronger than latex;	Contraceptive effectiveness and STD protection not as high as with male condom; couples may

continued

effectiveness is a measure of a contraceptive method's ability to prevent a pregnancy when the method is used precisely as directed during every act of intercourse. *Use effectiveness,* however, refers to the effectiveness of a method in preventing conception when used by the general public. Use effectiveness rates take into account factors that lower effectiveness below that based on "perfect" use. Failure to follow proper instructions, illness of the user, forgetfulness, physician (or pharmacist) error, and a subconscious desire to experience risk or even pregnancy are a few of the factors that can lower the effectiveness of even the most theoretically effective contraceptive technique.

Effectiveness rates are often expressed as the percentage of women users of childbearing age who do not become pregnant while using the method for 1 year. For some methods the theoretical-effectiveness and use-effectiveness rates are vastly different; the theoretical rate is always higher than the use rate. Table 16.1 presents data concerning effectiveness rates, advantages, and disadvantages of many birth control methods.

Selecting Your Contraceptive Method

In this section, we discuss some of the many factors that should be important to you as you consider selecting a contraceptive method. (Completing the Personal Assessment on page 509 will help you to make this decision.)

Those who wish to exercise a large measure of control over their fertility can consider the following:

- It should be safe.
- It should be effective.
- It should be reliable.

Method	Estimated Effectiveness		Advantages	Disadvantages
	Theoretical	Use		
			provides some STD protection; silicone-based lubrication provided; useful when male will not use a condom	be unfamiliar with a device that extends outside the vagina; more expensive than male condoms
IUD ParaGard (copper T) Mirena (progestin)	99%+ 99%+	99%+ 99%+	Easy to use; highly effective in preventing pregnancy; does not interfere with coitus; repeated action not needed	May increase risk of pelvic inflammatory disease (PID) and infertility in women with more than one sexual partner; not usually recommended for women who have never had a child; must be inserted by health care personnel; may cause heavy bleeding and pain in some women
Combined pill (estrogen-progestin) Minipill (progestin only)	99%+ 99%+	92%+ 92%+	Easy to use; highly effective in preventing pregnancy; does not interfere with coitus; regulates menstrual cycle; reduces heavy bleeding and menstrual pain; helps protect against ovarian and endometrial cancer	Must be taken every day; requires medical examination and prescription; minor side effects such as nausea or menstrual spotting; possibility of cardiovascular problems in a small percentage of users
Contraceptive ring (estrogen + progestin)	99%+	92%+	Easty to use after learning how to insert; remains in place 3 weeks	Like other hormonal methods, does not protect against STDs; requires physician prescription; possibility of cardiovascular problems in a small percentage of users
Contraceptive patch (estrogen + progestin)	99%+	92%+	Easy to apply; must change weekly for 3 weeks	No STD protection; requires physician prescription; possibility of cardiovascular problems in a small percentage of users
Depo-Provera	99%+	97%+	Easy to use; highly effective for 3-month period; continued use prevents menstruation	Requires supervision by a physician; administered by injection; some women experience irregular menstrual spotting in early months of use
Tubal ligation	99%+	99%+	Permanent; removes fear of pregnancy	Surgery-related risks; generally considered irreversible
Vasectomy	99%+	99%+	Permanent; removes fear of pregnancy	Generally considered irreversible

Adapted from Hatcher RA, et al. *Contraceptive Technology,* 18th ed. New York: Ardent Media, 2004.

- It should be reversible.
- It should be affordable.
- It should be easy to use.
- It should not interfere with sexual expression.

TALKING POINTS The method of birth control your partner prefers doesn't allow for spontaneous sex. How would you explain that this decreases your enjoyment?

Current Birth Control Methods

Abstinence

Abstinence as a form of birth control has gained attention recently on college campuses. This method is as close to 100 percent effective as possible. There have been isolated reports in medical literature of pregnancy without sexual intercourse, usually involving ejaculation by the male near the woman's vagina. Avoiding this situation should raise the effectiveness of abstinence to 100 percent.

Abstinence as a form of birth control has additional advantages in that it gives nearly 100 percent protection from sexually transmitted diseases, it is free, and it does not require a visit to a physician.

However, some concerns exist about the effectiveness of educational programs that encourage abstinence. In a study of 12,000 adolescents published in 2005, Yale and Columbia University researchers found that teenagers who "pledged virginity until marriage" were more likely to participate in oral sex and anal sex than were nonpledging teens who had not had sexual intercourse. (Both oral and anal sex carry risks of STD transmission.) Additionally, the researchers found that teens who pledged abstinence were less likely to use condoms during their first sexual intercourse and less likely to be tested for STDs than were nonpledging teens.[1] Abstinence works effectively only when it is broadly defined (to include many sexual behaviors) and used correctly and consistently. Abstinence is a challenging proposition for many adolescents and young adults.

Withdrawal

Withdrawal, or **coitus interruptus,** is the contraceptive practice in which the erect penis is removed from the vagina just before ejaculation of semen. Theoretically this procedure prevents sperm from entering the deeper structures of the female reproductive system. The use effectiveness of this method, however, reflects how unsuccessful the method is in practice (see Table 16.1).

Strong evidence suggests that the clear preejaculate fluid that helps neutralize and lubricate the male urethra can contain *viable* (capable of fertilization) sperm.[2] This sperm can be deposited near the cervical opening before withdrawal, which explains the relatively low effectiveness of this method. Furthermore, withdrawal does not protect users from the transmission of sexually transmitted diseases (STDs). It should never be considered a reliable contraceptive approach.

Periodic Abstinence

Five approaches are included in the birth control strategy called **periodic abstinence:** (1) the calendar method, (2) the Standard Days method, (3) the basal body temperature (BBT) method, (4) the Billings cervical mucus method, and (5) the symptothermal method.[3] All five methods attempt to determine the time a woman ovulates. Figure 16-1 shows a day-to-day fertility calendar used to calculate fertile periods. Most research indicates that an ovum is viable for only about 24–36 hours after its release from the ovary. (After they are inside the female reproductive tract, some sperm can survive

---

Key Terms

coitus interruptus (withdrawal) (**co** ih tus in ter rup tus) a contraceptive practice in which the erect penis is removed from the vagina before ejaculation

periodic abstinence birth control methods that rely on a couple's avoidance of intercourse during the ovulatory phase of a woman's menstrual cycle; also called *fertility awareness* or *natural family planning*

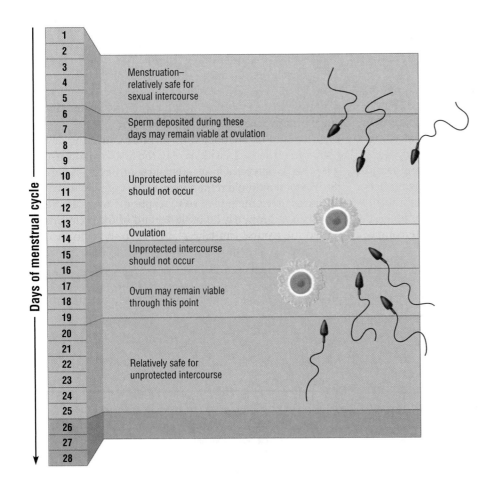

Days of menstrual cycle

Day	
1–5	Menstruation– relatively safe for sexual intercourse
6–9	Sperm deposited during these days may remain viable at ovulation
10–13	Unprotected intercourse should not occur
14	Ovulation
15–16	Unprotected intercourse should not occur
17–19	Ovum may remain viable through this point
20–28	Relatively safe for unprotected intercourse

Figure 16-1 Periodic abstinence (fertility awareness or natural family planning) can combine use of the calendar, basal body temperature measurements, and Billings mucus techniques to identify the fertile period. Remember that most women's cycles are not consistently perfect 28-day cycles like those shown in most illustrations.

up to a week.) When a woman can accurately determine when she ovulates, she must refrain from intercourse long enough for the ovum to begin to disintegrate. Fertility awareness, rhythm, natural birth control, and natural family planning are other terms for periodic abstinence. Remember that periodic abstinence methods *do not* provide protection against the spread of STDs, including HIV infection.

Periodic abstinence is the only contraceptive method endorsed by the Roman Catholic Church. For some people who have deep concerns for the spiritual dimension of their health, selecting a method other than periodic abstinence may entail a serious compromise of beliefs.

The **calendar method** requires close examination of a woman's menstrual cycle for the last 6–12 cycles. Records are kept of the length (in days) of each cycle. A *cycle* is defined as the number of days from the first day of bleeding of one cycle to the first day of bleeding of the next cycle.

To determine the days she should abstain from intercourse, a woman should subtract eighteen from her shortest cycle; this is the first day she should abstain from intercourse. Then she should subtract 11 from her longest cycle; this is the last day she must abstain from intercourse (see Changing for the Better above).[4]

The *basal body temperature method* requires a woman (for about three or four successive months) to take her body temperature every morning before she rises from bed. A finely calibrated thermometer, available in many drugstores, is used for this purpose. The theory behind this method is that there is a distinct correlation between body temperature and the process of ovulation. Around the time of ovulation, the body temperature rises at least 0.4° Fahrenheit and remains elevated until the start of menstruation. The woman is instructed to refrain from intercourse during the interval when the temperature change takes place.

Drawbacks of this procedure include the need for consistent, accurate temperature readings and the realization that all women's bodies are different. Some women may not fit the temperature pattern projection because of biochemical differences in their bodies. In addition, body temperature can fluctuate. Temperature kits cost about $5–$8 in drugstores.

The newest periodic abstinence approach is called the *Standard Days method*. This method is appropriate only for women who have menstrual cycles that are consistently between 26 and 32 days long. It is not to be used by women who have variable cycles that are shorter than 26 days or longer than 32 days. Having had just one cycle in the past year shorter than 26 days or longer than 32 days should encourage a woman NOT to use the Standard Days method. She should meet with her health care provider and discuss an alternative method.

To use this method, women must count the days of their menstrual cycle, with day 1 as the first day of menstrual bleeding. Women can have intercourse on days 1–7. On days 8–19, women should refrain from penis/vaginal intercourse or use a barrier method of contraception. Days 8–19 are the fertile days. From day 20 until the end of the cycle, unprotected intercourse can take place.[4] Keep in mind that the Standard Days method does not protect against the transmission of STDs.

The *Billings cervical mucus method* (also called the *ovulation method*) is another periodic abstinence technique.

Key Terms

calendar method a form of periodic abstinence in which the variable lengths of a woman's menstrual cycle are used to calculate her fertile period

Generally used with other periodic abstinence techniques, this method requires a woman to evaluate the daily mucous discharge from her cervix. Users of this method become familiar with the changes in both appearance (from clear to cloudy) and consistency (from watery to thick) of their cervical mucus throughout their cycles. Women are taught that the unsafe days are when the mucus becomes clear and is the consistency of raw egg whites. Such a technique of ovulation determination must be learned from a physician or family planning professional.

The *symptothermal method* of periodic abstinence combines the use of the BBT method and the cervical mucus method.[4] Thus, some family planning professionals consider the symptothermal method a combination of all of the periodic abstinence approaches.

Those who wish to practice one of these periodic abstinence methods should consult a professional to learn how to chart their menstrual cycle and detect the physical signs that help predict the "unsafe" days. Besides the lack of protection against STDs, the periodic abstinence methods have the following potential problems:

- Partner may be uncooperative.
- Couple may take risks during "unsafe" days.
- Record-keeping may be poor.
- Illness and lack of sleep can affect body temperature.
- Vaginal infections and douches change mucus.
- Method cannot be used if the woman has irregular periods or temperature patterns.

Vaginal Spermicides

Spermicides are agents that are capable of killing sperm. When used alone, they offer a moderately effective form of contraception for the woman who is sexually active on an infrequent basis. Modern spermicides are generally safe (but see precaution below), reversible forms of contraception that can be obtained without a physician's prescription in most drugstores and supermarkets. Spermicides are

> **Key Terms**
>
> **spermicides** chemicals capable of killing sperm

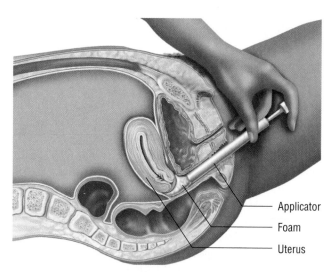

Applicator
Foam
Uterus

Figure 16-2 Spermicidal foams and suppositories are placed deep into the vagina in the region of the cervix no longer than 30 minutes before intercourse.

relatively inexpensive. Applicator kits cost about $8, and refills cost around $4–$8 (see Figure 16-2).

Spermicides, which are available in foam, cream, jelly, film, or suppository form, are made of water-soluble bases with a spermicidal agent in the base. Spermicides are commonly used with other contraceptives, such as diaphragms, cervical caps, and condoms.

Spermicides are not specific to sperm cells; they also attack other cells. Until recently, nonoxynol-9, the most commonly used spermicidal agent, was thought to protect women from developing **pelvic inflammatory disease (PID).** Health professionals believed that nonoxynol-9 provided this protection by attacking and killing pathogens which caused various STDs.

However, the latest research indicates that nonoxynol-9 is not very effective in killing other pathogens. Nonoxynol-9 may actually *increase* the likelihood of disease transmission, including HIV transmission, because it can cause skin irritations and abrasions in a small percentage of users.[5] These irritated areas and abrasions can provide the avenue for passage into the bloodstream.

For this reason, couples should not depend on vaginal spermicides to stop the spread of infections from person to person. Condoms, when used consistently and correctly, provide much better disease protection and contraceptive effect than spermicides used alone. The latest research also indicates that condoms coated with nonoxynol-9 do not have enough of the spermicide to serve as a back-up contraceptive if the condom breaks.[6] Thus, some health centers and family planning agencies have stopped distributing condoms with nonoxynol-9 in the lubricant. If you and/or your partner have concerns

Choosing not to have children gives couples more time and money to pursue other interests.

about your use of spermicides, you should seek advice from your physician or health center.

Condoms

Colored or natural, smooth or textured, straight or shaped, plain or reservoir-tipped, dry or lubricated—the latex condom is approaching an art form. Nevertheless, the familiar **condom** remains a safe, effective, reversible contraceptive device. All condoms manufactured in the United States must be approved by the FDA.[7]

| Key Terms |

pelvic inflammatory disease (PID) a generalized infection of the pelvic cavity that results from the spread of an infection through a woman's reproductive structures

condom a latex shield designed to cover the erect penis and retain semen upon ejaculation; "rubber"

Vaginal Contraceptive Film

A unique spermicide delivery system developed in England is vaginal contraceptive film (VCF). Vaginal contraceptive film is a sheet containing nonoxynol-9 that is inserted over the cervical opening. Shortly after insertion of the VCF, it dissolves into a gellike material that clings to the cervical opening. The VCF can be inserted up to an hour before intercourse. Over the course of several hours, the material will be washed from the vagina in the normal vaginal secretions.

This spermicide is a nonprescription form of contraception that is as effective as other spermicidal foams and jellies. Users should be aware that the nonoxynol-9 spermicide may not be as effective against STDs as was formerly thought. A box of 12 sheets costs about $12.

Vaginal contraceptive film

For couples who are highly motivated in their desire to prevent a pregnancy, the effectiveness of a condom can approach that of an oral contraceptive. A condom can be nearly 100 percent effective when used with contraceptive foam. For couples who are less motivated, the condom can be considerably less effective. Condoms cost from 25¢ to $2.50 each.

The condom offers a measure of protection against sexually transmitted diseases. For both the man and the woman, chlamydial infections, gonorrhea, HIV infection, and other STDs are less likely to be acquired when the condom is used correctly (see Changing for the Better on page 495). Some lubricated condoms also contain a spermicide. However, recent research indicates that the use of the spermicide nonoxynol-9 may irritate tissues in some users and actually increase the likelihood of disease transmission. Also, the small amount of spermicide present in the condom's lubricant is not enough to consistently prevent conception if the condom should break. Current recommendations are to use dry condoms or lubricated condoms without spermicide. Also, any additional lubricants used should be water-based lubricants.

The FDA has approved two types of nonlatex condoms. The polyurethane male condom and the polyurethane female condom are available as one-time-use condoms (see the Star box on page 497).[3] These condoms are good alternatives for people who have an allergic sensitivity to latex, estimated to be up to 7 percent of the population.[8] Also, they are thinner and stronger than latex condoms and can be used with oil-based lubricants. Currently, these condoms are believed to provide protection against STDs that is close to that of latex condoms. The contraceptive effectiveness of the polyurethane condoms remains somewhat less than that of the male latex condom.[9,10]

Diaphragm

The **diaphragm** is a soft rubber cup with a springlike metal rim that rests in the top of the vagina. The diaphragm covers the cervical opening (Figure 16-3). During intercourse

Male condoms

> **Key Terms**
>
> **diaphragm** a soft rubber cup designed to cover the cervix

Figure 16-3   A: Spermicidal cream or jelly is placed into the diaphragm. **B:** The diaphragm is folded lengthwise and inserted into the vagina. **C:** The diaphragm is then placed against the cervix so that the cup portion with the spermicide is facing the cervix. The outline of the cervix should be felt through the central part of the diaphragm.

the diaphragm stays in place quite well and cannot usually be felt by either partner.

The diaphragm is always used with a spermicidal cream or jelly placed inside the cup and around the rim. When used properly with a spermicide, the diaphragm is a relatively effective contraceptive, and when combined with the man's use of a condom, its effectiveness is even greater. The diaphragm must be inserted before intercourse. It should provide effective protection for 6 hours. If this time interval extends beyond 6 hours, some clinicians recommend that additional spermicide be placed in the vagina. Use of additional spermicide with multiple acts of intercourse is optional. After intercourse, the diaphragm must be left in place for at least 6 hours before it is removed. Because of the risk of toxic shock syndrome (TSS), the diaphragm must not remain in the vagina longer than 24 hours.[4] It is always best to ask a health care provider for specific instructions.

Diaphragms must always be fitted and prescribed by a physician.[11] The cost of obtaining a diaphragm and keeping a supply of spermicide may be higher than that of other methods. Typically, it costs $15–$75 for a diaphragm and $4–$8 for the spermicidal cream or jelly. An examination may cost between $50 and $200, but it will be less at family planning clinics. Also, a high level of motivation to follow the instructions *exactly* is important.

Diaphragms and other vaginal barrier methods (such as the cervical cap) do not provide reliable

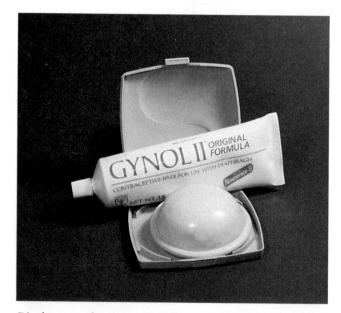

Diaphragm and contraceptive jelly

protection against STDs and HIV infection. Recent concerns about the spermicide nonoxynol-9 should prompt users to ask their physicians to recommend which spermicidal cream or jelly to use with diaphragms. If you are concerned about possible HIV infection, either avoid sexual activity or use a latex condom.

I have used condoms a few times, but I was always in a hurry and never read the small print instructions. My current partner asked me if "I knew what I was doing" the last time we had intercourse. What do I need to know to use condoms more effectively?

These simple directions for using condoms correctly, in combination with your motivation and commitment to regular use, should provide you with reasonable protection:

- Keep a supply of condoms at hand. Condoms should be stored in a cool, dry place so that they are readily available at the time of intercourse. Condoms that are stored in wallets or automobile glove compartments may not be in satisfactory condition when they are used. Temperature extremes are to be avoided. Check the condom package for the expiration date.
- Do not test a condom by inflating or stretching it. Handle it gently and keep it away from sharp fingernails.
- For maximum effectiveness, put the condom on before genital contact. Either the man or the woman can put the condom in place. Early application is particularly important in the prevention of STDs. Early application also lessens the possibility of the release of preejaculate fluid into the vagina.
- Unroll the condom on the erect penis. For those using a condom without a reservoir tip, a 1/2-inch space should be left to catch the ejaculate. To leave this space, pinch the tip of the condom as you roll it on the erect penis. Do not leave any air in the tip of the condom.
- Lubricate the condom if this has not already been done by the manufacturer. When doing this, be certain to use a water-soluble lubricant and not a petroleum-based product such as petroleum jelly. Petroleum can deteriorate the latex material. Other oil-based lubricants, such as mineral oil, baby oil, vegetable oil, shortening, and certain hand lotions, can quickly damage a latex condom. Use water-based lubricants only!
- After ejaculation, be certain that the condom does not become dislodged from the penis. Hold the rim of the condom firmly

against the base of the penis during withdrawal. Do not allow the penis to become flaccid (soft) while still in the vagina.
- Inspect the condom for tears before throwing it away. If the condom is damaged in some way, immediately insert a spermicidal agent into the vagina or consider using emergency contraception (see page 502).

Cervical Cap

The **cervical cap** is a small, thimble-shaped device that fits over the entire cervix. The cap is held in place by suction rather than by pushing against anatomical structures (Figure 16-4). As with the diaphragm, the cervical cap is coated with spermicide and prevents the sperm from reaching the egg. The cap carries no major health risks and is nearly equal to the diaphragm in effectiveness, although it can be slightly less effective for women who have already had a child.

The cervical cap is filled ⅓ full of spermicide before being placed snugly around the base of the cervix. The cap provides effective protection for 48 hours, no matter how

> **Key Terms**
>
> **cervical cap** a small, thimble-shaped contraceptive device designed to fit over the cervix

Figure 16-4 After the spermicidal cream or jelly is placed in the cervical cap, the cap is inserted into the vagina and placed against the cervix.

Lea's Shield

many times intercourse occurs. Use of additional spermicide with repeated acts of intercourse is optional. Leave the cap in place for at least 6 hours after intercourse.[4] It is always best to ask a health care provider for specific instructions.

The cervical cap comes in just four sizes and thus may be difficult to fit for some women.[4] A physician must prescribe the cervical cap and show the woman how to use it. With new concerns about the use of the spermicide nonoxynol-9, women are advised to ask their physicians which contraceptive or cream or jelly they should use with their cervical cap. The cost of a cervical cap is similar to that of a diaphragm.

Lea's Shield and FemCap

The two newest barrier methods for women were approved by the FDA in 2002. Both methods are used

How to insert the FemCap

with a spermicide. *Lea's Shield* is a reusable oval device made of silicone rubber that fits closely over the cervix. An attached loop helps in the removal from the vagina. The Lea's Shield works much like a diaphragm, but it has a central air valve that permits air to move out from beneath the shield and permit a closer fit. This device comes in only one size and must be prescribed by a physician. The first year, use effectiveness of this device (85 percent) is about the same as that for diaphragms (84 percent).[12]

The *FemCap* is a reusable hat-shaped silicone rubber cap that completely covers the cervix. Coated with spermicide, the FemCap's brim fits snugly against the deep vaginal walls. An attached strap helps in the removal of this device. The FemCap must be prescribed by a physician and comes in three sizes. Among women who have never been pregnant or given birth vaginally, the first year use effectiveness of this device is 86 percent. Costs for these new devices are similar to those for diaphragms and caps.[12]

Contraceptive Sponge

The **contraceptive sponge** is a small, pillow-shaped polyurethane device containing nonoxynol-9 spermicide. The sponge is dampened with tap water and inserted deep into the vagina to cover the cervical opening. This device provides contraceptive protection for up to 24 hours, regardless of the number of times intercourse

> **Key Terms**
>
> **contraceptive sponge** a small, pillow-shaped contraceptive device that contains a spermicide; placed deep in the vagina to cover the cervical opening

Cervical cap

Mirena IUD

occurs. After the last act of intercourse, the device must be left in place for at least 6 hours. Once removed, the sponge must be discarded. The sponge must not be left in place for longer than 24 or 30 hours because of the risk of toxic shock syndrome. Used alone, the sponge does not provide reliable protection against STDs and HIV infection. Consult your physician if you are concerned about the use of nonoxynol-9 spermicide. In women who have not given birth to children, the contraceptive effectiveness of the sponge is similar to that of the diaphragm.

The sponge has an interesting history. Before its removal from the market in 1995, the sponge was the most popular female over-the-counter contraceptive in the United States. The sponge came off the market because the manufacturer decided it was too expensive to retool the manufacturing plant to meet governmental safety regulations. The removal of the sponge prompted the TV sitcom show *Seinfeld* to develop an episode in which the character Elaine Benes purchased as many sponges as she could before they disappeared from the New York City marketplace. She then used her sponges sparingly and only with men she judged to be "spongeworthy."[13]

The company that originally manufactured the sponge sold the rights to Allendale Pharmaceuticals. In 2001, Allendale applied for FDA approval to start manufacturing and selling the sponge in the United States. In early 2005, the FDA granted its approval. It was anticipated that by the fall of 2005, the sponge would again be on drugstore shelves in the United States. Interestingly, the sponge had been available in Canada for a couple of years. Sponges are expected to cost between $2.50 and $3.00 and come in packs of three.[13]

Intrauterine Device (IUD)

The **intrauterine device (IUD)** is the most popular reversible contraceptive method in the world, although the number of users in the United States is relatively small. The IUD is a safe, highly effective method of birth control. IUDs work by preventing sperm from fertilizing ova or by preventing a fertilized ovum from implanting in the uterus.

Two types of IUDs are available in the United States: a T-shaped one containing the hormone progestin (Mirena) and a T-shaped one wrapped with copper wire (ParaGard). The Mirena IUD works by thickening cervical mucus, inhibiting sperm survival, and producing a thin endometrial lining that will not support a fertilized ovum. The ParaGard works by releasing copper ions that impair sperm function and prevent fertilization.[4] The Mirena IUD substantially reduces menstrual flow, but the ParaGard may increase menstrual flow. About 20 percent of women who use the Mirena IUD stop having their periods altogether.[14]

Key Terms

intrauterine device (IUD) a small, plastic, medicated or unmedicated contraceptive device that prevents pregnancy when inserted in the uterus

The Female Condom

The Reality female condom is a soft, loose-fitting polyurethane sheath containing two polyurethane rings. Reality is inserted like a tampon and lines the inner contours of the vagina. The larger ring remains outside the vagina, and the external portion of the condom provides some protection to the labia and the base of the penis. Reality is coated on the inside with a silicone-based lubricant. Additional lubricant is provided for the outside of the sheath. This lubricant does not contain a spermicide. Female and male condoms should not be used at the same time since they might adhere to each other and cause slippage or displacement. The contraceptive effectiveness of the female condom is not as high as that of the male condom. However, as people become more familiar with using the female condom, its effectiveness may increase. Each female condom costs about $2.50.

Female condom

The Mirena provides highly effective contraceptive protection for 5 years and the ParaGard for 10 years.

Only a skilled physician can prescribe and insert an IUD. As with many other forms of contraception, IUDs do not offer protection against STDs, including the AIDS virus.[11]

The IUD is inserted into the uterus by a trained clinician. Along with a physical examination, the physician will ask several questions about the woman's lifestyle, and she should be honest about her sex life, because the IUD is not for all women. Women who have multiple partners or woman who do not practice safe sex might be advised not to use the IUD. The IUD can be an acceptable form of contraception, especially for women who are in their middle to late reproductive years, unable to take birth control pills, have a stable, monogamous relationship, and are not at risk for STDs.

For many years, the public has been concerned about two potentially serious side effects: *uterine perforation* (in which the IUD embeds itself into the uterine wall) and pelvic inflammatory disease (PID, a widespread infection of the abdominal cavity). Recent research, however, indicates that these events rarely happen, especially when the IUD is inserted by a skilled clinician. Between 2 and 10 percent of IUD users experience *expulsion* (muscular contractions which force the IUD out of the uterus) within the first year of use.[4]

As Table 16.1 indicates, IUDs are very effective birth control devices, surpassed in effectiveness only by abstinence, sterilization, and hormonal (pill, injection, ring, patch) contraceptives. The cost for an IUD ranges from

$175–$400, which includes an exam, insertion, and a follow-up visit.[12]

Oral Contraceptives

Developed in the 1950s, the **oral contraceptive pill** provides the highest effectiveness rate of any single reversible contraceptive method used today. Worldwide, more than 100 million women are currently using oral contraceptives.[4]

Use of the pill requires a physician's examination and prescription. Because oral contraceptives are available in a wide range of formulas, follow-up examinations are important to ensure that a woman is receiving an effective dosage with as few side effects as possible. Matching the right prescription with the woman may require a few consultations.

All oral contraceptives contain synthetic (laboratory-made) hormones. The typical *combined pill* uses both synthetic estrogen and synthetic progesterone in each of 21 pills. With *triphasic pills,* the level of estrogen remains constant, but the level of progestin varies every 7 days. In

---

Key Terms

oral contraceptive pill a pill taken orally, composed of synthetic female hormones that prevent ovulation or implantation; "the pill"

Oral contraceptives

2003 the FDA approved a new oral contraceptive (Seasonale) that contains active hormones for 84 days (12 weeks) followed by 1 week of pills containing inactive ingredients.[3] Women using this contraceptive pill would expect to have only four menstrual periods each year. This pill could become a highly popular choice for women. As with many forms of contraception, *oral contraceptives do not protect against the transmission of STDs, including HIV infection.* Also, the use of antibiotics may lower the pill's contraceptive effectiveness.

Oral contraceptives function in several ways. The estrogen in the pill tends to reduce ova development. The progesterone in the pill helps reduce the likelihood of ovulation (by lowering the release of luteinizing hormone). The progesterone in the pill also causes the uterine wall to develop inadequately and helps thicken cervical mucus, thus making it difficult for sperm to enter the uterus.

The physical changes produced by the oral contraceptive provide some beneficial side effects in women. Because the synthetic hormones are taken for 21 days and then are followed by **placebo pills** or no pills for 7 days, the menstrual cycle becomes regulated. Even women who have irregular cycles immediately become "regular." Because the uterine lining is not developed to the extent seen in a non-pill-taking woman, the uterus is not forced to contract with the same amount of vigor. Thus menstrual cramping is reduced, and the resultant menstrual flow is diminished. Research indicates that oral contraceptive use can provide protection against anemia, PID, noncancerous breast tumors, acne, recurrent ovarian cysts, ectopic pregnancy, endometrial cancer, endometriosis, and ovarian cancer.[4]

The negative side effects of the oral contraceptive pill can be divided into two general categories: (1) unpleasant and (2) potentially dangerous. The unpleasant side effects

generally subside within two or three months for most women. A number of women report some or many of the following symptoms:

- Tenderness in breast tissue
- Nausea
- Mild headaches
- Slight, irregular spotting
- Weight gain
- Fluctuations in sex drive
- Mild depression
- More frequent vaginal infections

TALKING POINTS You've tried two different types of oral contraceptives and had unpleasant side effects with both. Your doctor says you should consider another birth control method, but you disagree. How could you talk with her about this in a matter-of-fact way?

The potentially dangerous side effects of the oral contraceptive pill are most often seen in the cardiovascular system. Blood clots, strokes, hypertension, and heart attack seem to be associated with the estrogen component of the combined pill. However, when compared with nonusers, the risk of dying from cardiovascular complications is only slightly increased among healthy young oral contraceptive users. Users of oral contraceptives are statistically more likely than are nonusers to develop cervical cancer. However, cervical cancer is also related to human papillomavirus (HPV) and unprotected intercourse with multiple partners. Additionally, over 50 scientific studies have determined that oral contraceptive use has little, if any, effect on the development of breast cancer, even among women with a family history of breast cancer.[4]

Most health professionals agree that the risks related to pregnancy and childbirth are much greater than those associated with oral contraceptive use. Certainly, a woman who is contemplating the use of the pill must discuss all of the risks and benefits with her physician. (For a discussion of the male oral contraceptive, see Learning from Our Diversity on page 500.)

There are some **contraindications** for the use of oral contraceptives. If you have a history of blood clots,

---

Key Terms

placebo pills (pla **see** bo) pills that contain no active ingredients

contraindications factors that make the use of a drug inappropriate or dangerous for a particular person

Learning from Our Diversity

The Male Contraceptive Pill

Having males be responsible for the medical control of fertility would be a big shift in the sexuality responsibility roles for men and women. Forty-five years after the breakthrough of the female contraceptive pill, researchers are gaining confidence that a version of a male contraceptive pill will be commercially available in the not-too-distant future, perhaps between 5 and 10 years.[1]

For decades, difficulties have surrounded the development of a male contraceptive pill. Although many people believe that the primary reason for the slow development was the fact that the researchers were male, the most plausible explanations deal with male physiology. The typical male ejaculate contains 300–500 million sperm cells. A contraceptive method that is over 99% effective would still leave thousands and thousands of sperm cells available. In contrast, female contraceptives must block the viability of only one egg each cycle, arguably an easier task.

The drug being tested that blocks sperm development is actually a female hormone. While it is effective at blocking sperm production, it also reduces the amount of testosterone that the male produces. Without adequate levels of testosterone, the male sex drive diminishes considerably. For this reason, researchers are testing the effects of replacement androgen, often in the form of an injection or an implant. It is also possible that a slow release patch, similar to the nicotine replacement patch, could be used in the future.

Critics claim that a safe, effective, and inexpensive form of male contraception already exists in the form of a vasectomy. They argue, why not use an approach that already has shown its effectiveness for years? Besides, are women going to trust a man who claims he is using an oral contraceptive pill? Would the pill also have to make a man's eyeballs turn blue as proof that he was using an effective method? When would a woman know that a man is being truthful? Unfortunately, the track record for honesty among couples in sexual relationships isn't particularly good.

Within the next decade, the obstacles that prevent a safe and effective male contraceptive pill from being manufactured may be overcome. But questions will still remain, especially for women, since after all is said and done, they will always be the ones who must bear the brunt (as well as the joy) of pregnancy, labor, and childbirth.

[1]Health news: Will men use a contraceptive pill? Will women trust them? InteliHealth Online, August 29, 2000, www.intelihealth.com/enews?296075.

---

migraine headaches, liver disease, a heart condition, high blood pressure, obesity, diabetes, hepatitis, cirrhosis, breast cancer, or if you are too young to have started consistent menstrual cycles, the pill probably should not be your contraceptive choice. Providing a physician with a complete and accurate health history is important before a woman starts to take the pill.

Two additional contraindications continue to draw considerable attention by the medical community. Cigarette smoking and advancing age are highly associated with an increased risk of potentially serious side effects. Increasing numbers of physicians are not prescribing oral contraceptives for their patients who smoke. The risk of cardiovascular-related deaths is greatly enhanced in women over age 35. The risk is even higher in female smokers over 35. The data are quite convincing.[4]

For the vast majority of women, however, the pill, when properly prescribed, is safe and effective. Careful scrutiny of one's health history and careful follow-up examinations when a problem is suspected are essential elements that can provide a good margin of safety. Monthly pill packs cost $20–$35 at drugstores and less at clinics. An exam may cost $35–$125.[12]

Minipills

Some women prefer not to use the combined oral contraceptive pill. Thus to avoid some of the potentially serious side effects of the combined pill, some physicians are prescribing **minipills.** These oral contraceptives contain no estrogen—only low-dose progesterone in all pills in the 28-day pill pack. The minipill seems to work by thickening cervical mucus, preventing ovulation, and producing a thin endometrial lining.[4] The effectiveness of a minipill is slightly lower than that of the combined pill. *Breakthrough bleeding* and **ectopic pregnancy** are more

---

> ### Key Terms
>
> **minipills** low-dose progesterone (progestin) oral contraceptives
>
> **ectopic pregnancy** a pregnancy in which the fertilized ovum implants at a site other than the uterus, typically in the fallopian tubes

The NuvaRing contraceptive ring is a flexible ring about 2⅛ inches in diameter. When inserted into the vagina, it delivers a low dose of hormones similar to those found in oral contraceptives.

common in minipill users than in combined-pill users. The cost of minipills is similar to that of combined pills.

Injectable Contraceptives

Depo-Provera is a highly effective (99 percent+) injectable progestin contraceptive that provides protection for 3 months. This hormone shot works primarily by preventing ovulation and thickening the cervical mucus to keep the sperm from joining the egg.

The most common side effects of Depo-Provera are irregular bleeding and spotting followed by *amenorrhea* (the absence of periods).[4] In particular, new users of Depo-Provera report occasional breakthrough bleeding as the most common unpleasant side effect.[4] When the woman's body adjusts to the presence of this drug, breakthrough bleeding diminishes, and the most common side effect is amenorrhea. This is understandable, because the drug inhibits ovulation. Many women consider amenorrhea to be a desirable effect of Depo-Provera use. Women who stop using Depo-Provera may experience infertility for a period of up to one year.[4] The cost of Depo-Provera ranges from $30 to $75 per injection.[12]

Contraceptive Ring

One of the newest contraceptives on the market is the vaginal **contraceptive ring** (NuvaRing). Available by prescription, NuvaRing is a thin polymer ring (2⅛ inches in diameter and ⅛ inch thick) that contains synthetic estrogen and progestin. Users insert this device deep into the vagina

where it remains for 3 weeks. At the end of the third week, the device is removed for a week and the woman has her period. The NuvaRing provides effective contraception (99 percent + effective when used perfectly) for the entire 4-week time frame.

The ring functions in a manner similar to the oral contraceptive pill: it reduces the chances of ovulation and thickens cervical mucus. Women who use the ring cannot at the same time use cervical caps or diaphragms as a backup method. The contraceptive ring does not protect against sexually transmitted diseases, including the virus that causes HIV/AIDS. The costs of the contraceptive ring are about $30–$35 per month for the device and $35–$125 for the exam.[12]

Contraceptive Patch

In 2002 the Ortho Evra **contraceptive patch** became available to women. This patch contains continuous levels

---

Key Terms

contraceptive ring thin, polymer contraceptive device containing estrogen and progestin; placed deep within the vagina for a 3-week period

contraceptive patch contraceptive skin patch containing estrogen and progestin; replaced each week for a 3-week period of estrogen and progestin delivered from a 1¾-inch square patch that is applied weekly to one of four areas on the woman's body: the buttocks, abdomen, upper chest (front and back, excluding the breasts), or upper outer arm.[21] The patch remains attached even while a woman bathes, swims, or exercises. After 3 weeks of patches, the woman uses no patch for the fourth week, during which time the woman has her period. The patch functions in a manner similar to the oral contraceptive pill. Like all hormonal measures of contraception, the patch does not protect against sexually transmitted diseases, including the virus that causes HIV/AIDS. The patch costs about $30–$35 per month. The exam may cost $35–$125.[12]

Emergency Contraception

Emergency contraception is designed to prevent pregnancy after unprotected vaginal intercourse such as when a condom breaks, when a couple uses no method of contraception, or when someone forces another to have intercourse. This method is also called postcoital or "morning after" contraception. (Emergency contraception is not the "abortion pill" or RU-486.) Emergency contraception is available in two forms: emergency hormonal contraception and the insertion of an IUD. Both forms of contraception can be prescribed (or carried out) by a physician.

As of May 2005, six states (Alaska, California, Hawaii, Maine, New Mexico, and Washington) had enacted laws that permit a pharmacist to provide emergency contraception to customers in the absence of a prescription by a physician. However, the pharmacist is required to act within a collaborative agreement with a physician or under state-approved protocols.[15]

Emergency hormonal contraception involves the use of one or two doses of certain oral contraceptives. Currently, only one FDA-approved oral contraceptive (Plan B) is available for emergency contraception, although physicians may prescribe other oral contraceptives for this purpose. (Previn, an FDA-approved combined estrogen-progestin pill was withdrawn from the market in 2004.) Plan B is a progestin-only pill whose first dose should be taken as soon as possible (but not later than 120 hours or 5 days) after unprotected intercourse. A second pill follows 12 hours after the first pill. This approach to emergency contraception reduces the risk of pregnancy after unprotected intercourse by 89 percent.[4]

The most commonly reported side effects of emergency hormonal contraception are nausea and vomiting. About 25 percent of users of progestin-only pills experience nausea, and 10 percent experience vomiting. Users of combined estrogen-progestin pills tend to experience more episodes of nausea and vomiting. The use of antinausea medication can help offset the nausea and vomiting. Some women also report fatigue, breast tenderness, abdominal pain, headaches, and dizziness. These side effects subside within a day or two after treatment.[4] Costs for Plan B are estimated to be $8–$35.[12]

A copper-releasing IUD is a less commonly used, but highly effective, form of emergency contraception. To function as an emergency contraceptive, however, the ParaGard IUD must be inserted within 5 days of unprotected intercourse.

Sterilization

All the contraceptive mechanisms or methods already discussed have one quality in common: they are reversible. Although microsurgical techniques are providing medical breakthroughs, **sterilization** should still be considered an irreversible procedure.[16] When you decide to use sterilization, you no longer control your own fertility because you will no longer be able to produce offspring.

Therefore, couples considering sterilization procedures usually must undergo extensive discussions with a physician or family planning counselor to identify their true feelings about this finality. People must be aware of the possible changes in self-concept they might have after sterilization. If you are a man who equates fertility with masculinity, you may have trouble accepting your new status as a sterile man. If you are a woman who equates motherhood with femininity, you might have adjustment problems after sterilization. Some people later regret not being able to have children. Sterilization does not protect one against STDs, including HIV infection.

The male sterilization procedure is called a *vasectomy*. Accomplished with a local anesthetic in a physician's office, this 20- to 30-minute procedure consists of the surgical removal of a section of each vas deferens. After a small incision is made through the scrotum, the vas deferens is located and a small section removed. The remaining ends are either tied or *cauterized* (Figure 16-5A).

Immediately after a vasectomy, sperm may still be present in the vas deferens. A backup contraceptive is recommended until a physician microscopically examines

---

Key Terms

emergency contraception contraceptive measures used to prevent pregnancy within 5 days after unprotected intercourse; also called post-coital or "morning after" contraception

sterilization generally permanent birth control techniques that surgically disrupt the normal passage of ova or sperm

Figure 16-5 The most frequently used forms of male and female sterilization. **A:** Vasectomy. **B:** Tubal ligation

a semen specimen. This examination usually occurs about six weeks after the surgery. After a vasectomy, men can still produce male sex hormones, get erections, have orgasms, and ejaculate. (Recall that sperm account for only a small portion of the semen.) Some men even report increased interest in sexual activity because their chances of impregnating a woman have been virtually eliminated.

What happens to the process of spermatogenesis within each testicle? Sperm cells are still being produced, but they are destroyed by specialized white blood cells called phagocytic leukocytes.

The future may hold a reversible form of vasectomy, as researchers experiment with injecting a plug-forming material into the vas deferens, with the intention that the plug could be removed at a later date if desired. The cost of a vasectomy ranges from $350–$1,000.[12]

The most common method of female sterilization is called *tubal ligation*. During this procedure, the fallopian tubes are cut and the ends tied back. Some physicians cauterize the tube ends to ensure complete sealing (Figure 16-5B). The fallopian tubes are usually reached through the abdominal wall. In a *minilaparotomy*, a small incision is made through the abdominal wall just below the navel. The resultant scar is small and is the basis for the term *band-aid surgery.*

Female sterilization requires about twenty to thirty minutes, with the patient under a local or general anesthetic. The use of a laparoscope has made female sterilization much simpler than in the past. The laparoscope is a small tube equipped with mirrors and lights. Inserted through a single incision, the laparoscope locates the fallopian tubes before they are cut, tied, or cauterized.

When a laparoscope is used through an abdominal incision, the procedure is called a *laparoscopy.*

In 2002, a new method of female sterilization was approved by the FDA. This is a nonincision approach (the Essure coil), whereby a physician inserts a small, soft metallic coil into the vagina, through the cervix and directly into each fallopian tube. This procedure is done under local anesthetic and takes about one half-hour. Once inserted, the coils encourage scar tissue growth that eventually blocks the fallopian tubes. If the tubes are obstructed, sperm are blocked from meeting the ovum. After 3 months, a woman returns to her physician for an X-ray test that determines whether the tubes are fully obstructed. During these first 3 months, couples must use another form of birth control. Cramping is the most common side effect. In rare cases, Essure coils can be expelled or perforate the fallopian tube.[3] Reports indicate that Essure has a 99.8 percent effectiveness rate.[12]

Women who are sterilized still produce female hormones, ovulate, and menstruate. However, the ovum cannot move down the fallopian tube. Within a day of its release, the ovum will start to disintegrate and be absorbed by the body. Freed of the possibility of becoming pregnant, many sterilized women report an increase in sex drive and activity.

Female sterilization is very effective, with failure rates of only 1 to 2 per 1,000 procedures. The complications tend to be few and minor, and there appear to be no serious long-term side effects. Tubal ligation costs $1,500–$6,000.[12]

Two other procedures produce sterilization in women. *Ovariectomy* (the surgical removal of the ovaries) and *hysterectomy* (the surgical removal of the uterus) accomplish sterilization. However, these procedures are used to remove diseased (cancerous, cystic, or hemorrhaging) organs and are not primarily considered sterilization techniques.

TALKING POINTS You and your husband have children. And you'd like to stop taking the pill for health reasons. Your husband says you're pressuring him to have a vasectomy. How can you keep the dialogue going in a cooperative way?

Abortion

Regardless of the circumstances under which pregnancy occurs, women may now choose to terminate their pregnancies. No longer must women who do not want to be pregnant seek potentially dangerous, illegal abortions. On the basis of current technology and legality, women need never experience childbirth. The decision will be theirs to make.

Abortion is a highly controversial, personal decision—one that needs serious consideration by each woman. On the basis of the landmark 1973 U.S. Supreme Court case *Roe v. Wade*, the United States joined many of the world's most populated countries in legalizing abortion within the following guidelines:

1. For the first 3 months of pregnancy (first trimester), the decision to abort lies with the woman and her doctor. Most abortions are performed in the first trimester.
2. For the next 3 months of pregnancy (second trimester), state law may regulate the abortion procedure in ways that are reasonably related to maternal health.
3. For the last weeks of pregnancy (third trimester) when the fetus is judged capable of surviving if born, any state may regulate or even prohibit abortion except where abortion is necessary to preserve the life or health of the mother.

In 2002, 1.29 million women made the decision to terminate a pregnancy in the United States.[17] Thousands of additional women probably considered abortion but elected to continue their pregnancies.

First-Trimester Abortion Procedures

The first trimester consists of the first 13 weeks (91 days) of pregnancy. During the first 49 days after a woman's last menstrual period, a woman has two options for terminating a pregnancy: *vacuum aspiration* or *medication abortion*. Once 63 days have passed, only vacuum aspiration is an abortion option.

Vacuum Aspiration   There are two common methods of performing vacuum aspiration abortions. Both procedures can be performed in a physician's office or in a hospital. Both procedures require **dilation** of the cervix. The method used depends on how long the woman has been pregnant. Together, these methods represent the most widely used abortion procedures in the United States. In 1999, 96 percent of all abortions in the United States were performed through aspiration procedures.[4]

The **manual vacuum aspiration (MVA)** procedure can be performed in the earliest part of the first trimester, from the time a woman knows she is pregnant and up to 10 weeks after her last period. After a physician injects a local anesthetic into the cervix, dilators can be used to enlarge the cervical opening. The physician then inserts a small tube into the uterus and applies suction with a handheld instrument. By rotating and moving this small tube across the uterine wall, the physician can empty the uterus. A return visit to the physician is an important follow-up procedure.[4]

After the first month of pregnancy and throughout the first trimester, physicians typically select **dilation and suction curettage (D&C)** (frequently called *vacuum aspiration*) as the abortion procedure of choice. D&C is similar to the MVA, but the clinician uses a vacuum machine rather than a manually operated suction instrument. The clinician tends to use more sedation for the woman, in addition to the local cervical anesthetic. The cervix is stretched open with dilators that gradually enlarge the opening to permit the insertion of a tube into the cervix. This tube is attached to a vacuum machine that empties the uterus with gentle suction. If the physician believes that additional endometrial tissue remains in the uterus, he or she can use a **curette** to scrape the wall of the uterus. A subsequent visit to the clinician is an important follow-up procedure. Costs range from $350–$700.[12]

Key Terms

abortion induced premature termination of a pregnancy

dilation gradual expansion of an opening or passageway, such as the cervix

manual vacuum aspiration (MVA) the abortion procedure performed in the earliest weeks after a pregnancy is established

dilation and suction curettage (D & C) (kyoo re **taage**) a surgical procedure in which the cervical canal is dilated to allow the uterine wall to be scraped; vacuum aspiration

curette a metal scraping instrument that resembles a spoon, with a cup-shaped cutting surface on its end

Medication Abortion Mifepristone (RU-486) and methotrexate are drugs that can be used to induce a **medication abortion** during the first trimester of pregnancy. RU-486 was developed in France in the 1980s and has been widely used in Europe. Finally, after years of testing in the United States, the FDA gave approval to the so-called "abortion pill." The pill is being marketed under the name Mifeprex and is available only through physicians. The cost of using mifepristone is about the same as the cost of first-term surgical procedures, or about $350–$650.[12]

Under the FDA's regimen, women must use mifepristone within 49 days of their last menstrual period. Mifepristone blocks the action of progesterone and causes the lining of the uterus to break down. Women take three pills at the first doctor visit and then return 48 hours later to take a second drug, misoprostol, which causes menstruation to occur, usually within about 5 hours.

A third visit to a physician is necessary to ensure that the woman is recovering well from medical abortion. Physicians will want to make certain that there is no infection or excessive bleeding and that the uterus is fully emptied. Over a decade of research studies have indicated that the use of mifepristone is around 95 percent effective, when used during the first 7 weeks of pregnancy.[18]

Methotrexate is a drug used since the 1950s for cancer treatment. Physicians have found that it is effective in inducing an early-term medication abortion. Typically, a woman receives an injection of methotrexate and, during an office visit 3 to 7 days later, receives misoprostol, usually through vaginal suppositories. The fetal contents are expelled, generally within 12 hours. A third visit to the physician is necessary to ensure that the woman is recovering well and that the abortion is complete. Costs of a medication abortion range from $350–$650.[12] If these and other new drugs continue to gain favor with women and their physicians, it is likely that more women will use physicians' offices, rather than abortion clinics, for abortion services.

Second-Trimester Abortion Procedures

When a woman's pregnancy continues beyond the 13th week of gestation, termination becomes a more difficult matter. The procedures at this stage become more complicated and take longer to be completed.

Dilation and Evacuation Between 13 and 16 weeks of pregnancy, the abortion method of choice is **dilation and evacuation (D&E).** Some physicians use this method up through 20 weeks or more of pregnancy.[4] The D&E is a more involved surgical procedure than is D&C and generally requires greater dilation of the cervix, larger medical

Uterus
Amniotic sac
Vacuum unit
Suction tube
Speculum

Figure 16-6 During dilation and evacuation, the cervix is dilated and the contents of the uterus are aspirated (removed by suction). This procedure is used to perform abortions through 20 weeks' or more gestation.

instruments (including forceps), suction, and curettage. (See Figure 16-6.) Some women may be given a general anesthetic during D&E procedures. After D&E, a return visit to the clinician is an important follow-up procedure.

In the 1970s and the 1980s, it was not uncommon for women reaching the end of the second trimester of pregnancy to undergo an abortion using a **hypertonic saline procedure** or a *prostaglandin procedure*. In the saline procedure, a strong salt solution was injected directly into the amniotic sac. This caused the uterine contents to dehydrate and be expelled from the uterus within 24–36 hours. In the prostaglandin procedure, an injection or a vaginal suppository of prostaglandin was administered. The prostaglandin produced strong uterine contractions that expelled the fetal contents. Both of these procedures are rarely used today.[4] The D&E remains the abortion method of choice for the second trimester.

Key Terms

medication abortion an abortion caused by the use of prescribed drugs

dilation and evacuation (D&E) second-trimester abortion procedure that requires greater dilation, suction, and curettage than do first-trimester vacuum aspiration procedures

hypertonic saline solution a salt solution with a concentration higher than that found in human fluids

Third-Trimester Abortion Procedures

If an abortion is required in the latter weeks of the gestational period, a surgical procedure in which the fetus will be removed or a procedure in which the entire uterus is removed (hysterectomy) can be undertaken. As you can imagine, these procedures are more complicated and involve longer hospitalization, major abdominal surgery, and an extended period of recovery.

In the late 1990s, the United States House of Representatives and the U.S. Senate voted to ban a rarely used third-trimester abortion procedure referred to as intact D and E (dilation and extraction). Lawmakers believed that this procedure, also called *partial-birth abortion,* was too gruesome to be permitted. President Clinton vetoed this ban, and because the Senate failed to override his veto, the ban on partial-birth abortion did not become federal law.

At the state level, however, many individual state governments had already passed laws banning partial-birth abortions. On June 30, 2000, the U.S. Supreme Court invalidated a Nebraska law that prohibited this procedure. This ruling called into question the constitutionality of other existing states' laws concerning this third-trimester procedure.

Despite the tenuous nature of most state laws that banned partial-birth abortion procedures, President George W. Bush signed into law a federal ban passed in 2003 by the U.S. Congress. However, in 2004, this federal ban on partial-birth abortions was declared unconstitu-tional by three district courts because it shared the same constitutional flaws that the U.S. Supreme Court found in the 2000 Nebraska law that was struck down. These flaws included (a) not having an exception for the woman's health and (b) having language so broad as to potentially cover other abortion procedures.[19]

At the time of this writing (May 2005), 26 states have passed bans on partial-birth abortions that apply throughout pregnancy. Eighteen of these bans have been specifically blocked by a court, and 7 remain unchallenged but are likely to be unenforceable because they do not permit a health exception for the woman. Only Ohio's partial-birth abortion ban throughout pregnancy has been challenged and upheld by a court.[19] (For the current status of laws pertaining to partial-birth abortion, go to www.guttmacher.org.)

A Final Word

In the heat of passion, people often fail to think rationally about the potential outcomes of unprotected sex. Therefore, the time to prepare for the romantic moment is *before* you are in a position where you don't want to think about the possibility of an unintended result. If you choose to be sexually active, find a form of protection that works well for you and use it consistently. If you choose not to be sexually active, realize that this is a viable choice that can be 100 percent effective.

Taking Charge of Your Health

- Use the Personal Assessment on page 509 to help you determine which birth control method is best for you.

- If you have a partner, discuss your personal preferences with him or her.

- Talk to your doctor about the health aspects of different types of birth control before making your decision.

- Find out as much as you can about the newest types of contraception (Seasonale, NuvaRing, Mirena, Lea's Shield, Essure, and Evra).

- Think about your likelihood of becoming pregnant or contracting an STD, and discuss with your partner how you might handle these possibilities if they should occur.

SUMMARY

- *Birth control* refers to all of the procedures that can prevent the birth of a child.
- *Contraception* refers to any procedure that prevents fertilization.
- Each birth control method has both a theoretical effectiveness rate and a use effectiveness rate. For some contraceptive approaches, these rates are similar (such as hormonal methods), and for others the rates are very different (such as condoms, diaphragms, and periodic abstinence).
- Many factors should be considered when deciding which contraceptive is best for you.
- Recent research indicates that the spermicide nonoxynol-9 may increase the spread of STDs among some users.
- Sterilization is usually considered an irreversible procedure.
- The birth control pill is safe and effective for the vast majority of women, but it does not protect against sexually transmitted diseases.
- Among the newest contraceptives are "the ring" and "the patch."
- Female condoms are currently available in drugstores without a prescription.
- The contraceptive sponge has returned to the U.S. market.
- Two types of IUDs are available: a hormone-containing IUD and a copper-wrapped IUD.
- Emergency contraception is safe and effective in preventing pregnancy when used within 5 days of unprotected intercourse.
- Currently, abortion remains a woman's choice under the guidelines of the 1973 *Roe v. Wade* decision and various state restrictions.
- The FDA has approved the drug mifepristone (RU-486) to induce a medication abortion during the first trimester of pregnancy.
- Abortion procedures vary according to the stage of the pregnancy.

REVIEW QUESTIONS

1. Explain the difference between the terms *birth control* and *contraception*. Give examples of each.
2. Explain the difference between theoretical and use effectiveness rates. Which is always higher?
3. Identify some of the factors that should be given careful consideration when selecting a contraceptive method. Explain each factor.
4. What is periodic abstinence? Identify and describe each of the five approaches to this birth control strategy.
5. Describe how vaginal spermicides work and how effective they are as a contraceptive.
6. What are the current concerns over the use of the spermicide nonoxynol-9?
7. What are the differences between the diaphragm and the cervical cap?
8. What are the two types of IUDs that are available in the United States?
9. How do minipills differ from the combined oral contraceptive pills?
10. What is emergency contraception? For what circumstances might this be used?
11. In what form is Depo-Provera delivered to a woman?
12. How does the contraceptive ring (NuvaRing) differ from the contraceptive patch (Evra)?
13. Describe the various sterilization procedures.
14. Identify and describe the different abortion procedures that are used during each trimester of pregnancy.
15. In which trimester of pregnancy are most abortions performed?
16. What is a medication abortion?

ENDNOTES

1. Bruckner H, Bearman P. After the promise: The STD consequences of adolescent virginity pledges. *Journal of Adolescent Health* (36) 271–278, 2005.
2. McAnulty RD, Burnette MM. *Exploring Human Sexuality: Making Healthy Decisions* (2nd ed.). Boston: Allyn and Bacon, 2004.
3. Crooks RL, Baur K. *Our Sexuality* (9th ed.). Belmont, CA: Wadsworth, 2005.
4. Hatcher RA, et al. *Contraceptive Technology* (18th ed.). New York: Ardent Media, Inc., 2004.
5. WebMD Medical News. *Warning for spermicide nonoxynol-9* (January 17, 2003), www.my.webmd.com, September 15, 2003.
6. Davis JL. *Spermicide Promotes HIV*, WebMD Medical News (September 26, 2002), www.webmd.com.
7. Allgeier ER, Allgeier AR. *Sexual Interactions* (5th ed.). New York: Houghton Mifflin, 2000.
8. DeNoon D. *Best Condoms Still Latex*, WebMD Health (March 21, 2003), www.my.webmd.com.
9. Planned Parenthood Federation of America. *Your Contraceptive Choices*, www.plannedparenthood.org, September 10, 2003.
10. Steiner MJ, et al. Contraceptive effectiveness of a polyurethane condom and a latex condom: a randomized controlled trial. *Obstetrics and Gynecology* 101(3): 539–547, 2003.
11. Strong B, DeVault C, Sayad BW, Yarber WL. *Human Sexuality: Diversity in a Contemporary America* (5th ed.). New York: McGraw-Hill, 2005.
12. Planned Parenthood Federation of America. *Health Info: Birth Control*, www.plannedparenthood.org, May 10, 2005.
13. Weise E. Contraceptive sponge is back, but why did it leave? *USA Today*, p. 7D, April 25, 2005.

14. Berlex Laboratories Web Site. *What Is Mirena?*, www.mirena-us.com, May 10, 2005.

15. The Alan Guttmacher Institute. *State Policies in Brief: Access to Emergency Contraception* (May 1, 2005), www.agi-usa.org.

16. Kelly GF. *Sexuality Today: The Human Perspective* (8th ed.). New York: McGraw-Hill, 2006.

17. The Alan Guttmacher Institute. *Facts in Brief: Induced Abortion in the United States* (May, 2005), www.agi-usa.org.

18. Creinin MD, et al. Mifepristone and misoprostol and methotrexate/misoprostol in clinical practice for abortion. *American Journal of Obstetrics and Gynecology* 188(3):664–669, 2003.

19. The Alan Guttmacher Institute. *Facts in Brief: Bans on "Partial-Birth" Abortion* (May 1, 2005), www.agi-usa.org.

personal assessment

Which birth control method is best for you?

To assess which birth control method would be best for you, answer the following questions, and check the interpretation below.

Do I: *Yes*   *No*

1. Need a contraceptive right away?   _____   _____
2. Want a contraceptive that can be used completely independent of sexual relations?   _____   _____
3. Need a contraceptive only once in a great while?   _____   _____
4. Want something with no harmful side effects?   _____   _____
5. Want to avoid going to the doctor?   _____   _____
6. Want something that will help protect against sexually transmitted diseases?   _____   _____
7. Have to be concerned about affordability? _____   _____
8. Need to be virtually certain that pregnancy will not result?   _____   _____
9. Want to avoid pregnancy now but want to have a child sometime in the future?   _____   _____
10. Have any medical condition or lifestyle that may rule out some form of contraception?   _____   _____

Interpretation

If you have checked *Yes* to number:

1. Condoms and spermicides may be easily purchased without prescription in any pharmacy.
2. Sterilization, oral contraceptives, hormone rings, patches, or injections, cervical caps, and periodic abstinence techniques do not require that anything be done just before sexual relations.
3. Diaphragms, condoms, or spermicides can be used by people who have coitus only once in a while. Periodic abstinence techniques may also be appropriate but require a high degree of skill and motivation.
4. IUD use should be carefully discussed with your physician. For most women, IUDs are quite safe. Sometimes the use of oral contraceptives or hormone products results in some minor discomfort and, on rare occasions, may have harmful side effects.
5. Condoms and spermicides do not require a prescription from a physician.
6. Condoms help protect against sexually transmitted diseases. Nonoxynol-9 may increase STD transmission in some users. No method (except abstinence) can guarantee complete protection.
7. Be a wise consumer: check prices, ask pharmacists and physicians. The cost of sterilization is high, but there is no additional expense for a lifetime.
8. Sterilization provides near certainty. Hormone-based contraceptives, IUDs, or a diaphragm-condom-spermicide combination also give a high measure of reliable contraceptive protection. Periodic abstinence, withdrawal, and douche methods should be avoided. Outercourse may be a good alternative.
9. Although it is sometimes possible to reverse sterilization, it requires surgery and is more complex than simply stopping use of any of the other methods.
10. Smokers and people with a history of blood clots should probably not use oral contraceptives or other hormone approaches. Some people have allergic reactions to a specific spermicide or latex material. Some women cannot be fitted with a diaphragm or cervical cap. The woman and her health care provider will then need to select another suitable means of contraception.

To Carry This Further . . .

There may be more than one method of birth control suitable for you. Always consider whether a method you select can also help you avoid an STD. Study the methods suggested above, and consult Table 16.1 to determine what method may be most appropriate.

chapter seventeen

Becoming a Parent

Chapter Objectives

On completing this chapter, you will be able to:

▍ describe the impact that having a baby can have on a couple.

▍ differentiate between the procedures involved in *human cloning* and *therapeutic cloning.*

▍ point out the challenges that can come when stepfamilies are created.

▍ identify physiological obstacles and aids to fertilization.

▍ identify the changes that take place in intrauterine development during each of the three trimesters of pregnancy.

▍ indicate the various activities that take place during each of the three stages of childbirth.

▍ discuss the complications that can take place during pregnancy and childbirth.

▍ list some of the reasons why couples might want to use genetic and prenatal counseling.

▍ identify the causes and treatment options for infertility.

▍ differentiate between surrogate parenting, foster parenting, and adoption.

Eye on the Media

TV Personality Encourages Gay and Lesbian Adoption

Rosie O'Donnell has worn a number of hats in her relatively brief career. She has been a comedian (in comedy clubs and on TV sitcoms such as *Will and Grace*), a film actress (*A League of Their Own, Sleepless in Seattle,* and others), a Broadway actress (*Grease*), and a television talk show host (*Rosie O'Donnell Show*). O'Donnell's talk show ran from 1996 until 2002, had many loyal followers, and won numerous Emmy Awards.[1] She was dubbed the "Queen of Nice" for her straightforward frankness and good sense of humor.[2]

O'Donnell has always been one to speak out on issues of personal and political importance, often with an unabashedly liberal stance. On her talk show, she encouraged political discussions on issues such as gun control and welfare reform. An issue of particular importance to O'Donnell was child advocacy.

When she heard about the difficulties a gay couple in Florida had over the adoption of a foster child, she felt it was time to speak out. In a March 2002 interview with Diane Sawyer on *Primetime Thursday,* O'Donnell revealed not only that she was a parent of adopted children but also that she was a lesbian. O'Donnell's "coming out" about her sexual orientation was directly related to her desire to spread the word about the large number of foster children in the United States. These foster children need good parents, and O'Donnell believes that many gay and lesbian persons would be great parents, if given the chance.

Through the medium of television, O'Donnell has now become a major public advocate for legislation that favors gay and lesbian adoption. She has been with her life partner, Kelli Carpenter, since 1998. On November 29, 2002, Carpenter gave birth to the couple's fourth child. Carpenter and O'Donnell were married in 2004 in San Francisco, but the legal status of that wedding is doubtful, after rulings by the Supreme Court in California.[2] In the future, as state legislatures review proposals related to adoption by gays and lesbians, look for Rosie O'Donnell to be a vocal advocate for change.

[1]Bateman GW. *Rosie O'Donnell,* www.glbtq.com/arts/odonnell_r.html, May 21, 2005.
[2]A&E Television Network. *Rosie O'Donnell,* www.biography.com/search/article.jsp?aid=9542144, May 21, 2005.

Although birth control is especially important for many young couples, most couples eventually want to have children and raise a family. In the past, couples had their children very soon after either high school or college. Now the trend seems to be to wait longer before having children. Most likely, educational, economic, contraceptive, and occupational factors have laid the groundwork for this trend. To the relief of many people, medical research indicates that women over the age of 30 or 35 are quite able to have healthy babies. (See Learning from Our Diversity on page 514.)

Parenting Issues for Couples

Before deciding to have children, couples should frankly discuss the effects that pregnancy and a newborn child will have on their lives (see Discovering Your Spirituality on page 512). In addition, anyone who is sexually active should consider these same issues, because very few contraceptive methods are 100 percent effective all the time, and pregnancy can result from nearly any act of intercourse. For those students contemplating single parenthood, we ask that you consider these issues as they relate to your particular situation and to excuse our consistent use of plural pronouns. In any event, couples should discuss some or all of the following basic considerations:

- What effect will pregnancy have on us individually and collectively?
- Why do we want to have a child?
- What effect will a child have on the images we have constructed for ourselves as adults?
- Can we afford to have a child and provide for its needs?
- How will the responsibilities related to raising a child be divided?

- How will a child affect our professional careers?
- Are we ready now to accept the extended responsibilities that can come with a new child?
- How will we rear our child in terms of religious training, discipline, and participation in activities?
- Are we ready to part with much of the freedom associated with late adolescence and the early young adult years?
- How will we handle the possibility of being awakened at 6 o'clock or earlier each morning for the next few years?
- What plans have we made in the event that our baby (or fetus) has a serious birth defect?
- Are we capable of handling the additional responsibilities associated with having a disabled child?
- Are we comfortable with the thought of bringing another child into an already overcrowded, violent, bigoted, and polluted world?

If these questions seem strikingly negative in tone, there is indeed a reason for this. We believe that all too frequently the "nuts and bolts" issues related to childbearing and parenting are ignored or at least are placed on the back burner. Of course, future parents will consider how cute and cuddly a new baby will be, how holidays will be enhanced with a new child, and how pleased the grandparents will be; however, we consider these issues to be secondary to the serious realities of having a child enter your lives. (Complete the Personal Assessment on page 531 to explore your feelings about parenting.)

 TALKING POINTS If you think you would like to have children some day, would you feel comfortable discussing these issues with your partner? How would you start the conversation?

For many young couples, the rewards of raising a family outweigh the stress that inevitably accompanies parenthood.

Parenthood Expands Personal Growth

Becoming a parent is almost always an exciting experience. Through 9 months of pregnancy, anticipation of the baby increases on a daily basis. What sex will the baby be? How much hair will he or she have? How large will the baby be? Will the baby be a healthy child? Will the labor and delivery go smoothly? How will the household be changed as a result of the baby? How will the parents interact with each other after the baby enters the picture?

All these parental thoughts are centered on the baby and its presence. This is natural. Carrying a pregnancy to term and adjusting to the new baby are exciting, challenging, and exhausting experiences for the parents. There are times when new parents wonder how they ever got themselves into this situation. But there are many more times when parents are likely to be immensely thankful and proud to be parents of a newborn child.

Sometimes as we watch the growth and development of a newborn baby, we fail to think about the opportunities parenthood provides for the parents themselves to grow and develop. Parenthood presents an extra dimension to the lives of most parents. Although one can see this extra dimension in a number of ways, perhaps the most noticeable change is in the depth and quality of human relationships.

Perhaps most easily seen is the connection between mother and child. Living together, sharing nutrients (ideally only good ones), and protecting each other for 9 months forges a spiritual bond between mother and child that remains for a lifetime. They experience labor and delivery in a way unique to themselves. Although fathers may be able to sense how strong this bond is, they never can fully understand or feel how close this mother-child connection is and how strong it tends to remain. *Parenthood is a life-altering experience for a woman.*

After becoming parents, fathers also tend to forge close, intimate bonds with their children, but these bonds are more likely related to the interactions they experience with the children as they grow and develop. Sometimes to their surprise, fathers find out that they have marvelous capabilities to adjust to the new demands a baby presents. Many fathers develop unexpected talents at nurturing their children. Perhaps because of this, more and more fathers are choosing to stay at home and raise their children, while their spouse works to support the family financially. This arrangement was virtually unheard of just three decades ago. *Indeed, parenthood is also a life-altering experience for a man.*

Parenthood encourages men and women to expand their focus from themselves (and their careers, their interests, their friends) to a broader spectrum of other people. This spectrum will certainly include the child, but also health care providers, teachers, school officials, their child's friends, the friends' parents and perhaps religious leaders, law enforcement personnel, and sports coaches. Parents will be required to expand their communication skills, their patience, and their insights as they try to raise their children the best way they can. Through this struggle comes added personal growth for the parents.

A final area in which parenthood offers a new dimension for the parents concerns the intimate bond between the parents themselves. Although it doesn't always happen (and the divorce statistics tell a compelling story), the process of conceiving a child, birthing a child, and raising a child to adulthood can make two people grow together in a way unmatched by any other experience. Older adult couples will often say that their most significant shared experience was raising their children. Many agree that it was through this experience that they gained a depth of understanding about each other that enriched their lives and established their most intimate connection. *In this sense, parenthood is a spiritual, life-altering experience for the parents.*

Human Cloning: An Ethical Dilemma

Today's most controversial issue related to parenting is reproduction through **human cloning.** With the 1997 breakthrough cloning of the Scottish sheep Dolly, the possibility of human cloning emerged within the scientific community. To clone a human, the procedure would involve the following steps:[1]

- Doctors would surgically retrieve an egg from the female donor.

- The nucleus of this egg would be removed.

- A cell is taken from a cloning subject (a male or female).

- Through an electrical jolt, the cloning subject's cell is fused with the **enucleated egg.** This creates a clonal zygote. Shortly after, this clonal zygote divides over and over and develops into a clonal embryo.

- The clonal embryo is implanted in the womb of a surrogate mother.

- After nine months, a genetically matched reproduction of the cloning subject is born.

Key Terms

human cloning the replication of a human being

enucleated egg an ovum with the nucleus removed

Although this step-by-step process may seem simple, it has never been accomplished with human subjects. In fact, it took scientists 277 attempts to produce Dolly, the cloned sheep.[1] The technical expertise to clone humans has not been fully developed, although some scientists believe it could be on the near horizon, if public policy would fully support this area of research.

However, public policy currently does not support human cloning. Several countries and a few states have passed laws banning human cloning.[1] The U.S. Food and Drug Administration (FDA) has warned researchers that any attempts at human cloning must first get FDA approval, which the FDA claims will not be forthcoming. Both the American Society for Reproductive Medicine and the National Academy of Sciences have voiced their opposition to human cloning.[2] Many public opinion polls have indicated that Americans are overwhelmingly against the use of cloning to produce babies.[3]

However, the potential use of a particular type of cloning has received much more popular public support in America. This is the use of cloning to reproduce body parts, tissues, and specific organs for use in medical transplant procedures. A baby is never reproduced in this cloning procedure.[2] In organ and tissue cloning, sometimes called **therapeutic cloning,** the clonal embryo is not implanted into a surrogate mother, but allowed to grow (divide) into a number of premature cells called **stem cells.** These stem cells have the potential to grow into any kind of body cell.

Theoretically, scientists could develop techniques that would cause these stem cells to grow into tissues or organs that would match the tissues or organs in the person who donated the genetic material. Because of this genetic match, these cloned organs would not be rejected after the transplant surgery. In essence, this technology permits a person's own body to be a human repair kit. Some predict that, in the not too distant future, scientists will be able to grow replacement organs like hearts, livers, and skin and replacement neurons for persons who suffer from Parkinson's or Alzheimer's disease.

In May 2005, South Korean cloning scientist Dr. Hwang Woo-suk published reports that he had successfully taken the DNA from a sick patient's skin cells and injected this DNA into the stem cells taken from donated human embryos that had been cloned. These stem cells supposedly then evolved into new skin cells that were a genetic match with the original patient's skin cells. However, in December 2005, Dr. Hwang acknowledged that he had fabricated his data, but maintained that he still had the ability to create patient-specific stem cells.[4]

There are those who wonder if cloning represents "science gone mad." Some believe that any kind of cloning is unethical because it interferes with nature. Altering a woman's eggs, reprogramming cells, and tampering with embryos is something that is *simply wrong.* Regardless of the position you take on this issue, you can expect to see more scientific advances regarding cloning, especially therapeutic cloning.

Becoming a Parent through a Stepfamily

Some people will become parents through a marriage in which one or both adult partners bring children from a previous relationship.[5] This newly constituted household is called a *stepfamily.*

Although some people call this a blended family, the Stepfamily Association of America believes the preferred term is a stepfamily. Children in stepfamilies do not lose their individual identities and instantly "blend" into a new family while losing attachments to the parent who is not a part of the new marriage. Things are rarely that smooth. If both parents remarry, a child may become a member of two stepfamilies and, perhaps, face even more obstacles concerning family loyalty. It is natural for children to wonder where they fit in or where they belong. Calling a newly constituted family a blended family may set up too many unrealistic expectations for children and adults and make adjustments more difficult. For example, children may balk when told that they are to consider their new family to be the family that deserves all their attention and loyalty.[5]

It is beyond the scope of this chapter to outline the challenges (and joys) that come with becoming a parent through a stepfamily arrangement. The Stepfamily Association of America, a nonprofit support group for persons involved in stepfamily relationships, indicates that for stepfamilies to be successful, parents should:

- Nurture and enrich the couple relationship.
- Reveal and understand emotions.
- Have realistic expectations.
- Develop new roles.
- Seek support and see the positive.

> **Key Terms**
>
> **therapeutic cloning** the use of certain human replication techniques to reproduce body tissues and organs
>
> **stem cells** premature cells that have the potential to turn into any kind of body cell

Learning from Our Diversity

Pregnancy and Parenting After 40

Women who become pregnant in their 40s are not a new phenomenon. Many young people and baby boomers today were delivered by mothers who were 40 or more years old. What is new is women becoming pregnant for the first time at an age when many women begin menopause.

The reasons for the delay are several. Some couples may have tried to conceive for years and only succeeded when in their 40s. Other women and couples delayed pregnancy in order to build their careers, travel, or become more financially secure. In addition, fertility technology, such as in vitro fertilization, microsurgery, and the use of donor eggs or sperm, have finally given many couples the baby they long wanted.

The trend of later childbearing began in the late 1970s, when better-educated baby-boom women began entering the workforce. For women 40 to 44, the rate of first babies increased from 0.3 to 1.4 per 1,000, still a small percentage but a significant jump.[1]

The common belief that men can father babies well into middle age is supported not only by anecdotal evidence (such as Tony Randall, Larry King, and Michael Douglas), but also recent research that shows that sperm function in older men does not differ significantly from that of younger men.[2]

Women traditionally were discouraged from becoming pregnant for the first time in their forties because of the health risks to the mother and the risk of birth defects for the baby. It is true that women 40 and older suffer more complications during childbirth, and the risk of having a baby with Down syndrome or another genetic abnormality increases as a mother ages.[1]

The chances of having a cesarean delivery are about 40% higher than in a younger woman.[3] The number of women over 40 with gestational diabetes and high blood pressure is higher, and many have more difficulty with labor and deliver babies that are underweight or premature. In addition, the risk of fetal death is higher in women over 35 years old.[4]

Women who want to have a baby should use this information to prevent the problems, however, rather than let it discourage them from having a baby at all, researchers say.

Women who want to start families in their 40s should consider the following points:

- Infertility can become a problem with age, but fertility drugs such as Clomid or treatments such as in vitro fertilization can help.
- The rate of miscarriage is higher among older women, so immediate prenatal care is vital.
- Early genetic testing can ease the fears about birth defects. Tests can reveal the presence of Down syndrome, Tay-Sachs disease, cystic fibrosis, and sickle-cell anemia.
- Cesarean sections are more common in older mothers.

On the plus side, another study recently reported that women who are able to give birth after age 40 (not including those who become pregnant through the use of fertility treatments) may be "slow to age" and live longer.[1] This can be good news to older moms who wonder whether they will have the energy to chase a toddler.

[1] Blackburn B. Moms starting families in 40s test odds. *USA Today* 1997; Sept 24:14A.
[2] Haidl G, Jung A, Schill WB. Aging and sperm function. *Hum Reprod* 1996; 11(3):558–560.
[3] Later age pregnancy. Preparing for the happy, healthy event of after 40. *Health Oasis*, Mayo Clinic, 1998. www.mayohealth.org/mayo/9708/htm/aged_p.htm
[4] Fretts RC et al. Increased maternal age and risk of fetal death. *N Engl J Med* 1995; 333(15):953–957.

Throughout the merging of families into stepfamilies, clear communication, honest feelings, and a positive attitude about one's new role can help the process run more smoothly. It is quite possible that new family relationships can be wonderful experiences for all involved.

Parenting across Cultures

In their recent text *Transcultural Health Care,* Purnell and Paulanka describe the various ways ethnic groups in America tend to view babies and young children.[6] In the Amish culture, children are seen as gifts from God and are enthusiastically welcomed into families. Amish families have an average of seven children per family and, unlike in other ethnic groups in America, this fertility pattern has not changed for the past century. Large families prize children because they are not only gifts from God, but they are also valuable resources on low-tech, labor-intensive family farms.

Children are considered a blessing to Jewish families. Children are to be afforded an education that prepares them for progress in society as well as increased understanding of their Jewish heritage. To that end, many Jewish children attend public school but also attend Hebrew school a couple of afternoons each week during the school year. Jewish children play important roles in most of the holiday celebrations and religious services. Parents are expected to treat their children fairly and to be flexible, caring, and attentive to discipline.[6]

Although there is much change taking place as Chinese increase their assimilation into the United States, many Chinese American families still hold on to Chinese traditions. Children are highly valued, but the number of children in a family tends to be small, perhaps because of

China's one-child rule. Independence is usually not fostered, and parents make many decisions for the children even into young adulthood. Teens are expected to work hard in school, score well on exams, and help with chores around the home.[6]

In discussing Arab Americans' views of children, Purnell and Paulanka write that high fertility rates tend to be favored because of the belief that "God decides family size" and because families follow Islamic dictates regarding birth control, treatment of infertility, and abortion. Procreation is considered the primary reason for a marriage, since it enhances family strength. As with a number of cultures around the world, pregnancy tends to occur early in the marriage, and the preference for boys over girls is a reality. The sex of a child can be a great concern for the pregnant woman, and observers will often note the way in which the mother "carries" her baby during the pregnancy (girls are thought to be carried high and boys to be carried low).[6]

Pregnancy: An Extension of the Partnership

Pregnancy is a condition that requires a series of complex yet coordinated changes to occur in the female body. This chapter follows pregnancy from its beginning, at fertilization, to its conclusion, with labor and childbirth. Fathers-to-be share many of the joys and worries of pregnancy and childbirth.

Physiological Obstacles and Aids to Fertilization

Many sexually active young people believe that they will become pregnant (or impregnate someone) only when they want to, despite their haphazard contraceptive practices. Because of this mistaken belief, many young people do not consistently use contraceptives. Young adults must remember that, to ensure the survival of our species, our bodies were designed to promote pregnancy. It is estimated that about 85 percent of sexually active women of childbearing age will become pregnant within one year if they do not use some form of contraception.[7]

With regard to pregnancy, each act of intercourse can be considered a game of physiological odds. Obstacles exist that may reduce a couple's chance of pregnancy, including the following.

Obstacles to Fertilization

1. *The acidic level of the vagina is destructive to sperm.* The low pH of the vagina kills sperm that fail to enter the uterus quickly.

The surface of an ovum is penetrated by sperm at fertilization.

2. *The cervical mucus is thick during most of the menstrual cycle.* Sperm movement into the uterus is more difficult, except during the few days surrounding ovulation.
3. *The sperm must locate the cervical opening.* The cervical opening is small and may not be located by most sperm.
4. *Half of the sperm travel through the wrong fallopian tube.* Most commonly, only one ovum is released at ovulation. The two ovaries generally "take turns" each month. The sperm have no way of "knowing" which tube they should enter. Thus it is probable that half will travel through the wrong tube.
5. *The distance sperm must travel is relatively long compared with the tiny size of the sperm cells.* Microscopic sperm must travel about seven or eight inches after they are inside the female.
6. *The sperm's travel is relatively "upstream."* The anatomical positioning of the female reproductive structures necessitates an "uphill" movement by the sperm.
7. *The contoured folds of the tubal walls trap many sperm.* These folds make it difficult for sperm to locate the egg. Many sperm are trapped in this maze.

There are also a variety of aids that tend to help sperm and egg cells join. Some of these are listed next.

Aids to Fertilization

1. *An astounding number of sperm are deposited during ejaculation.* Each ejaculation contains about a teaspoon of semen.[8] Within this quantity are between

Figure 17-1 After its release from the follicle, the ovum begins its week-long journey down the fallopian tube. Fertilization generally occurs in the outermost third of the tube. Now fertilized, the ovum progresses toward the uterus, where it embeds itself in the endometrium. A pregnancy is established.

200 and 500 million sperm cells. Even with large numbers of sperm killed in the vagina, millions are able to move to the deeper structures.

2. *Sperm are deposited near the cervical opening.* Ejaculation into the vagina by the penis places the sperm near the cervical opening.

3. *The male accessory glands help make the semen nonacidic.* The seminal vesicles, prostate gland, and Cowper's glands secrete fluids that provide an alkaline environment for the sperm. This environment helps sperm be better protected in the vagina until they can move into the deeper, more alkaline uterus and fallopian tubes.

4. *Uterine contractions aid sperm movement.* The rhythmic muscular contractions of the uterus tend to cause the sperm to move in the direction of the fallopian tubes.

5. *Sperm cells move rather quickly.* Despite their tiny size, sperm cells can move about one inch per hour. Powered by sugar solutions from the male accessory glands and the whiplike movements of their tails, sperm can reach the distant third of the fallopian tubes in less than 8 hours as they swim in the direction of the descending ovum.

6. *After they are inside the fallopian tubes, sperm can live for days.* Some sperm may be viable for up to a week after reaching the comfortable, nonacidic environment of the fallopian tubes. Most sperm, however, will survive an average of 48–72 hours. Thus they can "wait in the wings" for the moment an ovum is released from the ovary (Figure 17-1).

7. *The cervical mucus is thin and watery at the time of ovulation.* This mucus allows for better passage of sperm through the cervical opening when the ovum is most capable of being fertilized.

Signs of Pregnancy

Aside from pregnancy tests done in a professional laboratory, a woman can sometimes recognize early signs and symptoms. The signs of pregnancy have been divided into three categories.

Presumptive Signs of Pregnancy

Missed period after unprotected intercourse the previous month

Nausea on awakening (morning sickness)

Increase in size and tenderness of breasts

Darkening of the areolar tissue surrounding the nipples

Think you might be pregnant? A home pregnancy test is simple to do and can give you an accurate answer in 2 to 5 minutes.

Improved technology has made the urine home pregnancy test about as accurate as blood tests—99 percent under perfect conditions— although in actual use it may be less than that.*

Using a woman's urine, a home pregnancy test detects the presence of human chorionic gonadotropin (hCG), a hormone produced only during pregnancy. The tests contain monoclonal antibodies, which are molecules coated with a substance that bonds to the pregnancy hormone. If the hormone is present, a colored stripe, dot, or other symbol appears in the test windows. The tests also contain "control" windows to indicate whether the device has functioned properly.

Although the makers of today's tests say their products can detect hCG as soon as the very day a missed period was supposed to begin, they also advise taking the test again a few days later to confirm the result. If the result is positive, see a doctor as soon as possible.

*Williams RD. Healthy pregnancy, healthy baby. *FDA Consumer,* March–April 1999; 33(2):18–22.

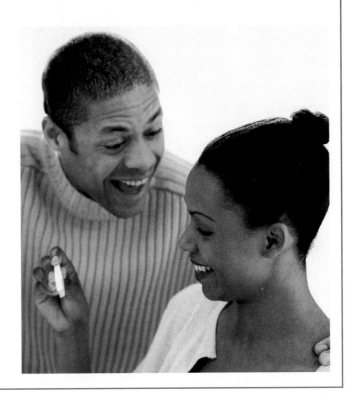

Probable Signs of Pregnancy

Increase in the frequency of urination (the growing uterus presses against the bladder)

Increase in the size of the abdomen

Cervix becomes softer by the sixth week (detected by a pelvic examination by a clinician)

Positive pregnancy test (see the Star box)

Positive Signs of Pregnancy

Determination of a fetal heartbeat

Feeling of the fetus moving (quickening)

Observation of the fetus by ultrasound or optical viewers

Agents That Can Damage a Fetus

A large number of agents that come into contact with a pregnant woman can affect fetal development. Many of these (rubella and herpes viruses, tobacco smoke, alcohol, and virtually all other drugs) are discussed in other chapters of this text. The best advice for a pregnant woman is to maintain close contact with her obstetrician during pregnancy and to consider carefully the ingestion of any over-the-counter (OTC) drug (including aspirin, caffeine, and antacids) that could harm the fetus.

Pregnant women should also avoid exposure to radiation. Such exposure, most commonly through excessive X-rays or radiation fallout from nuclear testing, can irreversibly damage fetal genetic structures. In addition, pregnant women should avoid Accutane, a drug prescribed for the treatment of cystic acne that can severely damage the fetus.

Intrauterine Development

Intrauterine development takes place over the course of three **trimesters.** Most pregnancies last from 38–42 weeks. For purposes of illustration, we will consider each trimester to be 13 weeks. The growth and development during these trimesters occurs in a typical pattern for most pregnancies.

> **Key Terms**
>
> **trimester** a 3-month period; human pregnancies encompass three trimesters

The fetus at 16 weeks' gestation within the amniotic sac

First Trimester

The first 13-week trimester starts at conception, when the egg and sperm unite to form a structure called the **zygote.** The zygote, or fertilized egg, undergoes a series of cellular changes as it grows and makes its week-long journey down the fallopian tube to the uterus. About the 10th day after conception, the zygote, now called a **blastocyst,** imbeds itself into the endometrial lining of the uterus. From the end of 2 weeks after conception until the end of the 8th week, the growing structure is called an **embryo.** After 8 weeks and until the birth, it is called a **fetus.**

The first trimester is characterized by rapid cellular growth. By the end of the first trimester, the fetus weighs only about 1 oz., yet most body organs are formed and the fetus can move.[9] It is currently thought that about half of all pregnancies end in **spontaneous abortion** during the early weeks of the first trimester, usually before the woman realizes she is pregnant. These miscarriages usually result from a genetic defect or a serious developmental problem.

Second Trimester

The second trimester is characterized by continued growth and maturation. During this time, the organs continue to grow and physicians can hear the fetal heartbeat with a stethoscope. The bone structures are fully evident during the second trimester. The fetus starts to look more and more like an infant.

Additionally, the mother's breast weight increases by about 30 percent because of the deposition of 2–4 pounds of fat. This fat serves as a reserve energy source for the mother should she decide to nurse her baby. For this reason, good maternal nutrition is essential during the second trimester.[9]

Third Trimester

The third trimester is another critical time for the developing fetus. At the beginning of this trimester, the fetus generally weighs 2–3 pounds. Over the final 13 weeks of gestation, the fetus will double in length and multiply its weight by up to five times.

This is also the time when the fetus absorbs considerable amounts of the minerals iron and calcium from the mother. For this reason, the mother must maintain sound eating patterns and avoid her body's depletion of mineral stores, perhaps by taking a vitamin and mineral supplement containing iron, which would reduce her risk of developing anemia during the final trimester.[9]

Childbirth: The Labor of Delivery

Childbirth, or *parturition,* is one of the true peak life experiences for both men and women. Most of the time, childbirth is a wonderfully exciting venture into the unknown. For the parents, this intriguing experience can provide a stage for personal growth, maturity, and insight into a dynamic, complex world.

During the last few weeks of the third trimester, most fetuses move deeper into the pelvic cavity in a process called *lightening.* During this movement, the fetus' body rotates and the head begins to engage more deeply into the mother's pelvic girdle. Many women report that their babies have "dropped."

Another indication that parturition may be relatively near is the increased reporting of *Braxton Hicks contractions.*[10] These uterine contractions, which are of mild intensity and often occur at irregular intervals, may be felt throughout a pregnancy. During the last few weeks of pregnancy (*gestation*), these mild contractions can occur more frequently and cause a woman to feel as if she is going into labor **(false labor).**

Key Terms

zygote a fertilized ovum

blastocyst early stage of the developing life form that imbeds into the endometrial lining of the uterus

embryo developmental stage from the end of the second week after conception until the end of the eighth week

fetus developmental stage from the beginning of the ninth week after conception until birth

spontaneous abortion any cessation of pregnancy resulting from natural causes; also called a miscarriage

false labor conditions that resemble the start of true labor; may include irregular uterine contractions, pressure, and discomfort in the lower abdomen

A First Stage

Placenta

Umbilical cord

Uterus

Cervical opening

Birth canal

Uterine contractions thin the cervix and enlarge the cervical opening.

Figure 17-2 Labor, or childbirth, is a three-stage process. During effacement and dilation, the first stage **A**: the cervical canal is gradually opened by contractions of the uterine wall. The second stage **B**: delivery of the fetus, encompasses the actual delivery of the fetus from the uterus and through the birth canal. The delivery of the placenta, the third stage **C**: empties the uterus, thus completing the process of childbirth.

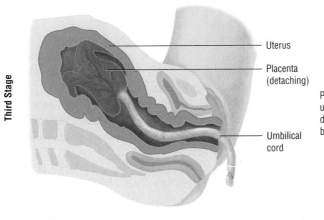

B Second Stage

Perineum

Uterine contractions are aided by mother's voluntary contractions of abdominal muscles.

Fetus moves through dilated cervical opening and birth canal.

C Third Stage

Uterus

Placenta (detaching)

Umbilical cord

Placenta detaches from uterine wall and is delivered through the birth canal.

Labor begins when uterine contractions become more intense and occur at regular intervals. The birth of a child can be divided into three stages: (1) effacement and dilation of the cervix, (2) delivery of the fetus, and (3) expulsion of the placenta (Figure 17-2). For a woman having her first child, the birth process lasts an average of 12–16 hours. The average length of labor for subsequent births is much shorter—from 4–10 hours on the average. Labor is very unpredictable: Labors that last from 1–24 hours occur daily at most hospitals. (See Considering Complementary Care on page 520 for a discussion of midwifery.)

For the past century, most of the women in the United States who went into labor followed a fairly standard procedure. This included a trip to the hospital and a lengthy wait in a labor room. The actual birth then took place in a delivery room, which was a surgical room equipped to handle most medical emergencies. Doctors and nurses were always close by to watch the expectant mother and to track the high-tech monitors.

This scenario is rapidly changing with the increased use of midwives, many of whom help deliver babies within hospital settings, at free-standing birthing centers, or in the homes of the pregnant women. Two types of nurse-midwives are certified by the American College of Nurse-Midwives (ACNM). A Certified Nurse-Midwife (CNM) is trained and certified in the two disciplines of nursing and midwifery, while the Certified Midwife (CM) has training and certification in midwifery. All Certified Nurse-Midwives have baccalaureate degrees and 72 percent also have master's or doctoral degrees.[1]

Both CNMs and CMs operate within a framework of a health care system that provides for consultation, collaborative management, or referral to additional medical care according to the health needs and condition of the pregnant woman. If the woman needs specialized help during the pregnancy or emergency care during labor, certified midwives do not hesitate to access the traditional medical system.

Since 97 percent of midwife deliveries take place within hospitals, this care is usually easily attainable. Presently, less than 3 percent of midwife-assisted births occur at free-standing birthing centers or in private homes.

For many years, the traditional medical establishment discounted the use of midwives, believing that midwives were incapable of providing professional prenatal care and birthing assistance to women. However, this position has softened considerably. Indeed, most pregnancies and births follow a natural, standard pattern in which trained midwives can function in a very cost-effective, low-tech, patient-friendly manner.

Today, over 10 percent of all births in the United States are attended by midwives. In the year 2002, certified midwives attended 307,527 births. With certified midwifery training programs in place at some of the most prestigious universities in the country (for example, Vanderbilt University, Baylor College of Medicine, the University of Michigan, and Yale University), this trend will likely continue.

[1] American College of Nurse-Midwives. *Basic Facts about Certified Nurse-Midwives,* www.midwife.org, May 21, 2005.

Stage One: Effacement and Dilation of the Cervix

In the first stage of labor the uterine contractions attempt to thin (*efface*) the normally thick cervical walls and to enlarge (*dilate*) the cervical opening.[11] These contractions are directed by the release of prostaglandins and the hormone oxytocin into the circulating bloodstream. In women delivering their first babies, effacement will occur before dilation. In subsequent deliveries, effacement and dilation usually occur at the same time.

The first stage of labor is often the longest. The cervical opening must thin and dilate to a diameter of 10 centimeters before the first stage of labor is considered complete.[12] Often this stage begins with the dislodging of the cervical mucous plug. The subsequent *bloody show* (mucous plug and a small amount of blood) at the vaginal opening may indicate that effacement and dilation have begun. Another indication of labor's onset may be the bursting or tearing of the fetal amniotic sac. "Breaking the bag of waters" refers to this phenomenon, which happens in various measures in expectant women.

The pain of the uterine contractions becomes more intense as the woman moves through this first stage of labor. As the cervical opening effaces and dilates 0–3 centimeters, many women report feeling happy, exhilarated, and confi-

dent. In the early phase of the first stage of labor, the contractions are relatively short (lasting 15–60 seconds) and the intervals between contractions range from 20 minutes to 5 minutes as labor progresses. However, these rest intervals will become shorter and the contractions more forceful when the woman's uterus contracts to dilate 4–7 centimeters.

In this second phase of the first stage of labor, the contractions usually last about 1 minute each, and the rest intervals drop from about 5 minutes to 1 minute over a period of 5–9 hours.

The third phase of the first stage of labor is called *transition*. During transition, the uterus contracts to dilate the cervical opening to the full 10 centimeters required for safe passage of the fetus out of the uterus and into the vagina (birth canal).[13] This period of labor is often the most painful part of the entire birth process. Fortunately, it is also the shortest phase of most labors. Lasting 15–30 minutes, transition contractions often last 60–90 seconds each. The rest intervals between contractions are short and vary from 30 to 60 seconds.

An examination of the cervix by a nurse or physician will reveal whether full dilation of 10 centimeters has occurred. Until the full 10-centimeter dilation, women are cautioned not to "push" the fetus during the contractions. Special breathing and concentration techniques help many women cope with the first stage of labor.

Stage Two: Delivery of the Fetus

When the mother's cervix is fully dilated, she enters the second stage of labor, the delivery of the fetus through the birth canal. Now the mother is encouraged to help push the baby out (with her abdominal muscles) during each contraction. In this second stage the uterine contractions are less forceful than during the transition phase of the first stage and may last 60 seconds each, with a 1- to 3-minute rest interval.

This second stage may last up to 2 hours in first births.[8] For subsequent births, this stage will usually be much shorter. When the baby's head is first seen at the vaginal opening, *crowning* is said to have taken place. Generally the back of the baby's head appears first. (Infants whose feet or buttocks are presented first are said to be delivered in a *breech position*.) After the head is delivered, the baby's body rotates upward to let the shoulders come through. The rest of the body follows quite quickly. The second stage of labor ends when the fetus is fully expelled from the vagina. In the past, deliveries were often performed with an *episiotomy*, a surgical incision of the **perineum** intended to prevent lacerations (tearing) during delivery.

Immediately after the birth, and again 5 minutes later, the newborn's physical health frequently is evaluated by obstetrical assistants using the Apgar score system. The baby will be judged (rated either 0, 1, or 2) on five criteria including appearance (color), pulse, response to foot stimulation, muscle tone, and respiration. After 5 minutes, 98 percent of infants score 7 or above. An Apgar score of less than 5 after 5 minutes indicates the possibility of a serious defect.

Newly delivered babies often look "unusual." Their heads are often cone-shaped as a result of the compression of cranial bones that occurs during the delivery through the birth canal. Within a few days after birth, the newborn's head assumes a much more normal shape. Most babies (of all races) appear bluish at first until they begin regular breathing. All babies are covered with a coating of *vernix*, a white, cheeselike substance that protects the skin.

Stage Three: Delivery of the Placenta

Usually within 30 minutes after the fetus is delivered, the uterus again initiates a series of contractions to expel the placenta (or *afterbirth*). The placenta is examined by the attending physician to ensure that it was completely expelled. Torn remnants of the placenta could lead to dangerous hemorrhaging by the mother. Often the physician manually examines the uterus after the placenta has been delivered.

After the placenta has been delivered, the uterus continues with mild contractions to help control bleeding and start the gradual reduction of the uterus to its normal, nonpregnant size. This final aspect of the birth process is called **postpartum.** External abdominal massage of the lower abdomen seems to help the uterus

Ultrasound scans are used to check the growing fetus for possible abnormalities, as well as size, development, position, and many other factors.

contract, as does an infant's nursing at the mother's breast. (For suggestions for successfully breast-feeding your baby, see Changing for the Better on page 522.)

Cesarean Deliveries

A **cesarean delivery** (cesarean birth, C-section) is a procedure in which the fetus is surgically removed from the mother's uterus through the abdominal wall. This type of delivery, which is completed in up to an hour, can be performed with the mother having a regional or a general anesthetic.

In 2003, the percentage of deliveries by cesarean section reached an all-time high of 27.6 percent.[14] The increasing use of cesarean deliveries is questioned by some medical experts, although others point to the need for this kind of delivery when one or more of the following factors are present:

- The fetus is improperly positioned.
- The mother's pelvis is too small.
- The fetus is especially large.

Key Terms

perineum in the female, the region between the vulva and the anus

postpartum the period after the birth of a baby during which the uterus returns to its prepregnancy size

cesarean delivery (si **zare** ee an) surgical removal of a fetus through the abdominal wall

My older sister is 7 months pregnant and wondering if she should try to breastfeed her new baby. I think it's a good idea, but I want to give her some sound reasons. Any ideas?

There are numerous benefits to breastfeeding. Among the most important is that it provides antibodies while the infant's immune system is still immature. Breastfeeding decreases the incidence of diarrhea and respiratory disease and reduces the risk of food allergies and intolerances. Breastfeeding establishes the habit of eating in moderation and, thus, decreases the possibility of obesity in later life. Breast milk is bacteriologically safe, always fresh and ready to be used, inexpensive, and facilitates bonding between mother and baby. For the mother, nursing enhances uterine recovery and decreases the risk of ovarian cancer and premenopausal breast cancer.[1]

Breastfeeding is a perfectly natural function, so every new mother should be able to do it instinctively, right? Well, not necessarily. Occasionally little problems occur, and reviewing some of the basic advice before beginning can make it a little smoother:[2]

- Begin as soon after birth as you can, when the baby's sucking instinct is strongest. Begin in the delivery room if possible.
- Don't allow the hospital's regulations or wishes to come between you and your baby. Arrange to room with your baby.

- When you are ready to begin, find a comfortable position.
- Position your baby facing your nipple.
- Support your breast with your free hand, gently tickle the baby's lips with your nipple, then let your baby take the initiative.
- Be sure the baby latches onto the areola as well as the nipple, or the baby will not compress the milk glands. This can cause soreness and cracking of the skin.
- Be sure the breast does not block the baby's nose.
- Watch the baby's cheek for the steady rhythm that indicates the baby is suckling.
- If your baby holds onto the breast after he or she has finished suckling, do not pull the nipple out abruptly to avoid injuring it. Instead, break the suction first by putting a finger into a corner of the baby's mouth or depressing the breast to admit some air.

InfoLinks

www.lalecheleague.org

[1]Wardlaw GM, Hampl JS, Disilvestro RA. *Perspectives in Nutrition*, 6th ed. New York: McGraw-Hill, 2003.
[2]La Leche League International. *When You Breast-Feed Baby: The First Weeks.* La Leche League, 1993.

- The fetus shows signs of distress.
- The umbilical cord is compressed.
- The placenta is being delivered before the fetus.
- The mother's health is at risk.

Although a cesarean delivery is considered major surgery, most mothers cope well with the delivery and post-surgical and postpartum discomfort. The hospital stay is usually a few days longer than for a vaginal delivery. The mother can still nurse her child and may still be able to have vaginal deliveries with later children. More and more hospitals are allowing the father to be in the operating room during cesarean deliveries. Fortunately, research indicates that early **bonding** between child, mother, and father can still occur with cesarean deliveries. Cesarean deliveries are much more expensive than vaginal deliveries.

Complications in Pregnancy and Childbirth

Most women progress through pregnancy and delivery without complications, but once in a great while something goes wrong. Complications are usually the result of genetics, an environmental factor (such as the use of drugs or alcohol by the mother), or some combination of these (see the Star box on page 523). Pregnant women should remember that the following complications are unusual if they are consuming a healthy diet, avoiding agents that can damage a fetus, such as alcohol and drugs, and following their doctor's recommendations. (See Changing for the Better on page 524.)

- *Ectopic pregnancy:* This is a pregnancy in which the embryo implants outside the uterus, most often in a fallopian tube. It can be serious and even life threatening, especially if not discovered early, but treatment can remove most of the risk for the mother while preserving future fertility.

> ### Key Terms
>
> **bonding** important initial recognition established between the newborn and those adults on whom the newborn will depend

Testing for Birth Defects

Many women undergo tests during pregnancy to check for birth defects, genetic disorders, and other problems.* A few of the most common tests are ultrasound scans, the alpha-fetoprotein (AFP) test, amniocentesis, and chorionic villi sampling (CVS). Each of these can be helpful in diagnosing problems, but the tests are not necessary for every pregnancy. Check with your doctor about what tests, if any, are appropriate for you.

Ultrasound—Ultrasound technology uses high-frequency sound waves to form pictures of the fetus on a computer screen. The test can verify a due date, determine causes of bleeding, check the overall health, development, sex, and position of the baby, measure the amniotic fluid, and check the condition of the placenta. There are no known risks from the tests, and many women have one or two ultrasounds in routine pregnancies. However, there is little scientific evidence that normal pregnancies benefit from ultrasound tests.

Alpha-Fetoprotein Screening (AFP)—A simple blood test that poses no risk to the fetus, AFP screening measures the levels of alpha-fetoprotein in the mother's blood. Abnormal levels can indicate a brain or spinal cord defect, the presence of twins, a miscalculated due date, or an increased risk of Down syndrome. Because AFP levels can be elevated for a number of reasons, a positive test is usually repeated or followed up by other tests before a diagnosis is made. Very few women with elevated AFP levels are found later to have babies with birth defects.

Amniocentesis—This test examines the cells shed by the fetus into the surrounding amniotic fluid. Performed about 16 weeks into pregnancy, the test involves inserting a long, thin needle through the mother's abdomen to extract fluid from the womb. The cells must be cultured in a laboratory and it may take up to a month for test results to be ready. The test is a reliable indicator of chromosomal abnormalities such as Down syndrome or genetic disorders such as Tay-Sachs disease, Hunter's syndrome, and others. While usually safe, amniocentesis can trigger cramping, leakage of amniotic fluid, and vaginal bleeding, and it may increase the risk of miscarriage by about 0.5–1 percent. The test is done only on women at increased risk of having babies with genetic disorders or to assess the maturity of the baby's lungs in the last trimester.

Chorionic Villi Sampling (CVS)—Performed between 10 and 12 weeks of pregnancy, CVS can detect the same genetic abnormalities as amniocentesis. It involves inserting a catheter or needle into the womb and extracting some of the chorionic villi (cells from the tissue that will become the placenta). The chorionic villi contain the same chromosomes as the fetus. The test is relatively safe, but it has a greater risk of miscarriage than amniocentesis. While there has been some concern that the test itself may be associated with limb deformities, many geneticists believe that CVS performed between 10 and 12 weeks of pregnancy does not increase that risk.

*Williams RD. Healthy pregnancy, healthy baby. *FDA Consumer,* March–April 1999; 33(2):18–22.

- *Miscarriage:* Early miscarriage is very common, occurring in as many as half of all conceptions, often passing unnoticed by the woman. It is usually related to a chromosomal abnormality or other problem in the fetus. Late miscarriage, on the other hand, is usually related to the mother's condition, her exposure to drugs or other toxins, or problems of the placenta.

- *Gestational diabetes:* This is a temporary condition in which the mother's body does not produce enough insulin to handle the increased blood sugar of pregnancy. Symptoms include unusual thirst, frequent urination, and fatigue. If treated, it is not a threat to the mother or baby.

- *Hyperemesis gravidarum:* This term literally means "excessive vomiting during pregnancy." This is a very unusual condition that is more serious than typical morning sickness. If untreated, it can result in malnutrition, dehydration, or damage to the fetus. It can be treated, however, with measures ranging from rest and antacids to hospitalization if necessary.

- *Preeclampsia (pregnancy-induced hypertension; toxemia):* This is a condition in which the woman's blood pressure becomes elevated during pregnancy; it occurs in one of every 10–20 pregnancies, and if untreated, preeclampsia can be serious and even life threatening. Fortunately, physicians almost invariably identify the disease if the mother is receiving regular prenatal care, and a poor outcome is rare. Treatment depends on the severity of the disease and can include an immediate induction of labor or hospitalization of the mother until the fetus is sufficiently developed to survive outside the uterus.

- *Eclampsia:* The final stage of preeclampsia, this disease is very unusual when the mother is receiving regular prenatal care. Symptoms include convulsions and coma. Treatment includes preventing convulsions and inducing labor or performing a cesarean delivery as soon as possible.

- *Intrauterine growth retardation (IUGR):* This term is used to describe insufficient growth of the fetus, which can occur because of genetic factors, maternal disease, or fetal malnutrition. With regular prenatal care, this condition can be identified and reversed.

- *Premature rupture of the membranes (PROM):* Rupture of the chorionic membranes, often called "breaking of the water," can occur prematurely. Infection is a risk because the protective membrane has been broken. Doctors typically try to delay delivery as long as possible up to about 37 weeks.

- *Premature labor:* Labor that begins after the fetus is considered viable and before term, at about 37 weeks, is called *premature labor*. It carries a variety of risks, but in many cases premature labor can be halted, and the mother can carry the baby to term. Quick medical attention is paramount.

- *Fetal distress:* This term describes a category of fetal problems, in particular a lack of oxygen caused by any of a variety of factors. The treatment usually is immediate delivery, by cesarean if necessary.

 TALKING POINTS Are there people in your life that you can comfortably ask, "What was it like to go through labor and delivery?" Will you feel open enough to express any personal concerns you might have about your own fears of this process?

Genetic and Prenatal Counseling

Genetic and prenatal counseling are two of the most beneficial advances in medical technology. Genetic counselors can provide timely, accurate, and complete information to patients, while maintaining the attitude that the patient's values should guide the decisions.

You should seek genetic counseling *before* attempting to conceive a child if you or your partner fall into any of the following categories:[15]

- History of multiple spontaneous abortions
- Consanguinity (partners are related by blood)
- Birth defect, possible genetic condition, neuromuscular or neurologic condition, or abnormalities of physical sexual development in the patient or families
- Ethnic background with increased risk of recessive genetic disease
- Maternal age of 35 or more years at delivery
- Paternal age of 55 or more years
- Positive maternal test for Down syndrome or trisomy 18
- Positive maternal test for an open neural tube defect
- Carrying a gene for a recessive disease that is more common in some ethnic populations

- Exposure to a known or suspected **teratogenic agent** (capable of causing birth abnormality)

The genetic counselor might use a variety of methods for gathering information about the couple, including DNA testing, other medical tests, medical records, family histories, and autopsy reports. When couples receive genetic counseling before conception and learn that they have a high risk of conceiving a child with birth defects, they then have a variety of options still open to them, such as artificial insemination by a donor, ovum donation, and adoption.

In addition, some couples can also reduce the risk of birth defects by changing their behavior or diet. For example, taking folic acid supplements has been shown to reduce the risk of neural tube defects. Abstaining from alcohol during pregnancy eliminates the risk of fetal alcohol syndrome. Stopping smoking reduces the risk of fetal intrauterine growth retardation, placental abruption (premature detachment of the placenta from the uterine wall), and fetal death. Women with the disease phenylketonuria who eliminate phenylalanine from their diet before pregnancy drastically reduce the risk of mental retardation in their children.[15]

If you have already become pregnant, you still should work with your physician to identify risk factors in your first prenatal visit, to allow time for tests to be conducted and medical records to be reviewed. Tests commonly performed for those at risk are chorionic villi sampling (CVS) and amniocentesis.

In the second trimester, tests commonly performed include targeted ultrasound and screening for Down syndrome, trisomy 18, and open neural tube defects. Couples who learn of an increased risk through a second-trimester test tend to be significantly more anxious than those who learned of the risk earlier in the pregnancy. In general, couples should attempt to receive genetic counseling and testing while they still have the legal option to terminate the pregnancy.

 TALKING POINTS You have a concern that makes you want to get genetic and prenatal counseling, but your partner balks at this suggestion. How can you get a dialogue going so that you can change his or her mind about this?

Infertility

Most traditional-age college students are interested in preventing pregnancy. However, increasing numbers of other people are trying to do just the opposite: They are trying to become pregnant. It is estimated that about one in six couples has a problem with *infertility*. These couples wish to become pregnant but are unsuccessful.

Causes of Infertility

What causes infertility? About 40 percent of infertility problems are attributed to male factors and about 40 percent are explained by female factors. Approximately 10 percent of the problems stem from a combination of female and male factors, while the remaining 10 percent come from unknown origins.[16]

Problems of infertility that may come from males include low sperm count, inability of the sperm to move properly, or structural abnormalities of the sperm. Female factors related to infertility center on lack of ovulation and obstructions in the fallopian tubes.

Enhancing Fertility

A number of approaches can be used to increase sperm counts. Among the simple approaches are the application of periodic cold packs on the scrotum and the replacement of tight underwear with boxer shorts. When a structural problem reduces sperm production, surgery can be helpful. Most experts (reproductive endocrinologists) suggest that couples have intercourse at least a couple of times in the week preceding ovulation. Frequent intercourse tends to lower sperm counts, so couples should not have sex more than every 36 hours.[17]

Artificial Insemination

Men can also collect (through masturbation) and save samples of their sperm to use in a procedure called *artificial insemination by partner*. Near the time of ovulation, the collected samples of sperm are deposited near the woman's cervical opening. In a related procedure called *artificial insemination by donor*, the sperm of a donor are used. Donor semen is screened for the presence of pathogens, including the AIDS virus.

Surgical Remedies

Causes of infertility in women center mostly on obstructions in the reproductive tract and the inability to ovulate. The obstructions frequently result from tissue damage (scarring) caused by infections. Chlamydial and gonorrheal infections often produce fertility problems. In certain women the use of IUDs has produced infections and PID; both of these increase the chances of infertility.

Key Terms
teratogenic agent any substance that is capable of causing birth defects

Other possible causes of structural abnormalities include scar tissue from previous surgery, fibroid tumors, polyps, and endometriosis. A variety of microsurgical techniques may correct some of these complications.

One of the most recent innovative procedures involves the use of **transcervical balloon tuboplasty.** In this procedure a series of balloon-tipped catheters are inserted through the uterus into the blocked fallopian tubes. After they are inflated, these balloon catheters help open the scarred passageways.

When a woman has ovulation difficulties, pinpointing the specific cause can be very difficult. Increasing age produces hormone fluctuations associated with lack of ovulation. Being significantly overweight or underweight also has a serious effect on fertility. However, in women of normal weight who are not approaching menopause, it appears that ovulation difficulties are caused by failure of synchronization between the hormones governing the menstrual cycle. Fertility drugs can help alter the menstrual cycle to produce ovulation. Clomiphene citrate (Clomid), in oral pill form, or injections of a mixture of luteinizing hormone (LH) and follicle-stimulating hormone (FSH) taken from the urine of menopausal women (Pergonal) are the most common fertility drugs available. Both are capable of producing multiple ova at ovulation.

Assisted Reproductive Technology (ART)

For couples who are unable to conceive after drug therapy, surgery, and artificial insemination, the use of one of four assisted reproductive technologies (ART) can be helpful. One option is *in vitro fertilization and embryo transfer (IVF-ET).* This method is sometimes referred to as the "test tube" procedure. Costing around $10,000 per attempt, IVF-ET consists of surgically retrieving fertilizable ova from the woman and combining them in a glass dish with sperm. After several days, the fertilized ova are transferred into the uterus. IVF-ET accounts for 98 percent of all ART procedures.[18]

A second test tube procedure is called *gamete intrafallopian transfer (GIFT).* Similar to IVF-ET, this procedure deposits a mixture of retrieved eggs and sperm directly into the fallopian tubes.

Fertilized ova (zygotes) can also be transferred from a laboratory dish into the fallopian tubes in a procedure called *zygote intrafallopian transfer (ZIFT).* One advantage of this procedure is that the clinicians are certain that ova have been fertilized before the transfer to the fallopian tubes. GIFT and ZIFT combined account for fewer than 2 percent of ART procedures.[18]

The fourth (and newest) procedure is *intracytoplasmic sperm injection (ICSI).* This is a laboratory procedure in which a single sperm cell is injected into a woman's retrieved egg. The fertilized egg is then transplanted into the woman's uterus. The cost and technical expertise involved in ICSI make it a seldom-used procedure for infertile couples.

Surrogate Parenting

Surrogate parenting is another option that has been explored, although the legal and ethical issues surrounding this method of conception have not been fully resolved. Surrogate parenting can take several forms. Typically, an infertile couple makes a contract with a woman (the surrogate parent), who will then be artificially inseminated with semen from the expectant father. In some instances the surrogate receives an embryo from the donor parents. The surrogate carries the fetus to term and returns the newborn to the parents. In some cases, women have served as surrogates for their close relatives. Because of the concerns about true "ownership" of the baby, surrogate parenting may not be a particularly viable or legal option for many couples.

Options for Infertile Couples

The process of coping with infertility problems can be an emotionally stressful experience for a couple. Hours of waiting in physicians' offices, undergoing many examinations, scheduling intercourse, producing sperm samples, and undergoing surgical or drug treatments place multiple burdens on a couple. Knowing that other couples are able to conceive so effortlessly adds to the mental strain. Fortunately, support groups have been established to assist couples with infertility problems. (Some of these groups are listed in the Star box on page 527.)

What can you do to reduce the chances of developing infertility problems? Avoiding sexually transmitted diseases is one crucial factor. Barrier methods of contraception (condom, diaphragm) with a spermicide reportedly cut the risk of developing infertility in half. The risk from multiple partners should encourage responsible sexual activity. Men and women should avoid working around hazardous chemicals or using psychoactive drugs. Being overweight or underweight, smoking, and heavy alcohol consumption are risk factors that reduce one's fertility.[19] Maintaining overall good health and having regular medical (and, for women, gynecological) checkups are good ideas. Because infertility is directly linked with advancing age, couples may not want to indefinitely delay having children.

Key Terms

transcervical balloon tuboplasty the use of inflatable balloon catheters to open blocked fallopian tubes; a procedure used for some women with fertility problems

Where to Find Help for Infertility and Adoption

These agencies can provide you with information about infertility and give referrals to specialists in your area:

American Society for Reproductive Medicine
1209 Montgomery Highway
Birmingham, AL 35216-2809
(205) 978-5000

www.asrm.com

Planned Parenthood Federation of America
434 West 33rd Street
New York, NY 10001
(800) 230-7526

www.plannedparenthood.org

RESOLVE
7910 Woodmont Ave.
Suite 1350
Bethesda, MD 20814
(301) 652-8585

www.resolve.org

These agencies can provide help to prospective adoptive parents:

The National Adoption Center
1500 Walnut Street, Suite 701
Philadelphia, PA 19102
1-800-TO-ADOPT

www.adopt.org

The National Council for Adoption
225 N. Washington Street
Alexandria, VA 22314-2561
(703) 299-6633

www.ncfa-usa.org

The North American Council on Adoptable Children
970 Raymond Ave. Suite 106
St. Paul, MN 55114
(651) 644-3036

www.nacac.org

Adoption

For couples who have determined that biological childbirth is impossible, adoption offers an alternative. Adopted children currently represent about 2 percent of all children in the United States.

As the supply of adoptable infants has decreased, young women considering putting their babies up for adoption have gained new leverage. Couples determined to adopt a healthy infant have increasingly turned to independent adoptions arranged by a lawyer, or they may negotiate directly with the birth mother. Independent adoptions now surpass those arranged by social service agencies.

Adoption is now a viable option for most adults. In the past, many states permitted only wealthy, heterosexual, young or midlife married couples to adopt children or become foster parents. Now, in many states, single persons can legally adopt children. Single gay and lesbian persons also can adopt. (See Eye on the Media about Rosie O'Donnell on page 510.) Same-sex couples may also adopt in many areas of the country. (Visit the nonprofit organization www.familieslikeours.org Web site for more information.)

The most important factors in adoption seem to be the ability of the adopting person or couple to be able to provide a stable, safe, and positive environment with sufficient space for the child. Adequate income is important, but being wealthy is not a requirement. (To find out more about adoption, visit www.naic.acf.hhs.gov, www.adopt.org, and www.davethomasfoundation.org.)

Foster Parenting

The number of children in foster care who are waiting to be reunited with their biological parents or awaiting adoption has risen steadily since the mid-1980s. Experts attribute the rise to family problems caused by parental drug abuse, unemployment, alcoholism, and other difficulties. Currently about one-half million children a year spend time in foster homes.

Like adoption, foster parenting has presented a variety of ethical and legal issues, especially the debate between "the best interests of the child" and parental rights.

TALKING POINTS You have tried for a couple of years to get pregnant, and now you are ready to consider some of the newest options to increase the chances of conception. Your partner seems unwilling to spend much money for these high-tech procedures. You are ready to spend some of your retirement savings in this effort. How can you and your partner best come to an agreement on this issue?

Taking Charge of Your Health

- Use the Personal Assessment on page 531 to help you think about your feelings about parenting.

- Talk to your partner (or roommate) about any ethical concerns that you think might be involved in human cloning.

- With the accuracy that exists with home pregnancy tests, do you envision yourself ever using one?

- If you are pregnant or think you might be pregnant, challenge yourself to avoid any agents that might damage your fetus.

- If you plan to become a parent one day, choose lifestyle behaviors that will enhance (not reduce) your fertility.

SUMMARY

- Couples have many important issues to discuss before deciding to have children.
- Having children through human cloning raises many ethical issues.
- Parents in stepfamilies face challenges as children merge into different living arrangements.
- Several physiological factors can be either aids or obstacles to fertilization.
- Women can often recognize the presumptive and probable signs of pregnancy; a physician can determine positive signs of pregnancy.
- Expectant fathers can experience many of the same symptoms and emotions as expectant mothers.
- Pregnant women, and women attempting to become pregnant, should avoid agents that can damage the fetus, including all drugs (prescription, over-the-counter, and illicit), tobacco smoke, and alcohol.

- The 9 months of pregnancy can be divided into three trimesters. The fetal growth and development during each trimester is unique.
- Childbirth takes place in three distinct stages: effacement and dilation of the cervix, delivery of the fetus, and delivery of the placenta.
- Complications during pregnancy and delivery are varied and can be caused by genetics, environmental factors, or a combination of these.
- Regular prenatal care is vital and can help prevent or reverse complications of pregnancy.
- Genetic and prenatal counseling can provide much information to prospective parents.
- For couples with fertility problems, numerous strategies can be used to help conception take place.

REVIEW QUESTIONS

1. What important issues should couples discuss before they decide to have children?
2. What is the difference between human cloning and therapeutic cloning?
3. How would you define the term *stepfamily*?
4. What are some obstacles and aids to fertilization presented in this chapter? Can you think of others?
5. What are the presumptive, probable, and positive signs of pregnancy?
6. Briefly describe the changes in intrauterine development during each trimester.
7. Identify and describe the events that occur during each of the three stages of childbirth. Approximately how long is each stage?

8. Who should seek genetic counseling? How can the counselor assess the couple's risk of having a child with birth defects?
9. What is meant by the term *genetic and prenatal counseling*?
10. List and describe several complications that can occur during pregnancy and delivery.
11. What can be done to reduce chances of infertility?
12. Explain the IVF-ET, GIFT, ZIFT, and ICSI procedures.
13. What options do couples have when they cannot conceive a child?

ENDNOTES

1. Bonsor K. *How Human Cloning Will Work,* www.science. howstuffworks.com/human-cloning.htm, September 24, 2003.
2. DeNoon D. *Cloning FAQs and Fiction,* www.my.webmd. com/content/article/57/66221.htm, September 24, 2003.
3. Warner J. *Most Americans Against Human Cloning,* www.my.webmd.com/content/article/59/66746.htm, September 24, 2003.
4. *Cloning scientist: Forgive me.* www.cnn.com (11 January 2006), accessed 17 January 2006.

5. Stepfamily Association of America. *Stepfamily Fact Sheet,* www.stepfamilies.org, September 23, 2003.

6. Purnell LD, Paulanka BJ. *Transcultural Health Care: A Culturally Competent Approach* (2nd ed.). Philadelphia: F. A. Davis, 2003.

7. Hatcher RA et al. *Contraceptive Technology* (18th ed.). New York: Ardent Media, Inc., 2004.

8. Hyde JS, DeLameter JD. *Understanding Human Sexuality* (9th ed.). New York: McGraw-Hill, 2006.

9. Wardlaw GM, Hampl JS, Disilvestro RA. *Perspectives in Nutrition* (6th ed.). New York: McGraw-Hill, 2003.

10. Allgeier EA, Allgeier AR. *Sexual Interactions* (5th ed.). New York: Houghton Mifflin, 2000.

11. LeVay S, Valente SM. *Human Sexuality.* Sunderland, MA: Sinauer Associates, Inc., 2003.

12. Kelly GF. *Sexuality Today: The Human Perspective* (8th ed.). New York: McGraw-Hill, 2006.

13. Strong B, DeVault C, Sayad BW, Yarber WL. *Human Sexuality: Diversity in Contemporary America* (5th ed.). New York: McGraw-Hill, 2005.

14. Hamilton BE, Martin JA, Sutton PD. Births: Preliminary data for 2003. (CDC: National Center for Health Statistics) *National Vital Statistics Reports* 53(9), November 23, 2004, p. 6.

15. Kuller JA, Chescheir NC, Cefalo RC. *Prenatal Diagnosis and Reproductive Genetics.* St. Louis: Mosby-Year Book, 1996.

16. McAnulty RD, Burnette MM. *Exploring Human Sexuality: Making Healthy Decisions* (2nd ed.). Boston: Allyn & Bacon, 2004.

17. WebMd. *Health Guide A–Z: Infertility—Home Treatment,* www.my.webmd.com/content/healthwise/130/32439, October 2, 2003.

18. WebMd. *A Couple's Guide: Trying to Conceive,* www.my.webmd.com/content/article/73/87996, October 3, 2003.

19. RESOLVE. *Preserving Your Fertility: Risk Factors,* www.resolve.org/, October 8, 2003.

personal assessment

How do you feel about parenting?

Respond to each of the following items based on your own opinions about parenting. Circle the letters that best match your response.

SA   **Strongly agree**
A   **Agree**
U   **Undecided**
D   **Disagree**
SD   **Strongly disagree**

1. One cannot parent successfully without, at the same time, being a generally successful adult member of the community.   SA   A   U   D   SD
2. It is inappropriate to view parenting as a method of achieving immortality.   SA   A   U   D   SD
3. Parenting requires that one be willing to make major personal sacrifices for the benefit of the child.   SA   A   U   D   SD
4. Parenting adds a large measure of vitality to an adult's life.   SA   A   U   D   SD
5. Parenting demands greater creativity than any other adult pursuit.   SA   A   U   D   SD
6. A person who cannot comfortably make decisions for others should not consider parenting.   SA   A   U   D   SD
7. A family cannot exist in the absence of children.   SA   A   U   D   SD

To Carry This Further . . .

After completing this personal assessment, join three of your classmates in comparing and discussing your responses. What suggestions were made to help increase your awareness of all that parenting involves?

Consumer and Safety Issues

Part Six includes chapters on consumer health and safety. The decisions you make in each of these areas can have a profound effect on your well-being in each dimension of your health.

1. **Physical Dimension**
   The physical dimension of health is directly influenced by consumer decisions, such as the physician you choose. And, of course, it is crucial to learn how to protect yourself from physical harm caused by intentional or unintentional injury.

2. **Emotional Dimension**
   The effect of an overcrowded, highly industrialized society on your emotional health is often evident. Yet an even more powerful influence is the potential for violence or unintentional injury. Many people who are rape survivors or victims of other crimes feel fearful or angry for years afterward. Those who have behaved violently themselves may find that the knowledge of their actions erodes their emotional health.

3. **Social Dimension**
   Good health care consumers are made, not born. The decisions you make about your health are shaped by many people. Your doctor, for example, may give you information about behavior change, or your insurance agent may offer you several managed care options from which to choose. Effective interaction with these professionals and many other people can help you meet your health care needs.

4. **Intellectual Dimension**
   Understanding violence-related issues and consumer options requires critical thinking skills. Isolating causes of safety-related problems and devising workable solutions are complex tasks. In addition, you must be able to analyze a number of variables to make difficult decisions about your health.

5. **Spiritual Dimension**
   Nurturing our spirituality and caring for the well-being of others are inextricably intertwined. As we search for solutions to complex social and health-related issues, we must often make difficult decisions: For example, will we someday deny health insurance coverage to persons based on the existence of high-risk health behaviors such as tobacco use and a sedentary lifestyle? Or, might we someday legally define smoking by parents as a form of child abuse? To build a better world for future generations may be the most serious challenge to our spiritual commitment to serve others.

6. **Occupational Dimension**
   Your occupational health can be enhanced by making sound decisions about your health care and personal safety. For example, choosing a health care provider who emphasizes prevention and positive behavior change will promote your overall well-being and minimize the number of days you are unable to work because of illness. In addition, avoiding intentional and unintentional injuries will allow you to perform at your peak.

chapter eighteen

Becoming an Informed Health Care Consumer

Chapter Objectives

On completing this chapter, you will be able to:

▌ identify several sources of reliable health information available to American consumers.

▌ be able to discuss health information found on the Internet with your health care provider.

▌ explain the role of the primary care physician as it relates to diagnosis, treatment, screening, consultation, and prevention.

▌ compare and contrast the medical training received by doctors of medicine with that received by doctors of osteopathy.

▌ explain the subtle but important differences between alternative medicine, integrative medicine, and complementary medicine.

▌ write a letter to your state legislator encouraging increased funding for home health care in your state, discussing both the advantages and disadvantages of these services in comparison to nursing home care.

▌ identify hospitals in your community and categorize them as public, voluntary, or private.

▌ describe the student health insurance plans available at your college or university, with details on deductibles, copayments, fixed indemnity, and exclusions.

▌ talk to friends and family about their level of satisfaction with their own health care coverage.

▌ evaluate the health claims of various dietary supplements.

Eye on the Media

The Internet—Your Health Superstore

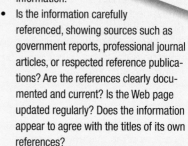

According to data collected by the Pew Internet & American Life Project (July 16, 2003), approximately 93 million Americans use the Internet as a source of health-related information. Most frequently, online users seek information regarding specific medical problems, followed by information regarding aspects of treatment and longer term management of these problems. The use of the Internet for health-related purposes is, however, not a daily occurrence for most Americans with Internet access. When the Internet is used for this purpose, women are more likely to be seeking information than are men, and they most often do so for other persons (spouses, children, and friends). If you are not already, it is highly probable that you too will be an online consumer of health-related information, products, or services.

The biggest challenge for you as a health consumer is determining the credibility of the information you find on the Internet. How can you know that this information (and accompanying products or services) is trustworthy and that the persons responsible for the information, products, or services are motivated by concern for your health and well-being rather than just by profit? Recognized authorities offer these guidelines to help you:

• Who does the Web site belong to? Is it sponsored by an institution of higher education, a professional society, a government or not-for-profit agency, or a recognized pharmaceutical company? If not, who is responsible for the information? Remember, virtually anyone can develop a web

page and begin disseminating information.

• Is the information carefully referenced, showing sources such as government reports, professional journal articles, or respected reference publications? Are the references clearly documented and current? Is the Web page updated regularly? Does the information appear to agree with the titles of its own references?

• Does the content of the information seem to have a critical or negative bias toward a particular profession, institution, or treatment method? Does the information discredit others more than it supports its own position?

• Are "significant breakthroughs" promised in a way that suggests that only this source has the "ultimate answer" to certain problems? Does this answer involve throwing out your prescriptions, going against your physician's orders, or considering suicide as a way of escaping the pain and difficulties associated with your illness?

If you are skeptical about the credibility of any health care information you find online, submit the information to a respected health care professional or organization for assessment. If you and your physician find suspicious information or fraudulent health claims, report this to the Federal Trade Commission. Today, most health care practitioners feel comfortable with well-informed patients. Many will welcome the

Health care providers often evaluate you by criteria from their areas of expertise. The nutritionist knows you by the food you eat. The physical fitness professional knows you by your body type and activity level. In the eyes of the expert in health consumerism, you are the product of the health information you believe, the health-influencing services you use, and the products you consume. When you make your decisions about health information, services, and products after careful study and consideration, your health will probably be improved. However, when your decisions lack insight, your health, as well as your pocketbook, may suffer.

Health Information

The Informed Consumer

As mentioned in *Eye on the Media* on page 534, the Pew Charitable Trust's on-going study of Internet use (Internet & American Life Project)[1] provides current information on health-related Internet use. The breadth of this interest is informative. Of the 93 million Americans who conducted health-related searches, 63 percent of the searchers sought information pertaining to specific conditions and problems, 47 percent to treatment and management of conditions, 44 percent to nutrition and diet, 36 percent to exercise and fitness, 34 percent to prescription medications and over-the-counter (OTC) products, and 28 percent to alternative treatments. Further, 25 percent sought information regarding health insurance, 17 percent investigated environmental health issues, and 10 percent pursued sexual health information. Among the 16 areas searched, only 8 percent sought information pertaining to drug and alcohol use, whereas 6 percent investigated information pertaining to smoking cessation, the area least visited.

In light of the breadth of these interest areas and the complexity associated with each, it is very likely that most people turn to a variety of sources for the information and access that they seek. Some sources are easily accessed, while others are more difficult to find but perhaps contain more appropriate information. In the section that follows you will be introduced to several sources of health-related information. (Complete the Personal Assessment on page 563 to rate your own skills as a consumer of health-related information, products, and services.)

Sources of Information

Your sources of information on health topics are as diverse as the number of people you know, the number of publications you read, and the number of experts you see or hear. No single agency or profession regulates the quantity or quality of the health-related information you receive. Readers will quickly recognize that all are familiar sources and that some provide more accurate and honest information than others.

Family and Friends

The accuracy of information you get from a friend or family member may be questionable. Too often the information your family and friends offer is based on "common knowledge" that is wrong. In addition, family members or friends may provide information they believe is in your best interest rather than facts that may have a more negative effect on you.

Unfortunately, some family members and friends today also might give biased health information because they are participating in a pyramid-type sales organization that sells health products. Some people might urge you to use a particular line of food supplements or vitamins or even ask you to join their sales team.

Advertisements and Commercials

Many people spend much of every day watching television, listening to the radio, and reading newspapers or magazines. Because many advertisements are health oriented, these are significant sources of information. The primary purpose of advertising, however, is to sell products or services. One newer example of this intertwining of health information with marketing is the "infomercial," in which a compensated studio audience watches a skillfully produced program that trumpets the benefits of a particular product or service. In spite of the convincing nature of these infomercials, however, the validity of their information is often questionable. This was the case in 2000 when the FTC ordered the producers of The Enforma System for weight loss—*Fat Trapper* and *Exercise in a Bottle*—to repay customers $10 million for having used spurious information in selling their product.

In contrast to advertisements and commercials, the mass media routinely offer public service messages, as mandated by the FCC, that give valuable health-related information. For example, the FCC ordered antismoking public-service announcements on television following the release of the first Surgeon General's Report on Smoking and Health (1964). These ads were powerful players in fostering a significant drop in smoking during the late 1960s and the 1970s.

Labels and Directions

Federal law requires that many consumer product labels, including all medications and many kinds of food (see Chapter 5), contain specific information. For example, when a pharmacist dispenses a prescription medication, he or she must give a detailed information sheet describing the medication.

Many health care providers and agencies give consumers informative information about their health problems or printed directions for preparing for screening procedures. Generally, information from these sources is accurate and current and is given with the health of the consumer foremost in mind.

Folklore

Because it is passed down from generation to generation, folklore about health is the primary source of health-related information for some people.

The accuracy of health-related information obtained from family members, neighbors, and coworkers is difficult to evaluate. As a general rule, however, one should exercise caution relying on its scientific soundness. A blanket dismissal is not warranted, however, because folk wisdom is occasionally supported by scientific evidence. In addition, the emotional support provided by the suppliers of this information could be the best medicine some people could receive. In fact, for some ethnic groups, indigenous health care is central to overall health care. For example, within the Chinese American community, practitioners of traditional healing arts represent primary health care. Even though many Americans would consider this form of care "folk medicine," it is highly valued and trusted by those who find it familiar. Additionally, what would be considered folklore represents important sources of dependable and valid health information to members of this ethnic group.

Testimonials

People eagerly want to share information that has benefited them. Others may base their decisions on such testimonials. However, the exaggerated testimonials that accompany the sales pitches of the medical quack or the "satisfied" customers appearing in advertisements and on commer-

cials and infomercials should never be interpreted as valid endorsements.

Mass Media

Health programming on cable television stations, stories in lifestyle sections of newspapers, health care correspondents appearing on national network news shows, and the growing number of health-oriented magazines are sources of health information in the mass media.

In terms of the public's priority for specific media sources of health information, a gradual evolution is occurring. As recently as 1999, television, followed by magazines and newspapers, were the three principal sources of health-related news for American adults.[2] Now, with more than 110 million Americans having cable or phone access, these traditional sources of information are gradually losing popularity to the Internet. Most likely this trend will continue until a new information-sharing technology moves into the mainstream of American life.

Health-related information in the mass media is generally accurate, but it is sometimes presented so quickly or superficially that its usefulness is limited. The consumer who wants more complete coverage of a health topic might acquire it by subscribing to a cable channel devoted partly or entirely to health-related programming, such as the Discovery Health Channel or The Learning Channel.

Practitioners

The health care consumer also receives much information from individual health practitioners and their professional associations. In fact, today's health care practitioner so clearly emphasizes patient education that finding one who does not offer some information to a patient would be difficult. Education improves patient **compliance** with health care directives, which is important to the practitioner and the consumer.

Another important development in the trend toward patient education is the evolution of the hospital as an educational institution. Because the American Medical Association advocates patient education activities in hospitals, wellness centers, and other health facilities, it now refuses to endorse health products with its logo, which would create a conflict of interest.

Online Computer Services

We have already discussed the rapidly growing utilization of the Internet as a primary source of health-related

---

Key Terms

compliance willingness to follow the directions provided by another person

---

information. We have even, in a sense, concluded that you are or would be one of those users. This assumption may not, however, be as predictable as we believe. In fact, a study reported in 2003 concluded that the use of the Internet for accessing health-related information had been overstated in previous studies, perhaps by a factor of three.[3] In yet another study in which persons who were unable to afford Internet access were provided it at no cost, less than 25 percent accessed health information.[4] A similarly low level of Internet use was reported for persons who were afflicted with one of five major adult chronic conditions—although those who did access information about their illnesses reported that it was very helpful.[5]

In spite of these somewhat conflicting research results regarding the Internet as a principal source of the health information, an important question remains to be answered:

How should health-related information gleaned from the Internet be used, particularly when communicating with health care providers? Howard LeWine, MD, offers the following suggestions:

- Inform your health care provider that you are accessing the Internet for information related to your particular area of concern. Know the name of the site you're using; your provider might already be familiar with the site, or wish to access it in preparation for your discussion.

- Do not bombard your provider with questions whenever you come across information that might be related to your health concern. Keep notes and discuss all of your findings at one time.

- Be prepared to *discuss* your information with your provider; don't use Web information to second-guess his or her position. Bear in mind that health concerns are too complex to generalize from the kind of one-size-fits-all information provided by even the most reliable Web sites, and they must be evaluated on a case-by-case basis by a physician who has actually examined you.

- Always recognize that health-related information involves knowledge from many disciplines and uses highly technical language; media-based sources may grossly oversimplify in an effort to be accessible to lay persons.

 TALKING POINTS A family member considers herself good at diagnosing health problems. Since she hasn't been wrong in years, she no longer relies on physicians. What questions could you ask her to point out the dangers associated with her approach?

Health Reference Publications

A substantial portion of all households own or subscribe to a health reference publication, such as the *Encyclopedia of Complementary Health Practices,* the *Physicians' Desk Reference* (PDR), or a newsletter such as *The Harvard Medical School Health Letter* or *The Johns Hopkins Medical Letter: Health after 50.* Some consumers also use personal computer programs and videocassettes or CDs featuring health-related information.

Reference Libraries

Public and university libraries continue to be popular sources of health-related information. One can consult with reference librarians and check out audiovisual collections and printed materials. More and more of these holdings can be accessed through the home computer.

Consumer Advocacy Groups

A variety of nonprofit consumer advocacy groups patrol the health care marketplace. These groups produce and distribute information designed to help the consumer recognize questionable services and products. Large, well-organized groups, such as The National Consumers' League and Consumers Union, and smaller groups at the state and local levels champion the right of the consumer to receive valid and reliable information about health care products and services.

Voluntary Health Agencies

Volunteerism and the traditional approach to health care and health promotion are virtually inseparable. Few countries besides the United States can boast so many national voluntary organizations, with state and local affiliates, dedicated to improving health through research, service, and public education. The American Cancer Society, the American Red Cross, and the American Heart Association all are voluntary (not-for-profit) health agencies. Consumers can, in fact, expect to find a voluntary health agency for virtually every health problem. College students should also note that volunteerism on their part, perhaps with a health agency like the Red Cross or the AHA, is both a personally satisfying experience and an activity viewed favorably by potential employers.

Government Agencies

Government agencies are also effective sources of information to the public. Through meetings and the release of information to the media, agencies such as the Food and Drug Administration, Federal Trade Commission, United States Postal Service, and Environmental Protection Agency publicize health issues. Government agencies also control the quality of information sent out to the buying public, particularly through labeling, advertising, and the distribution of information through the mail. The various divisions of the National Institutes of Health regularly release research findings and recommendations to clinical practices, which in turn reach the consumer through clinical practitioners.

Despite their best intentions, federal health agencies are often less effective than the public deserves. A variety of factors, including inadequate staff, poor administration, lobbying by special interest groups, and political pressures prevent these federal agencies from enforcing consumer-protection legislation. As a result, the public is left with a sense of false confidence in the consumer protection provided by the federal government.

State governments also distribute health-related information to the public. State agencies are primary sources of information, particularly in the areas of public health and environmental protection. (For an example of health care activism at work, see Learning from Our Diversity on page 539.)

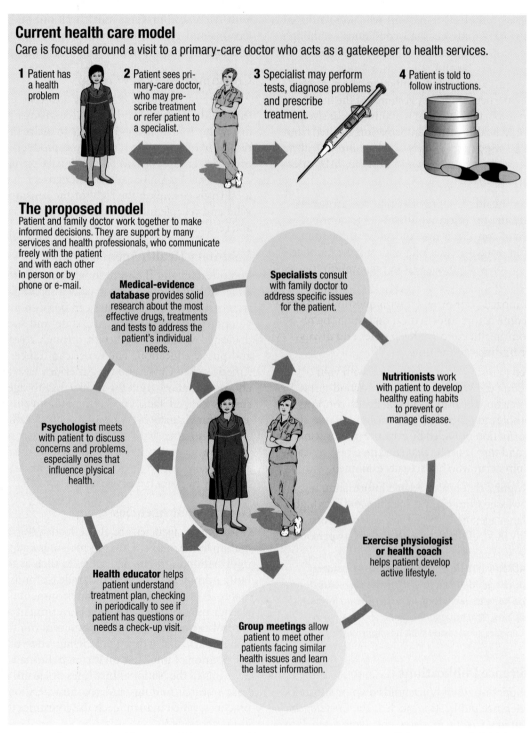

Current health care model
Care is focused around a visit to a primary-care doctor who acts as a gatekeeper to health services.

1 Patient has a health problem

2 Patient sees primary-care doctor, who may prescribe treatment or refer patient to a specialist.

3 Specialist may perform tests, diagnose problems and prescribe treatment.

4 Patient is told to follow instructions.

The proposed model
Patient and family doctor work together to make informed decisions. They are support by many services and health professionals, who communicate freely with the patient and with each other in person or by phone or e-mail.

Medical-evidence database provides solid research about the most effective drugs, treatments and tests to address the patient's individual needs.

Specialists consult with family doctor to address specific issues for the patient.

Nutritionists work with patient to develop healthy eating habits to prevent or manage disease.

Psychologist meets with patient to discuss concerns and problems, especially ones that influence physical health.

Exercise physiologist or health coach helps patient develop active lifestyle.

Health educator helps patient understand treatment plan, checking in periodically to see if patient has questions or needs a check-up visit.

Group meetings allow patient to meet other patients facing similar health issues and learn the latest information.

Compare the current health care model in the United States to a proposed model of health care.

Qualified Health Educators

Health educators work in a variety of settings and offer their services to diverse groups. Community health educators work with virtually all of the agencies mentioned in this section; patient educators function in primary care settings; and school health educators are found at all educational levels. Health educators are increasingly being employed in a wide range of wellness-based programs in community, hospital, corporate, and school settings.

Health Care Providers

The sources of health information just discussed can greatly help us make decisions as informed consumers. The choices we make about physicians, health services, and medical payment plans reflect our commitment to remaining healthy and our trust in specific people who are trained in keeping us healthy. (Refer to Changing for the Better on pages 540 and 541 for tips on choosing a physician and a hospital.)

Why We Consult Health Care Providers

Most of us seek care and advice from medical and health practitioners when we have a specific problem. A bad cold, a broken arm, or a newly discovered lump can motivate us to consult a health care professional. Yet *diagnosis* and *treatment* are only two reasons that we might require the services of health care providers.

We also might encounter health practitioners when we undergo *screening.* Screening most often involves a

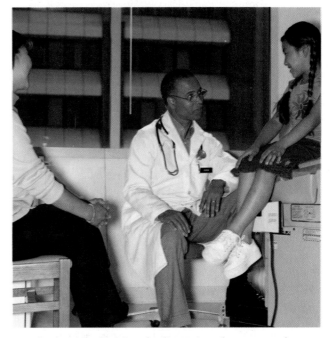

We often consult physicians for diagnosis and treatment of common ailments.

cursory (or noninvasive) collection of information that can quickly be compared to established standards often based on gender, age, race, or the presence of preexisting conditions. Your earliest experience with screening may have been in elementary school, where physicians, nurses, audiologists, and dentists sometimes examine all children for normal growth and development patterns. As an adult, your screening is more likely to be done on an individual basis by a physician's staff as a routine portion of every office visit when they collect baseline information such as height, weight, and blood pressure measurements. You may also encounter community-based screening when you stop at your local shopping mall's health fair and have your blood pressure taken or cholesterol checked. In both settings, the extent to which your data becomes incorporated into a larger data pool determines whether this screening is community-based or simply personally informing. Although screening should be considered much less precise than actual diagnosis, screening serves to identify people who should seek further medical examination.

Consultation is a fourth reason that knowledgeable consumers seek health care providers. A consultation is the use of two or more professionals to deliberate a person's specific health problem or condition. Consultations are especially helpful when **primary care health providers,** such as family practice physicians, gynecologists, pediatricians, internists, and general practice dentists, require the opinion of specialists. Using additional practitioners as consultants can also help reassure patients who may have doubts about their own condition or about the abilities of their physician.

Prevention is a fifth reason we might seek a health care provider. With the current emphasis on trying to stop problems before they begin, using health care providers for prevention is becoming more common. People want information about how to prevent needless risks and promote their health, and they seek such advice from physicians, nurses, dentists, exercise physiologists, patient educators, and other health promotion specialists.

When prevention becomes a routine component of your personal health care, you will annually receive, in addition to the baseline measurements of height, weight, and blood pressure, more in-depth assessments such as a blood chemistry assessment, lipid profile, and cardiogram.

Key Terms

primary care health providers health care providers who generally see patients on a routine basis, particularly for preventive health care

Women will also likely receive a ViraPap test, breast examination, mammography, and pelvic examination, while men will likely receive a Prostate Specific Antibody (PSA) test, digital prostate examination, and testicular examination.

Physicians and Their Training

In every city and many smaller communities, the local telephone directory lists physicians in a variety of medical specialties. These health care providers hold the academic degree of Doctor of Medicine (MD) or Doctor of Osteopathy (DO).

At one time, **allopathy** and **osteopathy** were clearly different health care professions in terms of their healing philosophies and modes of practice. Today, however, MDs and DOs receive similar educations and engage in very similar forms of practice. Both can function as primary care physicians or as board-certified specialists. Their differences are in the osteopathic physician's greater tendency to use manipulation in treating health problems. In addition, DOs often perceive themselves as being more holistically oriented than MDs are.

Medical and osteopathic physicians undergo a long training process. They usually take 4 years of initial undergraduate preparation with a heavy emphasis on the sciences—biology, chemistry, mathematics, anatomy, and physiology. Most undergraduate schools have preprofessional courses of study for students interested in medical or osteopathic schools.

After they are accepted into professional schools, students generally spend 4 or more years in intensive training that includes advanced study in the preclinical medical sciences and clinical practice. When they complete this phase of training, the students are awarded the MD or DO degree and then take the state medical license examination. Most newly licensed physicians complete a residency at a hospital. Residency programs vary in length from 3 to 4 years. When they conclude their residency programs, including board-related examinations, physicians are granted board-certified status. In addition to state and specialty board certification, comprehensive national certification of physicians is a frequently discussed possibility. At this time, no nationally required and all-encompassing certification of physician competency is required. Note, however, that with the advent of the Internet, something approaching this type of information is available through Web sites such as *HealthGrade*, described in Changing for the Better, on page 540.

Communication between Patients and Their Health Care Providers

In the complex world of modern health care, it is of critical importance that patients communicate important information to their health care providers and, in turn, that

---

Key Terms

allopathy (ah **lop** ah thee) a system of medical practice in which specific remedies (often pharmaceutical agents) are used to produce effects different from those produced by a disease or injury

osteopathy (os tee **op** ah thee) a system of medical practice in which allopathic principles are combined with specific attention to postural mechanics of the body they understand as fully as possible the information they receive from their providers. Below are 10 valuable suggestions from the Joint Commission on Accreditation of Healthcare Organizations and the U.S. Government's Agency for Healthcare Research and Quality.

- Take part in every decision about your health care.

- If you are not prepared to ask questions on your behalf, ask a family member or friend to fill this role for you.

- Tell your physician and pharmacist about every drug you are taking, including prescription drugs, OTC drugs, vitamins, supplements, and herbal products—bring them with you.

- Make certain that you get the results of every test, and understand what they mean.

- If you do not hear about test results, never assume that everything is all right. Call your doctor and ask.

- Whenever possible, choose a hospital where many patients receive the same procedure that you are to receive. Ask your physician or the hospital for the numbers of procedures performed.

- Ask hospital personnel if they have washed their hands before they begin touching you.

- If you are having surgery, make sure that you, your physician, and your surgeon all agree on what will be done during the operation.

- Insist that your surgeon write his or her initials or words such as "yes" or "this side" on the part of the body to be operated on. Put "no" on the opposite body part.

- When you are discharged, ask your doctor to explain your treatment plan, including changes in medications, restrictions on activity, and additional therapies you will need.

In many situations involving medical care, carefully communicated comments and questions between providers and patients can be the basis of the successful resolution of a health problem, as opposed to unnecessary delay, pain, discomfort, or even death.

Complementary, Alternative, and Integrative Care Practitioners

In addition to medical and osteopathic physicians, several other forms of health care offer alternatives within the large health care market. Included within this group of complementary or alternative forms of practice are chiropractic, acupuncture, homeopathy, naturopathy, herbalism, reflexology, and ayurveda.[6] (Also, see Considering Complementary Care on page 543 for a discussion on therapeutic touch.) Although the traditional medical community has long scoffed at these fields of practice as ineffective and un-

scientific, many people use these forms of health care and believe strongly that they are as effective as (or more effective than) allopathic and osteopathic medicine. As a result of this belief, today many physicians are better informed about complementary care methods and more comfortable discussing them with patients. Following are brief descriptions of some of the more popular of these complementary care fields and the practitioners that function within them. (Also reread Considering Complementary Care on page 13 of Chapter 1, which discusses the controversial nature of various fields of complementary or alternative care.)

Chiropractic

Historically (and, to varying degrees, today) the underlying premise of chiropractic is that misalignment or subluxation of the spinal (vertebral) column is the primary cause of illness, and, thus, its realignment is the appropriate treatment for illness. Accordingly, chiropractic medical practice is primarily limited to vertebral adjustments, where manual manipulation of the spine its used to correct misalignments. Recent studies have shown that **chiropractic** treatment of some types of low-back pain can be more effective than conventional care.[7] With about 50,000 practitioners in the United States, chiropractic is the third-largest health profession, used by 15 to 20 million people. Some chiropractors use only spinal manipulation, whereas others use additional medical technologies, including dietary supplementation and various noninvasive technologies similar to those used by physical therapists and athletic trainers, including massage.

In spite of the fact that chiropractors undergo nearly the same number of years of training as do primary care physicians and take courses closely aligned with those taken by physicians, current laws restrict the scope of chiropractic practice to noninvasive techniques initially consistent with the original theoretical basis of their discipline, "one cause—one cure of all illnesses and diseases." In 1998 the National Center for Complementary and Alternative Medicine established a Comprehensive Center for Chiropractic Research (the 11th alternative medical field to receive such a center) to establish scientific standards for the study of chiropractic effectiveness.[8] Research is ongoing at five sites. Should careful study of chiropractic demonstrate limited effectiveness, beyond the area of low-back pain, then chiropractic medicine is likely to remain a user-friendly, highly popular but highly limited approach to health care. There is, however, a current trend of including chiropractic physicians within

---

Key Terms

chiropractic manipulation of the vertebral column to relieve misalignments and cure illness

Therapeutic Touch (Biofield Therapy)

The biofield (or energy field) is believed by therapeutic touch practitioners to dwell within and immediately surround the body. For thousands of years, practitioners of biofield therapy, as exemplified by therapeutic touch, have attempted to identify irregularities or contractions in this electrical field and through appropriate touching (or near-touching of the body), restore its appropriate configuration. Once the biofield is aligned appropriately, the negative forces that have been disruptive to the physical and emotional balance required for healthful living are released. A second perception of biofield therapies is that through manipulation of the biofield a pathway or entry point is established that allows other health modalities, such as medications, to influence the restoration of the holistic balance needed for good health.

Practitioners of biofield therapies, including healing touch, therapeutic touch, and SHEN (Specific Human Emotional Nexus) therapy, describe their practice as noninvasive, deeply relaxing, gentle, and both safe and effective. Treatment sessions are usually conducted in a quiet and relaxed location, with the patient fully clothed and lying on a softly padded table or in bed. Sessions generally last from several minutes to an hour, often including a period of dialogue between the patient and the practitioner, and may be delivered for several days or for only a day or two.

Sessions may be delivered within a hospital (before or following surgery) or in the home following discharge from the hospital. Therapeutic touch is generally an adjunct therapy to more conventional therapies, given in conjunction with cancer treatment or during postsurgical recovery or as part of the treatment to alleviate the anxiety associated with traumatic injury recovery. Nurses are the most likely practitioners of therapeutic touch and related therapies in the hospital setting. In fact, it is in nursing journals that the most literature related to the practice is found. When therapeutic touch is used in a wellness-oriented manner, it is most often delivered by a certified practitioner. This is often a nurse practicing in a fee-for-service manner, a chiropractor, a naturopathic physician, or a psychologist.

The scientific literature regarding the effectiveness of therapeutic touch is very difficult to interpret. This is largely because of the difficulty of establishing double-blind experiments to study a therapeutic approach (that is, experiments in which neither practitioner nor patient knows whether the actual therapy versus a sham therapy is being delivered). A second difficulty is the problem of quantifying the outcome of the therapy. At this point it appears that therapeutic touch is somewhat effective in reducing anxiety, enhancing mood, improving sleep, and producing a higher level of relaxation among patients experiencing various emotionally traumatic medical treatments, such as breast cancer surgery. Its efficacy in enhancing holistic health and a sense of wellness is based largely on self-reported improvement and various inventories designed to assess feeling states.

Acupuncture has received increasing acceptance within the Western medical community.

allopathic medical groups, principally to treat those conditions clearly associated with postural injuries or conditions. If chiropractic physicians can accept this slightly subordinate role for the foreseeable future, while seeing their discipline evolve in the direction of osteopathic medicine (even transforming their schools into schools of osteopathic medicine), then chiropractic may move out of complementary/alternative/integrative medicine into the mainstream.

Acupuncture

Acupuncture is, for Americans, the most familiar component of the 3,000-year-old Chinese medical system. This system is based on balancing the active and passive forces within the patient's body to strengthen the qi ("chee"), or life force. The system also employs herbs, food, massage, and exercise.

> **Key Terms**
>
> **acupuncture** insertion of fine needles into the body to alter electroenergy fields and cure disease

Acupuncturists place hair-thin needles at certain points in the body to stimulate the patient's qi. These points are said to correspond to different organs and bodily functions and, when stimulated, help the body's own defenses fight illness. More specifically, the scientific communities suggest that acupuncture speeds up the electrical conductivity within the central and peripheral nervous systems, enhances the production of biological opiates, and alters the production of specific neurotransmitters within various areas of the nervous system.[9]

Of all the Chinese therapies, acupuncture is the most widely accepted in the West. Researchers have produced persuasive evidence of acupuncture's effectiveness with treating low-back pain, adult postoperative pain, nausea and vomiting associated with chemotherapy, and pain following dental surgery. Acupuncture may also be effective in other areas such as addiction, headache, menstrual pain, fibromyalgia, osteoarthritis, and tennis elbow.[10] However, because of the difficulty of conducting double-blind research that involves the insertion of needles, acupuncture research is challenging to design, thus its use may remain largely complementary.

Reflexology

Reflexology uses principles similar to those of acupuncture but focuses on treating certain disorders through massage of the soles of the feet. To date, however, there is relatively little data regarding its effectiveness, when evaluated under carefully controlled conditions. However, among reflexology studies available through the National Library of Medicine (Pubmed), three reflect the uncertainty of its role in integrative medical care. In a recent Korean study, foot reflexology, in four sessions of 40 minutes each, was given to a group of women undergoing breast cancer chemotherapy. In comparison to a control group, those receiving reflexology reported less nausea, vomiting, and fatigue.[11] A study conducted in Israel found that active reflexology therapy versus a sham (calf area massage) was beneficial in alleviating motor, sensory, and urinary difficulties in persons with multiple sclerosis.[12] In contrast, a Danish study in which middle ear infections in children were treated exclusively with reflexology versus antibiotics found reflexology to be ineffective as a treatment modality.[13] The National Center for Complementary and Alternative Medicine has yet to fund carefully controlled research into the effectiveness of reflexology.

Homeopathy

Widely accepted in Europe, **homeopathy** is the leading alternative therapy in France. Homeopathy uses infinitesimal doses of herbs, minerals, or even poisons to stimulate the body's curative powers. The theory on which homeopathy is based, the *law of similars*, contends that if large doses of a substance can cause a problem, tiny doses can trigger healing. A few small studies showed homeopathy

to be at least somewhat effective in treating hay fever, diarrhea, and flu symptoms, but members of the scientific community call the studies flawed or preliminary and suggest that the placebo effect was occurring. Much more informative, however, are reports from three meta-analysis studies, funded by the National Center for Complementary and Alternative Medicine, involving the reassessment of 240 individual studies, in which it was concluded that major methodology weaknesses existed in most studies of homeopathy conducted to date. It was further concluded that on the basis of these studies there was no strong evidence in favor of homeopathy over conventional treatment methods. The Center recommended that larger, more carefully controlled studies be conducted.[14] Since the report on homeopathic medication was released by the National Center for Complementary and Alternative Medicine, recent studies continue to experience methodological difficulties, principally related to the small sample sizes used by researchers.[15]

An interesting dimension to the marketing of homeopathy as an effective alternative to conventional medical care relates to the contention of some homeopathy physicians that the "molecular essence" of their homeopathic medicines can be sent via the Internet, thus allowing treatment to occur through cyberspace.

Naturopathy

The core of naturopathic medicine is what Hippocrates called *medicatrix naturae*, or the healing power of nature. Proponents of **naturopathy** believe that when the mind and the body are in balance and receiving proper care, with a healthy diet, adequate rest, and minimal stress, the body's own vital forces are sufficient to fight off disease. Getting rid of an ailment is only the first step toward correcting the underlying imbalance that allowed the ailment to take hold, naturists believe. Correcting the imbalance might be as simple as rectifying a shortage of a particular nutrient, or as complex as reducing overlong work hours, strengthening a weakened immune system, and identifying an inability to digest certain foods.

Naturopathy was popular in the 19th century and began a comeback in the 1970s in the Pacific Northwest, spurred by the back-to-nature themes of the counterculture. In

---

Key Terms

reflexology massage applied to specific areas of the feet to treat illness and disease in other areas of the body

homeopathy (hoe mee **op** ah thee) the use of minute doses of herbs, minerals, or other substances to stimulate healing

naturopathy (na chur **op** ah thee) a system of treatment that avoids drugs and surgery and emphasizes the use of natural agents to correct underlying imbalances some states, naturopaths are licensed, and health insurance plans must cover treatment they provide.

Herbalism

Herbalism may be the world's oldest and most widely used healing form. Herbalists make herbal brews for treating a variety of ills, such as depression, anxiety, and hypertension. In some cases, scientific research supports the herbalists' beliefs. For example, studies have found St. John's wort to be more effective than a placebo and one of the older tricyclic antidepressants in alleviating mild depression, and that garlic reduces cholesterol and blood pressure, while black cohosh (a member of the buttercup family) and soy can relieve hot flashes and other menopause symptoms.

However, the potential side effects of many dietary supplements have raised questions about the dangers associated with particular herbs, especially of products containing ephedra, a stimulant used to enhance athletic performance or stimulate weight loss.[16] The Food and Drug Administration began to consider taking increased control over the testing and safety of all dietary supplements following the ephedra-related death of Baltimore Orioles pitcher Steve Belcher in February 2003; more than 150 deaths have been linked to the supplement. In December 2003, after extensive studies, the FDA officially banned the sale and use of ephedra and implemented the ban in April 2004.[17] However, most supplements are not studied in this manner, and virtually no regulation of the supplements industry currently exists.

Key Terms

herbalism an ancient form of healing in which herbal preparations are used to treat illness and disease

Herbal supplements such as ginseng may be beneficial to some, but consumers should be informed about potential side effects as these products are not required to carry warning labels.

Ayurveda

Even older than Chinese medicine, India's **ayurveda** takes a preventive approach and focuses on the whole person. This system employs diet, tailored to the patient's constitutional type, or dosha; herbs; yoga and breathing exercises; meditation; massages; and purges, enemas, and aromatherapy. Practitioners of ayurveda report success in treating rheumatoid arthritis, headaches, and chronic sinusitis.

If you would like to consult a practitioner in one of the alternative disciplines but you don't know where to start, see Changing for the Better on page 545 for some tips on choosing a provider in alternative medicine.

At the urging of many people in both the medical and complementary health care fields, the National Institutes of Health requested federal funding to establish a scientific center for the study of alternative medical care. Today the National Center for Complementary and Alternative Medicine assembles information about alternative approaches to medical care and provides a framework for well-controlled research into the effectiveness of each approach. Double-blind studies, so called because neither the participants nor the researchers know which treatment each participant is receiving, are being conducted. The first substantial recommendation regarding an alternative form of care, acupuncture, was released in 1998.

It will be interesting to note whether all the branches of complementary medical care will want their theories of treatment and prevention tested under the rigorous criteria used by the National Center for Complementary and Alternative Medicine and to see how they respond if the results are not favorable.

Restricted-Practice Health Care Providers

We receive much of our health care from medical physicians. However, most of us also use the services of various health care specialists who also have advanced graduate-level training. Among these professionals are dentists, psychologists, podiatrists, and optometrists.

Dentists (Doctor of Dental Surgery, DDS) deal with a wide range of diseases and impairments of the teeth and oral cavity. Dentists undergo undergraduate pre-dental programs that emphasize the sciences, followed by 4 additional years of study in dental school and, with increasing frequency, an internship program. State licensure examinations are required. As with physicians, dentists can also specialize by completing a postdoctoral master's degree in fields such as oral surgery, **orthodontics,** and **prosthodontics.** Dentists are also permitted to prescribe therapy programs (such as the treatment of temporo-mandibular joint [TMJ] dysfunction) and drugs that pertain to their practices (primarily analgesics and antibiotics).

As discussed in Chapter 2, *psychologists* provide services to help patients understand behavior patterns or perceptions. More than 40 states have certification or licensing laws that prohibit unqualified people from using the term *psychologist*. The consumer should examine a psychologist's credentials. Legitimate psychologists have received advanced graduate training (often leading to a PhD or EdD degree) in clinical, counseling, industrial, or educational psychology. Furthermore, these practitioners will have passed state certification examinations and, in many states, will have met further requirements that allow them to offer health services to the public. Psychologists may have special interests and credentials from professional societies in individual, group, family, or marriage counseling. Some are certified as sex therapists.

Unlike psychiatrists, who are medical physicians, psychologists cannot prescribe or dispense drugs. They may refer to or work collaboratively with medical physicians about clients who might benefit from drug therapy.

Key Terms

ayurveda (ai yur **vey** da) traditional Indian medicine based on herbal remedies

orthodontics a dental specialty that focuses on the proper alignment of the teeth

prosthodontics a dental specialty that focuses on the construction and fitting of artificial appliances to replace missing teeth

Podiatrists are highly trained clinicians who practice podiatric medicine, or care of the feet (and ankles). Although not MDs or DOs, doctors of podiatric medicine (DPM) treat a wide variety of conditions related to the feet, including corns, bunions, warts, bone spurs, hammertoes, fractures, diabetes-related conditions, athletic injuries, and structural abnormalities. Podiatrists perform surgery, prescribe medications, and apply orthotics (supports or braces), splints, and corrective shoes for structural abnormalities of the feet.

Doctors of podiatric medicine follow an educational path similar to that taken by MDs and DOs, consisting of a 4-year undergraduate preprofessional curriculum, 4 additional years of study in a podiatric medical school, and an optional residency of 1 or 2 years. Board-certified areas of specialization include surgery, orthopedics, and podiatric sports medicine. Hospital affiliation generally requires board certification in a specialized area.

Optometrists are eye specialists who primarily treat vision problems associated with **refractory errors.** They examine the eyes and prescribe glasses or contact lenses to correct visual disorders. Additionally, optometrists prescribe prescription medications, such as antibiotic drops for application in the eye. Optometrists sometimes attempt to correct certain ocular muscle imbalances with specific exercise regimens. Optometrists must complete undergraduate training and additional years of coursework at one of sixteen accredited colleges of optometry in the United States or two Canadian colleges before taking a state licensing examination.

Opticians are technicians who manufacture and fit eyeglasses or contact lenses. Although they are rarely licensed by a state agency, they perform the important function of grinding lenses to the precise prescription designated by an optometrist or ophthalmologist (physicians who have specialized in vision care). To save money and time, many consumers take an optometrist's or ophthalmologist's prescription for glasses or contact lenses to optician-staffed retail stores that deal exclusively with eyewear products.

Nurse Professionals

Nurses constitute a large group of health professionals who practice in a variety of settings. Their responsibilities usually depend on their academic preparation. Registered nurses (RNs) are academically prepared at two levels: (1) the technical nurse, and (2) the professional nurse. The technical nurse is educated in a 2-year associate degree program. The professional nurse receives 4 years of education and earns a bachelor's degree. Both technical and professional nurses must successfully complete state licensing examinations before they can practice as RNs.

In light of the important role that nurse professionals play in today's health care system, it is worrisome that a significant shortage of nurses exists. On the basis of enrollment data for nursing programs in this country, and the number of nurses who have apparently left the workforce for various reasons, the current shortage of registered nurses is estimated to be 110,000. Projecting through 2012, it is estimated that 1.1 million new and replacement openings for nurses will exist in the United States,[18] a need that will most likely not be met.

Compounding the shortage of nurses is an equally acute shortage of nursing faculty to staff the nursing education programs that currently exist. As can be imagined, the demand for nurses has increased salaries, generated competition between health care institutions to recruit nurses, and increased the nurse-to-patient ratio to dangerously high levels in many areas of the country. In this final regard, it is estimated that as many as 20,000 unnecessary deaths that occur annually in American hospitals and nursing facilities can be attributed to the shortage—about one-fifth of all deaths attributed to medical errors.[19]

Many professional nurses continue their education and earn master's and doctoral degrees in nursing or other health-related fields. Some professional nurses specialize in a clinical area (such as pediatrics, gerontology, public health, or school health) and become certified as *advanced practice nurses* (APNs). Currently four APN fields, including nurse midwives, nurse anesthetists, nurse practitioners, and nurse case managers, can be found in larger communities. Working in close association with physicians, APNs perform an array of diagnositic, treatment, and administrative activities once limited to physicians. The ability of these highly trained nurses to function at this level gives communities additional primary care providers and frees physicians to deal with more complex cases. With the expansion of managed care, the role of APNs is growing. This increases access to medical care and allows physicians to use their time more cost effectively.

Licensed practical nurses (LPNs) are trained in hospital-based programs that last 12 to 18 months. Because of their brief training, LPNs' scope of practice is limited. Most LPN training programs are gradually being phased out.

Allied Health Care Professionals

Our primary health care providers are supported by a large group of allied health care professionals, who are often responsible for highly technical services and procedures.

Key Terms

refractory errors abnormal patterns of light wave transmission through the structures of the eye

These professionals include respiratory and inhalation therapists, radiographic technologists, nuclear medicine technologists, pathology technicians, general medical technologists, operating room technicians, emergency medical technicians, physical therapists, occupational therapists, cardiac rehabilitation therapists, dental technicians, physician assistants, and dental hygienists. Depending on the particular field, the training for these specialty support areas can take from 1 to 5 years of postsecondary school study. Programs include hospital-based training leading to a diploma through associate, bachelor's, and master's degrees. Most allied health care professionals must also pass state or national licensing examinations.

Self-Care/Home Care

The emergence of the **self-care movement** suggests that many people are becoming more responsible for maintaining their health. They are developing the expertise to prevent or manage many types of illness, injuries, and conditions. They are learning to assess their health status and treat, monitor, and rehabilitate themselves in a manner that was once thought possible only through a physician or some other health care specialist.

The benefits of this movement are that self-care can (1) reduce health care costs, (2) provide effective care for particular conditions, (3) free physicians and other health care specialists to spend time with other patients, and (4) increase interest in health-related activities.

Self-care is an appropriate alternative to professional care in three areas. First, self-care may be appropriate for certain acute conditions that have familiar symptoms and are limited in their duration and seriousness. Common colds and flu, many home injuries, sore throats, and non-allergic insect bites are often easily managed with self-care. That said, there are some symptoms that might seem somewhat familiar that should not be responded to through self-care, but rather by seeing a physician promptly. These include feeling of pressure or squeezing in the chest, a sudden severe headache, markedly blurred vision, difficulty talking or walking, dizziness and confusion, blood in urine or stool, unrelieved depression, and a cough with a yellow-green discharge. Self-care might be useful at some point, but not until the symptoms have been evaluated by a physician.

A second area in which self-care might be appropriate is therapy. For example, many people administer injections for diabetes mellitus, allergies, and migraine headaches and continue physical therapy programs in their homes. Asthma and hypertension are also conditions that can be managed or monitored with self-care.

A third area in which self-care has appropriate application is health promotion. Weight loss programs, physical conditioning activities, smoking cessation, and stress-reduction programs are particularly well suited to self-care (see Discovering Your Spirituality on page 549).

A potential fourth area in home care, self-diagnosis, is emerging, and not without some concern. Perhaps beginning with the thermometer, progressing to the home pregnancy test and the mail-in HIV diagnostic kit, today in-home genetic testing is available. These genetic screening tests are readily available and consist of a swab that is used to obtain a scraping of cells from the inner cheek and a mail-in envelope. Upon processing cells for their DNA, persons can obtain a genetic profile as it relates to specific disease predispositions. Principal concerns associated with the use of these tests are the shortcutting of primary care physicians (although some brands require physician consent) and the absence of genetic counselors to work with clients after they receive the results of their tests. Currently, in-home genetic screening tests cost $200–$400. A specific genetic screening test for the presence of the BRCA cancer tumor suppressor gene (see Chapter 11) has raised concerns in both Europe and this country regarding public policy, as well as patent law.[20]

As the U.S. population ages, it is becoming increasingly common for family members to provide home care to older relatives. As the number of frail older people increases, home care can significantly reduce the need for institutional care. Home care also can be delivered by home health care specialists. In fact, this form of care is proving so cost-effective that some insurance programs, including *Medicare* and *Medicaid,* cover portions of the cost of home health care for older adults. (See the sections on Medicare and Medicaid on page 552.)

With the rapid development of the home health care industry during the 1980s and 1990s, concerns mounted about the lack of regulation over aspects of the industry, particularly the background and training of personnel, and existence of fraud in the billing of services to Medicare and Medicaid. Although personnel issues remain to some degree, the financial aspects of professional home care have been addressed at the federal level. In 1999 the Healthcare Integrity and Protection Data Bank was established to better supervise the billing by home health care providers for services covered under Medicare and Medicaid.

A decision to provide family-based home care, particularly for older adults, is often made for admirable and

---

Key Terms

self-care movement the trend toward individuals' taking increased responsibility for prevention or management of certain health conditions

Good Health—What's It Worth, Now and Later?

The average life expectancy for women in the United States today is 80 years. For men, it's 76 years. That's a dramatic change from just a few generations ago. Thanks to tremendous advances in medical science and technology, many people are enjoying healthy, happy, and spiritually fulfilling lives well into their final years.

But this longevity comes with a price tag. It means that making healthful choices every day—including eating a balanced diet, getting exercise and adequate rest, and making opportunities for emotional and spiritual expression—takes on new importance. If you're going to live 10 "extra" years, what do you want to do with that time? Probably many of the things you're doing now, plus some different ones. Are you going to be able to meet the challenge—healthwise?

Taking charge of your health right now, when you're young and healthy, can be one of the most empowering things you do. By consciously choosing a healthy lifestyle—limiting your intake of alcohol,

avoiding drugs and cigarette smoking, and limiting your sexual partners—you are building the foundation for good health in your later years.

If you should ever have a serious health problem, you'll be better equipped to handle it if you're used to taking care of yourself. You'll feel comfortable being involved in your treatment decisions and doing whatever you can to control the quality of your life. You'll see your health crisis as a challenge you need to deal with, instead of viewing yourself as a helpless victim.

Taking charge of your own health—by being an informed health care consumer, by choosing a healthy lifestyle, and by fostering a positive attitude—brings a sense of peace. It's knowing that you're doing everything you can to take care of yourself. It's enhancing the quality of your life today and preparing for an active and rewarding tomorrow.

---

understandable reasons, including love for the relative who needs care and the high cost of professional home care and institutional care. For the millions of families who have made this decision, providing home health care can be highly rewarding. It also can be very demanding, however, because of the needs and limitations of the person who requires care and the compromises the caregivers must make.[21] Particularly when a spouse or family decides to provide care without the assistance of professional caregivers, they can jeopardize their own health long before the recovery or death of the person for whom they are caring. Even when their physical stamina seems unaffected, factors such as fatigue, emotional strain, postponement of personal and family goals, loss of social contact, and even physical abuse of caregivers by those receiving care can be substantial.

Health Care Facilities

Most of us have a general idea of what a hospital is. However, all hospitals are not alike. They usually fall into one of three categories—private, public, or voluntary. *Private hospitals* (or proprietary hospitals) function as profit-making hospitals. They are not supported by tax monies and usually accept only clients who can pay all their expenses. Although there are some exceptions, these hospitals are generally smaller than tax-supported public hospitals. Commonly owned by a group of business investors, a large hospital corporation, or a group of physicians, these hospitals sometimes limit their services to a few specific types of illnesses.

Public hospitals are supported primarily by tax dollars. They can be operated by government agencies at the state level (such as state mental hospitals) or at the federal level (such as the Veterans Administration Hospitals and various military service hospitals such as the National Naval Medical Center in Bethesda, Maryland). Large county or city hospitals are frequently public hospitals. These hospitals routinely serve indigent segments of the population. They also function as *teaching hospitals*.

The most commonly recognized type of hospital is the *voluntary hospital*. Voluntary hospitals are maintained as nonprofit public institutions. Often supported by religious orders, fraternal groups, or charitable organizations, these hospitals usually offer a wider range of comprehensive services than do private hospitals or clinics. Voluntary hospitals are supported by patient fees (covered by health insurance), Medicare reimbursement, and Medicaid and public assistance reimbursement.

In the last decade, hospitals, particularly private and voluntary hospitals, have expanded their scope of services. Today hospitals often operate *wellness centers,* stress centers, cardiac rehabilitation centers, chemical dependence programs, health education centers, and satellite centers for well-baby care and care for the homeless. During the 1990s two trends were observed in terms of hospital organization and ownership: the acquisition of small hospitals (such as county hospitals and smaller community hospitals) by larger regional hospitals and the reorganization of voluntary hospitals as for-profit hospitals. Both trends reflected the rapid movement of medical care in the direction of *managed care,* the term referring to the more profit-focused, cost-efficient, and third-party-controlled care reflective of the application of corporate strategies to the delivery of health care services. Whether these trends will be as obvious in the current decade is uncertain, as the federal government looks more critically at managed care and the dissatisfaction of the public and the medical community with its restrictive approach to delivering health care services.

Other health care facilities include clinics (both private and tax-supported), nursing homes (most of which are private enterprises), and rehabilitation centers. Rehabilitation centers are often supported by charitable organizations devoted to the care of chronically ill or handicapped people, orthopedically injured people, or burn victims.

In recent years, many private, 24-hour drop-in medical emergency and surgical centers have appeared. These clinics have their own professional staffs of physicians, nurses, and allied health professionals. They compete directly with larger hospital-based facilities. Some clinics specialize in women's health needs, including gynecological care, prenatal care, and childbirth services.

Another health-care provider is the *hospice*. Hospices provide prescribed medical care (most often palliative or comfort care) for patients who have been deemed terminal by their health care provider. Although some hospices are housed within hospitals and provide in-hospital care, most provide home-based care, thus allowing the terminal patient the opportunity to die in familiar surroundings and in the presence of loving family members or friends. Many hospice models can be found within the United States, including those operated by hospitals (in-hospital care and/or home-based care), for-profit companies, charitable organizations, and those affiliated with religious bodies.

Although you might have no direct experience with hospice services, you may recall that Terri Schaivo died in a hospice setting. The highly charged aspect of that particular person's life and death, however, should not distract from your appreciation of the compassionate care and dignity of death supported by virtually all hospices. (For an in-depth discussion of the Schaivo case, see Chapter 21.)

Regardless of the type of health care institutions in which you seek services, both you and the institutions have legally binding rights that structure your relationship. Table 18.1 details both your rights as a patient and their rights as a licensed health care facility.

Table 18.1 Patients' Institutional Rights

Regardless of the type of institution in which you are a patient, you have a variety of rights. These are intended to protect you from unnecessary harm and financial loss. The hospital too can expect your cooperation as a patient.

As a patient, you can expect all of the following from the institution:

- To be treated with respect and dignity
- To be afforded privacy and confidentiality consistent with federal and state laws, institutional policies, and the requirements of your insurance carrier
- To be provided services on request, as long as they are reasonable and consistent with appropriate care
- To be fully informed of the identity of the physicians and staff providing care
- To be kept fully updated about your condition, including its management and your prognosis for recovery
- To be informed of any experimental or other research/educational projects that may be utilized in your treatment and to refuse such treatment
- To have the opportunity to specify advance directives (a living will, a life-prolonging statement, or the appointment of a health care representative) in order to facilitate health care decisions
- To receive an explanation of your bill for services regardless of the source of payment
- To present a complaint and receive a response about any aspect of your care or treatment and to have your complaint taken seriously
- To be involved in ethical considerations that arise during the course of your care

The institution can expect you, as a patient:

- To keep all appointments
- To provide all background information pertinent to your condition
- To treat hospital personnel with respect
- To ask questions and seek clarification about matters that affect you
- To follow the treatment prescribed by your physician
- To be considerate and respectful of other patients and to ensure that your visitors are considerate and respectful as well
- To satisfy your financial obligation to health care providers through the provision of insurance information and by arranging credit where applicable

As a patient, you may at any time:

- Refuse treatment
- Seek a second opinion
- Discharge yourself from the institution

Health Care Costs and Reimbursement

There are many avenues for receiving health care. However, being able to pay for quality care is one of the greatest concerns of the American public. In 2003 (the last year for which statistics are available) nearly 45 million American were without health insurance for the entire year.[22] Some believe that adding those people who lacked coverage for a portion of the year to the preceding figure would result in a total number of 75 million people with less than full health care. No age group is more likely to be uncovered than are young adults between 18 and 24 years of age. American Indians and Alaskan Natives are the two racial groups least likely to have health insurance.[22] Employed persons, regardless of age or race, who work in the service sector and lack benefits, such as food workers, and the self-employed often find access to individual health insurance policies too expensive. Approximately 11.5 percent of all American children lack access to the fullest range of health services owing to a lack of health insurance.[22]

Regardless of category, people in this country who lack health insurance are truly living "dangerously." Furthermore, Americans are less optimistic today about their ability to maintain adequate health insurance coverage, find reasonably priced health care, and afford long-term home-based or nursing home care than ever before. Unfortunately, the word *crisis* is appropriate to use when talking about our ability to afford high-quality health care today.

In addition to the availability of health insurance, the simple cost of health care is a major concern, even for those who have access to health insurance. It is estimated that in 2002 Americans spent $1.553 trillion on health care,[23] and by 2013 this expenditure will increase to $3.358 trillion.[24] Stated another way, in 2002 Americans incurred an average of $5,241 per person in health care-related costs.[25] This amount is expected to increase to $7,100 per person by the year 2007. No developed country spends a greater percent of its gross domestic product on health care than does the United States.

As a result of factors such as the high cost of modern medical technology, an emphasis on long life at any cost, the growing number of older people with chronic conditions that require expensive long-term care, and the AIDS epidemic, controlling the cost of medical care is one of the most complex problems facing the nation. Nevertheless, more than 40 different plans have been advanced since 1990 to respond to this problem. These range from only modest changes in the current system, to tax-credit strategies and mandatory employment-based insurance, to a federally controlled national health plan. Today government officials seem to be particularly interested in lowering the cost of prescription drugs for older Americans. Three models have received close attention. The first assigns some aspects of prescription drug coverage to Medicare, while the second relates to the development of prescription drug plans by the pharmaceutical industry, for those who qualify on the basis of need. The third model assigns an increased role for the health insurance industry in negotiating lower drug prices for its senior members. Both the first and second models, in various forms, are now in operation.

In December 2003, President Bush signed the Medicare Prescription Drug Improvement and Modernization Act. Hailed as an answer to rising drug costs for seniors, the act was widely criticized as still being too costly for many seniors.

Health Insurance

Health insurance is a financial agreement between an insurance company and an individual or group for the payment of health care costs. After paying a premium to an insurance company, the policyholder is covered for specific benefits. Each policy is different in its coverage of illnesses and injuries. Merely having an insurance policy does not mean that all health care expenses will be covered. Most health insurance policies require various forms of payments by the policyholder, which includes deductible amounts, fixed indemnity benefits, coinsurance, and exclusions. In 2000 Americans spent $372.8 billion on private health insurance, and they are expected to spend $643.4 billion by 2007.[26]

A *deductible* amount is an established amount that the insuree must pay before the insurer reimburses for services. For example, a person or family may have to pay the first $200 of the year's medical expenses before insurance begins providing any coverage.

A policy with *fixed indemnity* benefits will pay only a specified amount for a particular procedure or service. If the policy pays only $1,000 for an appendectomy and the actual cost of the appendectomy was $1,500, then the policy owner will owe the health care provider $500. A policy with full-service benefits, which pays the entire cost of a particular procedure or service, may be worth the extra cost.

Policies that have *coinsurance* features require that the policy owner and the insurance company share the costs of certain covered services, usually on a percentage basis. One standard coinsurance plan requires that the policyholder pay 20 percent of the costs above a deductible amount, and the company pays the remaining 80 percent.

An *exclusion* is a service or expense that is not covered by the policy. Elective or cosmetic surgery procedures, unusual treatment protocols, prescription drugs, and certain kinds of consultations are common exclusions. Illness and injuries that already exist at the time of purchase (preexisting conditions) are often excluded. In addition, injuries incurred during high-risk activities (ice hockey, hang gliding, mountain climbing, intramural sports) might not be covered by a policy.

Health insurance can be obtained through individual policies or group plans. Group health insurance plans usually offer the widest range of coverage at the lowest price and are often purchased cooperatively by companies and their employees. In 2004, companies with health insurance benefits spent on average $7,289 for each employee's family health insurance plan—an 11.8 percent increase over 2003 costs.[27] Fortunately, no employee is refused entry into a group insurance program. However, when employees leave the company, their previous group coverage can follow them for a prescribed period of time only, usually 18 to 24 months. Today, as many large American companies continue to lay off employees, the eventual loss of health insurance becomes a serious personal and family crisis.

Individual policies can be purchased by one person (or a family) from an insurance company. These policies are often much more expensive than group plans and may provide much less coverage. Still, people who do not have access to a group plan should attempt to secure individual policies, because the financial burdens resulting from a severe accident or illness that is not covered by some form of health insurance can be devastating. Many colleges and universities offer annually renewable health insurance policies that students can purchase. (Changing for the Better on page 553 gives the consumer some questions to consider before purchasing a health insurance policy.)

Medicare

Since it was established in 1965, *Medicare* has been a key provider of health coverage for the nation's elderly. Medicare is a federally funded health insurance program for persons 65 years of age and older, as well as for persons of any age who have particular disabilities or permanent kidney failure. Funding for Medicare comes primarily from federal payroll taxes and is administered by the Health Care Financing Administration, within the Department of Health and Human Services.

In its current configuration Medicare is divided into two portions. Part A helps pay for care while in hospitals, as well as for care in skilled nursing facilities and hospice care, and for some home health care. Persons become eligible for Part A coverage on turning 65, on the condition of having paid Medicare taxes while working.

Part B is an optional portion of Medicare that can be chosen at the time of becoming eligible for Part A, or at selected times following initial eligibility. Unlike Part A, there is a monthly charge for Part B coverage. Currently that charge is $78.20 per month but is subject to annual adjustment.[28] Part B helps pay for doctor's services, outpatient hospital care, and some other medical services not covered under Part A, including physical and occupational therapy, medical devices, and some home health care. Routine dental and vision care are not included.

Because of the universal nature of Medicare Part A and the affordable monthly charge for Part B, group health insurance plans to which many retirees belong require that Medicare be the "first payer" for services, thus allowing the group plan to be responsible for only that portion of health-related charges not covered by Medicare.

The Medicare Prescription Drug Improvement and Modernization Act of 2003 (now referred to as Part D) provides new prescription coverage options for Medicare recipients. Beginning in 2006, it provides prescription coverage through third-party providers for a premium of about $35 per month. After meeting an annual deductible of $250, Medicare covers 75 percent of the costs of prescription drugs, up to $2,250 per year; there is then a gap in coverage until out-of-pocket expenses reach $3,500 in a single year, at which point Medicare kicks in again and covers 95 percent of further costs for the remainder of the year. The Medicare prescription drug program is expected to cost the Medicare system $724 billion during the first decade of its existence.

Medicaid

Unlike Medicare, a program that is almost exclusively for persons 65 or older, *Medicaid* is a program designed to assist in meeting the health care needs of qualified persons regardless of age. Also unlike Medicare, which is a federal program entirely funded through Medicare tax withholdings (Part A), user-paid elected enrollment fees (Part B), and the new Part D, Medicaid is a federal- and state-funded program administered by each of the individual states.

Qualification for receiving Medicaid assistance can be perplexing. Federal Medicaid law sets mandatory eligibility standards, while optional eligibility standards allow each state to tailor many aspects of the program to fit its unique needs. Central to the majority of the federally mandated eligibility standards is the current Federal Poverty Level (FPL), as well as the standards related to the Aid to Families with Dependent Children (AFDC) program and the Temporary Assistance to Needy Families (TANF) program. Optional eligibility standards allow states to define some aspects of eligibility for pregnant women, disabled children, certain working disabled persons, and those designated as Medically Needy.

Federally mandated Medicaid services are wide ranging and include hospital services, physician services, laboratory/X-ray procedures, immunizations, family planning services, home health care services, transportation for medical care services, and nursing home services. This final service is of critical importance to older adults in that it pays for the majority of nursing home care required by this age group. Optional services, which are under state control, include prescription drugs, rehabilitation and physical therapy services, prosthetic devices, vision services, hearing services, and dental services, to include a few.

Health Maintenance Organizations

Health maintenance organizations (HMOs) are health care delivery plans under which health care providers agree to meet the covered medical needs of subscribers for a prepaid amount of money. For a fixed monthly fee, enrollees are given comprehensive health care with an emphasis on preventive health care. Enrollees receive their care from physicians, specialists, allied health professionals, and educators who are hired (group model) or contractually retained (network model) by the HMO.

Managed care, and HMOs in particular, was a reaction to the sharply climbing costs of health care that began in the 1980s. Businesses, which paid a large portion of health care costs through employee-benefit plans, complained that no one in the health care loop had an incentive to control costs. Employers complained that consumers paid only a deductible and a small copayment, giving them little cause to question prices; doctors faced little financial oversight; and insurance companies merely rubber-stamped the bills.

When HMOs presented an alternative, employers began offering their workers incentives to select HMOs over traditional fee-for-service coverage and thus attempted to rein in the runaway costs of health care. HMOs now cover nearly 70 million Americans. Increases in membership continued until 2000, when many HMOs that participated in Medicare supplement plans discontinued participation and, thus, discontinued service to their previously enrolled older adult members. The escalating cost of prescription medications was the principal factor in this decision. In all HMOs the annual cost of membership continues to rise, particularly for persons enrolled in the for-profit HMOs. This increase reflects the rising cost of services that must be provided to members.

HMOs are usually the least expensive but most restrictive type of managed care. The premiums are 8–10 percent lower than those for traditional plans, they charge no deductibles or coinsurance payments, and copayments are $15–$20 per visit. However, you are limited to using the doctors and hospitals in the HMO's network, and you must get approval for treatments and referrals.

In theory, HMOs were to be the ideal blend of medical care and health promotion. Today, however, many observers are concerned that too many HMOs are being too tightly controlled by a profit motive in which physicians are being paid large bonuses to *not* refer patients to specialists or are prevented by "gag rules" from discussing certain treatment options with patients because of their costs to the HMOs.

Concerns, in addition to the "gag rules" mentioned above, have also arisen over the years. Among these have been concerns related to the right of members to sue their HMOs for medical negligence, the provision of better ob-gyn coverage, and the development of a more efficient mechanism to appeal denial of services. However, in the last regard, in 2004 the Supreme Court ruled that HMO patients could not use more permissive state laws to sue HMOs for damages resulting from their refusal to approve particular medical services.

In spite of the problems just mentioned, HMOs remain, in theory, more cost-efficient than the traditional fee-for-service healthcare model. Cost containment is achieved, in part, because most of the medical services within a group model HMO are centralized, there is little duplication of facilities, equipment, or support staff. Central filing of records gives all the HMO physicians access to a single file for each client. This saves time, administrative costs, and the overlapping of care. Many HMOs also routinely use health-promotion activities.[29]

Other new approaches to reducing health costs are independent practice associations (IPAs) and preferred provider organizations (PPOs). An IPA is a modified form of an HMO that uses a group of doctors who offer prepaid services out of their own offices and not in a central HMO facility. IPAs are viewed as "HMOs without walls." A PPO is a group of private practitioners who sell their services at reduced rates to insurance companies. When a policyholder chooses a physician who is in that company's PPO network, the insurance company pays the entire physician's fee less the deductible and copay amounts. When a policyholder selects a non-PPO physician, the insurance company pays a smaller portion of that physician's fee. Today, more than 80 percent of Americans with health benefits are enrolled in a managed care plan (HMO, IPA, or PPO). In some areas of the country, such as California, Oregon, and Washington, over 90 percent of persons with benefits are in managed care plans.

Extended or Long-Term Care Insurance

With the aging of the population and the greater likelihood that nursing home care will be required (at nearly $61,685 per year in 2004 for a semiprivate room), insurers have developed extended care policies.[30] When purchased at an early age (by mid-50s), these policies are much more affordable than if purchased when a spouse or family member will soon require institutional care. However, not all older adults will need extensive nursing home care, so an extended or long-term care policy could be an unnecessary expenditure.

Access to Health Care

With 45 million (or perhaps more) Americans lacking any health insurance and with nearly a quarter of those with insurance being underinsured, Americans are finding it increasingly difficult to access their country's highly sophisticated health care system. The unemployed poor, working poor, and minorities have the most difficulty accessing health care. African Americans, Hispanic Americans, and Native Americans have the worst health status of all Americans, yet they receive the fewest health care services. Even for older Americans with Medicare, gaping holes exist in the types of care covered (for example, glasses and hearing aids are not covered) and the prices of prescription medications far exceed the coverage provided. Thus, in America in the 21st century, people are expressing growing concern about the extent to which their health care needs will be met. As political opposition remains strongly against a national health care system, the United States joins South Africa to make them the only two major industrialized nations lacking a comprehensive and unified approach to meeting the health care needs of their populations.

Health-Related Products

As you might imagine, prescription and over-the-counter (OTC) drugs constitute an important part of any discussion of health-related products.

Prescription Drugs

Caution: Federal law prohibits dispensing without prescription. This FDA warning appears on the labels of approximately three-fourths of all medications. Prescription drugs must be ordered for patients by a licensed practitioner. Because these compounds are legally controlled and may require special skills in their administration, the public's access to these drugs is limited.

Although the *Physicians' Desk Reference* lists more than 2,500 compounds that can be prescribed by a physician, only 200 drugs make up the bulk of the nearly 3,215 million new prescriptions and refills dispensed by online, mail-order, supermarket, mass-market, corporate, and independent pharmacies in 2003.[31] Total retail prescription sales of $203.1 billion for 2003 represent a 10 percent increase over the previous year's sales. This upward trend reflects in large part the greater variety of prescription medications being prescribed each year by physicians. It is projected that by the year 2012 approximately $446 billion will be spent on prescription medications.[32] The rapid expansion of online pharmacies now occurring is unlikely to influence the number of prescriptions filled, though their presence will likely affect the sales of "brick and mortar" drugstore chains.

Research and Development of New Drugs

As consumers of prescription drugs, you may be curious about the process by which drugs gain FDA approval. The rigor of this process may be the reason that only about 100 new drugs are approved annually.

The nation's pharmaceutical companies constantly explore the molecular structure of various chemical compounds in an attempt to discover important new compounds with desired types and levels of biological activity. Once these new compounds are identified, companies begin extensive in-house research with computer simulations and animal testing to determine whether clinical trials with humans are warranted. Of the 125,000 or more compounds under study each year, only a few thousand receive such extensive preclinical evaluation. Even fewer of these are then taken to the FDA to begin the evaluation process necessary to gain approval for further research with humans. When the FDA approves a drug for clinical trials, a pharmaceutical company can obtain a patent, which prevents the drug from being manufactured by other companies for the next 17 years.

The $500+ million price tag for bringing a new drug into the marketplace reflects this slow, careful process. If the 7 years of work needed to bring a new drug into the marketplace go well, a pharmaceutical company enjoys the remaining 10 years of legally protected retail sales. Today new "fast-track" approval procedures at the FDA are progressively reducing the development period, particularly for desperately needed breakthrough drugs like those used to treat AIDS. Concern was expressed in 2000 that this "rush to approval" forced the FDA to utilize the services of independent evaluators, many of whom had ties to the pharmaceutical industry that would have influenced their assessments of a drug's readiness for marketing.

A recent example of problems stemming from the FDA's approval process was seen in the later months of 2004 and the early months of 2005, when three extremely popular (and highly profitable) nonsteroidal anti-inflammatory drugs, used in the management of osteoarthritis, were called into question regarding their role in the development of heart disease. Of the three drugs in question (Vioxx, Celebrex, and Bextra), Vioxx was pulled from the market in September of 2004 when heart problems were reported among some longer term users. Similar questions were quickly raised about Celebrex and Bextra, since all three drugs belong to the class of drugs called Cox-2 inhibitors. In response to rising levels of concern within the medical community and the general public, the FDA formed an advisory board to look at all safety-related information in the possession of the manufacturers. After three days of consideration, the 32-member advisory board issued its findings—all three drugs were deemed safe enough for continued sales. New concern immediately arose, however, when it was learned that 10 of the 32 board members had financial interests in one or both of the manufacturers of the medication under review.

The response of the FDA to its advisory board's finding, however, resulted in a compromise[33]—the continued absence of Vioxx from the market and a request that

Pfizer, the manufacturer of Bextra, discontinue sale of its product. Celebrex was allowed to continue being sold, but in conjunction with "Black Box" labeling warning physicians and patients about the potential risks associated with use of the product. However, even in the face of the FDA's more restrictive response, critics continue to see the FDA drug approval (and follow-up) process as being too dependent on the pharmaceutical industry for information and cooperation to truly protect the American consumer.

An additional area of concern related to the research and development of prescription medications includes the extent to which the pharmaceutical industry will continue to voluntarily use children (and pregnant women) in reassessment of drug dosages initially determined for adult men and nonpregnant women.

Generic versus Brand-Name Drugs

When a new drug comes into the marketplace, it carries three names: its **chemical name,** its **generic name,** and its **brand name.** While the 17-year patent is in effect, no other drug with the same chemical formulation can be sold. When the patent expires, other companies can manufacture a drug of equivalent chemical composition and market it under the brand name drug's original generic name. Because extensive research and development are unnecessary at this point, producing generic drugs is far less costly than is developing the original brand name drug. Nearly all states allow pharmacists to substitute generic drugs for brand name drugs, as long as the prescribing physician approves. For those interested in viewing all of the current approved generics, the FDA updates each month its Generic Drug Approvals list.[34]

 TALKING POINTS Your mother insists on using the brand-name drug that she has used for years to control her arthritis pain, even though her doctor has prescribed a generic version that has recently become available. What might you say to help her consider the less expensive option?

Key Terms

chemical name name used to describe the molecular structure of a drug

generic name common or nonproprietary name of a drug

brand name specific patented (proprietary) name assigned to a drug by its manufacturer

The Attraction of Canadian Prescription Drugs

On a weekday morning automobiles pull into the parking lot of an Indianapolis shopping mall, car doors open, and within a few minutes fifty or more people are waiting. In a few minutes they are joined by a comfortable new motor coach. The bus fills quickly and soon departs for a 5-hour drive to Windsor, Canada, via Detroit. Yet another "drug run" is under way to the closest point in Canada in order that Hoosier senior citizens can purchase American-made prescription medication in a foreign country more cheaply than at home. A comparison of prices gives credence to the sensibility of making this exhausting daylong trip. For example, a 90-pill supply of the prescription drug Zocor, used to lower blood cholesterol, costs more than $350 at an American pharmacy; in Canada, a patient can purchase the same amount of the same medication for $140.

Why are drugs manufactured in this country, that are in compliance with the rigorous safety and effectiveness standards of both Canada and the United States, priced more cheaply in Canada than in the United States? The answer to that question reflects the buying power of Canada's provincial health care programs that have forced American manufacturers to set lower Canadian wholesale prices in order to compete in their group-sales driven marketplace. A far less "structured" health care marketplace in this country, in combination with a "supportive" FDA and FTC, has allowed the American pharmaceutical industry to charge wholesale prices considerably higher than those charged to our "neighbor to the north." Thus, a disproportionate portion of the profit made by the American pharmaceutical industry comes from the pockets of its own citizens; while those in

a foreign country enjoy the benefits of our technology. Understandably, a similar trip northward is planned for the next week.

As popular as these trips are, they may soon have run their course. Three reasons seem applicable: (1) The FDA has issued a warning that medications obtained in Canada may be less safe than those sold in the United States, perhaps even counterfeit in some cases; (2) passports are required for all Americans to reenter the country from having visited either Canada or Mexico, even if visiting for less than a day; and (3) the new Medicare drug program (Part D) will help a large percentage of older adults secure needed medications at a more affordable price. Additionally, several states have formulated various plans to purchase medications from the United Kingdom and Europe for persons served by their respective Medicaid programs.

In recent years the pharmaceutical industry has actively attempted to extend the patent protection on several of the most profitable drugs on the market because their period of protected sales is expiring. In some cases the manufacturers have appealed directly to Congress for waivers to the current patent law, contending that they need the additional time to recoup research and development costs. This reason seems highly questionable to some people in light of the $4.35 billion spent by the drug industry in 2004 for advertising, most of which was directed to consumers through skillfully crafted televisions commercials (such as those for erectile dysfunction drugs). In addition to direct appeals to Congress, other manufacturers have quietly "layered" additional patents onto their products to prevent manufacturers of generic versions from using the same shape or color used in brand name versions, even though the chemical formulations are no longer protected. In another approach, manufacturers of highly profitable brand name drugs have offered to pay manufacturers of generic drugs to not make generic versions of their products once the patent protection has expired.

Today a variety of reference books are available to inform consumers about the availability of generic drugs and the prescription drugs that they can legally be substituted for. *Mosby's Drug Consult* series is a widely used reference focusing on both brand name drugs and

generic equivalents. Updated annually, this publication is currently available in the 2006 edition.[35]

Over-the-Counter Drugs

When people are asked when they last took some form of medication, for many the answer might be, "I took aspirin (or a cold pill, or a laxative) this morning." In making this decision, people engaged in self-diagnosis, determined a course for their own treatment, self-administered their treatment, and freed a physician to serve people whose illnesses are more serious than theirs. None of this would have been possible without readily available, inexpensive, and effective OTC drugs.

Although 2,500 prescription drugs are available, there are perhaps as many as 300,000 different OTC products, routinely classified into 26 different families. Like prescription drugs, nonprescription drugs are regulated by the FDA. However, for OTC drugs, the marketplace is a more powerful determinant of success.

The regulation of OTC drugs is based on a provision in a 1972 amendment to the 1938 Food, Drug, and Cosmetic Act. As a result of that action, OTC drugs were placed in three categories (I, II, and III) based on the safety and effectiveness of their active ingredient(s). Today, only category I OTC drugs that are safe, effective, and truthfully labeled are to be sold without

Dietary Supplements and the Self-Care Movement

Currently, more than 60 million Americans are using an array of vitamins, minerals, herbal products, hormones, amino acids, and glandular extracts in their quest for improved health. People turn to dietary supplements rather than the dietary recommendation discussed in Chapter 5 for many reasons, including concern over their own morbidity and mortality, dissatisfaction with today's impersonal health care system, distrust in the safety of the food supply, and people's increasing inability to control other aspects of life. As a result, we are now spending an estimated $12 billion annually on dietary supplements—many of which appear unnecessary and some of which may be unsafe and ineffective. Recall that dietary supplement makers are not required to submit evidence of safety or effectiveness to the Food and Drug Administration, as is the case with prescription medications and, to a lesser degree, the OTC products.

In spite of the lack of available data on safety and effectiveness, the traditional medical community is showing increasing interest in the potential benefits of dietary supplements. A growing number of teaching hospitals are establishing departments of complementary medicine, and medical students are learning about the documented role (to the extent that it is known) that these supplements can play in promoting health. Additionally, major international pharmaceutical companies are beginning to market dietary supplements. The reputation and resources of these companies are likely to generate more carefully controlled research into the safety and efficacy of these products. However, the extent to which the National Center for Complementary and Alternative Medicine (within the National Institutes of Health) will undertake carefully controlled studies of dietary supplements remains uncertain. Until studies have been completed, the public should be aware that only three supplements have received approval from the FDA to include specific health claims on their labels. These include folic acid and its ability to facilitate neural tube closure, calcium and its contribution to the prevention of osteoporosis, and a highly qualified claim for omega-3 fatty acids in the reduction of cardiovascular disease.

Using the Internet to comparison shop is one way of becoming a wise consumer of health care products and services, such as insurance policies and medications.

prescription. The FDA's drug-classification process also allows some OTC drugs to be made stronger and some prescription drugs to become nonprescription drugs by reducing their strength through reformulation. Whether the reformulation of a prescription drug into an OTC formulation is always to the consumer's advantage is questionable. For example, in 2003 Prilosec, a drug for reducing esophageal reflux disease, became available over the counter. Although Prilosec as an OTC drug is less expensive than it was as a prescription product, it is now no longer covered by health insurance. The loss of insurance coverage (usually 80 percent of the price once deductibles are met) makes the medication as expensive, if not more expensive, than it was initially, at least for patients who have prescription coverage. Of course, by being an OTC, a doctor appointment and resultant prescription are not required, but even this savings will soon be offset by the lack of insurance coverage if the medication is used over a long period of time.

Like the label shown in Figure 18-1, current labels for OTC products reflect FDA requirements. The labels must clearly state the type and quantity of active ingredients, alcohol content, side effects, instructions for appropriate use, warning against inappropriate use, and risks of using the product with other drugs (polydrug use). Unsubstantiated claims must be carefully avoided in advertisements of these products. In addition, under new labeling laws, following the controversy associated with Cox-2 medication, the use of Black Boxes will be required when it is known that OTC medications hold risks, particularly when used in combination with other medications. When used on a routine basis, OTC medications should be carefully discussed with a physician or a pharmacist.

Drug Facts

Active Ingredient (in each tablet)   **Purpose**
Chlorpheniramine maleate 2 mg   Antihistamine

Uses temporarily relieves these symptoms due to hay fever or other upper respiratory allergies:

   ■ sneezing ■ runny nose ■ itchy, watery eyes ■ itchy throat

Warnings

Ask a doctor before use if you have
■ glaucoma ■ a breathing problem such as emphysema or chronic bronchitis
■ trouble urinating due to an enlarged prostate gland

Ask a doctor or pharmacist before use if you are taking tranquilizers or sedatives

When using this product
■ you may get drowsy ■ avoid alcoholic drinks
■ alcohol, sedatives, and tranquilizers may increase drowsiness
■ be careful when driving a motor vehicle or operating machinery
■ excitability may occur, especially in children

If pregnant or breast-feeding, ask a health professional before use.
Keep out of reach of children. In case of overdose, get medical help or contact a Poison Control Center right away.

Directions

adults and children 12 years and over	take 2 tablets every 4 to 6 hours; not more than 12 tablets in 24 hours
children 6 years to under 12 years	take 1 tablet every 4 to 6 hours; not more than 6 tablets in 24 hours
children under 6 years	ask a doctor

Other information
■ store at 20-25° C (68-77° F) ■ protect from excessive moisture

Inactive ingredients D&C yellow no. 10, lactose, magnesium stearate, microcrystalline cellulose, pregelatinized starch

Figure 18-1 The FDA now requires over-the-counter drugs to carry standardized labels, such as the one at left.

Health Care Quackery and Consumer Fraud

A person who earns money by marketing inaccurate health information, unreliable health care, or ineffective health products is called a fraud, a **quack,** or a charlatan. **Consumer fraud** flourished with the old-fashioned medicine shows of the late 1880s. Unfortunately, consumer fraud still flourishes. You need look no further than large city newspapers to see questionable advertisements for disease cures and weight loss products. Quacks have found in health and illness the perfect avenues to indulge in **quackery**—to make maximum gain with minimum effort.

When people are in poor health, they may be afraid of becoming disabled or dying. So powerful are their desires to live and avoid suffering that people are vulnerable to promises of health improvement or a cure. Even though many people have great faith in their physicians, they also want access to experimental treatments or products touted as being superior to currently available

Key Terms

quack a person who earns money by purposely marketing inaccurate health information, unreliable health care, or ineffective health products

consumer fraud marketing of unreliable and ineffective services, products, or information under the guise of curing disease or improving health; quackery

quackery the practice of disseminating or supplying inaccurate health information, unreliable health care, or ineffective health products for the purposes of defrauding another person therapies. When tempted by the promise of help, people sometimes abandon traditional medical care. Of course, quacks recognize this vulnerability and present a variety of "reasons" to seek their help. (See Changing for the Better above.) Gullibility, blind faith, impatience, superstition, ignorance, or hostility toward professional expertise eventually carry the day. In spite of the best efforts of agencies at all levels, no branch of government can protect consumers from their own errors of judgment that so easily play into the hands of quacks and charlatans.

Regardless of the motivation that leads people into consumer fraud, the outcome is frequently the same. First, the consumer loses money. The services or products are grossly overpriced, and the consumers have little recourse to help them recover their money. Second, the consumers often feel disappointed, guilty, and angered by their own carelessness as consumers. Far too frequently, consumer fraud may lead to unnecessary suffering.

Becoming a Skilled Health Care Consumer

After reading this discussion of health information, services, and products, you should be a wiser, more prepared consumer. However, information alone is not enough. Consider these six suggestions to help you become a more skilled, assertive consumer:

1. *Prepare yourself for consumerism.* In addition to offering this personal health course, your university may offer a course on consumerism. Libraries and bookstores offer trade books on a variety of consumer topics. Consumer protection agencies can guide you in some subjects. Government agencies also may help you in your choices.

2. *Comparison shop.* In our free-enterprise system, virtually every service or product can be duplicated on the open market. Very few items or services are one-of-a-kind. Take the time to study your choices before you purchase a product or service.

3. *Insist on formal contracts and dated receipts.* Under the consumer laws in most states, you have a limited time in which to void a contract. Formal documentation of your actions as a consumer will give you the maximum protection available.

4. *Obtain written instructions and warranties.* Be certain of the appropriate use of any product you purchase. If you use a product inappropriately, you might void its warranty. Be familiar with what you can reasonably anticipate from the products and services you buy. In addition, be aware that a written warranty supersedes any verbal assurances a salesperson might make.

5. *Put your complaints in writing.* A carefully constructed record of your complaints is vital. Accurate records of the names and addresses of all companies and people with whom you have done business will enable you to document your actions as a consumer.

6. *Press for resolution of your complaints.* As a consumer, you are entitled to effective products and services. If your consumer complaints are not resolved, you have legal recourse through the courts. You should not hesitate to assert your rights, not only for your

own sake, but for consumers who might later become victims.

Consumerism is an active relationship between you and a provider. If the provider is competent and honest and you are an informed and active consumer, both of you will profit from the relationship. However, if the provider is not competent or honest, you can protect yourself by employing the preceding six suggestions.

Taking Charge of Your Health

- Keep yourself well informed about current health issues and new developments in health care.
- Analyze the credibility of the health information you receive before putting it into practice.
- Select your health care providers by using a balanced set of criteria (see pages 540 and 541).

- Explore alternative forms of health care, and consider using them as a complement to traditional health care.
- In selecting a health care plan, compare various plans on the basis of several key factors, not simply cost (see page 553).
- Assemble a complete personal/family health history as soon as possible. Be sure

to include information from older family members.
- Comply with all directions regarding the appropriate use of prescription and OTC medications.

SUMMARY

- Sources of health information include family, friends, commercials, labels, the Internet, and information supplied by health professionals, as well as others.
- Physicians can be either Doctors of Medicine (MDs) or Doctors of Osteopathy (DOs). They receive similar training and engage in similar forms of practice.
- Although alternative health care providers, including chiropractors, naturopaths, herbalists, and acupuncturists, meet the health care needs of many people, systematic study of these forms of health care is only now under way.
- Restricted-practice health care providers play important roles in meeting the health and wellness needs of the public.
- Nursing at all levels is a critical health care profession. Advanced practice nurses represent the highest level of training within nursing.
- Self-care is often a viable approach to preventing illness and reducing the use of health care providers.
- Our growing inability to afford health care services has reached crisis proportions in the United States.

- More than 45 million Americans, not just the poor, have problems getting health care. Minorities have the most limited access to health care services of all Americans.
- Health insurance is critical to our ability to afford modern health care services.
- HMOs provide an alternative way of receiving health care services, although the influence of the profit motive in their operation is a concern.
- Medicare and Medicaid are governmental plans for paying for health care services.
- The development of prescription medication is a long and expensive process for pharmaceutical manufacturers. The cost of prescription medication is the most rapidly increasing aspect of health care affordability.
- OTC products have a role to play in the treatment of illness, but their safe use is based on following label directions.
- Critical health consumerism, including avoiding health quackery, requires careful selection of health-related information, products, and services.

REVIEW QUESTIONS

1. Determine how you would test the accuracy of the health-related information you have received in your lifetime.
2. Identify and describe some sources of health-related information presented in this chapter. What factors should you consider when using these sources?
3. Describe the similarities between allopathic and osteopathic physicians. What is an alternative health care practitioner? Give examples of the types of alternative practitioners.
4. What are the theories underlying acupuncture and ayurveda?

5. Describe the services that are provided by the following limited health care providers: dentists, psychologists, podiatrists, optometrists, and opticians. Identify several allied health care professionals. What levels of training and expertise exist within nursing?
6. In what ways is the trend toward self-care evident? What are some reasons for the popularity of this movement?
7. How do private, public, and voluntary (proprietary) hospitals differ?

8. What is health insurance? Explain the following terms relating to health insurance: deductible amount, fixed indemnity benefits, full-service benefits, coinsurance, exclusion, and preexisting condition.

9. What is a health maintenance organization? How do HMO plans reduce the costs of health care? What are IPAs and PPOs?

10. What do the chemical name, brand name, and generic name of a prescription drug represent? How long is the patent protection for a prescription medication?

11. What role do Medicare and Medicaid play in meeting the health care needs of the American public? Which portion of Medicare is universal? What elective options does Medicare offer?

12. What are the three criteria that must be met by an OTC drug?

13. What is health quackery? What can a consumer do to avoid consumer fraud?

ENDNOTES

1. *Internet Health Resources.* Pew Internet & American Life Project. 2003. www.pewinternet.org/.

2. The National Council on the Aging. Media sources of health info. As reported in *USA Today.* 1999. 26 October, 9d.

3. Baker L, et al. Use of the Internet and e-mail for health care information: Results from a national survey. *JAMA.* 2003. 289(18):2400–2406.

4. Wagner TH, et al. Free internet access, the digital divide, and health information. *Med Care.* 2005. 43(4):415–420.

5. Wagner TH, et al. Use of the Internet for health information by the chronically ill. *Prev Chronic Dis.* 2004. 1(4):A13. Epub 2004 September 15.

6. Sierpina VS. *Integrative Health Care: Complementary and Alternative Therapies for the Whole Person.* Philadelphia: F. A. Davis, 2001.

7. National Center for Complementary and Alternative Medicine. *About Chiropractic and Its Use in Treating Low-Back Pain.* Research Report. February 2004. www.nccam.nih.gov/health/chiropractic/chiropractic.pdf.

8. National Center for Complementary and Alternative Medicine. *Chiropractic Consortium Becomes OAM's Eleventh Research Center.* NIH News Release. March 1998. www.nccam.nih.gov/news/19972000/030398.htm.

9. National Center for Complementary and Alternative Medicine. *Acupuncture: Mechanism of Action.* September 2003. www.nccam.nih.gov/health/acupuncture/#nccam.

10. National Center for Alternative and Complementary Medicine. *Acupuncture.* December 2004. www.nccam.nih.gov/health/acupuncture/.

11. Yang JH. The effects of foot reflexology on nausea, vomiting and fatigue of breast cancer patients undergoing chemotherapy. *Taehan Kanho Hakhoe Chi.* 2005. 35(1):177–185.

12. Siiev-Ner I, et al. Reflexology treatment relieves symptoms of multiple sclerosis: a randomized controlled study. *Mult Scler.* 2003. 9(4):356–361.

13. Kholler M. Children with ear disorders who are treated by reflexologists or general practitioners. *Ugeske Laeger.* 2003. 165(19):1994–1999.

14. National Center for Complementary and Alternative Medicine. *Questions and Answers about Homeopathy.* 2003. www.nih.gov/health/homeopathy/index.htm#al.

15. Jascobs J, et al. Homeopathy for menopausal symptoms in breast cancer survivors: A preliminary randomized controlled trial. *J Altern Complement Med.* 2005. 11(1):21–27

16. Shekelle PG, et al. Efficacy and safety of ephedra and ephedrine for weight loss and athletic performance: A meta-analysis. *JAMA.* 2003. 289(12):1537–1545.

17. FDA Statement. *FDA Announces Rule Prohibiting Sale of Dietary Supplements Containing Ephedrine Alkaloids Effective April 12.* April 12, 2004. www.fda.gov/bbs/topics/NEWS/2004/NEW01050.htm.

18. Department for Professional Employees. *Nurses: Vital Signs.* AFRL-CIO. 2004. www.dpeaflcio.org/policy/factsheets/fs_2004_nurses.htm.

19. Aiken LH, et al. Hospital nurse staffing and patient mortality, nurse burnout, and job satisfaction. *JAMA.* 2002. 288(16):1987–1993.

20. Paradise J. European opposition to exclusive control over predictive breast cancer testing and the inherent implications for U.S. patent law and public policy: A case study of the Myriad Genetics' BRCA patent controversy. *Food and Drug Law J.* 2004. 59(1):133–154.

21. Sanders S. Is the glass half empty or full? Reflections on strain and gain in caregivers of individuals with Alzheimer's disease. *Soc Work Health Care.* 2005. 40(3):57–73.

22. National Coalition on Health Care. Health insurance coverage. 2004. www.nchc.org/facts/coverage.shtml.

23. U.S. Census Bureau. *National Health Expenditures by Type: 1900–2002 (No. 115).* Statistical Abstract of the United States: 2004–2005.

24. U.S. Census Bureau. *National Health Expenditures— Summary, 1960–2002, and Projections, 2003–2013 (No. 114).* Statistical Abstract of the United States: 2004–2005.

25. U.S. Census Bureau. *Health Services and Supplies—Per Capita Consumer Expenditures by Object: 1990 to 2002. (No. 117).* Statistical Abstract of the United States: 2004–2005.

26. Health Care Financing Administration. *Personal Health Care Expenditures Amounts, and Average Annual Percent Change, Percent Distribution, and Per Capita Amounts, by Source of Funds for Selected Calendar Years 1970–2007.* Table 2a. November 2000. www.chfa.gov/stats/NHE-proj/t02b.htm.

27. The Kaiser Family Foundation and Health Research and Education Trust. *Employer Health Benefits: 2004 Annual Survey.* 2004. www.kff.org.

28. Centers for Medicare & Medicaid Services. *Medicare and You—2005.* U.S. Department of Health and Human Services. 2005. Pub No. CMS-10050.

29. McKenzie JF, Pinger RR, Korwcki JE. *An Introduction to Community Health* (5th ed.). Boston: Jones & Bartlett.

30. The MetLife Mature Market Institute. *The MetLife Market Survey of Nursing Home & Home Care Costs—September 2005.* www.MatureMarketInstitute@metlife.com.

31. U.S. Census Bureau. *Retail Prescription Drug Sales: 1995–2003 (No. 122).* Statistical Abstract of the United States: 2004–2005.

32. Centers for Medicare & Medicaid Services. *National Health Care Expenditure Amounts, and Average Annual Percent of Change by Type of Expenditure (Table 2).* 2002. U.S. Department of Health and Human Services. www.hhs.gov/statistics/nhe/projections-2002/t2a.asp.

33. U.S. Food and Drug Administration. *FDA Regulatory Actions for the Cox-2 Selective and Non-Selective Non-Steroidal Anti-Inflammatory Drugs (NSAIDs). 2005. Questions and Answers.* www.fda.gov/cder/drug/infopage/COX2/COX2qa.htm.

34. Center for Drug Evaluation and Research. *Generic Drug Approvals.* 2005. U.S. Food and Drug Administration. www.fda.gov/cder/ogd/approvals/default.htm.

35. *Drug Consult 2006: The Comprehensive Reference for Generic and Brand Name Drugs.* 2006. St. Louis: Mosby's Drug Consult, Mosby, 2006.

As We Go to Press

Does "wiring" a hospital make it a more effective institution for providers, patients, and families? A study was conducted that compared hospitals with highly developed computer accessibility to those with limited accessibility. Using data from a list of the 100 Most Wired Hospitals and similar data from hospitals not on the list, the study identified interesting differences in patient and physician practices. In the area of patient services, it found that patients able to access test results, renew prescriptions, schedule appointments, and request advice from physicians online were three to four times more likely to engage in these activities than patients who were required to use other means of communication. With respect to physicians, use of online access to clinical guidelines and the ability to order patient services (laboratory, radiography, and pharmacy) before patient admission, led these doctors to schedule such patient services two to three times more frequently than physicians who were required to use other modalities, such as the phone or fax.

Perhaps the most interesting observation involved patient surveillance by physicians using office or home computers in a secure manner. In hospitals on the Most Wired Hospitals list, physicians used this technology to monitor patients in intensive care units, in postsurgical units, and on general medicine floors. Physicians who could monitor patients only via a telephone call or by direct observation were less inclined to engage in patient monitoring than were those in high-tech institutions.

personal assessment

Are you a skilled health consumer?

Circle the selection that best describes your practice. Then total your points for an interpretation of your health consumer skills.

1 Never
2 Occasionally
3 Most of the time
4 All of the time

1. I read all warranties and then file them for safekeeping.

   1   2   3   4

2. I read labels for information pertaining to the nutritional quality of food.

   1   2   3   4

3. I practice comparative shopping and use unit pricing, when available.

   1   2   3   4

4. I read health-related advertisements in a critical and careful manner.

   1   2   3   4

5. I challenge all claims pertaining to secret cures or revolutionary new health devices.

   1   2   3   4

6. I engage in appropriate medical self-care screening procedures.

   1   2   3   4

7. I maintain a patient-provider relationship with a variety of health care providers.

   1   2   3   4

8. I inquire about the fees charged before using a health care provider's services.

   1   2   3   4

9. I maintain adequate health insurance coverage.

   1   2   3   4

10. I consult reputable medical self-care books before seeing a physician.

   1   2   3   4

11. I ask pertinent questions of health care providers when I am uncertain about the information I have received.

   1   2   3   4

12. I seek second opinions when the diagnosis of a condition or the recommended treatment seems questionable.

   1   2   3   4

13. I follow directions pertaining to the use of prescription drugs, including continuing their use for the entire period prescribed.

   1   2   3   4

14. I buy generic drugs when they are available.

   1   2   3   4

15. I follow directions pertaining to the use of OTC drugs.

   1   2   3   4

16. I maintain a well-supplied medicine cabinet.

   1   2   3   4

YOUR TOTAL POINTS _____

Interpretation

16–24 points	A very poorly skilled health consumer
25–40 points	An inadequately skilled health consumer
41–56 points	An adequately skilled health consumer
57–64 points	A highly skilled health consumer

To Carry This Further . . .

Could you ever have been the victim of consumer fraud? What will you need to do to be a skilled consumer?

chapter nineteen

Protecting Your Safety

Eye on the Media

Images of Terrorism: The World Trade Center Disaster

Where were you on the morning of September 11, 2001? How did you hear the news about the terror attacks on New York and Washington? The entire nation stood stunned as TV cameras captured a passenger jet crashing into one of New York's twin towers, followed a few minutes later by a second plane that hit the second tower. Soon after, it was reported that a third plane had hit the Pentagon, and a fourth had crashed in a field in Pennsylvania.

Most of the day's horrors were captured by television cameras, as well as by a few film crews who happened to be filming in Manhattan that day. Americans watched in horror as networks played and replayed footage of each plane hitting the World Trade Center, and of the fires that ensued; they saw office workers running for their lives and witnessed firefighters and other rescue workers going back into buildings that were clearly unsound to guide people out of the burning towers. And finally, they saw the two towers crumble to the ground.

For three full days the major TV networks suspended their regular programming to cover the disaster in depth. No commercials, no sitcoms, no soap operas, and no David Letterman or Jay Leno for days. When Letterman returned to the air, it wasn't to tell jokes but to have Dan Rather talk about the tragic events, and viewers saw the normally staunch newsman's eyes fill with tears. When *Saturday Night Live* featured New York Mayor Rudolph Giuliani, it was as a respected guest, not as a target for a spoof. By Saturday morning the cartoons were back—for the children. In fact, many networks geared toward children—most notably PBS— tailored their programming to offer them more comforting fare, and provided special public service announcements advising parents on how to help their children feel safe despite their own uncertainty.

In the weeks and months that followed, the media helped provide a sense of unity to a vast, grieving nation. But the constant coverage of the tragedy and its aftermath— including footage of the attacks, and of rescue workers searching the rubble of Ground Zero for the bodies of their fallen comrades—took a toll on many people watching. People lost sleep and felt depressed. Some worried about having to get on an airplane again. Young children had an especially difficult time— wondering why this happened and whether *they* would be victims of a terrorist attack. Some children touched buildings to make sure they were "safe" before going inside.

Today, Americans are acutely aware of the possibility of terror attacks on our soil. The international news media regularly report on anti-American sentiments in Middle Eastern countries. The Department of Homeland Security continually evaluates the national threat level, with a system ranging from Code Green (low) to Code Red (severe). When the national threat level was raised from Yellow (elevated) to Orange (heightened) in December of 2003, it was major news. Many media outlets—especially the 24-hour news channels—report on the nation's state of alert

In recent years, several high-profile violent crimes have been the subject of intense media scrutiny and public outrage: the killings of Matthew Shepard and James Byrd, Jr., and the terrorist attack on the World Trade Center in New York City, for example, have received exhaustive media coverage. Heinous sexual assaults and murders of children—Megan Kanka, JonBenet Ramsey, and Girl X in Chicago—have also generated much attention and angered the public. The killing of students and a teacher at Columbine High School by two students shocked the nation and caused residents of Littleton, Colorado, to wonder sadly what had happened to their "safe" community.

Domestic violence directed at women and children is all too common, and many people fear becoming a random victim of a homicide, robbery, or carjacking. Law enforcement officials contend that gang activities and hard-core drug involvement are significant factors that have led to violent behavior in our society.

Although violence may seem to be focused in urban areas, no community is completely safe. Even people who live in small towns and rural areas now must lock their doors and remain vigilant about protecting their safety. Crime on college campuses, much of which is a direct result of alcohol use, remains a threat. (For tips on avoiding becoming a victim of a violent crime, see Changing for the Better on page 566.)

For some students the content in this chapter may be the most important information in this textbook. Becoming a victim of violent behavior or sustaining an unintentional injury can harm your health as much (or more than) any of your own unhealthy behavior. The goal of this chapter is to help you understand the scope of violence and unintentional injury in our society and learn what you can do to avoid becoming a victim. (Complete the Personal Assessment on page 589 to see whether you are adequately protecting your own safety.)

Reducing Risk Factors

Many factors influence your risk of suffering an injury or becoming a victim of crime. Some of these you cannot change. For example, the greatest percentage of violent crimes tend to be committed by, and suffered by, the young. This risk is multiplied for those who are young and African American, and for those who live in an area with gang activity.

However, you *can* affect many of the other risk factors for injury or crime, as you will learn throughout this chapter. For example, alcohol plays a major role in driving, motorcycle, and boating accidents. You can reduce your risk of accidents by avoiding alcohol and drugs while you enjoy these activities. Likewise, boxes throughout this chapter will show you how to avoid becoming a victim of date rape, how to avoid accidents in your car, and how to maintain a safe and comfortable home.

Intentional Injuries

Intentional injuries are injuries that are committed on purpose. With the exception of suicide (which is self-directed), intentional injuries reflect violence committed by one person acting against another person. Criminal acts that result in intentional injuries include homicide, robbery, rape, sexual assault, aggravated assault (assault with a weapon), and simple assault. These acts may be carried out in the context of interpersonal or domestic violence, gang violence, hate crimes, or terrorism. Each year in the United States, intentional violence results in nearly fifty thousand deaths and another 2 million nonfatal injuries.[1]

In 2003, more than 24 million crimes were committed against U.S. residents age 12 and older, according to data collected in the National Crime Victimization Survey. Of these, one in four (5.4 million) was a violent crime (rape, sexual assault, robbery, aggravated assault or simple assault).[2] The good news is that these figures continue the downward trend in criminal victimization that began in 1994. The 2003 rate is less than half the 1994 rate.[3]

> **Key Terms**
>
> **intentional injuries** injuries that are purposely committed by a person

Homicide

Homicide, or murder, is the intentional killing of one person by another. Sadly, the United States leads the industrialized world in homicide rates. The 2002 murder rate, however, was 5.6 per 100,000 inhabitants. Fortunately, this rate reflects a decline since 1991, when the homicide rate was 9.8 per 100,000 population.[4]

Criminal justice experts are trying to pinpoint why U.S. homicide rates are dropping. No single answer has emerged but speculation centers on better community policing efforts; the 1994 passage of the broad Federal Crime Bill; legislation, such as the Brady Law; and a variety of tough state laws, such as the "three strikes and you're out" provision, that mandate life sentences without parole for repeat violent offenders. If recent incarceration rates do not change, an estimated 1 in 20 people (5.1 percent) will serve time in a state or federal prison. The chances of going to prison are higher for men (9 percent) than for women (1.1 percent).[5]

One clear trend is the extent to which illegal drug activity is related to homicide. A variety of research studies from large cities indicate that 25–50 percent of all homicides are drug related.[6] Most of these murders are associated with drug trafficking, including disputed drug transactions. For the country taken as a whole, this figure is much lower. For 2003, only 4.6 percent of homicides were drug related.[7] However, statistics reveal that high percentages of both homicide assailants and victims have drugs in their system at the time of the homicide.[6]

Key Terms

homicide the intentional killing of one person by another person

---

Another clear trend is that handguns are the weapons of choice for homicides. It was the proliferation of handguns and their use in violent crimes that led to the passage of the Brady Law.

Domestic Violence

Family life in the 21st century is a far cry from that portrayed in the popular 1950s and 1960s television shows like "The Donna Reed Show," "Father Knows Best," and "The Adventures of Ozzie and Harriet." The composition of families has changed considerably. In the 1950s a common family pattern included children being raised by both parents. Generally, the father was the income earner and the mother stayed at home and managed the growing family.

Today, family patterns are much more complex. Children are more frequently being raised in blended families or in families headed by single parents. In 2003 there were 10 million single-mother families in the United States and 2 million single-father families.[8] A much higher percentage of women are employed outside the home. Because of pressing family economic concerns, many children take care of themselves during after-school hours. Sociologists indicate that families, and the individuals in those families, are under more stress than ever. Nonetheless, reports of some types of family violence have decreased in recent years. Yet domestic violence remains a serious concern in our society.

Intimate Partner Violence

Intimate partner violence (IPV) refers to violence committed against a domestic partner. Most often the victims are women, and a significant percentage of these women are spouses or former spouses of the assailant. IPV can include murder, rape, sexual assault, robbery, aggravated assault, and simple assault. Violent acts that constitute abuse range from a slap on the face to murder.

A 2001 report released by the Bureau of Justice Statistics revealed encouraging findings. The report indicated that intimate nonlethal violence had declined 48 percent since 1993, from a rate of 5.8 nonfatal intimate victimizations per 1,000 persons to just 3 per 1,000 persons. The rate of decline was greater for female victims (49 percent) than for male victims (42 percent).[9] Two reasons have been proposed for this decline in intimate partner violence: better services for families at risk, and an improving economy during the period covered by the report.[10] Actually, rates of IPV began to edge upward in 2001, perhaps as a result of rising unemployment.

Murders by intimates in 2000, the most recent year for which statistics are available, reached the lowest levels since 1976. In 2000 1,687 murders were reported among intimate partners, whereas nearly 3,000 such murders took place in 1976. As has been the case for many years, three of every four victims of intimate murder were females.[10]

The most vulnerable female victims are African American and Hispanic, live in large cities, are young, unmarried, and are from lower socioeconomic groups. However, these trends do not mean that only women from these classifications are vulnerable to violent behavior. Men and women across all economic, racial, and age categories are potential victims.

One of the real difficulties related to intimate violence is the vast underreporting of this crime to law enforcement authorities. The U.S. Department of Justice estimates that about half of the victims of intimate violence do not report the crime to police. Too many victims view their violent situations as private or personal matters and not actual crimes. Despite painful injuries, many victims view the offenses against them as minor. Even psychological abuse, the least frequently reported form of intimate violence, can lead not only to feelings of loss of control and emotional dysfunction, but also to a wide array of physical health problems. Victims of psychological abuse are twice as likely as others to report chronic pain, spastic colon, irritable bowel syndrome, infections, and migraine headaches.[11]

Of course, it is easy to criticize the victims of intimate violence for not reporting the crimes committed against them, but this may be unfair. Why do women stay in these relationships? Many women who are injured may fear being killed if they report the crime. Women may also fear for the safety of their children. Women who receive economic support may fear being left with no financial resources.

However, help is available for victims of intimate abuse. Most communities have family support or intimate violence hot lines that abused people can call for help. Communities are establishing shelters where abused women and their children can seek safety while their cases are being handled by the police or court officials. If you are being abused or know of someone who is the victim of intimate violence, do not hesitate to use the services of these local hot lines or shelters. Also, check the resources listed in the Health Reference Guide at the back of this text.

TALKING POINTS A close friend confides that her boyfriend sometimes "gets rough" with her. She's afraid to talk to him about it because she thinks that will make things worse. What immediate steps would you tell her to take?

Key Terms

intimate partner violence violent victimization committed by current or former spouses, boyfriends, or girlfriends

Maltreatment of Children

Like many cases of intimate partner violence, **child maltreatment** tends to be a silent crime. It is estimated nearly one million children are victims of child abuse and neglect each year.[12] Some children are victims of repeated crimes, and since many victims do not report these crimes, the actual incidence of child abuse is difficult to determine.

Child maltreatment includes child abuse and child neglect. Children are abused in various ways. Physical abuse reflects physical injury, such as bruises, burns, abrasions, cuts, and fractures of the bones and skull. Sexual abuse includes acts that lead to sexual gratification of the abuser. Examples include fondling, touching, and various acts involved in rape, sodomy, and incest. Psychological abuse is another form of child abuse. Certainly, children are scarred by family members and others who routinely damage their psychological development. However, this form of abuse is especially difficult to identify and measure.

Child neglect is failure to provide a child with adequate clothing, food, shelter, and medical attention. The incidence of child neglect is approximately three times the incidence of physical abuse and about seven times the incidence of child sexual abuse. Child maltreatment deaths are more often associated with child neglect than with any type of abuse.[12] Educational neglect, such as failure to see that a child attends school regularly, is one of the most common types of child neglect. Each form of abuse can have devastating short- and long-term consequences for the child.

Research studies in the various areas of child maltreatment reveal some interesting trends. Abused children are much more likely than are nonabused children to grow up to be child abusers. Abused children are more likely to suffer from poor educational performance, increased health problems, and low levels of overall achievement. Abused children are significantly more likely than are nonabused children to become involved in adult crime and violent criminal behavior. Finally, neglected children's rates of arrest for violence were almost as high as those of physically abused children.[13]

It is beyond the scope of this book to discuss in detail how to reduce child abuse. However, the violence directed against children can likely be lessened through a combination of early identification measures and violence prevention programs. Teachers, friends, relatives, social workers, counselors, psychologists, police, and the court system must not hesitate to intervene early in cases of suspected child abuse. In fact, every adult is responsible for reporting suspected child abuse and neglect. To do so, persons should call their local police department or Child Protective Services (within the Department of Public Welfare) and request assistance in filing a report. So long as the report is filed in good conscience (without malice)

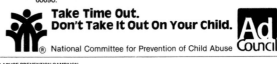

12 alternatives to lashing out at your child.

The next time everyday pressures build up to the point where you feel like lashing out — STOP! And try any of these simple alternatives.

You'll feel better . . . and so will your child.

1. Take a deep breath. And another. Then remember you are the adult . . .
2. Close your eyes and imagine you're hearing what your child is about to hear.
3. Press your lips together and count to 10. Or better yet, to 20.
4. Put your child in a time-out chair. (Remember the rule: one time-out minute for each year of age.)
5. Put yourself in a time-out chair. Think about why you are angry: is it your child, or is your child simply a convenient target for your anger?
6. Phone a friend.
7. If someone can watch the children, go outside and take a walk.
8. Take a hot bath or splash cold water on your face.
9. Hug a pillow.
10. Turn on some music. Maybe even sing along.
11. Pick up a pencil and write down as many helpful words as you can think of. Save the list.
12. Write for parenting information: Parenting, Box 2866, Chicago, IL 60690.

Take Time Out. Don't Take It Out On Your Child. Ad Council

® National Committee for Prevention of Child Abuse

Figure 19-1   Alternatives to hitting your child

there will be no negative ramifications for the person filing. The later the intervention, the more likely that the abuse will have worsened. When an individual has abused once, he or she is likely to do it again.

Violence prevention programs can help parents and caregivers learn how to resolve conflicts, improve communication, cope with anger, improve parenting skills, and challenge the view of violence presented in movies and television. These programs may help to stop violence before it begins to damage the lives of young children. Figure 19-1 provides simple alternatives parents can choose to avoid hitting a child.

Key Terms

child maltreatment   the act or failure to act by a parent or caretaker that results in abuse or neglect of a child or that places the child in imminent risk of serious harm

Maltreatment of Elders

Among the nation's 35 million adults 65 years of age and older, between 1 and 2 million have been injured, exploited, or otherwise mistreated.[14,15] Particularly vulnerable are women over the age of 75 years. Nearly half (47 percent) of the abusers are the children of the victims, and 85 percent are family members.[16]

Many older adults are hit, kicked, attacked with knives, or denied food and medical care; others are robbed of their Social Security checks and automobiles. These crimes probably reflect a combination of factors, particularly the stress of caring for failing older people by middle-aged children who also face the additional demands of dependent children and careers. In many cases, the middle-aged children were themselves abused, or there may be a chemical dependence problem. The alternative, institutionalization, is so expensive that it is often not an option for either the abused or the abuser.

Although protective services are available, abuse of older adults is frequently unseen and unreported. In many cases, the older adults themselves are afraid to report their children's behavior because of the fear of embarrassment that they were not good parents to their children. Regardless of the cause, however, abuse of older adults must be reported to the appropriate protective service so that intervention can occur.

Violence at College

A recent report has summarized violent victimization of college students. Perhaps the most important finding was that college campuses are a relatively safe place to be. College students (ages 18–24 years) experience less violence than do nonstudents in the same age group. Violence rates have declined for both groups since 1995, when rates were 88 per 1,000 for college students and 102 per 1,000 for nonstudents. The 2002 rates are 41 and 56, respectively.[17]

During the period 1995–2002, simple assault (assault without a weapon) accounted for 63 percent of the violent victimizations, whereas rape/sexual assault accounted for 6 percent. Males were about twice as likely to be victims of violence as women were. About 93 percent of the crimes occurred off campus, 72 percent occurred at night, and 41 percent of victims perceived that the offenders were using alcohol or drugs at the time of the offense.[17]

Gangs and Youth Violence

In the last 30 years, gangs and gang activities have been increasingly responsible for escalating violence and criminal activity. Before that time, gangs used fists, tire irons, and occasionally, cheap handguns ("Saturday night specials") as tools of enforcement. Now, gang members do not hesitate to use more lethal semiautomatic weapons.

Sixty-six percent of gang members live in large cities (more than 25,000 population),[18] where many socially alienated, economically disadvantaged young people live. Convinced that society has no significant role for them, gang members can receive support from an association of peers that has well-defined lines of authority. Rituals and membership initiation rites are important in gang socialization. Gangs often control territories within a city. Frequently, gangs are involved in criminal activities, the most common of which are illicit drug trafficking and robberies. In the late 1990s, gang-related murders and drive-by shootings contributed to the high death rate among young people and especially inner-city youth. In 1999 the rate of gang-related murders of young persons reached, on average, 24 deaths every two days—the equivalent of a classroom of dead young persons (below the age of 20) every other day. Perhaps no single example of youth violence, with a measure of gang affiliation included, is more vivid than the April 20, 1999, shootings that occured at Columbine High School in Littleton, Colorado. On that day Eric Harris and Dylan Klebold, dressed in their gang-affiliated black trench coats, entered their high school and began a planned and systematic gun and bomb rampage that resulted in the deaths of fourteen students and one teacher. To this day, no one is certain why Harris and Klebold, and their closest friends, felt such anger toward and sense of disenfranchisement from their classmates and community.

It is not only older male teenagers and young adults who are members of today's gangs. Law enforcement officials see younger people (ages 12, 13, and 14) joining gangs. Some gangs have recently included young women as members, and some cities report a growing number of all-female gangs. Some female gangs are reported to be every bit as ruthless as the male gangs. Only about 6 percent of gang members were female in 2000.[18]

Attempting to control gang and youth violence is particularly expensive for communities. When you consider that for every gang-related homicide, there are about one hundred nonfatal gang-related intentional injuries, it becomes obvious that gang violence is an expensive health care proposition. Furthermore, gang and youth violence takes an enormous financial and human toll on law enforcement, the judicial system, and corrections departments.

Fortunately, the recent decline in murders and other serious crimes also applies to gang-related crimes. Once again, some observers credit more aggressive police tactics for the decline. Some of the tactics being used to meet this problem are the aggressive "quality of life" policing in some cities and President Clinton's COPS program (Community Oriented Policing Services) to hire new police officers and put them on foot patrols, where they become acquainted with residents. Others believe that the drop in

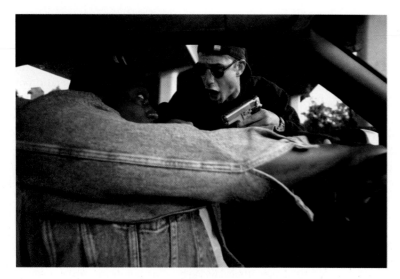

The prevalence of firearms in American society—especially among young men—is especially troubling. Guns are involved in more than half of all homicides and suicides, and are often used during violent crimes such as robberies and carjackings.

crime should be attributed to factors such as a stronger economy and the fading of the crack market. In Boston, a campaign aimed at youth gangs offered summer jobs to gang members, combined with threats of federal prison sentences for gun violence. In a 2-year period since that time, no youngsters under 17 have been shot and killed in Boston. Regardless, reducing gang and youth violence will be a continuing challenge for the nation in the 21st century.

Gun Violence

Guns are being used more widely than ever in our society and in other parts of the world. The fatality rate for gun injuries is 30 percent higher than the fatality rate for injuries of all causes (less than 1 percent).[19] More than 60 percent of the homicides and 55 percent of the suicides committed each year in the United States involve the use of guns. As previously mentioned, gun violence is a leading killer of teenagers and young men, especially African American men, and the use of semiautomatic assault weapons by individuals and gang members is common. Colleges and universities are not immune to gun violence. A recent study found that 4.3 percent of college students had a working firearm at college. Of these, nearly half stated that they had the gun for protection.[20] Accidental deaths of toddlers and young children from loaded handguns is another dimension of the violence attributable to guns in our society. In addition, guns are often used in **carjackings.**

The proliferation of firearm use has prompted serious discussions about the enactment of gun control laws. For years, gun control activists have been in direct battle with the National Rifle Association (NRA) and its congressional supporters. Gun control activists want fewer guns manufactured and greater controls over the sale and possession of handguns. Gun supporters believe

that such controls are not necessary and that people (the criminals) are responsible for gun deaths, not simply the guns. This debate will certainly continue.

Bias and Hate Crimes

One sad aspect of any society is how some segments of the majority treat certain people in the minority (see Learning from Our Diversity on page 571). Nowhere is this more violently pronounced than in **bias and hate crimes.** In 2003 more than half (52.3 percent) of all single-bias hate crimes were motivated by racial bias, followed by religious bias (16.4 percent), sexual orientation (16.4 percent), ethnic/national origin bias (14.2 percent), and disability bias (0.5 percent). Victims of hate crimes are often verbally abused, their property is damaged or destroyed, and too frequently they are physically attacked. Two recent hate-motivated killings shocked the nation. One case involved the beating death of Matthew Shepard, a gay college student who was taken from a Wyoming bar, driven to a rural area, tied to a fence post, and savagely beaten to death. Aaron McKinney, one of the two men accused in the

---

Key Terms

carjacking a crime that involves a thief's attempt to steal a car while the owner is behind the wheel; carjackings are usually random and unpredictable, and they frequently involve handguns

bias and hate crimes criminal acts directed at a person or group solely because of a specific characteristic, such as race, religion, sexual orientation, ethnic background, or other difference

Learning from Our Diversity

Violence against the Disabled

No one is totally free from the risk of senseless violence—children, adults, or college students. No single group, however, is a more tragic target of violence than the disabled. Despite the protective efforts of laws such as the Fair Housing Amendments Act, the Americans with Disabilities Act, and the Rehabilitation Act, the disabled remain an easily victimized segment of the population.

Because of the high level of vulnerability that disabled persons face, national advocacy groups, such as All Walks Of Life, are working to assist the disabled, their caregivers, and the general population in reducing the risk of violence to this group. However, much can also be accomplished on an individual basis. If you are an able-bodied college student, you can probably implement the following suggestions on your campus:

- Encourage your disabled peers to remain vigilant by staying tuned in to their environment. Remind them that simply because they appear disabled does not guarantee that they will be protected from harm.
- Support your disabled friends in the challenges imposed by their limitations, particularly when they are in unfamiliar environments or experiencing unusual situations.
- Suggest that your peers with disabilities carry, or wear a personal alarm device. Such devices, also frequently carried by able-bodied

students, can be purchased in bookstores or sporting goods stores.
- Remind your disabled friends to inform others about their schedule plans, for example, when they will be away from school and when they are likely to return.
- Encourage people with disabilities to seek the assistance of an escort (security personnel) when leaving a campus building or a shopping mall to enter a large parking area.
- Be an advocate for your disabled friends. For example, if residence hall room doors do not have peepholes at wheelchair height, find out if the doors can be modified.

One additional approach remains controversial. That is the teaching of self-defense techniques to people with disabilities. Groups that advocate instruction to the disabled in the martial arts, such as judo, remind us that "doing nothing will produce nothing." Others contend that a limited ability to use a martial art leads to a false sense of confidence that encourages a disregard for other forms of protection. They further argue that if disabled persons try to counter aggression with ineffectively delivered martial arts techniques, they may anger their attacker and actually increase the aggression against themselves.

---

killings, based his defense on "gay panic," contending that he was traumatized by a homosexual advance as a young child. A second case that shocked the nation was that of James Byrd, Jr., a 49-year-old African American man who was accosted by two white men as he walked along a rural roadway in Texas. After being beaten, spray-painted black, and chained to the rear of a pickup, Byrd was then dragged behind the truck for an extended distance. The trauma Byrd experienced was so severe that he was decapitated and his torso dismembered.

Typically, the offenders in bias or hate crimes are fringe elements of a larger society who believe that the mere presence of someone with a racial, ethnic, sexual orientation, or religious difference is inherently bad for the community, state, or country. Examples of groups commonly known to commit bias and hate crimes in the United States are skinheads, the Ku Klux Klan, and other white supremacist groups. Increasingly, state and federal laws have been enacted to make bias and hate crimes serious offenses.

With a small but growing presence of neo-Nazi groups in Europe and clear evidence that ethnic cleansing took place in Kosovo, Bosnia, Serbia, Croatia, Rwanda, Iraq, Darfur, and the former Soviet Union, bias and hate crimes are a worldwide problem. The recent push on college campuses to promote multicultural education and

the celebration of diversity may help today's generation of college graduates understand the importance of tolerance and inclusion and avoid bigotry and exclusion.

Stalking

In recent years the crime of **stalking** has received considerable attention. Stalking refers to an assailant's planned efforts to pursue an intended victim. Most stalkers are male. (One notable exception was the convicted female stalker of talk show host David Letterman.) Many of these stalkers are excessively possessive or jealous and pursue people with whom they formerly had a relationship. Some stalkers pursue people with whom they have had only an imaginary relationship.

Some stalkers have served time in prison and have waited for years to "get back" at their victims. In some cases, stalkers go to great lengths to locate their intended

---

Key Terms

stalking a crime involving an assailant's planned efforts to pursue an intended victim

Putting Fear in Perspective

Your neighbor, an elderly adult, stays locked in her house all day, afraid to open the door to anyone. Too many hours of watching local TV news, you think. But it's not just older people who are living in fear. Parents, women, gays, and minorities are all looking over their shoulders.

Some parents who walked to school when they were children wouldn't think of letting their kids do that. What about child molesters and kidnappers? A young woman at a party guards her drink all night—afraid that someone might put a drug in it. She's afraid of being raped. The gay person who goes to his old neighborhood to visit his grandmother feels uneasy. Is it his imagination, or are people looking at him in a threatening way? An African American man walking down the street hears a racial slur. Should he ignore it, or stop and say something?

All of these situations call for caution. If you're a parent, you need to be careful about your child's safety. But your child can walk to school—accompanied by you, another parent, or an older child. If you're a woman, you can keep an eye on your drink at a party without making that the focus of your attention. If you're a gay man who feels uncomfortable in an unfamiliar part of town, stay focused on where you're going. Walk quickly and confidently, without being intimidated. If you're a minority member who's being taunted, keep your dignity and remain calm.

Putting fear in perspective takes practice. First, stay reasonable. Recognize that acts of violence represent the extreme elements of society. There's a good reason you probably haven't met many (or any) murderers, robbers, or rapists. They make up a small segment of society. The people you usually encounter, who are basically good, represent the large majority. Second, be aware. Pay attention to what's going on around you. See things in a neutral way. If you do, you'll realize when an argument is about to turn into a fistfight or worse. Third, use common sense. Don't put yourself at risk, but don't stop living. You can't build your life around avoiding a potential act of violence. Fourth, trust your senses. If someone is walking too close to you and you feel uncomfortable, cross the street and go into a store. Last, practice what-if situations. For example, what would you do if you were in your car at a stoplight and someone held a gun up to your window? Considering your possible actions ahead of time, without dwelling on them, is one way of preparing yourself for real-life threats.

Living in fear is something that happens gradually—as fear takes control of a person's life. But that doesn't need to happen to you. You can take control of fear in a healthy, positive way—to build a life of rich experiences balanced by caution and good sense.

---

victims and frequently know their daily whereabouts. Although not all stalkers plan to batter or kill their victims, their presence and potential for violence are enough to create an extremely frightening environment for the intended victim and family. (See Discovering Your Spirituality above about putting your fear into perspective.)

Fortunately, since 1990 virtually all states have enacted or tightened their laws related to stalking and have created stiff penalties for stalkers. In many areas the criminal justice system is proactive in letting possible victims of stalking know, for example, when a particular prison inmate is going to be released. In other areas, citizens are banding together to provide support and protection for people who may be victims of stalkers.

A recent report indicates that about 13 percent of college women are stalked in a given year.[22] If you think you are or someone you know is being stalked, contact the police (or a local crisis intervention hot line number) to report your case.

 TALKING POINTS You suspect that someone is stalking you, but your friends think you're being dramatic. How would you get objective advice on what to do?

Sexual Victimization

Ideally, sexual intimacy is a mutual, enjoyable form of communication between two people. Far too often, however, relationships are approached in an aggressive, hostile manner. These sexual aggressors always have a victim—someone who is physically or psychologically traumatized. *Sexual victimization* occurs in many forms and in a variety of settings. In this section we briefly look at sexual victimization as it occurs in rape and sexual assault, sexual abuse of children, sexual harassment, and the commercialization of sex.

Rape and Sexual Assault

As violence in our society increases, the incidence of *rape* and *sexual assault* correspondingly rises. The victims of these crimes fall into no single category. Survivors of rape and sexual assault include young and old, male and female. They can be mentally retarded people, prisoners, hospital patients, or college students. We are all potential victims, and self-protection is critical. Table 19.1 deals with the myths surrounding rape.

Sometimes a personal assault begins as a physical assault that may turn into a rape. Rape is generally considered a crime of sexual aggression in which the victim is

Table 19.1 Rape: Myth versus Fact

Only women are raped.	Nearly 10 percent of rape victims (19,670) in 2003 were males.
Most rapists are strangers.	Seventy-four percent of male victims and 70 percent of female victims describe the offender as a nonstranger (intimate, other relative, or friend/acquaintance).
Most rapes occur in streets, alleys, and deserted places.	Ninety percent of rapes occur in living quarters—60 percent in the victim's residence.
Rapists are easily identified by their demeanor or psychological profile.	Most experts indicate that rapists do not differ significantly from nonrapists.
Rape is an overreported crime.	Only one in five rapes is reported.
Rape happens only to people in low socioeconomic classes.	Rape occurs in all socioeconomic classes. Each person, male or female, young or old, is a potential victim.
There is a standard way to avoid rape.	Each rape situation is different. No single method to avoid rape can work in every potential rape situation. Because of this we encourage personal health classes to invite speakers from a local rape prevention services bureau to discuss approaches to rape prevention.

forced to have sexual intercourse. Current thought concerning rape characterizes this behavior as a violent act that happens to be carried out through sexual contact. (See Changing for the Better on rape awareness on page 574.)

Psychiatrists and psychologists have long contended that the psychodynamic underlying the act of rape is that of a deviant urge to control and dominate others that is in no way related to the fulfillment of sexual desire. They support this contention by pointing out that rapists often experience impotence during the rape, that rapists are emotionally aroused by images of violent behavior directed toward people, and that rapists choose as victims those people whom they perceive to be most vulnerable. These traits are viewed by mental health professionals as being largely unrelated to sexually based needs.

In stark contrast to this approach, two evolutionary biologists have proposed that rape is an extreme expression of the evolutionary urge to reproduce common to all males.[23] According to the authors, their controversial theory in no way excuses rape, nor does it speak against the incarceration of rapists, but rather it suggests an alternative interpretation of rape's underlying causation that might eventually lead society to determine more effective ways to prevent the crime from occurring. Although thought provoking, this interpretation is unlikely to change many minds about the heinous nature of the act.

Acquaintance and Date Rape

Sexual victimization can occur in relationships. *Acquaintance rape* refers to forced sexual intercourse between individuals who know each other. *Date rape* is a form of acquaintance rape that involves forced sexual intercourse by a dating partner. Studies on a number of campuses

suggest that about 20 percent of college women report having experienced date rape; a recent report from the Bureau of Justice Statistics puts the figure at about 3 percent per year. This figure includes completed and attempted rapes.[22] A higher percentage of women report being kissed and touched against their will. Alcohol is frequently a significant contributing factor in these rape situations. (See Chapter 8 concerning alcohol's role in campus crime.) Some men have reported being psychologically coerced into intercourse by their female dating partners. In many cases the aggressive partner will display certain behaviors that can serve as warning signs (see Changing for the Better on page 575).

In addition to alcohol as an adjunct to acquaintance rape or date rape, the use of additional drugs such as rohypnol (roofies), ketamine hydrochloride (Special K), and gamma-hydroxybutyrate (GHB) (see Chapter 7) are playing a greater role in date rapes reported on or near college campuses. Because of the inconspicuous nature of these drugs, they are easily incorporated into drinks without intended victims knowing it. The effects of these drugs are disinhibition, increasing confusion (including the inability to give sexual consent), relaxation of voluntary muscles, and eventual unconsciousness.[24] The amnestic effect of these drugs reduces the ability of victims to supply information important in the apprehension of date rapists.

Psychologists believe that aside from the physical harm of date rape, a greater amount of emotional damage may occur. Such damage stems from the concept of broken trust. Date rape survivors feel particularly violated because the perpetrator was not a stranger; it was someone they initially trusted, at least to some degree. Once that trust has been broken, developing new relationships with other people becomes much more difficult for the date rape survivor.

Nearly all survivors of date rape seem to suffer from *posttraumatic stress syndrome.* They can have anxiety, sleeplessness, eating disorders, and nightmares. Guilt concerning their own behavior, self-esteem, and judgment of other people can be overwhelming, and the individual may require professional counseling. Indeed, all students should be aware of the risk of date rape.

Sexual Abuse of Children

One of the most tragic forms of sexual victimization is the sexual abuse of children. Children are especially vulnerable to sexual abuse because of their dependent relationships with parents, relatives, and caregivers (such as babysitters, teachers, and neighbors). Often, children are unable to readily understand the difference between appropriate and inappropriate physical contact. Abuse may range from blatant physical manipulation, including fondling, to oral sex, sodomy, and intercourse.

Because of the subordinate role of children in relationships involving adults, sexually abusive practices often go unreported. Sexual abuse can leave emotional scars that make it difficult to establish meaningful relationships later in life. For this reason, it is especially important for people to pay close attention to any information shared by children that could indicate a potentially abusive situation. Most states require that information concerning child abuse be reported to law enforcement officials.

Sexual Harassment

Sexual harassment consists of unwanted attention of a sexual nature that creates embarrassment or stress. Examples of sexual harassment include unwanted physical contact, excessive pressure for dates, sexually explicit humor, sexual innuendos or remarks, offers of job advancement based on sexual favors, and overt sexual assault. Unlike more overt forms of sexual victimization, sexual harassment may be applied in a subtle manner and can, in some cases, go unnoticed by coworkers and fellow students. Nevertheless, sexual harassment produces stress that cannot be resolved until the harasser is identified and forced to stop. Both men and women can be victims of sexual harassment.

Sexual harassment can occur in many settings, including employment and academic settings. On the college campus, harassment may be primarily in terms of the offer of sex for grades. If this happens to you, think carefully about the situation and document the specific times, events, and places where the harassment took place. Consult your college's policy concerning harassment. Next, you should report these events to the appropriate administrative officer (perhaps the affirmative action officer, dean of academic affairs, or dean of students). You may also want to discuss the situation with a staff member of the university counseling center.

If harassment occurs in the work environment, the victim should document the occurrences and report them to the appropriate management or personnel official. Reporting procedures will vary from setting to setting. Sexual harassment is a form of illegal sex discrimination and violates Title VII of the Civil Rights Act of 1964.

In 1986 the United States Supreme Court ruled that the creation of a "hostile environment" in a work setting was sufficient evidence to support the claim of sexual harassment. This action served as an impetus for thousands of women to step forward with sexual harassment allegations. Additionally, some men are also filing sexual harassment lawsuits against female supervisors.

I've heard that there are warning signs for date rape. What signs should I be alert for?

First, consider your partner's behaviors. Many, but not all, date rapists show one or more of the following behaviors: a disrespectful attitude toward you and others, lack of concern for your feelings, violence and hostility, obsessive jealousy, extreme competitiveness, a desire to dominate, and unnecessary physical roughness. Consider these behaviors as warning signs for possible problems in the future. Reevaluate your participation in the relationship.

Below are some specific ways both men and women can avoid a date rape situation.

Men

- *Know your sexual desires and limits.* Communicate them clearly. Be aware of social pressures. It's OK not to score.
- *Being turned down when you ask for sex is not a rejection of you personally.* Women who say no to sex are not rejecting the person; they are expressing their desire not to participate in a single act. Your desires may be beyond control, but your actions are within your control.
- *Accept the woman's decision.* "No" means "No." Don't read other meanings into the answer. Don't continue after you are told "No!"
- *Don't assume that just because a woman dresses in a sexy manner and flirts that she wants to have sexual intercourse.*

- *Don't assume that previous permission for sexual contact applies to the current situation.*
- *Avoid excessive use of alcohol and drugs.* Alcohol and other drugs interfere with clear thinking and effective communication.

Women

- *Know your sexual desires and limits.* Believe in your right to set those limits. If you are not sure, STOP and talk about it.
- *Communicate your limits clearly.* If someone starts to offend you, tell him so firmly and immediately. Polite approaches may be misunderstood or ignored. Say "No" when you mean "No."
- *Be assertive.* Often men interpret passivity as permission. Be direct and firm with someone who is sexually pressuring you.
- *Be aware that your nonverbal actions send a message.* If you dress in a sexy manner and flirt, some men may assume you want to have sex. This does not make your dress or behavior wrong, but it is important to be aware of a possible misunderstanding.
- *Pay attention to what is happening around you.* Watch the nonverbal clues. Do not put yourself into vulnerable situations.
- *Trust your intuitions.* If you feel you are being pressured into unwanted sex, you probably are.
- *Avoid excessive use of alcohol and drugs.* Alcohol and other drugs interfere with clear thinking and effective communication.

Not surprisingly, this rising number of complaints has served as a wake-up call for employers. From university settings to factory production lines to corporate board rooms, employers are scrambling to make certain that employees are fully aware of actions that could lead to a sexual harassment lawsuit. Sexual harassment workshops and educational seminars on harassment are now common and serve to educate both men and women about this complex problem.

Violence and the Commercialization of Sex

It is beyond the scope of this book to explore whether sexual violence can be related to society's exploitation or commercialization of sex. However, sexually related products and messages are intentionally placed before the public to try to sway consumer decisions. Do you believe that there could be a connection between commercial products, such as violent pornography in films and magazines, and violence against women? Does prostitution lead directly to violence? Do sexually explicit "900" phone numbers or pornography on the Internet cause an increase in violent acts? Can the sexual messages in beer commercials lead to acquaintance rape? What do you think?

Identity Theft

In today's cashless, wired society, we make several transactions each day in which personal information is transferred: we write checks, pay bills online, use credit and debit cards for purchases, and withdraw cash from ATMs; we might be asked to provide a social security number when we write a check, or give our phone number or address when we shop at a particular store. Each of these transactions provides an opportunity for thieves to obtain your personal information and use it fraudulently.

Identity theft has been on the rise since the early 1990s. Thieves have many ways of obtaining personal data, including stolen mail (or mail diverted with a "change of address" form); sorting through garbage for discarded bills or receipts that include account numbers;

Key Terms

identity theft a crime involving the fraudulent use of a person's name, social security number, credit line, or other personal financial or identifying information

Being aware of your surroundings when using an ATM is important for personal safety.

posing as a landlord or employer to obtain people's credit report; stealing records—either electronically (hacking) or physically removing them—from offices where the victim is a customer, patient, student, or employee. Thieves use falsely obtained names, addresses, and social security numbers to open credit card accounts and bank accounts, purchase cell phone services, and secure loans to buy automobiles and other big-ticket items. They might even avoid paying taxes by working under false social security numbers, or use your identity for other purposes—if they are arrested, for example. Identity thefts can drain a person's bank account and ruin their credit rating before a person knows they've become a victim. Often the crime is not discovered until a person wants to make a major purchase—such as a house or a car—that requires a credit check.

There are several steps that you can take to avoid becoming a victim of identity theft. The most important step involves ordering copies of your credit reports each year to make sure that there are no fraudulent accounts in your name.[25] Other steps are outlined in the Star box on page 577.

Campus Safety

Although many of the topics in this chapter are quite unsettling, students and faculty must continue to lead normal lives in the campus environment despite potential threats to our health. The first step in being able to function adequately is knowing about these potential threats. You have read about these threats in this section on intentional injuries; now you must think about how this information applies to your campus situation.

The campus environment is not immune to many of the social ills that plague our society. At one time the university campus was thought to be a safe haven from the real world. Now there is plenty of evidence to indicate that significant intentional and unintentional injuries can happen to anyone at any time on the college campus.

For this reason, you must make it a habit to think constructively about protecting your safety. In addition to the personal safety tips presented earlier in this section, remember to use the safety assistance resources available on your campus. One of these might be your use of university-approved escort services, especially in the evenings as you move from one campus location to another. Another resource is the campus security department (campus police). Typically, campus police have a 24-hour emergency phone number. If you think you need help, do not hesitate to call this number. Campus security departments frequently offer short seminars on safety topics to student organizations or residence hall groups. Your counseling center on campus might also offer programs on rape prevention and personal protection.

If you are motivated to make your campus environment safer, you might wish to contact an organization that specifically focus on campus crime. Safe Campuses Now is a nonprofit student group that tracks legislation, provides educational seminars, and monitors community incidents involving students. (For information about Safe Campuses Now, including how to start a chapter on your campus, call 706-354-1115. Visit the Web page for Safe Campuses Now, www.uga.edu\safecampus. This organization is located at the University of Georgia. We encourage you to become active in making your campus a safer place to live.)

Unintentional Injuries

Unintentional injuries are injuries that have occurred without anyone's intending that any harm be done. Common examples include injuries resulting from car crashes, falls, fires, drownings, firearm accidents, recreational accidents, and residential accidents. Each year,

---

Key Terms

unintentional injuries injuries that have occurred without anyone's intending that harm be done

Reducing Your Risk for Identity Theft

The Federal Trade Commission outlines several steps to minimize your risk for identity theft:

- Order a copy of your credit report from each of the three major credit bureaus, and review it carefully to make sure it's accurate.

- Place passwords on your credit card, bank and phone accounts. Avoid obvious passwords such as birthdays, mother's maiden name, or social security numbers.

- Keep personal information in your home secure. Be vigilant about guarding your mail and your trash; use a document shredder when discarding sensitive papers like credit card bills. Make sure your home computer has firewall protection.

- Ask about information security procedures in your workplace or at your school.

- Carefully read all your bills to make sure that you recognize all purchases and charges.

- Do not give out your personal information. Be especially wary of e-mail and phone solicitations requesting such information.

- Watch your wallet. Be wary of pickpockets, and carry only the identification and credit cards you need. Do not carry your social security card with you unless it is absolutely necessary.

- If you are a victim of identity theft, visit the FTC's Web site (www.consumer.gov/idtheft/) for valuable information on how to file a complaint and restore your credit.

Source: Federal Trade Commission. *ID Theft: When Bad Things Happen to Your Good Name.*

---

unintentional injuries account for about 100,000 deaths and 27 million visits to hospital emergency departments.[26]

Unintentional injuries are very expensive for our society, both from a financial standpoint and from a personal and family standpoint. Fortunately, to a large extent it is possible to avoid becoming a victim of an unintentional injury. By carefully considering the tips presented in the safety categories that follow, you will be protecting yourself from many preventable injuries.

Since this section of the chapter focuses on a selected number of safety categories, we encourage readers to consider some additional ones (see Considering Complementary Care below). To review important points in the area of first aid skills, consult Appendix 1 in this text. Finally, we

---

Considering Complementary Care

Safety and Health Care Decisions

In today's complex world of health care, four generalizations regarding the interfacing of traditional allopathic health care and complementary health care can be made. First, as adults age, they are increasingly likely to be under the care of several health care providers, in addition to their primary care physician. In fact, many middle-aged and older adults may be seeing three or more specialists, such as cardiologists, rheumatologists, and endocrinologists, in addition to their family physician or internist. As a result, these individuals may be taking multiple prescription medication simultaneously. Second, over 40 percent of adults report that they are using complementary care, including taking a vast array of dietary supplements. Third, less than 20 percent of adults mention the use of such complementary health care to their physicians, and an even smaller percentage of physicians question patients about their use of complementary health care. Fourth, despite its $50 million budget and newly designated independent status, the National Center for Alternative and Complementary Medicine has yet to carefully evaluate the effectiveness and safety of all the many forms of health care and the vast array of dietary supplements available in the marketplace.

When these factors are combined, the potential for unanticipated and dangerous drug interactions exists. It is, therefore, imperative that patients proactively inform their physicians about the type and extent of complementary health care they are using. It is equally important that physicians ask their patients about any alternative forms of care being received and any dietary supplements being taken. When this information is not taken into consideration in the patient's plan of care, the complementary care itself may become a negative factor. Therefore, until a great deal more is understood about complementary medical care procedures and the nature of prescription medication-dietary supplement interactions, the use of complementary care should be limited to preventive and palliative measures. In addition, such care should be discontinued during periods of treatment with prescription medications and chemotherapeutic agents or prior to undergoing surgery.

Should I Have a Watch Dog?

Some people feel safer with an animal companion around. Others have had bad experiences with pets and find them a nuisance and expensive as well. Does keeping a dog increase one's personal safety? And if so, what kind of dog is best . . . a *watch* dog? . . . a *guard* dog?

The difference between watch dogs and guard dogs is that a watch dog will bark to alert owners of an approaching stranger, but will not usually attack. The sound of a barking dog may be enough to deter an intruder. A guard dog may also deter by barking, but is also "large enough to intimidate and, if necessary, attack an intruder."[1]

If your planning to obtain a watch dog, you should be aware that some breeds are better that others. According to PetPlace.com, the American Eskimo, Boston terrier, Chihuahua, French bulldog, Pekingese, and Irish setter are among those breeds that make good watch dogs.

However, there are several disadvantages to owning a dog. There are considerable veterinary expenses involved as well as the cost of dog food. Also, there is the question of what to do with your dog when you need to be away for a few days and cannot take the dog with you. Between 6 and 8 million dogs and cats enter animal shelters each year, many of them surrendered by their owners who no longer want them or are unable to care for them. More than half of these animals are euthanized. Everyone must carefully consider both the cost and the responsibilities involved in ownership before acquiring a pet.[2]

Perhaps the biggest concern is safety. In 2001 an estimated 4.7 million dog bites occurred in the United States, and approximately, 799,700 of those required medical care.[3] Research has shown that the majority (80 percent) of bites incurred by those under 19 years of age were inflicted by a family dog

(30 percent) or a neighbor's dog (50 percent). Also, during 1997–1998, 75 percent of fatal dog bites were inflicted on family members or guests on the family's property.

Therefore, one should carefully consider the safety advantages and disadvantages of dog ownership. If you decide that owning a dog is right for you and your family, do some research and make sure that the dog you select is a safe one.

[1]PetPlace Staff. Top Watch Dogs: Breeds that protect the family. www.PetPlace.com/.
[2]The Humane Society of the United States. *HSUS Pet Overpopulation Estimates,* www.hsus.org.
[3]Centers for Disease Control and Prevention. Nonfatal dog bite-related injuries treated in hospital emergency departments—United States, 2001. Morbidity and Mortality Weekly Report 52(26):605–610. 2003. www.cdc.gov/mmwr/preview/mmwrhtml/mm5226a1.htm.

---

encourage you to take a first aid course from the American Red Cross. American Red Cross first aid courses incorporate a significant amount of safety prevention information along with the teaching of specific first aid skills.

Residential Safety

Many serious accidents and personal assaults occur in dorm rooms, apartments, and houses. As a responsible adult, you should make every reasonable effort to prevent these tragedies from happening. One good idea is to discuss some of the following points with your family or roommates and see what cooperative strategies you can implement:

- Fireproof your residence. Are all electrical appliances and heating and cooling systems in safe working order? Are flammable materials safely stored?
- Prepare a fire escape plan. Install smoke or heat detectors.
- Do not give personal information over the phone to a stranger.
- Use initials for first names on mailboxes and in phone books.
- Install a peephole and deadbolt locks on doors.

- If possible, avoid living in first floor apartments. Change locks when moving to a new place.
- Put locks on all windows.
- Require repair people or delivery people to show valid identification.
- Do not use an elevator if it is occupied by someone who makes you feel uneasy.
- Be cautious around garages, laundry rooms, and driveways (especially at night). Use lighting for prevention of assault.

Some people report feeling safer at home with a dog. Statistics on whether dogs actually improve safety are hard to come by, but one should consider several factors before acquiring a dog for protection (see the Star box above).

Recreational Safety

The thrills we get from risk taking are an essential part of our recreational endeavors. But a significant number of injuries occur in recreational settings. For example, bicycle riding accounted for more than 411,000 emergency department visits in 2002.[26] Some injuries occur because we fail to consider important recreational safety information. Do some of the following recommendations apply to you?

Wearing proper safety gear—including a helmet—is an essential safety measure when biking or skating. Obeying traffic laws and using proper hand signals are equally important.

- Seek appropriate instruction for your intended activity. Few skill activities are as easy as they look.
- Make certain that your equipment is in excellent working order.
- Involve yourself gradually in an activity before attempting more complicated, dangerous skills.
- Enroll in an American Red Cross first aid course to enable you to cope with unexpected injuries.
- Remember that alcohol use greatly increases the likelihood that people will get hurt.
- Protect your eyes from injury (see Changing for the Better on page 580).
- Learn to swim. Most drowning victims are people who never intended to be in the water.
- Obey the laws related to your recreational pursuits. Many laws are directly related to the safety of the participants.
- Be aware of weather conditions. Many outdoor activities turn to tragedy with sudden shifts in the weather. Always prepare yourself for the worst possible weather.

Bicycle Safety

With a little common sense and a few precautions, bicycling can be a very safe and enjoyable aerobic activity. Remember these key points:

- Wear a helmet. More than any other precaution, wearing a helmet is paramount and can save your life.
- When cycling at night or when visibility is poor, wear brightly colored reflective clothing.
- Use hand signals so drivers around you know what you plan to do.

- Obey traffic signals just like any other vehicle on the road. You have a right to bicycle on the road, but you also have the same responsibilities as other vehicles. Don't run stop signs or red lights!
- Brake carefully, and use both hand brakes at the same time. Using only the front brake can send you over the handlebars, and using only the back brake can cause a skid. On long downhills or in wet weather, gently tap the brakes to retain control. Be especially careful in wet weather, when wet brake pads are not very helpful.

Boating Safety

Most boating deaths result from drowning, when the victim was not wearing a personal flotation device (PFD). Of the 481 boaters who drowned in 2003, most could have been saved if they had been wearing a PFD, according to the U.S. Coast Guard. Eighty-six percent of the victims in fatal boating accidents are not wearing life jackets.[27]

The other major cause of boating accidents and fatalities is "operator error," including (1) inattention, not looking in the direction in which one is moving, (2) carelessness, going out in bad weather or water conditions or while intoxicated, and (3) speeding. In particular, intoxication is a factor in more than half of all boating accidents. Too many casual boaters assume that rules of boating safety do not apply to them. Every boater should learn how to handle high winds, storms, whitecaps, rough waters, and heavy boat traffic. Most boat dealers can give you information about PFDs, "rules of the road," and Coast Guard safety regulations.

Even some experienced boaters tend to go too fast. Some modern watercraft tend to climb out of the water at higher speeds, and less hull in the water means less stability. With less stability, the boat tends to rock from side to side, and this rocking is a warning that you are about to lose control.

I've heard that more than a million people suffer eye injuries each year in the United States. What can I do to protect my eyes on an everyday basis?

In the Home

- Make sure that all spray nozzles are directed away from you before you pull the handle.
- Read instructions carefully before using cleaning fluids, detergents, ammonia, or harsh chemicals. Wash your hands thoroughly after use.
- Use grease shields on frying pans to protect your eyes from splattering.
- Wear appropriate goggles to shield your eyes from fumes and splashes when using powerful chemicals.
- Use opaque goggles to avoid burns from sunlamps.

In the Workshop

- Think about the work you will be doing, and protect your eyes from flying fragments, fumes, dust particles, sparks, and splashing chemicals *before* you begin work.
- Read instructions carefully before using tools and chemicals, and follow precautions for their use.
- Protect yourself by wearing safety goggles.

Around Children

- Remember your child's age and responsibility level when you buy toys and games. Avoid projectile toys such as darts and pellet guns, which can hit the eye from a distance.
- Supervise children when they are playing with toys or games that can be dangerous.
- Teach children the correct way to handle items such as scissors and pencils.

In the Yard

- Keep everyone away when you use a lawnmower. Don't let anyone stand on the side or in front when you mow the lawn.
- Pick up rocks and stones before mowing. These objects can shoot out of the blades, rebound off curbs or walls, and cause severe injury to the eye.

- Make sure that pesticide spray-can nozzles are pointed away from your face.
- Avoid low-hanging branches.

Around the Car

- Sparks and fumes can ignite easily and explode. Battery acid can cause serious eye injuries.
- Put out all cigarettes and matches before opening the hood of the car. Use a flashlight, not a match or lighter, to look at the battery at night.
- Keep protective goggles next to your jumper cables and wear them.
- Wear protective goggles during auto body repairs when grinding metal or striking metal against metal.

When You Jump-Start a Car

- Make sure the cars are not touching each other.
- Make sure that the jumper-cable clamps never touch each other.
- Never lean over the battery when attaching cables.
- Attach the positive (red) cable to the positive terminal of the dead battery first; then attach the other end of the positive cable to the good battery. Attach the negative (black) cable to the negative terminal of the good battery, then attach the other end of the negative cable to a grounded area on the engine away from the negative terminal of the dead battery. *Never attach a cable to the negative terminal of the dead battery.*

In Sports

- Wear protective safety glasses, especially for sports such as tennis, racquetball, squash, baseball, and basketball.
- Wear protective caps, helmets, or face protectors when appropriate, especially for sports such as ice hockey.

Around Fireworks

All fireworks can be dangerous to people of all ages.

- Never allow children to ignite fireworks.
- Do not stand near others when lighting fireworks.

InfoLinks

www.elvex.com

Firearm Safety

In 2003, 29,778 people died of firearm injuries in the United States. Of these, 16,859 were firearm-related suicides, 11,599 died as a result of homicides committed with a firearm, another 752 died from firearm-related accidents, 394 died from legal interventions and 197 died from discharged firearms where intent was not determined.[28]

Most homicides are, in fact, committed using firearms, with handguns accounting for the vast majority of murders. (Shotguns and rifles tend to be more cumbersome than handguns and thus are not as frequently used in murders, accidents, or suicides.)

More than half of all murders result from quarrels and arguments between acquaintances or relatives. With many homeowners arming themselves with handguns for protection against intruders, it is not surprising that more than half of all gun accidents occur in the home. Children are frequently involved in gun accidents, often after they discover a gun they think is unloaded. On a positive note in this regard, youth gun deaths have declined significantly since the mid-1990s. In 1994, tragically, 5,833 children and adolescents died from firearm injuries. This number declined to 3,593 youth gun-related deaths in 1997 and 3,180 in 1998.[29] Firearm deaths declined further in 2003, as homicide dropped out of the top 15 leading causes of death.[28]

Handgun owners are reminded to adhere to the following safety rules:

- Consider every gun to be a loaded gun, even if someone tells you it is unloaded.
- Never point a gun at an unintended target.
- Keep your finger off the trigger until you are ready to shoot.
- When moving with a handgun, keep the barrel pointed down.
- Store your gun and ammunition safely in separate locked containers. Use a trigger lock on your gun when not in use.
- Never play with guns at parties. Never handle a gun when intoxicated.
- Make certain that your gun is in good mechanical order.
- Take target practice only at approved ranges.
- Load and unload your gun carefully.

- If you are a novice, enroll in a gun safety course. Your local police, sheriff, or fire department may offer such a course.
- Educate children about gun safety and the potential dangers of gun use. Children must never believe that a gun is a toy.
- Make certain that you follow the gun possession laws in your state. Special permits may be required to carry a handgun.

 TALKING POINTS You do not have a firearm in your home, but you're not sure whether your neighbors do, and your child enjoys playing at their house. How might you go about asking your neighbor if they have a gun in their home?

Motor Vehicle Safety

The greatest number of injury deaths in the United States occur on highways and streets. Young people (ages 16–24 years) are more likely to be involved in a fatal motor vehicle crash than persons of any other age (Figure 19-2). The most dangerous times to drive are 12 midnight to 3 A.M. on Saturdays and Sundays.[30] If the driver has been drinking and is driving a subcompact car or motorcycle, the likelihood of a fatal crash is even more pronounced.

Motor vehicle crashes also cause disabling injuries. With nearly two million such injuries each year, all college students should be concerned about avoiding motor vehicle crashes. With this thought in mind,

Figure 19-2 Driving is a dangerous activity for those under age 25. What could be done to reduce the number of driving fatalities among this age group?

Number of Fatal Motor Vehicle Crashes According to Age of Driver

Crashes per 100,000 drivers

Age	Crashes
16–20	63
21–24	45
25–34	32
35–44	26
45–54	22
55–64	20
65–74	19
75–up	26

Cell Phone Safety While Driving

Cell phones that fit easily into a pocket or purse are being used in every place imaginable, including restaurants, theaters, subways, parks, golf courses, and, of course, in cars. And it's in cars that the use of cellular phones is most controversial. A variety of studies and reports indicate a four- to nine-fold increase in the potential for car crashes associated with the driver's use of a cell phone. In July 2001, the state of New York passed the country's first *statewide ban* on the use of hand-held cellular phones while driving. Violators of this ban are subject to a $100 fine for the first offense. Since then, at least 24 other states have passed laws regulating cell phone use while operating a motor vehicle.*

Research suggests the use of a cell phone decreases driver concentration and delays driver reaction time. The use of mounted, hands-free phones may improve safety, although the safety benefit has been controversial. Experts in traffic safety are careful to point out that there are too many other factors associated with driving to make it fair to blame behind-the-wheel phone use for all or most accidents. These complicating factors include adverse weather conditions, the structural integrity of the cars, the age and health of the drivers, radio, CD, or cigarette use, and interactions between drivers and passengers. The influence of other drivers on the road must also be considered.

If you must use your cell phone in a car, consider these common sense rules: Get off the main road to a safe parking area to make your call, especially if the call is an important one or one that might upset you. If you must talk while driving, opt for a hands-free phone. Dial when your car is stopped. Keep calls very brief. Don't try to dial or talk in heavy traffic. Keep your eyes on the road. (Or, let a passenger make the call!)

*Governor's Highway Safety Association. Cell Phone Restrictions—State and Local jurisdictions, 2003 www.statehighwaysafety.org/html/stateinfo/cellphone_laws.

Consistent use of safety restraints during childhood can help make buckling up a life-long habit.

we offer some important safety tips for motor vehicle operators:

- Make certain that you are familiar with the traffic laws in your state.

- Do not operate an automobile or motorcycle unless it is in good mechanical order. Regularly inspect your brakes, lights, and exhaust system.

- Do not exceed the speed limit. Observe all traffic signs.

- Always wear safety belts, even on short trips. Require your passengers to buckle up. Always keep small children in child restraints.

- Never drink and drive. Avoid horseplay inside a car.

- Be certain that you can hear the traffic outside your car. Keep the car's music system at a reasonable decibel level. (See the Star box concerning cell phone use while driving.)

- Give pedestrians the right-of-way.

- Drive defensively at all times. Do not challenge other drivers. Refrain from drag racing.

- Look carefully before changing lanes.

- Be especially careful at intersections and railroad crossings.

- Carry a well-maintained first aid kit that includes flares or other signal devices.

- Drive even more carefully during bad weather.

- Do not drive when you have not had enough sleep.

In spite of the best efforts that people make to prevent motor vehicle crashes, when they occur there is, of course, not only damage to property but also the very real possibility of injury and even death. Also affected are family members and friends who pay an emotional price as they experience the loss of companionship when people for

Distractions and Safe Driving

Max Jones was a very popular youth soccer coach who was tragically killed when his car left the road while he was driving to an early morning practice. His family and his players and their parents were all devastated when they heard the news. It was only later, after the funeral, when several of Max's close friends were chatting, that someone mentioned how Max would drive with a cup of coffee between his legs. Then another friend noted that Max had a habit of picking up fast food on his way to soccer practice. He would sometimes eat a breakfast sandwich and drink coffee while driving. His friends began to wonder whether these distractions could have contributed to Max's crash.

A recent research study found that drivers are distracted an average of 16 percent of the time with activities that take their attention away from the road and their driving environment. Activities such as manipulating vehicle controls (air conditioning or windows), music/audio controls or talking to a child or baby in the car distracted drivers. Approximately three-fourths of those observed ate or drank something. Searching or reaching for an object while driving was also observed in a majority of the drivers who were observed. Forty percent were observed reading, writing or grooming while the vehicle was moving.

To lower your risk of injuring yourself or others avoid distractions while driving. Do not eat or drink while driving. If you are driving alone, make sure you have all of the vehicle's controls set appropriately before you embark on your trip. Use highway rest stops wisely to eat, read maps, arrange music, and reorganize the inside of your car so that you won't be distracted while at the wheel.

Source: Stutts J, Feaganes J, Rodgman E, Hamlett C, Meadows T, Reinfurt D, Gish K, Mercadante M, Staplin L. *Distractions in Everyday Driving.* Washington, DC: AAA Foundation for Traffic Safety, 2003.

---

whom they care a great deal have been in serious motor vehicle crashes. The effects of motor vehicle-related injuries and injury deaths are also felt in the workplace where they result in economic losses of employers and employees alike.

 TALKING POINTS You're in a car with a friend when another driver starts tailgating you very closely. Your friend, who is driving, slows down to annoy the tailgater. How would you convince your friend that his action is dangerous?

Motorcycle Safety

Some emergency-room physicians call motorcycles "murder-cycles" because of their experience with motorcycle crash victims. The statistics support this grim view. With the death rate for motorcycles at 34 per 100 million vehicle miles of travel compared to a death rate for cars of 1.3, motorcycles are 26 times more deadly.[30, 31]

If you choose to ride a motorcycle, you can improve your chances of avoiding injury or death by following these suggestions:

- Most important of all, wear a helmet. A variety of studies have supported the effectiveness of helmets in preventing head injuries. Warriors and athletes have worn helmets for centuries to protect themselves from head injuries. Modern examples include construction workers, football players, race car drivers, and military aircraft pilots.

- Wear boots, gloves, and heavy clothing to protect your skin from serious injury when you slide on pavement in a crash.

- Get proper training, such as the Motorcycle Safety Foundation course offered in some states.

- Your risk increases in wet weather. Consider whether a ride in the rain is necessary.

- Do not ride after taking medication that can affect your alertness or performance.

- Never ride after drinking alcohol or taking drugs. About half of motorcyclists killed in accidents had alcohol in their blood.

- Ride defensively. Remember that many drivers do not see you or may not give you the right-of-way you deserve.

For all the reasons discussed in conjunction with automobile accidents, motorcycle accidents can influence the well-being of a wide array of people. However, because of the very high probability of serious injury and death associated with these accidents, the distress suffered by family, friends, witnesses, and coworkers may be even more extensive.

Home Injury Prevention for Children and Elders

Approximately one person in ten is injured each year at home. Children and elders spend significantly more hours each day in a home setting than do young adults and adults. These groups are at greater risk of unintentional injury at home. (See Changing for the Better on page 584). Here are some important tips to remember. Can you think of others?

Making Your Home Safe, Comfortable, and Secure

I think that my apartment is reasonably safe, but I'm wondering if I can make it better. Any tips on home safety?

Entry

- Install a deadbolt lock on the front door and locks or bars on the windows.
- Add a peephole or small window in the front door.
- Trim bushes so burglars have no place to hide.
- Add lighting to the walkway and next to the front door.

Bedroom and Nursery

- Install a smoke alarm and a carbon monoxide detector.
- Humidifiers can be breeding grounds for bacteria; use them sparingly and follow the manufacturer's cleaning instructions.
- In the nursery, install pull-down shades or curtains instead of blinds with strings that could strangle a child.

Living Room

- Secure loose throw rugs or use ones with nonskid backing.
- Cover unused electrical outlets if there are small children in the home.
- Provide additional lighting for reading, and install adjustable blinds to regulate glare.

Kitchen

- Install ceiling lighting and additional task lighting where food is prepared.
- Keep heavy objects on bottom shelves or countertops; store lightweight or seldom-used objects on top shelves.
- Promptly clean and store knives.
- Keep hot liquids such as coffee out of children's reach, and provide close supervision when the stove or other appliances are in use.
- To avoid foodborne illness, thoroughly clean surfaces that have come into contact with raw meat.

Bathroom

- A child can drown in standing water; keep the toilet lid down and the tub empty.
- Clean the shower, tub, sink, and toilet regularly to remove mold, mildew, and bacteria that can contribute to illness.
- Store medications in their original containers in a cool, dry place out of the reach of children.
- Add a bath mat or nonskid strips to the bottom of the tub.
- Add grab bars near the tub or shower and toilet, especially if there are older adults in the home.
- Keep a well-stocked first aid kit equipped with bandages, first aid ointment, gauze, pain relievers, syrup of ipecac, and isotonic eyewash; include your physician's and a nearby emergency center's phone numbers.

Stairway

- Add a handrail for support.
- Repair or replace flooring material that is in poor condition.
- Add a light switch at the top of the stairs.
- If there is an older adult in the home, add a contrasting color strip to the first and last steps to identify the change of level.

Fire Prevention Tips

- Install smoke detectors on every level of your home.
- Keep fire extinguishers handy in the kitchen, basement, and bedrooms.
- Have the chimney and fireplace cleaned by a professional when there is more than one-fourth inch of soot accumulation.
- Place space heaters at least 3 feet from beds, curtains, and other flammable objects.
- Don't overload electrical outlets, and position drapes so that they don't touch cords or outlets.
- Recycle or toss combustibles, such as newspapers, rags, old furniture, and chemicals.
- Plan escape routes and practice using them with your family.

For Everyone

- Be certain that you have adequate insurance protection.
- Install smoke detectors appropriately.
- Keep stairways clear of toys and debris. Install railings.
- Maintain electrical and heating equipment.
- Make certain that family members know how to get emergency help.

For Children

- Know all the ways to prevent unintentional poisoning.
- Use toys that are appropriate for the age of the child.
- Never leave young children unattended, especially infants.
- Keep any hazardous items (guns, poisons, and so on) locked up.
- Keep small children away from kitchen stoves.

For Elders

- Protect elders from falls by removing damaged carpet, improving lighting near stairs, installing handrails, and repairing broken walks, steps, and porches.

- Be certain that elders have a good understanding of the medications they may be taking. Know the side effects.
- Encourage elders to seek assistance for home repairs.
- Make certain that all door locks, lights, and safety equipment are in good working order.

For young children who are mostly at home and elders whose dependence on homes is often an issue of restricted mobility and a sense of insecurity, homes should be dependably safe environments. Implementing the suggestions made in this section can help make a home safer.

Taking Charge of Your Health

- Use the Personal Assessment on page 589 to determine how well you manage your own safety.
- Assess your behaviors and those of your dating partners for signs of potential date rape by reviewing the Changing for the Better box on page 575.
- Check you residence for the safety strategies listed on page 584. Make the necessary changes to correct any deficiencies.
- Review the motor vehicle safety tips on page 581. If you need to make changes to your car or your driving, begin working on them at once.
- Check the recommendations for recreational safety on page 578 and put them into practice. Be assertive about using these measures when you are participating in activities with others.
- Find out about the security services available on your campus, and take advantage of them. Post the 24-hour-help phone number in your room and carry it with you.
- Minimize your risk for identity theft by taking the steps outlined in the Star box on page 577.

SUMMARY

- Everyone is a potential victim of violent crime.
- Each year in the United States, intentional injuries cause nearly 50,000 deaths and millions of additional nonfatal injuries.
- The national rate of serious crimes such as murder, rape, and robbery has been falling in recent years.
- Homicide is the leading cause of death for young male African Americans. Handguns are the weapon of choice for homicides.
- About half of all homes in the United States have a gun, for a total of about 230 million guns.
- In spite of changes in family structure, fatal and nonfatal, intimate partner violence has declined since 1993.
- Forms of child maltreatment include child abuse and child neglect. Child neglect is the most common form.
- Bicyclists and motorcyclists can best protect their safety by wearing helmets.

- Bias and hate crimes, as well as the crime of stalking, are increasingly recognized as serious, violent acts.
- Rape and sexual assault, acquaintance rape, date rape, and sexual harassment are forms of sexual victimization in which victims often are both physically and psychologically traumatized.
- The use of date rape drugs is a reality on today's college campuses.
- Unintentional injuries are injuries that occur without anyone intending that harm be done.
- The numbers of fatal and nonfatal unintentional injuries are exceedingly high.
- Recreational activities such as boating, bicycling, hunting, and simply being active at home place people at an increased level of risk.

REVIEW QUESTIONS

1. Identify some of the categories of intentional injuries. How many people are affected each year by intentional injuries?
2. What are some of the most important facts concerning homicide in the United States? How are most homicides committed?
3. Identify changes in the traditional family structure in America. What factors contribute to domestic violence?
4. What reasons might explain why so many women do not report domestic violence?
5. Aside from the immediate consequences of child maltreatment what long-term problems do many abused and/or neglected children face?
6. List some examples of groups that are known to have committed bias or hate crimes.
7. Explain some of the myths associated with rape. How can date rape be prevented?
8. What are the date rape drugs now appearing on college campuses, and how are they employed by rapists?

9. Identify some examples of behaviors that could be considered sexual harassment. Why are employers especially concerned about educating their employees about sexual harassment?

10. Identify some common examples of unintentional injuries. Point out three safety tips appropriate for safe bicycling, boating, firearm use, and driving automobiles and motorcycles. How can you make your home a safer environment?

11. In what ways can individuals protect themselves from identity theft?

ENDNOTES

1. Center for Disease Control and Prevention, National Center for Injury Prevention and Control, WISQARS (Web-Based Injury Surveillance Query and Reporting Systems), March 7, 2005, www.cdc.gov/ncipc/wisqars.

2. Bureau of Justice Statistics. *National Crime Victimization Survey: Criminal Victimization 2003.* U.S. Department of Justice, NCJ 205455, September 2004.

3. Bureau of Justice Statistics. U.S. Department of Justice, Office of Justice Programs, *National Crime Victimization Survey Violent Crime Trends, 1973–2003,* www.ojp.usdoj. gov/bjs/glance/tables/viortrdtab.htm.

4. Bureau of Justice Statistics. *Homicide Trends in the U.S., Long-Term Trends,* U.S. Department of Justice, Office of Justice Programs, November 2004, www.ojp.usdoj.gov/bjs/ homicide/tables/totalstab.htm.

5. Bureau of Justice Statistics. *Criminal Offenders Statistics: Lifetime Likelihood of Going to State or Federal Prison,* U.S. Department of Justice, November 2000.

6. Bureau of Justice Statistics. U.S. Department of Justice, Office of Justice Programs, *Homicide Trends in the United States,* November 21, 2002.

7. Bureau of Justice Statistics. U.S. Department of Justice, Office of Justice Programs, *Drug Use and Crime,* January 2005, www.ojp.usdoj.gov/bjs/dcf/duc.htm.

8. U.S. Census Bureau. *America's Families and Living Arrangements: 2003.* Washington, DC: 2004.

9. Bureau of Justice Statistics. U.S. Department of Justice, Office of Justice Programs, *Crime Data Brief, Intimate Partner Violence, 1993–2001,* NCJ 197838, February 2003.

10. McKenzie JF, Pinger RR, Kotecki JF. *An Introduction to Community Health* (5th ed.). Boston: Jones & Bartlett, 2005.

11. Coker AI, et al. Physical Health Consequences of Physical and psychological intimate partner violence. *Arch Fam Med* 9(5):451–457, 2000.

12. United States Department of Health and Human Services, Administration of Children, Youth and Families. *Child Maltreatment 2002.* Washington, DC: U.S. Government Printing Office, 2004, www.acf.hhs.gov/programs/cb/ publications/cm02/cm02.pdf.

13. National Institute of Justice. *The Cycle of Violence Revisited.* Washington, DC: U.S. Department of Justice, Office of Justice Programs, NIJ, Research in Progress Seminar Series, February 1996.

14. U.S. Census Bureau. *The 65 Years and Over Population: 2000, Census 2000 Brief.* U.S. Department of Commerce, Economics and Statistics Administration, 2001, www.census.gov/prod/2001pubs/c2kbr01-10.pdf.

15. National Research Council. *Elder Mistreatment: Abuse, Neglect, and Exploitation in an Aging America.* Washington, DC: The National Academies Press, 2003.

16. Office for Victims of Crime, Statistical Overviews. *Elder Abuse and Neglect.* Washington, DC: U.S. Department of Justice, Office of Justice Programs, 2001, www.ojp.usdoj. gov/ovc/ncvrw/2001/stat_over_7.htm.

17. Bureau of Justice Statistics. *Special Report: Violent Victimization of College Students, 1995–2002.*Washington, DC: U.S. Department of Justice, Office of Justice Programs, NCJ 206836, January 2005.

18. Office of Juvenile Justice and Delinquency Prevention. *OJJDP Fact Sheet: National Youth Gang Survey Trends from 1996 to 2000.* Washington, DC: U.S. Department of Justice, Office of Justice Programs, 2002.

19. Centers for Disease Control and Prevention. *Surveillance for Fatal and Nonfatal Firearm-Related Injuries—United States, 1993–1998.* Morbidity and Morality Surveillance Summaries 50(ss02):1–32, 2001.

20. Miller M, Hemenway D, Wechsler H. Guns and gun threats at college. *J AM Coll Hlth* 51(2):57–65.

21. Federal Bureau of Investigation. *Hate Crime Statistics— 2003.* Washington, DC: November 2004, www.fbi.gov/ ucr/03hc.pdf.

22. National Institute of Justice. *The Sexual Victimization of College Women.* U.S. Department of Justice, Bureau of Justice Statistics, Washington, DC, 2001.

23. Thornhill R, Palmer CT, Wilson M. *A Natural History of Rape.* Boston: MIT Press, 2000.

24. Schwartz RH, Milteer R, LeBeau MA. Drug-facilitated sexual assault ("date rape"). *South Med* 93(6):558–561, 2000.

25. Federal Trade Commission. ID THEFT: *When Bad Things Happen to Your Good Name.* www.consumer.gov/ idtheft_2002.

26. National Safety Council. *Injury Facts, 2004 Edition.* Itasca, IL, 2004.

27. U.S. Coast Guard. *Boating Statistics–2003.* www.uscgboating.org/statistics/boating_statistics_2003.pdf.

28. Hoyert DL, Kung HC, Smith BL. *Deaths: Preliminary Data for 2003.* National Vital Statistics Reports 53(15):1–48.

29. *Deaths: Final Data for 1998.* National Center for Health Statistics. November 2000, www.cdc.gov/nchs/data/nvsr/ nvs48_11.pdf.

30. National Highway Traffic Safety Administration. *Traffic Safety Facts 2003.* Washington, DC, U.S. Department of Transportation. DOT HS 809 775, 2005.

31. Shankar U. *Motorcyclist Fatalities: An Update.* National Highway Traffic Safety Administration, presented at the International Traffic Records Forum, Nashville, TN, July 26, 2004.

Every person should be aware of the steps to take to guard against identity theft, but sometimes when it occurs it is beyond an individual's control. In October 2004, it was revealed that the database of Choice-Point Inc., a national provider of identification and credential verification services, had been breached. In February 2005, the company announced that personal information of as many as 145,000 people had been compromised. By March 2005, new information came forth that this was not the first time ChoicePoint Inc. had been victimized by criminals.

Consumers concerned about whether such a security breach may have harmed their credit rating can contact one of the major credit rating companies—Equifax, Experian, or Transunion. These companies usually offer a free trial period, or they may provide help in case you have had your identification stolen.

personal assessment

How well do you protect your safety?

This quiz will help you measure how well you manage your personal safety. For each item below, circle the number that reflects the frequency with which you do the safety activity. Then, add up your individual scores and check the interpretation at the end.

3   I regularly do this

2   I sometimes do this

1   I rarely do this

1. I am aware of my surroundings and do not get lost.

   3   2   1

2. I avoid locations in which my personal safety would be compromised.

   3   2   1

3. I intentionally vary my daily routine (such as walking patterns to and from class, parking places, and jogging or biking routes) so that my whereabouts are not always predictable.

   3   2   1

4. I walk across campus at night with other people.

   3   2   1

5. I am careful about disclosing personal information (address, phone number, social security number, my daily schedule, etc.) to people I do not know.

   3   2   1

6. I carefully monitor my alcohol intake at parties.

   3   2   1

7. I watch carefully for dangerous weather conditions and know how to respond if necessary.

   3   2   1

8. I do not keep a loaded gun in my home.

   3   2   1

9. I know how I would handle myself if I were to be assaulted.

   3   2   1

10. I maintain adequate insurance for my health and my property.

   3   2   1

11. I keep emergency information numbers near my phone.

   3   2   1

12. I keep my first aid skills up to date.

   3   2   1

13. I use deadbolt locks on the doors of my home.

   3   2   1

14. I use the safety locks on the windows at home.

   3   2   1

15. I check the batteries used in my home smoke detector.

   3   2   1

16. I have installed a carbon monoxide detector in my home.

   3   2   1

17. I use adequate lighting in areas around my home and garage.

   3   2   1

18. I have the electrical, heating, and cooling equipment in my home inspected regularly for safety and efficiency.

   3   2   1

19. I use my car seat belt.

   3   2   1

20. I drive my car safely and defensively.

   3   2   1

21. I keep my car in good mechanical order.

   3   2   1

22. I keep my car doors locked.

   3   2   1

23. I have a plan of action if my car should break down while I am driving it.

   3   2   1

24. I use appropriate safety equipment, such as flotation devices, helmets, and elbow pads, in my recreational activities.

   3   2   1

25. I can swim well enough to save myself in most situations.

   3   2   1

26. I use suggestions for personal safety each day.

   3   2   1

TOTAL POINTS _____

Interpretation

Your total may mean that:

72–78 points	You appear to carefully protect your personal safety.
65–71 points	You adequately protect many aspects of your personal safety.
58–64 points	You should consider improving some of your safety-related behaviors.
Below 58 points	You must consider improving some of your safety-related behaviors.

Although no one can be completely safe from personal injury or possible random violence, there are ways to minimize the risks to your safety. Scoring high on this assessment will not guarantee your safety, but your likelihood for injury should remain relatively low. Scoring low on this assessment should encourage you to consider ways to make your life safer. Refer to the text and this assessment to provide you with useful suggestions to enhance your personal safety. Which safety tips will you use today?

chapter twenty

The Environment and Your Health

Chapter Objectives

On completing this chapter, you will be able to:

▍identify several environmental factors that can impact your personal health in either positive or adverse ways.

▍explain how your personal health is influenced by different environmental factors on several scales, including personal environment, the community and regional environment, and the global environment.

▍describe specific actions that you can take to minimize health risks associated with your personal environment—your home, your automobile, your workplace.

▍describe the distinction between a "point source" versus a "nonpoint source" of community/regional air or water pollution.

▍detail several specific actions that you can take to minimize environmental health risks at the community and regional level.

▍describe several global environmental health issues, and offer several actions that you might take to foster positive change.

Eye on the Media

Hype Versus Useful Information

An obscure scientist, an expert in an arcane subdiscipline of climatology, stands in front of his peers at a scientific conference and predicts a major shift in global climate. His warnings are brushed off by the powers-that-be. Within a month there are several massive polar hurricanes encircling the northern hemisphere of Earth. Within the following two weeks, the northern half of the United States is buried under ice and uninhabitable. Tens of millions of Americans are dead from storms and temperatures that dip to $-150°$ F. The survivors have moved to Mexico, probably permanently. Within two hours, *The Day After Tomorrow* has brought the complex, long-term process of global climate change to a tidy conclusion. Television pundits predict that the movie will raise public awareness of this looming environmental problem. A few weeks later the issue has fallen off the public radar.

"The Media" is one of the most powerful forces in American society, and its influence extends across most of the Earth's human population. As large multinational corporations have come to control many media producers, information and news are increasingly being filtered for their entertainment value. That which is deemed sufficiently interesting to be entertaining is often hyped, with the most titillating aspects repeated over and over. Information that is deemed uninteresting is simply ignored.

The "entertainment filter" of many media producers often does not interact well with issues of environmental health. Many environmental problems are complex and affect human health in subtle ways over long time periods. For example, likely effects of global climate change include expansion of tropical diseases into more northern latitudes, increased frequency of droughts and heat waves, gradual depletion of freshwater supplies, and extinctions of many species that cannot adapt to the changes. Compared to killer super polar storms and massive glaciers that appear in two weeks, these real-life issues have entertainment value similar to watching grass grow. The U.S. population is being exposed to hundreds, if not thousands of chemicals that have not been tested for human toxicity. They are found in our air, water, and food supply. They are found in our body fluids and hair. Some have been shown to cause cancer and birth defects in experimental animals. The U.S. Environmental Protection Agency estimates that air pollution in major U.S. cities contributes to thousands of deaths due to respiratory and cardiovascular disease each year. In the last 20 to 30 years, cancer rates in the U.S. population have increased substantially, while fertility of men as measured by sperm counts has been declining by 1–3 percent per year. When was the last time you heard anything about these issues on the evening news or read about them in a newspaper or magazine?

On the positive side, it has never been easier to obtain information about environmental health issues. The Internet provides a widely accessible means to obtain information on any topic. Just type a few words into the Google search line and you have more information at your finger tips than you can handle. Detailed reports from the U.S. Environmental Protection Agency and Centers for Disease Control can be copied from their Web sites to your computer in seconds.

When you "Google" an environmental health issue, you need to exercise some judgment about what you read. Environmental advocacy groups, industrial groups, liberal and conservative think tanks all have their Web presence, where they promote their perspectives. The mainstream news media has self-correcting mechanisms; when someone makes inaccurate statements in public, someone else exposes the mistake. Similar mechanisms have not yet been fully developed for the Internet. When an industry group or environmental group criticizes some change in environmental regulations, you need to understand their motivations to assess the validity of their claims.

Another weakness of replacing professional news outlets with self-directed information searches on the Internet is that you need to know there is something you want to research before the process can even begin. If the mainstream news media is not talking about environmental health issues, how will you know what to type in the Google search line? We tend to seek information about topics that concern us. Without adequate news coverage we remain ignorant, blissfully or otherwise. As our lives become progressively more complex and busy, we rely more heavily on the news media to help us identify issues of importance. When news is screened for its entertainment value, environmental health issues are often ignored on the evening news. By the time an environmental health issue become "entertaining," the damage is often already done. No wonder that "The Environment" is not perceived as a high-priority issue when we elect our leaders.

Environmental issues are important concerns for many college-age students as they perceive disturbing trends that may affect their future health and well-being. News programs regularly present the latest bad news about environmental problems such as over-population, pollution, global warming, damage to the ozone layer, loss of wilderness to economic exploitation, and endangered species. Movies such as *Water World, Blade Runner, Batman, The Matrix,* and *The Day After Tomorrow* depict various fictional futures that are dismal environmental disasters. Some college students join environmental organizations that work to clean up litter, encourage recycling, regulate pollution emissions, control human population growth, and protect endangered species and natural areas. Others feel there is nothing they can do about such monumental environmental issues. They lose hope for a future where the world will be a good place to live and raise a family, and may become depressed and apathetic. The impact of environmental quality on your health is influenced by both the nature of your environment and your intellectual, emotional, social, and spiritual responses to that environment.

Your **environment** includes a range of conditions that can influence your health, such as the availability of resources (oxygen, water, food) and environmental characteristics, such as temperature, humidity, toxins, allergens, pathogens, noise, and radiation. Conditions in your environment operate across a wide range of spatial scales, from the air immediately surrounding your body to the global earth, air, and ocean system. Your physical health is influenced primarily by your *personal environment*, comprised of conditions immediately around your body, in the home, neighborhood, and workplace. However, this personal environment is influenced by conditions in the larger *community* and *regional environment,* including such conditions as air pollution and water pollution. These local and regional conditions are influenced by conditions of the *global environment,* such as climate and solar radiation.

Your health can be influenced by changes in environmental conditions at the home/workplace, community/region, or global levels. Excessive noise in the workplace or neighborhood can significantly affect your sense of well-being and your ability to work effectively. High ozone levels in the air of your community can limit your ability to enjoy outdoors activities and cause or exacerbate asthma. Environmental conditions in a particular community and region can enhance or limit opportunities for various types of employment, and so affect occupational health. Few people ever visit a tropical rain forest, wilderness area, or whale sanctuary, but many feel their emotional and spiritual well-being is diminished when they hear these remote places are threatened or destroyed.

The goal of this chapter is to help you identify aspects of your environment that can significantly affect various dimensions of your health, and to suggest ways that you

---

Key Terms

environment the physical conditions (temperature, humidity, light, presence of substances) and other living organisms that exist around your body

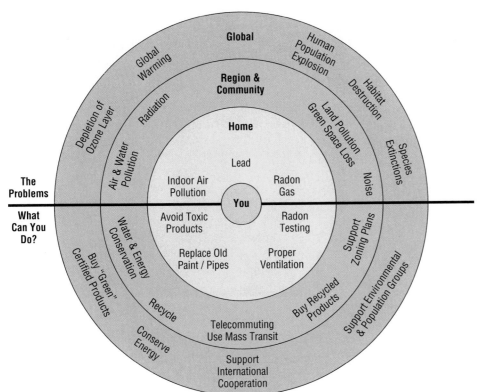

Figure 20-1 Spatial scales of environmental health risks and appropriate personal responses to environmental problems

can exert some level of personal control over these environmental influences. The range of options for personal action to improve your environment include altering personal behaviors and buying habits, becoming involved in the political process related to environmental issues, and supporting various nongovernmental organizations that work to address major environmental problems. Different specific environmental conditions and personal responses will be important at the various spatial scales of your environment (home/workplace, community/region, and global). Figure 20-1 displays a range of environmental problems that exist at various spatial scales of your environment, and a range of personal responses that might be appropriate at each level.

The Personal Environment: Home, Neighborhood, Workplace

On average you spend about 90 percent of your time indoors,[1] in your home, workplace, local stores, and entertainment venues. The indoor air you breathe, the water you drink from the tap on your sink, and the radiation and noise in your immediate surroundings are environmental factors that have the most direct and obvious impact on your health. Some indoor environmental problems cause immediate and obvious health effects,

such as headaches, dizziness, nausea, or allergic reactions. Other kinds of environmental problems act in subtle, cumulative ways over many years, causing major health problems such as cancer or neurological damage that may not become apparent until permanent damage is done.

Of all the different environmental influences that can affect your health, you have the greatest degree of control over factors in your personal environment. You are responsible for maintaining the appliances in your home so that they do not produce excessive air pollution. You have a great degree of control over the amount of ventilation you have in your home, allowing you to vent pollutants out from the indoor environment. You choose which products you will purchase and bring into your home, and can avoid products that may expose you to toxic chemicals. You can choose to not smoke tobacco, and to insist that others do not smoke in your home or workspace. In your personal environment, you can identify sources of health risk and have them removed from your home or notify those responsible for environmental safety at your workplace.

In this section you will learn to identify important environmental health risks in your personal environment, learn the effects of these environmental factors on your health, and see what you can do to minimize associated risks of health problems.

Protecting your family from environmental hazards begins at home. Have your home tested for radon gas, lead paint, asbestos, and other household pollutants, and take the necessary steps described in your text to reduce their impact on your family's health.

Indoor Air Quality

Indoor air quality within buildings can be influenced by a wide range of factors, including ventilation, humidity, gases given off by building construction materials, furniture and flooring materials, and combustion by-products from stoves and furnaces. When there is a problem with one or more of these factors, people in the affected building can experience a wide range of symptoms, from headaches and itchy eyes to unconsciousness and death. This section covers some of the most important health risks associated with indoor air quality.

Carbon Monoxide

Carbon monoxide is a highly toxic gas that is colorless, odorless, and tasteless, and so is not detectable by the unaided senses. Average levels in homes without gas stoves vary from 0.5 to 5 parts per million (ppm). Levels near properly adjusted gas stoves are often 5 to 15 ppm, and those near poorly adjusted stoves may be 30 ppm or higher.[1] The various sources of indoor carbon monoxide also produce nitrogen oxides and small particulates that contribute to indoor air pollution.

Health effects of carbon monoxide vary from mild discomfort to death, due to interference with oxygen transport by the blood. At low concentrations (1 to 70 ppm), effects of carbon monoxide are barely noticeable by most people. Persons who suffer from heart disease may feel chest pain. At concentrations between 70 to 150 ppm, your vision and coordination may be impaired and you may suffer from headaches, dizziness, mental confusion, and/or nausea. Regular exposure to these levels in the home or workplace can cause flulike symptoms that

rapidly disappear after you leave the location where you are exposed.[1] At very high concentrations (> 150 ppm), carbon monoxide poisoning can render you unconscious and then kill you.[2] Nitrogen oxides produced along with carbon monoxide can cause irritation to the eyes, nose, and throat, and impair respiratory function. Small particulates produced by these same sources irritate and damage lung tissues.

You can minimize your exposure to carbon monoxide and risk of poisoning by keeping all appliances that burn gas or other fuels in proper working order (to ensure complete combustion) and ensuring proper ventilation. You should have your gas-burning furnace and stove regularly inspected and repaired, as necessary. You should use the manufacturer-specified fuel in space heaters, and ensure proper ventilation of space heaters, woodstoves, charcoal and gas grills, and fireplaces, as directed by the manufacturer. You should avoid letting your car idle inside a garage, especially if it is attached to your home.[1] Never spend any long period of time close to the exhaust

Religious Perspectives on Human-Environment Relationships

In an article written by Lynn White (published in *Science*, 1967), he states that the root of all modern environmental problems can be found in Judeo-Christian (including Islamic) scripture. According to scripture of these religious traditions, the purpose of all of creation was to meet the needs and uses of humankind. This established a dualism (human versus not-human) that did not exist in earlier religions that perceived divinity in all of creation. Other passages in the Bible include statements that humankind should "go forth and multiply" and "subdue the Earth." These passages are often cited by those who seek a religious basis to justify unchecked human population growth and environmental destruction in pursuit of human goals. White proposed that the Judeo-Christian dualism encourages exploitation and dominion over nature by humans, resulting in the many environmental problems facing us today.

Earth-based religions of many indigenous cultures of the world (pre-Christian Europe, Native American, African religions) believed that many or all aspects of the natural world were manifestations of one or more gods. Humans were perceived as being at the mercy of these powerful, sometimes petty and vindictive natural forces, and often performed religious rituals to gain favors or atone for sins against Nature. Many of these cultures appear to have lived in ecological balance with their environment. Whether this balance was the consequence of their religious beliefs, their small populations, their limited technologies, or the combination of these factors is unknown.

Modern day Earth-based religions include Paganism, Wicca, Druidism (a resurrection of pre-Roman European Celtic religious traditions), and Goddess religions. These modern versions of ancient traditions also worship the natural world as a manifestation of the energy of God or Creation. People who follow these religious traditions are often dedicated to protecting the environment.[1]

Traditional Hinduism also lacks the distinction between humankind as separate from the rest of Creation. Hindus believe that humans, gods, and nature are all parts of a single organic whole. Many religious rituals serve to appease Mother Earth and seek forgiveness for any violations of Nature. Any abuse of Nature is considered a sacrilegious act.[2]

While traditional Earth-based and Hindu religious traditions encouraged followers to live in ecological balance with their environment, many of these cultures now face a modern dualism: economic development versus environmental protection. In their efforts to develop a modern economic system in India, many Hindus have abandoned traditional beliefs. In recent decades India has suffered from the same environmental degradation as many other developed nations. In recent decades some Native American groups have made environmentally destructive management decisions in the interest of economic development on their reservations. In many cases these environmentally destructive decisions occur in the context of grinding poverty and a breakdown in traditional social systems. All too often, the economic benefits from such decisions are short-lived, while the environmental damage lasts for generations.

In the Islamic tradition, humankind is considered the most favored of God's creation, and all the rest of Creation is deemed subservient to human needs and uses. However, Islamic tradition also holds that all living things in Nature are partners of humankind, deserving of respect and their own existence. Passages in the Qur'an (Koran) state that it is the duty of humankind to deal with the environment and other species in a loving, caring, and respectful manner. Islamic tradition also stipulates that humankind should be good stewards of natural resources and should not pollute clean waters with their wastes. Muslims are encouraged to put the common good ahead of personal benefit and to be moderate in consumption, including the use of natural resources. Taken together, these passages from the Qur'an encourage Muslims to protect and manage their environment for the common good.[3]

While the Judeo-Christian and Islamic religious traditions have scriptural passages that could be seen as justifying environmentally destructive behavior, they also have distinctly environment-friendly teachings. All three of these religious traditions revere the biblical Old Testament, wherein God created the heavens and Earth, the land and waters, the plants and animals, and humankind. At the end of each day of creation, the Bible states that God saw each of his creations was "good." Some theologians interpret these statements to mean that the Creator valued all aspects of creation, not just humankind. In subsequent biblical passages, several references are made regarding human responsibility to be "good stewards" over the other parts of Creation.

The National Religious Partnership for the Environment is an umbrella organization for Christians and Jews who believe that protecting the environment is a mandate well-founded in their scriptural traditions.[4] This association of religious congregations works to increase awareness of the environmental message in the Bible and the Torah. A main objective of this association is to enhance the activity of its members in the political process in support of environmental protection. For people who are committed to protecting the environment and dedicated to their Judeo-Christian religion, this organization offers a community of like-minded people working toward similar goals.

[1] *Pagan and Earth-Based Religions.* www.beliefnet.com/index/index_10015.html.
[2] Adhopia, A. 2001. *Hinduism Promotes Environmental Protection.* www.indianest.com/analysis/018.htm.
[3] Alhilaly, TH. 1993. *Islam and Ecology.* www.ummah.com/islam/taqwapalace/fitness/microcosmpage2.html.
[4] National Religious Partnership for the Environment. www.nrpe.org.

vent of a gas engine. Recent news reports have described several deaths of young people who were "body surfing" by holding on to the back of a power boat. They inhaled the exhaust from the engine, were rendered unconscious by carbon monoxide poisoning, and died before proper medical treatment could be obtained.

Installing a carbon monoxide detector will let you monitor levels of this gas in your home, and will sound an alarm if levels exceed safety standards. Every year, 300 people in the United States die from carbon monoxide poisoning.[3] In many cases, improperly maintained furnaces or incorrectly used space heaters vent carbon monoxide into the home. If this occurs while the occupants are sleeping, they may never wake up. A carbon monoxide alarm can prevent this tragedy from happening to you.

Volatile Organic Compounds

Volatile organic compounds (VOCs) are emitted from products such as paint, paint stripper, cleaning solvents, wood preservatives, aerosol sprays, cleaners, disinfectants, insect repellents and pesticides, air fresheners, stored fuels and automotive products, hobby supplies such as wood glue, and recently dry-cleaned clothing. Formaldehyde is a specific VOC that commonly enters the indoor environment due to emissions from pressed wood products (hardwood plywood wall paneling, particleboard, fiberboard)

and furniture made with these pressed wood products. Urea-formaldehyde foam used for home insulation can emit this gas into the indoor environment.[4] Studies have found that levels of several VOCs average two to five times higher indoors than outdoors. During and for several hours immediately after certain activities, such as paint stripping, levels of VOCs may be 1,000 times background outdoor levels.[4]

The health effects of volatile organic compounds will vary, depending on which specific substance is involved. Immediate effects of many VOCs include irritation to the eyes, nose, and throat, headaches, loss of coordination, and/or nausea. Longer term exposure to some VOCs can result in damage to the liver, kidney, and central nervous system. Some VOCs have been shown to cause cancer in animals, and some are suspected or known to cause cancer in humans.

There are several ways you can limit your exposure to toxic volatile organic compounds. First, you can minimize your use of products that contain these substances by

Key Terms

volatile organic compounds (VOC) a wide variety of chemicals that contain carbon and readily evaporate into the air choosing cleaning supplies, paints, and glues that do not contain VOCs. For example, you could use latex interior house paint rather than an oil-based paint. If you must use a product that contains VOCs, use it in accordance with manufacturer's directions and provide for plenty of ventilation to reduce levels indoors. If you want to strip the paint off that antique cabinet, do it in the backyard or garage (with the door open) instead of in the family room. Never mix household care products, as this may result in chemical reactions that emit toxic VOCs.[4] Also, you should buy only as much of the VOC-containing product as you will need for your current project and dispose of the unused portion in an appropriate manner as soon as possible. Many communities have regularly scheduled and advertised "Tox-Away Days." You can drop off these toxic household products at specified locations for proper disposal. Never simply pour these products down the sink or storm drain, since this will pollute local waterways and may be illegal.

Tobacco Smoke

Secondhand tobacco smoke is an indoor air pollutant widely recognized as a major health risk, especially for children. For example, this pollutant can increase the risk for acute asthma attacks that require hospital emergency care. There is some evidence that regular exposure to tobacco smoke increases the risk of developing asthma in the first place.[5] Exposure to tobacco smoke in the home is also associated with increased risk of Sudden Infant Death Syndrome (SIDS), childhood bronchitis, pneumonia and ear infections, cardiovascular disease, and cancer. The health effects of indoor tobacco smoke are covered in more detail in Chapter 9.

Asbestos

Asbestos is a building material that was widely used for insulation, floor tiles, and for its fire retardant and noise-dampening properties. Health effects of asbestos exposure include cancers of the lung and abdomen, and irreversible scarring of the lungs that can result in reduced respiratory function. These dire effects most commonly occur only after many years of exposure, usually in the workplace.[6] When the serious health risks associated with exposure to asbestos became known, governmental agencies banned several asbestos products, and manufacturers voluntarily limited other uses of asbestos. Today, asbestos is most commonly found in older buildings, including homes, schools, and factories. The greatest risk of exposure to asbestos occurs when insulation, floor tiles, and other asbestos-containing substances deteriorate with age, or are damaged during building renovation or repair. These activities release the microscopic asbestos fibers into the air, from which they are inhaled into the lungs. However, intact and undisturbed, asbestos-containing products are relatively safe.[6]

You can minimize your risk of exposure to inhaled asbestos fibers by leaving undamaged asbestos-containing materials alone, and by hiring qualified contractors to remove damaged asbestos. Before you remodel an old house, you should determine whether or not asbestos is present. If so, do not try to do the remodeling yourself. Never cut, rip, or use a sander on any material that contains asbestos. Some oven mitts, ironing board pads, and woodstove gaskets contain asbestos; you should follow manufacturer's recommendations for replacing and disposing of such materials as they become worn.[6]

Lead

Lead is a toxic metal that was widely used in house paint, as a gasoline additive, and in plumbing solder for metal pipes. As the health consequences of lead toxicity became better know, several of these uses of lead were banned, including lead-based house paint and leaded gasoline. However, lead is a very stable substance that remains in the environment today, long after its use was banned.

Lead exposure most commonly occurs in older homes, built before 1970. Many of these homes contain substantial amounts of lead-based paint, and older metal plumbing may contain lead solder. In late 1991, more than 10 years after lead-based paint was banned, the Secretary of the U.S. Department of Health and Human Services called lead, "the number one environmental threat to the health of children in the United States."[7] Exposure to lead from old paint occurs when the paint breaks down into paint flakes and dust, which are then inhaled or swallowed by children. Lead can also leach from solder in old plumbing and be ingested when people drink tap water.[7]

While lead additives in gasoline were banned by 1990, lead from automobile exhaust fumes was already deposited in soils and can still be found in high concentrations near major highways and city streets. Airborne dust from dirt tracked into the house on shoes can transfer this contaminant to the indoor environment.

Lead has serious health effects when ingested or inhaled, especially for children. Lead can affect virtually all organ systems of the body, but is particularly damaging to the nervous system, kidneys, and blood. *Acute lead toxicity* (blood lead level greater than 80 micrograms per deciliter) can lead to convulsions, coma, and death. However, blood lead levels as low as 10 micrograms per deciliter in children can delay physical and mental

---

Key Terms

asbestos a term used to refer to a class of minerals that have a fibrous crystal structure development, lower IQ, reduce attention span, and increase behavioral problems.[7]

You can minimize your exposure to lead by replacing deteriorated lead house paint and lead soldered plumbing, and by keeping your home clean of roadside dirt that may be contaminated with residual lead from automobile exhaust. If the lead-based paint in your old house is in good condition, leave it alone; it does not pose a hazard *if it is intact.* However, if the old paint is flaking or producing paint dust, you should have it removed by a contractor that is certified for lead abatement. Do not try to remove lead-based paint yourself, as you may inhale large amounts of paint dust or volatilized lead.

If you are exposed to lead contamination, eating a balanced diet that is rich in calcium and iron can reduce the effects of lead toxicity.[7] If you live in an older house with metal plumbing, you should have the tap water tested for lead. Lead is not readily excreted by the body, and will tend to accumulate over time. There are chelating drug treatments that help the body to excrete lead and reduce toxicity effects, but they have adverse side effects and are generally used only to treat acute lead toxicity.[8]

Biological Pollutants

There are many sources of **biological air pollutants** within your personal environment. Disease-causing viruses and bacteria (common cold, flu, measles) are put into the air when infected people or animals sneeze or cough. Contaminated central air handling systems can be breeding grounds for mold, mildew, and bacteria and can then distribute these contaminants throughout the home. *Humidifier fever* is associated with exposure to toxins produced by microorganisms that can grow in ventilation systems.[9] *Legionnaire's disease* is a sometimes fatal pneumonialike disease caused by bacteria that grow in moist indoor environments, such as air conditioning systems, cooling towers, showers, and whirlpool spas.[10] Some people have allergic reactions (itchy eyes, runny nose, sneezing, coughing, stuffy chest, shortness of breath, headache, and/or dizziness) to spores from mold that grows on moist surfaces inside buildings. Some research indicates that exposure to indoor mold can more than double your risk of developing adult onset asthma.[5] Pollen from plants around the home or workplace can cause allergic reactions (hay fever) in many people. Household pets, rats, mice, and cockroaches are sources of saliva, urine, feces, and skin dander that can also stimulate strong allergic reactions.[9]

You can minimize your exposure to biological indoor air pollutants by maintaining the relative humidity in your home within the range of 30–50 percent. This will minimize the growth of many microorganisms that can cause health problems. Control indoor air humidity by installing exhaust fans in bathrooms and kitchens (major sources of water vapor), venting places where water vapor accumulates (attics, basements, and crawl spaces), and using air conditioning or a dehumidifier. You should also eliminate standing water, rugs that have been damaged by leaks or floodwater, and any other wet surfaces.[9]

To minimize allergic reactions to biological indoor air pollutants, you should regularly clean and vacuum your home. While this will not completely eliminate dust mites, pollen, and animal dander, cleaning can substantially reduce the amounts of these allergens and the severity of allergy symptoms. Allergic individuals should leave the house while it is being vacuumed because this may temporarily increase airborne levels of mite allergens and other biological contaminants. You should also try to keep your house free of rodents and cockroaches as these pests are sources of potent allergens.[9]

Radon

Radon is an environmental health risk that seeps into buildings from the soil surrounding their foundation. It is invisible, odorless, and tasteless, and can be detected only by using radon detectors. Uranium, the source of radon, can be found in most parts of the world, and this element is present in rock and soil in parts of all 50 states of the United States. Once radon is produced by decay of uranium, this gas moves through the ground to the air above. Some radon gas may dissolve into groundwater. When radon undergoes radioactive decay, it emits radiation in the form of alpha particles and other byproducts that are also radioactive. These radioactive byproducts can attach to dust and other particles in the air and these particles can be inhaled.

It is estimated that indoor radon is at a level sufficient to increase risk of lung cancer in one of every 15 homes in the United States.[11] The U.S. Surgeon General has warned that exposure to radon gas is the second leading cause of lung cancer in the United States. The National Academy of Sciences estimates that radon exposure causes about 15,000 lung cancer deaths in the United States every year.[12] This risk from radon is especially high for cigarette smokers. Lung damage is caused by radioactive particles formed as by-products from decay of radon that are inhaled and trapped deep within the lungs. As the particles continue the radioactive decay process, they emit bursts of energy

┌─ **Key Terms** ─────────────────────────────────

biological air pollutants living organisms or substances produced by living organisms that cause disease or allergic reactions, including bacteria, molds, mildew, viruses, dust mites, plant pollen, and animal dander, urine, or feces

radon a naturally occurring radioactive gas that is emitted during the decay of uranium in soil, rock, and water

└──

that damage adjacent lung tissue. There are no obvious short-term effects from this damage, but with long-term exposure this damage can cause lung cancer.[12] There is some evidence that consuming water that is contaminated by radon gas can increase the risk of stomach cancer. The National Academy of Sciences estimates consumption of radon in drinking water causes 19 stomach cancer deaths per year in the United States.[13]

The key to minimizing the health risk of radon exposure is to have your home tested. You can purchase an inexpensive "do-it-yourself" test kit in some hardware stores and other retail outlets. If you can't find a radon test kit locally, you can purchase one from the National Safety Council's Radon Hotline (800-767-7236). After the kit is exposed to the air in your home for a specified time period, it must be returned to a laboratory for analysis.

If unsafe levels of radon are detected in your home, you should work with a contractor who is certified to install a radon reduction system in your home. This will often involve installing a venting system just below the concrete slab of the house foundation. This venting system will intercept the radon gas before it enters your home and vent it outside the home where it can be dissipated by wind. You should also have cracks in the slab, basement walls, or foundation of the home repaired to reduce seepage of radon gas through these spaces. However, just sealing the cracks, without installing the belowground venting system, does not adequately reduce indoor radon levels. If you live in a region where high radon levels are common and you plan to build a new home, you should work with your contractor to install radon-resistant features during construction. The average cost to install radon-resistant features in an existing home is $800–$2,500. The average cost to install radon-resistant features in a new home during construction is $350–$500 (a 128–400 percent savings).[11] For a map of radon risk zones in the United States, see www.epa.gov/iaq/radon/zonemap.html.

Nonionizing Radiation

Nonionizing radiation includes various forms of electromagnetic radiation that cannot break chemical bonds but may excite electrons (ultraviolet radiation) or heat biological materials (infrared, radio frequency, and microwave radiation). Common sources of nonionizing radiation are sunlight, electrical devices, electric power transmission lines, and cell phones. Most adverse health effects of nonionizing radiation are associated with heating tissues, resulting in burns.

Some experts have proposed that certain forms of nonionizing radiation may have more serious health effects, including increased risk of cancer. A small number of studies have documented DNA damage in brain cells of rats exposed to high levels of radiofrequency radiation (RFR) similar to that emitted by cell phones. However, other animal studies did not find similar effects. Large-scale studies of brain cancer incidence among people who do and do not use cell phones have also failed to document a link between RFR and increased incidence of brain cancer in humans.[14,15] However, cell phones are a relatively new technology, and there has not been sufficient time to study effects of long-term exposure to RFR. As people use cell phones more, beginning at an increasingly younger age, some suggest that it may be prudent to reduce exposure to RFR from these devices.[16] This can be easily done by using a headset attachment to the cell phone so that there is greater distance between the cell-phone transmitter and the brain. The intensity of RFR from cell phones decreases significantly over even small distances to levels so low that they are very unlikely to be a health risk.

Another common source of nonionizing radiation in the human environment is electricity flowing through wires and electronic devices, and electricity transmission lines. A few studies have suggested that exposure to nonionizing radiation around electric devices such as microwave ovens, televisions, tanning lamps, electric blankets, and electricity transmission lines may slightly increase risk for some cancers.[17,18,19] However, the vast majority of studies have failed to find any increased risk of adverse health effects associated with household electronics or living near power lines. (For a comprehensive review of the scientific literature, go to the Web site of J. E. Moulder, professor of radiation oncology at the Medical College of Wisconsin, www.mcw.edu/gcrc/cop/powerlines-cancer-FAQ/toc.html#C55.)

Drinking Water

The safety of drinking water in your home is affected by environmental factors both in the home or neighborhood and in the larger community. The water supply for rural homes is often a well that draws from groundwater, and can be much affected by environmental conditions around the home and neighborhood. In urban areas a municipal water supply system draws from rivers or lakes and then treats the water to make it safe to drink. The community/regional environment plays the dominant role in determining the safety of water from municipal suppliers. However, municipal water can be contaminated by the personal environment as it passes through pipes in the home. Environmental health issues relating to drinking water as influenced by conditions in your home and

---

Key Terms

nonionizing radiation forms of electromagnetic radiation that cannot break chemical bonds but may excite electrons or heat biological materials

Tap water is a key source of pollutants in the home.

neighborhood will be covered here. Issues related to municipal water supply are presented later in this chapter.

Approximately 23 million people in the United States obtain their drinking water from groundwater (that is, from private wells), streams, or cisterns that collect rainwater.[20] These households are responsible for ensuring the safety of their own drinking water. Private drinking water supplies that rely on surface waters, or wells that tap shallow groundwater layers, are at risk of contamination by pathogens from home septic systems, contaminants from leaking underground fuel storage tanks, improper disposal of various household chemicals (cleaners, automotive fluids, and pesticides), and agricultural chemicals applied to surrounding farm fields.

Nitrate from agricultural fertilizer that leaches into shallow groundwater supplies poses a widespread health risk in rural areas. The U.S. Geological Survey estimates that 10–20 percent of groundwater sources of drinking water may have levels of nitrate contamination that pose risks to human health. Excessive consumption of nitrate in contaminated drinking water can cause serious illness and death. Nitrate interferes with the oxygen-transport function of the blood (methemoglobinemia). This effect is most pronounced in children, resulting in "blue-baby" syndrome.[21] Nitrate can also cause reproductive problems and is linked to development of several types of cancer.

Rural wells contaminated by nitrate may also have high levels of other agricultural chemicals. Some researchers have suggested that agricultural pesticides and herbicides can contribute to the development of testicular cancer and reduced sperm production in men, breast cancer in women, and nervous system disorders in children.[22]

Leaching of substances from pipes in the plumbing of older homes is another potential source of contamination to drinking water in the home.[23] Metallic pipes can release toxic metals such as lead and copper into the water. Polyvinyl chloride (PVC) pipes manufactured before 1977 may release toxic vinyl chloride into the water. Vinyl chloride is a known human carcinogen.

Leaching of toxic substances from pipes into the drinking water supply is most problematic in small diameter pipes (less than a 2-inch diameter), with high water temperatures, and when the water is stagnant in the pipes for long periods (more than 24 hours).[23] A relatively easy way to reduce contaminants from household plumbing in your drinking water is to regularly flush fresh water through the plumbing. Let the water run from the tap for a couple of minutes before taking water to drink, especially first thing in the morning and if you have been away from home for long time periods. In some cases it may be advisable to replace the old plumbing, but this can be very expensive.

Private water supplies should be tested annually for nitrate and **fecal coliform bacteria.** If you suspect there may be a problem with radon or pesticide contamination, you may need to test your water even more frequently.[14] Testing generally requires that you send samples of your water to a laboratory that tests water quality. You can get a listing of local certified laboratories from your local or state public health department. Some local health departments test private water for free. A private laboratory will charge $10–$20 to perform a nitrate and bacteria test. Testing for pesticides or organic chemicals may cost from several hundred to several thousand dollars. Most laboratories mail back the sample results within a few days, or several weeks if the analyses are more complex. The results indicate the concentrations of contaminants and indicate whether each contaminant exceeds a drinking water quality standard.

If your drinking water contains contaminants that exceed safety standards, you should retest the water supply immediately and contact your public health department for assistance. High bacteria concentrations can sometimes be easily controlled by disinfecting a well. Water filters may also remove some contaminants. However, other problems may require a new source of water, such as a deeper well. Alternatively, you may need to rely on bottled water until a new water source can be obtained.[20] You can obtain technical assistance with residential drinking water supply problems from the organization Farm*A*Syst/Home*A*Syst (see the Web sites www.uwex.edu/farmasyst or www.uwex.edu/homeasyst).

Noise

Noise can be defined as any undesirable sound. What constitutes "undesirable sound" will vary from one person to the next, but it often involves loud sounds that occur at irregular intervals and are not controllable by the listener.[24] In the personal environment of the home, neighborhood, and workplace, noise may include overly loud music, barking dogs, motorcycles and cars with broken or missing muffler systems, loud machinery, appliances and power tools, airplanes flying overhead, and train whistles.

The health effects of environmental noise depend on the intensity, frequency, and nature of the noise. Excessively loud noise can cause physical damage to sensory tissues in your ears, resulting in partial or total hearing loss that can be temporary or permanent. This physical damage will depend on both the intensity (as measured in decibels) and the duration of exposure to the loud noise. For example, sitting in front of the speaker column at a large rock concert, with noise levels at 120 decibels for over 2 hours, can result in immediate pain and long-term or permanent

hearing loss. Ironically, the tissues that are damaged by excessively loud sounds are those responsible for hearing high frequency sounds associated with normal conversation, not the tissues that actually hear the damaging sound. Loud noise sources rob you of one of your most important senses, the ability to hear the unamplified human voice.

Even noise at lower levels can cause adverse health effects. The American Speech-Language-Hearing Association reports that low level noise can elevate blood pressure, reduce sleep, cause fatigue, and disturb digestion. These physical effects of low level noise can impact emotional, intellectual, social, and occupational health. Effects reported by the World Health Organization include increased frustration and anxiety, impaired ability to concentrate, reduced productivity and ability to learn, and increased absenteeism and accidents. These effects of noise can increase your feeling of stress and diminish your ability to tolerate minor irritations; you may exhibit anger and aggression that are out of proportion to the immediate source of your irritation.[24] This antisocial behavior may have negative consequences in your personal relationships and occupational health.

A common source of long-term exposure to loud sound that causes hearing loss in many young people is amplified music. Occasional loud rock music at 110–120 decibels may cause only temporary damage. However, daily exposure to such sound levels will cause permanent hearing loss. A number of aging rock stars have admitted to significant hearing loss that they attribute to standing in front of huge amplifiers night after night. Many rock musicians performing today stand behind the main speaker columns or wear ear protection. Jacking up the volume in your headphones, or the powerful amplifier in your car stereo, may be fun today, but is it worth a lifetime of incessant ringing in your ears and diminished hearing later in life? (See Changing for the Better on page 602 for tips on reducing health risks associated with noise pollution.)

The Community and Regional Environment

The community and regional environment is made up of the outdoor air you breathe, local rivers and lakes that provide water and recreation opportunities, surrounding

---

Key Terms
fecal coliform bacteria a category of bacteria that live within the intestines of warm-blooded animals; the presence of these bacteria is used as an indicator that water has been contaminated by feces

lands (urban, industrial, suburban, rural, agricultural, natural communities), and all the people and other species that live in these areas. A wide range of human activities can degrade this community environment in ways that affect personal health. Air, water, and land pollution include many substances that have significant negative effects on physical health. Loss of natural areas and other recreational and aesthetic "green space" to roads, cities, and industrial development can adversely affect your perceived quality of life, with negative effects on emotional and spiritual health. Degraded environmental conditions in many communities discourage new economic development and may limit occupational health.

While you can exert some influence on the environmental conditions in your community, the influence of any one individual is usually small. Your control over how the community environment affects your personal health is often limited to controlling your exposure to known health risks, such as contaminated water and land, or outdoor air pollution. You can also choose to reduce your own contributions to community/regional air, water, and land pollution through conservation of energy and water and recycling solid waste.

Because one person cannot have a significant impact on community environmental problems, many people join organizations that work to improve the environment and quality of life in their community. By working with others of like mind in the political process and in environmental organizations, you become "part of the solution" to major environmental problems that can affect your health and that of your family. For many people, getting involved in solving local environmental problems can provide significant benefits to emotional and spiritual health.

In this section you will learn about aspects of the community and regional environment that can affect your health, and what you can do to exert some level of personal control over these environmental influences.

Air Pollution

Air pollution includes substances that naturally occur in the air (pollen, microbes, dust, sea salt, volcanic ash) and substances produced by human activities (engine exhaust, ozone, various volatile organic compounds, and acid rain). In this section on community and regional environmental influences on health, we focus on those components of air pollution that are produced within a specific region and that have substantial health effects within that community or region.

The primary sources of human-caused air pollutants are various kinds of internal combustion engines associated with electric power plants, industry, and transportation (trucks, automobiles, and farm/construction equipment). Oil refineries and chemical production factories also contribute to air pollution in some communities. Electric power stations, industrial facilities, and chemical factories are classified as *point sources* that produce large amounts of pollution from a single location. Automobiles, trucks, heavy construction/farm equipment, gas stations, lawn mowers, and charcoal grills are *nonpoint sources* of air pollutants. Individually, nonpoint sources produce relatively small amounts of pollution, but when added together account for a large proportion of community air pollution.

Key Terms

air pollution refers to a wide variety of substances found in the atmosphere that can have adverse effects on human health, crop productivity, and natural communities

Smog over Los Angeles, California

Air pollutants that are directly produced by internal combustion engines include *carbon monoxide, nitrogen dioxide, sulfur dioxide, polycyclic aromatic hydrocarbons,* and *particulate matter.* Carbon monoxide is a toxic gas that impairs respiration, as described under indoor air quality in the previous section. Nitrogen and sulfur oxides interact with water vapor in the air to form small particulates (diameter < 2.5 μm) that are inhaled into the deepest parts of the lungs. These substances can damage lung tissues, reduce lung capacity, cause coughing and chronic bronchitis, and make worse such ailments as hypersensitivity to allergens, asthma, emphysema, and heart disease. The U.S. Environmental Protection Agency estimates that over 70 million people in the United States live in counties where levels of small particulate air pollutants exceed human health standards for at least some part of the year.[25] It has been estimated that small-particulate air pollution causes as many as 50,000 to 100,000 premature deaths in the United States per year.[26]

Polycyclic aromatic hydrocarbons (PAHs) are widespread air pollutants from fossil fuel combustion in vehicles and residential furnaces, and from environmental tobacco smoke. These substances have been shown to be carcinogenic to both test animals and humans. Several new studies indicate that PAHs can cross the placenta and cause adverse health effects on a developing human fetus.[27,28] Increased maternal exposure to PAHs was associated with lower birth weight, smaller head circumference, and reduced birth length of newborn children.[27] A study of 867 mothers and 822 newborns living in large cities in the United States, Poland, and China documented a significant association between maternal exposure to PAHs and PAH-linked DNA damage in newborns that is associated with increased risk of cancer.[28] This type of DNA damage was detected in 42 percent and 61 percent of two groups of newborns in New York City (where PAH exposure was lowest), 71 percent of newborns in Krakow, Poland, and 80 percent of newborns in Tongliang, China (where PAH exposure was highest). Higher levels of DNA damage were also associated with higher PAH exposure. The prevalence and amount of DNA damage did not differ between mothers and their babies, despite the fact that fetal exposure was only 10 percent that of the mother. This indicates that the developing fetuses are 10 times more susceptible to DNA damage from PAHs than adult mothers are.[28]

Tropospheric ozone is another important regional air pollutant that is linked to chemicals in exhaust fumes from internal combustion engines. This substance is produced when hydrocarbons, nitrogen oxides, and other small particle matter chemically interact in the presence of sunlight. The result is a brownish haze over affected cities, often called *smog.*

Ozone levels are particularly high in locations with warm, sunny climates (Southern California) and where natural vegetation produces volatile organic compounds that contribute to the photochemical process that produces ozone (eastern United States). The U.S. Environmental Protection Agency estimates that over 110 million people in the United States live in counties where ozone levels exceed human health standards for at least some

---

Key Terms

polycyclic aromatic hydrocarbons (PAHs) air pollutants from fossil fuel combustion

tropospheric ozone ozone comprises three oxygen atoms that are bound into a single molecule; tropospheric ozone refers to this substance as it occurs in the lower layer of the atmosphere, close to the ground

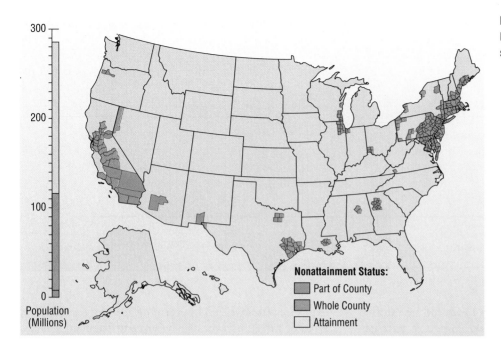

Figure 20-2 Counties classified by EPA as in "nonattainment" of ozone standards in the year 2003.

300 —

200 —

100 —

0 —

Population (Millions)

Nonattainment Status:
- Part of County
- Whole County
- Attainment

part of the year.[25] Most of these people live in Southern California and near the East Coast between Virginia and southern Maine (see Figure 20-2).

Inhalation of ozone can cause lung damage that reduces lung capacity. This is a particular health risk to individuals who suffer from asthma, emphysema, or heart disease. On days when ozone concentrations are highest, local hospital emergency room visits associated with respiratory distress increase from 10–20 percent.[29] There is also some evidence that childhood exposure to ozone can actually cause children to become asthmatic.[29,30]

Air toxics are a diverse collection of hazardous air pollutants produced mainly by electric power plants and industrial sources that constitute a widespread environmental health risk in the United States. When lifetime cancer risks for all carcinogenic air toxics are combined, 200 million people in the U.S. live in counties where that risk exceeds 10 in one million, and 20 million people live in areas where the risk exceeds 100 in one million.[33] However, these risk estimates are based on a lifetime of exposure to toxic air pollutant levels as they were last inventoried in 1996. With continued progress on reducing toxic air pollution, risks associated with air toxics might be expected to decrease in the future. Since Congress passed the Clean Air Act in 1970, substantial progress has been made in reducing most human-caused air pollution in the U.S. However, further reduction of air pollution poses serious technological and/or economic challenges, and efforts to strengthen regulations often face tough political opposition. For more information about air toxics, go to the U.S. EPA Web site www.epa.gov/ttn/atw.

Unfortunately, the degree to which you can control your own exposure to regional air pollution and the associated health risks is limited. In many larger urban areas, where air pollution levels are highest, weather reports in newspapers and on television often include information about air pollution. This is because weather conditions have a strong influence on air pollution levels. Hot, dry weather promotes tropospheric ozone formation. When there is little wind, or when there is limited vertical mixing of the atmosphere, air pollutants are not dispersed and can accumulate to dangerous levels near the ground. If you live in a large city, you should pay attention to air pollution information. This information is often conveyed in color-coded alerts. A "yellow" air pollution alert means people who suffer from respiratory or cardiac diseases, or hypersensitivity to allergens, should stay indoors. An "orange" air pollution alert indicates that everyone should limit their outdoor activities to the minimum possible.

You can also help to lower air pollution levels by limiting contributions from your own automobile, lawn mower exhaust, and charcoal grill. You can carpool, use

> **Key Terms**
>
> **air toxics** a class of 188 toxic air pollutants identified by the U.S. Environmental Protection Agency as known or suspected causes of cancer or other serious health effects, such as reduced fertility, birth defects, or adverse environmental effects

mass transit, or telecommute (work at home via a computer network) to reduce air pollution associated with automobile exhaust. You can fill your car gas tank, mow your lawn, and use your grill during the cooler evening hours to reduce your contribution to tropospheric ozone. You can conserve electricity to reduce emissions of air toxics, sulfur and nitrogen oxides, and particulates from electric power plants. In areas of the United States where air pollution is especially problematic, local laws may require that you do some of these things on days when conditions result in a "pollution emergency."

Water Pollution

Humankind has had a very schizophrenic relationship with our rivers and lakes. Water is an essential resource for all living things on our planet, including humans and the plants and animals we use for food. We also value our rivers and lakes for the recreational opportunities and aesthetic benefits they provide. Yet for decades, we used these water bodies as convenient dumps for our sewage and industrial wastes.

The problem of water pollution came to national attention on a day in 1968 when children playing with matches set on fire chemical pollutants that covered the Cuyahoga River in Ohio. The subsequent public outcry resulted in major national legislation, including the Clean Water Act of 1972 and the Safe Drinking Water Act of 1974. Since then, substantial progress has been made in reducing water pollution and insuring safe drinking water supplies.

The job of cleaning rivers and lakes in the United States is not complete, and people who come in close contact with contaminated waters or fish from these areas are still at risk for a variety of health problems. Water pollutants in surface waters come from obvious point sources (sewer overflows, confined livestock feedlot operations, sometimes called "factory farms") and from nonpoint sources such as water runoff from urban streets and agricultural areas that carries various chemicals and animal waste into local rivers. In some areas, water drainage from mines carries toxic metals into nearby streams. Toxic air pollutants can be deposited into water bodies in rainfall. Some of the most troublesome water pollutants in the United States today are described below.

Biological water pollutants from untreated sewage and drainage from leaking home septic systems include various species of disease-causing viruses, bacteria, and protozoa found in rivers and lakes. These organisms cause diseases that are at best uncomfortable (diarrhea) and at worst potentially lethal (dysentery, hepatitis, typhoid fever, and cholera). In the late 1800s, diseases associated with drinking water contaminated by biological pollution were the third leading cause of death in the United States.[32]

The largest sources of biological water pollutants in surface waters of the United States today are overflows from combined septic and storm sewers during heavy rainfall events, and animal wastes that are carried by runoff of rainfall from agricultural areas. While much has already been done to eliminate biological contamination from municipal sewer systems, billions of dollars are still required to dig up old combined sewer systems and replace them with separate systems for sewage and storm water runoff. As large animal "factory farms" have become more common in rural America, government agencies have established regulations for the proper handling of the huge amounts of animal sewage that are generated. Even so, violations of regulations and occasional accidents result in contamination of local surface waters with animal waste.

At present, your personal risk of exposure to biological water pollution in the United States is relatively small. Public health departments monitor local surface waters for the presence of fecal coliform bacteria in every county in the United States. While they may or may not cause illness or disease, the presence of fecal coliform organisms is an indicator that water has been contaminated by sewage. All municipal drinking water systems, and many private households, in the United States treat their water to kill pathogenic organisms. By the end of the 20th century, deaths due to water pathogens in the drinking water supply were very rare in the United States.[32]

A wide variety of other **toxic pollutants** can be found in surface and groundwater sources of drinking water. These substances include naturally occurring toxic elements (such as arsenic and mercury) produced by breakdown of minerals in certain kinds of rock. Various human activities produce a wide range of toxic chemicals that find their way into surface waters of the U.S., including metals, solvents, plastics, and PCBs (polychlorinated biphenols). Some toxic substances have both natural and human-caused sources, including arsenic and mercury.

Agricultural pesticides can be significant toxic water pollutants in parts of the United States where large areas of land are used for crop production. These chemicals include insecticides, fungicides, and herbicides to kill organisms that consume or compete with crop plants. While these chemicals are applied to croplands, they are often carried into local streams and rivers by runoff of rainfall.

> ### Key Terms
>
> **biological water pollutants** disease-causing organisms that are found in water
>
> **toxic pollutants** substances known to cause cancer or other serious health effects

While the dumping of toxic substances into surface waters is now illegal, some of these toxins are very stable and can be found in large quantities in the sediments of rivers and lakes that were polluted before 1972. Cleaning up these toxic sediments can be very costly. A recent decision to dredge and dispose of PCB-contaminated sediments in the Hudson River near Albany, New York, will cost hundreds of millions of dollars.

Health effects of agricultural chemicals and other toxic substances depend on the specific chemical.[32] Taken as a group, these substances have been linked to adverse effects on the blood, liver, spleen, kidney, adrenal gland, thyroid gland, reproductive system (fertility), and cardiovascular system. Some are known or suspected human *carcinogens* (substances that cause cancer), *mutagens* (substances that cause cell mutations), or *teratogens* (substances that cause birth defects). Obvious health effects that occur immediately after exposure to high concentrations of these substances include nausea, fatigue, headache, skin and eye irritation, or tremors. The risks for these adverse immediate health effects are greatest for workers who come in direct contact with the concentrated chemicals. More insidious are health effects such as cancer and birth defects that develop slowly, imperceptibly, after long-term exposure to low concentrations of these chemicals in the environment.

Many toxic chemicals and pesticides also have adverse consequences for natural systems, causing declines and extinctions of species and degradation of biological communities and ecosystems. For example, DDT was a widely used insecticide that has been blamed for the near extinction of many large bird species, including eagles, hawks, falcons, condors, and pelicans. While this was not a direct impact on human physical health, many people felt that the decline of these and other wildlife species diminished their emotional and spiritual health.

The best way for you to minimize physical health risks posed by consuming biological or toxic contaminants is to be well informed. Read the annual water quality report from your municipal water supplier. If your water supplier fails to meet health standards, consider drinking bottled, boiled, or filtered water until the supplier fixes the problems.

The U.S. Environmental Protection Agency has set **maximum contaminant level (MCL)** standards for the amounts of the biological pollutants, pesticides, and toxic chemicals that are allowed in municipal drinking water supplies.[25] MCLs are set at levels that minimize human health risks, but also take into account the limits of available treatment technology and the costs of meeting the standards. Municipal water suppliers are required to report any violations of MCLs to state and federal environmental agencies.

Many municipal water suppliers will provide consumers with annual reports that list the amounts of biological contaminants, agricultural pesticides, and toxic substances that are detected in their water. If your supplier does not provide a report, you can access the supplier's annual report to the U.S. Environmental Protection Agency at www.epa.gov/safewater/dwinfo.htm. These reports list the mean and range (minimum and maximum) concentrations for all regulated contaminants for all samples analyzed in a year. Look at the maximum value to determine if your water system occasionally fails to adequately remove any regulated contaminants.

You can also be exposed to toxic substances by eating contaminated fish or wild game. Some toxic substances, such as mercury and PCBs, accumulate to high levels in the bodies of shellfish, fish, and waterfowl. This problem can occur even in remote, apparently pristine areas if there are natural sources of toxic substances such as mercury. People who regularly consume wild food animals from contaminated waters may be at high risk of adverse health effects.

To reduce health risks associated with consuming wild game, you should be aware of health advisories for consuming contaminated fish or game. These advisories are often stated in terms of limits on how much fish or meat should be consumed in a specified time period. Pregnant women should be especially careful of consuming shellfish, fish, or wild game; mercury and PCBs can cause birth defects in the fetus they carry. These health advisories are usually issued by the public health department or state agencies responsible for fish and game.

You can also be exposed to waterborne pollutants, with associated health risks, as a result of recreational activities, such as swimming, boating, and backpacking. You can limit your personal risk of exposure to health risks from contaminated water by being aware of "Don't swim" warnings for your local rivers and lakes, usually issued by the public health department. If you are backpacking in an apparently pristine wilderness area, never assume that crystal clear water in the mountain stream is safe to drink. Backpackers should always filter, boil, or chemically treat drinking water to kill pathogens that may be present even in such remote water sources.

 TALKING POINTS How can you approach your political representatives about environmental policy? What are some effective ways of keeping health-related environmental issues on the national agenda?

Key Terms

maximum contaminant level (MCL) the highest concentration of a contaminant that is allowed in drinking water, as established and regulated by the U.S. Environmental Protection Agency

Finding someplace to put our garbage will continue to present a major environmental and health dilemma as we progress through the 21st century. Solid waste buried in landfills can pollute the surrounding air and water, creating health risks for people and wildlife that live in the surrounding areas.

Land Pollution

We do not physically consume land or soil the way we do air and water, but pollution of land can still result in serious adverse health effects. Disposal of toxic wastes often involves burying them in the ground. When done with proper safeguards, this disposal method can isolate these dangerous materials so they can do no harm to humans or natural systems. If done improperly, these toxic pollutants leach into groundwater or are carried into surface waters by the runoff of rain, where they cause serious ecological problems and pose significant human health risks.

Occasionally, housing developments are built on top of old toxic waste disposal sites, and the residents are exposed to toxic substances by inhaling or swallowing contaminated dust and soil, drinking contaminated water, or through chemicals leaching into their basements. One of the worst cases of such a mistake was the infamous Love Canal incident in New York State during the 1970s.[33] Schools and housing developments were built near an abandoned waste disposal site, into which many different toxic chemicals and sewage had been deposited. Children swimming in contaminated water holes suffered from skin lesions. Families living in the houses had children born with birth defects. In the end, the state of New York bought the homes and moved the families to other locations. While toxic waste disposal is now strictly regulated, and old toxic waste dumps are being cleaned up under the EPA Superfund program, there remain thousands of sites like Love Canal around the United States. These toxic waste sites are ticking time bombs waiting for ignorant or unscrupulous developers and unwary homebuyers.

Most land pollution today is associated with the disposal of **solid waste.** *Municipal solid waste* consists of everyday items such as product packaging, grass clippings, furniture, clothing, bottles, food scraps, newspapers, appliances, paint, and batteries. Other solid waste produced by business and industry includes waste tires, concrete, asphalt, bricks, lumber, and shingles from demolished buildings, and *sewage sludge* (solids remaining after wastewater treatment). In 1999 the U.S. population produced 230 million tons of solid waste, or about 4.6 pounds of waste per person per day (or 1,680 pounds per person per year).[34]

Municipal sanitation departments and private disposal companies are very efficient at removing these wastes from our homes and businesses and putting them someplace where we don't see them. These waste disposal locations include sanitary landfills (wastes are compacted and buried under soil), ocean dumping in garbage barges (with trash sometimes escaping to wash up on beaches), and incinerators (where solid wastes are burned).[33]

While out-of-sight often means out-of-mind, these solid wastes do not "go away," they accumulate. Many municipal and regional sanitary landfills are reaching their capacity and must be closed. No one wants a new landfill

Key Terms

solid waste pollutants that are in solid form, including nonhazardous household trash, industrial wastes, mining wastes, and sewage sludge from wastewater treatment plants

The High-Tech Revolution and E-Waste

The high-tech revolution has a hidden dark side, mountains of accumulating obsolete electronic equipment that contain large amounts of toxic substances. During the period from 1997 to 2007, it is estimated that over 500 million computers must be disposed of. These computers will contain 6.2 billion pounds of plastic, 1.6 billion pounds of lead, 3 million pounds of cadmium, 1.9 million pounds of chromium, and 632,000 pounds of mercury. Lead, cadmium, chromium, and mercury are highly toxic metals, and can cause a wide range of severe health effects if they end up in the air, drinking water, or food supply.[1,2]

Computers contain over 1,000 different substances, many of which are toxic. This makes recycling a complex, labor-intensive process that can cost more than the value of the recycled materials. Only 6 percent of obsolete computers disposed of after 1998 were recycled. The remainder was deposited in landfills across the country. It is estimated that 70 percent of heavy metals such as lead and mercury going into U.S. landfills today comes from electronic waste. Several states, including California and Massachusetts, have banned disposal of computer monitors in landfills to protect groundwater.[1]

While recycling of computers is seen as the ideal solution to the problem of waste disposal, it is estimated that 50 percent to 80 percent of computers "recycled" before the year 2002 were actually shipped to poor Asian countries.

Workers in these countries disassemble computers to recover useful materials for very low wages and with minimal or no protection from the toxic materials to which they are exposed. These countries have weak or poorly enforced environmental regulations, so materials that cannot be recycled are dumped into rivers or burned in open air pits. These practices expose the recycling workers and surrounding local populations to toxic substances. In one city in China, river water had 190 times the pollution levels allowed under World Health Organization standards, and drinking water had to be transported from 18 miles away.[1]

The practice of shipping toxic computer waste to underdeveloped countries is now banned by an international treaty, but the United States is the only developed nation that has not ratified this treaty. The "free market" justification for the practice of shipping toxic computer waste to underdeveloped countries is that this provides jobs and helps poor people. The question is whether or not it is moral to give poor people the choice between poverty or poisons?[1]

Given that the use of computers and electronics will only increase in the future, many argue that we must develop environmentally responsible computer recycling systems. In 2002 Rep. Mike Thompson introduced The Computer Hazardous-Waste Infrastructure Program (CHIP) Act that would require the Environmental Protection Agency to help set up computer recycling across the United States. The program would be funded by a fee of up to $10 on all retail sales of desktop and laptop PCs and computer monitors. Similar legislation is also appearing in many state legislatures. The electronics industry does not favor charging consumers a fee on new computers, but rather wants to charge consumers the fee when they return their old computers to the manufacturer. Some computer manufacturers are already initiating computer take-back programs. However, development of a comprehensive national strategy for responsibly addressing the computer waste problem continues as of this writing.

The other, and perhaps most important, approach to the computer waste problem is to develop electronic equipment that is less toxic and more easily recycled. This will require development of, and investment in, new technologies. In our free market system, this will happen only when the electronics manufacturers must share the cost of dealing with computer waste.

[1]Puckett J, et al: *Exporting Harm: The High-Tech Trashing of Asia.* The Basal Action Network and Silicon Valley Toxics Coalition, 2002.
[2]U.S. Environmental Protection Agency: *WasteWise Update: Electronics Reuse and Recycling.* 2003. www.epa.gov/wastewise/pubs/wwupda14.pdf.

located near their home, so it is politically and legally difficult to locate new landfills. Sometimes wealthy states pay to export their solid wastes to landfills in poorer states that have weaker environmental regulations. Sometimes, toxic wastes are shipped to poor underdeveloped countries with no environmental regulations. However, even these poorer countries are beginning to realize that accepting toxic wastes in return for money does not serve their long-term best interests and some have banned this practice.

As we run out of places to dump our solid waste, some have proposed that we burn it in large incinerators. However, many concerns have been raised about incinerators because they can release toxic substances into the atmosphere. Furthermore, the ash from these incinerators contains concentrated toxic chemicals in forms that can easily leach into ground and surface waters.

Most of the potential health effects of land pollution have already been described in this chapter under the topics of air and water pollution. Most human exposure to pollutants that are deposited on land occurs when those toxic substances end up in the air or water. You can limit your risk of these health effects by being aware of where solid wastes are disposed, both at the present time and in the past. You should be particularly aware of proximity to a local landfill or waste disposal site if your water source is a private well that draws from groundwater that might be contaminated. Municipal water systems are required to regularly monitor their water for pollutants.

If your water comes from a private well, it is very much in your best interests to do likewise.

You can reduce your personal contribution to the solid waste problem of your community by following the Three R's: Reduce, Reuse, Recycle. You can reduce the amount of solid waste you produce by consuming less and accepting less packaging materials on the products you buy. You can compost your yard waste for use as a mulch and fertilizer in flower beds, or use a lawn mower with a mulching blade to eliminate grass clippings and leaves in the autumn. Reusing items such as bottles, zipper-closure storage bags, cloth shopping bags, and cloth diapers reduces the amount of solid waste you throw away each week. Many items in typical household trash (newspapers and magazines, aluminum and steel cans, glass bottles, and many plastic containers) can be recycled and the materials used to make new products. Diverting these solid wastes away from the landfill toward reuse can greatly reduce the solid waste problem of your community. However, recycling will only work if you also buy products that are made from recycled materials, such as recycled paper and plastic "wood" products.

Loss of Green Space

Loss of **green space** represents another kind of land pollution that can affect your quality of life and health. In many parts of the United States, green space is being converted to housing developments, shopping malls, industrial sites, and highways. Hundreds of large, brightly lit signs along the highways pollute the visual environment. Wildlife species disappear from your community and surroundings as their habitats are destroyed.

While development of green space for human uses may provide job opportunities and be beneficial for your occupational health, it can also detract from recreational and aesthetic aspects of your community. If you find that you must travel farther and longer from home or work to find a safe and enjoyable location to jog or bicycle, you may exercise less often. Your sense of "quality of life" is diminished when you no longer see wild animals in your backyard or you feel that your community is becoming ugly. Many people feel their emotional and spiritual health are diminished when formerly green space is converted to asphalt parking lots and commercial buildings.

Some communities have created land-use (zoning) plans that allow for economic development while protecting recreational and aesthetic values in their communities. These zoning plans can be controversial, as they try to balance the rights of private property owners with the welfare of the entire community. You can contribute toward protecting environmental quality in your community by supporting land-use planning and enforceable zone laws that protect green space while allowing for responsible economic development.

Ionizing Radiation

Radiation is a general term that refers to various forms of energy that are emitted by atoms and molecules when they undergo change, including radio waves, infrared waves, visible light, ultra-violet waves, X-rays, and gamma rays. Each kind of radiation has different effects on biological materials and health. **Ionizing radiation** causes damage to biological structures such as DNA that can result in serious adverse health effects. Ionizing radiation is produced by nuclear reactions, and sources include medical X-rays, naturally occurring radioactive minerals such as uranium, various radioactive materials used by industry, nuclear reactors and their waste products, and nuclear bomb explosions.

The health effects of exposure to X-rays and gamma radiation depend on many factors, including the duration, type and dose of radiation, and your individual sensitivity. Heavy exposure to these forms of radiation can occur if you are near a nuclear bomb blast or downwind of a major nuclear reactor accident. In such cases, exposure can cause *radiation sickness,* including intense fatigue, nausea, weight loss, hair loss, fever, bleeding from the mouth, and compromised immune system, usually resulting in death.

On April 26, 1986, a major nuclear reactor accident at the Chernobyl nuclear power plant in the Soviet Union exposed hundreds of thousands of people to nuclear radiation. It has been estimated that 10,000 miners and soldiers who sealed the damaged nuclear reactor immediately after the accident died of radiation sickness. Families exposed to the radioactive fallout from the explosion have had an increased occurrence of birth defects and cancer. A much less severe accident in 1979 at the Three Mile Island nuclear power plant in eastern Pennsylvania released radioactive gases into the atmosphere. Subsequent studies suggest that people who lived in the surrounding community at the time of the accident have higher rates of some cancers than does the general population. However, no significant

---

Key Terms

green space areas of land that are dominated by domesticated or natural vegetation, including rural farmland, city lawns and parks, and nature preserves

ionizing radiation electromagnetic radiation that is capable of breaking chemical bonds, such as X-rays and gamma rays increase in mortality rate was found in a long-term study of this affected population.[35]

Exposure to lower levels of nuclear radiation can cause damage to eyes, skin, and reproductive organs and may result in birth defects in children. Since September 11, 2001, government officials have warned about the possibility of terrorists using *"dirty bombs,"* whereby conventional explosives are combined with radioactive materials. The resulting dispersion of radioactive matter by the conventional bomb blast and wind would contaminate land well beyond the area affected by the blast.

In the coming years, huge amounts of radioactive waste must be permanently stored where it cannot escape into our environment. Nuclear reactors that generate 20 percent of the U.S. electricity supply have been accumulating highly radioactive wastes on-site. During this time, the U.S. government has been working to develop appropriate technologies and sites to store these wastes permanently. The most likely location is in underground salt caves below Yucca Mountain, Nevada. Various technologies have been developed to contain nuclear wastes. However, nuclear wastes will be extremely toxic for thousands of years, and no one knows if our technologies will be able to contain them until they become harmless.

A major health concern raised about the U.S. nuclear waste disposal program is the need to transport large quantities of highly radioactive waste by truck or train across the United States. Much research has been done to devise containers that can withstand the worst imaginable wreck. Nonetheless, many people do not want these wastes to be transported through their community. However, the current situation is not safe either. Hundreds of tons of high-level radioactive waste are dispersed across the country in shallow, water-filled temporary holding tanks adjacent to nuclear power plants. This problem will get only worse as older nuclear power plants are retired and hundreds of tons of concrete and steel that are somewhat radioactive must be disposed of.

The Global Environment

The global environment is made up of the atmosphere, oceans, continental land masses, and all the living organisms that exist on Earth. Interactions among these components of the global environment influence the characteristics of solar radiation at the ground level, climate (temperature, precipitation, seasonal variation), production of food plants and animals, availability of freshwater, energy requirements for heating and cooling of human habitations, the geographic distribution of diseases, the composition of natural communities (deserts, tundra, rain forest), and the survival and extinction of species.

Some of the characteristics of the global environment have obvious and direct effects on human physical health, such as the presence of disease-causing organisms or solar UV radiation that can increase the risk of skin cancer. Other effects of the global environment on personal health are less well documented, such as the adverse effects on emotional or spiritual health associated with the extinction of species or destruction of beautiful natural communities. Many scientists warn that the global environment is being degraded by the combined forces of ever more powerful technology being used by a rapidly increasing global human population. In this section we briefly describe major concerns regarding the global environment and how these might affect personal health. We end this section and the chapter with some thoughts about how you can take some degree of personal control over these global environmental problems and their influence on your health.

Human Population Explosion

Many scientists warn that the human population is increasing at a rate that cannot be sustained by the resources of the Earth. (See Figure 20-3.) There are currently over 6 billion people in the global human population, and this is projected to increase to over 10 billion in the next 50 years. It took all of human history until 1830 for the global population to reach 1 billion people. It took only 25 years, between 1975 and 1999, to increase from 4 to 6 billion. Every year the world's population grows by about 78 million people, with 97 percent born into the poorest countries.[36]

To grasp the implications of this expansion of the human population, consider the vast problems we face with the current population, including depletion of natural resources (freshwater, food, and oil), air and water pollution, conflict and political upheaval, starvation, and destruction of natural communities. Now imagine trying to solve these problems in the 21st century with twice as many people trying to make a living and raise a family on the same Earth.

The effects of the human population explosion on personal health depend on who you are and where you live. Many of the poorer nations of Asia, Africa, and South America will not be able to feed their people; starvation and associated diseases will be major health problems for these populations. Growing populations in dry regions are exceeding their freshwater supply, and hundreds of millions of people must drink from contaminated water sources. Every year, 5 million children die from waterborne diarrhea diseases associated with unsanitary drinking water.[36] By 2025, 2.5 billion people may live in regions where available freshwater is insufficient to meet their needs.

Figure 20-3 Growth of the Earth's human population

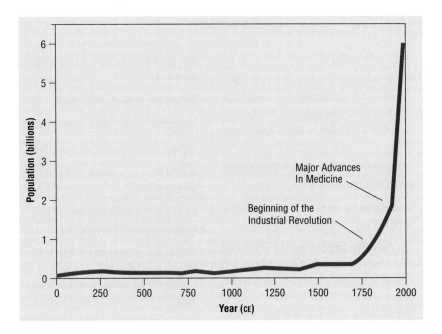

In many extremely poor countries, hungry people will destroy most or all of the remaining natural communities (tropical rain forests, African savanna) in vain efforts to grow food on lands that are not suited for agriculture. Over-cultivation of farmlands to meet the demand for food has already degraded the fertility of a land area equivalent to that of the United States and Canada combined.[36] Hungry people who live on oceanic islands often destroy their coral reefs trying to make a living by using dynamite or cyanide to catch fish. In Africa hungry people hunt wild game for food, putting more and more species at risk of extinction.

Competition among nations for limited supplies of water and oil is often a root cause of political tensions, terrorism, and war. Political upheaval in the Middle East, recent terrorist attacks on U.S. targets, and the war in Iraq can be partially explained by competition for scarce resources (water, land, and oil). The genocide that killed hundreds of thousands in Rwanda in 1994–1995 has been traced to inequitable distribution of land and associated hunger in some parts of that country.[37] Many fear that such social instability and strife will be the inevitable result of competition for scarce resources, associated with excessive human population growth and overconsumption of limited resources.

The solutions to the human population growth problem are simple in theory, but often complex in their implementation. Basic population ecology theory states that the rate of population growth can be reduced if: (1) women have fewer children over their lifetime and (2) if they delay the start of their reproduction. A some-what counterintuitive pattern is that population growth rate slows when infant survival rate is increased by better health care. It has been documented in many countries that women choose to have fewer children if they are confident that the children they do have will survive. Where infant mortality is high, women will often choose to have more children than they want or can afford as a "bet hedge" to ensure that at least some will live to adulthood.

Simply providing education opportunities to girls can have major and long-lasting effects that act to reduce population growth. Girls who have the opportunity to go to school and become educated delay having their first child; educated women have half the pregnancies of their uneducated sisters.[36] Educated women are more likely to be able to find employment outside the home. This has two effects: working women are too busy to care for large numbers of children, and women with an independent income have greater status and influence in deciding how many children they will have. Of course, universal access to birth control information and affordable contraception are also needed to allow women to have only as many children as they desire.

While this combination of commonsense actions can drastically reduce future human population growth, these proactive initiatives are often held hostage to political and cultural controversies. The sad result is that human populations may ultimately be controlled by increased death rates associated with starvation, disease, and war, rather than reduced birth rates.

Organizations Related to Environmental and Population Control Concerns

Population Issues

The organizations listed below provide material and informational support to women and men worldwide who seek to protect their reproductive health and to control their family size.

United Nations Family Planning Organization: www.unfpa.org

International Planned Parenthood Federation: www.ippf.org

The Population Institute: Provides information on the social and environmental consequences of rapid population growth, and advocacy for governmental support of voluntary family planning programs. www.populationinstitute.org

Environmental Political Advocacy Groups

The private environmental organizations listed below use the political and legal system to promote responsible use of the Earth's ecosystems and resources, and to provide information to the public about a full range of environmental issues. Some also employ scientists, policy analysts, and lawyers in support of lobbying

and litigation in support of environmental protection.

Sierra Club: www.sierraclub.org

Wilderness Society: www.wilderness.org

National Wildlife Federation: www.nwf.org

Natural Resources Defense Council: www.nrdc.org

Environmental Defense Fund: www.environmentaldefense.org

The League of Conservation Voters: A political action organization that provides information to voters on the voting records of politicians regarding environmental issues. This organization also campaigns to elect candidates who support environmentally responsible policies. www.lcv.org

Conservation of Natural Communities and Endangered Species

The Nature Conservancy: Uses private donations to purchase, protect, and manage important natural communities and habitats in the United

States and throughout the world (116 million acres worldwide, as of 2003). www.nature.org

World Wildlife Fund: Privately funded organization that works to protect endangered species and threatened habitats around the world, and to reduce pollution and climate change. www.panda.org

Sources of Environmental Information

World Resources Institute: A privately funded "think tank" that compiles environmental and economic data from around the world and publishes environmental policy analyses to promote a worldwide transition to an ecologically sustainable, socially just society. www.worldwatch.org

U.S. Environmental Protection Agency: The agency within the U.S. federal government responsible for monitoring environmental quality and enforcing environmental laws and regulations. This agency provides a wide range of environmental information to the public. www.epa.gov

Global Climate Change

A wide range of human activities add **greenhouse gases** to the atmosphere that trap heat and cause a net gain of energy and increase in temperature in the Earth system. This increase in global temperature is called the "Greenhouse Effect" or "Global Warming." Human-caused sources of greenhouse gases include both industrial and agricultural activities, including the burning of fuels, conversion of natural communities (grasslands, forests, and wetlands) to human uses, and methane emissions from large herds of cattle, flooded rice fields, and leaks from natural gas pipelines.

There is clear evidence that the concentration of greenhouse gases in the atmosphere has increased substantially since the beginning of the Industrial Revolution in the late 1700s. The average concentration of carbon dioxide in the atmosphere has increased 31 percent during this time period. Atmospheric methane, tropospheric ozone, and nitrous oxide concentrations have increased by 151 percent, 35 percent, and 17 percent, respectively.[38]

Most of the increase in atmospheric carbon dioxide is associated with burning of fossil fuels.[39]

There is growing evidence that increases in atmospheric greenhouse gases are associated with changes in global climate. Chemical analyses of gas bubbles in glacial ice core samples from the polar ice caps indicate that atmospheric carbon dioxide and methane concentrations have been closely related to changes in global temperature through several cycles of ice ages and warm periods

---

Key Terms

greenhouse gases a category of gases in the atmosphere that allow solar radiation to pass through the atmosphere to the Earth but then trap the heat that is radiated from the Earth back toward space; greenhouse gases include water vapor, carbon dioxide, methane, nitrous oxide, and tropospheric ozone during the past 420,000 years; when carbon dioxide and methane concentrations increased, so did atmospheric temperature.[40] Coincident with the current increase in atmospheric concentrations of greenhouse gases, average global surface temperature was higher during the decade of the 1990s than at any other time in the historical record of weather data.[38]

Many scientists around the world believe that the changes in global climate described above are the first evidence of global climate change related to human activities. However, there is still controversy regarding the relative contributions of humans versus natural processes, and whether or not this warming trend is a short-term phenomenon or the beginning of a long-term trend.

Because climate is such a fundamental characteristic of the environment, global warming is expected to have diverse and widespread effects, including melting of the polar ice caps, rising sea level, inundation of coastal areas (including major coastal cities), and increased frequency and severity of hurricanes and other destructive weather events. Effects of climate change on human health include increased heat stress in tropical and subtropical areas, loss of life in storms and floods, expansion of the range of disease-carrying insects (such as mosquitoes) from subtropical regions into temperate regions (such as the United States), increased abundance of waterborne pathogens, decreased air and water quality, and decreased food availability associated with severe weather and water shortages.

Ecological effects of global warming include increased frequency of wildfires and insect pest outbreaks that destroy forests, and widespread death of coral reefs associated with higher water temperature. Many scientists project large scale decline and extinction of species that cannot adapt to changes in climate and cannot migrate to more suitable areas because of barriers associated with human roads, cities, and farms. These ecological changes could adversely impact emotional and spiritual health as cherished natural wonders are degraded or disappear entirely under the onslaught of climate changes.

The primary means proposed for reducing and reversing global warming associated with human activities is to reduce the burning of fossil fuels such as oil and coal and increase the proportion of our energy needs that are met by other technologies. Many suggest that a combination of energy conservation, increased efficiency of automobiles and electrical appliances, and a gradual shift to alternate power sources for cars (fuel cells and/or hydrogen) and electricity (photovoltaic cells, wind turbines, geothermal energy, nuclear power) can get this job done. These transitions will require major shifts in the national and global economies, continuing innovation and technology development, and many small changes in everyday life of humans on planet Earth.

Your ability as an individual to take personal responsibility for addressing the global warming problem is limited, but all good things must start with individuals willing to do the right thing. You can reduce your personal contribution to global warming by conserving electricity at home, driving the most fuel-efficient automobile that meets your needs, using mass transit where available, recycling/reusing, and purchasing appliances that are rated as highly efficient. As technologies improve, you may someday be able to contribute to the electricity needs of your home using photovoltaic roof coverings and solar or geothermal energy for heating and cooling. Using compact fluorescent lighting is more expensive initially than standard lighting, but less costly over the long run. Fluorescent lighting uses much less electricity and has a much longer life span than standard incandescent light bulbs. Government action will be required to support widespread conservation practices in industry and business. You could join and be active in environmental organizations that work to address global warming. When politicians see their constituents want to protect our common global environment, they may find the political will to do the right thing.

 TALKING POINTS How can you encourage your children to develop sound habits regarding their environment and their personal health? What changes can you make in your own habits to serve as a better example for them?

Stratospheric Ozone Depletion

The *stratospheric ozone layer* is a concentration of ozone molecules located about 10 to 25 miles above the Earth's surface. This "ozone layer" contains about 90 percent of the planet's ozone. Stratospheric ozone is a naturally occurring gas formed by the interaction of atmospheric oxygen and components of solar radiation.

Unlike tropospheric (low-elevation) ozone, which has many adverse health and ecological effects, the stratospheric ozone layer has beneficial health effects by protecting living organisms on the Earth's surface from harmful solar ultraviolet (UV) radiation. For people, overexposure to UV rays can lead to skin cancer, cataracts (clouding of the lens of the eye), and weakened immune systems. Increased UV can also lead to reduced crop yield and disruptions in the ocean's food chain.

It has been well-documented that chemical reactions between stratospheric ozone and certain human-made air pollutants can significantly reduce the ozone layer, causing increased UV radiation at the Earth's surface. The chemicals that cause ozone depletion include chlorofluorocarbons or CFCs (used as coolants in many air conditioning and refrigeration systems, in insulating foams,

When you buy sunglasses, look for the UV-protection rating.

and as solvents), halons (used in fire suppression systems), and methyl bromide (used in pesticides). When these substances are released to the atmosphere and rise to the stratosphere, they release either chlorine or bromine molecules. One chlorine molecule can destroy 100,000 ozone molecules, and these substances can remain in the atmosphere for years.[41]

The vast majority of this depletion of the ozone layer occurs in the atmosphere above the north and south polar regions. In one year, ozone levels above Antarctica decreased by 60 percent. While the polar "ozone holes" allow the greatest amount of UV radiation to reach the ground in these sparsely populated areas, the ozone layer above the United States has decreased by 5–10 percent. These decreases in the stratospheric ozone layer have been associated with as much as a 50 percent increase in UV radiation at the ground level in Antarctica.[41]

The world community has worked to eliminate the use of ozone-depleting chemicals. For example, a complete ban on the production of halons and CFCs went into effect in the mid-1990s. As the amounts of ozone-depleting chemicals in the atmosphere decrease, the ozone layer will recover to natural levels by the year 2050.[41]

To limit your risk of skin cancer and other UV-related health problems, limit your exposure to direct sunlight, and when you are outside you should wear sunscreen on exposed skin. You should also wear sunglasses that are rated as eliminating over 95 percent of UV radiation. During months when the polar ozone holes are larger, you may want to further restrict your exposure to direct sunlight.

 TALKING POINTS Your sister is a sun worshipper who loves the look of a deep, dark tan. How might you persuade her to protect her skin from the rays of the sun?

Loss of Natural Habitats and Species Extinctions

On every continent, an exploding human population armed with increasingly powerful technology is altering or completely taking over the habitats of other species that share our planet. Sixteen to 23 percent of the total land surface of Earth has been converted entirely for human uses, including row crop fields, grazing lands, and urban/industrial areas. As much as 40–50 percent of the land surface has been transformed or degraded by human activities.[42] Only 20 percent of the original forest cover on Earth remains ecologically intact and able to support its full complement of species, mostly in the northern parts of Canada and Siberia.[43] As much as 30 percent of the African continent is at risk for **desertification,** mainly due to overgrazing by livestock, excessive brush and tree cutting for fuel, and inappropriate agricultural practices.[44]

The worldwide human population currently uses 50 percent of the Earth's freshwater runoff, 70 percent of which is used for agricultural irrigation. In some major river drainages—for example, the Colorado River in the southwest United States—water diversion is so great that no water reaches the ocean. Dams for electric power generation, flood control and irrigation have affected all but 6 percent of rivers in the world.[43]

Human impact on the biosphere is not limited to the land. Sixty percent of the human population lives within 100 km of an ocean coast, and humans consume 25–35 percent of the energy flow in coastal ocean waters. As of 1995, 22 percent of all ocean fisheries for human consumption were overexploited (resulting in population crashes of the targeted fish species), and another 44 percent were being exploited at their maximum sustainable level. In addition, 27 million tons of nontargeted fish species are caught, killed, and dumped back into the ocean each year, constituting 33 percent of the total catch.[42] In Indonesia, with the largest coral reef system in the world, 70 percent of the reefs have been severely degraded by dynamite fishing. Worldwide, 30 percent of all coral reefs have been destroyed by human activities, pollution, and coral bleaching that may be associated with global warming. Coastal water pollution has been linked to increased frequency of harmful algae blooms that cause extensive fish kills, massive "dead zones" where nothing

Key Terms	
desertification a process that converts lands that historically supported grasslands, shrublands, or dry forest to nonproductive desert	

else can live, and increased risk of shellfish poisoning for humans who eat seafood.[42]

The cumulative effects of all these human-caused changes to the Earth's land and oceans have increased the species extinction rate by 100 to 1,000 times over rates estimated for the period before human domination. The primary causes of these extinctions are habitat loss due to human transformations of land and water and overharvesting of species by humans.[43]

The effects on personal health associated with worldwide loss of natural communities and species extinctions are highly variable from person to person. Pharmaceutical companies have found many substances produced by species in various natural communities to be useful sources of drugs to treat human illnesses. A well-known example is Taxol, a substance derived from an endangered tree species found in the old-growth forests of the U.S. Pacific Northwest that is a potent drug to fight breast cancer. As the richness of species on Earth is depleted by extinction, we lose a wealth of genetic material that could be of great importance to human health. The degradation and loss of natural ecosystems also undermines the systems that function to make Earth a livable planet, contributing to such problems as global climate change, freshwater shortages, and increased frequency of destructive flooding.

Some have proposed that human evolution predisposes us to desire green spaces and diverse biological systems; this is called the *biophilia hypothesis*.[45] That is, we are most happy when we are surrounded by natural beauty. Many have written about the human psychological benefits from natural communities. John Muir, a famous early environmentalist in the United States, wrote:

> Climb the mountains and get their good tidings.
> Nature's peace will flow into you as sunshine flows into trees.
> The winds will blow their own freshness into you, and the storms their energy, while cares drop off like autumn leaves.

Wallace Stegner wrote a passage that appears in the Wilderness Act passed by the U.S. Congress in 1964 to protect areas of intact ecosystems in the United States for the enjoyment of future generations:

> It was a lovely and terrible wilderness, such a wilderness as Christ and the prophets went out into; harshly and beautifully colored, broken and worn until its bones are exposed, its great sky without a smudge or a taint from Technocracy, and in hidden corners and pockets under its cliffs, the sudden poetry of springs. Save a piece of country like that intact, and it does not matter in the slightest that only a few people every year will go into it. That is precisely its value . . . We simply need that wild country available to us, even if we never do more than drive to its edge and look in. For it can be a means of reassuring ourselves of our sanity as creatures, a part of the geography of hope.

Both Muir and Stegner refer to the psychological benefits that humans derive simply from the knowledge that

Recycling glass, paper, and metal can reduce land pollution and consumption of natural resources.

natural communities and wildlife species still exist, as they always have, somewhere on our planet. Now, try to imagine how you would feel about a world completely dominated and degraded by a massive human population; no great herds of caribou, zebra, and wildebeest moving like a tide across the landscape; no wolves, lions, tigers, or elephants to excite the imagination; no Monarch butterflies sipping nectar in your backyard on their migration from Maine to Mexico; no dolphins and orcas playing in the ocean waves; no humpback whales singing in the depths; no great, ancient trees stretching out of sight toward a clear blue sky; no expansive grasslands rippling in the breeze as far as the eye can see; the sky and waters tainted with pollution; the climate itself hostile to human civilization. The effects of such a dark and dismal world on the human psyche are unimaginable. The thought of forever losing the natural wonders of our planet could have profound adverse consequences for emotional, psychological, and spiritual well-being. For many, the thought of such a dark future can cause anger, frustration, depression, hopelessness, and despair.[46]

How can you or any one person exert any degree of personal control over such a great and complex threat to your physical, emotional, and spiritual health? Let's start with the little things: conserve energy, recycle and reuse what you can, limit your consumption of the world's resources to what you need, and join together with others of

Is Organic Food Good for the Environment?

Certified "organic" food in the United States is produced under guidelines set out by the Organic Foods Production Act. The guidelines in this law stipulate materials and practices that enhance the balance of natural systems and that integrate parts of the farming system into an ecological whole.

The primary goal of organic agriculture is to optimize the health and productivity of interdependent communities of soil life, plants, animals, and people. Organic farmers that produce grain, fruits, and vegetables may not use synthetic pesticides or fertilizers. Meat producers must feed their livestock only organically produced feedstuffs. In addition, many organic meat producers forgo the use of growth hormones and antibiotics that stimulate livestock growth rates. While organic foods have not been shown to be any more nutritious than non-organic food, organic foods have fewer chemical residues that may adversely impact human health.[1]

The description of organic food above suggests that organic farming practices are good for the environment. Organic farming puts far less pollution into local water and air, and fewer chemicals into the food supply. Local farmers can often make greater profits through direct sales of organic produce to local cooperatives or other consumer-supported agriculture organizations. This may help to preserve local green space against encroachment by suburban developers. Hence, organic farming can certainly be good for the local community environment.

Whether or not organic farming is good for the global environment is an open question. While organic farms produce less pollution, they also produce less food per acre. Lower production per acre, higher labor costs, and the small number of organic farmers often make organic foods an expensive luxury for the well-to-do. Many environmentalists call for a widespread shift from chemical-dependent agriculture to more ecologically sustainable organic farming. However, it is doubtful that organic farming on existing agricultural lands could feed the current human population of 6 billion people. A worldwide shift to organic farming would likely require an expansion of agricultural lands into national parks, nature preserves, and wilderness areas. This loss of natural habitats would result in massive species extinctions.[2] On the other hand, there is some uncertainty as to whether or not intensive, chemical-dependent agricultural systems will provide a sustainable food supply. Chemical fertilizers can replace lost nutrients, but can't repair compacted soil, nor replace eroded topsoil. Pesticides and herbicides can control pests and weeds now, but these species are already displaying signs of increased resistance that may prevent control in the future.

At the moment, your personal choices to buy organically grown, locally produced foods are probably most beneficial to your local environment, and may benefit your personal health. It is much less clear whether or not a widespread shift to organic farming would be beneficial to the larger global environment.

[1]Cable News Network Interactive. *In-Depth: Organic Food.* 1998. www.cnn.com/HEALTH/indepth.food/organic/index.html.
[2]Center for Global Food Issues. *Growing More Food per Acre Leaves More Land for Nature.* 2002. www.highyieldconservation.org.

---

like mind to provide political and financial support to organizations that are working to solve these big problems (see the photo on page 615 and the listing in the Star box on page 612). If you want to make a bigger personal commitment to solving global environmental problems, you could limit your own family size to no more than two children. For a list of many more ways you can help to preserve a healthy environment, go to the Web site www.earthshare.org/ get_involved/earth_saving_tips.html, and take a look at Changing for the Better on page 617.

Another way you can reduce the negative environmental effects of your personal consumption of natural resources is to "buy green" when you can (see Considering Complementary Care above). There are often multiple ways to meet human needs for food, clothing, and shelter, some of which are very destructive and degrade the natural heritage of the Earth. In recent years, environmental organizations have begun certification programs so that the consumer can identify which products are produced by "Earth-friendly" means (for more information, go to the Web site www.newdream.org/buygreen/). Examples of such products include sustainably harvested timber, shade-grown coffee, and organic food and cotton. Often these products are more expensive, as the means of their production lack the efficiency of mechanized, chemically dependent, environmentally destructive production systems. When you "buy green," you support Earth-friendly producers and may reduce the economic push to destroy more natural communities and species. Many "buy green" organizations also work to improve the economic conditions of small rural villages where the producers of their products live. These efforts at economic development are often associated with improved education opportunities that lead to reduced birth rates, slowing global human population growth that is the root cause for many environmental problems.

The combined actions of 6 billion people making personal choices will determine the future of the Earth's environment and thus the future of humankind on Earth. The solutions to the great environmental problems looming in the future begin with you, today. Your positive actions and faith in fellow humans to do the right thing will not only benefit the future but also enhance your emotional well-being in the present.

Taking Charge of Your Health

- Protect yourself from ultraviolet light. Always wear sunscreen, and make sure your sunglasses filter out UV rays.
- Have your home tested for radon, and install a radon reduction system if necessary.
- Install a water filtration device to remove contaminants from your drinking water.
- Keep your car in proper running condition to reduce the amount of noise and air pollution it produces.

- Reduce your personal impact on the environment by reducing your consumption of energy and recycling and reusing what you can, and using Earth-friendly products in your home.
- Take personal action on environmental issues using the suggestions outlined in Changing for the Better above.

SUMMARY

- Your environment contains a wide range of substances, living organisms, and forms of energy that may substantially impact one or more dimensions of your personal health.
- Environmental influences on personal health operate over a wide range of spatial scales, from the personal spaces of your home and workplace, to the common spaces of your community and region, to the global environment that supports all life on Earth.
- The most direct environmental risks to your physical health are related to the presence of toxic substances or pathogenic organisms (pollutants) in the air and water of your personal and community environments.
- You can exert the greatest degree of control over your exposure to pollutants within the personal environment of your

home and workplace. You can identify environmental health risks in your personal environment, and then eliminate or reduce these risks by changing your buying habits and eliminating pollutant sources.
- Air pollution in major urban areas can cause significant adverse health effects, especially for people who suffer from respiratory or cardiac disease.
- While you have no control over community air pollution, you can limit your exposure to these toxic substances by being aware of daily pollution levels and by restricting your outdoor activities when these levels are high.
- Much progress has been made in reducing community water pollution, but water in many rivers and lakes still contains chemicals and pathogens that can adversely affect your health.

- You should seek out information about any health advisories for wild foods you obtain from local rivers, and advisories regarding recreational use of those rivers.
- The U.S. Environmental Protection Agency monitors and regulates the quality of drinking water from municipal water suppliers, but it is up to you to ensure the safety of your drinking water if it comes from a private well.
- Improper disposal of toxic solid wastes in landfills designed for household waste is a major source of regional surface and groundwater pollution.
- You should never dispose of toxic household products (batteries, automotive fluids, pesticides, oil-based paint products) by simply putting them in the household trash or pouring them down a drain. Take them to specially designated toxic disposal locations.
- Loss of green space in your community and regional environment, associated with urban sprawl and unregulated land development, can diminish your perceived quality of life, and reduce opportunities for exercise, which is important for maintaining good physical health.
- While you have limited personal control over the environment of your community and region, you can still work to enhance your environment by joining others of like mind in groups that advocate environmental protection through the democratic political process.
- At the current rate of human population growth, most scientists of the world warn of increased starvation and disease, decreased standards of living, and increased conflict over progressively decreasing supplies of natural resources.
- Human population growth can be substantially slowed by simply providing girls and women opportunities to become educated and gainfully employed, and access to contraception.
- Pollutants produced by humans are responsible for changes in the atmosphere that are altering climate patterns and allowing harmful solar radiation to reach the surface of the Earth.
- Changes in the global environment have potential to increase risks to human health, and to significantly harm many other species and natural communities.
- While individuals can do little to address global environmental problems, the solutions all start with individual choices about family size, resource consumption, and political candidates. The best path to a livable future for humankind is to do your part and have faith that others will do theirs.

REVIEW QUESTIONS

1. What is radon, and what are the health risks associated with it? What actions can you take to minimize the health risks of radon?
2. Identify the sources and the potential health effects of the following common indoor air pollutants: carbon monoxide, volatile organic compounds, and biological pollutants such as mold, mildew, pollen, and pet dander. Describe actions you could take to minimize health risks from these pollutants.
3. What health risks are associated with lead and asbestos? What actions can you take to minimize these risks?
4. Describe actions you should take to safeguard drinking from a well on your own property.
5. Define the concept of "noise" in a way that clarifies how a particular type of music could be noise to some but not noise to others.
6. What are the physical and emotional health effects of noise? What actions could you take to minimize the health risks of noise?
7. Describe the distinction between a "point source" versus a "non-point source" of community/regional air or water pollution. Which type of pollution source do you think is most easily controlled? Explain your answer.
8. Tropospheric ozone and small particulate matter are community and regional air pollutants that have been linked to serious health risks. For each of these substances, describe the main human sources, the effect(s) on human physical health, and what actions you could take to minimize your own risk of adverse health effects from these air pollutants.
9. What are "air toxics" and where do you think you are most likely to be exposed to these substances? What do you think you could do to minimize your personal health risk from air toxics?
10. What is "biological water pollution" and what is the main source of this pollution in your community's rivers, streams, and/or lakes? What are the health risks associated with biological water pollution? What can you do to minimize the risk to your personal health from this type of pollution?
11. Who is responsible for ensuring the safety of your drinking water if the source is a municipal water company? What can you do to minimize any health risks associated with your drinking water in this circumstance?
12. What is the main health risk associated with land pollution from solid waste landfills? What can you do to minimize your personal contribution to this type of pollution?
13. What is "green space," and why is it important to your personal health? What personal actions could you take to protect green space in your community or region?
14. Which do you think is the best plan for dealing with radioactive wastes from U.S. nuclear reactors: storing it on the site of the reactor or shipping it across the country to the Yucca Mountain underground storage facility? Explain your answer in terms of the health risks posed by each option.
15. What policies should the U.S. foreign aid agencies implement in poor underdeveloped countries to help them reduce their population growth rate? Explain how these policies would work toward this goal.

16. Global warming and stratospheric ozone depletion are large-scale changes in the global environment with uncertain, but potentially significant, health consequences. For each of these global changes, describe the cause(s) of environmental change, the potential health effects, and what might be done to minimize these effects.

17. Loss of natural habitats and species extinctions are major ecological problems, but do these phenomena represent any risk to *your* personal health? Your answer should reflect your own perceptions, and should provide some explanation for your assessment.

18. A well-known environmentalist slogan is, "Think globally, but act locally." Based on what you've learned in this chapter, describe how you think this slogan applies to your personal actions in response to environmental health risks.

ENDNOTES

1. *U.S. Environmental Protection Agency. Healthy Buildings, Healthy People: A Vision for the 21st Century. 2003.* www.epa.gov/iaq/hbhp/index.html.

2. Consumer Product Safety Commission. *Carbon Monoxide Questions and Answers.* CPSC Document #466. 2003. www.cpsc.gov/cpscpub/pubs/466.html.

3. U.S. Environmental Protection Agency. *The Senseless Killer.* 2003. www.epa.gov/iaq/pubs/senseles.html.

4. U.S. Environmental Protection Agency. *The Inside Story: A Guide to Indoor Air Quality.* 1995. www.epa.gov/iaq/pubs/insidest.html.

5. Thorn J, et al. Adult-onset asthma linked to mold and tobacco smoke exposure. *Allergy* 56: 287–292, 2001.

6. U.S. Environmental Protection Agency. *Sources of Indoor Air Pollution: Asbestos.* 2003. www.epa.gov/iaq/asbestos.html.

7. U.S. Environmental Protection Agency. *Sources of Indoor Air Pollution: Lead (Pb).* 2003. www.epa.gov/iaq/lead.html.

8. U.S. Department of Health and Human Services, Public Health Service, Agency for Toxic Substances and Disease Registry. *Case Studies in Environmental Medicine: Lead Toxicity.* 1995. www.atsdr.cdc.gov/HEC/HSPH/caselead.html.

9. U.S. Environmental Protection Agency. *Sources of Indoor Air Pollution: Biological Pollutants.* 2003. www.epa.gov/iaq/biologic.html.

10. Centers for Disease Control. *Legionellosis: Legionnaire's Disease (LD) and Pontiac Fever.* 2001. www.cdc.gov/ncidod/dbmd/diseaseinfo/legionellosis_g.htm.

11. National Safety Council. *Radon.* 2002. www.nsc.org/ehc/radon.htm.

12. National Academy of Sciences. *Biological Effects of Ionizing Radiation (BEIR) VI Report:* The health effects of exposure to indoor radon. 1998. National Academy Press. http://books.nap.edu/books/0309056454/html/.

13. National Academy of Sciences. *Risk Assessment of Radon in Drinking Water.* 1999. www.nap.edu/books/0309062926/html/index.html.

14. Foster KR. Are mobile phones safe? Institute of Electrical and Electronic Engineers (IEEE), *Spectrum Online* 37(8), 2000.

15. U.S. Food and Drug Administration. Cell Phone Facts: Consumer Information on Wireless Phones. 2002. www.Fda.gov/cellphones/qa.html#25.

16. Health effects of radiofrequency exposure: A review. *Environmental Health Perspectives* 112 (17), 2004.

17. UK Childhood Cancer Study Investigators. Childhood cancer and residential proximity to power lines. *Brit J Cancer* 83: 1573–1580, 2000.

18. Savitz DA, Loomis DP. Magnetic field exposure in relation to leukemia and brain cancer mortality among electric utility workers. *Amer J Epidemiology* 141(2): 123–128, 1995.

19. Greenland S, Sheppard AR, et al. A pooled analysis of magnetic fields, wirecodes, and childhood leukemia. *Epidemiology* 11: 624–634, 2000.

20. U.S. Environmental Protection Agency. *Water on Tap: A Consumer's Guide to the Nation's Drinking Water.* 2003. www.epa.gov/safewater/wot/howsafe.html.

21. *Factsheet on: Nitrate/Nitrite.* 2002. www.epa.gov/safewater/dwh/t-ioc/nitrates.html.

22. Gray LE, Ostby J. Effects of pesticides and toxic substances on behavioral and morphological reproductive development: Endocrine versus no-endocrine mechanisms. *Toxicology and Industrial Health* 14: 159–184, 1998.

23. U.S. Environmental Protection Agency. *Permeation and Leaching.* 2003. www.epa.gov/safewater/tcr/pdf/permleach.pdf.

24. Bell PA. Noise, pollution, and psychopathology. In Ghadirian A, Lehmann HE (Eds.). *Environment and Psychopathology.* New York: Springer, 1993.

25. U.S. Environmental Protection Agency. *Draft Report on the Environment: Outdoor Air Quality.* 2003. www.epa.gov/indicators/roe/html/roeAirOut.htm.

26. Dockery DW, Pope CA III. Acute respiratory effects of particulate air pollution. *Annual Review Public Health* 15: 107–132, 1994.

27. Perera F, et al. Effects of transplacental exposure to environmental pollutants on birth outcomes in a multiethnic population. *Environmental Health Perspectives* 111 (2): 201–205. 2003

28. Perera F, et al. DNA damage from polycyclic aromatic hydrocarbons measured by Benzo[a] pyrene-DNA adducts in mothers and newborns from northern Manhattan, the World Trade Center area, Poland, and China. *Cancer, Epidemiology Biomarkers & Prevention* 14: 709–714. 2005.

29. U.S. Environmental Protection Agency. *Asthma Triggers— Related Topics—Ozone.* 2003. www.epa.gov/iaq/asthma/triggers/ozone.html.

30. McConnell R, Berhane K, Gilliland F, London S, Islam T, Gauderman WJ, Avol E, Margolis H, Peters J. Asthma in exercising children exposed to ozone. *The Lancet* 359: 386–391, 2002.

31. U.S. Environmental Protection Agency. *The National Air Toxics Assessment.* 2002. www.epa.gov/ttn/atw/nata.

32. U.S. Environmental Protection Agency. *Drinking Water and Your Health, What You Need to Know, List of Drinking Water Contaminants & MCLs.* 2003. www.epa.gov/safewater/mcl.html#1.

33. Beck EC. *The Love Canal Tragedy.* 2002. www.epa.gov/history/topics/lovecanal/01.htm.

34. U.S. Environmental Protection Agency. *Municipal Solid Waste: Basic Facts.* 2003. www.epa.gov/epaoswer/non-hw/muncpl/facts.htm.

35. Talbott EO, et al. Long-term follow-up of the residents of the Three Mile Island accident area: 1979–1998. *Environmental Health Perspectives* 111(3): 341–348, 2003.

36. The Population Institute. www.populationinstitute.org.

37. Gasana J. Remember Rwanda? *World Watch* 15(5): 24–33, 2002.

38. Intergovernmental Panel on Climate Change. *Climate Change 2001: Summary Report: Synthesis for Policy Makers.* 2001. www.ipcc.ch/pub/un/syreng/spm.pdf.

39. Bacastow R, Keeling DC. Atmospheric carbon dioxide and radiocarbon in the natural carbon cycle: II. Changes from AD 1700 to 2070 as deduced from a chemical model. In Woodwell GM, Pecan EV (Eds.). *Carbon and the Biosphere.* BHNL/CONF 720510, Springfield VA: National Technical Information Service, 1974.

40. Petit JR, et al. Climate and atmospheric history of the past 420,000 years from the Vostok ice core, Antarctica. *Nature* 399: 429–436, 1999.

41. U.S. Environmental Protection Agency. *The Science of Ozone Depletion.* 2003. www.epa.gov/docs/ozone/science/index.html.

42. Vitousek P, et al. Human domination of Earth's ecosystems. *Science* 277: 494–499, 1997.

43. World Resources Institute. 2003. www.wri.org.

44. United Nations. Food and Agriculture Organization. www.fao.org/desertification/default.asp?lang=en.

45. Wilson E. *Biophilia: The Human Bond with Other Species.* Cambridge, MA: Harvard University Press, 1984.

46. Gardner GT, Stern PC. *Environmental Problems and Human Behavior.* Boston: Allyn & Bacon, 1996.

personal assessment

Are you an environmentalist?

When asked, many people will say that they are an "environmentalist," including political leaders who are widely criticized for decisions perceived by others to be environmentally destructive. So what is an "environmentalist"? One definition of environmentalism is that it is an ideology that values and reveres Nature, and works to protect and preserve natural systems for both ethical reasons and because humankind depends on these systems for life. However, beyond this general statement environmentalists encompass a wide diversity of beliefs and practices. For some, their environmental beliefs are a form of religion, others function mainly in the political process, and some operate like terrorist groups who use violence to fight human economic development on behalf of Earth.[1] The wide diversity of beliefs and practices encompassed under "environmentalism" creates a situation where almost anyone could claim to be an environmentalist. Perhaps more useful criteria for determining if you are an environmentalist would be (1) your awareness of how various human activities create environmental health hazards or degrade natural systems; (2) your willingness to consider your own role in creating environmental problems; and (3) your willingness to act in ways that reduce your personal risk from environmental hazards and your contribution to the causes of these hazards. These three criteria define a hierarchy of commitment to environmental protection. First you have to know a problem exists. Then you have to recognize your own part in creating that problem. The last, and most difficult, step is that you must be willing to reduce or eliminate your contribution to environmental problems. Your answers to the following questions will help you think about where you really stand on protecting the environment for yourself, your community, and all the rest of life on Earth.

Awareness of Environmental Problems

1. Have you ever read the water quality assessment provided by the supplier of your drinking water?
2. If your drinking water is from a well, do you know about potential sources of contamination (landfills or other waste disposal sites, large agricultural areas, confined feedlot livestock operations) in your watershed?
3. If your drinking water supply is from a well, do you know if your water contains potentially harmful contaminants?
4. Do you know whether or not your community wastewater treatment system occasionally dumps raw sewage into the local river during high rainfall events?
5. If you use a gas furnace or kerosene space heater, do you know whether or not these appliances are functioning properly so as to maximize energy efficiency and minimize risks from indoor air pollution?
6. Have you ever made a note of air pollution alerts or information about high ultraviolet radiation published in a local newspaper or presented on a local TV news program?
7. Have you ever searched for information on air, water, and land pollution in your community?
8. When you eat fish, are you aware of health advisories regarding contaminants in fish (for example, mercury, PCBs) and recommendations that you limit the amount of the fish you consume?
9. When you purchase products, do you look at packaging materials for warnings that the product contains toxic chemicals?
10. When you listen to loud music, do you think about potential long-term damage to your hearing and the nuisance noise you create for your neighbors?
11. Do you know if your community (city, county, state) has a land-use management (zoning) plan?
12. When you see new economic developments (malls, superstores, warehouses, suburban housing developments) being constructed, do you wonder if wildlife habitat is being destroyed?
13. Do you know the proposed human causes of global warming and the potential consequences of this change in climate?
14. Do you know the causes and potential health effects of depletion of the stratospheric ozone layer?
15. Do you know the link between the wood you buy at a store like Menard's, Lowe's, and Home Depot and species extinctions?

Willingness to Consider Your Personal Environmental Impact

16. When you think about having a family of your own, do you worry about contributing to a rapidly growing human population that is responsible for widespread environmental degradation?
17. When you think about purchasing a vehicle, do you consider fuel efficiency more important than "image" sold by advertisers?
18. When you consider purchasing any product, do you consider the resources used, and pollution created, to produce that product?
19. When you purchase an electric appliance or a gas-powered device, do you consider energy efficiency?
20. When planning to build a new home, do you consider how your choices regarding location and amount of land could contribute to loss of green space and natural habitat?

21. When you use or dispose of household, yard, and automotive chemicals and fluids, do you consider that you may be contributing to local water pollution?

22. When you hear about global warming, do you recognize that your own use of electricity and gas-powered vehicles contributes to this problem?

23. Did you know that if you vent your home or automotive air conditioning system coolant while performing do-it-yourself maintenance, you are contributing to the depletion of the stratospheric ozone layer?

24. When you purchase lumber, do you wonder if the wood you are buying was harvested using environmentally sound practices, or if critical wildlife habitats or wilderness was destroyed to produce the lumber?

25. Do you consider how your vote in public elections can affect government policies that impact the environment?

Willingness to Alter Your Lifestyle to Protect Yourself and the Environment

26. Would you limit the number of your own children to one or two so as to reduce your contribution to the problem of global human population explosion?

27. When you purchase a vehicle, is energy efficiency your main concern?

28. Would you use mass transit to travel from home to work, if it were available, to reduce your contribution to local air pollution and need for paving more land to expand highways?

29. When you buy a home, would you seek to minimize the distance from work and schools to reduce gas consumption, minimize air pollution, and reduce demand for construction of new roads?

30. When you buy a home, would you look for a smaller, energy-efficient home to minimize your contribution to natural resource exploitation and pollution associated with energy consumption?

31. When you buy lighting, do you buy energy-efficient lights (compact fluorescent and LED lightbulbs) that are initially more expensive, but more efficient and less expensive over the long term?

32. When furnishing your home, would you seek out water-efficient toilets, faucets, and shower heads that conserve freshwater and reduce demands on wastewater treatment systems?

33. Do you set the thermostat in your home to cooler temperatures in winter and warmer temperatures in summer to conserve energy?

34. Would you invest money and effort to better insulate your home so as to reduce energy needed for heating and cooling?

35. When buying food, would you be willing to pay more for organically grown foods that were produced without the use of pesticides and fertilizers that pollute the surrounding environment?

36. Would you buy locally grown foods to support farmers (and their green spaces) in your community and reduce energy spent on long-distance transport?

37. When purchasing wood products, would you buy more expensive wood that is certified to have been harvested using environmentally sound practices?

38. Would you be willing to have something less than the perfect lawn to avoid using fertilizers and pesticides that contaminate local waterways?

39. Would you limit your personal consumption of material goods to mainly those things you need, so as to reduce exploitation of natural resources?

40. When you dispose of household chemicals, automotive fluids, and spent batteries, do you make the extra effort to be sure they do not end up polluting the environment, like taking them to a Tox-Away Day location?

41. Do you make the effort to recycle paper, glass, plastic, and metals?

42. When you make purchases, do you look for products made from recycled materials (for example, post-consumer recycled paper, "plastic wood," fleece clothing made from recycled plastic)?

43. Do you limit the noise that you produce (loud music, loud car or motorcycle engines, barking dogs) to reduce noise pollution in your neighborhood?

44. Do you contribute financial support to environmental groups that promote conservation and protection of natural resources through the legal and political systems?

45. When you consider candidates for public office, do you vote for the candidates who have strong records or position statements for environmental protection?

If the majority of your answers to questions 1 to 15 are "Yes," you are likely "environmentally aware." That is, you pay attention to news stories about environmental issues or have taken an environmental science course.

If most of your answers to questions 16 to 25 are "Yes," you are "environmentally conscious." That is, you are not only aware of the problems, but beginning to think about how these problems are related to your own lifestyle.

If the majority of your answers to questions 26 to 45 are "Yes," you are likely "environmentally active." That is, you are personally involved in efforts to address environmental problems through your own lifestyle choices and through the political process.

[1]Wikipedia (The Free Encyclopedia). www.wikipedia.org/wiki/Environmentalism.

part seven

Completing Life's Journey

This last part comprises a single chapter on a topic that inevitably affects each of us: dying and death. Traditional-age students may think that death will not touch their lives until they grow older. Yet many young people must face the reality of death much sooner, when a loved one is lost to an accident, a disease, suicide, or some other tragedy.

1. **Physical Dimension**

   Unless we die suddenly at a young age, most of us will enjoy years of good physical health before we begin a period of gradual decline. Eventually we may experience an extended period of failing health before dying of a chronic condition, such as heart disease. However, many people today experience their highest level of physical health late in life. An adequate activity level, weight management, smoking cessation, and moderation of alcohol use can increase the likelihood that an older adult will be able to enjoy good physical health well into his or her later years.

2. **Psychological Dimension**

   The process of dying and death can be emotionally draining for both the dying person and his or her loved ones. The death of a spouse, close friend, or child, especially when it is unexpected, can be emotionally taxing. The grieving person may feel anger, sadness, regret, and a range of other complex emotions. Indeed, coping with death can be a great challenge to the emotional stability of even the healthiest person.

3. **Social Dimension**

   The dying process and the event of a loved one's death offer opportunities for reaching out to others. In fact, many people who have had these experiences report that having a social support system was essential to maintaining their emotional balance during the ordeal. The families of people who are dying must also deal effectively with health care professionals, funeral directors, and estate executors.

4. **Intellectual Dimension**

   As in any other crisis, a strong intellect is a valuable resource during the dying and death process. Complex decisions about treatment options must be made. Loved ones may be left to sort out the finances of a family member who has died. These difficult situations require an ability to analyze many variables in order to make sound choices.

5. **Spiritual Dimension**

   Confronting the reality of death requires drawing on spiritual resources. Those who have a strong religious faith may find comfort in their beliefs, while others may find that their faith is shaken by the experience. Those who are not religious may look for other ways to find meaning in the event.

6. **Occupational Dimension**

   The dying process often unfolds slowly. A person who is terminally ill may have to continue working for months or even years before he or she becomes so ill that work is no longer possible. Clearly, such an illness can make work difficult. However, some people find that their job provides a welcome diversion as well as a social support network.

chapter twenty-one

Accepting Dying and Death

Chapter Objectives

On completing this chapter, you will be able to:

▌ Discuss dying in today's society.

▌ Explain the definitions of death.

▌ Describe the psychological stages of death.

▌ Explain advance health care directives.

▌ Describe coping with specific causes of death.

▌ Define *euthanasia.*

▌ Define *physician-assisted suicide.*

▌ Discuss near-death experiences.

▌ Discuss interacting with dying people.

▌ Discuss talking with children about death.

▌ Describe hospice care.

▌ Identify death rituals.

Eye on the Media

The Controversy Surrounding the Death of Terri Schiavo

Terri Schiavo's death became a legal battle, a media event, religious debate, and was even brought into the political spotlight. She was 26 years old when she had heart failure because of a chemical imbalance that may have been caused by an eating disorder. This left her severely brain damaged for 15 years. While she was in hospice care in a vegetative state, her husband and her parents were in a legal battle over whether to remove the feeding tube that was keeping her alive. If she had had a living will, this would have helped to make her wishes more clear, but it may not have precluded the legal debate. Advance directives such as living wills and durable powers of attorney for health care are legal documents that communicate the person's wishes about being kept alive with life support should they become incapacitated.

Both Terri Schiavo's husband and her parents claimed to know her end-of-life wishes, but none of them was named as her health care agent or proxy, giving a specific person the legal right to make this determination. Michael, her husband, stated that she had made casual comments about not wanting to be on life support if she were ever incapacitated. She had further stated to him that she didn't ever want to be a burden to him or her family. Her parents countered by saying that she was a devout Roman Catholic who believed in the sanctity of life. The publicity that this case received resulted in the America people becoming involved in this right-to-life battle, with a California businessman offering Michael Schiavo $1 million to walk away from Terri and allow her parents to have guardianship.

The tug of war that ensued between her family members, as well as the publicity surrounding her dying wishes, spurred thousands of people to consider completing living wills. In fact, the Aging with Dignity organization estimated that requests for advanced directives increased 10-fold because of the Schiavo case. They further reported that they distributed over 1 million copies of living wills since this case, and orders for more living wills continued to flood in at a rate of 200 an hour.

Bitter legal battles continued for 12 years between these families. The case was brought to the U.S. Supreme court six times and refused each time. The Governor of Florida, Jeb Bush, sided with the parents and lobbied to have the tube reconnected after it had been removed. Even President Bush became involved in this volatile case, signing a law allowing transfer of jurisdiction of the case from Florida state court to a U.S. District Court so that federal judges could review the case. Again, the judges stated that any action on their part would be improper. There was a great deal of public outcry, with some referring to her death as "judicial homicide."

Terri Schiavo remained in hospice care for 5 years. There were further disputes over who was allowed to be at her bedside when she died, because her husband prohibited her parents and brother from being in the room, saying he wanted her to have a peaceful environment for her death. Because she didn't

The primary goal of this chapter is to help people realize that accepting the reality of death can motivate us to live a more enjoyable, healthy, productive, and contributive life. Each day in our lives becomes even more meaningful when we have fully accepted the reality that someday we will die. We can then live each day to its fullest.

Our personal awareness of death can give us a framework from which to appreciate and conduct our lives. It helps us to prioritize our activities so that we can accomplish our goals (in our work, our relationships with others, and our recreation) before we die. Quite simply, death can help us to appreciate living.

Dying in Today's Society

Since the 1920s, the way people experience death in this society has changed. Formerly, most people died in their own homes, surrounded by family and friends. Young children frequently lived in the same home with their aging grandparents and saw them grow older and eventually die. Death was seen as a natural extension of life. Children grew up with a keen sense of what death meant, both to the dying person and to the grieving survivors.

Times have indeed changed. Today about 70 percent of people die in hospitals, nursing homes, and assisted living facilities, rather than in their own homes. The extended family is seldom at the bedside of the dying person.[1] Sometimes, frantic efforts are made to keep a dying person alive. Although medical technology has improved our lives, some people believe that it has reduced our ability to die with dignity. Some are convinced that our way of dying has become more artificial and less civilized than it used to be. The trend toward hospice care may be a positive response to this high-tech manner of dying.

Many families are forced to deal with death unexpectedly when a loved one dies in an accident or by violence. The emotions they feel are somewhat different from the ones normally evoked when a friend or relative dies of a disease or failing health in old age.

As the baby boomers age over the next 30 years, the number of people age 85 and older will more than double, to 9 million. This means that the topic of death and dying will become increasingly common and relevant for us all as we cope with the loss of our parents, grandparents, friends, and other family members.

Definitions of Death

Death was once easy to define. People were considered dead when a heartbeat could no longer be detected and when breathing ceased. Now, with the technological advances in medicine, especially emergency medicine, some patients who give every indication of being dead can be resuscitated. Critically ill people, even those in comas, can now be kept alive for years with many of their bodily functions maintained by medical devices, including feeding tubes and respirators.

Thus death can be a very challenging concept to define.[2] Many professional associations and ad hoc interdisciplinary committees have struggled with this problem and have developed criteria by which to establish death. Some of these criteria have been adopted by state legislatures, although there is certainly no consensus definition of death that all states embrace.

Clinical determinants of death measure bodily functions. Often judged by a physician, who can then sign a legal document called a *medical death certificate,* these clinical criteria include the following:

1. Lack of heartbeat and breathing.
2. Lack of central nervous system function, including all reflex activity and environmental responsiveness. This can often be confirmed by an *electroencephalograph* reading. If no brain wave activity is recorded after an initial measurement and a second measurement

after 24 hours, the person is said to have undergone *brain death.*

3. The presence of *rigor mortis,* indicating that body tissues and organs are no longer functioning at the cellular level. This is sometimes called *cellular death.*

The legal determinants used by government officials are established by state law and often adhere closely to the clinical determinants just listed. A person is not legally dead until a physician, *coroner,* or health department officer has signed a death certificate.

Psychological Stages of Dying

People who have a terminal illness undergo a process of self-adjustment. The stages in this process have helped form the basis for the modern movement of death education. Knowing these stages may help you understand how people adjust to other important losses in their lives.

Perhaps the most widely recognized name in the area of death education is Dr. Elisabeth Kübler-Ross. As a psychiatrist working closely with terminally ill patients at the University of Chicago's Billings Hospital, Kübler-Ross could observe the emotional reactions of dying people. In her classic book *On Death and Dying,* Kübler-Ross summarized the psychological stages that dying people often experience.[6]

- *Denial.* This is the stage of disbelief. Patients refuse to believe that they actually will die. Denial can serve as a temporary defense mechanism and can allow patients the time to accept their prognosis on their own terms.

- *Anger.* A common emotional reaction after denial is anger. Patients can feel as if they have been cheated. By expressing anger, patients can vent some of their fears, jealousies, anxieties, and frustrations. Patients often direct their anger at relatives, physicians and nurses, religious symbols, figures, and healthy people.

- *Bargaining.* Terminally ill people follow the anger stage with a bargaining stage. Patients who desperately want to avoid their inevitable deaths attempt to strike bargains—often with God or a church leader. Some people undergo religious conversions. The goal is to buy time by promising to repent for past sins, to restructure and rededicate their lives, or to make a large financial contribution to a religious cause (see Considering Complementary Care on page 630).

- *Depression.* When patients realize that, at best, bargaining can only postpone their fate, they may begin an unpredictable period of depression. In a sense, terminally ill people are grieving for their own anticipated death. They may become quite withdrawn and refuse to visit with close relatives and friends. Prolonged periods of silence or crying are normal components of this stage and should not be discouraged.

- *Acceptance.* During the acceptance stage, patients fully realize that they will die. Acceptance ensures a relative sense of peace for most dying people. Anger, resentment, and depression are usually gone. Kübler-Ross describes this stage as one without much feeling. Patients feel neither happy nor sad. Many are calm and introspective and prefer to be left either alone or with a few close relatives or friends.

The psychological stages of dying include two more important points. Just as each person's life is totally unique, so is each person's death. Unfolding deaths vary as much as do unfolding lives. Some people move through Kübler-Ross's stages of dying very predictably, but others do not. It is not uncommon for some dying people to avoid one or more of these stages entirely or to revisit a stage more than once.

The second important point about Kübler-Ross's stages of dying is that the family members or friends of dying people often pass through similar stages as they observe their loved ones dying. When informed that a close friend or relative is dying, many people also experience varying degrees of denial, anger, bargaining, depression, and acceptance. Because of this, as caring people we need to recognize that the emotional needs of the living must be fulfilled in ways that do not differ appreciably from those of the dying.[7]

Advance Health Care Directives

Because some physicians and families have difficulty supporting indirect euthanasia, many people are starting to use legal documents called *advance health care directives.*[5] One of these health care directives is the **living will.** This is a document that confirms a dying person's desire to be allowed to die peacefully and with a measure of dignity if a time should arise when little hope exists for recovery from a terminal illness or severe injury. All 50 states and the District of Columbia have living will statutes. The living will requires that physicians or family members carry out a person's wishes to die naturally, without receiving life-sustaining treatments.[5] About one-third of U.S. citizens have signed living wills. The Terri Schiavo case has drawn increased attention to health care advance directives, because she neither had a living will (see Figure 21-1) nor did she designate a health care agent. A bitter legal battle ensued between her husband and her parents regarding

Key Terms

living will a legal document that requires physicians or family members to carry out a person's wishes to die naturally, without receiving life-sustaining treatments

Figure 21-1 A sample living will.

whether to keep her on life support while she lay in a vegetative state for 15 years.

A second important document that can assist terminally ill or incapacitated patients is the **durable power of attorney for health care** document. This legal document authorizes another person (sometimes called a *health care agent* or *proxy*) to make specific health care decisions about treatment and care under specified circumstances, such as when patients are in vegetative states and cannot communicate their medical wishes. This document helps tell hospitals and physicians which person will help make the critical medical decisions. You can complete both a living will and a durable power of attorney for health care document.

Coping with Specific Causes of Death

Coping with Terminal Illness

Watching a family member or friend slowly die can bring mixed emotions, from being glad to have that person with you as long as possible to wishing that the person would

not have to suffer. It can be painful to see the person you know gradually slip away. In addition, he or she may become someone who seems more like a stranger to you and may not even recognize you or acknowledge your presence. Some people say that they are thankful for the time they have with this person and to be able to say good-bye. However, others may feel a false sense of hopefulness that the person is beating the illness only to feel shocked and devastated when the illness begins to progress at a faster rate. The research does suggest that we cope better with loss when we are expecting it, when we have time to prepare and take whatever action we feel necessary in response to it. In this way, a protracted illness can facilitate the ability to cope that people who experience loss through accidental death, natural disaster, suicide, or murder do not have.

> **Key Terms**
>
> **durable power of attorney for health care** a legal document that designates who will make health care decisions for people unable to do so

Coping with an Accidental Death, Natural Disasters, and Terrorism

Deaths that occur from natural disasters or accidental deaths bring some unique challenges. Accidental death is the number-one cause of death for 15- to 34-year-olds, and so college students may encounter this more often than terminal illnesses. Though any type of trauma or crisis is more difficult to deal with when it is unexpected, accidental death seems particularly devastating in that you are unprepared and shocked by the news. Often people have more trouble accepting this type of death because it is so unexpected that it seems unreal.

Death from natural disasters are typically uncommon and unlikely and so are even more difficult to comprehend and accept. We tend to cope better with events we can understand and explain. Yet this may be impossible to do with accidental deaths such as from a car accident or from incidents without a clear cause of death. Part of finding an explanation can also involve blaming someone: "I should have know he was too tired to drive." People can feel more vulnerable and fearful after accidents and disasters and become more hesitant in their day-to-day living. Things that you may not have questioned begin to seem potentially dangerous, such as going swimming after a friend has drowned or driving after a car accident.

Death associated with terrorism is something that Americans have not had to face, as other countries have, until 9/11. Since that time, Americans have felt less safe on their own soil and traveling abroad. People have changed their lifestyles in terms of the trips they take, having a survival kit at home, stockpiling food and water, and encountering stringent security. Organizations, hospitals, and government agencies are developing responses to bioterrorism and other types of terrorist attacks.

Coping with Death by Suicide

People react similarly to suicides as they do to accidental death, because both means of death are sudden and unexpected. Making sense of these types of death is difficult, and coping with a completed suicide brings the added burden of understanding the reason and motivation behind the death. If you hold religious beliefs that tell you committing suicide is a sin, this can lead to additional misunderstanding and anger. As with death by murder, this type of death is a crime, and so there are legal as well as religious and moral implications in accepting a person's decision to take his or her own life.

Family members frequently say they feel ashamed and embarrassed by the suicide because of these connotations. They worry that others will see them and their family as crazy. All these concerns usually mean that coping with death by suicide can be a longer process than coping with

Grief is even harder to bear when loss happens suddenly, such as when a person commits suicide or dies in an accident. Family members of victims of the terrorist attacks on September 11, 2001, comfort each other.

other types of death. It is helpful for people to understand the events that led up to and contributed to a person's choosing to take his or her life.

Chapter 2 discussed the warning signs and factors that contribute to suicide. Often people blame themselves for not seeing the warning signs or not acting on those they did see. There can also be a sense of feeling unimportant or unloved by this person because you tell yourself "if she really cared about me, she would have fought to stay with me and not left me." Survivors of suicide often feel abandoned and rejected. If your relationship with this person was distant, if you hadn't talked to him or her for awhile or you had recently had an argument, you may feel guilty and blame yourself, saying "if only I had been nicer or called her more often, this might not have happened."

Coping with Death by Murder

Shock, anger, guilt, confusion, and vulnerability are some of the emotions people commonly experience when they cope with a murder. Obviously, you don't expect murder to happen—certainly not to someone you know. It can be difficult to comprehend the taking of someone's life, which makes it even more difficult to accept such a loss. You may blame yourself for not protecting the victim in some way or not doing something to prevent it from happening. If the suspect hasn't been identified or apprehended, you may feel angry at the police for not doing more or feel frightened that you live in a world that seems suddenly very unsafe and frightening. If the murderer has been apprehended, it can take years before the trial is over, making it hard to have a sense of closure.

Euthanasia

There are two types of euthanasia: **indirect (passive) euthanasia** and **direct (active) euthanasia.** Indirect euthanasia is when people are allowed to die without being subjected to life-sustaining efforts such as being placed on life support. Examples of passive euthanasia include physicians' orders of "do not resuscitate (DNR)" and "comfort measures only (CMO)."

Indirect euthanasia is increasingly occurring in a number of hospitals, nursing homes, and medical centers. Physicians who withhold lifesaving techniques or drug therapy treatments or who disconnect life-support systems from terminally ill patients are practicing indirect euthanasia. Although some people still consider this form of euthanasia a type of murder, indirect euthanasia seems to be gaining legal and public acceptance for people with certain terminal illnesses—near-death cancer patients, brain-dead accident victims, and hopelessly ill newborn babies.

Direct euthanasia is when people are intentionally put to death. It is usually performed through the administration of large amounts of depressant drugs, which eventually causes all central nervous system functioning to stop. Although direct euthanasia is commonly practiced on house pets and laboratory animals, it is illegal for humans in the United States, Canada, and other developed countries. However, in 1992, the Netherlands became the first country to enact legislation that permits euthanasia under strict guidelines.

Physician-Assisted Suicide

In recent years, physician-assisted suicide has been the focus of some important news stories. In July 1997, the U.S. Supreme Court unanimously ruled that dying people have no fundamental constitutional right to physician-assisted suicide. In effect, this ruling left the decision to individual states to permit or prohibit physician-assisted suicide.

More than 30 states have enacted laws prohibiting assisted suicide, and many other states have essentially prohibited it through common law. Only the state of Oregon has passed a law, in 1994, that legalized assisted suicide, referred to as the Death with Dignity Act. This act allows doctors to prescribe fatal doses of barbiturates and other drugs to adults of sound mind who have less than 6 months to live. It requires the patient to be at least 18 years of age and of sound mind, make two oral and one written request for the medication with 15 days between the first request and the final one, consult with two physicians, and notify pharmacists and state health authorities before proceeding with physician-assisted suicide. A fatal drug is prescribed, and the patient may ingest it orally at his or her discretion, with or without the doctor present. It

Dr. Jack Kevorkian was convicted of murder in 1999. How do you stand on the issue of physician-assisted suicide?

remains illegal for physicians to administer lethal injections. To date, 70 people are known to have legally taken medication to hasten their death.

Even though physician-assisted suicide is legal in the state of Oregon, many physicians are unwilling to prescribe the lethal medication. Being confined to their bed or home, living a long way from a large urban area, experiencing difficulty finding a willing physician, dying before completing the requirements of the law, and encountering opposition from family and friends are some of the reasons why greater numbers of terminally ill patients are not obtaining medication to end their lives.

A second news story concerned the April 1999 Michigan conviction of Dr. Jack Kevorkian, a retired pathologist who had aided in the suicides of over 100 people. Kevorkian was convicted of second-degree murder and delivery of a controlled substance in the assisted suicide of Thomas Youk, a 52-year-old patient with Lou Gehrig's disease. This suicide had been televised on the CBS show *60 Minutes*. Kevorkian was sentenced to 10–25 years in prison and could be eligible for parole in 2007, when he will be 79 years old.[4]

> ### Key Terms
>
> **indirect (passive) euthanasia** allowing people to die without the use of life-sustaining procedures
>
> **direct (active) euthanasia** intentionally causing death

Near-Death Experiences

Death ends our physical existence. Perhaps this is the ultimate connection between death and our physical dimension of health. Many people believe that, in a positive sense, death brings a sense of relief and comfort—two qualities one may need most when one is dying. The classic work of Raymond Moody,[8] who examined reports of people who had near-death experiences, suggests that we may have less to fear about dying than we have generally thought.

In a comprehensive study of more than 100 people who had near-death experiences, Kenneth Ring[9] reported that these people shared a core experience. This experience was composed of some or all of the following stages:

1. A sense of well-being and peace
2. An out-of-body experience in which the dying person floats above his or her body and witnesses the activities that are occurring
3. A movement into extreme blackness or darkness
4. A shaft of intense light that generally leads upward or lies in the distance
5. A decision to enter into the light

Central to this experience is the need to decide whether to move toward death or to return to the body that has been temporarily vacated.

Experts do not agree whether near-death experiences are truly associated with death or more closely associated with the depersonalization that some people experience during particularly frightening situations. In a scientific sense, near-death experiences are impossible to prove. Science can neither verify nor deny the existence of out-of-body experiences.[1]

Regardless, for those who have had near-death experiences, simply knowing that death might not be such an unpleasant experience appears to be comforting. Most seem to have formed a more positive orientation toward living.[1]

Interacting with Dying People

Facing the impending death of a friend, relative, or loved one is a difficult experience. If you have yet to go through this situation, be assured that, as you grow older, your opportunities will increase. This is part of the reality of living.

Most counselors, physicians, nurses, and ministers who spend time with terminally ill people suggest that you display one quality when interacting with dying people: honesty. Just the thought of talking with a dying person may make you feel uncomfortable. (Most of us have had no training in this sort of thing.) Sometimes, to make ourselves feel less anxious or depressed, we may tend to deny that the person we are with is dying. Our words and nonverbal behavior reveal that we prefer not to face the truth. Our words become stilted as we gloss over the facts and merely attempt to cheer up both our dying friend and ourselves. This behavior is rarely beneficial or supportive—for either party.

As much as possible, we should attempt to be genuine and honest. We should not try to avoid crying if we feel the need to cry. At the same time, we can give dying people emotional support by allowing them to express their feelings openly. We should resist the temptation to try to pull someone out of the denial, anger, or depression. We should not feel obliged to talk constantly and to fill long pauses with idle talk. Sometimes nonverbal communication, including touching, may be much more appreciated than mere talk. Because our interactions with dying people help fulfill our needs, we too should express our emotions and concerns as openly as possible.

Talking with Children about Death

Because most children are curious about everything, we should not be surprised that they are also fascinated about death. From very young ages, children are exposed to death through mass media, adult conversations ("Aunt Emily died today," "Uncle George is very ill"), and their discoveries (a dead bird, a crushed bug, the death of a pet). The way children learn about death greatly affects their ability to recognize and accept their own mortality and to cope with the deaths of others.

Psychologists encourage parents and older friends to avoid shielding children from or misleading children about the reality of death. Young children need to realize that death is not temporary and is not like sleeping. Parents should make certain they understand children's questions about death before they give an answer. Most children want simple, direct answers to their questions, not long, detailed dissertations, which often confuse the issues. For example, when a 4-year-old asks her father, "Why is Tommy's dog dead?" an appropriate answer might be, "Because he got very, very sick and his heart stopped beating." Getting involved in a long discussion about "doggy heaven" or the causes of specific canine diseases may not be necessary or appropriate.

When a child suffers the loss of a near relative, informing the child is a painful task. Adults are usually present when a near relative dies, but children in Western societies are unlikely to be present at the time of death. In the death of a parent, the surviving parent usually must tell the child. The surviving parent sometimes tells the child the news much later, and often in a misleading form.

Two crucial pieces of information that help children to cope with death is that the person will never come back and the body has been buried or burned to ashes.[10] It is for this reason that children should be brought to funerals, so that they can better understand and accept death. Children's fantasies about death and burial can be more frightening to them than reality, especially if they are not told the truth about death. For example, a common tendency is to tell young children that the deceased has "gone to sleep." Since children tend to take things literally, they may develop a fear of going to sleep themselves, since they now associate sleeping with dying. Seeing the dead body at the funeral can dispel these myths.

People often hide their feelings of loss in an effort to be strong and protect children from emotional pain. However, it is good role modeling for children to see how adults mourn and grieve the loss of a loved one and that mourning assists with normalizing this part of the life cycle.

By telling children about the death of a loved one, using language that is age-appropriate, straightforward, and honest, you can help them to begin to learn that death is not something to be feared but something to be accepted. Sharing feelings, answering questions truthfully without too much detail, and giving him or her sympathy and support to cope with losses is the best gift you can give to a grieving child.

Death of a Child

Adults face not only the death of their parents and friends but perhaps also the death of a child. Whether because of sudden infant death syndrome (SIDS), chronic illness, accident, or suicide, adults are sometimes forced to grieve the loss of someone who was "too young to die."

Parents and children are bound by physical and emotional ties like no other relationship. When the tragic death of a young child severs that bond, the pain and anguish the parents feel can be too much to bear. Getting through such a traumatic experience can be one of life's toughest challenges.

Miscarriage

Most pregnancies progress to full term and result in the birth of a healthy child. However, researchers now believe that about one-third of pregnancies end in miscarriage. Since accurate home-pregnancy tests were developed, many women began learning early in the first trimester that they are pregnant. Thus, rather than mistaking the miscarriage for a late heavy menstrual period, more women now know that their pregnancy has ended. Most then go through a grieving process.

In addition, other couples may learn of complications that lead them to choose an elective abortion, or the baby may die during birth or during infancy. Though most people know that such things can happen, many believe that such tragedies happen only to others. When they face the death or potential loss of a child, parents often find their beliefs shaken and their faith tested.

Miscarriage can be especially difficult for the mother. She may think that something she did (or did not do) caused the miscarriage. The exact cause of a miscarriage may never be determined, and the woman needs to be reassured that she did not cause any abnormalities in the fetus.

A miscarriage can be painful and stressful for the woman. Physical symptoms may not occur when the baby dies but may be delayed for some time. Mild or moderate depression, sleeping difficulties, recurring images of the miscarriage, loss of appetite, and abdominal discomfort and cramping may occur weeks or months after a miscarriage. Not surprisingly, fathers can also experience similar symptoms of loss after a miscarriage.

Supportive comments acknowledging how painful their loss is can be helpful to the parents. If an unhealthy fetus is miscarried or aborted, sometimes people try to rationalize the loss for the parents by saying it was "nature's way" of preventing the birth of an imperfect child. Such comments are not only insensitive, but they also imply that the parents should be grateful that they lost the baby. Even seemingly innocent comments can cause pain in the wrong context.

Losing a Baby after It Is Born

Even after a baby is delivered, there are health risks. Sometimes newborn babies die. The support of family and friends is especially important when a couple is trying to recover from the death of a child. Friends and coworkers can help by acknowledging the death of the child and offering support. Often people will not mention the baby because they think that the parents will become upset, but not talking about the baby can cause greater pain for the parents. Calling to offer support or showing up in person can also help.

Parents often want to hold on to the memory of the child. Such feelings are normal and do not mean that the parents are clinging to their grief in an unhealthy way. Remembering the child can give a sense of meaning to parents' lives. Parents often do something constructive to help them remember their baby and accept this loss.

Putting together a scrapbook, donating the baby's clothes and toys to charity, writing memoirs, or setting up a place for remembrance can help the family keep memories of the baby.

Eventually the grief will lose its intensity. It may flare up again around "anniversaries" (the baby's due date or birthday, the date of the baby's death), but gradually things will become bearable. The family will be forever changed by the experience. The death of a child can change the parents' value system, and their spiritual beliefs may be challenged as well.

Sometimes parents become more protective and focused on their remaining children, creating a new set of problems. It is also not uncommon for parents to take their anger over their loss out on each other, sometimes resulting in so much distance, resentment, and bitterness that they eventually divorce.[12] So, how people come to terms with the loss of their child is important to the continued health and healing of the family unit.

Grieving for a Dead Child

Coping with the death of a child is particularly difficult because it seems so unnatural and wrong for a child to precede his or her parents in death. Experts agree that grieving adults, particularly the parents, should express their grief fully and proceed cautiously to return to normal routines. They can avoid many pitfalls. Adults who are grieving for dead children should do the following:

- Avoid trying to cope with grief by using alcohol or drugs.
- Make no important life changes. Moving to a different home, relocating, or changing jobs usually doesn't help parents deal any better with the grief they are experiencing.
- Share their feelings with others. Grieving adults should share their feelings, particularly with other adults who have experienced a similar loss. Group support is available in many communities.
- Avoid trying to erase the death. Giving away clothing and possessions that belonged to the child cannot erase the adult's memories of the child.
- Give themselves the time and space to grieve. On the anniversary of the child's death or on the child's birthday, family members should give themselves special time just for grieving.
- Don't attempt to replace the child. Do not quickly have another child or use the deceased child's name for another child.

For most adults, grief over the death of a child will require an extended time. Eventually, however, life can return to normal.

Learning from Our Diversity

Cultural Differences in Death Rituals

Death rituals vary considerably among ethnic and religious groups. Even within the broad categories of ethnic, racial, or religious distinction, differences exist in how groups of people dispose of their deceased. For example, funeral rituals may differ between Orthodox Jews and Conservative Jews. Furthermore, groups of people living in the United States may not be able to follow the traditional funeral rituals of their home countries because they lack the necessary resources and community support. However, some general cultural differences in funeral rituals can be seen in the following examples.

According to Purnell and Paulanka,[16] funeral rituals by the Amish are carried out in the deceased person's home. The church community takes care of the arrangements for visitors, relieving the grieving family of these tasks. In some Amish communities, a wakelike "sitting up" takes place in which family members are supported by friends throughout the night. The funeral itself is simple, with burial in an unadorned wooden coffin, often made by the local Amish carpenter. Children are encouraged to see death as a transition to a better life. Although the Amish clearly feel the pain of their loss, they often may not express this grief openly.

Muslim death rituals are based on their belief that death is the result of God's will. Death is foreordained. For Muslims (and for members of many other religious groups), life in this world is seen as a preparation for eternal life. At death, the deceased's bed is turned to face the Holy City of Mecca, and verses of hope and acceptance are read from the *Quran*. The dead body is washed three times by a Muslim of the same sex as the deceased and then it is wrapped in white material and buried as soon as possible, usually in a brick or cement-lined grave facing Mecca. Prayers are offered for the dead at the cemetery, at the mosque, or at the home. Unless the deceased is a husband or close relative, women usually do not attend the burial. Cremation is not practiced among Muslims.

In Judaism, death is seen as part of the life cycle.[16] Traditional Jews believe in an afterlife in which a person's soul continues to flourish. In this afterlife, people are judged by their actions in life. People who have lived righteous lives are likely to be rewarded in the next world. Judaism does not have a form of last rites; any Jew may ask for God's forgiveness.

At traditional Jewish funerals, the body is rarely embalmed, unless there are unusual circumstances causing burial to be delayed. Burial routinely takes place within a short time after death. Cosmetic restoration is used minimally, if at all. The body is wrapped in a shroud and placed in an unadorned wooden casket. Traditionally, flowers are not displayed at the funeral or at the cemetery. The funeral service is directed at honoring the deceased, while praising God and encouraging people to reaffirm their faith. Traditionally, a 7-day period of immediate mourning *(shiva)* takes place after the burial. After this period there are established mourning periods. For example, mourning for a relative typically lasts 30 days; for a parent, 1 year.[16]

Death of a Parent, Spouse, or Sibling

In some ways, coping with the death of a parent, spouse, or sibling is similar to coping with the death of a child. In each case, survivors must live with the significant loss of a family member. Each death produces some degree of emotional trauma for each survivor, followed by a period of grief. Gradually, the force of the grieving process lessens as the survivors put the death into a perspective that they can live with. Despite the similarities, there are some differences involving the death of a parent, spouse, or sibling.

Death of a Parent

The death of a parent can be especially difficult because parents have formed a foundation in most peoples' lives. In a sense, parents have always "been there." There is a sense of a loss of security that a parent provided for his or her children. A "safety net" for the children disappears. Perhaps for the first time, adult children genuinely see themselves as getting older. When a parent dies, the children realize they have become the new matriarchs and patriarchs, the leaders of their families.

When a parent dies, adult children are reminded of their own mortality.[11] It is not unusual for this realization to push adult children into serious reflection about their own lives. They may, for the first time, evaluate their lives to determine whether the dreams they had as young adults have materialized. This evaluation can be a positive experience for midlife adults, if it encourages them to refocus on the real priorities in their lives.

Some may consider the death of a mother to be more traumatic than the death of a father.[11] Perhaps this is because the mother traditionally has had the role of the primary nurturing caregiver in a family. From the mother's 9 months of pregnancy through a child's adult life, the maternal role produces a special bond between a mother and her child. Perhaps another reason why a mother's death is especially traumatic is the fact that men tend to die at younger ages than women do. Thus, a mother's death typically follows a father's death and leaves the adult child with the emptiness of "feeling orphaned."

Death of a Spouse

There is great variability in the way a person adapts to the death of a spouse depending on the length of the marriage (or relationship), the age of the person at death, the children from that marriage, financial resources, the vitality of the relationship, the manner in which the spouse died, and the health status of the widow or widower.

For many couples, the death of a spouse is the most traumatic of all deaths.[11] Some couples become so interconnected that the death of one leaves the survivor feeling utterly alone and not whole. A spouse's death might also create a single-parent family, thereby making day-to-day activities quite challenging for the survivor. Some couples may need to assume roles and responsibilities that are unfamiliar and difficult for them, such as handling finances and doing home repairs.

The death of a spouse can also result in the loss of a primary source of one's social interactions.[11] It is important for the remaining spouse to maintain a network of family and friends for social support and interaction. This social support will be crucial in determining how well the survivor will adjust to his or her new situation. Fortunately, there are support groups for recently widowed persons. These can be found in local communities through churches or social support agencies. Support groups also exist on the Internet, for those who wish to seek an online form of support.

Death of a Sibling

The death of a brother or a sister can be very difficult for the surviving sibling(s). It is common for children to feel great guilt for outliving their sibling. They may wonder why the death happened to the sibling rather than them. They may start to question their own mortality and feel more vulnerable to death themselves. Survivors may feel overwhelmed with guilt and believe that they, in some strange way, caused the death. For example, the surviving child who frequently had wished "that his brother was dead" (a common sibling rivalry wish) may believe that his wish caused the car accident that killed his brother.

The manner in which parents communicate and respond to the situation can help the surviving child come to terms with the sibling death. Parents need to keep the lines of communication open, listen to the child's concerns, avoid becoming overly protective of the child, and avoid attempting to re-create in the living child certain qualities of the deceased child.[11] Children must be allowed to express their feelings. Talking with mental health experts in the field of grief and bereavement can be especially helpful to children. Individual counseling sessions and group sessions are available in most communities.

Hospice Care for the Terminally Ill

The thought of dying in a hospital ward, with institutional furniture, medical equipment, and strict visiting hours, leaves many people with a cold feeling. Perhaps this thought alone has helped encourage the concept of **hospice care.** Hospice care is an alternative approach to dying for terminally ill patients and their families. The goal of hospice care is to maximize the quality of life of dying people and their family members. Popularized in England during the 1960s, yet derived from a concept developed during the Middle Ages (where hospitable lodges took care of weary travelers), the hospice helps people die comfortably and with dignity by using one or more of the following strategies:

Key Terms

hospice care (hos pis) an approach to caring for terminally ill patients that maximizes the quality of life and allows death with dignity

---

Hospice care allows terminally ill patients to spend their last days in a warm, homelike setting.

The grieving process consists of four phases, each of which varies in length and form in each individual. These phases are composed of the following:

1. *Internalization of the deceased person's image.* By forming an idealized mental picture of the dead person, the grieving person is freed from dealing too quickly with the reality of the death.
2. *Intellectualization of the death.* Mental processing of the death and the events leading up to its occurrence move the grieving person to a clear understanding that death has occurred.
3. *Emotional reconciliation.* During this third and often delayed phase, the grieving person allows conflicting feelings and thoughts to be expressed and eventually reconciled with the reality of the death.
4. *Behavioral reconciliation.* Finally, the grieving person can comfortably return to a life in which the death has been fully reconciled. The survivor reestablishes old routines and adopts new patterns of living where necessary. The grieving person has largely recovered.

The friends of a grieving person sometime make the mistake of encouraging a return to normal behavior too quickly. When friends urge the grieving person to return to work right away, make new friends, or become involved in time-consuming projects, they may be preventing necessary grieving. It is not easy or desirable to forget about the fact that a spouse, friend, or child has recently died.

- *Pain control.* Dying people usually are not treated for their terminal disease; they are given appropriate drugs to keep them free from pain, alert, and in control of their faculties. Drug dependence is of little concern, and patients can receive pain medication when they feel they need it.

- *Family involvement.* Family members and friends are trained and encouraged to interact with the dying person and with each other. Family members often care for the dying person at home. If the hospice arrangement includes a hospice ward in a hospital or a separate building (also called a hospice), the family members have no restrictions on visitation.

- *Multidisciplinary approach.* The hospice concept promotes a team approach.[12] Specially trained physicians, nurses, social workers, counselors, and volunteers work with the patient and family to fulfill important needs. The needs of the family receive nearly the same priority as those of the patient.

- *Patient decisions.* Contrary to most hospital approaches, hospice programs encourage patients to make their own decisions. The patient decides when to eat, sleep, go for a walk, and just be alone. By maintaining a personal schedule, the patient is more apt to feel in control of his or her life, even as that life is slipping away.

Another way the hospice differs from the hospital approach is in the care given to the survivors. Even after the death of the patient, the family receives a significant amount of follow-up counseling. Helping families with their grief is an important role of the hospice team.

The number of hospices in the United States has climbed quickly to more than 3,300. According to the National Hospice and Palliative Care Organization, hospices served at least 950,000 patients in 2003.[14] People seem to be convinced that the hospice system does work effectively. Part of this approval may be the cost factor. The cost of caring for a dying person in a hospice is usually less than the cost of full (inpatient) services provided by a hospital. Although insurance companies are delighted to see the lower cost of hospice care, many are still uncertain how to define hospice care. Thus not all insurance companies are fully reimbursing patients for their hospice care. Before you discuss the possibility of hospice care for members of your family, you may want to consider the extent of hospice coverage in your health insurance policy.

Grief and the Resolution of Grief

The emotional feelings that people experience after the death of a friend or relative are collectively called *grief*. *Mourning* is the process of experiencing these emotional feelings in a culturally defined manner. (See the Star Box above for more information about the grieving process.) The expression of grief is seen as a valuable process that gradually permits people to accept the loss of the deceased. Expressing grief, then, is a sign of good health.

Although people experience grief in remarkably different ways, most people have some of the following sensations and emotions:

- *Physical discomfort.* Shortly after the death of a loved one, grieving people display a similar pattern of physical discomfort. This discomfort is characterized by "sensations of somatic distress occurring in waves lasting from 20 minutes to an hour at a time, a feeling of tightness in the throat, choking with shortness of breath, need for sighing, and an empty feeling in the abdomen, lack of muscular power, and an intense

I know someone whose brother recently died. I want to help without getting in the way at this difficult time. What's the best approach?

Leming and Dickinson[1] report that the peak time of grief begins in the week after a loved one's funeral. Realizing that there is no one guaranteed formula for helping the bereaved, you can help by performing some or all of the following:

- Make few demands on the bereaved person; allow him or her to grieve.
- Help with the household tasks.
- Recognize that the bereaved person may vent anguish and anger and that some of it may be directed at you.
- Recognize that the bereaved person has painful and difficult tasks to complete; mourning cannot be rushed or avoided.

- Do not be afraid to talk about the deceased person; this lets the bereaved know that you care for the deceased.
- Express your own genuine feelings of sadness, but avoid pity. Speak from the heart.
- Reassure bereaved people that the intensity of their emotions is very natural.
- Advise the bereaved to get additional help if you suspect continuing severe emotional or physical distress.
- Keep in regular contact with the bereaved; let him or her know you continue to care about them.

subjective distress described as a tension or mental pain. The person soon learns that these waves of discomfort can be precipitated by visits, by mentioning the deceased, and by receiving sympathy."[15]

- *Sense of numbness.* Grieving people may feel as if they are numb or in a state of shock. They may deny the death of their loved one.
- *Feelings of detachment from others.* Grieving people see other people as being distant from them, perhaps because the others cannot feel the loss. A person in grief can feel very lonely. This is a common response.

- *Preoccupation with the image of the deceased.* The grieving person may not be able to complete daily tasks without constantly thinking about the deceased.
- *Guilt.* The survivor may be overwhelmed with guilt. Thoughts may center on how the deceased was neglected or ignored. Sensitive survivors feel guilt merely because they are still alive. Indeed, guilt is a common emotion.
- *Hostility.* Survivors may express feelings of loss and remorse through hostility, which they direct at other family members, physicians, lawyers, and others. Sometimes survivors may feel anger at the deceased

Several years ago, funeral homes wanted the public to feel they were not just focusing on the deceased but providing comprehensive service to the mourners. This sparked the concept of "after care," which refers to providing services to the family and friends of the deceased through the difficult times following the funeral. Funeral homes now offer counseling such as group meetings of widows or widowers where they can talk to one another about the difficulties they are having, especially during the holidays and special events of remembrance. They also coordinate special services in the cemetery or chapel during holidays such as Memorial Day or Mother's Day where everyone is invited and different ministers are invited to speak.

Some funeral homes offer seminars for the survivors on topics such as financial planning, cooking, auto and home repair, and parenting. Children are also provided supportive play therapy groups to give them a place to express their feelings of loss. Some advertise that they help with processing life insurance benefits, social security, and pension claims for deceased's family. They also act as a community referral and resource agency to assist other life transitions especially during the first year after the death. Thus the roles of funeral director and funeral home are expanding beyond helping to put the deceased to rest to also helping the survivors to live happy, fulfilling lives.

person, perhaps at the suddenness of the death, at leaving the survivor to deal with problems, or at abandoning the survivor. Such a feeling may cause the survivor to feel guilty and ashamed. Survivors should know that such hostility can be a normal part of grieving.

- *Disruption in daily schedule.* Grieving people often find it difficult to complete daily routines. They can suffer from an anxious type of depression. Seemingly easy tasks take a great deal of effort. Starting new activities and relationships can be difficult. Social interaction skills can be temporarily lost.
- *Delayed grief.* In some people, the typical pattern of grief can be delayed for weeks, months, and even years.

The grief process continues until the bereaved person can establish new relationships, feel comfortable with others, and look back on the life of the deceased person with positive feelings (see Changing for the Better on page 636). Although the duration of the grief resolution process varies with the emotional attachments one has to a deceased person, grief usually lasts for 18 months. One should seek professional help when grieving is characterized by unresolved guilt, extreme hostility, physical illness, significant depression, and a lack of other meaningful relationships. Trained counselors, physicians, and hospice workers can all play significant roles in helping people through grief.

Rituals of Death

Our society has established many rituals associated with death that help the survivors accept the reality of death, ease the pain associated with the grief process, and provide a safe disposal of the body. Our rituals give us the chance to formalize our good-byes to a person and to receive emotional support and strength from family members and friends. In recent years, more of our rituals seem to be celebrating the life of the deceased. In doing this, our rituals also reaffirm the value of our own lives. (See Learning from Our Diversity on page 633 for a discussion on cultural differences in death rituals.)

Most of our funeral rituals take place in funeral homes, churches, and cemeteries. Funeral homes (or mortuaries) are business establishments that provide a variety of services to the families and friends of the deceased. The services are carried out by funeral directors, who are licensed by the state in which they operate. Most funeral directors are responsible for preparing the bodies for viewing, filing death certificates, preparing obituary notices, establishing calling hours, assisting in the preparation and details of the funeral, selecting a casket, transporting mourners to and from the cemetery, and counseling the family. Although licensing procedures vary from state to state, most new funeral directors must complete one year of college, one year of mortuary school, and one year of internship with a funeral home before taking a state licensing examination.

Full Funeral Services

An ethical funeral director will attempt to follow the wishes of the deceased's family and provide only the services requested by the family. Most families want traditional, **full funeral services.** Three significant components of the full funeral services are as follows.

Embalming

Embalming is the process of using formaldehyde-based fluids to replace the blood components. Embalming helps preserve the body and return it to a natural look. Embalming permits friends and family members to view the body without being subjected to the odors associated with tissue decomposition. Embalming is often an optional procedure, except when death results from specific communicable diseases or when body disposition (disposal) is delayed.

Calling Hours

Sometimes called a *wake* or *visiting hours,* this is an established time when friends and family members can gather in a room to share their emotions and common experiences about the deceased. Generally in the same room, the body will be in a casket, with the lid open or closed. Open caskets assist some people to confirm that death truly did occur. Some families prefer not to have any calling hours.

Funeral Service

Funeral services vary according to religious preference and the emotional needs of the survivors. Although some services are held in a church, most funeral services today take place in a funeral home, where a special room might serve as a chapel. Some services are held at the graveside. Families may also choose to have a simple memorial service within a few days after the funeral. (Completing the Personal Assessment on page 643 will help you think about what kind of funeral arrangements, if any, you would prefer for yourself.)

Some families prefer to have a **memorial service** in addition to (or instead of) the full funeral services. The memorial service is usually a celebration of the life of the deceased person. This service may have elements of a religious service,

---

Key Terms

full funeral services all the professional services provided by funeral directors

memorial service a broad term for a ceremony that honors the life of a person who has died

People cope with death in many individual ways. Collectively these serve the diverse needs of society. As our society becomes more culturally diverse, funeral directors are becoming more familiar (and accommodating) with rituals used not only by dozens of Christian denominations but also with rituals for Buddhist, Hindu, and Muslim groups.

Increasingly, funeral directors indicate that there is no longer a set "conventional funeral service." Families mourn the loss of loved ones by developing their own customized funerals. For example, soft music, classical music, rap music, folk music, rock music, or ethnic music may be heard at calling hours (body visitation). Food and drinks (even alcoholic drinks) might be served during calling hours or after the service is performed. More and more families are choosing to display collages of pictures of the deceased person to allow the mourners to remember the life of the dead person.

One unconventional practice that is gaining popularity is the use of the "drive-through mortuary."[11] Mourners can save time by driving up to a funeral home's drive-through window. Without getting out of their car, they can view the body, sign the guest register, and pay their "respects." Although viewed by many as a callous approach, this option was probably inevitable in a society that seems to value squeezing more activities into less time.

With cremation on the rise in the United States, some companies are starting to capitalize on ways to use or display the cremated remains (ashes). Some of these approaches can only be characterized as high-tech. For example, one company will rocket into space a small container of your loved one's ashes. Other companies manufacture and sell display urns for ashes. These attractive urns can be placed in burial grounds, masoleum niches, or the survivor's home. Jewelry artisans are even producing customized "cremation jewelry" that allows you to carry the ashes of the deceased in a pendant around your neck. Some of this jewelry can cost up to $10,000.[11]

Another high-tech approach to death is the use of "electronic" memorials. These are Internet websites that people create to memorialize their deceased loved ones. They usually contain pictures of the person who died, a written life story or family history, and notes and written remembrances from relatives or friends. Some websites allow cybermourners to post condolence messages and share their grief online. "Virtual cemeteries" are websites that feature the posting of pictures and biographical information of the deceased, a chance for mourners to sign the guest book, and the option of leaving "digital flowers."[11]

Some cemeteries even are offering high-tech choices. Special grave markers store a small video monitor that can display up to 250 pages of information about the deceased person.[11] Thus, while standing at the grave site, a mourner can study the entire life of the person buried beneath their feet.

Other high-tech influences reflect the variety of ways that people cope with death. Many funeral homes now make videotapes that are sold to friends and relatives who cannot attend the funeral service. In some cases, digital cameras are used to transmit live video images of a funeral service over the Internet. As the world rapidly changes, so do the ways we handle death rituals.

---

with eulogies spoken by friends and relatives of the dead person. Frequently, the public is invited to attend a memorial service. A memorial service typically takes place weeks or months after a person's death, and follows the surviving family's earlier private funeral service. Thus, the body of the deceased person is rarely present at a memorial service.

Disposition of the Body

Ground Burial We dispose of bodies in one of four ways. Ground burial is the most common method. About 75 percent of all bodies undergo ground burial. The casket is almost always placed in a metal or concrete *vault* before being buried. The vault serves to further protect the body (a need only of the survivors) and to prevent collapse of ground because of the decaying of caskets. Most cemeteries require the use of a vault. See Table 21.2 for the costs involved in this type of burial.

Entombment A second type of disposition is *entombment*. Entombment refers to nonground burial, most often in structures called **mausoleums.** A mausoleum contains a series of shelves where caskets or urns of cremated remains can be sealed in vaultlike spaces called **niches.** Entombment also can take place in the floors, walls, or basements of buildings, especially in large, old churches. For example, the bodies of many famous British religious, cultural, and government leaders are entombed in the **crypts** of Westminster Abbey in London.

Cremation *Cremation* is a third type of body disposition. In the United States, 29 percent of all bodies are cremated.[17]

Key Terms

mausoleum (moz oh **lee** um) an above-ground structure, which frequently resembles a small stone house, into which caskets can be placed for disposition

niche a recessed area in a mausoleum where a casket can be placed

crypts burial locations generally in the walls, floors, or basements of churches

This practice is increasing. Generally both the body and casket (or cardboard cremation box) are incinerated so that only the bone ash from the body remains. The body of an average adult produces about 5–7 pounds of bone ash. These ashes then are placed in containers called *urns,* and then buried, entombed, or scattered, if permitted by state law. The itemized crematory fee ($500–$850) is much less than the fee for ground burial. Some families choose to cremate after having full funeral services.[18]

Anatomical Donation A fourth method of body disposition is *anatomical donation.* Separate organs (such as corneal tissue, kidneys, or the heart) can be donated to a medical school, research facility, or organ donor network. Certain states permit people to state on their driver's licenses that they wish to donate their organs. However, family consent (by next of kin) is also required at the time of death for organ or tissue donation to proceed. Recently, hospitals have been required by federal law to inform the family of a deceased person about organ donation at the time of his or her death. Thus anyone who wishes to donate organs at the time of death should discuss these wishes with his or her family as soon as possible so that family members will support the donation at the time of the individual's death.

The need for donor organs is much greater than our current supply (see the Star Box above and Table 21.1). For some, the decision to donate body tissue and organs is rewarding and comforting. Organ donors understand that their small sacrifice can help give life or improve the quality of life for another person. In this sense, their death can mean life for others. To become an organ donor, you must fill out a uniform organ donor card like the one in Changing for the Better on page 640.

Some people choose to donate their entire body to medical science. Often this is done through prior arrangements with medical schools. Bodies still require embalming. After they are studied, the remains are often cremated and returned to the family, if requested. Just as with an organ donation, those who wish to donate their bodies should discuss their wishes with family members beforehand so that their wishes can be carried out at the time of death.

Table 21.1 Sample Patient Waiting List for Organ Transplant from the United Network for Organ Sharing (UNOS)

Type of Transplant	Patients Waiting for Transplant
Kidney transplant	55,000
Liver transplant	18,434
Pancreas transplant	1,229
Cornea transplant	5,000
Kidney-pancreas transplant	2,478
Intestine transplant	187
Heart transplant	4,163
Heart-lung transplant	230
Lung transplant	3,819
Total	***Total Patients: 90,540**

Note: UNOS policies allow patients to be listed with more than one transplant center (multiple-listing), thus the number of registrations is greater than the actual number of patients. Waiting lists are updated weekly at www.unos.org/Newsroom/critdata_main.htm.

*Some patients are waiting for more than one organ, therefore the total number of patients is less than the sum of patients waiting for each organ.

Costs

The full funeral services offered by a funeral home costs upward of $4,000, with other expenses added to this price. Casket prices vary significantly, with the average cost between $1,500–$2,500. If the family chooses an especially

Planning an Organ Donation

I've thought about organ donation for a long time, and now I am ready. What steps do I need to take to do this?

Donating organs is one of the most compassionate, responsible acts a person can perform. Only a few simple steps are required:

1. You must complete a uniform donor card. Obtain a card from a physician, a local hospital, or the nearest regional transplant or organ bank.
2. Print or type your name on the card.
3. Indicate which organs you wish to donate. You may also indicate your desire to donate all organs and tissues.
4. Sign your name in the presence of two witnesses, preferably your next of kin.
5. Fill in any additional information (such as date of birth, city and state in which the card is completed, and date the card is signed).
6. Tell others about your decision to donate. Some donor cards have detachable portions to give to your family.
7. Always carry your card with you.
8. If you have any questions, you can call the United Network for Organ Sharing (UNOS) at 1-888-TXINF01, or visit this organization's Web site at www.unos.org.

Uniform Donor Card

Of _____
(print or type name of donor)

In the hope that I may help others, I hereby make this anatomical gift, if medically acceptable, to take effect upon my death. The words and marks below indicate my wishes.
I give: ☐ any needed organs or parts
        ☐ only the following organs or parts

_____
specify the organ(s), tissue(s), or part(s)

for the purposes of transplantation, therapy, medical research or education:
        ☐ my body for anatomical study if needed.
Limitations or special wishes, if any:_____

National Kidney Foundation

Please detach and give this portion of the card to your family.

This is to inform you that, should the occasion ever arise, I would like to be an organ and tissue donor. Please see that my wishes are carried out by informing the attending medical personnel that I have indicated my wishes to become a donor. Thank you.

Signature _____ Date _____

For further information write or call:
National Kidney Foundation
(800) 622 – 9010
1522 K Street NW Suite 825 Washington, DC
20005–1213 www. kidney.org

---

fancy casket, then the costs could spiral up to $10,000 or more. Costs that extend beyond these expenses include (should one choose them) those shown in Table 21.2. When all the expenses associated with a typical funeral are totaled, the average cost is $5,500–$7,000.

Regardless of the rituals you select for the handling of your body (or the body of someone in your care), most educators encourage people to prearrange their plans. Before you die, you can save your survivors a lot of misery by putting your wishes in writing. *Funeral prearrangements* relieve the survivors of many of the details that must be handled at the time of your death. You can gather much of the information for your obituary notice and your wishes for the disposition of your body. You can make prearrangements with a funeral director, family member, or attorney. Many individuals also prepay the costs of their funeral. By making arrangements before the need arises, you can

improve your own peace of mind. Currently about 30–40 percent of funerals are preplanned and prepaid. In the 1960s nearly all funerals were planned by relatives at the time of a person's death.

Table 21.2 Estimated Funeral Costs

Cemetery lot	$400–$1,200
Opening and closing of grave	$300–$800
Vault	$350–$1,000
Mausoleum space	$1,500–$5,000
Honorarium for minister	$75–$100
Organist and vocalists	$50–$75 each
Flowers over casket	$100+
Grave marker	$500–$1,500+
Hairstyling, cosmetology	$250
Embalming	$200
Refrigeration	$85 per day

Personal Preparation for Death

We hope that this chapter helps you to develop a new framework about death and form your own personal perspective on death and dying. Remember that the ultimate goal of death education is a positive one—to help you best use and enjoy your life. Becoming aware of the reality of your own mortality is a step in the right direction. Reading about the process of dying, grief resolution, and the rituals surrounding death can also help you accept that someday you too will die.

You can prepare for the reality of your own death in some additional ways. Preparing a will, purchasing a life insurance policy, making funeral prearrangements, preparing a living will, and considering an anatomical or organ donation (see Changing for the Better on page 640) are measures that help you to prepare for your death. At the appropriate time, you might also wish to talk with family and friends about your death. You may discover that an upbeat, positive discussion about death can help relieve some of your apprehensions and those of others around you.

Another suggestion to help you emotionally prepare for your death is to prepare your *obituary notice* or **eulogy.** Include all the things you would like to have said about you and your life. Now compare your obituary notice and eulogy with the current direction your life seems to be taking. Are you doing the kinds of activities for which you want to be known? If so, great! If not, perhaps you will want to consider why your current direction does not reflect how you would like to be remembered. How do you want to restructure your life to better fit your life's goals, meaning, and purpose?

Another suggestion to help make you aware of your eventual death is to write your own **epitaph,** an inscription on a grave marker or monument. Before doing this, you might want to visit a cemetery. Reading the epitaphs of others may help you develop yours.

To assist you in expanding and accepting your awareness of your own mortality, consider answering the following questions: (1) If I had only one day to live, how would I spend it? (2) What one accomplishment would I like to achieve before I die? (3) After I am dead, what two or three things will people miss most about me? By answering these questions and accomplishing a few of the tasks suggested in this section, you will have a good start on accepting your own death and understanding the value of life itself.

Key Terms

eulogy a composition or speech that praises someone; often delivered at a funeral or memorial service

epitaph an inscription on a grave marker or monument

SUMMARY

- Death is determined primarily by clinical and legal factors.
- Euthanasia can be performed through either direct or indirect measures.
- Currently, physician-assisted suicide is legal in only one state, Oregon.
- The most current advance health care directives are the living will and the durable power of attorney for health care.
- Denial, anger, bargaining, depression, and acceptance are the five classic psychological stages that dying people commonly experience, according to Kübler-Ross.
- Deaths of a child, parent, spouse, or sibling are especially difficult for survivors.
- The expression of grief is a common response that can be expected when a friend or relative dies. The grief process can vary in intensity and duration.

- When a parent dies, a child needs support and the truth, especially two crucial pieces of information: that the dead parent will never return and that the body has been buried in the ground or cremated.
- Death in our society is associated with many rituals to help survivors cope with the loss of a loved one and to ensure proper disposal of the body.
- In the past, most people died at home, whereas now the majority of people die in hospitals, nursing homes, and assisted-living facilities.
- The shortage of organ donations is the biggest problem facing people who need a transplant to save their lives.
- Hospice care is an alternative end-of-life health care option for terminally ill patients and their families.
- We dispose of bodies in four ways: ground burial, entombment, cremation, or anatomical donation.

REVIEW QUESTIONS

1. How does the experience of dying today differ from that in the early 1900s?
2. Identify and explain the clinical and legal determinants of death, and identify who establishes each of them.
3. Explain the difference between direct and indirect euthanasia.
4. What is physician-assisted suicide, and in what states is it legal?
5. How does a living will differ from a durable power of attorney for health care document? Why are these advance health care directives becoming increasingly popular?

6. Identify and explain the five psychological stages that dying people tend to experience. Explain each stage.
7. Identify and explain the four strategies that form the basis of hospice care. What are the advantages of hospice care for the patient and the family?
8. Define the term *grief*. Identify and explain the sensations and emotions most people have when they experience grief. When does the grieving process end?

9. What special impacts do the deaths of a parent, spouse, or sibling have on the survivors?
10. What purposes do the rituals of death serve? What are the significant components of the full funeral service?
11. What are the four ways in which bodies are disposed?
12. Define these terms: mausoleum, niche, crypt, vault, urn, eulogy, obituary, and epitaph.

ENDNOTES

1. Leming MR, Dickinson GE. *Understanding Dying, Death and Bereavement* (5th ed.). New York: Harcourt, 2001.
2. Kastenbaum RJ. *Death, Society, and Human Experience* (6th ed.). Boston: Allyn & Bacon, 1998.
3. Knapp D. *Oregon Assisted-Suicide Rate Stays Low,* www.cnn.com, February 24, 2000.
4. *The Kevorkian File,* http://rights.org/deathnet/open.html, June 15, 2000.
5. Partnership for Caring. *Facts about Advance Directives,* www.partnershipforcaring.org, October 10, 2000.
6. Kübler-Ross E. *On Death and Dying* (reprint ed.). Collier Books, 1997.
7. Kübler-Ross E. *To Live Until We Say Goodbye* (reprint ed.). Upper Saddle River, NJ: Prentice Hall, 1997.
8. Moody RA. *The Last Laugh: A New Philosophy of Near Death Experiences, Apparitions, and the Paranormal.* Hampton Roads, 1999.
9. Ring K. *Life at Death: A Scientific Investigation of the Near-Death Experience.* Coward, McCann and Geoghegan, 1980.
10. Bendiksen R, Fulton R (Eds). *Death and Identity* (3rd ed.). Charles Press, 1994.
11. DeSpelder LA, Strickland AL. *The Last Dance: Encountering Death and Dying* (5th ed.). Mayfield, 1999.
12. Staudacher, C. *Beyond Grief.* Oakland, CA: New Harbinger Publications, 1987.
13. Field MJ, Cassel CK (Eds.). *Approaching Death: Improving Care at the End of Life,* Institute of Medicine, National Academy Press, 1997.
14. National Hospice and Palliative Care Organization. *Facts and Figures on Hospice care in America,* www.nhpco.org, November 27, 2000.
15. Lindemann E. Symptomology and management of acute grief, in Fulton et al., *Death and Dying: Challenge and Change.* Boston: Addison-Wesley, 1978.
16. Purnell LD, Paulanka BJ. *Transcultural Health Care: A Culturally Competent Approach.* F.A. Davis, 1998.
17. Cremation Association of North America (CANA): *Updated 1999 Cremation Data by State and Predictors to 2000 and 2010,* www.cremationassociation.org, November 25, 2000.
18. Bowman J (Licensed Funeral Director). Personal correspondence, November 15, 2000.
19. United Network for Organ Sharing. *The Critical Organ Shortage,* www.unos.org, November 20, 2000.
20. Organ donors lives on the line, *St. Louis Post,* May 22, 2005.

As We Go to Press . . .

Cryonics: Challenging the Definition of Death

Over 100 legally deceased people are currently suspended in tanks of liquid nitrogen in the United States with thousands more making plans to join them. The legendary baseball Hall of Famer Ted Williams turned the spotlight on this alternative way of disposing of one's body—freezing it—when he had himself frozen. Cryonics involves embalming the body with a glycerin-based solution, cooling it under dry ice until it reaches minus 40°F, and then gradually lowering the body into a pool of liquid nitrogen until the body reaches minus 320°F. All cell movement ceases at this temperature. The cost for this process and storage ranges from $28,000 to $120,000 per person. The first patient to be frozen was in 1967.

Why would you want to freeze your body when you die? Some believe that the body can be thawed and the cause of death be reversed. Sound like a science fiction movie? Proponents of cryonics predict that diseases such as cancer will have cures sometime in the future, and so the deceased can be unfrozen and treated for whatever killed him or her in the first place. However, patients who are legally brain dead are not accepted for this procedure. Also, you can opt to freeze only your head (for some people, the brain is perceived as critical for revival). Freezing a severed head is less costly, around $40,000, and takes less effort to freeze and revive. In addition, it is thought that when future people develop the technology to bring you back to life, they will also have the technology to generate a new body for you based on your DNA. While it is rumored that Walt Disney was frozen, this has not been substantiated. However, a few well-known scientists have also been put into cryonic suspension. Dr. Eric Drexler, known as the father of nanotechnology, and Dr. Marvin Minsky, the founder of artificial intelligence research in the United States, are also frozen. Is this an option you would consider for your future?

personal assessment

Planning your funeral

In line with this chapter's positive theme of the value of personal death awareness, here is a funeral service assessment that we frequently give to our health classes. This inventory can help you assess your reactions and thoughts about the funeral arrangements you would prefer for yourself.

After answering each of the following questions, you might wish to discuss your responses with a friend or close relative.

1. Have you ever considered how you would like your body to be handled after your death?

   _____ Yes   _____ No

2. Have you already made funeral arrangements for yourself?

   _____ Yes   _____ No

3. Have you considered a specific funeral home or mortuary to handle your arrangements?

   _____ Yes   _____ No

4. If you were to die today, which of the following would you prefer?

   _____ Embalming   _____ Ground burial

   _____ Cremation   _____ Entombment

   _____ Donation to medical science

5. If you prefer to be cremated, what do you want done with your ashes?

   _____ Buried   _____ Entombed

   _____ Scattered

   _____ Other; please specify

6. If your funeral plans involve a casket, which of the following ones do you prefer?
   _____ Plywood (cloth covered)
   _____ Hardwood (oak, cherry, mahogany, maple, etc.)
   _____ Steel (sealer or nonsealer type)
   _____ Stainless steel
   _____ Copper or bronze
   _____ Other; please specify

7. How important is a funeral service for you?
   _____ Very important
   _____ Somewhat important
   _____ Somewhat unimportant
   _____ Very unimportant
   _____ No opinion

8. What kind of funeral service do you want for yourself?
   _____ No service at all
   _____ Visitation (calling hours) the day before the funeral service; funeral held at church or funeral home
   _____ Graveside service only (no visitation)
   _____ Memorial service (after body disposition)
   _____ Other; please specify

9. How many people do you want to attend your funeral service or memorial service?
   _____ I do not want a funeral or memorial service
   _____ 1–10 people
   _____ 11–25 people
   _____ 26–50 people
   _____ Over 51 people
   _____ I do not care how many people attend

10. What format would you prefer at your funeral service or memorial service? Select any of the following that you like:

	Yes	No
Religious music	_____	_____
Nonreligious music	_____	_____
Clergy present	_____	_____
Flower arrangements	_____	_____
Family member eulogy	_____	_____
Eulogy by friend(s)	_____	_____
Open casket	_____	_____
Religious format	_____	_____
Other; please specify	_____	_____

11. Using today's prices, how much do you expect to pay for your total funeral arrangements, including cemetery expenses (if applicable)?
    _____ Less than $4,500
    _____ Between $4,501 and $6,000
    _____ Between $6,001 and $7,500
    _____ Between $7,501 and $9,000
    _____ Above $9,000

To Carry This Further . . .

Which items had you not thought about before? Were you surprised at the arrangements you selected? Will you share your responses with anyone else? If so, whom?

appendix 1

First Aid

Accidents are the leading cause of death for people ages 1 to 37. Injuries sustained in accidents can often be tragic. They are grim reminders of our need to learn first aid skills and to practice preventive safety habits.

First aid knowledge and skills allow you to help people who are in need of immediate emergency care. They also can help you save yourself if you should become injured. We recommend that our students enroll in American Red Cross first aid and safety courses, which are available in local communities or through colleges or universities. In this appendix, we briefly present some information about common first aid emergencies. (Please note that our information is *not* a substitute for comprehensive American Red Cross first aid instruction.)

First Aid

- Keep a list of important phone numbers near your phone (your doctor, ambulance service, hospital, poison control center, police and fire departments).

- In case of serious injury or illness, call the appropriate emergency service immediately for help (if uncertain, call "911" or "0").

Common First Aid Emergencies

Specific Problem	What To Do
Asphyxiation Victim stops breathing and skin, lips, tongue, and fingernail beds turn bluish or gray.	Tip head back with one hand on forehead and other lifting the lower jaw near the chin. Look, listen, and feel for breathing. If the victim is not breathing, place your mouth over victim's mouth, pinch the nose, get a tight seal, and give 2 slow breaths. Do pulse check. If no pulse is detected, CPR must be administered (Note: Some states require CPR training for those who administer CPR). If there is a pulse but no breathing, give breaths once every 5 seconds for an adult, once every 3 seconds for a child, once every 3 seconds for infants (do not exaggerate head tilt for babies). Recheck pulse and breathing every minute.
Bleeding Victim bleeding severely can quickly go into shock and die within 1 or 2 minutes.	Use universal precautions. With the palm of your hand, apply firm, direct pressure to the wound with a clean dressing or pad. Elevate the body part if possible. Do not remove blood-soaked dressings; use additional layers, continue to apply pressure, and elevate the site.
Choking Accidental ingestion or inhalation of food or other objects causes suffocation that can quickly lead to death. There are over 3,000 deaths annually, mostly of infants, small children, and the elderly.	The procedure of giving abdominal thrusts is easy to learn; however, the correct technique must be learned from a qualified instructor. The procedure varies somewhat for infants, children, adults, pregnant women, and obese people.

continued

Specific Problem	What To Do
Hyperventilation A situation in which a person breathes too rapidly; often the result of fear or anxiety; may cause confusion, shortness of breath, dizziness, or fainting. Intentional hyperventilation before an underwater swim is especially dangerous, since it may cause a swimmer to pass out in the water and drown.	Have the person relax and rest for a few minutes. Provide reassurance and a calming influence. Having the victim take a few breaths from a paper bag (not plastic) may be helpful. Do not permit swimmers to practice hyperventilation before attempting to swim.
Bee Stings Not especially dangerous except for people who have developed an allergic hypersensitivity to a particular venom. Those who are not hypersensitive will experience swelling, redness, and pain. Hypersensitive people may develop extreme swelling, chest constriction, breathing difficulties, hives, and shock signs.	For nonsensitive people: Scrape stinger from skin and apply cold compresses or over-the-counter topical preparation for insect bites. For sensitive people: Get professional help immediately. Scrape the stinger from skin; position the person so that the stung body part is below the level of the heart; help administer prescribed medication (if available); apply cold compresses.
Poisoning Often poisoning can be prevented with adequate safety awareness. Children are frequent victims.	Call the poison control center immediately; follow the instructions provided. Keep syrup of ipecac on hand.
Shock A life-threatening depression of circulation, respiration, and temperature control; recognizable by a victim's cool, clammy, pale skin; weak and rapid pulse; shallow breathing; weakness; nausea; *or unconsciousness.*	Keep the victim calm; loosen tight clothing. Help the victim to a comfortable, reclining position with legs elevated 8–12 inches (*if there are head, neck, back, or internal injuries, do not move the person at all*; if breathing is difficult, help the person to sit or semi-recline). Prevent loss of body heat; cover if necessary. Do not give food or fluids. Seek further emergency assistance.
Burns Burns can cause severe tissue damage and lead to serious infection and shock.	Minor burns: immerse in cold water 10–15 minutes; dry; apply antibiotic agent and loose sterile dressing; do not apply butter or grease to burns. Major burns: immerse in cold water; cover affected area with sterile or clean dressings; do not try to clean the burn area or break blisters. Seek medical attention. Chemical burns: flood the area with running water.
Broken Bones Fractures are a common result of car accidents, falls, and recreational accidents.	Do not move the victim unless absolutely necessary to prevent further injury. Immobilize the affected area. Give care for shock while waiting for further emergency assistance.

Epilepsy: Recognition and First Aid

Seizure Type	What It Looks Like	Often Mistaken For	What To Do	What Not To Do
Convulsive Generalized tonic-clonic (also called grand mal)	Sudden cry, fall, rigidity, followed by muscle jerks, frothy saliva on lips, shallow breathing or temporarily suspended breathing, bluish skin, possible loss of bladder or bowel control, usually last 2–5 minutes; normal breathing then starts again; there may be some confusion and/or fatigue, followed by return to full consciousness	Heart attack Stroke Unknown but life-threatening emergency	Protect from nearby hazards Loosen ties or shirts collars Place folded jacket under head Turn on side to keep airway clear; reassure when consciousness returns Look for medical identification *after* seizure subsides or protective steps have been taken If single seizure lasted less than 5 minutes, ask if hospital evaluation wanted If multiple seizures, or if one seizure lasts longer than 5 minutes, seek medical attention	Don't put any hard implement in the mouth Don't try to hold tongue; it can't be swallowed Don't try to give liquids during or just after seizure Don't use artificial respiration unless breathing is absent after muscle jerks subside, or unless water has been inhaled Don't restrain
Nonconvulsive	This category includes many different forms of seizures, ranging from temporary unawareness (petit mal) to brief, sudden, massive muscle jerks (myoclonic seizures)	Daydreaming, acting out, clumsiness, poor coordination, intoxication, random activity, mental illness, and many others	Usually no first aid necessary other than to provide reassurance and emotional support If behavior during seizure places person in potentially hazardous situation (e.g., traffic, machinery), gently guide person away from hazard Medical evaluation is recommended	Do not shout at, restrain, or grab a person having a nonconvulsive seizure (unless danger threatens); do not expect verbal instructions to be obeyed

appendix 2

Body Systems

The Circulatory System

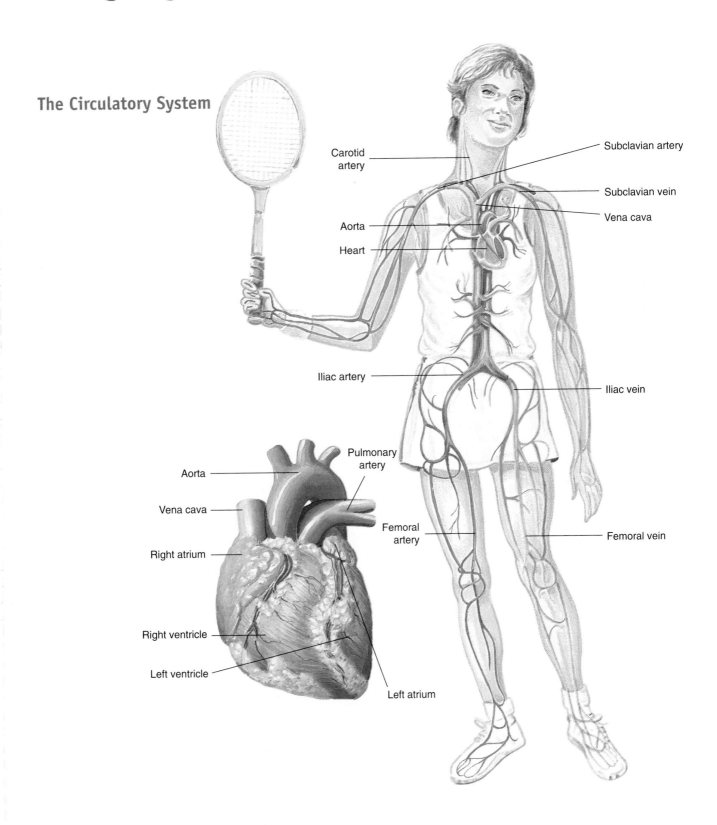

Carotid artery

Subclavian artery

Subclavian vein

Vena cava

Aorta

Heart

Iliac artery

Iliac vein

Aorta

Pulmonary artery

Vena cava

Right atrium

Femoral artery

Femoral vein

Right ventricle

Left ventricle

Left atrium

The Respiratory System

Nasal cavity

Larynx

Trachea

Right main bronchus

Left main bronchus

Right lung

Left lung

Capillary

Alveolar duct

Alveoli

Terminal end of bronchiole

The Muscular System

Sternocleidomastoid

Trapezius

Deltoid

Pectoralis major

Biceps

Triceps

Rectus abdominis

Rectus femoris

Sartorius

Gastrocnemius

Ligaments

The Skeletal System

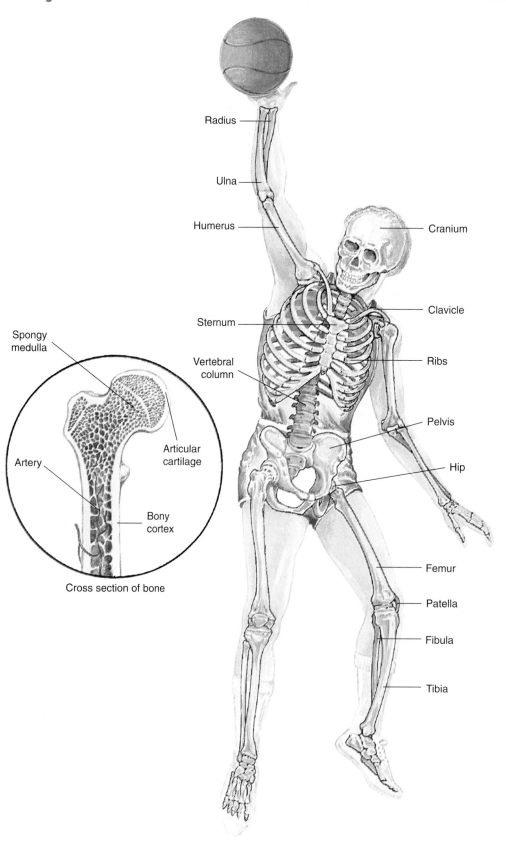

Radius

Ulna

Humerus

Spongy
medulla

Sternum

Vertebral
column

Artery

Articular
cartilage

Bony
cortex

Cross section of bone

Cranium

Clavicle

Ribs

Pelvis

Hip

Femur

Patella

Fibula

Tibia

The Nervous System

Brain

Optic nerve

Cervical nerve

Spinal cord

Cerebellum

Pons

Radial nerve

Ulnar nerve

Thoracic nerves

Lumbar nerves

Sacral nerves

Sciatic nerve

Tibial nerve

Nerve

Ganglion

Spinal cord

Meninges

Vertebra

Spinal cord detail

The Digestive System

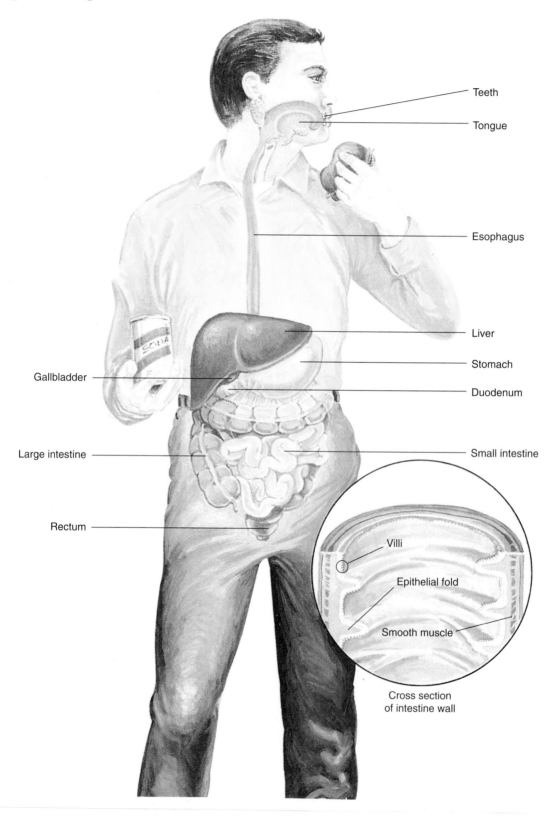

Teeth

Tongue

Esophagus

Liver

Stomach

Gallbladder

Duodenum

Large intestine

Small intestine

Rectum

Villi

Epithelial fold

Smooth muscle

Cross section
of intestine wall

The Urinary System

Cortex

Pelvis

Renal artery

Renal vein

Medulla

Ureter

Cross section of kidney

Kidney

Ureter

Bladder

Urethra

The Endocrine System

NOTE: Refer to Figures 14-2 and 14-3 for detailed anatomical illustrations of the reproductive systems.

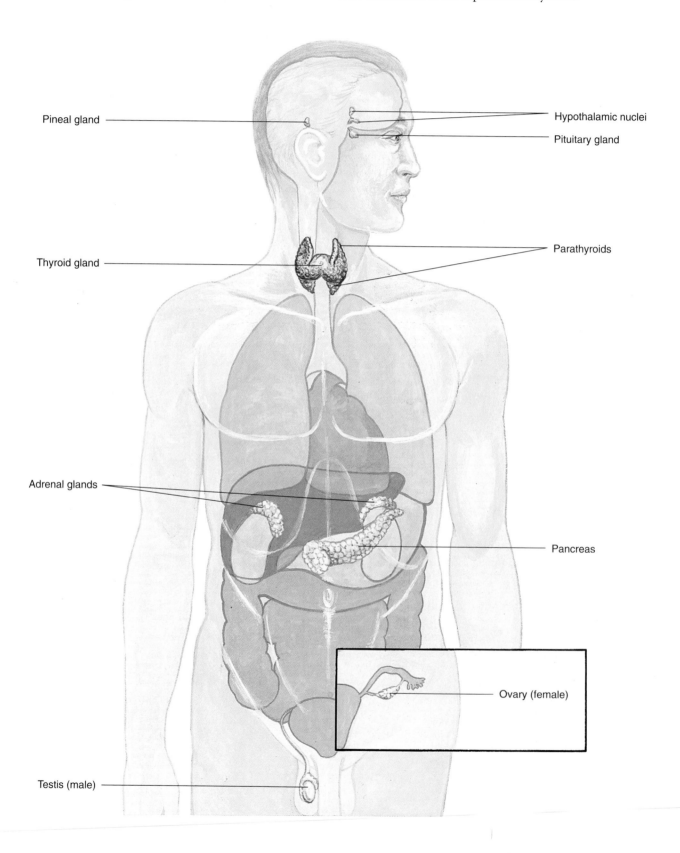

Pineal gland

Hypothalamic nuclei

Pituitary gland

Parathyroids

Thyroid gland

Adrenal glands

Pancreas

Ovary (female)

Testis (male)

appendix 3

Canadian Health

by Professor Don Morrow, The University of Western Ontario

Composed of 10 provinces and 3 territories, Canada is a huge geographic land mass with a relatively small population—some 30 million people. The population is mainly concentrated along the lower one-third of the country. Historically, relationships with its southern neighbor, the United States, have been good, although Canadians perceive themselves as distinctly different from Americans. The most obvious distinction is the bilingual nature of the country, English and French, with a significant concentration of the French-speaking population located in the province of Quebec. Unlike the United States, Canada has not experienced a major civil war. Still, escalating tensions over the potential for Quebec's separation from Canada's confederation to become a sovereign state have given rise to a great deal of discussion, reflection, and concern about nationhood and our current political structure. Clearly, the prospect of Quebec and succession threatens the integrity of Canada as a nation and as a society.

One unifying element in Canadian society has been its comprehensive program of national health insurance, in which coverage is provided to all citizens directly through government, without the involvement of insurance companies. The major responsibility for health care rests with the provinces, while the federal government has served as policymaker, along with assuming some direct health-care responsibilities for special populations such as Native Canadians, the three territories, and the military. The umbrella for Canadian health is a national health insurance program. The envy of many developed countries, this program represents a cost of about 10 percent of the gross domestic product; however, the expenses of maintaining the program have exceeded anyone's forecast. For example, in 1993 the total cost of the health-care system was some $55 billion, almost double the amount of just seven years earlier. Clearly, changes in concept, structure, and funding are needed if government is to continue offering any health-care system. This section outlines the history, nature, and future directions of health and health care in Canada. Further readings are listed at the end.

Historical Background

The first universal hospital insurance program in Canada was implemented in the province of Saskatchewan shortly after the end of World War II; by 1960 the other nine provinces had established similar programs, with federal legislation enacted for a national program in 1971 (Frankel et al. 1996; Pederson et al. 1994). In the early 1980s this federal, political infrastructure became the Canadian Health Promotion Directorate. Without question, the landmark federal initiative was the publication and dissemination in 1974 of the document titled *A New Perspective on the Health of Canadians*. The impact of this document nationally and internationally cannot be overstated. It received worldwide attention for its recasting of the concept of health toward what is now called *health promotion*. Whereas health traditionally had been equated with the health-care system, the *Perspective's* thrust was toward the broad concept of a *health field* that included all matters affecting health. This *health field concept* embraced four avenues or elements:

- health care organization: the "system" of health care
- the environment
- lifestyle
- human biology

Such a concept was radical for the mid-1970s. It challenged the prevalent and ingrained equation that level of health equals quality of medicine. While applauding Canada's health care system as "second to none in the world," the *New Perspective* underlined "ominous" counterforces threatening the standard of living, public health protection and advances in medical science; such counterforces as environmental pollution, city living, abuse of alcohol, tobacco, and other drugs, eating patterns, and sedentary habits of indolence were identified for concern and action. In effect, the *Perspective* paper provided a whole new way of conceptualizing health as much broader than the traditional "medical model" of health and health care that had been so strongly focused on disease and illness.

The Health Field Concept

Careful to recognize that "the provision of personal health services to the general public is clearly a matter of provincial jurisdiction," the 1974 document highlighted the existence of national health problems that know no provincial boundaries and that arise from causes embedded in the social fabric of the nation as a whole (page 6). To convince health professionals and the public alike, the *New Perspective* showed that major causes of illness, defined as number of hospitalization days, were diseases of the cardiovascular system, followed by accidents and violence, then mental illness; in turn these were directly related to the interplay of the four elements identified as the health field concept. Thus, ill health was shown to be the direct result of self-imposed risks like drug abuse, poor diet, and insufficient exercise as well as of careless driving, promiscuity, and so forth. Also tied to the health field concept were environmental problems such as urbanization, working conditions, rapid social change, and economic deprivation. The paradox so clearly illuminated in the *New Perspective* was that of lip-service agreement on the importance of research and prevention in health improvement, juxtaposed against the continued tendency to increase disproportionately the amount of money spent on existing illnesses and their treatment. The health field concept was characterized as comprehensive, as allowing for a workable system of analysis, and as bringing focus to neglected areas. The document's authors believed this reconfigured understanding of health would greatly assist in identifying factors that contribute to sickness/death and in determining actions that could improve the quality of health. In this regard the *New Perspective* offered 74 suggestions or proposals to analyze health care issues and to develop more effective health care policy.

Not only was the *New Perspective* document symbolic of major health reform, but it was also the first federal government articulation of a comprehensive and inclusive view of health that went far beyond the World Health Organization definition, "Health is a state of complete physical, mental, and social well-being and not merely the absence of disease and infirmity," so entrenched in health care systems worldwide. In reality, however, this 1974 perspective was ahead of its time; and it presented a viewpoint that challenged the status quo as represented by the Canadian medical establishment, the country's health care institutions, and the collective consciousness of Canadians themselves. It was just too easy to cling to the old equation of level of health = quality of medicine/health care. Moreover, economic prosperity and growth masked the significance of such threats to health as environmental and lifestyle factors. Further, it was widely held that the *New Perspective* was too narrow, and that it intended to "blame the victim" for health problems. What was needed, critics said, was a more socially oriented view of health and health education, one that accounted more directly for environmental and social factors, to place health in context in Canadian society.

The Ottawa Charter

Major indicators of change were witnessed in the early 1980s. The city of Vancouver in British Columbia, Canada's westernmost province, hosted a "Shifting Medical Paradigm Conference" in 1980; formulated to usher in a shift from the medical, disease-prevention/treatment model, this conference represented more of a challenge to Western medical tradition, rather than offering any concrete concept of health promotion. Of somewhat greater impact was the Toronto-based 1984 conference, "Beyond Health Care," which stressed the need for transitions in public health policy to promote healthy cities and communities (Pederson et al. 1994). The most important piece of health legislation or reform was produced in 1986 when the *Ottawa Charter for Health Promotion* was created after a conference on health promotion hosted in Ottawa, the nation's capital. Spiraling health-care costs were the major force behind the reform initiatives that resulted in the *Charter;* however, individual and agency initiatives in the spirit of health reform complemented the federal document.

The *Charter* took bold and needed steps to move the concept of health away from the treatment of illnesses and the attendant technologies toward a concept and policy that truly focused on health. Instead of trying to change the definition of health—so sacred to many health professionals—the *Charter* used the concept of *health promotion,* or "the process of enabling people to increase control over, and to improve their health." Health in this sense was perceived as a resource for everyday life, not the goal or objective of living. This concept underscored the importance of quality of everyday life in the process of health in preference to the traditional statistical emphasis on longevity or illness. Health promotion was envisioned in this document as a process rather than as a set of risk factor outcomes or as the "social work of medicine" (Pederson et al. 1994). Health promotion was not merely presented as the responsibility of the health-care sector but as an arena of shared personal and social resources and decisions. The *Charter* identified the fundamental conditions and resources for health:

- peace
- shelter
- education
- food
- income

- stable economic system
- sustainable resources
- social justice
- equity

In short, this set of Maslow-like conditions reflected the multifaceted nature of the concept of health. Moreover, the *Charter* gained worldwide attention for its identification and explanation of strategies for change:

- Build healthy public policy.
- Create supportive environments.
- Strengthen community action.
- Develop personal skills.
- Reorient health services.

Set against the action orientations of *advocate, enable,* and *mediate,* the prerequisites for health and the strategies for change were aligned for a new conceptual and realistic vision of health and its promotion. Once again Canada played a leadership role in framing and operationalizing the concept of health promotion, just as it had in changing the medical perception of health care in 1974 via the *New Perspective* document.

A Framework for Health Promotion

The World Health Organization and Health and Welfare Canada were responsible for hosting the 1986 Ottawa conference and establishing an action-oriented *Charter* that challenged participating organizations, governments, and individuals to pursue a "health for all" goal for the year 2000 and beyond. In the same year, the federal Minister for Health and Welfare, Jake Epp, took the *Charter*

out of the realm of abstract conceptualization by articulating and promoting a practical model to achieve the *Charter's* goal. It was called *A Framework for Health Promotion* and it is configured in the chart below.

Some explanation will be helpful. The *Framework* paper identified three major challenges that were not being addressed by current health policies and practices. First, disadvantaged groups had a significantly lower life expectancy, poorer health, and higher prevalence of disability than the average Canadian. Second, various forms of preventable diseases and injuries continued to undermine the health and quality of life of the citizenry. Third, the lack of support for chronically ill, disabled, or emotionally stressed people was pronounced and serious; improved coping mechanisms and support services were needed. Such challenges, the document stated, warranted mechanisms for relief. First, self-care, or the decisions and actions individuals take in the interests of their own health, was intrinsic to health promotion. Second, through mutual aid, people could help each other cope; and third, the creation of conditions and surroundings conducive to health was strongly recommended. These three strategies could be implemented in provinces, municipalities, and communities to enhance health.

The *Framework* received large-scale promotion and, like the 1974 federal document (*New Perspective*), it was criticized for being too vague in its strategies. Nonetheless, the *Framework* must be credited with targeting health promotion as the central focus of health reform and direction in Canada. Because health is constitutionally defined as a provincial concern, federal policy could serve only to stimulate, challenge, and frame new concepts and tactics for health. Together with the *Charter,* the *Framework* represented new commitments that both provoked

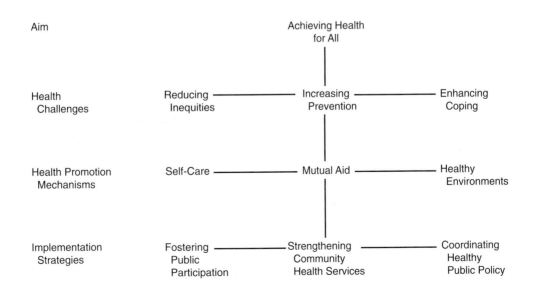

and empowered changes in health in line with the World Health Organization's enabling definition of health promotion defined in the *Charter* just described. If health promotion was to involve social responsibility, then the federal initiatives in 1986 did establish a new framework for health promotion. The challenge of "health for all" seems ambitious and lofty; however, if health can be perceived as an attitude and a process more than an end in itself, then the goal of health for all seems more realistic. Cost containment may well be an engine that drives health care reform in Canada, yet reform is absolutely necessary, as is the reduction of health expenditures everywhere.

Current Provincial Perspectives

The acid test of any policy initiative is, of course, its implementation. In 1988 the Canadian Public Health Association, inspired by the three key strategies presented in the *Framework* model, created the Strengthening Community Health Program with a view toward focusing and applying health promotion at the community level. This program had its roots in the Ottawa *Charter* and might best be examined by considering a cross-Canada description of health promotion during the late 1980s and early 1990s. Most of the material discussed in this section is synthesized from Pederson's comprehensive book, *Health Promotion in Canada* (1994). The intent here is to provide a brief overview of the provincial and community responses to federal policy and strategy.

On the west coast, the province of British Columbia has been successful in inducing some 100 communities to join a vibrant "healthy community" movement inspired directly by the *Framework* document. Government initiatives in that province are directed toward recognizing, promoting, and linking community actions that reflect health promotion activities such as community health plans, conferences, surveys, and educational programs. By contrast, in neighboring Alberta, we see conflicting perspectives about health promotion that range from full commitment at one extreme to the notion that it represents an unaffordable luxury. Nevertheless, the provincial government in Alberta stresses changes related to promoting healthy lifestyles and addressing health determinants.

Saskatchewan, the first province to adopt a universal hospital insurance program, has a decades-old health action strategy of creating coalitions through which communities have been encouraged and supported in health promotion activities with dramatic success. In 1992, this province's government released a major health reform initiative, *A Saskatchewan Vision for Health*, which is based on two principles for action: the concept of wellness as the goal of health services, and community control of health

service delivery. In the same year, the fourth prairie province, Manitoba, published its *Quality Health for Manitobans* paper to support health promotion for its 1 million inhabitants. Manitoba boasts seven strong healthy community projects based on a partners-for-health agreement between the government and the communities involved.

In central Canada, the most populous and arguably the most prosperous area of the country, responses to the *Charter* and the *Framework* are significantly different. The 10 million people in Ontario have seen lengthy policy statements on the province's *Nurturing Health* documents, but very little in the way of developments at the community or grassroots level of health reform. Instead the Ontario government seems intent on taking only the broad social view of health that is grounded in the determinants of health and the health care system. Quebec's 7 million people (about 80 percent of whom are French speaking) and their governing bodies have given only token acknowledgment to federal initiatives in health promotion. The province has had very few "champions" of the concept of health promotion and very little political pressure for reform. As a unit, the Atlantic provinces are victims of inequity because they live in a distinctly poorer economic environment. Many of the communities in these four provinces are single-industry towns. As a result, change is slow, and at best some of these provinces are just beginning to move toward the concept and practice of health promotion. Including the Yukon Territory, which is under direct federal health jurisdiction, it is evident that across Canada the contemporary trend is toward community or grassroots initiatives in health promotion. It will be helpful to examine the trends in health care as a means of viewing the community and provincial moves toward health reform in a larger context.

Health Practices and Health Status

As we have seen in our review of provincial programs, health care structures are rooted in the individual social ideologies of each province. Less evident is the effect of these programs on the actual health practices or health status of the Canadian population. If over $55 billion is currently spent on health care in Canada, it is useful to ascertain where the money is being spent in relation to health concepts, practices, and reform policies. In a recent publication, *The Sociology of Health and Health Care*, the authors point out that health care expenditures in Canada consume a greater proportion of our gross national product than is the case in most other industrialized nations. This information is critical in discussing and understanding Canadian health. Just over one-third of total provincial budgets are expended on health, and by far the majority (75 percent) of that money goes to institutional and physician services, that is, for health care itself, not for prevention or programs for change (Sutherland and Fulton, 1990). Canadian life expectancy in general has increased, but the reasons for the increase have less to do with improvements in health care and more to do with positive changes in standard of living related to living conditions, nutrition and nutritional practices, and decreases in the rate of infant mortality. Frankel and other authors are careful to point out that increased life expectancy carries greater risks for decreases in the quality of life; for example, life expectancy does not automatically imply disability-free life expectancy. If social class is isolated, no matter which measure of socioeconomic status is used, higher income earners and people working in more prestigious jobs experience lower mortality rates and longer life expectancy even when the latter is adjusted for quality measures. Overall, changes in longevity among the Canadian population do not necessarily mean proportional changes in health status. The converse of this statement is equally instructive; in countries like Hungary and Finland, where life expectancy has decreased in spite of costly health care systems, suicide and lifestyle risk have actually increased (Sutherland and Fulton, 1990). Thus, it is important to interpret longevity data in context with other measures or indicators of health and health status.

In this decade, cardiovascular diseases and cancer remain the most significant causes of death for both sexes from the age of 25 years onward (*Action Statement*). Mortality rates continue to be considerably higher for males than for females throughout the life span. The irony here is that females in Canada report higher rates of illness and higher rates of use of health services than do males (Frankel et al. 1996). Whether the latter tendency represents a cultural and/or gender difference in the approach to health behavior, it is a significant sex difference worthy of greater exploration and analysis. From a Canadian and a global perspective, it is critical to recognize the epidemic proportions of depression, anxiety, stress, loneliness, and insecurity (Sutherland and Fulton, 1990), all of which contribute to a decline in the quality of life and lifestyle—more evidence to underline the importance of health promotion that is beyond mere physical health or well-being.

Health workers make up about 8 percent of the Canadian labor force. Of that percentage, about three-quarters work in the nation's approximately 1,200 hospitals. The Canadian health care system constitutes the largest social service sector in the country, and it is the third largest employer in the nation (Frankel et al. 1996). Sutherland and others contend that since the 1970s, Canada has had "too many physicians." This is a debatable point when the stature of physicians is so elevated in our society and when hospitals themselves serve as such powerful symbols of wealth and power. What is remarkable and worthy of reconsideration is the rejection of "alternative" forms of health practitioners like naturopaths, homeopaths, and practitioners of Eastern forms of medicine (acupuncture, for example). Also, in spite of community-based health policy reforms, the whole notion of community health centers is slow to gain acceptance by traditional medical personnel, who perceive them as threatening to their power and independence. The concept of community health-care centers is based on a team or shared approach to health delivery, which challenges the current top-down approach. Community health centers support a variety of health-care personnel only some of whom are medical doctors, in order to serve health consumers. To date, only the province of Quebec has achieved significant inroads in establishing such centers (Frankel et al. 1996), solid evidence that health promotion may be more of a factor in that province than its perceived lack of compliance with either the *Charter* or the strategies of the *Framework* documents.

Action Statement for Health Promotion

Lifestyle, special environments, age, sex, wealth, power, institutional dominance, biological factors, and a wide variety of other variables interact in Canada, as they do elsewhere in the world, to characterize the status of health in any given time period or social grouping. And still the mirage of the importance of the health care system continues to overwhelm health care reform and to monopolize human and economic resources. To renew efforts toward greater health promotion, with optimal health as a goal, the Canadian Public Health Association in 1996 recommitted itself to the strategies of the *Charter* and the *Framework*. In July of 1996, the association published a working paper called *Action Statement for Health Promotion in Canada,* with the following introductory comment:

> This *Action Statement* is the product of a two-year consultation process involving more than 1,000 people. Participants in the process were mainly health professionals and volunteers who work to promote health. Other participants came from areas such as social services, education, recreation, environment and law enforcement. These people share the values and ways of working that define health promotion, even though they may not call themselves health promoters. Together we represent a community of shared purpose.

The Canadian Public Health Association is a group within the Population Health Directorate of the federal ministry, Health Canada. The *Action Statement* is a policy developed for provinces and health-care workers to consider and implement in local areas. Notice that paid professionals in the health care industry, such as physicians and hospital personnel, are conspicuous by their absence in this process of formulating an action statement. Instead it is a grassroots commitment based on shared values with respect to the goals of health promotion. The wisdom or necessity of not using health professionals/workers in strategic policy is not the issue here; instead it is important to examine the direction of this proposal and then to look at examples of what has been happening recently in health promotion in the country.

The *Action Statement,* significantly, represents a recommitment to the framework established in the 1986 *Charter* as a viable approach to health promotion; 10 years after the charter was published, the *Action Statement* refines the document's focus to the mid-1990s. Noting global trends with respect to the escalation of poverty levels, rapidly increasing unemployment, and economic decisions and practices that threaten the environment and consolidate wealth and power in private corporations with few legal responsibilities to the common good, the *Action Statement* recommends that priorities be set to affirm and share the vision and values of health promotion. The statement also calls for the creation of alliances across and between different community and health sectors; honing knowledge, skills, and the capacity to improve health; emphasizing political commitment and the development of healthy public policies; working to ensure that health system reform truly promotes health both inside and outside the health care system. Of major importance in this statement is the recognition that improving health is a vital component of human development. Instead of reiterating ill-health data, the *Action Statement* succinctly summarized the implications of that data in sifting out the following critical health determinants:

- healthy childhood development
- adequate incomes
- small gaps between the rich and poor
- absence of discrimination based on gender, culture, race, and sexual orientation
- lifelong learning opportunities
- healthy lifestyles
- meaningful work opportunities with some control over decision making
- social relationships that respect diversity
- freedom from violence or its threat
- freedom from exposure to infectious disease
- protection of humans from environmental hazard
- protection of the environment from human hazards

The *Action Statement* takes a refreshing approach to health status data by interpreting what it means to work toward health as a process with direction instead of merely reporting the state of ill health. Further, the statement recognizes that health promotion has a firm values base. For example, of the six value statements given in the document, one stresses the value that individual liberties must be respected with a priority given to the common good, and another stresses that individuals must be treated with dignity and respect. Although these might seem like obvious commonsense principles, explicitly recognizing and stating them provides some validation for perceiving health in its fullest sense: physical, emotional, mental, and spiritual.

Also important, relative to this *Action Statement,* is the learning gained from the 1986 commitment to health promotion. The document stresses that strategic principles must be understood in guiding the development and implementation of health promotion:

- Health promotion addresses health issues in social and environmental context.
- Health promotion supports a holistic approach to all aspects of healthy development.
- Health promotion requires a long-term perspective; time must be taken to create awareness and build understanding about health determinants.
- Health promotion supports a balance between centralized and decentralized decision making on policies affecting people.
- Health promotion is multisectional in that cooperation must be achieved between people and organizations to dovetail with program initiatives in the health sector.
- Health promotion draws on formal knowledge in the social, economic, political, medical, and environmental sciences and on personal experience.
- Health promotion emphasizes public accountability.

Apparently much has been learned about solidifying and implementing health promotion from a strategic perspective. In particular, it is recognized that, while change in health policy and behavior must come, it will come slowly; newer or "sexier" health initiatives are not the answer. Instead the *Action Statement* confirms health promotion from an empowerment perspective. Strategies require some concrete tactics for implementation, and the *Action Statement* supplies strong suggestions in that regard. Once again, the *Charter* is used as a springboard to reinvigorate specific thrusts in health promotion. With respect to advocating healthy public policy, the statement accurately highlights the shaping power of policies in determining how money, power, and material resources flow through institutions of health and thereby offer the determinants of health behavior and outcomes. During the past 10 years, the emphasis in policy making has been on support for creating and developing healthy lifestyles; more emphasis must now be placed on policies that create healthy living conditions and that give voice to society's least powerful groups. To that end, the *Action Statement* provides a comprehensive list of priorities and tactics for action in policy making.

Community Focus

Equally stressed in this 1996 document is the dominant and proven need to *strengthen communities* in the health promotion thrust. Because communities already share common space, identities, interests, and concerns through various agencies and activities, the *Action Statement* mentions several action priorities to provide community training opportunities, funding, support from/for community networks, and the development of evaluation methods for continued monitoring and improvement. The evidence is clear in Canada that changes in health promotion will not come from the institutionalized health care sector. The provincial initiatives toward health promotion described earlier demonstrate that change in the area of health promotion works best at the community, grassroots level. Related to this fact is the third tactic identified in the *Action Statement:* the absolute necessity to *reform health systems.* The document narrows its focus to two specific objectives: to shift the emphasis from treating disease to improving health; and to increase the effectiveness and efficiency of the health care system.

Both of these objectives form part of most provincial policy statements on health reform. Still, the reality of health system reform lags considerably behind the recognition that it is needed. Political debate and public attention tend to be focused on insured medical treatments and reducing the number of hospital beds; cuts in primary health care are widespread. For example, in Ontario, the *Toronto Daily Star* gave full-page coverage to the appointment of retired Queen's University former dean of medicine Duncan Sinclair to the chair of the province's Health Services Restructuring Committee (*TDS,* September 15, 1996). Sinclair's task, the article said, was to "shake up/down the Ontario hospital system" to rid the system of duplication and to "ensure there is a health care system for future generations." This is a prime example of praiseworthy reductions in cost but failure to address the broad determinants of health: closing hospitals is not the sole answer to health reform. Instead, according to the *Action Statement,* family- and community-based care must be improved with stronger health protection programs and access to client-centered primary health care services. To achieve real benefits from and by health promotion, the knowledge base about health determinants and regional health profiles must be increased and stronger alliances or coalitions must be fostered among different organizations that share the common goal of health promotion, and can effect real change in the broad determinants of health. Ultimately, as the *Action Statement* points out, if efforts to develop health promotion efforts in Canada are to succeed, they must be allied to similar efforts throughout the global community.

Current Initiatives and Future Directions

In Canada's health promotion survey in 1990, in which some 13,000 people across the country were interviewed regarding health status, practices, and beliefs, self-reports were compiled to assess the status of health promotion in the population. The respondents reported very little change in health status. The rich and the well educated were more likely to report good to excellent health status than those with less wealth and education. The same survey showed findings about social relationships, environmental health practices, personal health practices, alcohol and other drug use, nutritional practices, heart disease prevention, leisure time physical activity, cancer prevention practices, injury control and safety, sexual health, and dental health. The conclusion, once again, is that health education is absolutely critical as a catalyst for improvement in health behaviors.

Similarly, in 1991 Angus published an extensive "Review of Significant Health Care Commissions and Task Forces in Canada Since 1983–84," sponsored by the Canadian Medical Association. His finding? At the root of all of these commissions and reforms is the desire to rebalance and redirect the system in three important ways: toward greater emphasis on disease prevention and health promotion; toward community-based health-care alternatives; and toward greater accountability of the health-care system. Clearly, Canada has committed itself to the whole concept and implementation of health promotion. Is it working? This question is difficult to answer, because generalizations are impossible. The following section examines specific pockets of information and examples in an effort to find out if and how health promotion is being implemented in Canada.

The Implementation of Health Promotion

A positive sign of knowledge-based, applied research is the work of the Canadian Fitness and Lifestyle Research Institute (CFLRI). This organization's mission is to "enhance the well being of Canadians through research and communication of information about physically active lifestyles to the public and private sectors." The Institute seeks to understand active living by addressing fitness issues from the complementary perspectives of the health professions, the social and psychological sciences, and the physiological and biological sciences. In 1994 the CFLRI published its findings on "Health Promotion at Work: Results of the 1992 National Workplace Survey." The Institute recognized that because some 13 million Canadians are employed, the workplace is a very important environment and avenue for health promotion. Some 45,000 Canadian companies claim to have health promotion programs in place to varying degrees. The most popular lifestyle or health promotion intervention on the part of employees is in the realm of smoking cessation. Some 3,500 companies with 20 or more employees responded to the survey and provided information about such health determinants as stress, harassment, discrimination, financial uncertainty, conflicts at work, fatigue, and levels of physical activity. The survey data show that workplace health promotion efforts are increasing and expanding. Only businesses in Quebec were more likely to claim that health is the sole responsibility of the employee. Workplaces must continue to be targeted for health promotion and reform. Philosophically, however, such efforts run counter to the value system in a capitalist society. Capitalism is based on the values of material gain and inequality, reflected in most workplaces by the very fact of work and its goals. Health promotion, in contrast, is rooted in equality of opportunity and benefits as well as in the quality of everyday life rather than material ends or goals. This contradiction in values is one that must be resolved to functionally support and implement health promotion initiatives.

ParticipACTION

If data don't convince people—and the history of health data and ill-health data confirm that most people are not scared easily by statistical trends—then there must be alternatives to persuasion. In Canada, one of the most successful campaigns focused on healthy behavior has been ParticipACTION, a nongovernment movement to promote healthy lifestyles. Established in the early 1970s, this not-for-profit organization was initially commissioned by the federal government to campaign for improved fitness and lifestyle improvement. ParticipACTION's objective was to market physical fitness as one would market toothpaste or any other product. The organization used two key marketing strategies: (1) to employ modern marketing methods in advertising; and (2) to finance itself from the private sector, not the public purse. To implement the first strategy, the organization developed a four-cornered approach to marketing fitness: educate, motivate,

remind, and provide solutions about/for physical fitness. The group leans heavily on private corporations to achieve its goals and is distinguished by its clever use of advertising. In its 30-year history, ParticipACTION has had to compete with service agencies and charities like the United Way for advertising time and space. Annual reviews of its efforts show impressive cost-benefit ratios for its advertising. It is difficult to open any newspaper today and not find some small ad or teasing clip provided by this organization, which is highly effective in targeting the population at the grassroots level.

ParticipACTION also publishes *Active Living,* a national magazine that provides resource information to educators, health professionals, fitness leaders, and others in the broad spectrum of health interests in Canada. This publication and the efforts of ParticipACTION to involve itself in wider aspects of health and behavior change and information exchange are clear indicators of health promotion at work.

Food Guides and Eating Patterns

A growing body of evidence suggests that symptoms and causes of ill health are directly attributable to eating choices and patterns. Canada has long been famed for its *Food Guide to Healthy Eating,* a simple, one-sheet "recipe" for appropriate daily food selection from the four main food groups. Heavy marketing emphasis is placed on low-fat foods, reducing portion sizes, focusing on "grazing" foods, and becoming better consumers by paying attention to food labels. The Heart and Stroke Foundation of Canada, long committed to decreasing the incidence and prevalence of these disorders, actively promotes *heart-smart* foods, and has supported the publication of a heart-healthy cookbook.

Another excellent example of promoting health through healthier eating is a highly successful recipe book called *Looneyspoons: Low-Fat Food Made Fun,* written by two sisters in Ontario. Using the teasing style employed in ParticipACTION campaigns, the book taps into the day-to-day experiences and interests of ordinary people. Chapter titles include, "If You Bake It, They Will Come," and, "Meatless in Seattle." Straightforward low-fat tasty recipes are presented with lighthearted comments like, "Low-fat eating is for those who are thick and tired of dieting," and "Dieting is the penalty for exceeding the feed limit." Even the recipe titles have flair and appeal: "Pita-the-Great," "Scalloping Gourmet," "Mission Shrimpossible," and "Veal of Fortune" are a few examples. Such an innovative approach to healthy behavior through nutritious eating is a solid and useful response to serious problems like obesity and anorexia nervosa, which so negatively affect the health and health costs of Canadians.

Wellness

Newspapers in Canada carry stories regularly about communities hosting "health fairs," local gatherings at which the public has easy access to health care personnel, resources, and information. Similarly, educational curricula reflect growing trends toward teaching and learning about health. For example, the *Food Guide to Healthy Eating* is known to most elementary school children across Canada. In secondary schools, such as those in Ontario, the most senior course in physical education contains an entire, comprehensive section on "wellness" and "psychological and social development" related to a framework of holistic health education. Several universities have implemented wellness or well-being research; teaching and study centers patterned themselves after the phenomenally successful National Wellness Center in Stevens Point, Wisconsin, but with greater emphasis on the research component and mandate in postsecondary education.

Promoting Men's Health

In Canada, as in the United States and other Western Hemisphere countries, women are far more likely to seek help in matters of health than men—despite the fact that men have distinct health problems and earlier incidences of disease and premature death than do women. Part of the reason for this gender-based difference in response to health initiatives and reform lies in social conditioning; traditionally, men have been expected to be stoic, invulnerable, almost bulletproof in their day-to-day lives. Until recently, boys have been brought up to be self-reliant, to suppress "soft" emotions, and to "prove" their toughness through sports, hazardous jobs, war, and high-risk behaviors like workaholism, social isolation, and avoidance of intimacy. There are no clear answers to the dramatic difference in men's and women's responses to health promotion, but new approaches must be identified as the role of men in Canadian society continues to change.

A Regional Example

If health promotion is grounded in community-based programs and reform, then we must have evaluations and information bases for those communities. A comprehensive study, "Community Health and Well Being in Southwestern Ontario," recently was compiled to provide epidemiological information on the determinants of health and health status of the region, a community of some 1.5 million people, or about 13 percent of the province's total population. Results of this study show that the region has significantly higher rates of mortality from heart attacks and other cardiovascular diseases and diabetes. Hospitalization rates are at least 10 percent higher for these same problems than in

the rest of Ontario. The residents of this community smoke more, eat more fat, exercise less, and have more body fat than residents of Ontario as a whole—not surprising given the mortality and hospitalization findings presented above. The area has a higher proportion of seniors and residents aged 15 and over with less than a grade 9 education than do other parts of the province.

Significantly, the study found that the only factor that predicts life expectancy of a community is its poverty rate (not the number of hospital beds available or other traditional data); the higher the poverty level, the higher the rate of premature mortality. These findings are important for many reasons. First, they dramatically illustrate once again that health status does not equal health care. Further, they show that social environment, physical environment, and biological endowment (how well one chooses his/her parents!) all are determinants of health as is the individual's responses to those factors. Lifestyle factors, the study's authors stress, are not the sole or even the primary cause of poor health; rather, they are symptoms of a variety of social, psychological, and economic factors, perhaps the most important of which is low income. In fact, low income may be such a key health variable that it "may set off a domino effect on other health hazards." Community-based studies like this appear to contribute significantly to ongoing efforts toward health promotion and corresponding evaluation in Canada.

Summary

Health promotion is a slow process, but the changes occurring in health delivery and health behavior toward enhancement of quality lifestyles are rapid. The ability to diagnose symptoms from such sources as the Internet and its resources are a boon, as well as a challenge to traditional health procedures and forms of care. Clearly, changes in health cannot be the responsibility of government: individuals in communities must assume increasing responsibility for promoting health as a process, not a static end or achievable goal. In reality, health, like most forms of human behavior, is an attitude, one that is based on personal, social, and cultural values and practices. Until Canada or any other nation recognizes that fact, the achievement of true health will remain an elusive goal.

Sources and Further Reading

Action Statement for Health Promotion in Canada, Ottawa: Canadian Public Health Association, July, 1996.
Active Learning, September 1992, Volume 1, Number 4.
Alder, R., Vingilis, E., Mai, V., editors. London, Ontario: Middlesex-London Health Unit and the Faculty of Medicine, The University of Western Ontario, 1996.

Craig, C. L., Beaulieu, A., Cameron, C. *Health Promotion at Work: Results of the 1992 National Workplace Survey.* Ottawa: Canadian Fitness and Lifestyle Research Institute, 1994.

Crichton, A., Hsu, D., Tsand, S. *Canada's Health Care System: Its Funding and Organization.* Ottawa: Canadian Hospital Association, 1990.

Epp, J. *Achieving Health for All: A Framework for Health Promotion.* Ottawa: Health and Welfare Canada, 1986.

Frankel, G., Speechley, M., Wade, T. J. *The Sociology of Health and Health Care: A Canadian Perspective.* Toronto: Copp Clark Ltd., 1996.

Lazear, D. *Seven Ways of Knowing.* Palatine, IL: Skylight Publishing, 1991.

Ottawa Charter for Health Promotion. Ottawa: World Health Organization and Health and Welfare Canada, 1986.

Pederson, A., O'Neill, M., Rootman, I. *Health Promotion in Canada: Provincial, National and International Perspectives.* Toronto: W. B. Saunders Canada, 1994.

Podleski, J., Podleski, G. *Looneytoons: Low-Fat Food Made Fun.* Ottawa: Granet Publishing Inc., 1996.

Stephens, T., Fowler, G. D., editors. *Canada's Health Promotion Survey 1990: Technical Report.* Ottawa: Ministry of Supply and Services Canada, 1993.

Sutherland, R. W., Fulton, M. J. *Health Care in Canada: A Description and Analysis of Canadian Health Services.* Ottawa: The Health Group, 1990.

Canada's Food Guide to Healthy Eating

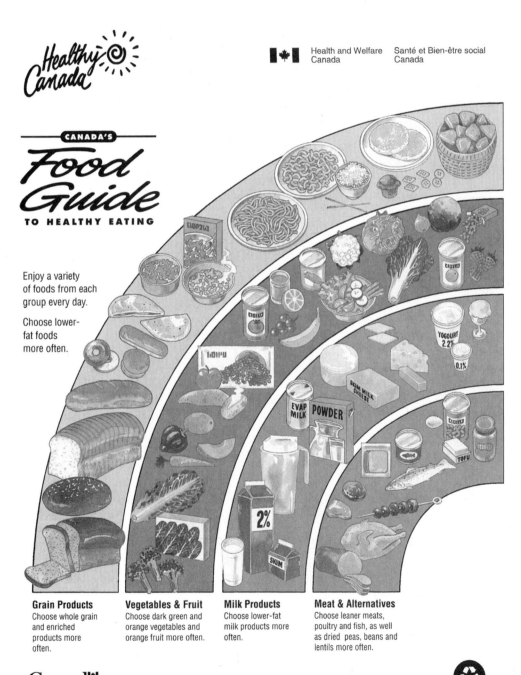

Healthy Canada

Health and Welfare Canada   Santé et Bien-être social Canada

CANADA'S Food Guide
TO HEALTHY EATING

Enjoy a variety of foods from each group every day.

Choose lower-fat foods more often.

Grain Products
Choose whole grain and enriched products more often.

Vegetables & Fruit
Choose dark green and orange vegetables and orange fruit more often.

Milk Products
Choose lower-fat milk products more often.

Meat & Alternatives
Choose leaner meats, poultry and fish, as well as dried peas, beans and lentils more often.

Canada

Different People Need Different Amounts of Food

The amount of food you need every day from the 4 food groups and other foods depends on your age, body size, activity level, whether you are male or female and if you are pregnant or breast-feeding. That's why the Food Guide gives a lower and higher number of servings for each food group. For example, young children can choose the lower number of servings, while male teenagers can go to the higher number. Most other people can choose servings somewhere in between.

Grain Products
5-12
SERVINGS PER DAY

1 Serving
1 Slice
Cold Cereal 30 g
Hot Cereal 175 mL 3/4 cup

2 Servings
1 Bagel, Pita or Bun
Pasta or Rice 250 mL 1 cup

Vegetables & Fruit
5-10
SERVINGS PER DAY

1 Serving
1 Medium Size Vegetable or Fruit
Fresh, Frozen or Canned Vegetables or Fruit 125 mL 1/2 cup
Salad 250 mL 1 cup
Juice 125 mL 1/2 cup

Milk Products
SERVINGS PER DAY
Children 4–9 years: 2–3
Youth 10–16 years: 3–4
Adults: 2–4
Pregnant & Breast-feeding Women: 3–4

1 Serving
MILK 250 mL 1 cup
Cheese 3"x1"x1" 50 g
2 Slices 50 g
175 g YOGOURT 3/4 cup

Other Foods

Taste and enjoyment can also come from other foods and beverages that are not part of the 4 food groups. Some of these foods are higher in fat or Calories, so use these foods in moderation.

Meat & Alternatives
2-3
SERVINGS PER DAY

1 Serving
Meat, Poultry or Fish 50-100 g
Fish 1/3–2/3 Can 50–100 g
1-2 Eggs
Beans 125-250 mL
TOFU 100 g 1/3 cup
Peanut Butter 30 mL 2 tbsp

Enjoy eating well, being active and feeling good about yourself. That's VITALIT

Glossary

A

abortion induced premature termination of a pregnancy.

absorption the passage of nutrients or alcohol through the walls of the stomach or intestinal tract into the bloodstream.

abuse any use of a legal or illegal drug in a way that is detrimental to health or well-being.

acquired immunity (AI) the major component of the immune system; forms antibodies and specialized blood cells capable of destroying pathogens.

acupuncture the insertion of fine needles into the body to alter electroenergy fields and treat disease.

acute has a sudden onset and a prompt resolution.

acute alcohol intoxication a potentially fatal elevation of BAC, often resulting from heavy, rapid consumption of alcohol.

acute rhinitis the common cold; the sudden onset of nasal inflammation.

adaptive thermogenesis the physiological response of the body to adjust its metabolic rate to the presence of food.

addiction compulsive, uncontrollable dependence on a substance, habit, or practice to such a degree that cessation causes severe emotional or physiological reactions.

additive effect the combined (but not exaggerated) effect produced by the concurrent use of two or more drugs.

adipose tissue tissue made up of fibrous strands around which specialized cells designed to store liquefied fat are arranged.

aerobic energy production the body's primary means of energy production, used when the respiratory and circulatory systems can process and transport sufficient oxygen to muscle cells to convert fuel energy.

agent the causal pathogen of a particular disease.

agoraphobia a fear of being in situations from which there is no escape or where help would be unavailable should an emergency arise; often associated with panic disorder.

air pollution refers to a wide variety of substances found in the atmosphere that can have adverse effects on human health, crop productivity, and natural communities.

air toxics a class of 188 toxic air pollutants identified by the U.S. Environmental Protection Agency as known or suspected causes of cancer or other serious health effects, such as reduced fertility, birth defects, or adverse environmental effects.

alarm stage the first stage of the stress response involving physiological, involuntary changes which are controlled by the hormonal and nervous system; the fight or flight response is activated in this stage.

alcoholism a primary, chronic disease with genetic, psychosocial, and environmental factors influencing its development and manifestations.

allopathy (ah **lop** ah thee) a system of medical practice in which specific remedies (often pharmaceutical agents) are used to produce effects different from those produced by a disease or injury.

alveoli(al **vee** oh lie) thin, saclike terminal ends of the airways; the site at which gases are exchanged between the blood and inhaled air.

amenorrhea cessation or lack of menstrual periods.

amino acids the building blocks of protein; manufactured by the body or obtained from dietary sources.

anabolic steroids(ann uh **bol** ick) drugs that function like testosterone to produce increases in weight, strength, endurance, and aggressiveness.

anal intercourse a sexual act in which the erect penis is inserted into the rectum of a partner.

anaerobic energy production the body's alternative means of energy production, used when the available oxygen is insufficient for aerobic energy production. Anaerobic energy production is a much less efficient use of stored energy.

androgyny (an **droj** en ee) the blending of both masculine and feminine qualities.

angina pectoris (an **jie** nuh **peck** tor is) chest pain that results from impaired blood supply to the heart muscle.

anorexia nervosa an eating disorder in which the individual weighs less than 85% of their expected weight, and has an intense fear of gaining weight; in females, menstruation ceases for at least 3 consecutive months; people with anorexia perceive themselves as overweight, even though they are underweight.

antagonistic effect the effect produced when one drug reduces or offsets the effects of a second drug.

antibodies chemical compounds produced by the body's immune system to destroy antigens and their toxins.

artificially acquired immunity (AAI) a type of acquired immunity resulting from the body's response to pathogens introduced into the body through immunizations.

asbestos a term used to refer to a class of minerals that have a fibrous crystal structure.

asphyxiation death resulting from lack of oxygen to the brain.

atherosclerosis the buildup of plaque on the inner wall of arteries.

attention deficit hyperactivity disorder (ADHD) an above-normal rate of physical movement; often accompanied by an inability to concentrate on a specified task; also called *hyperactivity*.

autoimmune disorders disorders caused by the immune system's failure to recognize the body as "self"; thus the body mounts an attack against its own cells and tissues.

axon the portion of a neuron that conducts electrical impulses to the dendrites of adjacent neurons; neurons typically have one axon.

ayurveda (ai yur **vey** da) traditional Indian medicine based on herbal remedies.

B

balanced diet a diet featuring selections from each of the food groups in the Food Guide Pyramid.

ballistic stretching a "bouncing" form of stretching in which a muscle group is lengthened repetitively to produce multiple, quick, forceful stretches.

bariatrician a physician who specializes in the study and treatment of obesity.

basal metabolic rate (BMR) the amount of energy (expressed in calories) the body requires to maintain basic functions.

basic needs deficiency needs that are viewed as essential and fundamental, including physiological safety, belonging, and love and esteem needs.

behavior therapy a behavior modification therapy based upon the learning principles of reinforcement therapy, stimulus-response, and conditioning responses to change behavior.

benign noncancerous; tumors that do not spread.

beta blockers drugs that reduce the workload of the heart, which results in angina pectoris.

beta endorphins mood-enhancing, pain-reducing, opiatelike chemicals produced within the smoker's body in response to the presence of nicotine.

bias and hate crimes criminal acts directed at a person or group solely because of a specific characteristic, such as race, religion, ethnic background, sexual orientation, or other attribute.

binge drinking the consumption of five drinks or more on one drinking occasion.

binge eating disorder an eating disorder formerly referred to as compulsive eating disorder; binge eaters use food in the same way to cope as bulimics do, but do not engage in compensatory purging behavior.

biological air pollutants living organisms or substances produced by living organisms that cause disease or allergic reactions, including

bacteria, molds, mildew, viruses, dust mites, plant pollen, and animal dander, urine, or feces.

biological water pollutants disease-causing organisms that are found in water.

biopsychological model a model that addresses how biological, psychological, and social factors interact and affect psychological health.

bipolar disorder a mood disorder characterized by alternating episodes of depression and mania.

birth control all of the methods and procedures that can prevent the birth of a child.

blackout a temporary state of amnesia experienced by an alcoholic; an inability to remember events that occur during a period of alcohol use.

blood alcohol concentration (BAC) the percentage of alcohol in a measured quantity of blood; BAC can be determined directly, through the analysis of a blood sample, or indirectly, through the analysis of exhaled air.

body image our subjective perception of how our body appears.

body mass index (BMI) a numerical expression of body weight based on height and weight; used to determine desirable body weight.

bolus theory a theory of nicotine addiction based on the body's response to the bolus (ball) of nicotine delivered to the brain with each inhalation of cigarette smoke.

bradycardia slowness of the heartbeat, as evidenced by a resting pulse rate of less than 60 beats per minute.

brand name the specific patented name assigned to a drug by its manufacturer.

bulimia nervosa an eating disorder in which individuals engage in episodes of binging, consuming unusually large amounts of food and feeling out of control, and engaging in some form of compensatory purging behavior to eliminate the food.

C

calcium channel blockers drugs that reduce the workload of the heart; used in the long-term management of angina pectoris.

calendar method a form of periodic abstinence in which the variable lengths of a woman's menstrual cycle are used to calculate her fertile period.

calipers a device used to measure the thickness of a skinfold from which percent body fat can be calculated.

calories units of heat (energy); specifically, one calorie (used here to mean *kilocalorie*) equals the heat required to raise one kilogram of water one degree Celsius.

carbohydrates chemical compounds composed of sugar units; the body's primary source of energy.

carbon monoxide a gaseous by-product of the incomplete combustion of natural gas, kerosene, heating oil, wood, coal, gasoline, and tobacco.

carcinogens environmental agents, including chemical compounds within cigarette smoke, that stimulate the development of cancerous changes within cells.

cardiac muscle specialized muscle tissue that forms the middle (muscular) layer of the heart wall.

cardiorespiratory endurance the ability of the heart, lungs, and blood vessels to process and transport oxygen required by muscle cells so that they can contract over a period of time. Cardiorespiratory endurance is produced by exercise that requires continuous, repetitive movements.

cardiovascular pertaining to the heart (cardio) and blood vessels (vascular).

carjacking a crime that involves a thief's attempt to steal a car while the owner is behind the wheel; carjackings are usually random and unpredictable, and they frequently involve handguns.

catabolizing the metabolic process of breaking down tissue for the purpose of converting it into energy.

CAT scan computerized axial tomography scan; an x-ray procedure designed to illustrate structures within the body that would not normally be seen through conventional x-ray procedures.

cellulite tissue comprised of fat cells intertwined around strands of fibrous connective tissue.

cerebrovascular occlusions (ser ee bro **vas** kyou lar) blockages to arteries supplying blood to the cerebral cortex of the brain; the most common type of stroke.

cervical cap a small, thimble-shaped contraceptive device designed to fit over the cervix.

chemical name the name used to describe the molecular structure of a drug.

chemoprevention cancer prevention using food, dietary supplements, or medications thought to bolster the immune system or reduce the damage caused by carcinogens.

child maltreatment the act or failure to act by a parent or caregiver which results in abuse or neglect of a child or which places the child in imminent risk of serious harm.

chiropractic manipulation of the vertebral col-umn to relieve malalignment and cure illness.

chlamydia the most prevalent sexually transmitted disease; caused by a nongono-coccal bacterium.

cholesterol a primary form of fat found in the blood; lipid material manufactured within the body, as well as derived from dietary sources.

chronic develops slowly and persists for an extended period of time.

chronic bronchitis persistent inflammation and infection of the smaller airways within the lungs.

chronic fatigue syndrome (CFS) an illness that causes severe exhaustion, fatigue, aches, and depression; mostly affects women in their thirties and forties.

chronic stress refers to remaining at a high level of physiological arousal for an extended period of time; it can also occur when an individual is not able to immedi-ately react to a real or perceived threat.

cilia (**sill** ee uh) small, hairlike structures that extend from cells that line the air passages.

circadian rhythms the internal, biological clock that helps coordinate physiological processes to the 24-hour light/dark cycle.

clinical depression a psychological disor-der in which individuals experience a lack of motivation, decreased energy level, fatigue, social withdrawal, sleep disturbance, disturbance in appetite, diminished sex drive, feelings of worthlessness, and despair.

club drug one of a variety of psychoactive drugs typically used at raves, bars, and dance clubs.

cognitive-behavioral therapy an action-oriented form of therapy that assumes that maladaptive, or faulty, thinking patterns cause maladaptive behavior and negative emotions; treatment focuses on changing an individual's thoughts or cognitive patterns in order to change his or her behavior and emotional state.

cohabitation sharing of a residence by two unrelated, unmarried people; living together.

coitus (**co** ih tus) penile-vaginal intercourse.

coitus interruptus (withdrawal) (**co** ih tus in ter **rup** tus) a contraceptive practice in which the erect penis is removed from the vagina before ejaculation.

cold turkey immediate, total discontinua-tion of use of a drug; associated withdrawal discomfort.

collateral circulation the ability of nearby blood vessels to enlarge and carry additional blood around a blocked blood vessel.

colonoscopy (co lun **os** ko py) examination of the entire length of the colon, using a flexible fiberoptic scope to inspect the structure's inner lining.

compliance willingness to follow the direc-tions provided by another person.

condom a latex shield designed to cover the erect penis and retain semen upon ejacula-tion; "rubber."

congestive heart failure inability of the heart to pump out all the blood that returns to it; can lead to dangerous fluid accumula-tions in veins, lungs, and kidneys.

consumer fraud the marketing of unreli-able and ineffective services, products, or information under the guise of curing disease or improving health; quackery.

contraception any method or procedure that prevents fertilization.

contraceptive patch contraceptive skin patch containing estrogen and progestin; replaced each week for a three-week period.

contraceptive ring thin, polymer contra-ceptive device containing estrogen and progestin; placed deep within the vagina for a three-week period.

contraindications factors that make the use of a drug inappropriate or dangerous for a particular person.

coronary arteries vessels that supply oxygenated blood to heart muscle tissues.

coronary artery bypass surgery a surgical procedure designed to improve blood flow to the heart by providing alternate routes for blood to take around points of blockage.

corpus luteum (kore pus **loo** tee um) the cellular remnant of the graafian follicle after the release of an ovum.

c-reactive protein a chemical compound found in the blood that is associated with inflammation; high levels are related to increased risk of coronary heart disease.

cross-tolerance transfer of tolerance from one drug to another within the same general category.

cruciferous vegetables (crew **sif** er us) vegetables that have flowers with four leaves in the pattern of a cross.

crystal methamphetamine a dangerous form of methamphetamine that quickly produces intense physical and psychological exhilaration when smoked.

cunnilingus (cun uh **ling** gus) oral stimula-tion of the vulva or clitoris.

cyanosis blue coloration of the lips, skin, and nail beds caused by inadequate oxygenation of the blood.

D

degenerative a slow but progressive deteri-oration of the body's structure or function.

dehydration abnormal depletion of fluids from the body; severe dehydration can be fatal.

dementia the loss of cognitive abilities, including memory and reason.

dendrite the portion of a neuron that receives electrical stimuli from adjacent neurons; neurons typically have several such branches or extensions.

dependence a general term that refers to the need to continue using a drug for psychological or physical reasons or both.

depressants a category of drugs that sedate the user by slowing central nervous system function; they produce tolerance and strong psychological and physical addiction in users.

desertification a process that converts lands that historically supported grasslands, shrub lands, or dry forest to nonproductive desert.

designated driver a person who abstains from or carefully limits alcohol consump-tion to be able to safely transport other people who have been drinking.

desirable weight the weight range deemed appropriate for people, taking into consider-ation gender, age, and frame size.

diaphragm a soft rubber cup designed to cover the cervix.

diastolic pressure (**dye** uh stol ick) the blood pressure against blood vessel walls when the heart relaxes.

dietary supplements nutrients taken in addition to those obtained through the diet; includes powdered protein, vitamins, and mineral extracts.

dilation the gradual expansion of an opening or passageway, such as the cervix.

dilation and curettage (D & C) (kyoo re taage) a surgical procedure in which the cervical canal is dilated to allow the uterine wall to be scraped.

dissonance a feeling of uncertainty that occurs when a person believes two equally attractive but opposite ideas.

distress stress that diminishes the quality of life; commonly associated with disease, illness, and maladaptation.

double-blind study a scientific study in which both the researchers and the study participants are said to be "blind" because neither group knows the makeup of the test and control groups during the actual course of the experiment; this information is revealed only at the study's conclusion.

drug any natural or artificial substance, other than food, that by its chemical or physical nature alters structure or function in the living organism.

drug synergism (**sin** er jism) enhancement of a drug's effect as a result of the presence of additional drugs within the system.

duration the length of exercise time of each training session; for aerobic fitness, 20–60 minutes is recommended.

dynamic therapy an intensive therapy based upon the belief that effective treatment must focus on the psychological forces underlying the individual's problems.

E

ectopic pregnancy a pregnancy in which the fertilized ovum implants at a site other than the uterus, typically in the fallopian tubes.

electrical impedence a method used to measure the percentage of body fat using a harmless electrical current.

embolism a potentially fatal condition in which a circulating blood clot lodges in a smaller vessel.

emergency contraception contraceptive measures used to prevent pregnancy within 72 hours after unprotected intercourse; also called post-coital or morning after contraception.

emotional intelligence the ability to understand others and act wisely in human relations and measure how well you know your emotions, manage your emotions, motivate yourself, recognize emotions in others, and handle relationships.

empowerment the nurturing of an individual's or group's ability to be responsible for their own health and well-being.

empty calories calories obtained from foods that lack most other important nutrients.

enriched the process of returning to foods some of the nutritional elements (B vitamins and iron) removed during processing.

enucleated egg an ovum with the nucleus removed.

environment the physical conditions (temperature, humidity, light, presence of substances) and other living organisms that exist around your body.

environmental tobacco smoke tobacco smoke, regardless of source, that stays within a common source of air.

enzymes organic substances that control the rate of physiological reactions but are not altered in the process.

epinephrine (epp i **neff** rin) a powerful adrenal hormone whose presence in the bloodstream prepares the body for maximal energy production and skeletal muscle response.

epitaph an inscription on a grave marker or monument.

erection the engorgement of erectile tissue with blood; characteristic of the penis, clitoris, nipples, labia minora, and scrotum.

ergogenic aids supplements that are taken by athletes to improve performance.

erotic dreams dreams whose content elicits a sexual response.

eustress (**yoo** stress) stress that enhances the quality of life.

exercise a subcategory of physical activity; it is planned, structured, repetitive, and purposive in the sense that an improvement or maintenance of physical fitness is an objective (Casperson, et al., 1985).

excitement stage initial arousal stage of the sexual response pattern.

exhaustion stage the point at which the physical and psychological resources used to deal with stress have been consumed.

exocrine glands glands whose secretions are released through tubes or ducts, such as sweat glands.

F

fat density the percentage of a food's total calories that are derived from fat; above 30% reflects higher fat density.

FDA Schedule I a list of drugs that have a high potential for abuse but have no medical use.

fecal coliform bacteria a category of bacteria that live within the intestines of warm-blooded animals; the presence of these bacteria is used as an indicator that water has been contaminated by feces.

fellatio (feh **lay** she oh) oral stimulation of the penis.

fermentation a chemical process whereby plant products are converted into alcohol by the action of yeast cells on carbohydrate materials.

fertility the ability to reproduce.

fetal alcohol syndrome (FAS) the characteristic birth defects noted in the children of some women who consume alcohol during their pregnancies.

fiber the plant material that cannot be digested; found in cereal, fruits, and vegetables.

fight-or-flight response the physiological reaction to a stressor that prepares the body for confrontation or avoidance.

fistula a fissure, break, or hole in the wall of an organ.

flaccid (**fla** sid) nonerect; the state of erectile tissue when vasocongestion is not occurring.

flexibility the ability of joints to function through an intended range of motion.

folacin (**foe** la sin) folic acid; a vitamin of the B-complex group; used in the treatment of nutritional anemia.

food additives chemical compounds intentionally added to food to change some aspect of it, such as color or texture.

food allergy a reaction in which the immune system attacks an otherwise harmless food or ingredient; allergic reactions can range from mildly unpleasant to life-threatening.

food intolerance an adverse reaction to a specific food that does not involve the immune system; usually caused by an enzyme deficiency.

foreplay activities, often involving touching and caressing, that prepare individuals for sexual intercourse.

frequency the number of exercise sessions per week; for aerobic fitness, 3–5 days are recommended.

FSH (follicle-stimulating hormone) a gonadotrophic hormone required for initial development of ova (in the female) and sperm (in the male).

functional foods foods capable of contributing to the improvement/prevention of specific health problems.

G

gaseous phase portion of tobacco smoke containing carbon monoxide and many other physiologically active gaseous compounds.

gateway drug an easily obtainable legal or illegal drug that represents a user's first experience with a mind-altering drug; this drug can serve as the "gateway" to the use of other drugs.

gender the general term reflecting a biological basis of sexuality; the male gender or the female gender.

gender adoption the long process of learning the behavior that is traditional for one's gender.

gender identification the achievement of a personally satisfying interpretation of one's masculinity or femininity.

gender identity recognition of one's gender.

gender preference emotional and intellectual acceptance of one's own gender.

general adaptation syndrome (GAS) sequenced physiological responses to the presence of a stressor, involving the alarm, resistance, and exhaustion stages of the stress response.

generalized anxiety disorder (GAD) an anxiety disorder that involves experiencing intense and nonspecific anxiety for at least six months, in which the intensity and frequency of worry is excessive and out of proportion to the situation.

gene replacement therapy an experimental therapy in which a healthy human gene is incorporated into a harmless virus to be delivered to cells that have an abnormal version of the gene.

generic name the common or nonproprietary name of a drug.

green space areas of land that are dominated by domesticated or natural vegetation, including rural farmland, city lawns and parks, and nature preserves.

greenhouse gases a category of gases in the atmosphere that allow solar radiation to pass through the atmosphere to the Earth, but then trap the heat that is radiated from the Earth back toward space; Greenhouse gases include water vapor, carbon dioxide, methane, nitrous oxide, and tropospheric ozone.

H

hallucinogens psychoactive drugs capable of producing hallucinations (distortions of reality).

health claims the liable statements attesting to a food's contribution to the improvement/prevention of specific health problems.

health maintenance organizations (HMOs) groups that supply prepaid comprehensive health care with an emphasis on prevention.

health promotion movement in which knowledge, practices, and values are transmitted to people for use in lengthening their lives, reducing the incidence of illness, and feeling better.

herbalism an ancient form of healing in which herbal preparations are used to treat illness and disease.

high-density lipoprotein (HDL) the type of lipoprotein that transports cholesterol from the bloodstream to the liver, where it is eventually removed from the body; high levels of HDL are related to a reduction in heart disease.

high-risk health behavior a behavioral pattern, such as smoking, associated with a high risk of developing a chronic illness.

holistic health a view of health in terms of its physical, emotional, social, intellectual, spiritual and occupational makeup.

homeopathy (hoe mee **op** ah the) the use of minute doses of herbs, minerals, or other substances to stimulate healing.

homicide the intentional killing of one person by another.

hormone replacement therapy (HRT) the use of medically administered estrogen to replace estrogen lost as the result of menopause.

host negligence a legal term that reflects the failure of a host to provide reasonable care and safety for people visiting the host's residence or business.

hot flashes temporary feelings of warmth experienced by women during and after menopause, caused by blood vessel dilation.

human cloning the replication of a human being.

human papilloma virus (HPV) sexually transmitted viruses, some of which are capable of causing precancerous changes in the cervix; causative agent for genital warts.

humanistic therapy a treatment approach based on the belief that people, left to their own devices, will naturally grow in positive and constructive ways.

hydrostatic weighing weighing the body while it is submerged in water.

hypercellular obesity a form of obesity that results from having an abnormally large number of fat cells.

hyperglycemia the condition of having an abnormally high blood glucose level.

hypertonic saline solution a salt solution with a concentration higher than that found in human fluids.

hypertrophic obesity a form of obesity in which there are a normal number of fat cells, but the individual fat cells are enlarged.

hypervitaminosis excessive accumulation of vitamins within the body; associated with the fat-soluble vitamins.

hypoglycemia the condition of having an abnormally low blood glucose level.

hypothyroidism a condition in which the thyroid gland produces an insufficient amount of its hormone, thyroxin.

hypoxia oxygenation deprivation at the cellular level.

I

ICSH (interstitial cell stimulating hormone) a gonadotropic hormone of the male required for the production of testosterone.

identity theft a crime involving the fraudulent use of a person's name, social security number, credit line, or other personal, financial, or identifying information.

immune system the system of cellular chemical elements that protects the body from invading pathogens and foreign protein and abnormal cells.

indoor air quality characteristics of air within homes, workplaces, and public buildings, including the presence and amount of oxygen, water vapor, and a wide range of substances that can have adverse effects on your health.

infatuation an often shallow, intense attraction to another person.

inhalants psychoactive drugs that enter the body through inhalation.

inhibitions inner controls that prevent a person from engaging in certain types of behavior.

insulin a hormone produced by the islet cells of the pancreas that is necessary for the normal utilization of glucose.

intensity the level of effort put into an activity; for aerobic fitness, 50–80% of heart rate range is recommended.

intentional injuries injuries that are purposefully committed by a person.

intimacy any close, mutual, verbal, or nonverbal behavior within a relationship.

intimate partner violence violent victimizations committed by current or former spouses, boyfriends, or girlfriends.

intrauterine device (IUD) a small, plastic, medicated or unmedicated contraceptive device that prevents pregnancy when inserted in the uterus.

ionizing radiation electromagnetic radiation that is capable of breaking chemical bonds, such as x-rays and gamma rays.

isokinetic exercises (eye so kin **et** ick) muscular strength training exercises in which machines are used to provide variable resistances throughout the full range of motion.

isometric exercises (eye so **met** rick) muscular strength training exercises in which the resistance is so great that the object cannot be moved.

isotonic resistance exercises muscular strength training exercises in which traditional barbells and dumbbells are used to provide variable resistances throughout the full range of motion.

L

learned helplessness a theory of motivation explaining how individuals can learn to feel powerless, trapped, or defeated.

learned optimism an attribution style, comprised of permanence, pervasiveness, and personalization; how people explain both positive and negative events in their lives, accounting for success and failure.

low-density lipoprotein (LDL) the type of lipoprotein that transports the largest amount of cholesterol in the bloodstream; high levels of LDL are related to heart disease.

lumpectomy a surgical treatment for breast cancer in which a minimal amount of breast tissue is removed; when appropriate, this procedure is an alternative to mastectomy, in which the entire breast and underlying tissue are removed.

luteinizing hormone (LH) (**loo** ten eye zing) a gonadotropic hormone of the female required for fullest development and release of ova; ovulating hormone.

Lyme disease a bacterial infection transmitted by deer ticks.

M

macrocytic anemia (mac roe **sit** ick uh **nee** mee a) the form of anemia in which large red blood cells predominate, but in which total red blood cell count is depressed.

mainstream smoke smoke inhaled and then exhaled by a smoker.

mania an extremely excitable state characterized by excessive energy, racing thoughts, impulsive and/or reckless behavior, irritability, and being prone to distraction.

masturbation self-stimulation of the genitals.

maximum contaminant level the highest concentration of a contaminant that is allowed in drinking water, as established and regulated by the U.S. Environmental Protection Agency.

medical abortion an abortion caused by the use of prescribed drugs.

medical power of attorney for health care a legal document that designates who will make health care decisions for people unable to do so for themselves.

menopause the decline and eventual cessation of hormone production by the female reproductive system.

metaneeds secondary concerns, such as spirituality, creativity, curiosity, beauty, philosophy, and justice, that can be addressed only after the basic needs are met.

metabolic rate (met uh **bol** ick) the rate or intensity at which the body produces energy.

metastasis (muh **tas** ta sis) the spread of cancerous cells from their site of origin to other areas of the body.

minipills low-dose progesterone oral contraceptives.

misuse the inappropriate use of legal drugs intended to be medications.

monogamous (mo **nog** a mus) a paired relationship with one partner.

mononucleosis ("mono") a viral infection characterized by weakness, fatigue, swollen glands, sore throat, and low-grade fever.

morbidity pertaining to illness and disease.

mortality pertaining to death.

MRI scan magnetic resonance imaging scan; an imaging procedure that uses a giant magnet to generate an image of body tissue.

mucus the clear, sticky material produced by specialized cells within the mucous membranes of the body; mucus traps much of the suspended particulate matter within tobacco smoke.

multifactorial requiring the interplay of many factors; refers to the cause of a disease or condition.

multiorgasmic capacity potential to have several orgasms within a single period of sexual arousal.

murmur an atypical heart sound that suggests a backflow of blood into a chamber of the heart from which it has just left.

muscular endurance the aspect of muscular fitness that deals with the ability of a muscle or muscle group to repeatedly contract over a long period of time; supported by the respiratory and circulatory systems.

muscular strength the aspect of muscular fitness that deals with the ability to contract skeletal muscles to a maximal level; the maximal force that a muscle can exert.

mutual monogamy a pattern of dating in which a person is involved exclusively with one partner.

myocardial infarction heart attack; the death of heart muscle as a result of a blockage in one or more of the coronary arteries.

N

narcolepsy a sleep-related disorder in which a person has a recurrent, overwhelming, and uncontrollable desire to sleep, often at inappropriate times.

narcotics opiates; psychoactive drugs derived from the Oriental poppy plant; narcotics relieve pain and induce sleep.

naturally acquired immunity (NAI) a type of acquired immunity resulting from the body's response to naturally occurring pathogens.

nature the innate factors that genetically determine personality traits.

naturopathy (na chur **op** ah thee) a system of treatment that avoids drugs and surgery and emphasizes the use of natural agents to correct underlying imbalances.

neuron a nerve cell.

neurotransmitters chemical messengers that transfer electrical impulses across the synapses between nerve cells.

nicotine physiologically active, dependence-producing drug found in tobacco.

nocturnal emission ejaculation that occurs during sleep; "wet dream."

nomogram a graphic means of finding an unknown value.

non-ionizing radiation electromagnetic radiation that cannot break chemical bonds, but may excite electrons (ultraviolet radiation) or heat biological materials (infrared, radio frequency, and microwave radiation).

nontraditional-age students administrative term used by colleges and universities for students who, for whatever reason, are pursuing undergraduate work at an age other than that associated with traditional college years (18–24).

norepinephrine (nor epp in **eff** rin) an adrenalin-like chemical produced within the nervous system.

nurture the effect that the environment, people, and external factors have on personality.

nutrient density quantity of selected nutrients in 1,000 calories of food.

nutrients elements in foods that are required for the growth, repair, and regulation of body processes.

O

obesity a condition in which a person's body weight is 20% or more above desirable weight as determined by standard height/weight charts.

obsessive-compulsive disorder an anxiety disorder characterized by obsessions—intrusive thoughts, images, or impulses causing a great deal of distress—and compulsions—repetitive behaviors aimed at reducing anxiety or stress that is associated with the obsessive thoughts.

oncogenes faulty regulatory genes that are believed to activate the development of cancer.

oral contraceptive pill a pill taken orally, composed of synthetic female hormones that prevent ovulation or implantation; "the pill."

orgasmic platform expanded outer third of the vagina, which grips the penis during sexual intercourse.

orgasmic stage the third stage of the sexual response pattern; the stage during which neuromuscular tension is released.

orthodontics a dental specialty that focuses on the proper alignment of the teeth.

osteoarthritis arthritis that develops with age; largely caused by weight bearing and deterioration of the joints.

osteopathy (os tee **op** ah thee) a system of medical practice in which allopathic principles are combined with specific attention to postural mechanics of the body.

osteoporosis loss of calcium from the bone, seen primarily in postmenopausal women.

outercourse sexual activity that does not involve intercourse.

overload principle the principle whereby a person gradually increases the resistance load that must be moved or lifted; this principle also applies to other types of fitness training.

overweight a condition in which a person's body weight is 1–19% above desirable weight.

ovolactovegetarian diet (oh voe **lack** toe veg a **ter** ee in) a diet that excludes all meat but does allow the consumption of eggs and dairy products.

ovulation the release of a mature egg from the ovary.

oxidation the process that removes alcohol from the bloodstream.

oxygen debt a physical state in which one's activity exceeds the body's ability to produce energy aerobically, causing the body to switch to anaerobic energy production. This produces an excess buildup of by-products, especially lactic acid, and a feeling of inability to "catch one's breath." Respiration and heart rate remain increased until the excess by-products are cleared and the body can return to aerobic energy production.

P

panic disorder an anxiety disorder characterized by panic attacks, in which individuals experience severe physical symptoms. These episodes can seemingly occur "out of the blue" or because of some trigger, and can last for a few minutes or for hours.

Pap test a cancer screening procedure in which cells are removed from the cervix and examined for precancerous changes.

particulate phase the portion of tobacco smoke composed of small suspended particles.

passively acquired immunity (PAI) a temporary immunity achieved by providing extrinsic antibodies to a person exposed to a particular pathogen.

pathogen a disease-causing agent.

pelvic inflammatory disease (PID) a generalized infection of the pelvic cavity that results from the spread of an infection through a woman's reproductive structures.

perfectionism a tendency to expect perfection in everything one does, with little tolerance for mistakes.

periodic abstinence birth control methods that rely on a couple's avoidance of intercourse during the ovulatory phase of a woman's menstrual cycle; also called fertility awareness or natural family planning.

periodontal disease destruction of soft tissue and bone that surround the teeth.

peripheral artery disease (PAD) atherosclerotic blockages that occur in arteries that supply blood to the legs and arms.

peritonitis (pare it ton **eye** tis) inflammation of the peritoneum, or lining of the abdominopelvic cavity.

permanence the first dimension of an individual's attribution style, related to whether certain events are perceived as temporary or long-lasting.

personality a specific set of consistent patterns of behavior and traits that helps to identify and characterize an individual; personality is comprised of thoughts, feelings, behaviors, motivation, instinct, and temperament.

personalization the final dimension of attribution style, related to whether an individual takes things personally or is more balanced in accepting responsibility for positive and negative events.

pervasiveness the second dimension of an individual's attribution style, related to whether they perceive events as specific or general.

pesco-vegetarian diet a vegetarian diet that includes fish, dairy products, and eggs along with plant foods.

physical activity any bodily movement produced by skeletal muscles that results in energy expenditure (Casperson, et al., 1985).

physical fitness a set of attributes that people have or achieve that relates to the ability to perform physical activity (Casperson, et al., 1985).

phenylpropanolamine (PPA) (**fen** ill **pro** pan **ol** ah meen) the active chemical compound still found in some over-the-counter diet products.

placebo pills (pla **see** bo) pills that contain no active ingredients.

placenta the structure through which nutrients, metabolic wastes, and drugs (including alcohol) pass from the bloodstream of the mother into the bloodstream of the developing fetus.

plateau stage the second stage of the sexual response pattern; a leveling off of arousal immediately before orgasm.

platelet adhesiveness tendency of platelets to clump together, thus enhancing the speed at which the blood clots.

platonic close association between two people that does not include a sexual relationship.

positive caloric balance caloric intake greater than caloric expenditure.

postpartum depression a form of depression that affects women in the weeks and months following childbirth.

post-traumatic stress disorder an anxiety disorder that sometimes develops following exposure to an extreme stressor involving threat of death or serious injury; symptoms include recurrent and distressing thoughts or nightmares about the event, emotional numbness, feelings of detachment, sleep disturbance, hypervigilance, and irritability.

potentiated effect a phenomenon whereby the use of one drug intensifies the effect of a second drug.

preventive or prospective medicine physician-centered medical care in which areas of risk for chronic illnesses are identified so that they might be lowered.

primary care health providers health care providers who generally see patients on a routine basis, particularly for preventive health care.

primary prevention measures intended to deter first-time drug use.

problem drinking an alcohol use pattern in which a drinker's behavior creates personal difficulties or difficulties for other people.

Prochaska's stages of change the six predictable stages—precontemplation, contemplation, preparation, action, maintenance, and termination—people go through in establishing new habits and patterns of behavior.

procreation reproduction.

procrastination a tendency to put off completing tasks until some later time, sometimes resulting in increased stress.

prophylactic mastectomy surgical removal of the breasts to prevent breast cancer in women who are at high risk of developing the disease.

prophylactic oophorectomy surgical removal of the ovaries to prevent ovarian cancer in women at high risk of developing the disease.

prostate-specific antigen (PSA) test a blood test used to identify prostate-specific antigen, an early indicator that the immune system has recognized and mounted a defense against prostate cancer.

prosthodontics a dental specialty that focuses on the construction and fitting of artificial appliances to replace missing teeth.

proteins compounds composed of chains of amino acids; primary components of muscle and connective tissue.

proto-oncogenes (pro toe **on** co genes) normal regulatory genes that may become oncogenes.

psychiatrist a medical doctor with specialized training in the diagnosis and treatment of psychological disorders through the use of biological and medical interventions.

psychoactive drug any substance capable of altering one's feelings, moods, or perceptions.

psychological health a broadly based concept pertaining to cognitive functioning in conjunction with the way people express their emotions, cope with stress, adversity, and success, and adapt to changes in themselves and their environment.

psychologist a doctoral level practitioner with specialized training in the diagnosis and treatment of psychological disorders through the use of psychotherapy.

psychoneuroimmunology the biomedical science field that studies the interrelationship of the mind, nervous system, and immune system and its influence on illness and disease.

psychosocial sexuality masculine and feminine aspects of sexuality.

psychosomatic disorders physical illnesses of the body generated by the effects of stress.

pulmonary emphysema an irreversible disease process in which the alveoli are destroyed.

purging using vomiting, laxatives, diuretics, enemas or other medications, or such means as excessive exercise to eliminate food.

R

radio frequency radiation electromagnetic radiation with frequency in the range of 3 kilohertz to 300 megahertz, emitted by cell phones, radios, communications transmitters, and other electronic devices.

radon a naturally occurring radioactive gas that is emitted during the decay of uranium in soil, rock, and water.

recessive inheritance pattern the inheritance of traits whose expression requires that they be carried by both biological parents.

reflexology massage applied to specific areas of the feet in order to treat illness and disease in other areas of the body.

refractory errors abnormal patterns of light wave transmission through the structures of the eye.

refractory phase that portion of the male's resolution stage during which sexual arousal cannot occur.

regulatory genes genes that control cell specialization replication, DNA repair, and tumor suppression.

resistance stage the second stage of a response to a stressor, during which the body attempts to reestablish its equilibrium or internal balance.

resolution stage the fourth stage of the sexual response pattern; the return of the body to a preexcitement state.

retinal hemorrhage uncontrolled bleeding from arteries within the eye's retina.

rheumatic heart disease chronic damage to the heart (especially the heart valves) resulting from a streptococcal infection within the heart; a complication of rheumatic fever.

rigor mortis the rigidity of the body that occurs after death.

risk factor a biomedical index such as serum cholesterol level, or a behavioral pattern such as smoking, associated with a chronic illness.

rubella German or 3-day measles.

rubeola (roo **bee** oh luh) red or common measles.

S

salt sensitive the term used to describe people whose bodies overreact to the presence of sodium by retaining fluid, thus increasing blood pressure.

satiety value (suh **TIE** uh tee) a food's ability to cause a feeling of fullness.

saturated fats fats that promote cholesterol formation; they are in solid form at room temperature; primarily animal fats.

schizophrenia one of the most severe mental disorders, characterized by profound distortions in one's thought processes, emotions, perceptions, and behavior; symptoms may include hallucinations, delusions, disorganized thinking, and/or maintaining a rigid posture and not moving for hours.

sclerotic changes (skluh **rot** ick) thickening or hardening of tissues.

seasonal affective disorder (SAD) a form of depression that develops in relation to the changes in the seasons.

secondary prevention measures aimed at early detection, intervention, and treatment of drug abuse before severe physical, psychological, emotional, or social consequences can occur.

secondary virginity the discontinuation of sexual intercourse after initial exploration.

self-actualization the highest level of psychological health—at which one reaches his or her highest potential and values truth, beauty, goodness, spirituality, love, humor, and ingenuity.

self-antigens the cells and tissues that stimulate the immune system's autoimmune response.

self-care movement the trend toward individuals taking increased responsibility for prevention or management of certain health conditions.

self-concept an individual's internal picture of him or herself; the way one sees oneself.

self-esteem an individual's sense of pride, self-respect, value, and worth.

self-fulfilling prophecy the tendency to inadvertently make something more likely to happen as a result of your own expectations and attitudes.

semen a secretion containing sperm and nutrients discharged from the urethra at ejaculation.

semivegetarianism a diet that significantly reduces but does not eliminate meat consumption and allows consumption of dairy products and eggs.

serial monogamy a pattern of dating in which a person is involved in a series of exclusive relationships, one after the other.

set point a genetically programmed range of body weight beyond which a person finds it difficult to gain or lose additional weight.

sex chromosomes the X and Y chromosomes that determine sex; chromosomes other than the autosomes.

sex flush the reddish skin response that results from increasing sexual arousal.

sexual fantasies fantasies with sexual themes; sexual daydreams or imaginary events.

sexually transmitted diseases (STDs) infectious diseases that are spread primarily through intimate sexual contact.

shingles painful fluid-filled skin erruptions along underlying sensory nerve pathways—due to reactivation of once-sequestered herpes zoster (chickenpox) virus.

shock the profound collapse of many vital body functions; evident during acute alcohol intoxication and other serious health emergencies.

sidestream smoke the smoke that comes from the burning end of a cigarette, pipe, or cigar.

skinfold measurement a measurement to determine the thickness of the fat layer that lies immediately beneath the skin; this measurement is used to calculate body composition.

sleep apnea a condition in which abnormalities in the structure of the airways lead to periods of greatly restricted air flow during sleeping, resulting in reduced levels of blood oxygen and placing greater strain on the heart to maintain adequate tissue oxygenation.

sliding scale a method of payment by which patient fees are scaled according to income.

smegma cellular discharge that can accumulate beneath the clitoral hood or the foreskin of an uncircumcized penis.

social phobia a phobia characterized by feelings of extreme dread and embarrassment in situations in which public speaking or social interaction is involved.

social worker a professional with a master's degree in social work; social workers provide both mental health and social services to the community and are the largest group of professionals to provide psychological services.

sodomy generally refers to anal or oral sex; a legal term whose definition varies from state to state.

solid waste pollutants that are in solid form, including non-hazardous household trash, industrial wastes, mining wastes, and sewage sludge from wastewater treatment plants.

solution-focused approach a goal-oriented counseling approach that helps clients change by looking for solutions rather than dwelling on problems.

specific phobia an excessive and unreasonable fear that causes anxiety and distress and interferes with a person's functioning.

spermatogenesis (sper mat oh **jen** uh sis) the process of sperm production.

spermicides chemicals capable of killing sperm.

stalking a crime involving an assailant's planned efforts to pursue an intended victim.

static stretching the slow lengthening of a muscle group to an extended stretch; followed by a holding of the extended position for a recommended time period.

stem cells premature cells that have the potential to turn into any kind of body cell.

sterilization generally permanent birth control techniques that surgically disrupt the normal passage of ova or sperm.

stimulants psychoactive drugs that stimulate the function of the central nervous system.

stress the physiological and psychological state of disruption caused by the presence of an unanticipated, disruptive, or stimulating event.

stressors factors or events, real or imagined, that elicit a state of stress.

stress response the physiological and psychological responses to positive or negative events that are disruptive, unexpected, or stimulating.

sudden cardiac death immediate death resulting from a sudden change in the rhythm of the heart.

synapse (**sinn** aps) the location at which an electrical impulse from one neuron is transmitted to an adjacent neuron; also referred to as a *synaptic junction*.

synergistic effect a heightened, exaggerated effect produced by the concurrent use of two or more drugs.

synesthesia a sensation of combining of the senses, such as perceiving color by hearing or perceiving taste by touching.

systemic (sis **tem** ic) distributed or occurring throughout the entire body system.

systolic pressure (sis **tol** ick) the blood pressure against blood vessel walls when the heart contracts.

T

tachycardia excessively rapid heartbeat, as evidenced by a resting pulse rate of greater than 100 beats per minute.

tar a chemically rich, syrupy, blackish-brown material obtained from the particulate matter within cigarette smoke when nicotine and water are removed.

target heart rate (THR) the number of times per minute the heart must contract to produce a cardiorespiratory training effect.

tertiary prevention the treatment and rehabilitation of drug-dependent people to limit physical, psychological, emotional, and social deterioration or prevent death.

test anxiety a form of performance anxiety that generates extreme feelings of distress in exam situations.

therapeutic cloning the use of certain human replication techniques to reproduce body tissues and organs.

titration (tie **tray** shun) the particular level of a drug within the body; adjusting the level of nicotine by adjusting the rate of smoking.

tolerance an acquired reaction to a drug in which the continued intake of the same dose has diminishing effects.

toxic shock syndrome (TSS) a potentially fatal condition caused by the proliferation of certain bacteria in the vagina that enter the general blood circulation.

trace elements minerals whose presence in the body occurs in very small amounts; micronutrient elements.

transcenders self-actualized people who have achieved a quality of being ordinarily associated with higher levels of spiritual growth.

transcervical balloon tuboplasty the use of inflatable balloon catheters to open blocked fallopian tubes; a procedure used for some women with fertility problems.

trans fatty acid an altered form of an unsaturated fat molecule in which the hydrogen atoms on each side of the double bond(s) are on opposite sides.

transient ischemic attack (TIA) (**tran** see ent iss **key** mick) strokelike symptoms caused by the temporary spasm of cerebral blood vessels.

transsexualism a sexual variation in which a person rejects his or her biological sexuality.

transvestism atypical behavior in which a person derives sexual pleasure from dressing in the clothes of the opposite gender.

tropospheric ozone ozone is comprised of three oxygen atoms that are bound into a single molecule. Tropospheric ozone refers to this substance as it occurs in the lower layer of the atmosphere, close to the ground.

tumor a mass of cells; may be cancerous (malignant) or noncancerous (benign).

type A personality a personality type that tends to be competitive, ambitious, and impatient; often associated with heart attacks and other stress-related conditions.

type B personality a personality type that tends to be more relaxed and patient.

U

unbalanced diet a diet lacking adequate representation from each of the food groups.

underweight a condition in which body weight is below desirable weight.

unintentional injuries injuries that have occurred without anyone's intending that harm be done.

unipolar disorder depressed state during which people experience periods of lack of motivation and other symptoms—depression.

urethra (yoo **ree** thra) the passageway through which urine leaves the urinary bladder.

V

vasectomy a surgical procedure in which the vasa deferens are cut to prevent the passage of sperm from the testicles; the most common form of male sterilization.

vegan vegetarian diet a vegetarian diet that excludes all animal products, including eggs and dairy products.

virulent (**veer** yuh lent) capable of causing disease.

vitamins organic compounds that facilitate the action of enzymes.

volatile organic compounds a wide variety of chemicals that contain carbon and readily evaporate into the air.

W

wellness the promotion and achievement of optimal health, including physical, emotional, social, spiritual, intellectual, and occupational well-being.

withdrawal illness an uncomfortable, perhaps toxic response of the body as it attempts to maintain homeostasis in the absence of a drug; also called *abstinence syndrome.*

X

xenotransplant a transplant of tissue from an animal, such as a pig, to a human recipient.

Y

Yerkes-Dodson Law a bell-shaped curve demonstrating that there is an optimal level of stress for peak performance. This law states that too little or too much stress is not helpful, while a moderate level of stress is positive and beneficial.

young adult years segment of the life cycle from ages 18 to 24; a transitional period between adolescence and adulthood.

Z

zero tolerance laws laws that severely restrict the right to operate motor vehicles for underage drinkers who have been convicted of driving under the influence of alcohol or any other drug.

zoonosis the transmission of diseases from animals to humans.

Credits

Chapter One: p. 4 (Star Box), Data from Yankelovich Monitor 1997, as reported in What is success? *USA Today* Jan 19:1A.

Chapter Two: p. 67 (Personal Assessment), Modified from Study Guide and Personal Exploration for *Psychology Applied to Modern Life: Adjustment in the 80s,* by Wayne Weitan. Copyright © 1983 by Wadsworth, Inc. Reprinted by permission of Brook/Cole Publishing, Pacific Grove, CA 93950.

Chapter Three: p. 97 (Personal Assessment), Modified from Holmes TH, Rahe RH: The social adjustment rating scale, *Journal of Psychosomatic Research* 11:213–218, 1967; p. 98 (Personal Assessment), Adapted with the permission of The Free Press, a Division of Simon and Schuster Adult Publishing Group, from *Never Good Enough: Freeing Yourself From the Chains of Perfectionism* by Monica Ramirez Basco, Ph.D. Copyright©1999 by Monica Ramirez Basco. All rights reserved.

Chapter Four: p. 103 (Figure 4-1), Data from *The Wirthlin Report,* Harris Interactive Inc. All rights reserved; p. 118 (Star Box),© 2005 American Academy of Orthopaedic Surgeons. Reprinted with permission from *Your Orthopaedic Connection,* the patient education Web site of the American Academy of Orthopaedic Surgeons, located at http://orthoinfo.aaos.org; p. 124 (Table 4.1), Prentice, WE: *Fitness for College and Life.* ed 5; New York, 1997, McGraw Hill; pp. 127–128 (Personal Assessment), Data from the National Fitness Foundation.

Chapter Five: p. 130 (Table 5.1), From Dietary Guidelines for Americans 2005, United States Department of Health and Human Services; p. 136 (Table 5.3), From Dietary Guidelines for Americans 2005, United States Department of Health and Human Services; p. 141 (Table 5.4) Data from the United States Department of

Agriculture; pp. 148–149 (Table 5.6), Data from Nutrition Action Newsletter, March 2005; pp. 154–155 (Figure 5-3), Data from US Food and Drug Administration and Wardlow G, Insel P: *Perspectives in Nutrition,* ed 3, St. Louis, 1986, Mosby.; p. 160 (Star Box), Duyff, RL. *American Dietetic Association Complete Food and Nutrition Guide,* 2nd ed., © John Wiley & Sons. This material is used by permission of John Wiley and Sons, Inc.; p. 173 (Personal Assessment), From *Nutrition for a Healthy Life,* Courtesy of March Leeds.

Chapter Six: p. 176 (Table 6.1), From Wardlaw G, Insel P, and Seyler M: *Contemporary Nutrition: Issues and Insights,* ed 2, St. Louis, 1994, Mosby; p. 177 (Star Box), Data from C. Everett Koop Foundation, American Diabetes Association; p. 180 (Table 6.2), Adapted from *Clinical Guidelines on the Identification, Evaluation, and Treatment of Overweight and Obesity in Adults: The Evidence Report,* National Institutes of Health; p. 182 (Table 6.4), Adapted from Najjar MF, Rowland M: Anthropometric reference data and prevalence of overweight, United States 1976–1980, Vital and Health Statistics, series 11, no 238, (PHS) 87–1688, Public Health Service, Washington, DC, 1987. US Government Printing Office; p. 192 (Table 6.5), Adapted from Guthrie H: *Introductory Nutrition,* ed 7, St. Louis, 1989, Mosby-Year Book, pp. 226–227; p. 193 (Figure 6-4), Opinion Research Institute for *Simply Lite Foods;* pp. 194–195 (Table 6.6), Adapted from Guthrie H: *Introductory Nutrition,* ed 7, St. Louis, 1989, Mosby; p. 198 (Table 6.7), USA Today. Copyright 2002. Reprinted with permission.

Chapter Seven: pp. 230–231 (Table 7.2), Modified from Muncie Star © 1987. Reprinted with permission; p. 247 (Personal Assessment), US Department of Education, A parent's guide to prevention.

Chapter Eight: p. 251 (Figure 8-1), Data from Core Institute: *2003 Statistics on alcohol and other drug use on American campuses,* Center for Alcohol and Other Drug Studies, Student Health Programs, Southern Illinois University at Carbondale, 2003; p. 253 (Figure 8-2), Data from Core Institute: *2003 Statistics on alcohol and other drug use on American campuses,* Center for Alcohol and Other Drug Studies, Student Health Programs, Southern Illinois University at Carbondale, 2003; p. 257 (Table 8.2), Reprinted from *Cecil Textbook of Medicine,* 18e, Wyngardener, JB, and Smith, LH, copyright 1988, with permission from Elsevier; p. 258 (Figure 8-3), Feldman, *Understanding Psychology,* 5e, 2002, McGraw-Hill; p. 260 (Figure 8-4), From Wardlaw G: *Perspectives in Nutrition,* ed 3, St. Louis, Mosby; p. 267 (Changing for the Better), Modified from brochure of the Indiana Alcohol Countermeasure Program; p. 277 (Personal Assessment), From *Are You Troubled by Someone's Drinking?,* 1980, by Al-Anon Family Group Headquarters, Inc. Reprinted by permission of Al-Anon Family Group Headquarters, Inc.

Chapter Nine: p. 279 (Table 9.1), Data from *MMWR* 2004, 52(53): 1277–1280; p. 280 (Table 9.2), Data from *MMWR* 1999, 48(45): 1034–1039 and *MMWR* 2000, 49(SS-2): 1–60; p. 290 (Table 9.3) Adapted from Mulcahy S., *The Toxicology of Cigarette Smoke and Environmental Tobacco Smoke, A Review of Cigarette Smoke and Its Toxicological Effects;* p. 305 (Table 9.5), USA Today. Copyright 2001. Reprinted with permission; p. 309 (Personal Assessment), Reproduced with permission of the American Cancer Society.

Chapter Ten: p. 313 (Figure 10-1) Data from American Heart Association, *Heart Disease and Stroke Statistics—2005 Update,* 2005; p. 314 (Table 10.1) Data from American Heart Association, *Heart Disease and Stroke Statistics—2005 Update,* 2005; p. 321

(Figure 10-3) Reproduced with permission, © 1988, American Heart Association: Heart Facts; **p. 324 (Figure 10-4)** 1990 *Heart Facts*, art by Donald O'Connor; **p. 335 (Personal Assessment)**, From Howard E: *Health Risks*, Tucson, 1985, Body Press.

Chapter Eleven: p. 340 (Figure 11-1), Data from National Cancer Institute: Horizons of cancer research, NIH Pub. No. 89-3011 © 1989; **pp. 345, 348, 354 (Changing for the Better),** American Cancer Society; **p. 359 (Changing for the Better),** Courtesy of the American Academy of Dermatology; **p. 367 (Personal Assessment),** American Cancer Society.

Chapter Twelve: p. 374 (Star Box) and **pp. 381, 386 (Changing for the Better),** ©Health Letter Associates, 1996, 1997 www.wellnessletter.com.

Chapter Thirteen: p. 408 (Table 13.2) Courtesy of United States Department of Health and Human Services, Centers for Disease Control and Prevention; **p. 409 (Table 13.3),** Courtesy of the National Institute of Allergy and Infectious Diseases; **p. 437 (Personal Assessment),** Centers for Disease Control and Prevention, Atlanta.

Chapter Fifteen: p. 483 (Personal Assessment), Modified from USA Today.

Chapter Sixteen: p. 487 (Table 16.1), Adapted from Hatcher et al., *Contraceptive Technology.* 17th rev. ed., 1998, Ardent Media, Inc; **p. 509 (Personal Assessment),** From Haas K, Haas A: *Understanding Sexuality,* 3rd ed., St. Louis, 1993, Mosby.

Chapter Eighteen: p. 540 (Changing for the Better), Pell, AR: *Making the Most of Medicare,* DCI Publishing, 1990, in *insynch,* Erie, PA Spring 1994, Erie Insurance.

Chapter Nineteen: p. 568 (Figure 19-1), Courtesy of the National Committee to Prevent Child Abuse, Chicago, IL; **p. 575 (Changing for the Better),** From the American College Health Association; **p. 580 (Changing for the Better),** Reprinted with permission of the American Academy of Ophthalmology, *Preventing Eye Injuries;* **p. 581 (Figure 19-2),** National Safety Council; **p. 584 (Changing for the Better),** Adapted from Pynoos J, Cohen E: *Creative ideas for a safe and livable home,* Washington DC, American Association of Retired Persons 1992, and Van Tassel D: *Home safe*

home, St. Louis, 1996, GenCare Health Systems.

Chapter Twenty: p. 604 (Figure 20-2), Environmental Protection Agency.

Chapter 21: p. 640 (Changing for the Better), The National Kidney Foundation Uniform Donor Card is reprinted with permission from the National Kidney Foundation, Inc. Copyright 2000, New York, NY.

Photo Credits

Chapter 1 Page 7: (top) Getty Images, (bottom) Ryan McVay/PhotoDisc/Getty Images; p.14: Digital Vision; p. 16: Geoff Manasse/PhotoDisc/Getty Images; p. 18: Joaquin Palting/PhotoDisc/Getty Images; p. 20: Keith Brofsky/PhotoDisc/Getty Images; p. 21: Don Farrall/PhotoDisc/Getty Images

Chapter 2 p. 42: Mel Curtis/PhotoDisc/Getty Images; p. 43: Buccina Studios/PhotoDisc/Getty Images; p. 51: Mel Curtis/PhotoDisc/Getty Images; p. 53: Michael Matisse/PhotoDisc/Getty Images; p. 55: PhotoDisc/Getty Images

Chapter 3 p. 75: Milton Montenegro/Getty Images; p. 77: © Image Source/Corbis; p. 79: (left) PhotoDisc/Getty Images, (right) The McGraw-Hill Companies, Inc./Andrew Resek, photographer; p. 82 © K. Solveig/zefa/Corbis; p. 87: Ryan McVay/PhotoDisc/Getty Images

Chapter 4 p. 101: Ryan McVay/PhotoDisc/Getty Images; p. 104: Ryan McVay/PhotoDisc/Getty Images; p. 111: Ryan McVay/PhotoDisc/Getty Images; p. 113: Ryan McVay/PhotoDisc/Getty Images; p. 118: (top & bottom) www.asicsamerica.com; (left) Courtesy Stewart Halperin; p. 119: (left) www.asicsamerica.com, (right) Courtesy Stewart Halperin; p. 127: Courtesy Stewart Halperin; p. 128: Courtesy Stewart Halperin

Chapter 5 p. 140: Ryan McVay/PhotoDisc/Getty Images; p. 144: PhotoLink/PhotoDisc/Getty Images; p. 145: PhotoDisc/Getty Images; p. 153: © Royalty-Free/Corbis; p. 160: F. Schussler/PhotoLink/PhotoDisc/Getty Images; p. 163: Ryan McVay/PhotoDisc/Getty Images

Chapter 6 p. 178: Suza Scalora/PhotoDisc/Getty Images; p. 179: (top) © David Barber/PhotoEdit, (bottom) © Custom Medical Stock Photo; p. 205: Ryan

McVay/PhotoDisc/Getty Images; p. 206: © Tony Freeman/PhotoEdit

Chapter 7 p. 223: Image100/Corbis; p. 233: Jack Star/PhotoLink/PhotoDisc/Getty Images; p. 237: (top) Doug Menuez/PhotoDisc/ Getty Images, (bottom) © The Cover Story/ Corbis

Chapter 8 p. 252: Jim Arbogast/PhotoDisc/Getty Images; p. 261: (top) George Steinmetz, (bottom) Courtesy Mothers Against Drunk Driving; p. 265: Doug Menuez/PhotoDisc/Getty Images

Chapter 9 p. 280: Emma Lee/Life File/PhotoDisc/Getty Images; p. 283: Jonnie Miles/PhotoDisc/Getty Images; p. 285: Jack Star/PhotoLink/PhotoDisc/Getty Images; p. 293: Courtesy Wayne Jackson; p. 294: © Custom Medical Stock Photo; p. 297: © Photick/Superstock

Chapter 10 p. 318: Karl Weatherley/PhotoDisc/Getty Images; p. 319: Ryan McVay/PhotoDisc/Getty Images; p. 328: Keith Brofsky/PhotoDisc/Getty Images

Chapter 11 p. 338: © Kevin Laubacher/Getty Images/Taxi; p. 356: © AP/Wide World Photos; p. 360: From Thibodeau G., Patton, K. *Anatomy and Physiology,* 3/e, St. Louis, 1996. Mosby

Chapter 12 p. 373: © Custom Medical Stock Photo; p. 375: © Custom Medical Stock Photo; p. 376: © Custom Medical Stock Photo; p. 377: © Custom Medical Stock Photo; p. 389: © Rufus F. Folkks/Corbis

Chapter 13 p. 409: Janis Christie/PhotoDisc/Getty Images; p. 416: © Touhig Sion/Corbis Sygma; p. 418: © Reuters/Corbis; p. 420: © Roger Ressmeyer/Corbis; p. 428: © Phototake; p. 429: © Custom Medical Stock Photo

Chapter 14 p. 444: Digital Vision/Getty Images

Chapter 15 p. 473: Ryan McVay/PhotoDisc/GettyImages; p. 475: (left) Buccina Studios/PhotoDisc/Getty Images, (right) Digital Vision/Getty Images

Chapter 16 p. 492: PhotoDisc/Getty Images; p. 493: (top) Courtesy Stewart Halperin, (bottom) Lisley Photographics; p. 494: © Laura J. Edwards; p. 496: © Joel Gordon; p. 497: Courtesy Stewart Halperin; p. 498: (left) © Laura J. Edwards, (right) Courtesy of Duramed Pharmaceuticals: Inc.; p. 499:

Courtesy of Alza Corp.; p. 501: Courtesy Organon USA

Chapter 17 p. 511: E. Dygas/PhotoDisc/ Getty Images; p. 515: © Science Photo Library/Photo Researchers, Inc.; p. 517: Digital Vision/Getty Images; p. 518: © Science Photo Library/Photo Researchers, Inc.; p. 521: Keith Brofsky/PhotoDisc/ Getty Images

Chapter 18 p. 539: Ryan McVay/PhotoDisc/ Getty Images; p. 543: Anthony Saint

James/PhotoDisc/Getty Images; p. 546: Mitch Hrdlicka/PhotoDisc/Getty Images; p. 557: Ryan McVay/PhotoDisc/Getty Images

Chapter 19 p. 570: Jack Star/PhotoLink/ PhotoDisc/Getty Images; p. 576: Ryan McVay/PhotoDisc/Getty Images; p. 579: Ryan McVay/PhotoDisc/Getty Images; p. 582: Ryan McVay/PhotoDisc/Getty Images

Chapter 20 p. 594: Digital Vision/Getty Images; p. 600: Nick Koudis/PhotoDisc/

Getty Images; p. 603: Kent Knudson/ PhotoDisc/Getty Images; p. 607: D. Falconer/ PhotoLink/PhotoDisc/Getty Images; p. 614: Digital Vision/Getty Images; p. 615: Tomi/ PhotoLink/PhotoDisc/Getty Images

Chapter 21 p. 628: AP/Wide World; p. 629: © John Freilich/Corbis Sygma

Index

drinking patterns of, 253*f*

drug use of, 221*t*

minority, 12

nontraditional-age, 11–12

ritalin and, 234

supporting responsible drinking, 265–266

traditional-age, 11

violence and, 549

colon cancer, 345

colonoscopy, 356

colorectal cancer, 355–357

Columbine High School, 569

combination drug effects, 228–240

combined pill, as method of birth control, 499

commercials. *See also* advertising; media

as health information source, 535

common cold, 409–410

communication

about birth control, 486

conflict resolution through, 472

developing, 43–44

between patient and health care provider, 541–542

for relationships, 478, 480

community environment, 601–610

community health promotion, 6

companionate love, 473, 474

complementary care

acupuncture, 543–544

acupuncture for alcoholism, 270

acupuncture for drug abuse, 242

antioxidant supplementation, 165

aphrodisiacs, 466

ayurveda, 546

biofeedback, 59, 89–90

biofield therapy, 543

chiropractic, 543

choosing practitioners of, 545

for common cold, 410

DHEA, 447

ergogenic aids, 120

herbal medicine for fertility, 491

herbalism, 545

homeopathy, 410, 544

hypnotism and smoking cessation, 304

ma huang, 200, 231

macrobiotic diet for cancer, 362

meditation to lower hypertension, 327

melatonin for sleep, 91

midwifery, 520

naturopathy, 544

organic food and environment, 616

practitioners of, 542–548

reflexology, 544

safety and, 577

for symptomatic irritable bowel disease, 387

terminal illness and, 630

therapeutic touch, 543

what is, 13

compulsion, in addiction process, 223–224

compulsive behavior. *See* obsessive-compulsive disorder (OCD)

conditioning, and physical fitness, 111

condoms, as method of birth control, 492–493, 495. *See also* female condom

conflict management, 44

conflict-habituated marriage, 476

confrontation, for drug dependence, 242

congenital abnormalities, 375–378

congenital heart disease, 330–331

congenital rubella syndrome, 330

congestive heart failure, 331

consultation, 539

consumer advocacy groups, as health information source, 537

consumer fraud, 558–559

contact inhibition, 340

contemplation stage, of change, 9

contraception. *See also* birth control

birth control *vs.*, 485

emergency, 502

oral, 498–500

selecting method of, 487–488

tobacco use and, 297–298

vaginal contraceptive film, 493

contraceptive patch, as method of birth control, 501–502

contraceptive ring, as method of birth control, 501

contraceptive sponge, as method of birth control, 497

contraindications, 500

controlled fasting, 196–197

convalescence stage, of infection, 402

Cookie Monster, 170

cooldown phase, of physical fitness, 111

coping strategies, 85–92

cord blood (stem) cells, 406

coronary arteries, 315

coronary artery bypass surgery, 324

coronary heart disease, 320–325

corpus luteum, 452

Coué, Emil, 89

counseling

genetic, 374

prenatal, 524–525

counselors, 59

couples therapy, 61–62

Couric, Katie, 356

Cowper's glands, 425, 447

CPR. *See* cardiopulmonary resuscitation

crabs, 431

crack cocaine, 234

C-reactive protein, 322

creativity, 46

cremation, 638–639

cremation jewelry, 638

crime and violence

alcohol-related, 262–263

at ATMs, 566

bias and hate, 570–571

preventing, 566

sexual, 572–575

Crohn's disease, 385–386

cross-dressing, 468

cross-tolerance, 226

cross-training, 120–121

shoes, 119

cruciferous vegetables, 144

cryonics, 630, 642

crypts, 638

crystal methamphetamine, 232

cultural factors, of obesity, 187

cunnilingus, 470

curette, 504

CVA. *See* cerebrovascular accidents

CVD. *See* cardiovascular disease

cyanosis, 376

cybermourners, 637

cystic fibrosis, 372–373

cystitis, 432

D

dancing, as aerobic exercise, 116

date rape, 575

depressants, 235

dating, 472–473

death. *See also* dying; suicide; terminal illness

accepting, 624–644

accidental, 628

of children, 631–632

coping with specific causes of, 627–628

cryonics, 630

intentional injuries, 565–572

intercourse, 470

    anal, 470–471

    painful, 465

internet

    addiction to, 60

    as health information source, 3, 536–537

    health products available through, 534

    online support groups, 337

    stress from, 68–69

intervention and treatment, in addiction
    process, 224

intimacy, 473

    nurturing, 14

intimate partner violence (IPV), 567

intracytoplasmic sperm injection (ICSI), 526

intrauterine development, 517–518

intrauterine device (IUD), as method of
    birth control, 497–498, 502

intrauterine growth retardation (IUGR),
    523–524

intrinsic asthma, 385

involuntary smoking, 299

ionizing radiation, 609–610

irradiation, of food, 157

irritable bowel disease, hypnosis for, 387

isokinetic exercise, 105

isometric exercise, 105

isotonic resistance exercise, 105

IUD. *See* intrauterine device

J

Johnson, Magic, 398

journaling, 38

Judaism, death rituals of, 633

K

Kaposi's sarcoma, 420

ketosis, 195

Kevorkian, Jack, 629

Klinefelter's syndrome, 371–372

L

labels

    food, 153, 154*f*, 157

    as health information source, 536

labia majora/labia minora, 448

labor, 518–524, 519*f*

lactose intolerance, 131

lactovegetarian diet, 164

land pollution, 607–610

laparoscopy, 503

Latin American diet pyramid, 159*f*

laughter, 42–43, 224

LDL. *See* low-density lipoproteins

lead, 597–598

learned helplessness, 47

learned optimism, 47–48

learning, stress and, 81

Lea's Shield, as method of birth control, 496

lesbians. *See* homosexuality

leukemia, 341

life expectancy. *See* longevity

lightening, in delivery, 518

limited food choice diets, 194*t*

lipoproteins, 322–323

liposuction, 202–203

listening skills, 43, 224

living will, 626, 627*f*

longevity

    keys to, 10

    men *vs.* women, 17

long-term care insurance, 554

loss of control, in addiction process, 224

love, 473–474

low back pain, and exercise, 114

low-calorie foods, 195–196

low-calorie, high-protein diet, 194*t*

low-carbohydrates, 129

low-density lipoproteins (LDLs), 322

low-fat foods, 134

low-impact aerobic activities, 116

LSD (lysergic acid diethylamide), 236

lumpectomy, 349

lung cancer, 342–344

    tissue changes associated with, 295*f*

lupus, 386–387

luteinizing hormone (LH), 452

lyme disease, 415

lymphatic cancer, 357–358

lymphoma, 341

lysing, 406

M

ma huang, 200, 231

macrobiotic diet, for cancer, 362

macronutrients, 138

macrophages, 404

Mad Cow Disease, 160

MADD. *See* Mothers Against Drunk Driving

magazines, as health information source, 2

magnetic resonance imaging (MRI) scan, 329

mainstream smoke, 299

maintenance stage, of change, 9

male contraceptive pill, as method of birth
    control, 499

male reproductive system, 444–448, 445*f*

malnutrition, 135

mammography, 345, 348–349, 365

managed care. *See* health insurance

mania, 53

manipulation, and nicotine dependence, 288

manual vacuum aspiration (MVA), 504

marijuana, 237–239

    effects of, 238*t*

marriage, 474–475, 477

    death of spouse, 634

    improving, 474

Maslow's hierarchy of needs, 45–47, 45*f*, 61

Master Settlement Agreement (MSA),
    279, 282

masturbation, 469

maternal immunity, 404

math anxiety, 79–80

mausoleums, 638

maximum containment level (MCL), 606

McDonald's, 148*t*, 149*t*, 150*t*

    as animal welfare reform activists, 160

    nondisclosure of ingredients, 163

McGuire, Mark, 120, 177

MCL. *See* maximum containment level

MDMA (ecstasy), 237

measles immunization, 407, 408*t*

meat, 144–145

media. *See also* advertising; television

    ads influencing drug use, 228

    advertising to gays and lesbians, 460

    AIDS in news, 398–399

    birth control and sexuality resources, 484

    fibromyalgia in, 369

    as health information source, 2–3, 536

    homosexual adoption, 510

    hype *vs.* useful information, 591–592

    hypertension in, 312

    internet support groups for chronic
        health conditions, 337

    low-carb advertising, 129

    Master Settlement Agreement (MSA),
        279, 282

    scare tactics about drugs, 220

    Schiavo controversy, 624–625

    sexual behavior, 440

    technological stressors, 68–69

    television ads for medications, 36–37

    television teaching about healthy food, 170

    TV ads targeting drunk driving, 250

stimulants, 230t, 231
stratospheric ozone depletion, 613–614
stress, 68–94, 85, 381
    benefits of, 76
    cardiovascular disease and, 320
    costs of, 75–76
    inoculation, 91
    learning and, 80–81
    managing, 85–92
    physical toll of, 75–76
    realistic perspective on, 92–93
    relieving, 86f
    resolving, 72f
    responding to, 70–72
    response, 74f
    sources of, 75
    of students, 76–85
    three stages of, 72–75
    what is, 69–70
stress management, 86–89
stress response, 70–72
stressors, 75
    physiological reactions to, 74f
    technological, 68
stretching, 106, 110, 111
stroke, 328. See also heart disease
    cause of, 329f
    diagnosis and treatment of, 329–330
    recognizing warning signs of, 330
student
    drinking on campus, 251–253
    stress of, 76–85
Students Against Destructive
    Decisions, 265
Students Against Drunk Driving
    (SADD), 265
sudden acute respiratory syndrome (SARS),
    418–419
sudden cardiac death, 292
suicide, 52–53, 65, 628
    alcohol-related, 263–264
    dos and don'ts of intervention, 54
    physician-assisted, 629
sun, cancer and, 358–360, 363
surgical interventions, for weight
    management, 201–203
surgical remedies, for infertility, 525–526
surgical treatments, for heart disease, 324
surrogate parenting, 526
sweeteners, 131, 146
symptothermal method, of birth
    control, 491

synapse, 222
synergistic effect, 228
synesthesia, 236
synthetic narcotics, 240
syphilis, 426t–427t, 430, 431
systemic, 386
systemic lupus erythematosus (SLE),
    386–387
systolic pressure, 325

T

T cells, 404, 405, 417
tachycardia, 332
tai chi chuan, 106
talipes (clubfoot), 375
tar, 291
target heart rate (THR), 108
teaching hospitals, 549
TEF. See thermic effect of food
television
    ads targeting drunk driving, 250
    as health information source, 2
    obesity and, 196
    weight loss and reality, 174–175
telomerase, 340
tenderpoint locations, 383f
tennis elbow, 124t
tennis shoes, 118
tension, 75
teratogenic agent, 525
teratogens, 606
terminal illness
    coping with death from, 628, 630
    hospice care for, 634–635
termination stage, of change, 9
termperature rules, for cooking, 156f
terrorism, 564, 628
tertiary prevention, 222
test anxiety, 78–79, 81
testes, 444
testicles, 444
testicular cancer, 355
testicular self-examination, 354
testimonials, as health information
    source, 536
testosterone, 120, 445–446
    androstendione and, 122
tetanus immunization, 407, 408t
tetrahydrocannabinol (THC), 238
THC. See tetrahydrocannabinol
therapeutic cloning, 513
therapeutic touch, 543

therapy. See also counseling
    biofield, 543
    cognitive-behavior, 61
    couples, 61–62
    dynamic, 61
    electroconvulsive, 51
    family, 61–62
    gene replacement, 372
    group, 62
    highly active antiretroviral, 423
    hormone replacement, 344, 351, 389,
        390, 454, 455
    humanistic, 61
    solution-focused, 61
thermic effect of food (TEF), 191
"30-Somethings," exercise for, 115
thorax, 314
THR. See target heart rate
thrombus, 329f
TIA. See transient ischemic attack
time management, 81–82, 83
titration, 284
tobacco use
    alcohol combined with, 298
    in American society, 279–284
    cancer and, 361
    cigarette smoking and college students,
        280–282
    current cigarette smoking by sex and
        state, 279t
    demographics of, 280–282
    dependence development from, 284
    early childhood intervention,
        289–290
    environmental health and, 597
    health effects of cigarette smoking, 292t
    heart disease and, 317
    illness and premature death from,
        291–296
    marketing of products, 282
    new product development, 301
    oral contraceptives and, 297–298
    patterns of cigarette smoking, 280t
    physiologically active compounds linked
        to, 290–291
    preventing teen, 288–289
    psycho social factors related to
        dependence of, 287–288
    in public places, 300
    question of rights of, 305
    quitting smoking, 301–305
    rejecting, 278–308

heart disease and, 317
hypertension and, 334
longevity of, 17
sexual response pattern of, 461–464
staying sober, 271
tobacco use causing infertility in, 296
using analgesic medications, 334
World Health Organization (WHO), health promotion initiative, 8
World No-Tobacco Day, 287

World Trade Center disaster, 564
wrinkling, premature, 296

X

xenotransplant, 390

Y

Yates, Andrea, 52
yeast infections, 431
Yerkes-Dodson Law, 76, 76*f*

yoga, 78
young adulthood
developmental tasks of, 13–15
reassessing plans of, 16

Z

zoonosis, 419
zygote, 518
zygote intrafallopian transfer (ZIFT), 526